This work is dedicated to Kirsten and my daughters, Laura and Caitlin. May you always maintain humility as your accomplishments meet the stars.

Bob Elling

In memory of my mother, Inge Nicholson, 1940–2000, whose love and support I miss very much. To my husband, Bob, whose support and inspiration drive me to continuously improve patient care in the field.

Kirsten Elling

My deepest thanks to Kirt and Bob for asking me to be part of this project. It was an honor to work with such close friends and respected colleagues. I truly appreciate their tolerance of my obsessive nature and attention to detail. As always, I am forever grateful to my wife, Diane, and children, Kara and Marc, for their gracious acceptance of my time needs. Thank you, our readers, for being inquisitive and asking, "Why?" Without you, our mission would have been doomed from the outset.

Mikel Rothenberg

About the Authors

Bob Elling, MPA, REMT-P

Bob has been involved in EMS since 1975 and is currently a faculty member for the Institute of Prehospital Emergency Medicine at Hudson Valley Community College in Troy, NY. Bob teaches in the EMT-Basic, Paramedic, and recertification courses. Bob has served as the Institute's Program Director and was responsible for providing leadership in the expansion of the Institute, accreditation of the paramedic program, as well as the development of the AAS: EMT-Paramedic degree.

Bob is also an active paramedic with the Town of Colonie EMS Department. Bob is a member of the NYS Department of Health EMS Bureau's Regional Faculty, as well as an American Heart Association national faculty member.

Bob is also a professor of EMS at the American College of Prehospital Medicine (Richardson University), which is a distance-learning college in Florida. He is a member of the *JEMS* editorial review board, as well as the author of many articles, video scripts, and books, including *Essentials of Emergency Care, First Responder Exam Preparation and Review, Emergency Care Student Workbook, Pocket Reference for the EMT-Basic and First Responder, Essentials of Emergency Care Instructor's Resource Manual,* and *MedReview for the EMT-Basic.* He is a contributing author for *Paramedic Care: Principles & Practice,* and a co-author of the National First Responder, Paramedic, and EMT-Intermediate curricula.

Bob has served as a paramedic and lieutenant for NYC EMS, the associate director for NYS EMS, education coordinator for PULSE: Emergency Medical Update, evaluation coordinator for REMO, and a firefighter–paramedic in Colonie throughout his 27-year EMS career.

Kirsten M. Elling, BS, REMT-P

Kirt Elling is a career paramedic who works in the Town of Colonie in upstate New York. She began work in EMS in 1988 as an EMT–firefighter and has been a national registered paramedic since 1991. She has been an EMS educator since 1990 and teaches basic and advanced EMS programs at the Institute of Prehospital Emergency Medicine in Troy, New York. Kirt serves as regional faculty of the NYS DOH, Bureau of EMS, and regional faculty of the American Heart Association, Northeast region. She has written numerous scripts for the EMS training video series *PULSE: Emergency Medical Update,* is a contributing author of the *Paramedic Lab Manual* for the IPEM, and an adjunct writer for the 1998 revision of the National Highway Traffic Safety Administration, EMT-Paramedic and EMT-Intermediate: National Standard curricula.

Mikel A. Rothenberg, M.D., Emergency Care Educator

Dr. Rothenberg, M.D., is a board-certified internal medicine specialist with a special interest in critical care and emergency medicine. He has served as an ICU/CCU director, as well as physician advisor for both air and ground ambulance services. He is a professor of Emergency Medical Services at the American College of Prehospital Medicine.

Dr. Rothenberg has written several medical, EMS, and legal books, numerous journal articles, and an Advanced Cardiac Life Support (ACLS) computer software program. He served as the executive editor of ACLS Alert, and wrote an Advanced Cardiac Life Support column on the Internet (Merginet).

Dr. Rothenberg's forte is putting complex topics into "plain English." This skill, combined with over 25 years of medical practice and 15 years of medicolegal consultation, makes his teaching and writing both informative and enjoyable for a wide variety of audiences. A strong advocate of personal growth and self-esteem building, Dr. Rothenberg speaks internationally, presenting courses on "plain English" medical topics.

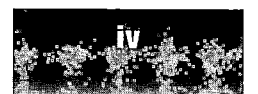

Why-Driven EMS Enrichment

Bob Elling, MPA, REMT-P

Kirsten M. Elling, BS, REMT-P

Mikel A. Rothenberg, M.D.

DELMAR

THOMSON LEARNING   Australia   Canada   Mexico   Singapore   Spain   United Kingdom United States

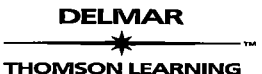

DELMAR

THOMSON LEARNING ™

Why-Driven EMS Enrichment
Bob Elling, Kirsten M. Elling, Mikel A. Rothenberg

Health Care Publishing Director:
William Brottmiller

Editorial Assistant:
Matthew Thouin

Production Editor:
Mary Colleen Liburdi

Executive Editor:
Cathy L. Esperti

Executive Marketing Manager:
Dawn F. Gerrain

Developmental Editor:
Darcy M. Scelsi

Channel Manager:
Jennifer McAvey

Library of Congress Cataloging-in-Publication Data
ISBN 0-7668-2507-8

NOTICE TO THE READER

Table of Contents

1. The Well-Being of the EMS Provider 1

2. EMS Systems, Roles, and Responsibilities 17

3. Illness and Injury Prevention 32

4. Medicolegal Issues 40

5. Ethical Issues for the EMS Provider 55

6. General Principles of Pathophysiology 59

7. Pharmacology 83

8. Medication Administration 91

9. Basic Cardiac Life Support 104

10. Life Span Development 113

11. Airway Management and Ventilation 129

12. History Taking and Therapeutic Communication 145

13. Techniques of Physical Examination 150

14. Patient Assessment Overview 158

15. Scene Size-Up and Initial Assessment 162

16. Focused History and Physical Examination:
    Medical Patient 172

17. Focused History and Physical Examination:
    Trauma Patient 178

18. Assessment-Based Management 185

19. Ongoing Assessment and Clinical Decision Making . 189

20. Communication 192

21. Documentation 201

22. Pulmonary and Respiratory 211

23. Cardiology 234

24. Neurology 253

25. Endocrinology 276

26. Allergies and Anaphylaxis 290

27. Gastroenterology and Urology 296

28. Toxicology 310

29. Environmental Conditions 324

30. Infectious and Communicable Diseases 340

31. Behavioral and Psychiatric Disorders 347

32. Hematology 355

33. Gynecology and Obstetrics 363

34. Trauma Systems and Mechanism of Injury 376

35. Hemorrhage and Shock 380

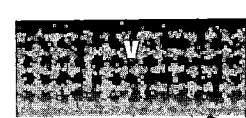

36 Soft Tissue Trauma 388

37 Burns 396

38 Head and Facial Trauma 407

39 Spinal Trauma 420

40 Thoracic Trauma.................................. 434

41 Abdominal Trauma................................ 449

42 Musculoskeletal Trauma.......................... 455

43 Neonatology...................................... 464

44 Pediatrics 474

45 Geriatrics: Abuse and Assault 491

46 The Challenged Patient 502

47 Acute Interventions with the Home-Care Patient.... 511

48 Ambulance Operations and Multiple Casualty
    Incidents 516

49 Rescue Awareness and Operations 537

50 Hazardous Materials: Issue Awareness............. 557

51 Crime Scene Awareness 567

52 Advanced Cardiac Life Support.................... 576

Standard Abbreviations

AAA abdominal aortic aneurysm
AAL anterior axillary line
ABC airway, breathing, and circulation
ABCD airway, breathing, circulation, defibrillation
Abd abdomen/abdominal
AC antecubital fossa
ACE angiotensin-converting enzyme
ACEP American College of Emergency Physicians
ACH acetylcholine
ACLS advanced cardiac life support
ACS acute coronary syndromes; American College of Surgeons
ACTH adrenocorticotropic hormone
AD affective disorders
ADA Americans With Disabilities Act
AED automated external defibrillator
AEIOU-TIPS alcohol, epilepsy, endocrine, exocrine, electrolytes, infection, overdose, uremia, trauma, temperature, insulin, psychoses, stroke, shock, space-occupying lesion, subarachnoid bleed
AF atrial fibrillation
AHA American Heart Association
AICD automatic internal cardiac defibrillator
AIDS acquired immunodeficiency syndrome

AL anterior-left lateral
ALS advanced life support; amyotrophic lateral sclerosis
ALTE apparent life-threatening event
AMA against medical advice
AMI acute myocardial infarction
AMP adenosine monophosphate
AMS altered mental status; acute mountain sickness
ANS autonomic nervous system
ANSI American National Standards Institute
A/O alert and oriented
AOI apnea of infancy
AOP apnea of prematurity
AP anterior–posterior
APCO Association of Public Safety Communications Officials
APE acute pulmonary edema
APGAR appearance, pulse, grimace, activity, reflex
ARDS adult respiratory distress syndrome
ASA aspirin
ASL American Sign Language
ATLS advanced trauma life support
ATP adenosine triphosphate
ATV automatic transport ventilator
AV atrioventricular

AVP arginine vasopressin
AVPU alert, verbal, painful, unresponsive

BAC blood alcohol content
BCLS basic cardiac life support
BiPAP biphasic positive airway pressure
BLS basic life support
BM bowel movement
BP blood pressure
bpm beats per minute
BS blood sugar; bowel sounds
BSA body surface area
BSI body substance isolation
BTLS basic trauma life support
BVM bag-valve-mask resuscitator

CA cancer
Ca calcium
CAAMS Commission on Accreditation of Air Medical Services
CABG coronary artery bypass graft
CAD computer-aided dispatch system; coronary artery disease
cAMP cyclic adenosine monophosphate
CB citizen band
CBF cerebral blood flow
CBT core body temperature
C-collar cervical collar
CCU Critical Care Unit

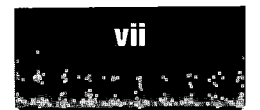

CDC Centers for Disease Control
CE continuing education
CEVO certified emergency vehicle operator
CHD coronary heart disease
CHF congestive heart failure
CISD critical incident stress debriefing
CISM critical incident stress management
Cl chloride
CMV cytomegalovirus
CNS central nervous system
CO carbon monoxide; cardiac output
CO₂ carbon dioxide
CONTOMS Counter Narcotic and Terrorism Operational Medical Support program
COPD chronic obstructive pulmonary disease
COT Committee on Trauma
CP chest pain
CPAP continuous positive airway pressure
CPR cardiopulmonary resuscitation
CQI continuous quality improvement
CRF chronic renal failure
CRT cardiac rescue technician
C-spine cervical spine
CSF cerebrospinal fluid
CT computed tomography
CTC color, temperature, and condition of skin; critical trauma care
CUPS critical, unstable, potentially unstable, stable
CVA cerebrovascular accident
CVC central venous catheter
CVP central venous pressure

D&C dilation and curettage
DA district attorney
DAN Divers Alert Network®
DCAP-BTLS deformity, contusion, abrasion, puncture/penetration, burn, tenderness, laceration, swelling
DCI decompression illness
DDC defensive driving course
DEA Drug Enforcement Agency
DAI diffuse axonal injury
DIC disseminated intravascular coagulation
Dig digoxin
DKA diabetic ketoacidosis
DLS dispatch life support

DMD Duchenne muscular dystrophy
DNA deoxyribonucleic acid
DNAR do not attempt resuscitation
DNR do not resuscitate
DOA dead on arrival
DOB date of birth
DOT Department of Transportation
DPE detailed physical examination
DPL diagnostic peritoneal lavage
DPT diphtheria, pertussis, tetanus
DTs delirium tremens
DVR demand-valve resuscitator
DVT deep vein thrombosis
Dx diagnosis

ECF extracellular fluid
ECG/EKG electrocardiogram
ED emergency department
EDD estimated due date
EEG electroencephalogram
EENT ears, eyes, nose, throat
EGTA esophageal-gastric tube airway
EID esophageal intubation detector
EJ external jugular vein
EMD emergency medical dispatcher
EMS emergency medical services
EMS-C Emergency Medical Services for Children
EMSS emergency medical services system
EMT-B emergency medical technician-basic
EMT-I emergency medical technician-intermediate
EMT-P emergency medical technician-paramedic
EOA esophageal obturator airway
EOM extraocular movements
EPA Environmental Protection Agency
EPI epinephrine
ER emergency room
ET endotracheal; endotracheal tube
ETA estimated time of arrival
ETC esophageal tracheal combitube
EtCO₂ end-tidal carbon dioxide
EtOH ethyl alcohol
EVOC Emergency Vehicle Operator Course

FAS fetal alcohol syndrome
FAX facsimile
FBAO foreign body airway obstruction
FCC Federal Communications Commission

Fe iron
FEMA Federal Emergency Management Agency
FH focused history
FHS follicle-stimulating hormone
FiO₂ fraction of inspired oxygen
FLSA Fair Labor Standards Act
FMLA Family and Medical Leave Act
FOIA Freedom of Information Act
FOIL Freedom of Information Law
FU follow up
FUO fever of unknown origin
Fx fracture

GAS general adaptation syndrome
GCS Glasgow Coma Scale
GI gastrointestinal
GSW gun shot wound
gtt/gtts drip/drops
GU genitourinary
GYN gynecology

H₂O water
HACE high-altitude cerebral edema
HAPE high-altitude pulmonary edema
HAV hepatitis A virus
hazmat hazardous material
Hb hemoglobin
HBV hepatitis B virus
Hct hematocrit
HCV hepatitis C virus
HDL high-density lipoprotein
HDV hepatitis D virus
HELP heat-escape lessening position
HEV hepatitis E virus
HF heart failure
HHNC hyperosmolar hyperglycemia nonketotic coma
HIV human immunodeficiency virus
HMO health management organization
HPI history of present illness
HPV human papilloma virus
HR heart rate
HTN hypertension
Hx history

IA initial assessment
IBS irritable bowel syndrome
IC incident commander
ICF intracellular fluid
ICHD Intersociety Committee on Heart Disease

ICP intracranial pressure
ICU intensive care unit
ID identification
IgE immunoglobulin
IM intramuscular
IMS incident management system
IO intraosseous
IPPB intermittent positive-pressure breathing
IQ intelligence quotient
IRB institutional review board
ISP internet service provider
IUD intrauterine device
IV intravenous
IVP intravenous medication push
IVPB IV piggyback

JVD jugular vein distention

K potassium
KCl potassium chloride
KE kinetic energy
KED Kendrick extrication device
KVO keep vein open

LDL low-density lipoprotein
LEA law enforcement agency
LLQ left lower quadrant
LMA laryngeal mask airway
LMP last menstrual period
LOC level of consciousness
LPN licensed practical nurse
LR lactated ringer's
LUQ left upper quadrant
LZ landing zone

MAL midaxillary line
MAP mean arterial pressure
MAST/PASG military antishock trousers/pneumatic antishock garment
MCI multiple casualty incident
MD muscular dystrophy; medical doctor
MDI metered dose inhaler
MI myocardial infarction
MMR measles, mumps, rubella
MODS multiple organ dysfunction syndrome
MOI mechanism of injury
MRI magnetic resonance imaging
MS mental status; musculoskeletal
MVA motor vehicle accident
MVC motor vehicle crash

N$_2$ nitrogen
Na sodium
NAIDS nonsteroidal anti-inflammatory drugs
NALS neonatal advanced life support
NFNA National Flight Nurses Association
NFPA National Fire Protection Agency; National Flight Paramedics Association
NG nasogastric
NHTSA National Highway Traffic Safety Administration
NIOSH National Institute of Occupational Safety and Health
NKA no known allergies
NPA nasopharyngeal airway
NPO nothing by mouth
NRB non-rebreather face mask
NREMT National Registry of Emergency Medical Technicians
NS normal saline
NSR normal sinus rhythm
NTG nitroglycerin
N/V nausea and vomiting

O$_2$ oxygen
Ob-gyn obstetrics and gynecology
OD overdose
OG orogastric
OPA oropharyngeal airway
OPQRST onset, provocation, quality, rest, relief, recurrence, severity, time of onset
OR operating room
OTC over the counter

P pulse
PA physician assistant
PAC premature atrial contraction
PaCO$_2$ partial pressure of carbon dioxide in arterial blood
PAD public access defibrillation
PALS pediatric advanced life support
PAR primary area of responsibility
PAT paroxysmal atrial tachycardia
PCC Poison Control Center
pCO$_2$ partial pressure of carbon dioxide
PCP phencyclidine
PCR prehospital care report
PE physical examination; pulmonary embolism
PEA pulseless electrical activity
PEARLA pupils equal and reactive to light and accommodation
PEEP positive end-expiratory pressure

PFD personal flotation device
pH potential of hydrogen
PHTLS Prehospital Trauma Life Support
PIAA personal injury auto accident
PID pelvic inflammatory disease
PKU phenykletonuria
PMH past medical history
PMI point of maximal impulse
PMS pulse, motor, and sensation; premenstrual syndrome
PND paroxysmal nocturnal dyspnea
PNI psychoneuroimmunology
PNS peripheral nervous system
PO per os (oral intake)
PO$_2$ partial pressure of oxygen
PPE personal protective equipment
PPV positive pressure ventilation
PR per rectum
PSAP public safety access point
PSVT paroxysmal supraventricular tachycardia
Pt patient
PTL pharyngeotracheal lumen airway
PTU propylthiouracil
PVC premature ventricular contraction

QA quality assurance
QI quality insurance

RAD radiation absorbed dose
RAS reticular activating system
RBC red blood cell
REM roentgen equivalent in man
RIBA recombiant immunoblot assay
RL Ringer's lactate
RLQ right lower quadrant
RMA refusal of medical assistance
RN registered nurse
ROM range of motion
RR respiratory rate
RSI rapid sequence induction
RTPA recombinant tissue plasminogen activator
RUQ right upper quadrant
RV right ventricular
Rx prescription

SA sinoatrial
SABA supplied-air breathing apparatus
SAMPLE signs, allergies, medication, past medical history, last meal, menses, events leading up to

SAR search and rescue
SARA Superfund Amendments and Reauthorization Act
SBS shaken baby syndrome
SCBA self-contained breathing apparatus
SCI spinal cord injury
SCIWORA spinal cord injury without radiographic abnormalities
SCUBA self-contained underwater breathing apparatus
SIDS sudden infant death syndrome
SL sublingual
SOB shortness of breath
SOP standard operating procedure
SpO$_2$ oxygen saturation of arterial blood measured by pulse oximetry
SQ/SC subcutaneous
SRS supplemental restraint system
SSKI supersaturated solution of potassium iodide

SSM system status management
START simple triage and rapid treatment
STD sexually transmitted disease
SUDS single unit diagnostic study
SUX succinylcholine
SV stroke volume
SVN small volume nebulizer
SVR systemic vascular resistance
SVT supraventricular tachycardia

TB tuberculosis
TBI traumatic brain injury
TCP transcutaneous pacer
TEMS Tactical Emergency Medical Support
TIA transient ischemic attack
TKO to keep open
TLCV translaryngeal cannula ventilation
TOT turned over to
TPA tissue plasminogen activator

UHF ultra-high frequency
ULQ upper-left quadrant
URI upper-respiratory infection
URQ upper-right quadrant
USFPA U.S. Fire Protection Administration
UTI urinary tract infection

V&T vehicle and traffic
VAD vascular access devices
VD venereal disease
VF ventricular fibrillation
VHF very high frequency
VS vital signs
VSD ventricular septal defect
VT ventricular tachycardia

WBC white blood cell
WPW Wolff-Parkinson-White syndrome

Preface

When I wandered inquisitively into an EMT course while at college some 27 years ago, I never could have predicted the wild and exciting ride that this career in EMS has taken me on! I feel very fortunate to have worked in the field for so long as an EMS provider, all the while serving in a number of different educational roles. Still, caring for sick people, holding their hand, wiping their brow, and helping to get them through the first hour of their crisis is a constant reminder of why I have enjoyed this career for so long.

In my travels these past years as New York's State Training Coordinator, as the educational coordinator for Emergency Medical Update, and as an EMS educator and author, I have met thousands of highly motivated EMS providers who continue to search for knowledge. These are the "why-driven" providers. Don't let the committees fool you. The EMS provider on the street does not want a dumbed-down curriculum, nor does the EMS educator in the classroom. EMS providers do not consider themselves "automatons" nor do they want to mindlessly follow treatment "cookbooks" without being a thinking cook. They not only want to know how, they also want to know why!

When a patient dies suddenly and everything seems to have been done quickly and correctly, the EMS providers want to know why he died and what else could possibly have been done to make a difference. When a patient who should have died, based on the severity of his injuries, makes it, again the EMS provider wants to know why. Want to frustrate an EMS provider? Let management come up with a new policy and forget to explain why! Have a young child die and don't allow the EMS provider in on the case review. They simply want to know why!

I remember a "pearl of wisdom" I picked up along the way that continues to be very true. Give me a list to memorize and I will forget it 10 minutes after the test. Explain to me why things are on the list and what the mechanism is that occurs to the patient, and I'll remember it forever! Each of the training curricula issued by the National Highway Traffic Safety Administration during the 1990s have used a format that includes a section called "enrichment." It is not surprising that this section is always left blank! When I saw this format, my first thought was, "Who is going to write the enrichment material?" Then, I instantly thought of my friend Mikel, who has the unique ability to break down tremendously complex concepts into understandable bits of knowledge. Of course, often the best educators are also very busy people and, in this case, Mikel's writing plate was rather full. So, after convincing Kirsten, my beloved partner, to help me with this project, we worked out a plan to write the enrichment book. We would write a large part of the book and Mikel would review every word and add his "Clinical Pearls," which are from his heart and hard-earned experience as a clinician, throughout the book. And of course, whenever our research ran astray, he always pulled us back to reality.

The focus of this book is on the patient and the provider. It is on the patient because he is the one who relies on EMS providers to be experts in what we do. It is on the provider because she wants to know much more than the minimum "core" information provided in EMS texts. Providers want to be enriched and want to know why. They want to be able to explain to their patients, their peers, their friends, and their family members the reasons why clinical conditions occur.

Probably the questions most often asked of us by fellow EMS educators were, "Is it a first responder book? Is it an EMT-Basic book? Is it an EMT-Intermediate book? Is it a paramedic book?" And the answer was always the same: yes, yes, yes, and yes. We have purposefully chosen to use the term "EMS provider" throughout the book. That is because this book is written for the why-driven EMS provider at any level of certification. When we introduce new concepts or use some of the "35 cent words" of medicine, we have tried to define them as we go. We have used the organizational format of the paramedic curriculum, with a few minor modifications (e.g., two life support chapters, 9 and 52) because we like the format and can envision some paramedic programs actually using this book to summarize their course and prepare for a state or national examination.

So, how can this book be best used? Read it from cover to cover, highlight it, scribble in the margins, and keep it nearby on your reference shelf. We anticipate that many instructors will find this book a helpful resource in preparing their classes. It may be particularly helpful to the experienced provider who is recertifying, be it by taking a class or an ongoing CME program. Because many conditions are concurrent, topics often overlap in this book.

Because this question and answer format lends itself to the addition of even more information as we all continue to expand our body of knowledge in EMS, we anticipate that future editions will involve many of your comments. So feel free to let us know what you like and what you think should be added in the future by corresponding with the authors at the e-mail address <BobElling@USA.net>. There is also a companion book to this text, called the *Paramedic Review,* that has multiple-choice review questions based on the paramedic-level material and curriculum objectives found in portions of this book.

So, enjoy the book. We hope you find many tidbits of information that help enrich your EMS education, as well as help you understand why.

See you in the streets!

Bob Elling

The Well-Being of the EMS Provider

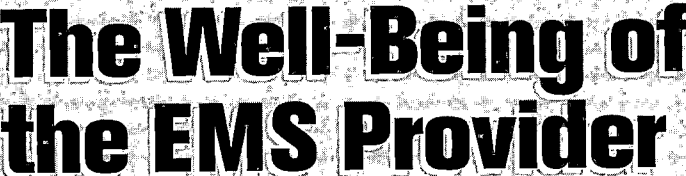

This chapter discusses you, the EMS provider. The focus is on *why* you must take care of yourself so you will be ready to do the job of an EMS provider. There are tips on health and fitness as well as suggestions on how to keep EMS a safe career. It may be heroic to say the patient comes first; however, the reality is that you must come first in order to provide any assistance to a patient!

Wellness and Taking Care of Number One

Q What is wellness and health?

A Wellness is defined as good health, especially as an actively sought goal or lifestyle. Health, defined by the World Health Organization, is not merely the absence of disease or infirmity; it is a state of complete physical, mental, and social well-being. It is important for all EMS providers to understand and implement lifestyle changes to enhance their personal wellness. Doing so will benefit the EMS provider personally in physical, mental, and emotional well-being, while aiding the EMS provider to serve as a role model or coach to others.

Q What are the components of wellness?

A The components of wellness include physical well-being and proper nutrition, as well as mental and emotional health (Table 1–1).

TABLE 1–1

Components of Wellness	
Component	Example
Physical	Strong back and knees for lifting.
Nutrition	Eat a properly balanced diet with vitamin supplements.
Mental	Able to empathize but not internalize stressful situations.
Emotional	Even tempered and well mannered to deal with chaos.

Q What are the components of wellness that are associated with proper nutrition?

A Proper nutrition involves an understanding of the nutrients the body needs (carbohydrates, fats, proteins, vitamins, minerals, and water), the food groups (sugar, fats, proteins, dairy products, vegetables, fruits, and grains), and the principles of weight control (eating in moderation, limiting fat consumption, and exercise).

Q How do diet and nutrition contribute to wellness?

A The standard American diet has long-term negative effects on the body. Eating too much animal food, fat, oil, and sugar and

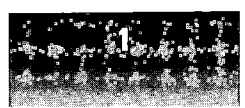

eating too few complex carbohydrates, such as fresh vegetables and fruits, whole grains and legumes, contributes to the development of degenerative diseases. These include the major killers like heart disease, diabetes, cancer, stroke, and obesity. This diet also contributes to a number of annoying conditions such as constipation, hemorrhoids, gout, osteoporosis, and tooth decay.

According to the Surgeon General's Report on Nutrition and Health, diet-related diseases account for over two-thirds of all deaths in the United States. To further complicate the diet of EMS providers, they often have rushed or interrupted meals with limited food choices.

■ What are some suggestions for an EMS provider on improving the diet at work?

A Some suggestions for better eating at work include:

- Adjust your food planning and shopping habits so you can eat more fresh foods.
- Stock your refrigerator and pantry with healthier foods.
- Plan and prepare better meals.
- Pack a small cooler full of fresh fruits and vegetables that you can take with you.
- Popcorn or pretzels make a great low-fat, low-calorie snack instead of chips or candy.
- Expand the range of foods from your normal choices.
- Instead of stopping for greasy fast food, a moderate-sized supermarket can offer dozens of types of nutritious foods that are already prepared.
- If you must go to a fast food restaurant, consider the alternative menu for low-fat meals.

■ What are some suggestions for the EMS provider on changing the intake of fats and switching to a healthier diet?

A Some suggestions for changing your diet include the following:

- Make small changes to your diet over an extended period of time rather than radical changes overnight. Making a slow transition is not only easier but is more likely to be effective.
- Cut back on fat intake. Try reading labels to see exactly how much fat is in each food.
- Switch to nonfat or low-fat dairy products and cheeses.
- Choose leaner cuts of meat.
- Eat less each meal by leaving some food on your plate and skipping the second helping.
- Drink more fluids before and during meals to prevent overeating at meals.

- Watch the calories, not just fat. Low- or no-fat foods often compensate for taste with increased calories.
- Don't limit your diet to only a few foods. Eating a variety of foods decreases the risk of missing essential vitamins and minerals.

■ So, should snacks be cut out completely?

A No! Actually, snacking will not make you fat unless you overdo it. It is too many calories and inactivity that makes you fat. Experts say that a 100 to 200 calorie snack eaten two to three hours before a meal will actually decrease your appetite for the meal. Other tips on snacks include:

- Use snacks to fill the voids between meals throughout the day.
- Do not think of snacks as extra treats. Think of them as a part of your food plan.
- Plan snacks ahead of time rather than a last minute raid of the icebox or snack machine.
- If you have a higher fat snack, make sure it fits into your overall fat and calorie count.
- Beware of the low-fat snacks that use sugar and calories for taste.
- Never snack when you are bored or anxious. Snack only when you are actually hungry.
- Try to eat higher fiber snacks for better dental health.
- Be prepared and have the proper snack foods on hand.
- Try to eat snacks when you are slightly hungry. Do not wait until you are starving because you will not be satisfied with only one snack in that case.

CLINICAL PEARL

Several "alternative" diets have received widespread publicity. The two most popular types involve either low fat/high carbohydrate (the "Ornish Diet" or variants thereof) or low carbohydrate/high protein (the "Atkins Diet" or variants thereof). Whether either is superior to the current recommendations is unclear. Investigators are presently comparing the two types of diets on a prospective basis.

■ What does it mean to be physically fit?

A Being physically fit involves a combination of aerobic conditioning, strength, speed, endurance, flexibility, balance, coordination, body composition, and attitude. Each person should develop personal fitness goals and consult with a personal physician before starting a very strenuous routine. New EMS providers beginning a fitness program may consider consulting with an athletic trainer. A considerable amount of information on this subject is available from the President's Council on Physical Fitness and Sports (call 202-690-9000).

Q. Where is a good place to start with a fitness program?

A. When beginning any fitness program, it is a good idea to obtain a baseline physical exam. Most EMS providers may work or volunteer for agencies that can provide the funds to obtain a good physical exam and health assessment from a physician. It is also a good idea to bring immunizations current at this time (Table 1–2). Baseline health records are helpful in the event an EMS provider becomes injured or ill while working. A physical examination by a physician will identify any specific limitations to consider in planning a fitness program.

TABLE 1–2

Immunizations for the EMS Provider	
Tetanus and Diphtheria	Polio
Rubella	Influenza
Measles	Hepatitis B
Mumps	Lyme disease
Chicken Pox	

Q. What are the benefits to the EMS provider of being physically fit?

A. The benefits of being physically fit include:

- A decrease in the resting heart rate and blood pressure, which comes from aerobic conditioning. When a person does aerobic activity for at least 20 minutes three or more times a week, the heart becomes a more efficient pump. Basically, the heart ejects a larger volume with each stroke and does not need to pump as often. Over a lifetime, decreased "wear and tear" on the heart adds up tremendously. There is less need for an increase in blood pressure, which may have serious long-term effects on the entire body. The oxygen carrying capacity of red bloods cells is also increased with exercise.

- An enhancement of one's quality of life by improving personal appearance and self-image and facilitating the maintenance of motor skills throughout life.

- Increased muscle mass and metabolism as well as increased resistance to injury.

- Avoidance of personal injury especially because EMS providers have such a high incidence of back injuries. All the lifting required by EMS work places the EMS provider at an increased risk for back injuries. Using proper lifting techniques and having good physical conditioning greatly reduce the chance of back injuries. Special attention should be given

to strengthening the abdominal and leg muscles, as these are the primary muscles used when lifting.

Q. How important is endurance to the EMS provider?

A. When responding to a patient having respiratory distress or chest pain involves having to climb one or several flights of stairs, the EMS provider should not be more short of breath than the patient! Routine aerobic exercise lasting at least 20 minutes, three times a week begins to improve the cardiac stroke volume of the heart while increasing physical endurance.

Q. Are there any benefits to exercise in addition to endurance and physical conditioning?

A. Yes! Besides the psychological aspect of feeling better about the way you look, there is a direct impact on brain function. To maintain intelligence, you must continually retrain the brain. Just as vision fades and hair disappears from the head, the human brain also deteriorates with age. The ability to recognize numbers in a test sequence starts to decline after age 25. Stimulating the central nervous system with physical activity may retard the loss of nerve cells in the brain by improving oxygenation of the brain.

Q. What are circadian rhythms and how do these cycles affect shift workers such as EMS providers?

A. Circadian rhythms are regular changes in mental and physical characteristics that occur in the course of a day (*circadian* is Latin for "around a day"). These biological cycles include hormonal and body temperature fluctuations, appetite and sleep cycles, and other bodily processes. When life patterns disrupt the circadian rhythms, such as jet lag from extensive time-zone travel and shift work, there are biological effects that can be stressful (Table 1–3) and disrupt normal sleep patterns.

Sleep deprivation is also common among people who work at night. This is because their schedules are at odds with powerful sleep regulating clues like sunlight. They often become uncontrollably drowsy during work and may suffer insomnia when they try to sleep.

TABLE 1–3

Effects of Shift Work on Circadian Rhythms
Shift workers have a higher incidence of:
Constipation
Diarrhea
Excessive Gas
Abdominal Pain
Heartburn
Peptic Ulcers

How much sleep does the average EMS provider need?

The average adult needs about eight hours of sleep a night until age 60, after which six hours may be adequate. Researchers estimate that there were at least 56,000 motor vehicle crashes annually between 1989 and 1993 due to driver drowsiness and fatigue. Major industrial accidents attributed partly to errors made by fatigued night-shift workers include the Exxon Valdez oil spill, and the Three Mile Island and the Chernobyl nuclear plant accidents. Some states have moved to legislate the maximum number of hours that resident physicians can work in the hospital. One study of residents working on the night shift found they were twice as likely as others to misinterpret hospital test results, which certainly has the potential to endanger patients.

If you must work the midnight shift and need to sleep during the day, how can you reduce the stress this causes?

Here are some tips to minimize the stress of trying to sleep during the day:

- Try sleeping in a cool, dark place that is similar to a nighttime environment.
- Establish an anchor time and stick to sleeping during your anchor time even on your days off. An anchor time is a time period you can rest without interruption. For example, if you work 9 P.M. to 5 A.M. and your anchor time is 8 A.M. to 12 noon, on workdays you sleep from 8 A.M. to 3 P.M.
- Try to relax by reading, watching TV, taking a bath, or listening to soothing music before going to bed.
- A small snack, not a big meal, before bedtime helps many people sleep. Foods such as milk or turkey meat have a natural sleep inducer called L-tryptophan in them.
- Try posting a "day sleeper" sign on your front door.
- Turn off the phone's ringer and lower the volume on the answering machine.
- Consider using special darkening blinds in the bedroom.
- Consider using earplugs or eye blinders.

What is addiction?

An addiction is a compulsive need for and use of a habit-forming substance such as alcohol, nicotine, cocaine, or heroin. Patients who are addicted have a well-defined physiological withdrawal from the substance that they are addicted to. Due to the stressful nature of their work, it is not uncommon for EMS providers to be at risk for substance abuse.

Why do people start smoking?

One of the most common reasons people start smoking is peer pressure. They continue to smoke due to the addicting effect of nicotine in tobacco.

What are the benefits of quitting smoking?

According to the American Lung Association (ALA), there are many benefits of smoking cessation. The ALA groups these benefits at different time intervals after your last cigarette:

- 20 minutes after quitting—blood pressure decreases, pulse rate drops, and the body temperature of the hands and feet increases.
- 8 hours after quitting—carbon monoxide levels in the blood drop to normal and oxygen levels in the body increase to normal.
- 24 hours after quitting—the chance of a heart attack decreases.
- 48 hours after quitting—the nerve endings start regrowing and the ability to smell and taste is enhanced.
- 2 weeks to 3 months after quitting—circulation improves, lung function increases, and walking becomes easier.
- 1 to 9 months after quitting—coughing, sinus congestion, fatigue, and shortness of breath decrease.
- 1 year after quitting—the excess risk of coronary heart disease is decreased to half that of a smoker.
- 5 to 15 years after quitting—stroke risk is reduced to that of people who have never smoked.
- 10 years after quitting—the risk of lung cancer drops to as little as one half that of continuing smokers. The risk of cancer of the mouth, throat, esophagus, bladder, ulcer, kidney, and pancreas decreases.
- 15 years after quitting—the risk of coronary heart disease is now similar to that of people who have never smoked.

CLINICAL PEARL

Even individuals who have been long-time smokers stand to benefit from quitting. The logic that "it's too late to stop because the damage has already been done," just doesn't fly. Newer data suggest that even heavy smokers show potentially significant improvement in both cardiac and pulmonary function after quitting.

Why is it so difficult to stop using nicotine?

Nicotine is a drug that causes addiction. In one study, researchers noted that 80 percent of women who wanted to stop smoking were unable to do so. Depending on the amount taken in, nicotine can act as either a stimulant or a sedative. Smokers often look forward to the first cigarette of the day because of the way brain cells respond to the first nicotine rush. This first nicotine intake of the day enhances the activity of dopamine-sensitive neurons in the brain. During the day, nerve cells become desensitized to nicotine. Smoking may become less pleasurable and smokers develop a tolerance to the drug requiring increasingly higher levels of nicotine for any pleasurable effect at all.

Withdrawal is difficult with nicotine. Even after years of nonsmoking, about 20 percent of ex-smokers still have occasional cravings for cigarettes. One study reported that 68 percent of all smokers wanted to quit and during a one-year period, a third of them tried seriously, but only 6 percent succeeded. People who keep trying, however, have a 50 percent chance of finally quitting. In any case, the attempts to quit are never a waste of time because the amount of smoking is reduced during these periods.

Researchers have been trying to identify those behaviors that can help predict why so many people fail to quit. Another study found that a consistent predictor of failure to quit was cheating during the first two weeks of withdrawal. Some people actually cheated even if they were wearing a patch. Typically, these cheaters were back smoking again in six months. On the other hand, nearly half of the people who didn't cheat during the first two weeks were still not smoking after six months.

How can an EMS provider stop smoking?

First and foremost the individual who is trying to quit must make a commitment to this goal. A plan for quitting should be supervised by a physician and assisted by family and coworkers as well as one of the many support groups that are available.

What is anxiety?

Anxiety is an uneasiness about future uncertainties.

What is the importance of personal time, meditation, or contemplation to injury prevention in the EMS provider?

As the saying goes, "Get a life!" EMS providers whose work, play, and vacations revolve solely around EMS activities are on a grim journey. No matter how involved and committed you are to EMS activities, you must take a break and do things that are different from work. Everyone needs a little time to himself or herself to put their life or significant emotional events into perspective. This is time to "recharge" the batteries. To some this comes in the form of a half hour on the front porch swing and to others this comes as a walk in the woods or running a few miles through the neighborhood. Some people have learned how to meditate, while others wind down from a busy day by watching a mindless TV show or a funny movie. Whatever you do that works for you is fine. However, we all need a little time in our day to wind down and contemplate the events of the day. Without this recharge time, the body is constantly stressed and is more apt to sickness and injury.

What is the importance of family, peer, and community networks to injury prevention in the EMS provider?

People who have a network of peers, family, and community members are not alone. It is helpful to be able to bounce ideas off others as well as have a backup to help you with life's chores. People who are depressed and have no support network are the ones most likely to commit suicide. Everyone needs to take a mental health day every once in a while, and with a support network there is someone to watch the kids or cover your shift or other responsibilities for the day.

CLINICAL PEARL

There has been a strong move in EMS and emergency medicine toward injury prevention. This is true for patients as well as the EMS providers. In these days of managed care, the prevention of problems is cost-effective for all sides.

What is the importance of freedom from prejudice toward good mental and emotional health in the EMS provider?

To be an excellent caregiver, you must be accepting of the many unique things that make cultures and individuals different. The best way you can do this is to educate yourself about other cultures. For example, different cultures have different views on acceptable social distances as illustrated in Table 1–4. Learn how to recognize the variations between cultures as positive differences.

The EMS provider should recognize the individual differences between people. It is part of your responsibility as an EMS provider to listen carefully to another person's story and work toward win-win solutions to problems rather than judging patients by some stereotype. Having an open and understanding attitude toward all people from all cultures will help improve your mental and emotional health.

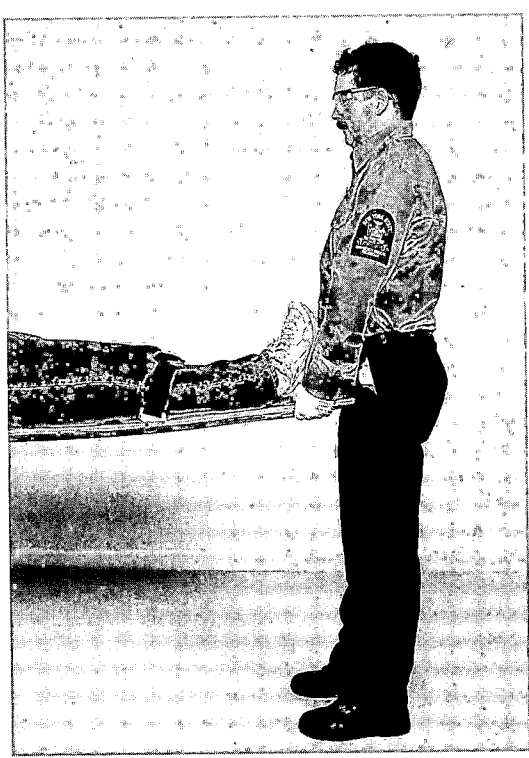

CLINICAL PEARL

Acceptance of diversity in our society is crucial for everyone, especially those providing public services.

TABLE 1-4

Varying Attitudes toward Social Distance

Group	Social Distance
African American	Close and personal
Asian American	Avoid physical closeness
European American	Often avoid close physical contact
Hispanic American	Close proximity is acceptable
Native Americans	Space is important and has no boundaries

Safety and Injury Prevention on the Job

Q **What are some of the ways an EMS provider can prevent injury by lifting properly?**

A The following are some tips to avoid injury when lifting patients:

- Know your limits.
- Only move a patient you can move safely.
- Do not be afraid to ask for more help rather than overextending your abilities and injuring yourself, your partner, or the patient.
- Be careful to look where you are walking or crawling. Whenever possible, move forward rather than backward.
- Take short steps when walking with a patient.
- Bend at the hips and knees, not at the back.
- Keep the load as close to your body as possible (Figure 1-1).
- Do not twist when lifting.
- Always have a secure base by positioning your feet as wide as your hips on firm, flat footing.

Q **What is the best way for an EMS provider to handle a hostile situation?**

A The best way to handle a hostile situation is to avoid it in the first place. If it cannot be avoided, always leave yourself an exit and bring in the radio. Call for police assistance and retreat if in

danger and there is a threat to you or your crew. Do not return until the police have arrived and secured the scene.

When entering any scene, the EMS provider should always be aware of potential weapons that may be present and available to the patient. Some weapons are not as obvious (e.g., bottles, bats, letter openers, and ashtrays).

Q **What are some safety practices in rescue situations that can prevent injury to the EMS provider?**

A To avoid injury at a rescue scene, always wear protective gear that is easily seen at night. Be especially careful of oncoming traffic, as it is not uncommon for drunk, drugged, or sleepy drivers to drive right into the collision scene. Watch your footing when going into the woods to pack out an injured camper. Train in rescue techniques and be aware of the safest way to do each procedure so as not to injure yourself or your partners. For example, use cribbing to stabilize an automobile on its side before trying to access the vehicle.

Q **What are some of the factors that contribute to safe vehicle operation to prevent injury to the EMS provider?**

A You can be extremely healthy and fit and have the best attitude about life, but if your partner takes unnecessary risks when

FIGURE 1-1 Proper lifting technique should be used to prevent injury to your back.

driving the emergency vehicle, your chances of being involved in a serious, often fatal, collision are greatly increased. Driving an emergency vehicle is serious business and should never be taken lightly! The following are some tips to consider that could save your life:

- Be properly trained, have experience, and know how to safely operate the ambulance. Consider taking an emergency vehicle operator course (EVOC).
- Understand the proper use of lights and sirens as well as the public's typical reactions. Also understand the limitations of these devices and that they do not guarantee you the right of way!
- Understand the profile of a typical ambulance collision (i.e., daytime, clear road conditions, dry roads with good visibility, occurring in an intersection). This is discussed in more detail in Chapter 48, Ambulance Operations and Multiple Casualty Incidents.
- Understand the safe ways to park your emergency vehicle at the scene of a collision to keep the patient and other EMS providers protected when working around the ambulance.
- Avoid the use of a police or fire department escort whenever possible.
- Use due regard for the safety of others and understand the legal implications of this "higher standard" of driving.
- Take extra precautions during inclement driving conditions to accommodate poor visibility and longer stopping distances.
- Cover the brake (foot off the accelerator and hovering over the brake) when approaching an intersection or any "iffy" driving situation to decrease the overall stopping distance of the vehicle. This technique helps to keep the driver more aware, and decreases the reaction time and the subsequent distance the vehicle would normally travel while the driver's foot is moving from the accelerator to the brake.
- Always drive with the headlights on to be seen more easily.
- Before proceeding through an intersection, make eye contact with the other drivers so they understand your intent and then cross one lane at a time.
- Always wear your seatbelt when driving and, whenever possible, in the patient compartment of the ambulance.
- Use proper child restraints when transporting children.

What strategies can my EMS agency develop to help eliminate ambulance collisions?

To develop strategies to eliminate ambulance collisions in your service area consider the following areas of emergency-vehicle operator training:

- Qualifications and license checks with the department of motor vehicles.
- Hands-on training.
- Knowledge of the standard operating procedures (SOPs).
- Knowledge of the streets in your community and the location of the hospitals.
- Familiarity with the ambulance size and weight, use of mirrors, braking distances, steering and turning radius, and speed controls.
- Knowledge of the proper reaction to emergency situations such as the loss of brakes, jamming of the throttle, a blowout of a tire, or loss of the power steering.
- Familiarity with the proper way to use the lights and siren and how to properly negotiate an intersection.
- Lots of driving experience with a vehicle that handles much differently than your 2,500-pound compact car.

For what emergency vehicle operation topics should each emergency service have an SOP?

Each agency should have an SOP for their drivers covering at least the following topics:

- How the agency qualifies drivers.
- Who is not allowed to operate your ambulances.
- What should happen when a collision has occurred.
- What are the review, investigation, and quality improvement processes for drivers who have been involved in a collision.
- The use of a spotter, someone properly placed behind the vehicle to guide the driver, for backing the vehicle.
- The use of seat belts in the ambulance and how to transport a child passenger under 40 pounds.
- What constitutes an emergency response and what exemptions may be taken under your state's law and under what conditions.
- A policy on prudent speed.
- A policy on traveling in the oncoming lane.
- A policy on how to negotiate an intersection.

What are the recommended considerations for using escorts when driving an emergency vehicle?

This is an easy one, the recommendation is not to use escorts! They are very dangerous because the public does not expect the second vehicle and begins to drive through the intersection just after the first emergency vehicle passes. If you follow too closely, there is an increased chance of a chain reaction collision when the first vehicle suddenly comes to a stop. The best way to avoid an escort is to know exactly how to get where you are going and when asked if you need one, say no!

It is good practice to tell following family members that they should not follow too closely behind your vehicle and that they are not permitted to go through red lights or stop signs just because your emergency vehicle is doing so. The safest thing to do is to make sure the family has directions to the hospital so they do not have to rely on following your ambulance to the hospital. A good idea is to print up business cards that have directions to the hospitals from various main intersections in your district. This direction card could be given to the family just prior to leaving the scene. Some agencies choose to put other important information on the flip side of the card, such as how to contact your customer service office, how to make a donation, or where to take a CPR course.

To prevent injury, what safety equipment and supplies should EMS personnel use at the scene of a crash?

Based on the types of injuries that occur at crash scenes, the most important safety equipment is a highly visible vest or turnout coat so the other drivers can see you! Other equipment that should be available and used at the scene of a rescue or collision includes:

- Body substance isolation (BSI) equipment such as latex disposable gloves, masks, and goggles.
- Head protection, such as a helmet.
- Eye protection, such as safety goggles or shields.
- Hearing protection as necessary.
- Respiratory protection as necessary.
- Gloves for protection from broken glass and hot objects.
- Heavy-duty boots for protection from the weather and heavy objects.
- Coveralls or a combination turnout coat and pants for protection from sharp objects and for visibility.
- Specialty equipment for specific types of rescue (e.g., self-contained breathing apparatus (SCBA), full-body harness, haz-mat suits).

Stress and the EMS Provider

What is stress?

Stress is defined as a factor that induces bodily or mental tension. When we speak of stress in EMS, we mean tension that results from the interaction of events, such as environmental stimuli, and the adjustment abilities of the individual. Although usually thought of as a negative factor (e.g., fear, depression, guilt, etc.), stress is a natural and necessary emotion and is experienced with positive events also.

What are the types of stress?

There are two types of stress: eustress and distress. Eustress is a good stress, a response to a positive event such as the excitement of being the center of attention at a surprise party. Distress is a bad stress, a negative response to an environmental stimulus such as the reaction to the death of a loved one.

What is GAS?

Early last century, Hans Selye postulated the existence of a nonspecific defense system initiated by stress called the *general adaptation syndrome* (GAS). Individuals suffering from a wide variety of physical disorders all seemed to share a common cluster of overt symptoms. Following his initial observation, Selye determined that illness was not the only event capable of eliciting this syndrome. He realized that this pattern of bodily responses was manifested whenever the internal or external environment of an organism was altered in some significant way. He reasoned that when environmental conditions change, the organism must adapt. The complete GAS process is a long-term physiological response pattern to adaptation. The response is mediated by cortisol release from the adrenal cortex. We now equate the stages of GAS with the processes and development of human stress. Selye outlined three phases of the syndrome:

1. Alarm reaction. The *alarm reaction* is analogous to Cannon's fight or flight response. It is the onset of the stress process. During the alarm reaction, the body reacts to a change in circumstances. It is as though a physiological alarm went off somewhere inside the body, suddenly mobilizing internal activity. During this phase, the body notes the environmental change and reacts by initiating its adaptive defenses. An environmental change can be internal or external (e.g., change in outside air temperature, a change in chemical balance within the body, standing in the shower when the hot water runs out, or tripping on a sidewalk and breaking your ankle). The alarm reaction is the body's first response to begin adapting to the new set of circumstances. Homeostasis is called into action.

2. Stage of resistance. The *stage of resistance* is a plateau phase of the response. During this stage, the body continues to adapt by actively using its homeostatic resources to maintain its physiological integrity and resist the changes imposed on it. This is the longest phase of the GAS. It may last for months, years, or even decades.

3. Stage of exhaustion. The *stage of exhaustion* occurs when one or more organ systems can no longer hold up under the increased workload of the adaptation effort. In this last phase, some facet of the human body's functioning fails. When one or more organ systems fail or become exhausted under the stress of adaptation, the organism can develop a disease of adaptation. Diseases of adaptation are the end result of GAS. At this point, stress manifests itself as a definable medical problem such as a heart attack, gastric ulcer, stroke, breakdown of the immune system, or diabetes. Such diseases of adaptation are also referred to as *stress-related diseases*.

[Q] What is the psychoneuroimmunologic response to stress?

[A] Psychoneuroimmunology (PNI) is the study of the interrelations between behavior, the neural and endocrine functions, and the immune system. PNI studies the connections between stress, physiological dysregulation, and health outcomes. Research supports the theory that emotional distress and the resultant neuroendocrine activation can induce immune system suppression. This suppression has significant implications for disease susceptibility and progression. Psychological stress is

TABLE 1–5

Effect of Stress on the Body

Organ Affected	Receptor Type	Response	Organ Affected	Receptor Type	Response
Eyes			**Intestine**		
Radial muscle of the iris	α_1	Pupillary contraction	Motility and tone	$\alpha_1, \alpha_2, \beta_1, \beta_2$	Decrease
Ciliary muscle	β_1	Relaxation for far vision	Sphincters	α_1	Contraction
Heart			Secretion	α_2	Inhibition
S-A node	β_1, β_2	Increased heart rate	**Gallbladder**		
Atria	β_1, β_2	Increased contractility and conduction velocity	**and Ducts**	β_2	Relaxation
A-V node	β_1, β_2	Increased conduction velocity	**Urinary Bladder**		
His-Purkinje system	β_1, β_2	Increased conduction velocity	Detrusor	β_2	Relaxation
Ventricles	β_1, β_2	Increased contractility	Trigone and sphincter	α_1	Contraction
Arterioles			**Ureters**		
Coronary	α_1, α_2	Constriction	Motility and tone	α_1	Increase
	β_2	Dilation	**Uterus**	α_1	Contraction (pregnant)
Skin and mucosa	α_1, α_2	Constriction		β_2	Relaxation (pregnant and nonpregnant)
Skeletal muscle	α_1	Constriction	**Male Sex Organs**	α_1	Ejaculation
	β_2	Dilation	**Skin**	α_1	
Cerebral	α_1	Constriction	Pilomotor muscles	α_1	Contraction
Pulmonary	α_1	Constriction	Sweat glands	α_1	Slight, localized secretion
	β_2	Dilation	**Spleen Capsule**	α_1	Contraction
Abdominal viscera	α_1	Constriction		β_2	Relaxation
	β_2	Dilation	**Liver**	α_1, β_2	Glycogenolysis
Salivary glands	α_1, α_2	Constriction	**Pancreas**		
Renal	α_1, α_2	Constriction	Acini	α (subtype unknown)	Decreased secretion
	β_1, β_2	Dilation	Islets	α_2	Decreased insulin and glucagon secretion
Systemic Veins	α_1, α_2	Constriction		β_2	Increased insulin and glucagon secretion
	β_2	Dilation			
Lungs			**Salivary Glands**	α_1	Thick, viscous secretion
Bronchial muscle	β_2	Relaxation		β (subtype unknown)	Amylase secretion
Bronchial glands	α_1	Inhibition			
	β_2	Stimulation	**Lacrimal Glands**	α (subtype unknown)	Secretion
Stomach					
Motility and tone	$\alpha_1, \alpha_2, \beta_2$	Decrease	**Adipose Tissue (fat)**	$\alpha_1, \beta_1, \beta_2$	Lipolysis
Sphincters	α_1	Contraction	**Juxtaglomerular Cells**	β_1	Increased renin secretion
Secretion	α_2	Inhibition			

able to alter the susceptibility of animals and humans to infectious agents, influencing the onset, course, and outcome of certain infectious pathologies. Data suggests that stress also affects cancer, HIV infection, autoimmune diseases (e.g., lupus, rheumatoid arthritis), neurodermatitis, asthma, and psoriasis.

Q **Because catacholamines are released during a stress reaction, what are the physiologic effects of catacholamines on the following: brain, cardiovascular, pulmonary, muscle, liver, adipose tissue, skin, skeleton, gastrointestinal (GI) and genitourinary (GU) systems, and lymphoid tissue?**

A The physiologic effects of catacholamines on these organs and systems and their receptors are summarized in Table 1–5. Often, but not always, parasympathetic (cholinergic) stimulation has opposite effects.

Q **What is the role of cortisol in the stress response?**

A Cortisol is secreted by the adrenal gland in response to adrenocorticotropic hormone (ACTH) secretion from the pituitary. Any physical or mental stress initiates release, though the exact mechanism is uncertain. Cortisol exerts the following effects on metabolism:

- Decreases protein stores in extrahepatic tissues. Amino acids are released into the blood, taken up by the liver, and converted into glucose and proteins.
- Increases blood glucose concentration and stimulates hepatic gluconeogenesis (production of new glucose) and impairs the utilization of glucose by peripheral tissues.
- Permits mobilization of fatty acids by epinephrine and growth hormone.

Q **What is the role of hormones in the stress reaction?**

A Two general types of hormones are released during the stress reaction, peptides (e.g., epinephrine, glucagon) and steroids (cortisol). Epinephrine and glucagon stimulate the sympathetic nervous system leading to a variety of effects, including increased blood sugar levels. Cortisol works as described previously. The net effect is an organism better equipped to handle stress. More nutrients are also available and the necessary systems are "activated" to process them quicker.

Q **What is the role of the immune system during a stress reaction?**

A Acutely, the fight or flight response triggers catecholamine release, leading to increased levels of available white blood cells.

Chronic physical or emotional distress and the resultant neuroendocrine activation can induce immune system suppression.

Q **What are the medical interventions for effective and ineffective coping with stress?**

A Sometimes stress is healthy. Studies have shown that moderate levels increase productivity. On the other hand, too much of anything is potentially harmful. There are a variety of medical techniques for dealing with stress. The most successful involve a combination of:

- Biofeedback.
- Patient education.
- Medication.
- Psychotherapy.
- Meditation.
- "Complementary" health therapy (e.g., aroma therapy, massage therapy).

Q **What are examples of factors that trigger the stress response?**

A Factors that can trigger a stress response include:

- Poor health or nutrition.
- The loss of something that is of value to the individual.
- An injury or the threat of an injury to the body.
- Ineffective coping.

Q **What are the physical signs and symptoms of stress?**

A The physical signs and symptoms of stress include:

- Chest tightness or pain.
- Heart palpitations.
- Cardiac rhythm disturbances.
- Difficulty breathing.
- Tachypnea.
- Nausea and vomiting.
- Profuse sweating and diaphoresis.
- Flushed skin.
- Sleep disturbances.
- Aching muscles and joints.
- Headache.

Q **What are the emotional signs and symptoms of stress?**

A The emotional signs and symptoms of stress include:

- Panic reactions.
- Fear.
- Anger.
- Denial.
- Feeling overwhelmed.

Q What are the cognitive signs and symptoms of stress?

A The cognitive signs and symptoms of stress include:
- Difficulty making decisions.
- Disorientation.
- Decreased level of awareness.
- Memory problems.
- Poor concentration.
- Distressing dreams.

Q What are the behavioral signs and symptoms of stress?

A The behavioral signs and symptoms of stress include:
- Crying spells.
- Hyperactivity.
- Withdrawal.
- Depression.
- Changes in eating habits.
- Increased smoking.
- Increased alcohol consumption.
- Changes in sleep patterns.

Q What are the general categories of stress causes in EMS?

A General causes of stress in EMS are categorized as environmental, psychosocial, and personality or emotional.

Q What are the causes of environmental stress in EMS?

A Environmental stress is often caused by:
- Siren noise.
- Inclement weather.
- Confined work spaces.
- Rapid scene response.
- Life and death decision making.

Q What are the causes of psychosocial stress in EMS?

A Psychosocial stress is often caused by:
- Family relationships.
- A spouse or significant other who doesn't understand what EMS work or training involves.
- Conflicts with supervisors and coworkers.
- Abusive patients or their family members.

Q What are the causes of personality and emotional stress in EMS?

A Personality and emotional stress is often caused by:
- The need to be liked.
- Personal expectations.
- Feelings of guilt.
- Feelings of anxiety.
- Feelings of incompetence.
- Response to the death or injury of a child or coworker.

Q What are the typical reactions to stress?

A The reactions to stress are individual and are affected by previous exposure to the stressor. They relate to your personal perception of the event. Experience can help in dealing with stress as well as using personal coping skills.

Q What are some ways people adapt to stress?

A Adaptation is a dynamic evolving process. It involves defenses and coping, problem-solving, and mastery skills. People develop defenses as a part of their personality, which assist in adjusting to stressful situations. Some people develop defenses such as distortion of the facts or denial.

Coping is an active process of confronting the stress or the cause of the stress. Information is gathered and used to change or adjust to a new situation.

Problem solving is viewed as a healthy approach to everyday concerns. It involves an analysis of the problem, the generation of options for action, and a determination of the proper course of action. Mastery at adaptation involves being able to see multiple options or potential solutions for challenging situations. This results from extensive experience with similar situations.

Q What are examples of techniques used to manage stress?

A Examples of techniques used to manage stress include reframing, controlled breathing, progressive relaxation, and guided imagery. Extensive volumes have been written on each of these techniques. For details on any of these techniques visit your local library or the "self-help" section of a local bookstore.

[Q] What are some tips to help control stress, rather than letting it control you?

[A] The following is a list by John Towler, Ph.D., of tips and techniques to reduce stress, reprinted with permission from his book *A Love Affair With Life*.

- Maintain a good sense of humor.
- Maintain the right eating habits.
- Set realistic goals for yourself.
- Understand stress, what it is, and how it works.
- Maintain a stable home.
- Learn and use relaxation skills.
- Get enough sleep.
- Write things down instead of relying on your memory.
- Don't put up with something that doesn't work right.
- Never let a computer know that you are in a hurry.
- Be prepared to wait.
- Relax your standards.
- Learn how to say "no."
- Find some time for yourself.
- Don't be a slave to the phone.
- Associate with Type B personality types instead of Type A's.
- Get organized.
- Always focus on the positives.
- Inoculate yourself against events.
- Get up and stretch.
- Eliminate destructive self-talk.
- Live one day at a time.
- Do something you enjoy every day.
- Exercise.
- Do something to improve your appearance.
- Become more flexible.
- Do one thing at a time.
- If you have something unpleasant to do, do it first thing in the morning.
- Learn to delegate.
- Do something nice for somebody else.

[Q] What is CISM?

[A] *Critical incident stress management* (CISM) is an organized process involving a network of peers and mental health professionals supporting EMS providers who have been involved in a critical incident. A CISM enables emergency personnel to vent feelings and facilitates an understanding of stressful situations.

[Q] What are the components of a CISM?

[A] The components of CISM include the following:

- Pre-incident training in stress recognition and management and how to activate the support network.
- On-scene support of distressed personnel at a major incident.
- Individualized consultation.
- A defusing after a large-scale incident.
- Mobilization services immediately after a large-scale incident.
- Critical incident stress debriefing 24 to 72 hours after an event.
- Follow-up mental health services.
- Specialty debriefings to nonemergency groups in the community (e.g., the families that witnessed the event).
- Support during routine discussions of an incident.
- Advice to command staff during large-scale incidents.

[Q] What are examples of situations where a CISM should be considered?

[A] The organizations that do CISM recommend that their services be considered in the following situations:

- Line of duty death or serious injury.
- Disaster situations.
- Emergency worker suicide.
- The death of an infant or child that affected EMS providers.
- Extreme threat to emergency workers.
- A prolonged incident that ends in a loss or success.
- Patients known to the EMS providers.
- Death or injury of a civilian caused by the EMS providers.
- Other significant events.

[Q] What are some of the indications that a coworker is experiencing a crisis-induced stress reaction?

[A] When an EMS provider has been exposed to any of the significant events listed previously, they may begin to have any of the following signs of excessive stress:

- Nausea, vomiting, or chills.
- Signs of gastrointestinal distress.
- Dry mouth, shakes, or headache.
- Vision problems or sleep disturbances.
- Confusion, shorter attention span, or memory problems.
- Poor concentration, difficulty making decisions, or distressing dreams.
- Anxiety, feeling overwhelmed, or feeling numb.
- Identifying with a victim, wanting to hide, or hopelessness.
- Increased smoking, drinking, or drug use.
- Excessive humor, crying spells, or withdrawal.

What are the key techniques for reducing crisis-induced stress?

The key techniques for reducing crisis-induced stress include:

- Plenty of rest.
- Replacing food and fluids.
- Limiting exposure to the incident.
- Alternating assignments.
- Post-incident defusings or debriefings.

Coping with Death and Dying

What are the stages of the grieving process?

Dr. Elizabeth Kübler-Ross is widely appreciated for her pioneering work in the field of grief, death, and dying. According to the Kübler-Ross model, the stages of the grieving process that the patient and their family go through include six specific steps. There is no timetable on how long it generally takes for someone to go through the steps; however, most do go through each. The steps, in order of occurrence, are:

1. Shock. This is a kind of numbness that acts as nature's insulation, cushioning the blow of the incident. The victim may experience physical sensations like feeling spaced-out or a knot in the stomach and no appetite.
2. Denial. This is the inability or refusal to believe the reality of the event. It is a defense mechanism, which involves the victim saying, "This is not happening to me." People do things like continuing to set a place at the dinner table for the deceased or refusing to visit the grave. Some people leave the deceased's room unchanged for quite a while. For most

people, keeping a few treasures and photos in view indefinitely is not denial but an affirmation of love.
3. Anger. This is due to frustration related to the inability to control the situation. The anger may be focused on anyone or anything. Anger is an emotion that must be expressed. One person screams in a private place. Another beats a mattress with a piece of hose. Another does hard exercise. Everyone should at least talk about it because holding in anger causes stress and sooner or later it comes out.
4. Bargaining. This is attempting to buy more time, trying to make deals to put off or change expected outcomes. This is the person who says, "Can I just have a few more minutes to do . . . ?"
5. Depression. Sadness and despair from the loss can lead to depression, withdrawal or retreating. Typically, when the numbness wears off and the rage has been exhausted, depression arrives. Some people describe the feeling as one of hopeless emptiness. Often it is the people who "seemed to take it so well" who hit bottom at a later time. This is the time when a friend who is willing to listen and not judge the victim's rambling and repetitive talk about the loss can be very helpful.
6. Acceptance. This is the realization of fate and obtaining a reasonable level of comfort with the anticipated outcome or loss. Some experts say families do not actually come to complete acceptance until a full year's worth of holidays have passed without the loved one's presence (e.g., Thanksgiving, Christmas, Chanukah, New Year's, birthday, and anniversary).

CLINICAL PEARL

It is not unusual for families to vent their anger toward EMS providers. Do not take this personally or argue with the person. As long as there is no perceived physical harm to you, allow them to express their feelings. Avoid expressing any opinions or judgments.

What are the needs of the EMS provider in dealing with death and dying?

After being involved in a call involving an unexpected death, the EMS provider also needs the support from friends and family following the incident. There has to be an opportunity to process the incident to prevent it from turning into cumulative stress. Some EMS providers tend to make light of everything, but eventually the stress will catch up to them.

What are the developmental considerations when dealing with death and dying?

Developmental considerations when dealing with death and dying can be broken into the following specifics for age groups:

- Newborn to age three—Children in this age group sense that something has happened in the family because people are crying and sad all the time. Children will realize there is extra activity in their house. Watch children for signs of eating or sleeping disruptions or irritability. Be sensitive to the child's needs and try to maintain some consistency in the routines and with significant people in the child's life.

- Three to six years old—This age group does not understand the concept of the finality of death. The child believes that the deceased will return and the child may continue to ask, "When will daddy be back home?" This child believes in magical thinking and may also think he is responsible for the parent "going away." The child may believe that everyone else he loves may leave also. Watch children for changes in behavior patterns with friends and at school, difficulty sleeping and eating. Try to emphasize to the child that he was not responsible for the death and reinforce that when people are sad they cry, which is normal and natural to do. Encourage the child to draw pictures of his feelings or talk about his feelings.

- Six to nine years old—These children are beginning to understand the finality of death. They will seek out detailed explanations for the death and want to understand the difference between a fatal illness and just being sick. This child may also be afraid that other significant people in her life may die as well and will be uncomfortable expressing feelings. She may act embarrassed when talking about death. Try to talk about normal feelings of anger, sadness, and guilt with the child and share your feelings about death. Do not be afraid to cry in front of the children. This gives the children permission to express their feelings.

- Nine to twelve years old—These children are aware of the finality of death and may want to know all the details surrounding the death. This child may try to "act like an adult," but then regress to an earlier stage of emotional response. Try to set aside time to talk about feelings and encourage sharing memories to facilitate the grief response with this child.

- Adolescents—These young adults should be watched closely without smothering them. They are old enough that they may have already been experimenting with drugs, alcohol, or cults. They may glamorize death or seek to "copycat" a suicidal gesture. Watch them for signs of depression and try to involve them in the family's grief response without undue embarrassment that may cause them to go off on their own.

- The elderly—They will be concerned about the other family members and further loss of independence and the costs.

How do you tell a child that someone he loves has died?

This is very difficult, but the first rule is to tell the truth and be straightforward. Do not distort reality by saying he has "gone to sleep" or "God took him." These phrases can lead to unnecessary fears. The assurance of love and support is the greatest thing a parent or family member can do for the grieving child.

Any other words of wisdom on helping children deal with grief?

It is wise to let the child participate in the family sorrow. If shielded she may feel rejected. Let the child see the family's grief and that it is okay to cry. It may be distressing to see dad cry over mom's death, but it is probably far more distressing for the child to see that "everything appears normal."

Try to protect the child from unnecessary burdens. Do not let others say, "You are now the man of the house" or "be brave." Having to take on more responsibility or put on a false front makes grieving more difficult.

Preventing Disease Transmission

This material is covered in detail in Chapter 30, Infectious and Communicable Diseases. This section deals with an overview of disease transmission prevention by the EMS provider.

Q **What are the most common types of pathogens EMS providers may be exposed to in the field?**

A EMS providers should be prepared to protect themselves from airborne pathogens (e.g., TB) and blood-borne pathogens (e.g., HIV, hepatitis B).

Q **What is an exposure?**

A An exposure is contact with a potentially infectious body fluid that may be carrying a pathogen. Examples of exposures can include:

- Respiratory secretions sprayed into the face.
- Bleeding onto the broken skin of an EMS provider.
- A needle stick or sharps injury.
- Coughing in the face of an EMS provider.
- Exposure to pus or secretions from an infected wound.

Q **What are the definitions of cleaning, disinfection, and sterilization?**

A The definitions are as follows:

- Cleaning—removal of the dirt on the surface of an object, usually with a cleaner or soap and water.
- Disinfection—cleaning the surface of objects with a specific agent designed to kill pathogens that may have come in contact with the object. There are three levels of disinfection: high, intermediate, and low. A high-level agent destroys all forms of microbial life except high numbers of bacterial spores. An intermediate-level disinfectant kills Mycobacterium tuberculosis, vegetative bacteria, most viruses, and most fungi, but not bacterial spores. A low-level disinfectant kills most bacteria, some viruses, and some fungi, but no Mycobacterium tuberculosis or bacterial spores.
- Sterilization—a process designed to kill all forms of microbial life including high numbers of bacterial spores. Instruments, such as a laryngoscope, can be gas sterilized or liquid sterilized by soaking for a specific period of time in an agent such as Cydex II®.

Q **What is BSI?**

A BSI is an acronym for *body substance isolation* procedures, which is a series of practices designed to prevent contact with body substances such as blood, urine, fecal material, vomitus, and so forth.

Q **What can the EMS provider do to be protected against air- or blood-borne pathogens?**

A To protect yourself from air- or blood-borne pathogens, follow work practices such as:

- Good personal hygiene habits, such as handwashing after every patient contact, and general cleanliness. It is always surprising in a public bathroom to see how many people do not even wash their hands after going to the bathroom!
- Maintain your immunizations. EMS providers should have up-to-date records of immunizations for tetanus, polio, hepatitis B, measles, mumps, rubella, and influenza.
- Obtain periodic TB screening. Most services recommend every six months if you are in direct contact with patients.
- Practice BSI. When appropriate, use gloves, mask, gown, eyewear, and other equipment to prevent exposure to pathogens.
- Proper cleaning and disinfection of materials and equipment. This includes the proper use of sharps containers, proper handling of laundry and any bedding that may have been exposed to body fluids. This also includes the proper labeling of exposured materials and equipment.
- Periodic risk assessment and ongoing exposed control training.

Q **How do periodic risk assessments and knowledge of the warning signs of cancer, cardiovascular disease, and infectious disease contribute to disease prevention?**

A When EMS providers are aware of the importance of periodic risk assessments and know the warning signs of cancer, cardiovascular disease, and infectious disease, they are not only able to prevent disease in their patients and family, but themselves as well.

Relating to cardiovascular disease, the EMS provider should consider the implications of the following:

- Cardiovascular endurance.
- Blood pressure.
- Body composition.
- Total cholesterol/high density lipoprotein (HDL) ratio—some physicians are prescribing medications called "sartans," such as Lipitor®, which decrease cholesterol and may cause a regression or prevention of atherosclerosis.
- Triglycerides.
- Estrogen use.
- Stress.

Relating to cancer, the EMS provider should consider the implications of the following:

- Dietary changes.
- Too much exposure to the sun.
- The need for regular examinations.
- The warning signs of cancer—see Chapter 6, General Principles of Pathophysiology.

Relating to infectious diseases, the EMS provider should consider the implications of the following:

- Personal hygiene.
- Using practices designed to limit occupational exposures (e.g., having the sharps container at the patient's side when the IV is started, not recapping sharps).
- Reporting exposures promptly.

What is involved in documenting and managing an exposure?

An exposure must be properly managed and taken very seriously. The following are steps to be taken in addition to following your service's exposure control plan:

- Wash the area of contact thoroughly and immediately.
- Document the situation in which the exposure occurred.
- Describe actions taken to reduce chances of infection.
- Comply with all required reporting responsibilities and time frames within your organization.
- Cooperate with the incident investigation.
- Check for TB status.
- Comply with the prophylaxis recommended by your service medical director or Infection Control expert.
- Make sure you are up to date on all the proper immunization boosters.
- Complete the required medical follow-up.

Special Thanks

John Towler, Ph.D., for the list of "Tips and Techniques to Help Control Stress," from his book, *A Love Affair with Life*, American College of Prehospital Medicine, 1998.

EMS Systems, Roles, and Responsibilities

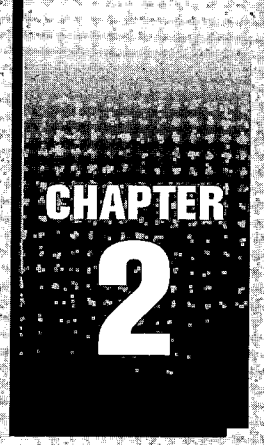

CHAPTER 2

T his chapter discusses the history of EMS development as well as the roles and respon-sibilities of the EMS provider. The focus is on *why* the EMS provider must have certain professional attributes for the roles they fulfill. A good understanding of the management of EMS systems, the history, and the role of Medical Control will help prepare the EMS provider for a career.

The History of EMS System Development

Q What were some of the milestones in the development of EMS systems nationally?

A The following history lesson gives some "perspective" as to how far we have evolved in such a short amount of time in EMS.

- The original "Good Samaritan," who provided medical assistance to a traveler at the side of the road, dates back to the biblical times.

- Some of the earliest known medical "protocols" were written on clay tablets in Mesopotamia approximately 4,000 to 5,000 years ago. In 1862, Edwin Smith purchased scrolls dating back to 1,500 B.C. that contained the "Book of Wounds," which explained the treatment of injuries such as fractures and dislocations with splints, dressings, and bandages and described solutions to clean wounds.

- In 1797, Jean Larrey, one of Napoleon's chief surgeons, was credited with developing the ambulances volantes (the flying ambulances) during the Napoleonic wars. The purpose was to triage and transport the injured from the field to aid stations.

- In 1855, Florence Nightingale helped to introduce hygienic standards into the military hospitals.

- Between 1861 and 1865, during the American Civil War, Clara Barton was the nurse responsible for coordinating service to the wounded at battlefield sites. She went on to become the founder of the American Red Cross.

- The first civilian ambulance service was started in Cincinnati in 1865. Within a few years, ambulance service was provided by the New York City Department of Health from Bellevue Hospital.

- In 1915, the first known medical air transport occurred during the retreat of the Serbian army from Albania.

- In the 1920s, many of the first volunteer rescue squads were organized in Roanoke, Virginia, and along the New Jersey coast.

- During World War I, the average evacuation time from the battle scene was 18 hours. In World War II, a system of transportation to echelons of care was created. This was a move in the right direction, but it still took the patient a considerable amount of time to reach definitive care.

- In the 1950s to 1960s, many of the urban hospital-based systems developed into municipal services. Many of the rural

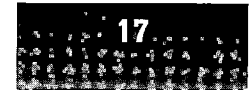

17

funeral homes developed into volunteer fire or ambulance services.

- In 1958, Peter Safar, M.D. demonstrated the effectiveness of mouth-to-mouth ventilation.

- In 1960, CPR was first shown to be an effective treatment method for cardiac arrest victims.

- The use of the helicopter was introduced during the Korean War and further perfected during the Vietnam conflict. It was not uncommon for patients to make it to the field hospital within 20 minutes of their injury. After stabilization, the patients were often transported within 48 hours to a hospital in the Philippines.

- In 1966, the white paper "Accidental Death and Disability: The Neglected Disease of Modern Society" by the National Academy of Sciences was published. This paper depicted a very poor emergency care system and was credited as the match that sparked the future development of modern EMS systems.

- In 1966, the Highway Safety Act was enacted. This landmark legislation created the U.S. Department of Transportation (DOT) as a cabinet level department. It also required the Secretary of the DOT, through their newly created EMS program, to develop a series of training programs to respond to the needs of patients injured on the highways.

- In 1968, the Secretary of DOT's Advisory Committee on Traffic Safety report on EMS was issued. Many of the early advanced life support pilot programs were developed with grants awarded as seed money during this period.

- During the years from 1968 to 1979, the DOT gave out over $140 million in matching 402 grants—traffic safety grants used for EMS development—to 10 DOT regions.

- In 1968, AT&T announced that 911 would be the universal emergency number and the first official call to 911 was placed on February 16, 1968, in Haleyville, Alabama.

- In 1969, the DOT published the first EMT–Ambulance curriculum.

- In September 1969, six Los Angeles County firefighters began their training to become paramedics. They may not have been the first as there were a number of cities in the country starting their programs around this time. However, with the assistance of Producer Jack Webb, of *Dragnet* fame, and Battalion Chief Jim Page the television show *Emergency* was born in LA County. Many dedicated career paramedics can trace their original passion for EMS to the prime-time TV series.

- In 1970, the National Highway Traffic Safety Administration (NHTSA) was established with DOT. NHTSA provides leadership to the EMS community and states as well as other federal agencies involved in EMS.

- In June of 1970, the first meeting of the Board of Directors of the National Registry of EMTs (NREMT) was convened.

- In 1973, the Emergency Medical Services Systems Act (PL-154) was enacted to begin to build "wall-to-wall" national EMS systems. The legislation defined 15 required EMS system components and emphasized a regional approach to trauma care. The Department of Health Education and Welfare awarded $182 million to 543 grantees between 1974 and 1979.

- In 1973, the Robert Wood Johnson Foundation appropriated $15 million to fund 44 regional EMS projects in 32 states and Puerto Rico.

- In May of 1973, the first National Conference on Standards for CPR was held in Washington, DC.

- In 1974, the DOT published the "KKK-A-1822" Federal Ambulance Specifications in an attempt to standardize the design of ambulances. These "specs" have been revised over the years and are now in a proposed fourth edition.

- In 1975, the National Association of EMTs was formed.

- In 1977, national educational standards for paramedics were first developed by NHTSA.

- In 1978, Jeff Clawson, M.D. revolutionized medical dispatch with the introduction of a system that involves prearrival instructions and dispatch according to medical priority protocols. He also started the emergency medical dispatcher (EMD) training throughout the country.

- In the 1980s, the federal deficit halted national funding and many national initiatives. The Omnibus Budget Reconciliation Act of 1981 shifted the categorical EMS system grants to block grants (Preventative Health and Health Services Block Grant). This greatly reduced federal control and allowed the states to disburse funds as they wished. States began to take a more prominent role in regulation and standard setting, which made national standardization difficult to attain. This shift in funding diminished efforts and a tremendous amount of momentum was lost. NHTSA began an effort to sustain the early effort of the Department of Health and Human Services with reduced funding and staff.

- In 1983, the American College of Surgeons identified the standard equipment to be carried on BLS ambulances.

- In 1983, the Emergency Medical Services for Children (EMS-C) Act was passed (PL-98-555). This Act was designed to improve the care of children. Over 40 states have received funding through this program.

- In 1986, the U.S. Department of Defense disseminated Directive No. 6000.10 on EMS, which required all technicians or hospital corpsman working in EMS or assigned to ambulance duty to obtain national registration.

- In 1988, the American College of Surgeons identified the standard equipment to be carried on ALS ambulances.
- The 1990s brought a new federal approach to health care cost cutting introducing managed care. Many services were consolidated. Many ambulance services merged to create large national ambulance services that could now be found on the stock market.
- In the 1990s, out of a need for a unified EMS voice, many of the national EMS organizations formed the EMS Alliance. This alliance caused NHTSA to decide to contract with the National Association of State EMS Directors and the National Association of EMS Physicians to develop a comprehensive review of EMS and prioritize an EMS agenda for the future.
- In 1990, the Trauma Care Systems Planning and Development Act (PL-101-590) was passed. This legislation was designed to encourage development of inclusive trauma systems and provide funding to states for trauma system planning, implementation, and evaluation. In 1995, Congress did not reauthorize funding for this program.
- The 1995 revision of EMT-Basic curriculum included the use of the automated external defibrillator, making it a skill taught to all levels of EMT, rather than reserved for only the advanced EMTs. This skill had been "piloted" by many states at the EMT-B level for most of the past 10 years so the timing was definitely right to move it into all curriculums. During the next few years, many states passed public access defibrillation laws that opened the door to laypersons becoming trained in the use of an automated external defibrillator (AED).
- In 1998, DOT published the revised EMT-Paramedic and EMT-Intermediate curriculums.

Q **What are some of the national groups that have played an important role in the development, education, and implementation of EMS?**

A There have been many national organizations that have played a role in the development of EMS as we know it today. Those organizations include:

- National Association of EMTs.
- National Association of Search and Rescue.
- National Association of State EMS Directors.
- National Council of State EMS Training Coordinators.
- National Flight Paramedic Association (NFPA).
- National Association of EMS Physicians.
- National Registry of EMTs.
- American Academy of Orthopaedic Surgeons.

- American Ambulance Association.
- American College of Emergency Physicians.
- American College of Surgeons, Committee on Trauma.
- American Heart Association.
- American Red Cross.
- American Trauma Society.
- American Society for Testing and Materials, Committee F30 on EMS.
- Committee on Accreditation of Educational Programs for the Emergency Medical Services Professions.
- Commission on Accreditation of Ambulance Services.
- International Critical Incident Stress Foundation.
- International Association of Fire Fighters.
- Continuing Education Coordinating Board for EMS.
- National Association of EMS Educators.
- National Academy for Emergency Medical Dispatch.
- Federal Emergency Management Agency, Emergency Management Institute.
- U.S. Dept. of Health and Human Services, Maternal and Child Health, Centers for Disease Control, and National Disaster Medical System.
- U.S. Department of Labor, Occupational Safety and Health Administration.

Q **What is the role of EMS standard-setting organizations?**

A EMS standard-setting groups (e.g., NHTSA, OSHA, NREMT, NFPA, state EMS agencies, Regional EMS Councils, and ambulance service and EMS educational program accrediting agencies) establish standards with input from the profession and the public. Most of these groups have a direct or indirect responsibility for ensuring that the public interest is served through standard development and implementation. The state agencies also have a regulatory function to protect the public from individuals who do not meet professional standards.

The Basics

Q **What is an EMS System?**

A An EMS system is a coordinated effort to bring together at least 10 key components to reduce out-of-hospital morbidity and mortality. The components of the emergency medical services system (EMSS) have evolved over the past 25 years from 15 essential components (EMSS Act of 1973) to 10 standard components (NHTSA Technical Assistance Program 1988):

- Facilities (e.g., hospitals).
- Transportation (e.g., ambulances, aircraft).
- Communication (e.g., radio, telephone).
- Human Resources and Training (e.g., First Responders, EMT-Basic, Paramedics).
- Resource Management (e.g., coordination of available services).
- Regulation and Policy (e.g., state laws and rules on equipment carried on vehicles).
- Evaluation (e.g., data analysis of how fast, how often, how accurate).
- Public Information and Education (e.g., who to call, how to call, what to do until EMS arrives).
- Medical Oversight (e.g., medical protocols and clinical prerogatives of field personnel).
- Trauma Systems (e.g., which hospitals are prepared to handle the most severe trauma patients).

What is meant by licensure of EMS providers?

Licensure is permission that is granted by a governmental authority to practice in a profession, business, or activity. Examples of licenses include: a driver's license, a fishing license, a boating license, a medical license, and in some states a paramedic license.

What is meant by certification of EMS providers?

A certification is a document testifying to the fulfillment of the requirements for practice in a field. This is usually used to refer to an action of a nongovernmental entity granting authority to an individual who has met predetermined qualifications to participate in an activity. An example is a CPR certification or a life guard certification.

What is meant by registration of EMS providers?

To register is to enroll one's name in a book of record. The National Registry of Emergency Medical Technicians (NREMT) registers EMS providers from across the U.S. The Registry is a not-for-profit, nongovernmental agency led by a board of directors representing many EMS organizations. The Registry administers a practical and written examination for each of the four national levels of out-of-hospital EMS training (i.e., First Respon-

der, EMT-Basic, EMT-Intermediate, and EMT-Paramedic). Currently, there are approximately 155,000 registered EMS providers and the NREMT's registration services are part of the licensure process in 39 states.

What are the nationally recognized levels of EMS training leading to licensure, certification, or registration?

The national levels of EMS training as described in the DOT curricula are outlined in Table 2–1.

> **CLINICAL PEARL**
>
> *Some states have added other provider levels such as cardiac rescue technician (CRT). The four national levels of care (FR, EMT-B, EMT-I, EMT-P) are standardized, at least in terms of the DOT curriculum.*

What is the role of the NREMT?

The National Registry is responsible for the following:
- Contributing to the development of professional standards.
- Verifying competency by developing and administering practical and written examinations.
- Simplifying the process of state-to-state reciprocity or credentialing. Reciprocity is the acceptance of one's education and training by another jurisdiction such as from state to state.
- Spreading the costs of exam development and validation across a larger user base than most states.

What are the forms of recertification generally available throughout the country?

Traditionally, the DOT has published a recertification curriculum that corresponds to each national level of care. The refresher training curriculum covers most of the material in the original training program but in less time. Some states continue to recertify their EMS providers by requiring the completion of a recertification course. Other states offer a "challenge" mechanism whereby the EMS provider can demonstrate competency through a written and practical examination.

Still other states use a form of continuing medical education that involves attendance at a series of lecture and skill reviews that cover the required topics of a refresher course over the certification period (two, three, or four years depending on the state).

In 1995, when the EMT-Paramedic curriculum and the EMT-Intermediate curriculum were published by NHTSA, they did not

TABLE 2-1

Comparison of Provider Levels

Provider	Training Hours	Clinical Field	Pre-requisites	Patient Assessment	Airway Management	Medical	Trauma	Special Considerations	Operations
First Responder	40	None	None	General assessment with vital signs	Manual maneuvers; Pocket mask	Initial stabilization; AED use	Basic stabilization; Bleeding control; Basic shock management; Limited splinting	Childbirth	Interaction with EMS System
EMT-Basic	110	Optional clinical. May include field ride-along on EMS unit.	CPR	Complete assessment	Oral airways; Oxygen	Assessment-based support; Assist with patient; Prescribed medical administration; AED use	Assessment and basic stabilization; Bleeding and shock management; Spinal immobilization; Traction splinting; Introduction to basic rescue	Pediatrics; Geriatrics; Behavioral emergencies	Inroduction to EMS System; Wellness; Vehicle operations
EMT-Intermediate	~250	Clinical and Field	EMT-B	History taking; Clinical decision making; ECG interpretation	Oral intubation; Combitube; or PtL airway	Advanced assessment and definitive pharmacological intervention; ECG monitoring and electrical therapy	Advanced assessment; Fluid replacement; Chest decompression	Intraosseous fluid replacement; Pharmacological interventions in behavioral emergencies; Geriatrics; Neonatal resuscitation; Obstetric emergencies	Wellness; Prevention research in EMS
EMT-Paramedic	~1200	Clinical and Field	EMT-B; Anatomy and Physiology	Comprehensive and diagnostic based	Nasal intubation; Surgical airway	Field diagnosis and advanced pharmacological intervention; Increased knowledge base of pathophysiology, 12-lead ECG monitoring, and cardiac pacing	Advanced assessment; Increased knowledge base of pathophysiology; Basic rescue techniques	Neonatology; Abuse and assault; Patients with special challenges; Acute intervention for chronic care patient	Wellness; Prevention and Public education research in EMS; Medical incident command; Hazardous materials; Crime scene awareness

From Walz, B., 2002. *Introduction to EMS Systems.* Albany, NY: Delmar Thomson Learning.

contain recertification curricula. Rather, NHTSA issued a lengthy position paper emphasizing the need for states to move toward recertification by using continuing education and adhering to a format similar to that used by the National Registry. Some states have already moved in the direction of shifting to continuing education recertification. As of the publication of this book, there is no published research demonstrating which method of recertification works the best to keep the EMS provider's skills and knowledge base up to date as well as reviewing changes in the practice of their level of certification.

Q **What is reciprocity and how do I find out if my state has reciprocity with another state?**

A The process of issuing credentials based on prior training in another state is referred to as reciprocity. Reciprocity is the legal recognition of training obtained in another state. Many states have

their own levels of EMS training. These state-specific levels often do not exactly relate to other states. For example, in New York State there is an advanced level called EMT-Critical Care Technician, which includes many of the skills of an EMT-Paramedic without the corresponding didactic knowledge. This is an example of a course that does not "travel well" if you move to another state.

When an EMT moves to another state, if he would like to gain certification in the new state of residence, he should contact the state EMS office. (Check out the National Association of State EMS Directors Internet Web site at <www.nasemsd.org> for the address of your state EMS Office.)

The four national levels of EMS training (FR, EMT-B, EMT-I, EMT-P) are based on the DOT curricula and are recognized by NREMT. Providers at these levels of training usually have less difficulty obtaining credentials when moving from state to state. This is especially true if you have taken the time to obtain a NREMT card as well as a state card.

🔲 What are the benefits of continuing education?

🅰 No study has shown that recertification by continuing education (CE) is any better or worse than taking a refresher course. However, there are benefits to continuing one's EMS education as a "lifelong" process. Attending CE increases the EMS provider's knowledge base and understanding of relevant EMS issues. It also refreshes knowledge and skills and introduces new material. CE is usually affordable in terms of time and money because it is often provided in a single day workshop. Most medical specialties require some form of CE for renewal of their credentials.

🔲 What is a profession?

🅰 A profession is a "calling" requiring specialized preparation and specific academic preparation. Professions usually involve a specialized body of knowledge or expertise. They are often self-regulating through a licensure or certification process that requires competence validation. They also often have CE or re-licensure requirements.

🔲 What is professionalism?

🅰 Professionalism is the conduct and qualities that characterize a profession. In EMS, examples of these qualities include the following:

- Empathy.
- Integrity.
- Self-motivation.
- Good practice ethic.
- Good appearance.
- Good personal hygiene.
- Good interpersonal communicator.
- Good time manager.
- Team player.
- Diplomatic.
- Respectful.
- Careful in delivery of service.
- Patient advocate.
- Self-confidence.

🔲 What is a health care professional?

🅰 A health care professional is one who conforms to the standards of a health care profession providing quality patient care.

Health care professionals work to instill pride in their profession by striving for high standards and earning the respect of others. There are high expectations by society of health care professionals both on and off duty.

CLINICAL PEARL

Although in certain occupations, such as athletics, accepting remuneration designates one as a "professional," EMS professionalism is more about attitude than the acceptance of fees for services. Remember, "professionalism" has more to do with your behavior and attitude than your paycheck!

🔲 How important is image to health care workers?

🅰 Image and your behavior in public are extremely important. EMS providers are very visible role models whose behaviors are closely observed. For example, you cannot say seatbelts are important to use without always using them yourself. EMS providers represent themselves; their peers; their EMS agency; and the state, county, city, or district EMS office when they interact in public.

🔲 What are ethics?

🅰 Ethics are moral principles of one's practice in their profession. For more information on this topic see Chapter 5, Ethical Issues for the EMS Provider.

🔲 What is peer review?

🅰 Constructive feedback by other EMS providers in a genuine effort to improve future performance is called peer review. Examples include a coworker providing tips on how to lift a patient out of a tight spot or reviewing each other's paperwork for better ways to document what was done on the call.

🔲 What is the single most important attribute of an EMS professional?

🅰 Although there are many important attributes of a health care professional, integrity is at the top of the list. This means honesty in all of your actions and words. This important attribute is assumed by the public to be a part of the responsibility of an EMS provider. Examples of behavior demonstrating integrity are always telling the truth, never stealing, and providing complete and accurate documentation.

What is empathy?

True empathy is best described in the words of an ancient Indian leader who said you can never have empathy until you have walked a mile in someone else's moccasins. Having empathy in emergency medicine means identifying with and understanding the feelings, situations, and motives of your patients. Empathy should be demonstrated to patients, their families, and other health care professionals. It is best to ask yourself, "How would I feel if this was happening to me?" Examples of behavior demonstrating empathy include:

- Showing caring and compassion.
- Being supportive and reassuring.
- Exhibiting a calm, compassionate, and helpful demeanor.
- Demonstrating an understanding of patient and family feelings.
- Demonstrating respect.

CLINICAL PEARL

There is a difference between "empathy" and "sympathy." Sympathy is less effective and involves actually "taking on" the patient's pain. Empathy acknowledges the patient's circumstances and how serious they are without the provider becoming emotionally involved.

What is meant by the professional attribute of self-motivation?

Self-motivation is the internal drive for excellence. Examples of this behavior include:

- Taking initiative to complete assignments.
- Taking initiative to improve and/or correct behavior.
- Taking on and following through on tasks without being prodded by constant supervision.
- Showing enthusiasm for learning and continuous improvement.
- Accepting constructive feedback in a positive manner.
- Taking advantage of all learning opportunities.

What is meant by the professional attribute of self-confidence?

Self-confidence is trust and reliance on oneself. To be a good EMS provider, you must be confident in your abilities and have a good understanding of your strengths and limitations. Examples of behavior demonstrating self-confidence include: an ability to trust your personal judgment, an awareness of your

ability to lift, and an awareness of when to call for additional assistance. Someone who is self-confident, not overly confident, knows when to call for backup or consult with Medical Direction rather than getting in over one's head.

CLINICAL PEARL

Most authorities agree that it's better to "call in the troops" early (and maybe not need them) than to call them in too late. This is a sign of self-confidence, not the lack of it!

Why is a good appearance and personal hygiene an important professional attribute for EMS providers?

The manner in which you walk and carry yourself is important! A neat and professional appearance, well groomed and clean, helps to instill confidence in the patients and their families. Patients do not appreciate an EMS provider with body odor or bad breath nor do they appreciate an EMS provider who has overdone their aftershave or perfume! Indeed, each EMS provider should look in the mirror and ask herself, "Do I look like a good role model of a health care professional?" The answer to that question is very subjective and up to you to make.

Why are good time-management skills an important professional attribute for EMS providers?

Good patient care involves good time-management skills. Trauma patients and evolving myocardial infarction (MI) patients do not have much time to spare while an inexperienced EMS provider fumbles with the basics. A good time manager is able to organize tasks to make maximum use of time. Prioritizing tasks is important especially when the patient's condition warrants a scene time of no longer than 10 minutes.

In addition, time management involves being punctual for meetings, appointments, and work shifts. EMS is a business that requires the employees to be present and prepared to work before the start of their shift because the calls do not wait.

Why are good teamwork and diplomacy important professional attributes for EMS providers?

Teamwork is the ability to work with others to achieve a common goal. In order for a patient to have a positive outcome, the EMS providers must work well as a team. The team includes the Emergency Medical Dispatcher (EMD), the public safety first responder agency personnel, the BLS and ALS personnel on the scene, Medical Direction, and the health care professionals at the receiving facility.

Diplomacy is tact and skill in dealing with people. Being a diplomat also involves saying and doing things that are considered "politically correct." When an EMS provider jumps up on the hood of a car at a collision and starts barking orders to the personnel on scene, this can come across as not treating them with respect. On the scene of a serious call, the EMS provider may "bully" his way through the call and in his own mind rationalize that the abusive behavior is in the patient's best interest. Yet, this type of behavior is not good for the system or patients when he finds cooperation and teamwork hard to come by on future calls. This is like the old saying you may win the battle but lose the war! Remember there is no "I" in "teamwork!"

Examples of behavior demonstrating teamwork and diplomacy include:

- Placing the success of the team above self-interest.
- Not undermining the team.
- Helping to support other team members.
- Showing respect for all team members.
- Remaining flexible and open to change.
- Communicating with coworkers in an effort to resolve problems.
- Disagreeing in private but never in public.

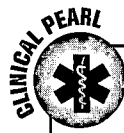

CLINICAL PEARL

The patient's bedside is no place for interprofessional disagreements.

Q Why is being a patient advocate an important professional attribute for EMS providers?

A Patients are at a disadvantage when thrust into the health care system due to a sudden illness or injury. Part of your responsibility as the EMS provider is to advocate for your patient. Sometimes, this means not just delivering the patients to the busy ED, but staying with them for a few minutes to ensure that the ED staff fully understands the extent of the mechanism of injury (MOI) or nature of the illness. This may involve describing the scene or the patient's residence environment. Some EMS agencies take a Polaroid® photo of the wrecked car to visually impress the ED staff with the MOI.

Yet, being a patient care advocate goes beyond just advocating for a specific patient. Becoming involved in the EMS system, EMS education, and EMS prevention efforts are also patient advocate activities. Are you involved in your Regional EMS Council or EMS agency's Quality Improvement (QI) Committee? Do you know about the proposed EMS legislation in your state?

Being a patient advocate doesn't mean becoming a zealot or becoming overbearing about your beliefs in safety and prevention issues. It is necessary to accept others' rights to differ from your

beliefs and to avoid imposing your beliefs on others. An educational approach is often effective. For example, a patient might tell you he doesn't wear a seat belt because he thinks it would be safer to be thrown clear of the wrecked car for fear it would burst into flames. In this case, rather than saying that is a stupid idea, tell him that less than 1 percent of car crashes involve a fire. Also tell him that the safest place to be is inside the vehicle compartment. If thrown clear, there is a 1,300 percent increased chance of neck injury or the chance of being run over by their own vehicle or the oncoming tractor trailer in the opposite lane!

Examples of behavior demonstrating patient advocacy include:

- Not allowing personal biases to impact on patient care (e.g., religious, ethical, political, social, legal).
- Placing the needs of patients, except safety, above your own self-interest (e.g., spending a few minutes at the hospital to be sure the patient gets checked in properly even if it means being a little late for a personal engagement after work).
- Protecting the patient's confidentiality.

Q Why is being careful in the delivery of service considered an important professional attribute for EMS providers?

A A good EMS provider pays attention to details. There may be times when the details are skipped due to the patient's injury severity, but most calls involve enough time for you to pay attention to things like wiping your feet before entering a patient's home, protecting their furniture from damage by your stretcher, or making sure the house is locked and the patient has the keys.

Another very important part of providing careful delivery of service is one's ability to critically evaluate performance and attitude. Examples of behavior demonstrating careful delivery of service include:

- Mastering and refreshing skills.
- Performing complete equipment checks each shift.
- Careful and safe ambulance operations.
- Following the standard operating procedure (SOP) of your agency and medical protocols.
- Following the orders of superiors.

Q Why is it necessary for EMS providers to be good communicators?

A Most of what EMS providers do involves communication skills. They talk on radios, talk to coworkers and other emergency service providers, and most importantly establish a rapport with patients so a history and assessment can be obtained.

Communication is the exchange of thoughts, messages, and information, which in EMS is a key part of the job. It is essential that the EMS provider be an effective communicator. This includes the ability to convey information to others both verbally and in writing as well as the ability to interpret verbal and written messages. Examples of behavior demonstrating good communication include: speaking clearly, writing legibly, listening actively, and adjusting communication strategies to various situations.

CLINICAL PEARL

Remember that nearly 97 percent of communication involves "body language." Try to make eye contact with the patient when you communicate.

How does professionalism apply to the EMS provider both on and off duty?

Because EMS providers are often looked up to by community members, it is important to live up to this professional standard both on duty and off. Examples include smoking or drinking and driving. If an EMS provider is seen smoking in public or drinking and driving, it sets a poor example. Some EMS organizations have very strict policies about wearing any uniform parts (e.g., shirts, hats, or jackets with logos on them) that identify your service when in establishments that serve alcohol because of the potential for poor public perception.

Medical Direction and Protocols

How important is Medical Direction to EMS agencies?

This is best answered by reviewing the American College of Emergency Physician's (ACEP) policy on Medical Direction of EMS (September, 1997). "ACEP believes that, because of rapidly changing technology and advances in EMS research, all aspects of the organization and the provision of basic (including first responder) and advanced life support emergency medical services (EMS) require the active involvement and participation of physicians. ACEP also believes that EMS must have an identifiable physician medical director at the local, regional or state level."

What are the roles and responsibilities of the Medical Director?

The primary role of the medical director is to ensure quality patient care. Responsibilities of the medical director should include:

- Involvement with the ongoing design, operation, evaluation, and revision of the EMS system from initial patient access to definitive patient care.
- Authority over patient care and the authority to limit immediately the patient care activities of those who deviate from established standards or do not meet training standards.
- The responsibility and authority to develop and implement medical policies and procedures.
- The EMS medical director's qualifications, responsibilities, and authority must be delineated in writing within each EMS system. The EMS system has an obligation to provide the EMS medical director with the resources and authority commensurate with these responsibilities.

What are protocols?

Protocols are guidelines for the management of specific patient presenting problems. Assessment-based protocols tend to be more complaint based (e.g., breathing difficulty, chest pain, altered mental status, etc.), whereas diagnosis-based protocols are for a specific presumptive field diagnosis (e.g., asthma, heat stroke, acute myocardial infarction [AMI], etc.).

Many protocols follow a national standard such as the American Heart Association ACLS guidelines. Some protocols are local and limited to problems or patients that only occur in a very specific environment such as protocols for exposure to certain chemicals used in manufacturing.

Most protocols involve specific medical treatments and as such come under the domain of medical direction. Many protocols have "stop lines" built into them. The EMS provider can provide care based on a standing order, but must contact medical direction for a verbal order before going beyond the stop line.

What is the role of the EMS physician in providing medical direction to the EMS provider?

The EMS physician's role has expanded over the past 10 years. Today, many BLS and ALS agencies have a medical director. The typical roles of the EMS physician include:

- Educating and training personnel.
- Participating in the personnel selection process.
- Participating in equipment selection.
- Developing clinical protocols in cooperation with expert EMS personnel and participating on the Regional Medical Authority.
- Participating in quality improvement and problem resolution.
- Providing direct input into patient care.
- Interfacing between EMS systems and other health care agencies.
- Advocating within the medical community.

- Serving as the medical conscience of the EMS organization.
- Providing both on-line (direct) and off-line (indirect) medical direction.

![Q] What is the benefit of on-line (direct) and off-line (indirect) medical direction?

![A] Potential benefits of on-line (direct) medical control include the ability to obtain real-time direction and orders. Off-line (indirect) medical control primarily relies on protocols. Some argue that protocols with appropriate "stop lines" are more efficient. Retrospective review, including prehospital care report (PCR) review and continuous quality improvement (CQI), is mandatory whether an EMS system uses direct control, indirect control, or a combination.

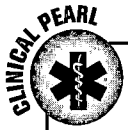

CLINICAL PEARL

> *There is not a single best system for every locality.*
> *Different approaches may be equally effective.*

![Q] What is the relationship between the physician on the scene, the ALS provider on the scene, and the medical control physician in most systems?

![A] Most systems have a policy on what to do when there is a physician on the scene. First, it is good to confirm that the person actually is a physician (medical doctor) and not a Ph.D. in Economics or something just as irrelevant to the patient's medical care. Next, it is good to determine whether the physician is actually the patient's physician. If so, they can take responsibility for the care of their patient. If the physician is just stopping by to render some assistance and not planning on accompanying the patient to the hospital, it is a good policy to be friendly and explain your plan of action. If the physician has any ideas that do not fit in with your protocols, explain what you are expected to do and suggest that the physician talk directly with your medical control physician.

If the physician wants to take over and is planning on going to the hospital, then contact your medical control so they can talk with the physician and you can work together to assist the patient with the least amount of visible controversy.

Specific Roles of the EMS Provider

![Q] What are the primary responsibilities of EMS providers?

![A] EMS providers are responsible for the following areas:

1. Preparation. They must be prepared with the proper training, well-maintained equipment, adequate supplies, good physical condition, and a positive mental and emotional attitude.
2. Response. They must respond in a safe and timely manner.
3. Scene assessment. They must safely determine the MOI and prevent harm to their crew, bystanders, and the patient.
4. Patient assessment. They must properly assess the patient using the recommendations contained in this book as well as their protocols and medical direction.
5. Recognize the injury or illness. They must properly prioritize the patient's needs.
6. Management. They must manage the patient following their protocols and interact with medical direction as required.
7. Appropriate disposition. They must determine the appropriate destination for the patient after considering factors such as: knowledge of the receiving facilities, hospital categorization and levels of care, and hospital resource and clinical capabilities that include:
   - ED, OR.
   - Post-anesthesia recovery room or surgical intensive care unit.
   - Intensive care units for trauma patients.
   - Cardiac.
   - Neurology.
   - Acute hemodialysis.
   - Burn specialization.
   - Acute spinal cord or head injury management.
   - Radiology.
   - Rehabilitation.
   - Clinical laboratory service.
   - Toxicology and hazmat decontamination.
   - Hyperbarics.
   - Reperfusion.
   - Pediatrics.
   - Psychiatric facilities.
   - Trauma centers.
   - High risk delivery.
8. Patient transfer. They must act as a patient advocate and be sure to brief the receiving hospital staff on the patient.
9. Documentation. They must provide a thorough, accurate PCR completed in a timely manner.
10. Returning to service. They must prepare the equipment and supplies for the next call, disinfecting and restocking as needed, and prepare the crew by debriefing or talking about the call so they can improve on the next one.

Q **What are the benefits of EMS providers teaching in their community?**

A There are four primary benefits to EMS agencies by having EMS personnel teach in the community:

1. Improving the health of the community regarding injury and illness prevention (see Chapter 3, Illness and Injury Prevention) and enhancing compliance with treatment regimes.

2. Ensuring appropriate utilization of resources by making sure the public knows when, where, and how to use EMS.

3. Improving the integration of EMS with other health care and public safety agencies through creating cooperative public education efforts. .

4. Enhancing visibility and a positive image of EMS providers and their agencies.

Q **What is citizen involvement in the EMS system?**

A Citizen involvement in EMS systems runs from knowing how to access EMS to obtaining the training and being willing to do bystander CPR to fundraising and lobbying for EMS improvements and funding to participating in EMS agency boards and regional EMS councils.

Q **How can EMS providers benefit the EMS system by supporting primary care to patients in the out-of-hospital setting?**

A As the roles of EMS providers expand in some communities, the "scope of practice" is also changing. Some EMS systems find it beneficial to utilize EMS providers in nontraditional programs such as community inoculation programs, injury prevention inspections, and patient checkup visits to enhance compliance with treatment regimes. The expanded scope pilots have been used to bring medically trained health care professionals to the patients when they are underserved or transportation alternatives are very costly. In some communities, this involves a nonhospital ED clinical provider and free-standing emergency clinics. Talk to your medical director about the status of EMS providers and primary care in the out-of-hospital setting in your community.

National EMS Issues

Q **What are the national issues affecting EMS and where can you learn more about them?**

A When NHTSA brought together many representatives from national organizations to develop the *EMS Agenda for the Future*,

the document that was developed identified 14 EMS system attributes to work on in the future:

1. Integration of health services.
   - Expand the EMS role in public health and involve EMS in community health monitoring activities.
   - Integrate and incorporate EMS with other health care providers and within provider networks to deliver quality care.
   - Be cognizant of the special needs of the entire population and incorporate health systems within EMS that address special needs.

2. EMS research.
   - Allocate federal and state funds for a major EMS system research thrust.
   - Develop information systems that provide linkage between various public safety services and other health care providers.
   - Develop academic institutional commitments to EMS-related research and collaborative relations between EMS systems, medical schools, and private foundations.
   - Interpret informed consent rules to allow for clinical and environmental circumstances inherent in conducting credible EMS research.
   - Develop involvement in and support of EMS research by all those responsible for EMS structure, processes, or outcomes and enhance the quality of EMS research.
   - Designate EMS as a physician subspecialty and as a subspecialty for other health professions, and include research-related objectives in the education processes of EMS providers and managers.

3. Legislation and regulation.
   - Authorize and sufficiently fund a lead federal EMS agency.
   - Pass and periodically review all state EMS enabling legislation that supports innovation and integration, and establishes and sufficiently funds an EMS lead agency that can provide technical assistance.
   - Establish and fund the position of state EMS medical director in each state and authorize state and local EMS lead agencies to act on the public's behalf in cases of threats to the availability of quality EMS to the entire population.
   - Implement laws that provide protection from liability for EMS field and medical direction personnel when dealing with unusual situations.

4. System finance.
   - Collaborate with other health care providers and insurers to enhance patient care efficiency and develop proactive financial relations between EMS, other health care providers, and health care insurers and provider organizations.

- Compensate EMS on the basis of a preparedness-based model, reducing volume-related incentives and realizing the cost of an emergency safety net.
- Provide immediate access to EMS for emergency medical conditions.
- Address relevant EMS issues within governmental health care finance policy (e.g., Medicare and Medicaid) and commit local, state, and federal attention and funds to continued EMS infrastructure development.

5. Human resources.
- Ensure that changes in the expectations of EMS personnel to provide health care services are preceded by adequate preparation and adopt the principles of the national *EMS Education and Practice Blueprint*.
- Develop a system of reciprocity for EMS provider credentials.
- Develop collaborative relations between EMS systems and academic institutions.
- Conduct EMS occupational health research and provide a system for critical incident stress management.

6. Medical direction.
- Formalize relations between all EMS systems and medical direction and appropriate sufficient resources to do so.
- Require appropriate credentials for all those who provide on-line medical direction and develop EMS as a physician and nurse subspecialty certification.
- Appoint state EMS medical directors.

7. Education systems.
- Ensure the adequacy of EMS education programs and conduct EMS education with medical direction.
- Update education core content objectives frequently so that they reflect patient EMS health care needs and incorporate research, quality improvement, and management learning objectives.
- Commission the development of national core contents to replace EMS program curricula.
- Seek accreditation for EMS education programs.
- Establish innovative and collaborative relations between EMS education programs and academic institutions so that EMS education is recognized as an academic achievement.
- Develop bridging and transition programs and include EMS-related objectives in all health professions' education.

8. Public education.
- Acknowledge that public education is a critical EMS activity and collaborate with other community resources and agencies to determine public education needs.
- Engage in continuous public education programs and educate the public as consumers.
- Explore new techniques and technologies for implementing public education and evaluate public education initiatives.

9. Prevention.
- Collaborate with community agencies and health care providers with expertise and an interest in illness and injury prevention.
- Support the Safe Communities concept and advocate for legislation that potentially results in injury and illness prevention.
- Develop and maintain a prevention oriented atmosphere within EMS systems and include the principles of prevention and its role in improving community health as part of EMS education core contents.

10. Public access.
- Implement 911 nationwide and provide emergency telephone service for those who cannot otherwise afford basic telephone service.
- Ensure that all calls to a public safety access point (PSAP), regardless of origin, are automatically accompanied by unique location identifying information and develop uniform cellular 911 service that reliably routes calls to the appropriate PSAP.
- Evaluate and employ technologies that attenuate potential barriers to EMS access.
- Enhance the ability of EMS systems to triage calls, and provide resource allocation that is tailored to patients' needs.

11. Communications systems.
- Assess the effectiveness of various personnel and resource attributes for EMS dispatching.
- Receive all calls for EMS using personnel with the requisite combination of education, experience, and resources to optimally query the caller, make a determination of the most appropriate resources to be mobilized, and implement an effective course of action.
- Promulgate and update standards for EMS dispatching.
- Develop cooperative ventures between communications centers and health providers to integrate communications processes and enable rapid patient-related information exchange.
- Determine the benefits of real time patient data transfer.
- Appropriate federal, state, and regional funds to further develop and update geographically integrated and functionally based EMS communication networks.
- Facilitate the exploration of potential uses of advancing communication technology by EMS and collaborate with pri-

vate interests to effect shared purchasing of communication technology.

12. Clinical care.
   - Commit to a common definition of what constitutes baseline community EMS care and subject EMS clinical care to ongoing evaluation to determine its impact on patient outcomes.
   - Employ new care techniques and technology only after it is shown to be effective.
   - Conduct task analyses to determine appropriate staff configurations during secondary patient transfers and eliminate patient transport as a criterion for compensating EMS systems.
   - Establish proactive relations between EMS and other health care providers.

13. Information Systems.
   - Adopt uniform data elements and definitions, and incorporate them into information systems. Develop systems that are able to describe an entire EMS event.
   - Develop mechanisms to generate and transmit data that are valid, reliable, and accurate.
   - Develop integrated information systems with other health care providers, public safety agencies, and community resources and provide feedback to those who generate data.

14. Evaluation.
   - Develop valid models for EMS evaluations that incorporate consumer input.
   - Evaluate EMS effects for multiple medical conditions.
   - Determine EMS effects for multiple outcome categories and cost effectiveness.

For more information on the *EMS Agenda For The Future* download the publication off the Internet Web site at <www.nhtsa.dot.gov/people/injury/ems>.

Continuous Quality Improvement and EMS Research

[Q] What are examples of areas where continuous quality improvement (CQI) can be helpful in an EMS system?

[A] A good CQI focuses on the system and not any specific individual. It is a process that is designed to uncover problems and provide solutions to solve those problems in any of the following areas of an EMS system:

- Medical direction.
- Financing.
- Training.
- Communication.
- Out-of-hospital treatment and transport.
- Interfacility transport.
- Receiving facilities.
- Specialty care units.
- Dispatch.
- Public information and education.
- Audit and quality assurance.
- Disaster planning.
- Mutual aid.

[Q] What is meant by the statement, "CQI must be a dynamic process?"

[A] Using the following steps, each component being evaluated in the EMS system has ongoing quality improvements:

- Delineate the system-wide problems identified.
- Elaborate on the causes of the problem.
- Develop the remedy for the problem.
- Lay out the plan to correct the problem.
- Enforce the plan of correction for the problem.
- Reexamine the problem.

[Q] How should CQI relate to research and continuing medical education?

[A] There is a direct connection between the three areas. The CQI process may have identified a problem. This problem is then researched and solutions to the problem are developed. Once the solutions are researched and the best solution is agreed upon, it can be implemented with all EMS providers using continuing medical education (CME). An example might be CQI turning up a large number of unrecognized esophageal intubations. Various solutions are researched. Implement a CME program using the solution that is most practical for your EMS agency. Then, the CQI process again reviews the intubations to see if the initial problem has actually been fixed by implementation of a new procedure or the use of a device such as an end-tidal CO_2 monitor, pulse oximeter, or esophageal intubation detector device (EIDD).

[Q] What is the importance of research to EMS?

[A] The benefits of research to EMS are many. Unfortunately, for many years, there was very little research and decisions were often based on "bells and whistles," tradition, "gut feelings," and the opinion of the bully pulpit. Today, many medical directors' first response to a new device, procedure, or medication is "show me the research!" Quality EMS research is beneficial to the future of EMS. Changes in professional standards, training, equipment, and procedures must be based on empirical data rather than "great ideas" or the gadget of the month.

EMS funding is beginning to be based on scientifically proving the value of EMS services. The anecdotes of the past no longer suffice. Reduced spending by managed care and governmental bodies has helped to speed up the financial impetus of tying funding to research or "results." More often, outcome studies are necessary to ensure continued funding for EMS system grants. In addition, research helps to enhance recognition and respect for EMS professionals.

CLINICAL PEARL

The current term for this movement is "evidence-based medicine." Until recently, trained EMS providers did not perform most out-of-hospital research. Even the most seasoned emergency physician or nurse should have field experience or assistance from those who do when performing research studies.

[Q] What is the EMS provider's role in data collection?

[A] Simply put, the role is to enthusiastically participate and honestly comply with the study requirements without negatively affecting patient care. In one city, the EMS providers participating in a study, where two medications were blindly administered on alternate days, were known to have tasted a drop of the medication to help them figure out which they were administering. A bias of this kind can negatively impact on what may be a very important research project.

[Q] What are the basic principles of research?

[A] Although it is beyond the scope of this book to teach statistics and basic research methods, the EMS provider should develop an understanding of the following research concepts:

- Value of peer review and publishing research.
- Types of research (descriptive, experimental, prospective, retrospective, and cross sectional).
- Populations to be researched.
- How to randomize and how to select a control group.
- How to select a sample using various methods (systematic, alternative times or days, or convenience sampling).

- Considerations for sampling error and selection bias.
- Specifying the parameters of the study and controlling nuisance variables.
- Blinding the study (single, double, or triple blind).
- Basic descriptive statistics and measures of central tendency (mean, median, mode, and standard deviation).
- Basic inferential statistical methods (the null hypothesis and a research hypothesis).
- Ethical considerations for research; the need for consent and approval for human research by a hospital institutional review board.
- The format of a research paper (introduction, methods, results, discussion, and conclusion).

[Q] What is the typical procedure for conducting research in EMS?

[A] Most research involves at least the following steps:
- Preparation of the question to be studied.
- Writing down the hypothesis.
- Deciding what should be measured and how best to do the measuring. Remember the yardstick should be appropriate so the results are useful.
- Describe the population to be studied.
- Identify the limitations of the study.
- Seek the necessary approvals to conduct the study. This may involve someone to fund the project or an institutional review board if there is research on human subjects involved.
- Obtain legal advice on how to obtain informed consent if that is a part of the study.
- Gather the data and if needed conduct pilot trials first. It is necessary to determine the appropriate sample size for the study.
- Analyze the data obtained, considering any pitfalls of interpreting the data.
- Determine what to do with the data you have uncovered. Should you publish it, present it at a conference or workshop, or consider follow-up studies?

[Q] What are some examples of out-of-hospital research?

[A] There are three general areas that the examples fall into:
1. Conclusions made based on scientifically sound procedures, techniques, and equipment (e.g., the decision of the American Heart Association to promote the links in the chain of survival).

2. Answering a clinically important question (e.g., should D5W be used for head-injured patients or how much sodium bicarbonate should be used in a cardiac arrest to counteract acidosis).

3. Providing results that lead to system improvements (e.g., repositioning units based on the location and frequency of calls to improve the average response time).

🔲 What is an example of a process for evaluating and interpreting research?

🅰 When an EMS provider picks up a journal or reads the headline in the local newspaper describing recent research findings, consider making a critical review of the study and asking the following questions:

- Was the research peer reviewed?
- What was the research hypothesis?
- Was the study approved by an institutional review board and conducted in an ethical manner?

- What population was being studied?
- What were the entry and exclusion criteria for the study?
- What method was used to draw a sample of patients?
- How many groups were the patients divided into?
- How were patients assigned into groups?
- What types of data were collected?
- Does it appear that there were enough patients enrolled in the study?
- Do there appear to be any confounding variables that are not accounted for in the study?
- Were the data properly analyzed?
- Is the conclusion of the author's logic based on the data analyzed?
- Does this study apply to the local EMS system and will the study results be replicated in different locations?
- Are patients in the study similar to those in the local EMS system?

Special Thanks

Emergency Medical Services Agenda For The Future, U.S. Department of Transportation, National Highway Traffic Safety Administration publication DOT HS 808 441, August 1996.
American College of Emergency Physicians, Medical Direction of EMS Policy 400192, September 1997.

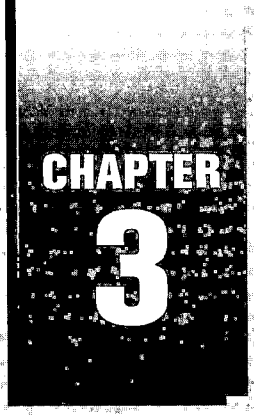

CHAPTER 3

Illness and Injury Prevention

This chapter discusses the epidemiology of disease and injury and the feasibility of EMS providers being involved in prevention activities. The focus is on *why* EMS providers should be involved in illness and injury prevention as well as offer strategies for involvement in community efforts to decrease morbidity and mortality.

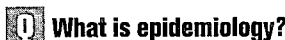

Epidemiology

Q What is epidemiology?

A Epidemiology is the study of the occurrence of disease.

Q What is the incidence of an injury or illness?

A The incidence is the number of times the injury or disorder occurs over a period of time.

Q What is the morbidity and mortality of a disease or injury?

A The morbidity is the extent of the sickness or injury. The mortality is the number of patients who die from the injury or disease.

Q What are the leading causes of death in the United States?

A The data used in this chapter are based on the most recently released version of the National Vital Statistics Reports. Because there is a lag in the time to compile data, all statistics are from the calendar year 1997. More recent data can be reviewed at the Centers for Disease Control's Internet Web page located at <www.cdc.gov/nchswww/about/major/dvs/mortdata.htm>.

There were 2,314,245 deaths in 1997, which is a rate of 864.7 deaths per 100,000 people. This is referred to as the crude death rate because it is strictly the actual number factored against the U.S. Census population data. A more informative statistic is the age-adjusted death rate that is designed to eliminate the distorting effects of the aging of the U.S. population. The age-adjusted rate was 479.1 per 100,000, which was a record low. The leading causes of death in 1997, ranked from highest age-adjusted rate to lowest, are shown in Table 3–1.

Q Do the causes of death differ when the data is subdivided by sex, age, and race?

A Yes, there are a number of differences in the causes of death in Table 3–1 when they are broken down by sex, age, and race. Following are some highlights from the 1997 data that are interesting to note:
- For ages 1–44, accidents were the leading cause of death.
- For ages 45–64, cancer was the leading cause of death followed by heart disease for those over 65 years of age.

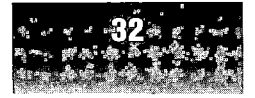

TABLE 3-1

Leading Causes of Death

Rank Cause	Percent	Age-Adjusted Rate
1. Diseases of the heart	31.4	130.5
2. Malignant neoplasms	23.3	125.6
3. Cerebrovascular diseases	6.9	25.9
4. Chronic obstructive pulmonary diseases	4.7	21.1
5. Vehicle accidents	4.1	30.1
6. Pneumonia and influenza	3.7	12.9
7. Diabetes	2.7	13.5
8. Suicide	1.3	10.6
9. Nephritis and nephrosis	1.1	4.4
10. Liver disease and cirrhosis	1.1	7.4
11. Alzheimer's disease	1.0	2.7
12. Septicemia	1.0	4.2
13. Homicide	0.9	8.0
14. HIV infection	0.7	5.8
15. Atherosclerosis	0.7	2.1

- When death rates for whites are compared to those of blacks, the leading causes of death are the same except in two age groups. In the 15–24 year olds, the leading cause was accidents in whites and homicide in blacks. In the 25–44 year olds, the leading cause was accidents in whites and HIV in blacks.

- The infant mortality rate was an all-time record low of 7.2 per 1,000 live births.

- Those who had never married had the highest mortality followed by those who were widowed or divorced.

- Higher education attainment was associated with a lower risk of death.

- The life expectancy for males is 73.6 years and for females is 79.4 years.

- It has been estimated that the lifetime cost of injuries is over $114 billion dollars.

- It is estimated that there are 19 hospitalizations and 254 emergency department visits for each injury death.

What is the effect of a patient's early release from the hospital on EMS services?

As the hospitals have moved toward doing more procedures on an out-patient basis and are decreasing the number of hospital stay days for the treatment of injuries and illnesses, the reliance on EMS has increased. This is, in part, a cost-cutting trend that is bound to continue. EMS services are expected to provide more care for patients who are being managed in the home setting. For more information review Chapter 47, Acute Interventions with the Home-Care Patient.

What is an injury?

Injury is defined as intentional or unintentional damage to a person resulting from acute exposure to thermal, mechanical, electrical, or chemical energy, or from the absence of essentials such as heat or oxygen.

What is injury risk?

Injury risk is defined as a real or potential hazardous situation that puts individuals at risk for sustaining an injury.

What is injury surveillance?

Injury surveillance is the ongoing systematic collection, analysis, and interpretation of injury data essential to the planning, implementation, and evaluation of public health practice. An important part of any injury surveillance program is the timely dissemination of the data to those who need to use it for prevention and control efforts.

What is the difference between primary, secondary, and tertiary prevention efforts?

Primary injury prevention is an effort to keep an injury from ever occurring (e.g., not allowing diving in the shallow end of a swimming pool to prevent spinal injuries). Secondary injury prevention includes those activities involved in the care of an injury that has already occurred to prevent it from getting worse (e.g., teaching the lifeguards and EMS personnel how to properly remove the potentially spine-injured diver from the pool immobilized on a long spine board). Tertiary injury prevention includes those activities involved in the rehabilitation of an injured person (e.g., preventing infections and making the patient's home accommodate any disability).

What is a "teachable moment"?

A teachable moment is the time after an injury has occurred when the patient and observers remain acutely aware of what has happened and may be more receptive to learning about how the injury or event could have been prevented (e.g., after the patient cracked the windshield with his head and sustained facial lacerations because he was unrestrained).

What is meant by the statistic "years of productive life?"

The years of productive life is the calculation that is done by subtracting age of death from the normal retirement age of 65.

Thus, someone who dies suddenly at the age of 25 is considered to have lost 40 years of productive life.

EMS Involvement in Prevention Activities

Q Why is it sensible for EMS providers to be involved in injury and illness prevention efforts in their communities?

A There are many good reasons why EMS providers should be involved in prevention efforts in their communities. Here are a few:

- EMS providers are distributed widely throughout the population.
- They often are a mirror image of the community's composition.
- In rural settings, the EMS providers may be the most medically educated individuals.
- There are over 600,000 EMS providers across the United States.
- They are often high-profile role models.
- They are often considered the advocate of the consumer.
- They are welcome in schools, nursing homes, and other environments.
- They are often thought of as the experts on injury and prevention.

Q What are some examples of opportunities for primary prevention that EMS providers can become involved in?

A There are many primary prevention activities that you can easily get involved with. Just pick the cause that best suits your interest or experience and start from there. Better yet, pick a group you have always wanted to know something about and stretch a little to learn about their cause. The following list will serve as some excellent examples of primary prevention opportunities for EMS provider involvement:

- Bicycle-related head injuries. In 1997, 813 bicyclists were killed in crashes with motor vehicles. Of these, 97 percent were not wearing helmets. There were an estimated 567,000 Americans who sustained a bicycle-related injury requiring care in the ED. The solutions to the problem include education, legislation, and distribution of helmets (Figure 3–1).

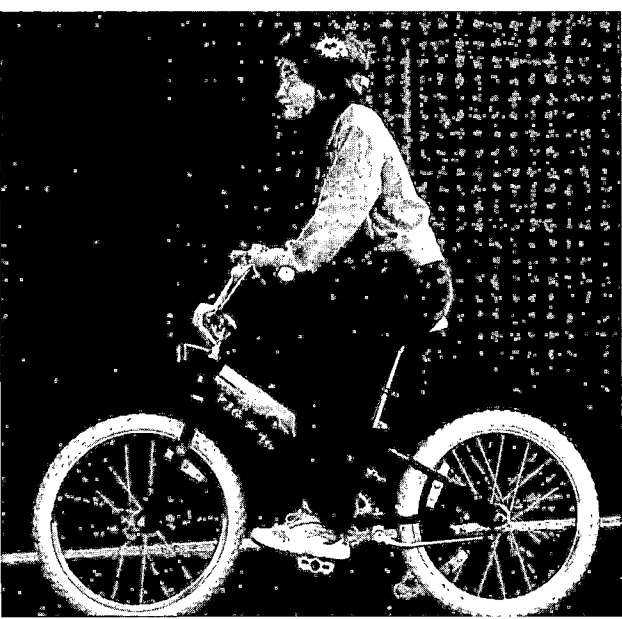

FIGURE 3-1 Children should always wear a helmet when riding a bike. *(Courtesy of Bob Elling)*

- Drowning. In 1997, nearly 1,000 children age 14 and under drowned. Children age 4 and under accounted for more than half of these deaths. The solutions to the problem include mandates for four-sided isolation fencing equipped with self-closing and self-latching gates, as well as requiring that personal flotation devices (PFDs) be worn whenever children or adults who cannot swim are near water. Public education is necessary. This includes recommendations such as never leave a child unsupervised in or around water in the home, and empty all containers after use and immediately store out of reach because many toddlers drown in filled buckets each year.

- Child passenger and motor vehicle safety. Motor vehicle crashes are the leading cause of death for 15 to 20 year olds, killing 3,387 in 1996 and injuring 373,000. The key strategy for reducing deaths from motor vehicles is getting adults in the vehicle to wear a seat belt and place all children in the appropriate size child safety seat. According to National Highway Traffic Safety Administration (NHTSA), over the past 10 years, safety belts have prevented some 55,600 deaths, 1,300,000 injuries, and saved more than $105 billion in economic costs. Many EMS services have been trained to assist the public by doing child restraint seat inspections because it is estimated that over 70 percent of the seats are not properly belted into the vehicles.

- Poisoning. In 1998, more than 1.1 million unintentional poisonings of children age 5 and under were reported to U.S. poison

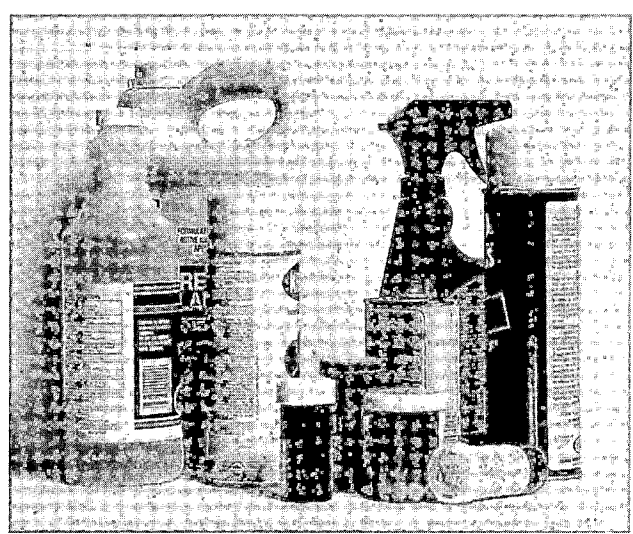

FIGURE 3-2 Household substances can be hazardous and poisonous.

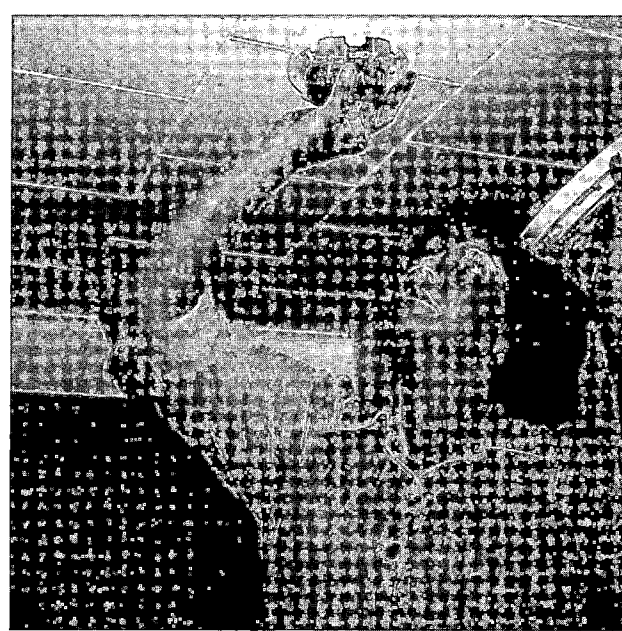

FIGURE 3-3 Batteries in smoke detectors must be changed at least annually.

control centers. With more than 90 percent of the poison exposures occurring in the home, the strategy is to educate the parents and older children to lock up the hazardous substances and label them appropriately (Figure 3–2). Legislation has been effective in this area such as the Poison Prevention Act (1970), which authorized the U.S. Consumer Product Safety Commission to require the use of child-resistant packaging for toxic substances used in and around the home.

- Fire safety. It is estimated that roughly 18,000 people are injured and 3,400 killed in home fires each year in the United States. The key strategy here is to get smoke alarms and carbon monoxide (CO) detectors into every home and get the residents to change the batteries on the alarms once a year (Figure 3–3). Other strategies include family fire escape plans practiced every six months, never smoking in bed, proper use of space heaters, keeping matches and lighters away from children, and knowing what to do if your clothing has caught on fire.

- Motorcycle safety. Approximately 2,000 motorcyclists are killed and more than 50,000 are injured in traffic crashes each year. The key strategies here are educating the riders about wearing a helmet and protective gear, not drinking and driving, and receiving training. Motorcycle safety courses are available by calling 1-800-446-9227.

- Playground safety. Every two-and-a-half minutes a child is injured on a playground in the United States. The key strategies are adult supervision and making sure that any surface they might fall onto is soft and padded. The best playgrounds have surfaces with at least six inches of mulch chips, pea gravel, fine sand, or shredded rubber to cushion a fall. Some EMS agencies have begun doing playground inspections looking for equipment in need of repair or with jagged edges and sharp points.

- Preventing falls. These injuries affect the very young and very old the worst. Childhood falls account for an estimated 2 million ED visits each year, while one in every three adults 65 years or older falls each year (more than 400,000). The strategies for prevention include metal grates on windows in high-rise buildings, grab bars near the toilet and bathtub, handrails and lights in all stairways, eliminating throw rugs and things that one could trip over from the floor, using safe baby products (cribs and highchairs) that do not tip over, and strapping toddlers into shopping carts. According to the American Academy of Pediatrics, using a baby walker is extremely dangerous because they are unstable and often fall down the stairs.

- Preventing strangulation and suffocation among infants and children. Approximately 50 babies suffocate or strangle each year after being trapped in an unsafe crib. Drawstrings on the hoods of sweaters can become entangled in playground equipment, fences, and furniture causing strangulation. Consider the curtains and blinds with draw cords in your own home. Another serious problem is children being left unattended in a vehicle during hot weather. Additional safety information to prevent choking, strangulation, and suffocation can be found at the following Internet Web sites: <www.aap.org/family/toybroc.htm>, <www.cpsc.gov>, <www.jpma.org/public/safe-sound.html>, <www.nsc.org/lrs/lib/fs/home/babyprf.htm>.

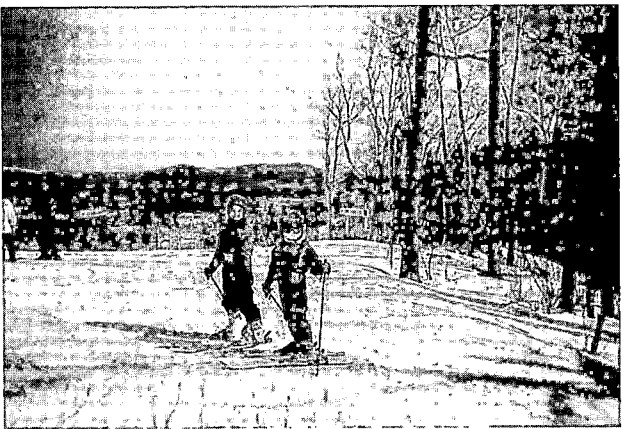

FIGURE 3-4 All skiers, especially children, should wear a helmet. *(Courtesy of Bob Elling)*

- Winter sports injury prevention. The U.S. Consumer Product Safety Commission estimates that 84,200 skiing injuries and 37,600 snowboarding injuries were treated in the ED in 1997. This includes 17,500 head injuries, many of which could have been prevented or lessened by wearing helmets. The key strategies for reducing skiing injuries are proper training, not using alcohol on the slopes, and always wearing a helmet (Figure 3–4).

- Firearm injuries and fatalities. In 1994, there were 38,505 firearm-related deaths in the United States. These included over 17,800 homicides and over 18,700 suicides. In 1990, firearm injuries cost over $20.4 billion, the majority of which is paid by the taxpayers. The key strategies are gun control; the proper storage, training, and licensing of handgun owners; and the need for trigger locks and loading indicators.

- Pedestrian safety. Each year approximately 82,000 pedestrians are injured in traffic crashes. This includes over 50,000 children who often sustain a serious brain injury. Key strategies include: teaching adults and children to cross only at intersections, to look left-right-left before crossing, and to wear reflective clothing after dark.

- Safe Railroad Crossings. Basically, the train can't stop fast enough to prevent a collision with a person or vehicle on the track. Recent Supreme Court decisions have held the railroads "not liable" for the failure of their crossings. The public has a responsibility to take appropriate and safe action here and should understand that.

- Drinking and driving. Drinking is one of the biggest contributors to highway deaths and injuries. Drinking and walking near traffic is unsafe also! Check out the information available from your governor's Traffic Safety Office, the National Highway Traffic Safety Administration, or your local police department.

- Preventing heart attacks. Check out the information available from the American Heart Association.

- Preventing stroke. Check out the information available from the American Heart Association.

- Hazards of smoking. Check out the information available from the American Lung Association.

PEARL

> *EMS providers are in an ideal position to be front-line advocates for injury and disease prevention. Other health care providers rarely have such an opportunity in out-of-hospital care.*

Leadership Activities

Q What are ways that EMS providers can lead in the area of illness and injury prevention?

A There are many ways EMS providers can make it acceptable and within the mission of the organization to be involved in prevention activities. Some administrators still have not realized the importance of prevention activities and that the tone of the organization should be set by the leaders in the agency. Employees need to be empowered to be involved in an effective injury and illness prevention program. The leaders not only need to say they are for prevention and their organization is involved in prevention efforts, they lead by example. For instance, the leaders can say they are pro-fitness and health, but if the administrators are obese, chain smokers, the message is marred by the true image of the leaders in the minds of the employees and the public.

Q What are some examples of areas where EMS leaders can promote illness and injury prevention in their service?

A To promote prevention in the EMS service, the leaders can do the following:

- Protect individual EMS providers from injury.
- Provide education to EMS providers.
- Support and promote the collection and utilization of injury data.
- Obtain resources for primary injury prevention activities.
- Empower individual EMS providers to conduct primary injury prevention activities.

How can the EMS leadership protect individual EMS providers from injury?

The best leaders tell their employees what objectives they want accomplished, provide the necessary training for their employees to accomplish the objectives, provide the necessary equipment and supplies to attain the objectives, allow the employees to accomplish the objectives, and then tell them how they did. Ways an EMS leader can protect individual EMS providers from injury involve the following:

- The leaders can develop sensible policies and procedures promoting safety during response, scene management, and transport.
- They can set an example.
- They can ensure that all EMS providers are provided appropriate equipment for eye, back, and skin safety (e.g., body substance isolation [BSI] precautions).
- They can ensure that the appropriate equipment is given to EMS providers to prevent communicable disease and chemical exposure.
- They can implement a safety program for their organization.
- They can utilize a safety officer at multiple casualty incidents.
- They can establish a wellness program for EMS providers in their organization.

> **CLINICAL PEARL**
>
> *The message is clear—education and action begins "at home." An EMS system must "practice what they preach" throughout the* entire *organization.*

What education can EMS leaders provide their organization's members to promote illness and injury prevention?

Start by educating all EMS providers in the fundamentals of injury prevention. If they are knowledgeable about strategies to prevent injury and practice them at home and work, other family members and community members will certainly benefit. Incorporate prevention education into both the primary and continuing EMS provider education. The EMS leader should seek out public and private sector specialty groups for specific education and training for their service's members.

How should the EMS leaders promote the collection and utilization of injury data?

Develop policies and promote the documentation of injuries by EMS providers. Consider developing a "dangerous sit-uation" report, within the bounds of patient confidentiality, that can be forwarded to the appropriate social service or public safety agency. An example might be reporting a dangerous condition at a local playground to the parks and recreation department so other children are not injured the way your patient was. It is also helpful to modify data collection tools so the prompt recording of data is feasible and realistic. EMS leaders should ensure that their agency contributes to local, state, and national surveillance systems so we all benefit from the data.

How can the EMS leaders obtain resources for primary injury prevention programs?

First, if prevention is part of the mission, budget for it or it will not get done. Seek out financial resources to sponsor injury prevention programs. This can include using bartering or "in-kind" services, developing fees to obtain equipment used for prevention activities, and publicizing events. Network with other injury prevention organizations to learn how they can help your organization and vice versa. Consider attending the meetings of local organizations requesting injury prevention assistance to learn how they can help you help them.

How can EMS leaders empower EMS providers to conduct primary injury prevention activities?

EMS leaders should start by learning about their people. Many of the talents needed for primary prevention already exist in the organization's most valuable treasure, its workforce. The EMS leader should identify and encourage interest and support whenever possible. Make it possible for employees to participate in prevention efforts by providing rotational assignments to the prevention programs and providing a salary for off-duty injury prevention activities. Provide rewards and remuneration for participation in the prevention program.

EMS Provider Injury Prevention Activities

What are some of the injuries or illnesses that EMS providers should be aware of as a part of the service prevention program?

Examples of injuries and illnesses that EMS providers should be aware of and watch for include:

- Infancy—issues involving mortality and morbidity as well as low birth weights.

- Childhood—intentional, unintentional, and alleged intentional events. Violent acts by the child to themselves or others.
- Adults—abuse, ignorance about or noncompliance with common safety practices.
- Geriatrics—abuse, neglect, and refusal to acknowledge changes in reaction times. Multiple medications and an inability to read the labels properly are major problems.
- Recreation—alcohol mixed with most activities.
- Work hazards—noncompliance with safety regulations, exposure to hazardous substances, substance abuse, or lack of adequate sleep.
- Day care centers—licensed and nonlicensed centers. Lack of proper supervision of children and inadequate training of staff often contribute.
- Early release from the hospital—patient is unsupervised or noncompliant with physician follow-up instructions.
- Discharge from urgent care, or other out-patient facilities—patient is unsupervised or noncompliant with follow-up instruction.
- Self-medication—stopping a medication regimen at the first sign of relief rather than completing the course of treatment; borrowing medications from other patients; improper storage and use of expired medications; over-medication, either accidental or purposeful.

Q What steps does the implementation of prevention strategies involve?

A Steps to implementing prevention strategies by EMS providers include the following:

- Preservation of the safety of the responding team.
- Patient care considerations.
- Recognizing signs and symptoms of exposure.
- Recognizing the need for outside resources.
- Documentation.
- On-scene education.
- Identifying resources needed.

Q What things should the EMS provider recognize exposure to?

A The EMS provider must be able to recognize exposure to hazardous materials, temperature extremes, vectors, communicable diseases, assault, battery, and structural risks.

Q What are examples of the concerns that should be documented as a part of a prevention program?

A The EMS provider should follow their agency's procedure for documenting prevention issues. Some agencies use a special incident report to document safety hazards. At a minimum, the EMS provider should document the primary care provided and primary injury data that includes: scene conditions, mechanism of injury (MOI), use of protective devices, absence of protective devices, risks overcome, and other information as required by the EMS agency.

Q What should the EMS provider be aware of as a part of the on-scene educational strategy of a prevention program?

A The EMS provider should gain a sense of whether the injury was caused by an event that could recur (e.g., the next time the patient travels without a seat belt or uses equipment without safety goggles). Try to use the concepts of effective communication, including:

- Recognizing the teachable moment.
- Being nonjudgmental.
- Being objective.
- Having a sense of timing.
- Taking into consideration ethnic, religious, and social diversity.
- Informing the patient, family members, or coworkers how they can prevent a recurrence.
- Informing individuals about use of protective devices.

Q What are examples of the resources that the EMS provider and EMS supervision should be aware of as a part of a prevention program strategy for the community?

A Resources should be available for each of the following situations:

- Access to specialty equipment or devices.
- Child protective services.
- Sexual abuse.
- Spousal abuse.
- Elder abuse.
- Food, shelter, or clothing.
- Employment.
- Counseling.

- Alternative health care (e.g., free clinics).
- Alternative means of transportation (e.g., bus, taxi, invalid coach).
- After-care services.
- Rehabilitation.
- Grief support.
- Immunization programs.

- Vector control.
- Disabled services.
- Day-care services.
- Alternative modes of education.
- Work-study program.
- Mental health resources and counseling.

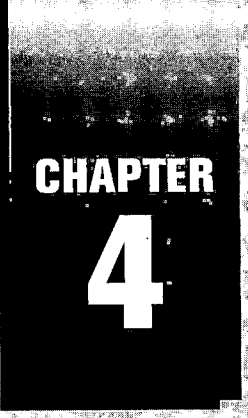

CHAPTER 4

Medicolegal Issues

This chapter discusses both basic and advanced aspects of legal issues affecting the out-of-hospital provider. The focus is on *why* you should be aware of the legal issues involved in out-of-hospital patient care and *why* you should protect yourself legally. The best way for a good EMS provider to avoid legal problems is to know the law and to practice good medicine. Being pleasant to the patient and the patient's family and always treating the patient and the patient's property with respect also goes a long way toward keeping you out of court!

Basic Definitions and Legal Concepts

Q What are the general types of law?

A There are many types of law that EMS providers encounter as a part of their practice. These include: legislative, administrative, common, criminal, and civil (tort).

Legislative law is made up of statutes voted on and passed by the legislature, be it a city council, county board, state legislature, or Congress. One example is a state's EMS Act. This Act defines which governmental agency takes the lead in supervising the EMS and issuing certifications. The state agency then promulgates specific regulations or codes (a form of administrative law) to implement the Act's provisions.

Administrative law is the body of rules and regulations made by governmental agencies such as the state EMS bureau or Department of Motor Vehicles. Often these rules contain the time period covered by a certification or licensure, equipment standards, the process for recertification, and penalties for breaking the EMS code. The EMS code is the code of rules and regulations that outline the specifics of the EMS law in each state.

Common law comes from the English legal system and consists of laws based on principles that have remained constant over time. Common law in the United States can be traced back to the time of the American Revolution.

> **CLINICAL PEARL**
>
> *"Case law" is often used in a court to decide pending cases. Small local court decisions are usually not used as precedents by higher state and federal courts. Even lower federal appellate decisions from one circuit court may not always be adopted or followed by another circuit court.*

Criminal law deals with wrongs against members of society such as homicide and rape. Federal, state, and local governments prosecute individuals for violating these laws. Violations are punished by fines or incarceration. An example is an EMS provider who intentionally hurts patients by withholding essential medication or treatment for the purpose of inflicting additional pain to "teach the patient a lesson."

Civil law, also called tort law, deals with noncriminal acts. A civil lawsuit is started in the court system to obtain damages, usually money, for the plaintiff. An example is a plaintiff suing an EMS provider for a breach of confidentiality that she believes caused harm to her reputation in the community.

An EMS provider may be requested to testify in several different types of civil lawsuits; for example, when a patient sues the town for injuries he claims to have been caused by an improperly maintained sidewalk. As a witness, you can be asked to describe the patient's injuries, your treatment, and your recollection of the condition of the sidewalk.

What is meant by the plaintiff and the defendant?

A party who brings an action against another person is called the plaintiff. The party being sued is called the defendant.

What is the difference between an administrative hearing, a trial court, and an appellate court?

An administrative hearing is a less formal process in which a judge and attorneys are present, but no jury. These hearings are usually used for administrative law actions such as the state EMS bureau charging an EMS agency with not having a properly equipped ambulance. The hearing process is quicker than a jury trial.

A trial court decides individual cases and may or may not have a jury. A jury is made up of six to twelve people, depending on the jurisdiction, type of case, and the specific court. The role of the jury, if one is used, is to decide the facts of the case presented by the competing sides through testimony and evidence. In civil cases, the jury also determines damages, such as money, for compensation, but the judge may modify the award. When there is no jury, the judge takes on both roles.

If a party to a legal action is not satisfied with the results of the case, the decision may be appealed to a higher court. With few exceptions, appellate court decisions are always based on the record of the first trial and do not involve a retrial or the introduction of new evidence. An appellate court decision can uphold the decision of the trial court, overrule it, or send it back (remand) to the lower court for various reasons.

PEARL

A successful appeal is based on an alleged error committed by the judge, jury, or other parties during the trial.

What is meant by a "jury of your peers?"

A "jury of your peers" is a jury panel composed of a selection of people from the community. An EMS provider accused of

harming a patient due to improper spinal immobilization is not entitled to a jury composed solely of EMS providers with similar experiences. Because the jury is selected by either the judge or the attorneys for each side, there is little chance of someone who knows about an EMS provider's roles and responsibilities being selected for the jury. Attorneys may oppose selecting fellow EMS providers to sit on the jury because they may be sympathetic to the defendant.

What is a grand jury?

A grand jury has more members than a typical trial jury and is convened to help decide if the district attorney (DA) or prosecutor has enough evidence to indict an individual to stand trial for a crime. An example of a case that may go to the grand jury is one involving allegations of wrongdoing during an ambulance collision. It is often the grand jury that decides if the DA will charge the driver of the ambulance for actions that may have caused injury, death, or property damages. The grand jury does not inflict penalties. Rather, they decide whether the case should go on or the charges should be dropped. This does not prevent patients or families from pursuing civil (tort) actions against an EMS provider or service.

What is negligence?

Deviation from the accepted standard of care is called negligence (e.g., providing an arterial tourniquet as the means of bleeding control for a relatively minor bleeding wound). This is also called malpractice when speaking of a failure to exercise an acceptable degree of professional skill or competence.

What four elements must the plaintiff prove to prevail in a malpractice (negligence) suit against an EMS provider?

A plaintiff who was less than satisfied with the care that he or a family member received can bring a civil action. This usually involves an allegation that the EMS provider was negligent in improperly providing care or failing to provide care. The objective of the plaintiff is to receive a financial award for the damage (injury or death) that was allegedly done by the defendant.

The plaintiff must prove the EMS provider had a duty to act, breached that duty to act, compensable damages occurred, and there was proximate cause. Proximate cause means that the damages were directly caused by the EMS provider's act of omission or commission.

It may be difficult to prove that the EMS provider's actions, or lack of appropriate actions, was directly responsible for the patient's injuries. Because jury verdicts could be in the millions of dollars, cases are sometimes settled rather than going to court.

🔘 Why do attorneys decide to settle a lawsuit out of court?

🅰 A decision to settle a case before enduring a trial often takes into consideration many factors such as the costs of damages and defending the suit, insurance company wishes, and the potential that a sympathetic jury may rule against the EMS provider on behalf of the injured plaintiff.

🔘 How does an EMS provider incur a "duty to act?"

🅰 A duty to act is a legal responsibility to provide service to the patient. If an EMS provider responds to a call with an EMS agency, the duty is not in question. If an EMS agency puts their service in the phone book and receives a call for assistance, they may be establishing a duty to the callers.

This duty may be unclear when you are not actually on duty; for example, if you stop in your personal vehicle at the scene of a collision on the highway. Then, you have a duty to act when you identify yourself as a trained EMS provider willing to help and begin to do so.

🔘 How might an EMS provider breach the duty to act and what are some examples?

🅰 A breach occurs if you have an established duty to act and do not comply with that duty (e.g., receiving an EMS call and refusing to respond). Malfeasance is doing a wrongful or unlawful act. Misfeasance is doing a legal act in a way that is harmful or causes injury. Nonfeasance is the failure to do a required act or duty; for example, if you did not provide care to a patient who needed it because you did not want to. Failure to provide CPR might be considered a breach of your duty if your protocols require that you do so.

🔘 What is an example of proximate cause and an error of commission or omission?

🅰 The plaintiff's attorney must prove that the primary or producing cause of the injury was the breach of a duty owed by the defendant. The jury analyzes the evidence to decide whether the plaintiff's injury was caused by the defendant's actions (e.g., improper removal from the swimming pool when spinal injury is suspected).

Errors of commission are inappropriate or incorrect actions such as improperly applying a traction splint or administering a medication or procedure that is beyond the scope of the EMS provider's training level. Errors of omission are appropriate treatments that were not administered to the patient. An example is deciding not to immobilize the spine of a patient who has the mechanism of injury (MOI) for a spine injury.

For example, assume you treated a patient involved in a motor vehicle collision who suffered a spinal injury resulting in paralysis. The patient may claim that your negligent treatment, not the initial accident, caused the injury. The question to the jury is really at what point did the injury transect the spinal cord. Was it during the collision or during the spinal immobilization of the patient?

Expert witnesses might testify that the standard of care before and after immobilization includes an assessment of the distal pulses and the motor and sensory function of all four extremities. The findings should be properly documented on the prehospital care report (PCR). Without documentation that procedures were actually done by the EMS providers, a jury may question whether or not you provided adequate care.

🔘 What is the concept of "gross negligence?"

🅰 Gross negligence involves willful, wanton, intentional, or reckless actions such as passing the ET tube down the esophagus to see how long it takes for the pulse oximeter to drop below 80. Another example of gross negligence is care provided by an intoxicated EMS provider. Yet another example would be an EMS provider giving the patient an excessive dose of Furosemide (a diuretic) just to enjoy watching the patient urinate all over him/herself.

🔘 What is a Good Samaritan law and does it effect licensed or certified EMS providers?

🅰 Many state laws provide legal protection and limited immunity from civil suit for individuals who stop at the scene of an accident to render first aid without any expectation of remuneration for their services. Specific laws differ from state to state. Sometimes, Good Samaritan laws may not cover EMS providers. In other situations, the EMS providers are covered under different statutes that are specific to their training level.

> **CLINICAL PEARL**
>
> *Regarding the statutes' application to EMS providers, Good Samaritan laws have not been thoroughly tested in most courts. Do not depend on them to protect you in case of a lawsuit.*

What is abandonment and how might an EMS provider be accused of abandonment?

Abandonment is the termination of an EMS provider–patient relationship before ensuring that a provider of equal or higher level will continue the care. An example is stopping at a roadside to offer assistance and then leaving the scene before turning the patient over to the arriving EMS providers. Another example is delivering a patient to a busy ED, placing the patient onto a stretcher in the hall, and leaving without giving a report to the triage nurse or ED physician.

What is false imprisonment?

Detaining a patient without their consent or legal authority is considered false imprisonment. This is one of the reasons why it is so important to get consent before taking the patient to the hospital. It may be construed as false imprisonment or kidnapping if the patient is taken against their will.

What is slander?

Slander is an act in which a person's character or reputation is injured by the false or malicious spoken words of another person. Spreading rumors not only can be a very vicious activity, but it can hurt the reputation of another person who could potentially sue for slander.

What is libel?

Libel is an act in which a person's character or reputation is injured by the false or malicious written words of another person. Writing graffiti or anonymous notes not only can be a very vicious activity, but it can hurt the reputation of another person who could potentially sue for libel.

What is a Medical Practice Act and how does it impact on out-of-hospital care?

A Medical Practice Act is legislation that governs the practice of medicine in a particular state. These laws also prescribe how and to what extent a physician may delegate authority to an EMS provider to perform medical acts.

What is meant by delegation of authority?

In the out-of-hospital arena, delegation of authority is the granting of medical privileges by a physician, either on-line (direct) or off-line (indirect), to an EMS provider to perform skills or procedures within the EMS provider's scope of practice.

What is the scope of practice?

The scope of practice is the range of duties and skills an EMS provider is expected to perform when necessary. This scope is usually set by state law or regulation and by local medical authorities.

What is meant by *res ipsa loquitur*?

This is a Latin phrase that means "the thing speaks for itself." This term is used in reference to malpractice in which the cause of the damages does not require any special expertise to detect—the negligence is evident to a layperson. An example would be when a surgeon leaves an instrument in the patient during surgery. These cases are rare in the EMS arena but it is possible that one could involve the improper use of equipment on an unconscious patient.

What is negligence per se?

Negligence per se is the unexcused violation of a statute. An example is an ambulance traveling through a red light at an excessive speed and injuring a pedestrian.

What is contributory negligence?

Contributory negligence arises when the actions of the plaintiff contribute to her own injury. As a result, the damages awarded the plaintiff may be reduced.

What happens when a lawsuit is filed?

As the saying goes, everyone is entitled to their day in court. Our society has become very litigious over the past 20 years and this trend certainly has begun to affect the EMS community. Knowing the most basic processes involved in civil litigation may be helpful to some EMS providers. Typical parts of the civil litigation process include:

- Investigation—after an incident occurs, the plaintiff's representative investigates to see what facts can be uncovered.
- Filing of a complaint—the plaintiff files a complaint with the court system that sets forth the allegations of the claims against the defendant.

- Serving of the defendant—the defendant is served with notice that there is a legal proceeding pending. This takes the form of a summons and a copy of the complaint. The summons directs the defendant to file an answer to the complaint within a certain number of days after service.

- Discovery phase—the pretrial phase where the opposing sides have an opportunity to obtain the facts and information from the other side in preparation for the trial. Discovery may involve releasing documents such as dispatch tapes, patient records, and PCRs. During the discovery phase, witnesses may be asked to make oral statements under oath called depositions. Both parties may demand written answers to a list of questions called interrogatories. This phase allows the opposing sides to formulate their theories of the case and how they will present them, and to prevent surprises at trial.

- The trial—is conducted in a county, state, or federal court.

- Verdict—the verdict is handed down by the judge or jury and determines whether liability has been proven. The verdict also indicates whether damages have been proven and the amount of money, if any, that was awarded.

- Settlement—at any time while the case is pending, an agreement may be made between the parties to settle the case.

What is governmental immunity?

Some states or localities have laws that grant immunity to governmental officials who act in good faith as a part of their duty to act. These laws are limited in scope and have been replaced in many jurisdictions. Check with your service's attorney to see if these apply in your community.

What is a statute of limitations?

The time limit within which a lawsuit may be filed is called the statute of limitations. The applicable time limits differ from state to state and also vary depending on the cause of action. For care involving minors, the statute includes the period until the minor reaches the age of majority (usually eighteen) in that particular state.

How long should records be maintained?

This is a good question to ask your service's attorney. Generally, seven years is a good period to save the records of interactions with adult patients. If the patient was a minor, it should be seven plus the number of years the child is away from the age of majority. Training records, OSHA training (e.g., instructor, objectives, topic taught, date, time, and attendance list), medical records, tax records, and quality assurance records may vary as to the amount of time they should be kept.

What are the typical characteristics of an effective PCR?

An effective PCR should be completed promptly, thoroughly, objectively, and accurately, and should maintain patient confidentiality. More specifics on the PCR are found in Chapter 21, Documentation.

What are the different types of consent?

There are four basic types of consent: expressed, informed, implied and involuntary.

- Expressed consent—the patient directly agrees, either verbally or nonverbally, to receiving care.

- Informed consent—is given after full disclosure, or explanation, of information to the patient.

- Implied consent—given for emergency intervention by a patient who is physically or mentally unable to provide expressed consent. This type of consent remains in effect for as long as the patient requires lifesaving treatments. This is also called the "emergency doctrine."

- Involuntary consent—mandated treatment by law for mental health evaluations or by law enforcement for patients under arrest.

Do patients have a right to decide what medical care and transport they will accept?

Yes, if the patient is of legal age or is an emancipated minor and is able to make a reasoned decision. They can also revoke consent at any time.

Patients must be properly informed by the EMS provider about the nature of the illness or injury, the treatment recommended, the risks of that treatment if there are any, alternate treatments and associated risks, and the dangers of refusing treatment. For example, "I would like to immobilize your arm with a padded board splint. Failure to immobilize the injury may cause the bone to break through the skin increasing the potential for infection, pain, and the length of time to set the fracture in the hospital."

Can an unemancipated minor refuse care?

No. This means that a parent or guardian must be contacted if the minor is involved in a medical emergency.

What is an emancipated minor?

In most states, a child must be treated as an adult if they are emancipated. Minors who are married, a parent themselves, or in the armed services are generally considered emancipated. Minors living independently and who are completely self-supporting are usually considered emancipated.

Can a patient refuse care?

Yes, a competent adult can refuse care. Children cannot legally refuse care without the agreement of their parent or guardian.

Is a refusal of medical assistance (RMA) legal?

Yes, if it is obtained in a proper manner with full disclosure to the patient of assessment findings, treatment recommendations, and the implications of refusal. Disclosure should be observed and documented by a credible witness.

What is the best way to document a patient's refusal of care or transport?

If the patient has an "alert" mental status, the EMS provider should follow the procedure outlined by the medical director. That procedure often includes the following steps:

- Try to convince the patient to accept the care and transport. Also, try using your partner to persuade the patient.
- Enlist the help of significant others or family members to help persuade the patient.
- Ensure that the patient is properly informed of the implication of her decision and the potential harm (e.g., failure to allow a rigid collar in this instance may lead to a permanent spine injury, or failure to be transported to the hospital in this instance may lead to death).
- Consult the medical director. It may be helpful to put the patient "online" with the physician.
- Have the patient and a credible disinterested witness (e.g., a police officer) sign a release-from-liability form.
- Advise the patient that he may call back to request additional assistance or transport.
- Attempt to get family or friends to stay with the patient. It is not a good idea to leave the patient alone if you really feel they should be transported to the hospital!
- Document the situation and the actions taken thoroughly on the PCR. Some EMS agencies read this documentation to the patient so they may initial it, and then have the patient sign the formal release with a witness present.

Should an intoxicated patient be allowed to refuse treatment or transport?

No. Persons with an altered mental status usually are not able to make a competent decision. However, can the EMS provider accurately say the patient is intoxicated? Because most EMS providers do not receive formal training to make such a judgment and they do not carry equipment to measure the percentage of alcohol in the blood (e.g., Breathalyzer), saying the patient is intoxicated is not appropriate. The ill patient may only be exhibiting behavior or signs and symptoms similar to intoxication.

Sometimes a patient may be quoted on the PCR as indicating exactly what substance they took and how much they consumed. Assistance from the police is recommended in these situations. Police can do a breathalizer test on a person to measure the level of intoxication. Remember that alcohol is highly volatile and excreted, in part, from the body through the pores in the skin. Thus, the fact that the patient smells of alcohol does not help the EMS provider distinguish whether that was "two beers" or "two six-packs of beer."

What recourse do you have if the patient refuses, but you feel care is really warranted?

Police intervention (protective custody) or medical control involvement (put the patient on the line with the physician) may be helpful. Sometimes a patient becomes unconscious during the refusal process. In that case you may evoke the emergency doctrine (implied consent) for management of life threats only.

What if a patient refuses some of your care, but accepts transport?

Some patients will not authorize certain treatments (e.g., rigid collar, spinal immobilization, or an IV). Try to explain why it is so important that the treatment be given and the consequences of it not being given. If they still say no after your attempts at explanation, then document the refusal and have the patient sign the PCR. Do not refuse to transport patients just because they refuse part of the offered treatment.

What is protective custody?

The police can, in most jurisdictions, take a person into protective custody for a limited amount of time if they feel the person may have a serious condition that could pose a life threat without the appropriate emergency care.

Can mental health or other health care professionals simply come and "take someone away" against their will?

Involuntary commitment requirements and procedures vary from state to state. Speak with your agency's attorney to learn what your state's laws are in this area. EMS providers are often put in a difficult position by family members who would like them to take the patient away against his will.

Can a mentally incompetent adult provide consent for care?

Consent for a mentally incompetent (mentally disturbed) patient must come from a legal guardian. The emergency doctrine applies if the legal guardian is not present or cannot be contacted.

What civil rights statutes are EMS employers responsible for complying with?

Services that employ EMS providers are responsible for complying with the Civil Rights Act (Title VII) of 1964, which is the federal law prohibiting discrimination based on race, color, religion, sex, or national origin. This Title also deals with discrimination based on pregnancy and sexual harassment. Title VII prohibits discrimination in employment in recruitment, hiring, promotions, training, salary, benefits, and firings. Discrimination based on sexual orientation and marital status is not covered under Title VII, but is covered under many state statutes.

What about the patient's civil rights?

EMS providers should not discriminate in providing service to patients because of race, color, religion, sex, or national origin or their ability to pay. All patients should be provided with the appropriate care regardless of their disease, condition, or injury.

Is an EMS provider actually an EMS provider when off duty or out of state?

Yes, but his ability to practice may be limited by the lack of medical control to give him the permission to practice advance modalities. The safest approach when confronted with a life-threatening medical emergency or injury outside your medical control region is to limit your care to lifesaving BLS treatment as a first responder and let the local EMS system respond in their usual manner.

What is governmental obstruction?

When a citizen gets in the way of an agent of the government who is performing their duties, especially when it involves protecting the public, that citizen may be violating a governmental obstruction provision of a state or local law. Some statutes impose harsh fines or jail time for obstructing or assaulting an EMS provider in the course of their duty.

What is filing a false instrument or record tampering?

Knowingly filing an incorrect document with a government agency is illegal. An example is lying about your age or prior convictions on the application for an EMT card. It is also illegal to change a permanent record that has been filed for the purpose of covering up inappropriate or incorrect actions. This is considered record tampering.

Is there a legal liability attached to the dispatching phase of an EMS incident?

Yes, most definitely. That is why it is strongly recommended that all dispatch agencies have training, protocols that are medically reviewed, ongoing quality assurance, and that all communication, both radio and telephone, be recorded.

Can an EMS provider honor a permission-to-treat form for a minor left with a babysitter?

This practice is questionable at best. It is suggested that the parent be contacted immediately and care only be given for life-threatening conditions.

What is an advance directive?

An advance directive is a document or order prepared at the request of the patient, an authorized family member or legal representative, or physician to ensure that certain treatment choices are followed at a time when the patient is unable to speak for herself.

What is a living will?

A living will is a type of advanced directive. It is a document that states the type of lifesaving medical treatment a patient wants or does not want to be employed in case of terminal illness, coma, or persistent vegetative state.

Q What is the Patient Self-Determination Act?

A This is a 1991 federal law that requires all hospitals and nursing homes to provide patients with information on advance directives and determine if each patient already has an advance directive in place.

Q What is a Health Care Power of Attorney?

A A durable power of attorney or health care proxy allows a person to designate an agent to act in cases where the person is unable to make decisions themselves.

Q What information must EMS providers keep confidential?

A To maintain the patient–EMS provider relationship, the information about patient history, assessment findings, and treatment rendered must remain confidential. Because EMS providers are invited into very private parts of patients' homes, whatever is observed should be kept in confidence. An exception to this is the necessary reporting of observations if required by law, such as a mandated report of suspected child abuse.

Q What information can be released about the patient by an EMS provider or his agency?

A Release of patient information requires written permission from the patient or legal guardian in all cases except the following:

- To other health care providers with a need to know to provide care to the patient.
- When a law requires the release of information (e.g., mandatory child abuse reporting).
- When a third party requires the information for billing.
- In response to a subpoena. Make sure that your service's attorney has established a policy on how employees are to respond to a subpoena.

Q Can the improper release of information or the release of inaccurate information result in liability?

A Yes, it can. This is an invasion of privacy. The release, without a legal mandate, of private information may expose the patient to notoriety, embarrassment, or ridicule. This is the case whether the information is true or not.

Q What is a "do not resuscitate" (DNR) order and must EMS providers follow it?

A Such an order is a directive to medical care providers not to perform any life-sustaining measures after respiratory or cardiac arrest. EMS providers should consult with their service medical director as to the state law and service policy for dealing with a DNR order in out-of-hospital care and what forms of this order are acceptable (e.g., specific document, bracelet, necklace). It is worth noting that this term is being changed to "do not attempt resuscitation" or DNAR.

Q What is meant by "comfort care?"

A Comfort care is patient management and care of the family that complies with the DNR order and advance directives. This is also called palliative care, which means to ease without curing.

Q Should EMS providers carry malpractice insurance?

A That is a personal decision that should include an analysis of the risk, costs, and any insurance provided by your agency. Clearly, anyone can be sued and hiring legal counsel to represent you is expensive. Most insurance policies do not cover punitive damages.

Q When is patient restraint allowed and what is meant by "humane restraints"?

A Restraint is appropriate with unruly or violent patients who may hurt themselves or the EMS providers. Law enforcement should be involved and humane restraint must be used. Humane restraints are not handcuffs; rather, the use of sheets, tape, or padded leather restraints are more acceptable to reduce the potential harm to the patient.

Q Does an EMS provider have a responsibility to resuscitate a potential organ donor?

A Although there is usually no legal responsibility, the EMS provider has an ethical responsibility to resuscitate all potential organ donors so that others may benefit from the organs. Each EMS agency medical director should establish a policy that guides EMS providers on how to handle these situations.

Q What responsibility does an EMS provider have at a crime scene to preserve evidence?

A The EMS provider has a responsibility at a crime scene to first and foremost protect herself and other EMS providers.

Next, your responsibility is to provide care for the patient and to notify law enforcement if they have not yet been dispatched to the scene. Observe and document any items moved or anything unusual at the scene. Protect potential evidence whenever possible (e.g., leave holes in clothing from bullet or stab wounds intact). Additional information on this topic can be found in Chapter 51, Crime Scene Awareness.

Why is it important that your PCR be completed promptly?

The PCR is an important part of the patient's record and a copy needs to go to the ED for the patient's chart. It should be completed while information is fresh in the EMS provider's mind. It also must be a record made "in the course of business" and not completed later.

What is meant by the phrase, "If you didn't write it down, you didn't do it."

It is presumed that your assessment findings and management are completely documented in the normal course of business. If you did not write it on the PCR within a reasonable time after caring for the patient, it is difficult to prove that you actually did additional assessment or patient management at a later time.

What types of EMS calls seem to produce the most lawsuits against EMS providers?

The calls with large malpractice costs often involve spinal injuries and pediatric long-term disabilities (e.g., problems during emergency delivery). Families of deceased patients often sue for an unexpected (wrongful) death if they believe the EMS provider may have had a direct or indirect role in their loved one's death.

What are examples of compensable physical or psychological damages that an EMS provider may be sued for?

In a malpractice suit, an EMS provider may be required to pay compensable damages such as medical expenses, lost earnings, and conscious pain and suffering.

What are punitive damages?

Punitive damages are designed to punish the defendant for the harmful actions. Not all states allow plaintiffs to seek punitive damages. If awarded, these are usually not covered by malpractice insurance.

Are personal notes you made on a call allowed in court?

They are allowed if relevant. Copies are made available to both parties.

Can information be added to the PCR after it has been turned in?

Once copies have been handed in, it is not good practice to add information to only one copy of the PCR. This additional information is best suited for inclusion on a special incident report. Check with your medical director to see exactly how she would like situations like this handled. Records should never be altered.

What are examples of situations requiring the completion of an incident report?

Each agency should have a policy that indicates when a special incident report is to be used. The agency's legal counsel should have input into the policy because she will be involved if legal representation is later needed. Examples of situations that may warrant a special incident report include infectious disease exposures, multiple casualty incidents, crimes affecting an EMS provider, collision of an emergency vehicle, injury to an EMS provider, missing narcotics, miscellaneous unusual incidents, and additions to the PCR.

What is meant by a PCR being completed thoroughly?

The PCR should be a complete record of the assessment, management, and other relevant facts. It should provide a clear picture of what occurred and not require additional explanation.

What is meant by a PCR being completed objectively?

The role of the EMS provider is to observe and document, not to make value judgments about the living conditions or social strata of the patient. Objective findings should be documented on the PCR. Objective findings are measurable, whereas subjective findings depend on the perceptions of the patient and EMS provider.

What is meant by the PCR being completed accurately?

The descriptions on the PCR should be as accurate as possible. Because the EMS provider may end up in court testifying using the documentation, he should avoid using jargon, especially that which gives a negative connotation (e.g., skell, frequent flyer, system abuser). Medical abbreviations are good to use provided they are standard abbreviations that can be found in most pocket references and are not your own. For a list of medical abbreviations consult a medical dictionary.

How can EMS providers best avoid lawsuits?

Always be respectful and pleasant to your patients, their families, and their property. Practice good medicine and be a competent caregiver. Accurately and clearly document the assessment and management of the patient on the PCR.

If you provide the right care to your patient, can you still be sued?

Absolutely!

What is the difference between a legal duty and an ethical responsibility?

The legal duties of the EMS provider are to the patient, medical director, and public and are based on generally accepted standards as well as laws or regulations. Ethical responsibility is morally desirable conduct of a professional. Additional information on ethics can be found in Chapter 5, Ethical Issues for the EMS Provider.

What mandatory reporting requirements do EMS providers have?

This varies from state to state, but usually EMS providers have a requirement to make a report or personally notify a mandated reporter (e.g., physician or nurse) in the receiving facility of cases that may involve:

- Child abuse or neglect.
- Elder or spousal abuse.
- Sexual assault.
- Gunshot and stab wounds.
- Animal bites.
- Communicable diseases.

What is the difference between "scope of practice" and "standard of care?"

Scope is the range of skills and knowledge the EMS provider is trained in. The standard of care is based on national standards

(e.g., American Heart Association guidelines), national curricula, and national testing standards (e.g., National Registry of EMTs), and the recognized treatment for patients in similar circumstances.

Are all "standards of care" national?

No, because EMS providers are physician extenders and physicians are licensed by states and not nationally. The EMS provider practicing in a large urban academic medical center is held to a standard of similar EMS providers. The EMS providers practicing in a small rural setting may be held to a different standard. The standard of care is not just based on the EMS provider's training, testing, and protocols, it also takes into consideration the setting, environment, and resources.

Are actions taken by quality assurance committees open to public review?

No. They should remain confidential; otherwise, obtaining objective participation from all involved in the process would be difficult. The problem usually lies with members of the committees who talk publicly about the committee's activities.

CLINICAL PEARL

> *Despite the long-held belief that "peer review" and quality assurance proceedings are not discoverable in a lawsuit, this is not always the case. Though we are unaware of any case involving EMS providers, physician peer review documents and hospital incident reports have been allowed into evidence in a few medical malpractice cases.*

What is the Freedom of Information Act (FOIA)?

The Freedom of Information Act (sometimes called the freedom of information law or FOIL request) makes certain types of information collected by public agencies available to the media, legal counsel, or the public on demand. The agency that is being requested to provide the information may charge a minimal fee for the duplication or preparation of the information and must provide the information within a reasonable time of its request.

Does patient care documentation come under FOIA?

No. The PCR is confidential information. The PCR can be subpoenaed, but is not accessible to the public or media by submitting a FOIA request. It may be possible to obtain dispatch records or other public documents that do not have specific patient names on them. Always check with legal counsel before releasing information.

Is the medical control physician liable for the care provided in the field?

Yes. The medical director's liability for out-of-hospital care falls into two categories:

- On-line or direct supervision—orders given over the radio or telephone to the EMS provider at the scene.
- Off-line or indirect supervision—authorization of EMS providers through protocols and standing orders.

Is the EMS provider liable for the actions of an EMT-Basic on his crew?

If the EMS provider is acting in a supervisory capacity, she may be held liable for the actions of an EMT-Basic. For example, an EMS provider may be liable for the actions of an EMT-Basic in training. The supervising EMS provider must provide direct observation, guidance, and feedback to the student and must supervise all of the student's actions. It is also the supervisor's duty to step in when needed to prevent the student from taking an action that could harm the patient.

What is the relationship between ALS providers and the medical director?

The Advanced Life Support (ALS) provider is the eyes and ears of the physician when on a call and as such is an extension of the physician's care. It is imperative that the EMS provider follows the on-line orders and off-line protocols. ALS providers administer advanced modalities as an extension of the physician and not as a licensed free agent.

Why must an EMS provider obtain consent from a patient to treat or transport?

All EMS providers must have patient consent to treat with the exception of the emergency doctrine for unconscious patients. Failure to obtain consent could cause problems.

Do patients have a right to know who you are and your level of training?

Yes. Always wear an ID tag or patch indicating the level of your training and your name. It is a good practice to introduce yourself to your patient by name and level of training.

What protection does the EMS provider have from assault or battery while performing his duties?

Some states or jurisdictions have made it a serious crime to assault or strike an EMS provider in the course of his duties.

What is sexual harassment in the workplace?

It is the perception of pressure for sexual favors in exchange for any form of special privileges or advancement on the job. In addition, any offensive behavior of a sexual nature (e.g., conduct, comments, posters, jokes, movies, or videos) can be classified as sexual harassment. The person who feels harassed has the right to file a complaint directly with the human resources office without making it known to the offending person. These complaints are taken very seriously.

What is the role of the Occupational Safety and Health Administration (OSHA) regarding EMS?

The Occupational Safety and Health Act of 1970 created OSHA within the Department of Labor. The purpose of OSHA is to:

- Develop standards and guidelines for employers and employees that reduce the incidence of deaths, injuries, and illnesses.
- Establish and maintain a reporting system for workplace injuries and illnesses.
- Encourage the improvement of existing safety and health programs.
- Develop an enforcement procedure for safety and health standards.

Who is covered under OSHA regulations?

All employers and their employees in the 50 states, the District of Columbia, and any U.S. territory are covered by either OSHA or an OSHA-approved state program. Exceptions are self-employed people, farms where only family members are employed, and employment by federal agencies. State and local government employees are often covered by a form of OSHA that may differ somewhat from state to state.

What are some examples of OSHA regulations that apply to EMS?

More is discussed in other chapters of this book, but examples of OSHA regulations include:

- Blood-borne Pathogens (29CFR 1910.1030).
- OSHA 200 (records of occupational injuries).
- OSHA 1910.134 (respiratory protection program).
- OSHA 1910.120 (hazardous waste operations and emergency response standard).
- OSHA 1910.1200 (hazard communications standard).
- OSHA 1910.132-138 (personal protective equipment).

Can OSHA violations result in a fine against the EMS agency?

Yes, some very serious fines in fact. Examples include:

- Serious violation ($1,500 to $7,000).
- Willful violation ($5,000 to $70,000).
- Repeat violation (up to $70,000).
- Failure to abate ($7,000 per day).

Must an EMS provider respond to a subpoena?

Yes. You should never ignore legal papers; consult with your attorney right away so you handle this properly. Once litigation has started, do not discuss the issues involved with anyone except your attorney or service management.

What is the Family and Medical Leave Act (FMLA)?

The FMLA is a federal law that requires employers to give employees up to 12 weeks of unpaid leave for certain family and medical reasons (e.g., family or personal illness or the birth or adoption of a child). The leave may also be paid if the person has the time accrued.

What is the Fair Labor Standards Act (FLSA)?

The FLSA is the federal law that regulates minimum wages and overtime in the workplace. In EMS, the law has an impact on issues such as on-call pay, comp time, long shifts, and overtime

pay. This law has been the subject of fierce debate due to an exemption to the overtime section of the law for fire department employees engaged in fire protection activities. In many instances, fire department employees involved in EMS duty have claimed their departments violated the overtime statute and sued their departments for back pay.

What is the Americans With Disabilities Act (ADA)?

The ADA is a federal law designed to protect qualified persons with disabilities from discrimination in employment, transportation, and public accommodation. Specifically, employers of 15 employees or more and all public employers of any size cannot discriminate against protected individuals in all aspects of employment (e.g., recruitment, hiring, promotions, training, salary, benefits, and firings).

Who is covered under the ADA?

A qualified individual is one who has a disability that limits one or more major life activities (e.g., walking, seeing, hearing, learning, or caring for oneself) and possesses the legitimate skill, experience, education, or other requirements of employment and can adequately perform the essential functions of the job with or without reasonable accommodations. Temporary disabilities, such as a fractured leg, are not covered under ADA. Those who use drugs illegally are not covered by ADA.

What should an EMS provider or EMS employer do if they have a question about an ADA issue?

Read the statute and consult with your agency's attorney.

Driving an Emergency Vehicle

What are courtesy lights and are there exemptions to the traffic (V&T) laws for their use during an emergency response?

Each state is different, but courtesy lights are usually green or blue, if blue is not an emergency light color. The use of a green or blue light does not give the motor vehicle operator any exemption from the State V&T laws, nor does it provide any immunity for your actions during its use. The green or blue light is called a courtesy light, which is requesting the right of way from other drivers during an emergency.

Q What is considered emergency vehicle operation?

A State laws do differ, but an emergency operation usually includes responding to or working at the scene of an accident, disaster, alarm of fire, or other emergency. Emergency operation does not include returning from such service.

Q Can emergency vehicles respond to a drill using emergency lights and sirens?

A No. In most states, the law only allows for the displaying of red (or blue) lights on authorized emergency vehicles when such vehicles are in an emergency operation. Many fire trucks and ambulances have been seen returning to station with the rear beacons on. This is an old practice that was useful to alert the public that there were firefighters on the back step. Today, this is not acceptable because riding the back step is too dangerous and keeping the lights on does nothing but confuse the other motorists.

Q When an ambulance is not operating as an emergency vehicle, are the operator and passengers required by state law to fasten their seat belts?

A That depends on how your state law is written. In many states, the law specifically excludes authorized emergency vehicles, which includes ambulances, from the mandatory use of seat belts for driver and front-seat passenger. The authorized emergency vehicle does not lose this status when it is not on an emergency operation. However, it is strongly recommended that all ambulance services develop a standard operating procedure (SOP) that includes the following: all operators and front-seat passengers must use seat belts, all patients being transported on the stretcher must be secured by two or more straps, all non-EMS personnel in the patient compartment must be belted in, and all EMS personnel in the patient compartment must use seat belts when they are not attending to the patient.

Q Are child restraining seats required when transporting a child in an ambulance?

A Child restraint laws usually exclude emergency vehicles. It is strongly recommended that all ambulance services develop a SOP to cover this issue.

If a child is taken along to the hospital and the child's own restraining device is available, he should be placed in the device and belted into the ambulance seat. If the child is the patient, she should be placed on an appropriately secured stretcher.

In the past much emphasis has been placed on a parent holding a child so the child feels less threatened and is more likely to stay calm. Though the EMS provider has a tendency to have a parent hold a small child during transport, it should be stressed how dangerous this practice is.

Q Do typical V&T laws require the emergency lights or siren to be used whenever a patient is being transported?

A Certainly not! The laws usually state that the driver, when involved in an emergency operation, may exercise the privileges set forth in the law. This clearly gives the option of not using emergency lights and siren on most calls. Most laws go on to say that whenever the driver of the authorized emergency vehicle exercises the privileges set forth in the law, at least one revolving emergency light visible from 500 feet in each direction must be on and an audible device as may be reasonably necessary must be sounded.

Q What is a true medical emergency and how does this relate to ambulance operation?

A A true medical emergency is one in which there is a high probability of death or serious injury to an individual or significant property loss, and action by the emergency vehicle operator may reduce the seriousness of the situation. If you are involved in an ambulance collision where property damage, injury, or loss of life occurs, your actions will be evaluated and judged. Was the situation a true emergency? And did you exercise due regard for the safety of others?

Q What does due regard mean and how does it affect the operation of an ambulance?

A An accepted definition of due regard is "a reasonably careful person performing similar duties and under the same circumstances would act in the same manner." In judging due regard, the following criterion is used: Was there enough notice of approach to allow other motorists and pedestrians to clear a path and protect themselves? If you do not give notice of the ambulance's approach until a collision is inevitable, you may not have satisfied the principle of due regard for the safety of others.

In determining whether or not an ambulance operator was exercising due regard in the use of signaling equipment, the following points should be considered:

• Was it reasonably necessary under all of the circumstances to use the signaling equipment?

• Was the signaling equipment actually used?

• Was the signal given audible or visible to the motorist and pedestrians?

What exemptions to the V&T laws do the lights and siren generally give an operator of an ambulance in the emergency mode?

The laws do differ from state to state, but the operator of an authorized emergency vehicle, when involved in an emergency operation, may typically exercise the following privileges:

- Stop, stand, or park despite the posted signage.
- Proceed past a steady red signal, a flashing red signal, or a stop sign, but only after slowing as may be necessary for safe operation.
- Exceed the maximum speed limits if he does not endanger life or property.
- Disregard regulations governing directions of movement or turning in specified directions.

Are there any conditions attached to these privileges?

Yes, usually there are conditions. These will vary from state to state. Ask your agency attorney or medical director for the specific conditions in your state.

Can an ambulance operator proceed through a stop sign or red light operating just the emergency lights and not the siren?

Usually not. Typical state laws say that the exemptions for authorized emergency vehicles apply only when audible signals are sounded and when the vehicle displays its emergency lights. Conservative and cautious use of emergency lights and sirens should be based on the medical priority of the patient as judged by the highest trained EMS providers on the crew (going to the hospital).

If the ambulance is involved in a collision en route to the hospital or on an EMS call is it necessary to stop?

Yes. There is usually no exemption to the provisions that mandate that the operator stop and exchange information immediately after an automobile collision resulting in property damage or personal injury. Immediate attention should go toward providing alternate ambulance transportation for the patient you were transporting, and determining if there are any new injuries from the collision that require attention.

Are family members allowed to follow the ambulance through red lights and exceed the maximum posted speed limit when following an ambulance to the hospital?

Definitely not! It is illegal and very dangerous for a private vehicle to attempt to use an emergency vehicle as an escort. This should be explained to the family members who you think will be following the ambulance to the hospital. In fact, you may want to discourage them from trying to keep up with the ambulance and make sure they have directions.

Does the use of emergency lights and sirens give the operator and ambulance service complete immunity during an emergency response?

Certainly not! Whenever exercising privileges during an emergency response, the operator assumes the extra burden of driving with due regard for others. In other words, the operator has the added responsibility to ensure that no one is injured and that no property becomes damaged because of her driving. Since the V&T law does not specify that normal motor vehicle operators must use due regard, the emergency vehicle operator will be held to a higher standard in the eyes of the law.

Who should determine whether the emergency mode is necessary from the scene to the hospital?

The highest medical authority attending the patient who will be going to the hospital should decide the severity of the patient's condition and the appropriate response mode to the hospital. Although the operator may be asked to drive in the emergency mode, this does not give the operator permission to drive in a reckless manner.

If the call was not a true emergency, but the operator believed that the call was a true emergency because of information provided to him by the medical authority attending the patient, the ambulance operator may be found to have acted in good faith and in a reasonable fashion.

What should an emergency vehicle operator do if other vehicles are not yielding the right of way during an emergency run?

Typical V&T laws require the general driving motorist to yield the right of way to an emergency vehicle with lights and siren sounding.

If someone does not yield, this does not give the emergency vehicle operator the right to recklessly run him off the road. This aggressive style of driving is a common cause of ambulance collisions. Instead, wait for a safe location to pass the vehicle or follow the vehicle in a safe manner.

Q **Does an Emergency Vehicle Operator Course (EVOC) or defensive driving course (DDC) provide any immunity from lawsuits or special credits from insurance carriers?**

A These courses do not give you any extra immunity. Courses such as these do provide you and your organization with training that may demonstrate that your agency has taken every effort possible to promote safe driving practices. Insurance carriers in many states are required by law to extend a rate or point reduction credit on personal automobile insurance for attending a state approved course. Sometimes insurance carriers extend this credit to an ambulance service's insurance policy after a minimum number of their operators have completed an approved course.

Q **Once an ambulance has arrived on the scene of an emergency and the patient's condition appears to be less than an emergency in the medical judgment of the attending EMS providers, is it illegal for the ambulance operator to proceed to the hospital with the emergency lights or siren?**

A Emergency operation is defined as the operation of an authorized emergency vehicle when the vehicle is engaged in transporting a sick or injured person or responding to or working at the scene of a collision. The scenario presented is a nonemergency situation and the use of emergency lights and sirens would not be authorized.

Q **There seems to be a rumor that some ambulance services' insurance policies state that they must use emergency lights and siren whenever the vehicle is on a call. Is there any truth to this rumor?**

A If a vehicle is merely in use and not responding to an emergency, sirens and emergency lights should not be in operation. Any insurance policy that requires emergency lights and sirens in nonemergency operation is contrary to traffic laws.

EMS Education

Q **What is the difference between a license and a certification?**

A A certification is the act of certifying or the state of being certified. A license is the permission granted by an authority to engage in an activity. A certificate is a document testifying that one has fulfilled certain requirements such as a course of instruction. Most states provide a certificate upon the completion of EMS provider training and passing a state examination. Physicians, nurses, PAs, and other health care professionals are required to be licensed. Some states license paramedics but not EMT-Basics. Licensure and certification depend on the appropriate state legislative or local health or EMS authority.

Q **Why have agencies such as the American Heart Association (AHA) gotten away from the term *certification*?**

A The AHA does not provide medical control for the interventions taught in Basic Cardiac Life Support (BCLS), Advanced Cardiac Life Support (ACLS), or Pediatric Advanced Life Support (PALS) courses. As such they do not certify or attest to the skill level of the provider. A card verifying successful completion of the course is provided to graduates. This means that the participant met a certain level of cognitive and performance standards at the end of the course. According to the AHA, "Successful completion of an AHA course does not warrant performance or qualify or authorize a person to perform any procedures on a patient." Actually, the newest version of the cards that are being issued say, "This is to certify completion of . . ."

Q **Can convicted felons become EMS providers?**

A That depends on the laws of the state agency that issues the license or certification. Most states have a process by which convicted felons may apply to the state agency and demonstrate that they have obtained a release from the probation and correctional system. The decision whether they are allowed to sit for the state examination depends on the law and policies of the state agency.

Q **Should an EMS instructor carry insurance?**

A That is a personal decision. It is worth asking who would provide a legal defense if you were to become involved in a lawsuit.

Q **What about insurance for the EMS educational institution?**

A This is recommended to cover injuries to students or faculty that may occur at the training facility. The AHA requires all community training centers to maintain insurance coverage.

Ethical Issues for the EMS Provider

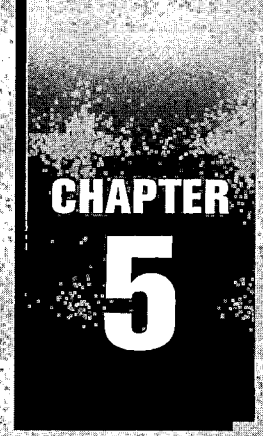

This chapter discusses ethics. The focus is on *why* you must be aware of ethical issues related to out-of-hospital patient care. The best way for a good EMS provider to stay out of the middle of an ethical dilemma is to think things through ahead of time and maintain a high degree of integrity.

Basic Definitions and Concepts

Q What is ethics?

A Socrates defined ethics as how one should live. Actually ethics comes from the Greek word "ethos," which means moral custom. Ethics is a system of principles governing moral conduct. Ethics involve larger issues than an out-of-hospital provider's practice.

Q What is the difference between an ethical decision and a moral decision?

A Morals relate to societal standards and ethics relate to personal standards. Acting in a lewd or crude manner might be considered immoral, whereas cheating on an examination is considered unethical.

Q What fundamental premise should underlie the EMS provider's ethical decisions?

A The fundamental question to ask yourself is, "What is in the patient's best interest?" Deciding what the patient wants should incorporate what the patient has said, what the patient has written, and family input.

Q What types of criteria are used in allocating scarce EMS resources?

A Three basic types of criteria are used for allocating scarce EMS resources: true parity, need, and earned. *True parity* is an attempt to compare all the variables in an effort to arrive at a similarity; that is, what is fair for everyone concerned. *Need* is based on an established criteria, the standard for which may be subjective. However, it is better for there to be an objective standard that those needing the resource can be measured against. Finally, *earned* is based upon an established criteria awarding points or value for things that have been done previously.

Q What are some ethical decisions involved in out-of-hospital resuscitations?

A It is sometimes an ethical decision whether or not to resuscitate when considering the patient's wishes and the presence or absence of an advance directive. Sometimes the family members do not agree, which presents an ethical dilemma. When in doubt, resuscitate.

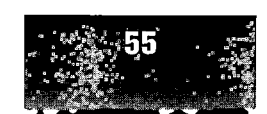

Q **What criteria govern following an advance directive in the field?**

A This varies somewhat from state to state. You should seek the advice of your medical director before being confronted with an advance directive. In general, appropriate documentation should be provided to the EMS provider on arrival so a decision can be made to withhold CPR. Once CPR has begun, either by first responders or members of your crew who were not aware that an advance directive existed, it may be local policy to contact medical control to obtain advice on ceasing the resuscitation. Some state laws provide protection for the EMS provider who begins CPR on a patient with a "do not attempt resuscitation" (DNAR) order. These laws cover circumstances where it was not clear the order was genuine or may have expired. There may also be a conflict between family members. This immunity from liability does not extend to a willful, wanton, or malicious disregard for the wishes of the patient.

Q **What global concepts should be considered when making an ethical decision?**

A Consider whether the decision you make will provide a benefit to the patient, avoid harm, and acknowledge the patient's autonomy. This is important to keep in mind in situations where you may have to talk the patient into going to the hospital. As a rule, it is always best to be honest and use terms the patient can easily understand so they can make a well-informed decision.

Q **How do EMS providers resolve ethical issues when global concepts are still in conflict?**

A Society attempts to resolve global ethical conflicts by creating laws protecting patient rights and using preplans, such as wills and advanced directives, to make patient wishes known. Within the EMS community, global ethical conflicts are resolved by established norms or standards of care, knowledge of research and treatment protocols, and prospective and retrospective reviews of medical decisions.

Q **How does the area of consent involve ethical decisions?**

A A fundamental element of the patient–physician relationship is that of a patient's right to make decisions on health care. This is stated in the American Medical Association Code of Medical Ethics.

Q **Does the area of implied consent involve ethical decisions?**

A Yes. Sometimes one has to wonder if the patient understood the decisions at hand. One might also wonder how an informed decision, based on options, could be in the patient's best interest. The best approach is to be honest and help the patient understand the ramifications of his decision in terms that are easily understood.

Q **What are some of the examples of ethical out-of-hospital decisions EMS providers are confronted with?**

A Examples of ethical decision making in EMS include:
- Defining a futile situation and who makes the decision (e.g., does a trauma patient have a mortal injury that does not warrant resuscitative measures).
- Deciding whether you should act as a good samaritan and stop to render assistance when not on duty.
- Dealing with patients who have no ability to pay may be an issue in some services.
- Providing services that are not "covered in the patient's health plan" but you feel are medically needed, patient "dumping" (issues of transportation and diversion).

Q **What types of ethical dilemmas can be a part of an out-of-hospital EMS provider's role as a physician extender?**

A Occasionally, the provider is given a physician order that she believes is contraindicated, medically acceptable but not in the patient's best interest, or medically acceptable but morally wrong.

Q **How can a refusal of medical assistance involve ethical decisions?**

A The extent to which you should persuade a patient to receive treatment or transport is vague at best and can involve an ethical decision. Be careful not to fall into the trap of making a value judgment; always act in the patient's best interest.

Q **How can decisions on where to transport a patient involve ethics?**

A In EMS systems with multiple hospitals and ill-defined transport protocols, the EMS provider can have a significant influence on the patient's decision about where to be transported. Is your decision based on the fastest trip because it is close to the end of the shift or is it based on your knowledge of the capabilities of the hospital choices you have? Consider this in all cases, "What would I do if this was my parent or child needing care for this presenting problem?"

Q. If witness to a coworker doing something unethical (e.g., making an error in administering a medication and then covering it up with a lie on the PCR), what should you do?

A. This is a personal decision that you should think through before it occurs! We suggest you keep the following two strong statements in mind:

- The EMT Code of Ethics as adopted by the National Association of EMTs in 1978:

Be it pledged as an Emergency Medical Technician, I will honor the physical and judicial laws of God and man. I will follow that regimen which, according to my ability and judgment, I consider for the benefit of patients and abstain from whatever is deleterious and mischievous, nor shall I suggest any such counsel. Into whatever homes I enter, I will go into them for the benefit of only the sick and injured, never revealing what I see or hear in the lives of men unless required by law.

I shall also share my medical knowledge with those who may benefit from what I have learned. I will serve unselfishly and continuously in order to help make a better world for mankind.

While I continue to keep this oath unviolated, may it be granted to me to enjoy life and the practice of the art, respected by all men, in all times. Should I trespass or violate this oath, may the reverse be my lot. So help me God.

- The following words were delivered by General Charles C. Krulak as a keynote speaker in a recent conference:

. . . Of all the moral and ethical guideposts that we have been brought up to recognize, the one that, for me, stands above the rest . . . the one that I have kept in the forefront of my mind . . . is integrity. It is my ethical and personal touchstone.

Integrity as we know it today . . . stands for soundness of moral principle and character, uprightness, honesty. Yet there is more. Integrity is also an ideal . . . a goal to strive for . . . and for a man or woman to "walk in their integrity" is to require constant discipline and usage. The word integrity itself is a martial word that comes to us from the ancient Roman army tradition. During the time of the twelve Caesars, the Roman army would conduct morning inspections. As the inspecting centurion would come in front of each legionnaire, the soldier would strike with his right fist the armor breastplate that covered his heart. The armor has to be strongest there in order to protect the heart from the sword thrusts and from arrow strikes. As the soldier struck his armor, he would shout "integritas," which in Latin means material wholeness, completeness, and entirety. The inspecting centurion would listen closely for the affirmation

and also for the ring that well-kept armor would give off. Satisfied that the armor sound and that the soldier beneath it was protected, he would then move on to the next man.

At the same time, the Praetorians or imperial bodyguard were ascending into power and influence. Drawn from the best "politically correct" soldiers of the legions, they received the finest equipment and armor. They no longer had to shout "integritas" to signify that their armor was sound. Instead, as they struck this breastplate, they would shout "Hail Caesar," to signify that their heart belonged to the imperial personage—not to their unit—not to an institution—not to a code of ideals. They armored themselves to serve the cause of a single man.

A century passed and the rift between the legion and the imperial bodyguard and its excesses grew larger. To signify the difference between the two organizations, the legionnaire, upon striking his armor would no longer shout "integritas" but instead would shout "integer" which means undiminished—complete—perfect. It not only indicated that the armor was sound, it also indicated that the soldier wearing the armor was sound of character. He was complete in his integrity . . . his heart was in the right place . . . his standards and morals were high. He was not associated with the immoral conduct that was rapidly becoming the signature of the Praetorian guards. The armor of integrity continued to serve the legion well. For over four centuries they held the line against the marauding goths and vandals. But by 383 A.D. the social decline that infected the Republic and the Praetorian guard had its effect on the legion.

As the fourth century Roman general wrote, "When, because of negligence and laziness, parade ground drills were abandoned, the customary armor began to feel heavy since the soldiers rarely, if ever, wore it. Therefore, they first asked the emperor to set aside the breastplates and mail and then the helmets. So our soldiers fought the goths without any protection for the heart and head and were often beaten by archers. Although there were many disasters, which led to the loss of great cities, no one tried to restore the armor to the infantry. They took their armor off, and when the armor came off—so too came their integrity." It was only a matter of a few years until the legion rotted from within and was unable to hold the frontiers . . . the Barbarians were at the gates.

Integrity . . . it is a combination of the words, "integritas" and "integer." It refers to the putting on of armor, of building a completeness . . . a wholeness . . . a wholeness in character. How appropriate that the word integrity is a derivative of two words describing the character of a member of the profession of arms.

The military has a tradition of producing great leaders that possess the highest ethical standards and integrity. It produces men and women of character . . . character that allows them to deal ethically with the challenges of today and to make conscious decisions about how they will approach tomorrow. However, as I mentioned earlier, this is not done instantly. It requires that integrity become a way of life . . . it must be woven into the very fabric of our soul. Just as was true in the days of the imperial Rome. You either walk in your integrity daily, or you take off the armor of the "integer" and leave your heart and soul exposed . . . open to attack.

My challenge to you is simple but often very difficult . . . wear your armor of integrity . . . take full measure of its weight . . . find comfort in its protection . . . do not become lax. And always, remember that no one can take your integrity from you . . . you and only you can give it away!

The biblical book of practical ethics—better known as the book of proverbs—sums it up very nicely, "The integrity of the upright shall guide them, but the perverseness of transgressors shall destroy them."

Special Thanks

National Association of EMTs for the EMT Code of Ethics.
General Charles C. Krulak for the excerpts from his speech.

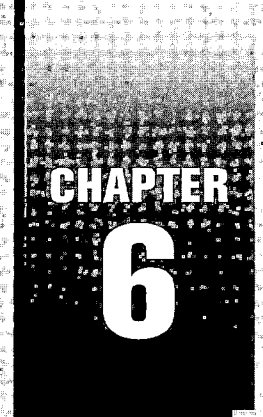

General Principles of Pathophysiology

CHAPTER 6

This chapter discusses the human body and the effects that disease has on it. The focus is on *why* patients present in a certain manner and *why* you need to respond in a certain way to the problems they present. An understanding of the human body's basic functions and normal compensatory responses to injury or disease is key to an EMS provider's preparation for the field. It is this background information that helps the EMS provider understand the impact of multiple diseases on the body, as is the case with many of the patients found in the field. To avoid duplication, particular disease conditions, which would fall into this area, are discussed in detail in the specific chapters they would fall under; for example, asthma, is covered in Chapter 22, Pulmonary and Respiratory.

The Basics

Q What is pathophysiology?

A Simply defined, it is the study of how normal physiological processes are altered by disease.

Q What is the correlation between pathophysiology and the disease process?

A Pathophysiology essentially delineates the mechanisms of disease processes. The body has a set of "checks and balances" that normally maintains balance (homeostasis). Disease results when the normal balance is altered. The greater an EMS provider's understanding of the connections between specific bodily systems and functions, the easier it is to understand disease processes.

Q What is the difference between a disease and a disorder?

A A disease is a change in anatomy or physiology that is considered abnormal. A disorder is an abnormality of function or a structural problem such as a bone disorder. Because these two terms are closely defined, they are often used synonymously.

Q What is the difference between pathology and pathologic?

A Pathology is the study of disease. Pathologic is a term that is used to describe the disease process or disease itself (e.g., fractures caused by a disease that weakens the bones are said to be pathologic fractures).

Q What is pathogenesis?

A Pathogenesis is a description of how a disease develops from its onset.

Q What is the etiology of an illness or disease?

A The etiology is the cause of the disease. If the cause is unknown, it is said to be idiopathic.

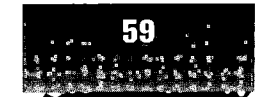

Q What is the difference between iatrogenic and nosocomial causes of a disease?

A Iatrogenic connotes any injury or illness caused or significantly contributed to by the actions of a health care provider. Nosocomial refers to infections acquired as a patient in the hospital. Although iatrogenic diseases require a specific action or lack of action, nosocomial infections may occur even if no inappropriate actions occurred.

Q What is the difference between the diagnosis and prognosis of a disease?

A A diagnosis is the identification of the cause of a medical problem, whereas the prognosis is the predicted outcome of the problem.

Q What is meant by remission and exacerbation of a disease?

A Remission is a period of time where the symptoms of a chronic disease are diminished or temporarily resolved. Exacerbation occurs when the symptoms become rapidly worse.

Q What are the seven causes of disease?

A Disease is primarily caused by heredity, trauma, inflammation, infection, neoplasm, nutritional imbalance, and impaired immunity.

> **CLINICAL PEARL**
>
> *Inflammation is a specific pathological reaction to a variety of stimuli, including infections. Not all infections result in inflammation, and not all inflammatory processes are caused by infection. Patients with rheumatoid arthritis, for example, may have severe joint inflammation, but no infection is present.*

Q What is a syndrome?

A A syndrome is a group of symptoms or conditions that may be caused by a disease or various related medical problems. A commonly known syndrome is Down syndrome, a combination of a specific physical appearance and some degree of mental impairment. These patients typically have a small flat skull, a short flat nose, wide set eyes, an epicanthus (a fold of skin on both sides of the nose), a protruding tongue, short broad hands, feet with a wide gap between the toes, underdeveloped genitalia, congenital heart defects, and below average height.

Cells and Cell Injury Patterns

Q What are the major types of tissues and their normal function in the body?

A There are four major tissue types:
1. Epithelial—covers the internal and external surfaces of the body, including the linings of vessels.
2. Connective—supports and binds other tissue types together.
3. Muscle—is characterized by its ability to contract.
4. Nervous—is characterized by its ability to conduct nerve impulses.

Q What is meant by cellular adaptation?

A When cells are exposed to adverse conditions, they go through a process of adaptation. In some situations, the cells change permanently; in others, they change their structure and function temporarily. Examples of adaptation types include atrophy, hypertrophy, hyperplasia, dysplasia, metaplasia, and neoplasia.

Q What is atrophy?

A Atrophy is a decrease in cell size leading to a decrease in the size of the tissue and organ. The actual number of cells remains unchanged. An example is a leg that has been in a cast for six weeks or more. After the cast is removed, it is not uncommon for the muscle to atrophy (Figure 6–1).

Q What is hypertrophy?

A Hypertrophy is an increase in the size of the cell leading to an increase in tissue and organ size. An example is the left ven-

Normal

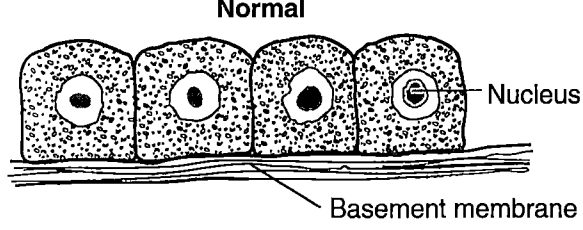

Atrophy

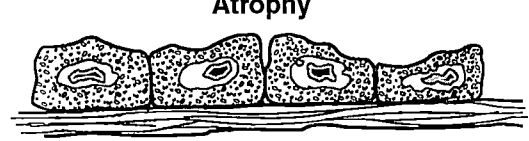

FIGURE 6-1 Normal cell versus atrophied cell.

Normal

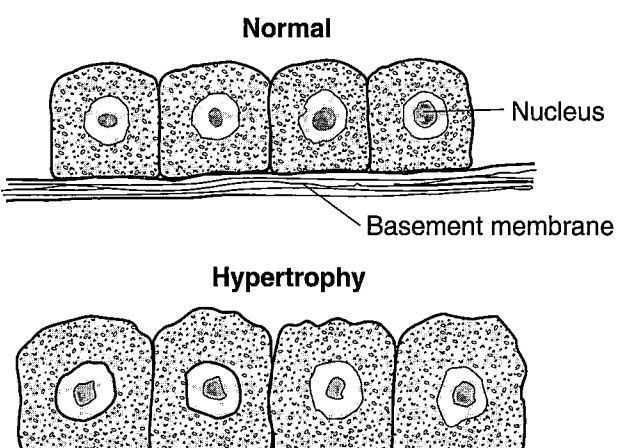

Nucleus

Basement membrane

Hypertrophy

FIGURE 6-2 Normal cell virus hypertrophied cell.

tricle of a patient who has diseased valves and arteries. Over time, the left ventricle muscle enlarges in size. This enlarged heart is also referred to as cardiomegaly. Hypertrophy occurs in the heart when one side (usually the left) has to compensate for a defect such as an acute myocardial infarction (AMI), high resistance pressures from hypertension, or atherosclerosis (Figure 6-2).

CLINICAL PEARL

> *Bodybuilding results in hypertrophy of muscles. Each cell becomes bigger though the total number of muscle cells remains the same.*

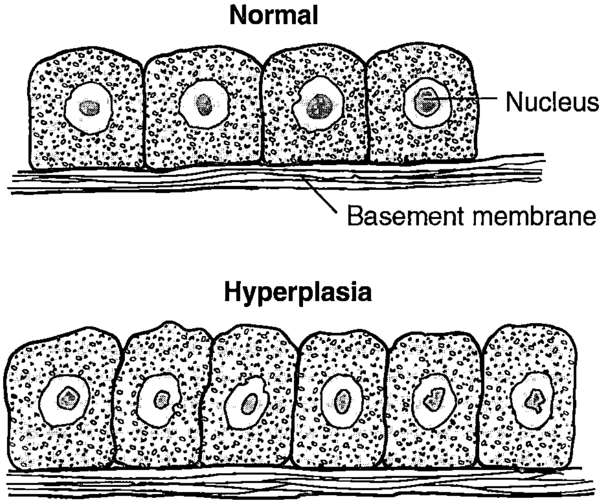

What is hyperplasia?

Hyperplasia is an increase in the actual number of cells often due to hormonal stimulation. This excess growth often causes tumors that may be malignant or benign (Figure 6-3).

CLINICAL PEARL

> *Benign prostatic hyperplasia is an increase in the number of prostate cells. This condition occurs commonly in men over 50 years old. It may be asymptomatic or result in urinary difficulty. Some experts feel that this disease is a precursor to prostate cancer.*

What is dysplasia?

Dysplasia is an alteration in the size and shape of cells as in a developing tumor (Figure 6-4).

CLINICAL PEARL

> *When a woman has a pap smear, cells from the cervix and vagina are obtained and examined under a microscope. Sometimes, dysplastic cells are seen. This may be an early sign of cervical cancer. Cervical dysplasia is treatable if diagnosed early.*

What is metaplasia?

Metaplasia is a cellular adaptation in which one cell changes to another type of cell. For example, changes in the lower esophagus from the normal squamous cell epithelium (flat, nonglandular) to columnar epithelium (columns, glandlike; more similar to

Normal

Nucleus

Basement membrane

Hyperplasia

FIGURE 6-3 Normal tissue versus hyperplasia.

Normal

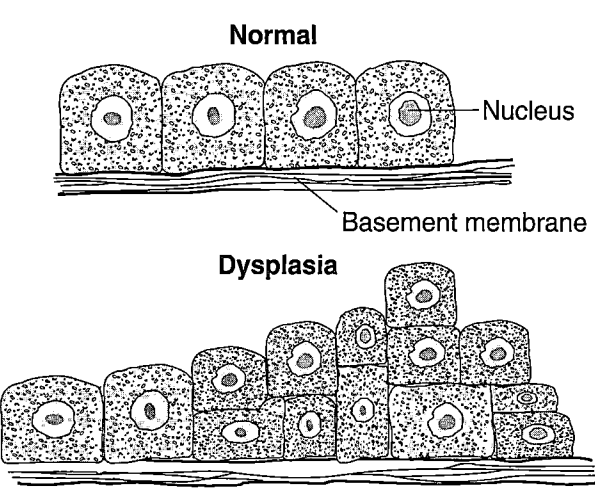

Nucleus

Basement membrane

Dysplasia

FIGURE 6-4 Normal tissue versus dysplasia.

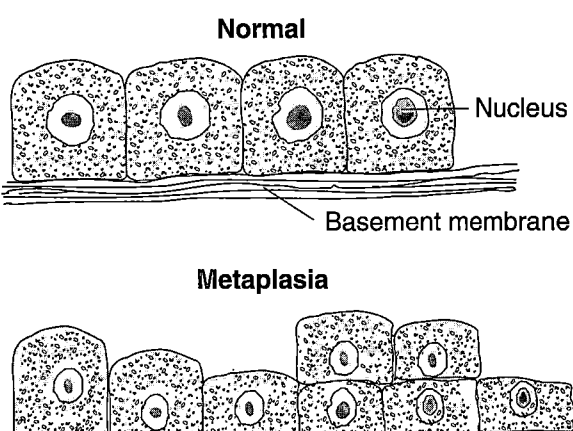

FIGURE 6–5 Normal tissue versus metaplasia.

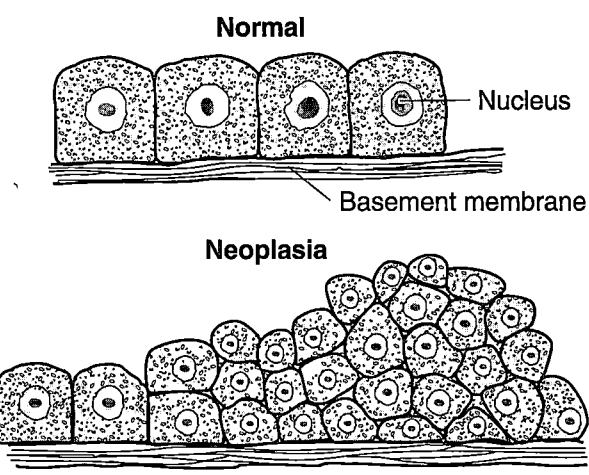

FIGURE 6–6 Normal tissue versus neoplasia.

stomach cells) results in Barrett's esophagus. This lesion is a response to acid reflux and has a high incidence of progression to cancer of the esophagus (Figure 6–5).

Q What is neoplasia?

A Neoplasia is the development of a new type of cell with an uncontrolled growth pattern (Figure 6–6). Neoplasia is a generic term for the growth of a new type of cell. These cells may be either benign or malignant.

Mechanisms and Effects of Cell Injury

Q What can cellular injury result from?

A Cellular injury may result from various different causes such as hypoxia (the most common cause), chemical injury, infectious injury, immunological injury, and inflammatory injury. Hypoxia is discussed in detail in Chapter 35, Hemorrhage and Shock.

Q What are the effects of chemical injury on the cell?

A Chemicals injure and ultimately destroy cells. Examples of chemical agents that cause cellular injury include poisons, lead, carbon monoxide, ethanol, and pharmacological agents. Chemical carcinogens, cancer-causing agents, can be found everywhere in our environment. The exposure of workers to various chemicals used in industry can lead to cancer. Examples include:

- Naphthylamine found in dyes can cause bladder cancer.
- Nickel ore miners have a high rate of nasal cancer.
- Asbestos (previously used in insulation) leads to lung cancer.
- Arsenic in insecticides leads to skin and lung cancer.
- Tobacco and cigarette smoke is the leading cause of lung cancer.

Q What are the effects of infectious injury on the cell?

A Infectious injury to the cells is caused by an invasion of either bacteria or viruses. The pathogenicity of these microorganisms is a function of their ability to reproduce within the human body. Bacteria may cause injury either by direct action on cells or by the production of toxins. Viruses often initiate an inflammatory response that leads to cell damage and patient symptoms.

Q What is virulence?

A Virulence measures the disease-causing ability of a microorganism. The disease-producing potential depends on the microorganism's ability to invade and destroy cells, produce toxins, and produce hypersensitivity reactions.

Q What factors affect the growth of bacteria within the body?

A The growth and survival of bacteria in the body depends on the effectiveness of the body's own defense mechanisms and the bacteria's ability to resist those mechanisms. The immune system helps to fight off foreign matter that the body perceives as harmful. A depressed immune system is present in many people:

newborn infants, elderly patients, diabetics, and people with cancer or other chronic diseases.

Many bacteria have a capsule that protects it from ingestion and destruction by phagocytes. Not all bacteria are encapsulated—*Mycobacterium tuberculosis* lacks a capsule, yet resists destruction. It may be transported by phagocytes throughout the body. Phagocytes are cells, such as white blood cells, that engulf and consume foreign material such as microorganisms and debris.

What substances produced by bacteria can injure cells?

Bacteria produce toxins. These are usually referred to as exotoxins or endotoxins. Bacteria such as *Staphylococci*, *Streptococci*, and tetanus secrete exotoxins into the medium surrounding the cell. Endotoxins are lipopolysaccharides that are part of the cell wall of gram-negative bacteria. When large amounts of endotoxins are present, the patient may experience septic shock.

When cells are injured, circulating white blood cells (WBCs) are attracted to the site. These WBCs release endogenous pyrogens that cause a fever to develop.

The body's most common reaction to the presence of bacteria is inflammation. Some bacteria have the ability to produce hypersensitivity reactions. The proliferation of microorganisms in the blood is called bacteremia or sepsis.

CLINICAL PEARL

Pyrogens act by affecting the hypothalamic thermo-regulatory center. Fever-reducing drugs, such as aspirin or acetaminophen, blunt the hypothalamic response to pyrogens.

What are the effects of a virus on the cell?

Viral diseases are the most common seen in humans. When a virus becomes an intracellular parasite, it takes over control of the metabolic processes of the host cell and uses the cell to help it replicate.

The protein coat that encapsulates most viruses protects them from phagocytosis. The replication of a virus occurs inside the host cell because viruses do not contain any of their own organelles. This causes a decreased synthesis of macromolecules that are vital to the host cell. As opposed to bacteria, viruses do not produce exotoxins or endotoxins.

There may be a symbiotic relation between a virus and normal cells that results in a persistent unapparent infection. Viruses have been known to evoke a strong immune response and can

rapidly produce an irreversible, lethal injury in highly susceptible cells as in the case in AIDS.

What is the difference between immunologic and inflammatory injury?

Inflammation is a protective response that can occur without bacterial invasion. Infection is the invasion of microorganisms causing cell or tissue injury that leads to the inflammatory response. The immune system provides protection for the body by providing defenses to attack and remove foreign organisms such as a bacteria or virus.

The cellular membranes are injured by direct contact with the cellular and chemical components of the immune or inflammatory process such as phagocytes, histamine, antibodies, and lymphokines. When cell membranes are altered, potassium leaks out of the cells and water flows inward.

CLINICAL PEARL

Inflammation is a common response to many different stimuli, including infection, immune responses, and trauma.

What are some examples of injurious genetic factors affecting the cell?

Examples of injurious genetic factors affecting the cell include chromosomal disorders (e.g., Down syndrome), premature development of atherosclerosis, and obesity (some cases). There are two ways an individual may develop an abnormal gene: (1) by mutation of the gene during meiosis, which affects the newly formed fetus, or (2) by heredity. In trisomy 21 (Down syndrome), the child is born with an extra chromosome, usually number 21.

What are examples of injurious nutritional imbalances?

Good nutrition is required to maintain good health and assist the cells in fighting off disease. Examples of nutritional disorders that can injure the cell as well as the organism include obesity, malnutrition, vitamin excess or deficiency, and mineral excess or deficiency. Any of these can lead to alterations in physical growth, mental and intellectual retardation, and even death in some circumstances.

What are some of the manifestations of cellular injury?

Manifestations of cellular injury occur at the microscopic and functional levels. Common microscopic abnormalities include:

- Cell swelling.
- Rupture of cell membranes.
- Rupture of nuclear membranes.
- Breakdown of nuclear material (chromosomes).

This damage often results in a change in cell shape and its function. Functional changes may include:

- Inability to use oxygen adequately.
- Development of intracellular acidosis.
- Accumulation of toxic waste products.
- Inability to metabolize nutrients.

Damage to and functional changes in individual cells often impact the entire organism.

The Cellular Environment

Q What is meant by the term "cellular environment"?

A The cellular environment includes:

- The distribution of cells throughout the body.
- Changes in cell distribution with aging.
- Changes in cell distribution with disease.
- The movement of water, sodium, and chloride in and out of cells.
- Acid–base balance in the cells and surrounding tissues.

Q What is the normal distribution of body fluids?

A The body consists primarily of water. About 50–70 percent of the total body weight is fluid. The average male is 60 percent and the average female is 50 percent fluid. Most (63 percent) of the body's fluid is in the cells and is called intracellular fluid (ICF). The remainder (37 percent) lies outside the cells and is called extracellular fluid (ECF). ECF is further broken down into the fluid that is between the cells (interstitual fluid), fluid inside the blood vessels (intravascular fluid), lymph, and transcellular fluid.

Q What is included in the category of transcellular fluid?

A Transcellular fluid includes the following components:

- Cerebrospinal fluid.
- Aqueous and vitreous humors in the eyes.
- Synovial fluid in joints.
- Serous fluid in body cavities (e.g., pleural fluid).
- Glandular secretions.

Fluid and Water Balance

Q How does the body balance water input and output?

A The average adult takes in about 2,500 ml of water a day. The stimulus to take in water arises in the hypothalamic thirst center. Most is by drinking (approximately 1,500 ml or 60 percent); another 30 percent comes from the water in foods, such as fruits; and the remaining 10 percent is a byproduct of cellular metabolism.

Most water is lost in the form of urine (approximately 1,500 ml or 60 percent), 28 percent is lost through the skin and lungs, 6 percent is lost in the feces, and 6 percent is lost through sweat. The amount of water loss through sweating is highly variable—in hot environmental conditions or during periods of rigorous exercise, it is possible to lose large amounts of fluid. These patients can become severely dehydrated if not properly hydrated before, during, and after the physical activity. Sodium ($Na+$), the major extracellular cation, is often lost along with water. This loss may affect nerve and muscle function, as well as ECF volume (see Chapter 29, Environmental Conditions).

Q What are the mechanisms by which water and dissolved particles move across cell membranes?

A The two general methods of water and dissolved particle movement are passive and active transport. *Passive transport* includes:

- Diffusion—the movement of a substance from an area of higher concentration to an area of lower concentration.
- Facilitated diffusion—a helper molecule within the membrane helps the movement of a substance from areas of higher concentration to areas of lower concentration.
- Osmosis—the movement of water in the body from areas of more water (and less solute) to areas of less water (and more solute).
- Filtration—the movement of water and a dissolved substance from an area of high pressure to an area of low pressure.

Active transport includes movement via "pumps" that require energy and move substances from an area of low concentration to an area of high concentration.

Q What specific terms relate to the ingestion of various substances by cells?

A There are several cell-specific ingestion processes:

- Endocytosis—when a cell membrane ingests substances.
- Phagocytosis—the engulfing of solid particles by a cell membrane.

- Pinocytosis—the engulfing of liquid droplets.
- Exocytosis—the secretion of cellular products from the cell.

[Q] How does water move between intracellular and extracellular fluids?

[A] Water moves between ICF and ECF by osmosis. This is also referred to as osmotic pressure. Osmotic pressure is the pressure that develops when two solutions of different concentrations are separated by a semipermeable membrane. When you compare two solutions, a solution with a higher solute concentration has a higher osmotic pressure and is referred to as *hypertonic*. The solution with a lower solute concentration has a lower osmotic pressure and is referred to as *hypotonic*. Solutions with equal solute concentrations are called *isotonic*. (See Figure 6–7.)

[Q] Does the distribution of body fluids change as we mature?

[A] The distribution of body fluids changes with age and varies with gender. The total body water, as a percentage of body weight, is summarized in Table 6–1:

TABLE 6–1

Percentage of Body Fluids		
AGE	MALE	FEMALE
10–18	59%	57%
18–40	61%	51%
40–60	56%	47%
OVER 60	52%	46%

[Q] How does plasma and interstitual fluid move?

[A] Water moves between plasma and interstitial fluid. Plasma makes up about 55 percent of the blood and is comprised of 91 percent water and 9 percent plasma proteins. The plasma proteins include:

- Albumin (maintains the osmotic pressure).
- Globulin.
- Fibrinogen and prothrombin (assists with clotting).

Starling's forces govern the movement of water between the vascular compartment and the interstitual space. Under normal conditions, the amount of fluid filtering outward through the arterial ends of the capillaries equals the amount of fluid that is returned to the circulation by reabsorption at the venous ends of the capillaries. This equilibrium state between the capillary and interstitial space is controlled by four forces: capillary hydrostatic pressure, capillary colloidal osmotic pressure, tissue hydrostatic pressure, and tissue colloidal osmotic pressure.

The role of these four forces is as follows:

1. Capillary hydrostatic pressure. This is the pressure pushing water out of the capillary into the interstitial space. Because the pressure is higher on the arterial end than the venous end, more water is pushed out of the capillaries on the arterial end and more is reabsorbed on the venous end.

2. Capillary colloidal osmotic pressure. This is osmotic pressure generated by dissolved proteins in the plasma that are too large to penetrate the capillary membrane.

3. Tissue hydrostatic pressure. This is the pressure that opposes the pushing of fluids from the capillary into the interstitial space.

4. Tissue colloidal osmotic pressure. This pressure pulls fluid into the interstitial space. Thus, capillary and membrane

Hypertonic solution

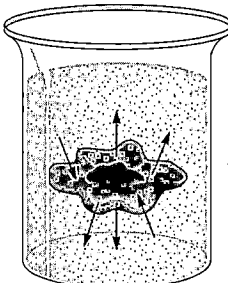

Hypotonic solution

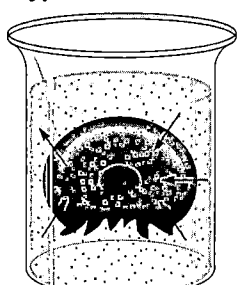

Water molecules

Isotonic solution

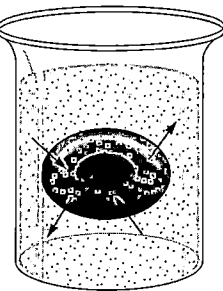

Hypertonic solution (seawater) a red blood cell will shrink and wrinkle up because water molecules are moving out of the cell.

Hypotonic solution (freshwater) a red blood cell will swell and burst because water molecules are moving into the cell.

Isotonic solution (human blood serum) a red blood cell remains unchanged, because the movement of water molecules into and out of the cell are the same.

FIGURE 6–7 Movement of water molecules in solutions of different osmotic pressure.

permeability plays an important role in the movement of fluid and the creation of edema in the surrounding tissues.

Abnormal Fluid Accumulations

What is the pathophysiology and clinical manifestation of edema?

Edema is the accumulation of excess fluid in the interstitial space. Peripheral edema (e.g., ankles and feet as shown in Figure 6–8) develops as a result of liver or heart failure. If the patient is bedridden, it may accumulate in the sacral area (sacral edema).

The healthy liver produces the protein albumin, which is responsible for the osmotic pressure of the blood. This pressure directly affects the movement of fluid, mostly water in the plasma, from the blood through the capillaries to the tissues and back into the blood. In the absence of osmotic pressure, the blood fluid leaks into the tissues and stays there. Decreased plasma albumin levels reduce osmotic pressure, causing edema in the feet and ankles.

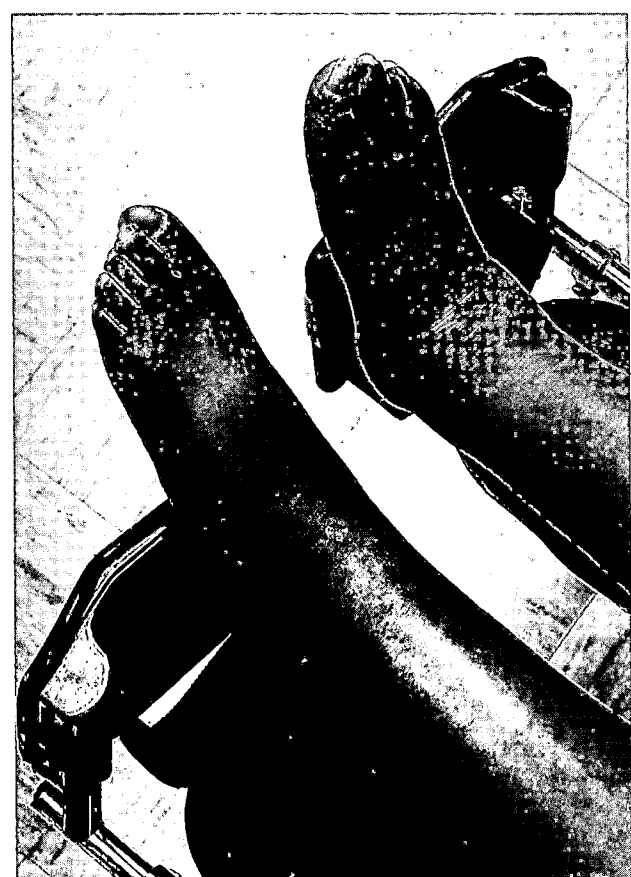

FIGURE 6–8 Edema.

Causes of edema include:

- Increased capillary pressure—arteriolar dilatation (e.g., allergic reaction and inflammation), venous obstruction (e.g., hepatic obstruction, heart failure, or thrombophlebitis), increased vascular volume (e.g., heart failure), increased levels of adrenocortical hormones, premenstrual sodium retention, pregnancy, environmental heat stress, and the effects of gravity from prolonged standing.
- Decreased colloidal osmotic pressure—decreased production of plasma proteins (e.g., liver disease, starvation, or severe protein deficiency), increased loss of plasma proteins (e.g., protein-losing kidney diseases, and extensive burns).
- Lymphatic vessel obstruction due to infection, disease of the lymphatic structures or their removal (e.g., mastectomy and removal of lymph nodes may lead to buildup of edema in the extremity).

The clinical manifestations of edema may be local at an injury site or generalized. It is also possible for a patient with left heart failure to have pulmonary edema for cardiac reasons, or edema may present following a near drowning, or a narcotic overdose. When there is excess fluid in the lungs (e.g., acute pulmonary edema [APE]), this fluid impairs the diffusion of oxygen into pulmonary capillaries making the patient hypoxic. Patients can literally drown in their own fluids if proper medications are not administered. (See Chapter 23, Cardiology, for more on APE)

What is ascites?

Ascites is fluid that accumulates in the peritoneal cavity. Patients who are bedridden tend to develop fluid in the sacral area of the back.

What is meant by pitting edema?

When edematous tissue, such as in the ankles, is compressed with a finger, the fluid is pushed aside causing a temporary impression or a "pit." This pit gradually refills but is referred to as *pitting edema*. Pitting edema can be significant in the patient with chronic heart failure.

What is the function of the sodium–potassium pump?

The ICF volume is controlled by the large amount of proteins and organic compounds that cannot escape through the cell membrane and by the sodium–potassium ion (Na+/K+) membrane pump. Most of the intracellular substances are negatively charged and attract many positively charged ions including potassium. Because all of these substances are osmotically active, they can pull water into the cell until it ruptures. The pump is responsible for keeping this situation in check by continuously removing three Na+ ions from the cell for every two K+ ions that are moved back into the cell. If the pump is impaired due to insufficient potassium in the body, sodium accumulates and causes the cells to swell.

CLINICAL PEARL

Some drugs, such as digitalis preparations, affect the sodium–potassium exchange pump. If toxic levels are reached in the blood, electrolyte imbalance leads to cardiac dysfunction and dysrhythmias.

Fluid and Electrolyte Balance

Q | What is tonicity?

A | Changes in water content can cause a cell to shrink or swell. *Tonicity* refers to the tension exerted on cell size due to water movement across the cell membrane. Solutions that body cells are exposed to are classified as isotonic, hypotonic, or hypertonic. Cells that are placed in an isotonic solution, which has the same osmolarity as ICF (280 mOsm/L), neither shrink nor swell. When cells are placed in a hypertonic solution (has a greater osmolarity than ICF), they shrink as the water is pulled out of the cell. When cells are placed in a hypotonic solution (has a lower osmolarity than ICF), they swell.

Q | What is the effect of administering sterile water to a patient intravenously?

A | Because sterile water is a hypotonic solution, the water enters the red blood cells causing them to swell and ultimately burst.

Q | Why is a hypertonic solution, such as mannitol, used to decrease cerebral swelling?

A | A hypertonic solution contains more solute than the interstitial or tissue fluid in the brain. This causes excess fluid to be drawn into the blood, decreasing the swelling within the brain.

Q | What is the significance of sodium balance in the body?

A | Sodium is the most common cation in the body. The average adult has 60 mEq of sodium for each kilogram of body weight (2.2 lbs = 1 kg). Most of the body's sodium is found in the ECF. A small amount is found in the ICF. When sodium enters the

cell, it is transported out of the cell by the sodium–potassium pump because a resting cell membrane is relatively impermeable to sodium. Sodium also plays an important role in the regulation of the body's acid–base balance (sodium bicarbonate).

Sodium is taken in with foods. As little as 500 mg/day meets the body's needs. In the United States, studies have shown that the average adult ingests between 6 and 15 grams of sodium per day. Sodium regulation occurs in the kidneys. When there is an excess, sodium is excreted into the urine. When the body levels are low, the kidneys reabsorb sodium.

Normally, only about 10 percent of the sodium is lost through the skin and GI tract. However, the loss due to diarrhea, vomiting, extensive burns, or fistula drainage can be considerable. Sweat loss increases greatly with vigorous exercise and exposure to a hot environment. A person sweating profusely can lose 30 grams of sodium a day. This is why some exercise physiologists recommend that athletes use sports drinks that replace electrolytes, such as sodium, when engaged in lengthy training.

Q | What is the significance of chloride balance in the body?

A | Chloride is an important anion (Cl–) that, when combined with sodium, makes table salt (NaCl). It assists in regulating the acid–base balance, especially the pH of the stomach, and is involved in the osmotic pressure of the ECFs. Table salt, milk, eggs, and meats all contain CL–.

Q | What is the role of the renin–angiotensin–aldosterone mechanism?

A | This complex feedback mechanism is responsible for the kidney's regulation of sodium in the body. Renin is a protein enzyme that is released by the kidney into the bloodstream in response to changes in blood pressure, blood flow, the amount of sodium in the tubular fluid, and the glomerular filtration rate.

When renin is released, it converts the plasma protein angiotensinogen to angiotensin I. In the lung, angiotensin I is converted rapidly to angiotensin II by the angiotensin converting enzyme. Angiotensin II is responsible for stimulating sodium reabsorption by the renal tubules. It also constricts the renal blood vessels, slowing kidney blood flow and decreasing the glomerular filtration rate. As a result, less sodium is filtered and more is reabsorbed.

Angiotensin II is also responsible for stimulating the secretion of the adrenal hormone, aldosterone. Aldosterone acts on the kidney to increase the reabsorption of sodium into the blood and the elimination of potassium in the urine. Besides angiotensin II, three other factors stimulate aldosterone release:

- Increased extracellular potassium levels.
- Decreased extracellular sodium levels.
- Release of adrenocorticotropic hormone (ACTH) from the pituitary gland.

The interaction of renin, angiotensin, and aldosterone regulates sodium and fluid levels in the body.

CLINICAL PEARL

Recently, angiotensin III was shown to result from the conversion of angiotensin II in the plasma. Though the mechanism of action is uncertain, angiotensin III also vasoconstricts and stimulates the release of aldosterone.

What are the implications of isotonic fluid volume deficits?

An isotonic fluid volume deficit is a decrease in ECF with proportionate losses of sodium and water.

What are the implications of isotonic fluid volume excesses?

An isotonic fluid excess represents a proportionate increase in both sodium and water in the ECF compartment. Common causes include kidney, heart, or liver failure.

What are the causes and manifestations of hypernatremia?

Hypernatremia is defined as a serum sodium level that is above 148 mEq/L and a serum osmolality greater than 295 mOsm/kg. It is caused by excess body water loss without a proportionate sodium loss. Hypernatremia manifestations include:

- Increased thirst.
- Oliguria or anuria (reduced or no excretion of urine).
- Skin that is dry and flushed.
- A tongue that is rough and fissured.
- Decreased tears and salivation.
- Agitation and restlessness.
- Headache.
- Decreased reflexes.
- Manic behavior.
- Seizures and coma.
- Tachycardia (weak and thready pulse).
- Hypotension.

What are the causes and manifestations of hyponatremia?

Hyponatremia is defined as a serum sodium level that is below 135 mEq/L and a serum osmolarity that is less than 280 mOsm/kg. It is caused by excessive sodium loss with less water loss. Causes may include excess sweating from hot environments or exercise, GI losses through vomiting, diarrhea, or diuresis. Hyponatremia manifestations include:

- Headache.
- Depression.
- Personality changes.
- Confusion.
- Apprehension and a feeling of impending doom.
- Lethargy and weakness.
- Stupor or coma.
- Anorexia, nausea, or vomiting.
- Abdominal cramps.
- Diarrhea.
- Pitting edema.

CLINICAL PEARL

Normal values vary from laboratory to laboratory. The previously discussed values are approximations. The normal range for lab tests is usually printed on the report form.

How do alterations in potassium affect the body?

Potassium is the major intracellular cation and is critical to many functions of the cell. Potassium is necessary for neuromuscular control, regulation of the three types of muscles (skeletal, smooth, and cardiac), acid–base balance, intracellular enzyme reactions, and maintenance of intracellular osmolality. Potassium (K+) levels may be normal, low (hypokalemia), or elevated (hyperkalemia).

Hypokalemia is defined as a decreased serum potassium level. The causes of hypokalemia include:

- Diet deficient in potassium.
- Inability to eat.
- Over administration of potassium-free parenteral solutions.
- Diuretic therapy (except potassium sparing diuretics).
- Increased mineralocorticoid levels (e.g., Cushing's disease).
- Diuretic phase of renal failure.
- Excessive vomiting or diarrhea.
- GI suctioning or draining of GI fistula.

- Excessive sweating.
- Treatment of diabetic ketoacidosis.
- Alkalosis (either metabolic or respiratory).

  The manifestations of hypokalemia include:

- Increased thirst.
- Polyuria, nocturia, urine of low osmolality and specific gravity.
- Anorexia, nausea, and vomiting.
- Abdominal distension.
- Paralytic ileus.
- Postural hypotension.
- Cardiac dysrhythmias.
- Increased sensitivity to digitalis toxicity.
- Muscle tenderness, cramps, weakness, or flaccidity (lack of normal tension).
- Paralysis or paresthesia.
- Confusion.
- Depression.
- Metabolic alkalosis.
- ECG changes may include a low T wave and a sagging S-T segment.

  Hyperkalemia is defined as an elevated serum potassium level. The causes of hyperkalemia include:

- Excess oral intake of potassium.
- Excess or rapid infusion of parenteral fluids containing potassium.
- Tissue crushing syndrome or major burns resulting in the release of intracellular potassium.
- Renal failure.
- Adrenal insufficiency (e.g., Addison's disease).
- Treatment with potassium sparing diuretics.
- Treatment with angiotensin converting enzyme inhibitors.

  The manifestations of hyperkalemia include:

- Paresthesia.
- Weakness and dizziness.
- Muscle cramps.
- Nausea and vomiting.
- Diarrhea.
- Intestinal colic.
- GI distress.
- ECG changes include: peaked T waves, depressed S-T segments, depressed P wave, and widening QRS complex.
- Cardiac arrest.

How do alterations in calcium affect the body?

The vast majority (99 percent) of the body's calcium is found in the bone. The purpose of calcium is to provide strength and stability for the collagen and ground substance that forms the matrix of the skeletal system. Calcium enters the body through the GI tract and is absorbed from the intestine by vitamin D. It is then stored in the bone and ultimately excreted by the kidney. Calcium (Ca) levels may be normal, low (hypocalcemia), or elevated (hypercalcemia).

Hypocalcemia is defined as a decreased serum calcium level. The causes include:

- Hypoparathyroidism.
- Resistance to the actions of parathyroid hormone.
- Hypomagnesemia.
- Vitamin D deficiency.
- Impaired ability to activate vitamin D, including liver and kidney disease.
- Medications that impair activation of vitamin D.
- Renal failure and hyperphosphatemia.
- Increased pH.
- Increased fatty acids.
- Rapid transfusion of citrated blood.
- Acute pancreatitis.

  The manifestations of hypocalcemia include:

- Decreased ionized calcium.
- Paresthesia.
- Skeletal muscle cramps.
- Abdominal spasms and cramps.
- Hyperactive reflexes.
- Carpopedal spasm.
- Tetany.
- Laryngeal spasm.
- Hypotension.
- Cardiac insufficiency.
- Failure to respond to drugs that act by calcium mediated mechanisms.
- Osteomalacia.
- Bone pain, deformities, and fractures.

  Hypercalcemia is defined as an increased serum calcium level. The causes include:

- Excess vitamin D.
- Excess calcium in the diet.
- Milk alkali syndrome (the ingestion of excess milk or calcium-containing antacids).

- Increased levels of parathyroid hormone.
- Malignant neoplasms.
- Prolonged immobilization.
- Thiazide diuretics.
- Lithium therapy.

    The manifestations of hypercalcemia include:

- Increased thirst.
- Polyuria.
- Flank pain.
- Signs of acute reversible renal insufficiency.
- Signs of kidney stones.
- Anorexia.
- Nausea and vomiting.
- Constipation.
- Muscle weakness and atrophy.
- Ataxia, loss of muscle tone.
- Lethargy.
- Personality and behavioral changes.
- Stupor and coma.
- Hypertension.
- Shortening of the Q-T interval.
- Atrioventricular block on ECG.

How do alterations in phosphate affect the body?

Phosphate is primarily an intracellular anion and is essential to many body functions. Phosphate levels may be normal, low (hypophosphatemia), or elevated (hyperphosphatemia). Hypophosphatemia is characterized by a decrease in phosphate levels. The causes include:

- Antacids.
- Severe diarrhea.
- Lack of vitamin D.
- Alkalosis.
- Hyperparathyroidism.
- Diabetic ketoacidosis.
- Renal tubular absorption defects.
- Alcoholism.
- Total parenteral hyperalimentation.
- Recovery from malnutrition.
- Administration of insulin and recovery from diabetic keto-acidosis.

    The manifestations of hypophosphatemia include:

- Intention tremor.

- Ataxia.
- Paresthesia.
- Hyporeflexia.
- Confusion.
- Stupor and coma.
- Seizures.
- Muscle weakness.
- Joint stiffness.
- Bone pain.
- Osteomalacia.
- Anorexia.
- Dysphagia.
- Hemolytic anemia.
- Platelet dysfunction with bleeding disorders.
- Impaired WBC function.

    Hyperphosphatemia is defined as an increased serum phosphate level. The causes include:

- Phosphate-containing laxatives.
- Phosphate-containing enemas.
- Intravenous administration.
- Massive trauma.
- Heat stroke.
- Seizures.
- Tumor lysis syndrome (from the death of tumor cells releasing their intracellular contents into the serum following chemotherapy).
- Potassium deficiency.
- Kidney failure.
- Hypoparathyroidism.

    The manifestations of hyperphosphatemia include:

- Paresthesias.
- Tetany.
- Hypotension.
- Cardiac dysrhythmias.

How do alterations in magnesium affect the body?

Magnesium is the second most abundant intracellular cation. About 50 percent of the body's magnesium is stored in the bones, 49 percent is contained in the body cells, and the remaining 1 percent is in the ECF. Serum levels may be normal, low (hypomagnesium), or high (hypermagnesemia).

    Causes of hypomagnesium include:

- Alcoholism.
- Malnutrition or starvation.

- Malabsorption.
- Small bowel bypass surgery.
- Parenteral hyperalimentation with inadequate amounts of magnesium.
- High dietary intake of calcium without concomitant amounts of magnesium.

The manifestations of hypomagnesemia include:

- Personality change.
- Athetoid (slow, snake-like twisting movements of the extremities) or choreiform (nervous twitching of the face) movements.
- Nystagmus (involuntary rapid eye movements).
- Tetany.
- Positive Babinski's (loss or diminished achilles tendon reflex).
- Positive Chvostek's (a spasm of the facial muscles following a tap on one side of the face over the facial nerve).
- Trousseaus's sign (a muscular spasm resulting from pressure applied to nerves and vessels of the upper arm).
- Tachycardia.
- Hypertension.
- Cardiac dysrhythmias.

Causes of hypermagnesium include:

- Renal failure.
- Excessive intake of magnesium-containing antacids.
- Adrenal insufficiency.

The manifestations of hypermagnesemia include:

- Fatigue, weakness, lethargy.
- Anorexia.
- Nausea.
- Constipation.
- Impaired renal function.
- Kidney stones.
- Dysrhythmias, bradycardia, cardiac arrest.
- Bone pain, osteoporosis.

Acid–Base Balance

Q | What is the significance of acid–base balance in the body?

A | The normal body functions depend on an acid–base balance that is regulated within a normal physiologic pH range from 7.35 to 7.45.

Q | What is pH?

A | pH is a measurement of the hydrogen ion concentration. A blood pH greater than 7.45 is called alkalosis and a blood pH of less than 7.35 is called acidosis. The mathematical formula for calculating pH is: $pH = -\log [H+]$. Log refers to the base 10 logarithm and $[H+]$ refers to the hydrogen ion concentration. Changes in the pH are exponential, not linear. Thus, a change in the pH from 7.40 to 7.20 results in a 10^2 or 100-fold change in the acid concentration. The Henderson–Hasselbach equation is used to discuss the relation between the pH. It is as follows: $pH = 6.1 + \log HCO_3 - /.03(PaCo_2)$.

Q | What is metabolic acidosis and when does it occur?

A | Metabolic acidosis is an accumulation of abnormal acids in the blood for any of several reasons (e.g., sepsis, diabetic ketoacidosis, and salicylate poisoning). Initially, the pCO_2 is not affected, but the pH is decreased. Later, the body compensates for the metabolic abnormality by hyperventilating, leading to excretion of CO_2 and a compensatory respiratory alkalosis. This is why patients with diabetic ketoacidosis often have Kussmaul respirations (deep, rapid sighing ventilations). They are hyperventilating to "blow off" CO_2 and decrease the acidosis.

Q | What is metabolic alkalosis and when does it occur?

A | Metabolic alkalosis is a less common condition in acute care, yet very common in chronically ill patients, especially those undergoing nasogastric suction. There is either a buildup of excess metabolic base (e.g., chronic antacid ingestion) or a loss of normal acid (e.g., through vomiting or nasogastric suctioning). The pH is high and the pCO_2 unchanged initially. Chronically, the body compensates by slowing ventilation and increasing the pCO_2, creating a compensatory respiratory acidosis.

Q | What is respiratory acidosis and when does it occur?

A | Respiratory acidosis occurs when CO_2 retention leads to increased levels of pCO_2. It also occurs in situations of hypoventilation (e.g., heroin overdose) or intrinsic lung diseases (e.g., asthma or COPD).

Q | What is respiratory alkalosis and when does it occur?

A | Excessive "blowing off" of CO_2 with a resulting decrease in the pCO_2 causes respiratory alkalosis. Though often called hyperventilation, many potentially serious diseases may be responsible (e.g., pulmonary embolism, AMI, severe infection, diabetic ketoacidosis) for increased ventilatory levels.

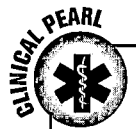

Always assume that any hyperventilating patient has a potentially serious underlying medical condition.

Causes of Disease

What are the typical disease-causing factors?

Diseases are caused by genetics, environmental factors, age, and gender. Genetic factors are those with which the patient is born and are passed on through his genes to future generations. Environmental factors include microorganisms, immunologic and toxic exposures, personal habits and lifestyle, exposure to chemical substances, physical environment, and the psychosocial environment.

Age and gender factors involve a combination of genetic and environmental factors, lifestyle, and anatomic or hormonal differences. The risk of a particular disease often depends on the patient's age. For example, newborns are at greater risk of disease because their immune systems are not fully developed. Girls in their early teens have a high risk for a difficult pregnancy. Women over the age of 40 are considered to have high risk pregnancies. The older we become the greater the risk of cancer, heart disease, stroke, and Alzheimer's disease.

Some diseases are more prevalent in men such as lung cancer, gout, and Parkinson's disease. Women are more likely to get osteoporosis, rheumatoid arthritis, or breast cancer. There are uncontrollable factors (e.g., genetics) that influence a disease process, yet there are many that can be controlled.

Individuals have control over their lifestyles. Behaviors such as smoking, drinking alcohol, poor nutrition (e.g., excessive fat, salt, and sugar and not enough fruits, vegetables, and fiber), lack of exercise, and stress can be modified to improve one's quality of life.

What is involved in analyzing disease risk?

Analyzing disease risk involves reviewing the rates of incidence (frequency of occurence), prevalence (number of cases in a particular population over time), and mortality (the number of deaths in a given population), as well as causal and noncausal risk factors.

What is meant by a familial disease?

A familial disease is one that runs in the family.

What is meant by a genetic disease?

A genetic disease is one that is passed through generations on a gene.

This section introduces many of the diseases found in the field. Many of the disorders are discussed in more detail in other chapters of this book (e.g., allergies in Chapter 26 and asthma in Chapter 22).

What is an allergy?

Allergies are an acquired hypersensitivity. First, the person is exposed or sensitized to the antigen. Repeated exposures cause a reaction by the immune system to the allergen. Signs and symptoms include redness, heat, swelling and itching, runny nose, coughing, sneezing, wheezing, and nasal congestion. This is a familial disease.

What is rheumatic fever?

Rheumatic fever develops following a streptococcal infection (e.g., strep throat) and is characterized by myocarditis and arthritis. The first occurrence may be mild, but subsequent episodes can cause scarring and deformity of the heart valves. Each year more than 2.1 million cases are reported and 5,000 deaths occur from the disease. Patients seem to have a genetic predisposition to this disease.

What is cancer and how prevalent is it?

Cancer is very prevalent. One in two men and one in three women will be diagnosed with cancer during their lifetime. Cancer includes a large number of malignant neoplasms. The prognosis often depends on the extent of its spread when found, metastases, and the effectiveness of treatment. The recognition of warning signs is key to finding cancer early. The American Cancer Society uses the acronym "CAUTION" to list the signs:

- Change in bowel or bladder habits.
- A sore that does not heal.
- Unusual bleeding or discharge.
- Thickening or lump development.
- Indigestion or difficulty swallowing.
- Obvious change in a wart or mole.
- Nagging cough or hoarseness.

Lung cancer is the leading cause of cancer deaths and second leading cause of cancer cases in males and females combined, accounting for a combined 171,500 cases and 160,100 deaths each year. Breast cancer is the leading type of cancer in women, and accounts for as many as 178,700 cases a year and 43,500 deaths each year. Colorectal cancer is the third leading type of cancer in both males and females, accounting for a combined 131,600 cases yearly and 55,500 deaths each year.

What is a drug-induced anemia?

Drug-induced hemolytic anemia is a hemolytic anemia that is characterized by an increased destruction of red blood cells. It occurs from a number of causes such as a Rh factor blood tranfusion reaction, a disorder of the immune system, or exposure to chemicals, such as benzene, and bacterial toxins. Hemolytic anemia following aspirin overdose or penicillin is rare; it is much more common, though still rare, with sulfa drugs for urinary tract infection, such as Septra® or Bactrim®.

What is hemophilia?

Hemophilia is a gender-linked hereditary bleeding disorder most commonly passed on from an asymptomatic mother to a male child. Hemophiliacs lack certain blood clotting proteins. Their disease may range from mild to severe. There is no cure for this disease. Patients may experience severe and prolonged bleeding from even a minor injury.

What is hematochromatosis?

Hematochromatosis is an inherited disorder of abnormal iron retention by the liver. Nearly one in every 250–300 people are affected. Eventually, patients develop liver damage. Management includes the weekly removal of blood to stabilize the iron levels (phlebotomy).

What is the significance of long Q-T syndrome?

Long Q-T syndrome is one of several inherited cardiac conduction system abnormalities resulting in a prolongation of the Q-T interval. Sometimes, these syndromes are associated with congenital hearing loss, asymmetric septal hypertrophy of the heart, or mitral valve prolapse. Patients are at risk for palpitations and ventricular dysrhythmias, especially torsade de pointes.

PEARL

Hereditary prolongation of the Q-T interval may occur by itself or may be associated with other diseases. Often, the first indication is finding a prolonged Q-T interval in a sibling of a young patient who died from sudden cardiac death. Beta-blockers decrease the Q-T interval and may help surviving at-risk relatives.

What are cardiomyopathies?

Cardiomyopathies are incurable diseases of the heart that ultimately lead to congestive heart failure, AMI, or death. The diseases cause the heart muscle to become thin, flabby, dilated, or enlarged. There are a number of disease forms. Some are idiopathic, others are common in alcoholics, and still others, such as hypertrophic cardiomyopathy, are hereditary.

PEARL

One of the most common, yet severe, cardiomyopathies is viral myocarditis. Victims often develop severe heart failure, requiring cardiac transplant to survive.

What is a mitral valve prolapse?

Mitral valve prolapse is also referred to as a floppy mitral valve; it occurs in 2.5 percent of males and 7.6 percent of females in the population. The cause is unknown, but it has been associated with Marfan's syndrome, osteogenesis imperfecta, and other connective tissue disorders, and with cardiac, hematologic, neuroendocrine, metabolic, and psychologic disorders. The mitral valve leaflets balloon into the left atrium during systole when under high ventricular pressure. Typical symptoms experienced by the patient include prolonged chest pain, weakness, dyspnea, fatigue, anxiety, palpitations, and lightheadedness. Management focuses on symptom relief and prevention of complications.

What is coronary heart disease?

Coronary heart disease (CHD), also called coronary artery disease (CAD), is a disease caused by impaired circulation to the heart. Typically, patients have occluded coronary arteries from atherosclerotic plaque buildup. The effects can range from ischemia to infarction and necrosis (death) of the myocardium. By definition, infarction results in death to at least some of the myocardium. This can lead to the patient having any one of a number of medical problems including angina, AMI, dysrhythmias, conduction defects, heart failure, and sudden death. Almost half of all cardiovascular deaths result from CHD. Notice in Figure 6–9 how the mortality rate from CHD compares to other causes of death. In a typical year, according to the Agency for HealthCare Policy and Research, CHD causes 487,490 deaths and 13,670,000 patients experience angina or AMI or both. Although the cause of atherosclerosis has not been determined with certainty, studies have identified a number of risk factors that can predispose the patient to CHD.

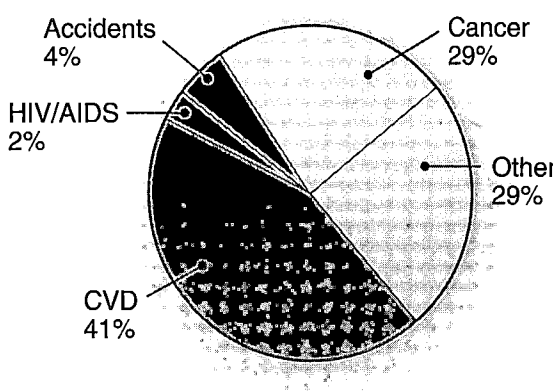

FIGURE 6–9 Cardiovascular disease (CVD) versus other disease mortality rates.

What are the risk factors for CHD?

The risk factors for CHD include the following:

- Hypercholesteremia. This is a major risk factor for atherosclerosis, but it is a factor that can be changed. Low-density lipoprotein (LDL) cholesterol (less than 35 mg/dL) is considered a positive factor and high-density lipoprotein (HDL) cholesterol (greater than 60 mg/dL) is considered a negative factor.

- Family history of premature CHD. The tendency to develop atherosclerosis has been shown to run in families. In addition, a significant risk factor for CHD development includes having a father who had an AMI or died suddenly before 55 years of age or a mother before 65 years of age.

- Cigarette smoking. This is a major risk factor closely linked with CHD development and sudden death. Fortunately, this is a risk factor that can be reversed by not smoking.

- Hypertension. High blood pressure (as defined by greater than 140/90 mm Hg or requiring antihypertensive medication) is another risk factor that can be controlled. It cannot, however, be cured.

- Age. This is an uncontrollable risk factor. The risk of CHD increases with males over 45 years of age and females over 55 years of age or who have experienced premature menopause without estrogen replacement therapy.

- Soft-risk factors. There are also a number of "soft" factors that have been shown to be associated with an increase in the risk of CHD, such as stress, obesity, and diabetes.

What is gout?

Gout is a disorder of protein metabolism that primarily affects males (approximately 95 percent). The onset is after 30 years of age and patients with chronic gout often have a uric acid accumulation in subcutaneous tissues. The disease leads to inflammation of the joints due to a metabolic problem in the breakdown of proteins. Uric acid crystals are deposited in joints, primarily the metatarsophalangeal joint of the big toe, causing symptoms of swelling, redness, heat, and pain in the joint. It is also not uncommon for these patients to develop kidney dysfunction and kidney stones. Treatment includes adjustments in the diet and anti-gout medication.

What are gallstones?

Gallstones, also referred to as cholelithiasis, are caused by the precipitation of substances contained in bile such as cholesterol and bilirubin. Three factors contribute to the formation of gallstones: (1) abnormalities in the composition of bile, (2) stasis of bile, and (3) inflammation of the gallbladder with many cholesterol gallstones. Gallstones may be asymptomatic. Stones cause symptoms when they obstruct the flow of bile. The small stones that are able to pass into the common duct produce indigestion and biliary colic. Biliary colic pain is sudden in onset and increases steadily to its maximum in approximately an hour. The pain is located in the upper-right quadrant or the epigastric area and may be referred to the back, above the waist, the right shoulder, or right scapula. The pain usually persists for two to eight hours followed by soreness in the upper-right quadrant. The larger stones can obstruct the flow of bile and cause the patient to turn jaundice (yellow colored).

What is obesity and why is it such a health problem?

Obesity is defined as an excess of adipose tissue. It is thought that the hormone leptin is responsible for informing the brain of the amount of adipose tissue in the body. The brain can then make adjustments in the energy intake or output. Leptin is found in the obesity gene and an increased linkage to this gene has been found in the massively obese. Other factors in the development of obesity include heredity; socioeconomic, cultural, environmental, psychologic influences; and activity levels. Two types of obesity have been described in the literature: upper-body obesity (central, abdominal, android, or male obesity) and lower-body obesity (peripheral, gluteal-femoral, gynoid, or female obesity). The obesity type is determined by dividing the waist by the hip circumference. A waist-hip ratio greater than 1.0 in men and 0.9 in women indicates upper-body obesity. The health risks associated with obesity include hypertension, hyperlipidemia, cardiovascular disease, glucose intolerance, insulin resistance, diabetes, gallbladder disease, infertility, and cancer of the endometrium, breast, prostate, and colon. Morbidly obese patients have respiratory function impairment and sleep apnea.

What is Huntington's disease?

Huntington disease is a rare hereditary disorder involving chronic progressive chorea (a nervous condition marked by spontaneous, rapid, purposeless, jerking movements), psychological changes, and dementia. Symptoms do not usually develop until patients are over 30 years of age and by then, they may have already passed the gene to their own offspring. The disease produces localized death of brain cells. There is no cure.

What is muscular dystrophy?

Muscular dystrophy (MD) is any of several genetic disorders that involve the progressive deterioration of skeletal muscles due to mixed muscle cell hypertrophy, atrophy, and necrosis. MD is a muscular disease and not thought to be a neurological disease. The most common forms of MD are Duchenne muscular dystrophy (DMD) and Becker's muscular dystrophy, which together affect one in every 3,000 live male births. Females are carriers of the disease. DMD is inherited as a recessive single gene defect on the X chromosome and transmitted from the mother to her offspring. Typically, the postural muscles of the hip and shoulder show effects around three years of age. The child usually is wheelchair bound by age 10. Death due to respiratory and cardiac muscle involvement usually occurs by young adulthood.

What is multiple sclerosis?

Multiple sclerosis (MS) is a demyelinating disease of the central nervous system. It is a major cause of neurological disability in young and middle-aged adults. The number of cases in the United States is approximately 300,000, involving twice as many women as it does men. Although MS is not directly inherited, there is a familial predisposition in some cases, suggesting a genetic influence on susceptibility. The manifestations of this disease include acute episodes of paresthesias, optic neuritis (e.g., visual cloudiness or pain on movement of the globe), diplopia, or gaze paralysis. Lhermitte's symptom (an electric-shock-like tingling down the back and onto the legs) is produced by flexion of the neck. Other symptoms may include abnormal gait, bladder and sexual dysfunction, vertigo, nystagmus, fatigue, speech disturbance, mood swings, depression, euphoria, inattentiveness, apathy, forgetfulness, and loss of memory.

What is Alzheimer's disease?

Alzheimer's disease is a disorder that affects approximately 4 million Americans. Cortical atrophy and a loss of neurons in the frontal and temporal lobes of the brain characterize Alzheimer's disease. Atrophy occurs and there is ventricular enlargement from the loss of brain tissue. Studies on the genetics of inherited early-onset Alzheimer's have been linked to mutations on

three genes. The manifestations of Alzheimer's disease follow three distinct stages:

- Stage 1—memory loss, lack of spontaneity, subtle personality changes, and disorientation to time and date.
- Stage 2—impaired cognition and abstract thinking, restlessness and agitation, wandering, inability to carry out activities of daily living, impaired judgment, inappropriate social behavior, lack of insight or abstract thinking, repetitive behavior, and a voracious appetite.
- Stage 3—indifference to food, inability to communicate, urinary and fecal incontinence, and seizures.

What is schizophrenia?

Schizophrenia is one of the most serious public health problems in the world, accounting for 25 percent of mental health admissions. The disease is one that affects the brain and has been linked to genetic factors. Common reasons for the schizophrenic to seek medical assistance include a worsening of their psychosis usually from stress or noncompliance with medications, suicidal behavior, violent behavior resulting from paranoid thinking, and extrapyramidal side effects of neuroleptic drugs.

CLINICAL PEARL

Only a portion of patients with symptoms related to mental disorders are aware of the problem. Remember that part of the disease process may involve a decreased awareness of reality.

What is a manic-depressive disorder?

Manic-depressive disorder, currently referred to as bipolar disorder, is characterized by episodes of mania (over-activity) usually interspersed with hypoactive periods and depression. Depressive episodes are more frequent than manic episodes. Manics feel "on top of the world," elated, energetic, and precarious, but quickly become argumentative and hostile when their plans are thwarted. The disorder is equally common in males and females. The course of this disorder is episodic with the duration and frequency varying greatly.

Pathophysiological Concerns at the Cellular Level

What is shock?

Shock is a clinical syndrome involving widespread cellular dysfunction due to the inadequate delivery of oxygen at the cellular level.

What are the five typical "types" of shock?

Shock has traditionally been broken down into five types: cardiogenic, hypovolemic, neurogenic, anaphylactic, and septic.

Is there a better way to classify shock?

Yes, the Weil-Shubin classification of shock utilizes a mechanistic view and breaks shock into the following four types:

- Two are central (cardiogenic and obstructive).
- Two are peripheral (hypovolemic and distributive).

What are examples of the causes of the four Weil-Shubin classifications of shock?

The causes of cardiogenic shock include:

- AMI.
- Ventricular septal defect.
- Hemodynamically significant dysrhythmias.
- Heart failure.

The causes of obstructive shock include:

- Vena cava syndrome or supine hypotension.
- Pericardial tamponade.
- A ball valve thrombus in the cardiac chambers.
- A pulmonary embolism in the pulmonary circulation.
- A dissecting aortic aneurysm.

The causes of hypovolemic shock include:

- Hemorrhage, either internal (e.g., ruptured spleen) or external.
- Plasma loss from burns or inflammation.
- Electrolyte loss from dehydration or diarrhea.
- Inflammation.
- Trauma.
- Anaphylaxis.
- Envenomation.

There are two subtypes of distributive shock:

- Low resistance—normal or high cardiac output, vasodilatation, and arteriovenous shunting. Causes include cervical spine transection, inflammation, peritonitis, and gram-negative shock in its early phase.
- High or normal resistance—cardiac output either normal or low, increased venous capacitance. Causes include barbiturate intoxication, ganglionic blockade, and gram-negative shock in its late phase.

What is multiple organ dysfunction syndrome (MODS)?

MODS is a new diagnosis (since 1975) that involves the progressive failure of two or more organ systems after severe illness or injury. The mortality rate is between 60 and 90 percent. MODS accounts for the major cause of death following septic, traumatic, and burn injuries. MODS can be classified as primary or secondary.

What is the difference between primary and secondary MODS?

Primary MODS is a direct result of an insult, such as a pulmonary contusion from striking the chest on the steering wheel during a collision. Secondary MODS develops as a part of a host response and is involved in the systemic inflammatory response syndrome (e.g., renal failure following the trauma).

What is the pathophysiology of MODS?

The pathophysiology of MODS includes the following events:

- An injury occurs or an endotoxin is released.
- Vascular endothelial damage, neuroendocrine response, and release of inflammatory mediators.
- Activation of the complement system. This is a defense system that produces numerous chemical mediators with differing roles. Various clinical disorders (e.g., capillary leak syndrome, septic shock, and multiple organ failure) are driven by an overactive complement system. The system activates phagocytes and can induce further inflammation and damage to the cells.
- Activation of the coagulation system. Due to endothelial damage, coagulation becomes uncontrolled. This results in microvascular thrombus formation and tissue ischemia.
- Activation of the kallikrein–kinin system, which releases bradykinin, a potent vasodilator. This contributes to low systemic resistance.
- Massive systemic immune, inflammatory, and coagulation responses. The combined effect of the three systems (complement, coagulation, and kallikrein–kinin) is a hyperinflammatory and hypercoagulable state that leads to edema formation, cardiovascular instability and hypotension, and clotting abnormalities.
- Vascular changes, including vasodilation, increase in capillary permeability, selective vasoconstriction, and microvascular thrombi.
- Maldistribution of systemic and organ blood flow. This results in a hyperdynamic circulation with increased venous return. There is a decrease in oxygen delivery to the tissues because of the shunting of blood past selected regional capillary beds

and the formation of interstitial edema due to permeability changes. Capillary obstruction occurs from microvascular thrombi and aggregation of inflammatory cells. The resultant ischemia contributes to the MODS.

- Hypermetabolism or a catabolic state is caused by the same hormonal responses that help conserve volume during shock by altering carbohydrate, fat, and lipid metabolism to meet the increased demand for energy. Over time, the combination of sympathetic drive and hyperdynamic circulation places excessive demands on the heart. The net result is the depletion of oxygen and fuel supplies.

- Tissue hypoperfusion causes tissue hypoxia. As the patient decompensates, decreased perfusion of the brain and coronary arteries causes cells to switch over to anaerobic metabolism. Lactic acid is produced, further impairing cellular function.

- The energy supply for the cells fails due to a decreased synthesis of adenosine triphosphate (ATP) and glucose. Energy failure leads to increased intracellular sodium and water and intracellular swelling. Increased intracellular calcium leads to lysosome rupture, releasing enzymes that further increase cellular permeability. Other enzymes such as histamine, serotonin, kinins, and prostaglandins are produced and all increase vascular permeability. This in turn increases the fluid loss back to the interstitium.

- Organ dysfunction due to decreased cardiac function and myocardial depression, renal failure, a failure of the smooth muscle of the vascular system, and the release of the capillary sphincters and vasodilation.

What is the clinical presentation of MODS?

The clinical presentation of MODS at about 24 hours post-resuscitation includes a low-grade fever due to the inflammatory response, tachycardia, dyspnea and adult respiratory distress syndrome (ARDS), altered mental status, hyperdynamic state, and a hypermetabolic state.

During a 14- to 21-day window, the patient exhibits renal and liver failure, and GI and immune system collapse. Finally, during the 21- and 28-day window, the patient sustains a cardiovascular collapse and death.

What is cellular metabolism impairment?

Cellular metabolism impairment involves the inability of the organism to properly use oxygen and glucose at the cellular level. Oxygen impairment may result from anerobic metabolism, which causes increased lactates and metabolic acidosis; decreased oxygen affinity for hemoglobin; decreased ATP; changes in the cellular electrolytes; cellular edema, making it difficult for oxy-

gen to make it from the blood to the cells; and release of lysosomal enzymes. Glucose impairment involves increased blood sugar, catacholamines, cortisol, growth hormone release, increased gluconeogenesis, increased glucoenolysis, and increased lipolysis.

The Immune System

What are the self-defense mechanisms of the body?

The human body has a complex system in place, called the immune system, that acts to fight off foreign substances and disease-causing agents. In addition, there are anatomic barriers and the normal inflammatory response.

What are the characteristics of an immune system response?

The immune system includes all of the structures and processes to mount a defense against a foreign agent. The immune system response can be broken down as follows:

- Specific or nonspecific immunity—nonspecific immunity protects the body against many different types of foreign agents, whereas specific immunity hones in on a particular foreign substance.

- Natural or native immunity—the immunity that you acquire either by getting the disease or receiving antibodies from your mother (also referred to as passive immunity). An example of naturally acquired immunity is chickenpox; you develop an immunity after having the disease. An example of a passively acquired immunity passed from mother to offspring is immunity to hepatitis A. Unlike active immunity that lasts a lifetime, passive immunity usually only lasts a short time, usually six months. If the infant is breast fed, the passive immunity time period can be extended a few months.

- Acquired immunity—is similar to natural immunity. You can acquire immunity in two ways. The first is by the injection of a vaccine, an antigen-bearing drug injected into a person to stimulate antibody production. The other way is by an injection of an immune globulin, actual antibodies obtained from another human or animal.

- Primary or initial immune response—the primary or initial immune response takes place during the initial exposure to a foreign substance. It may or may not result in clinical symptoms. Sometimes, the initial response of the body is to produce an antibody that causes symptoms on subsequent exposures.

- Secondary or anamnestic immune response—the body forms a "memory" for certain antigens (foreign substances). When exposed to the antigen a second time, a symptomatic reaction occurs.

- Humoral immune response—the type of immunity that involves antibodies. Antibodies are substances that react with a specific antigen (a foreign substance found in the body). B-cell lymphocytes synthesize antibodies.

- Cell-mediated immunity—T-cell lymphocytes are involved in this process. It is especially effective against pathogens, fungi, cancer cells, protozoan parasites, and foreign tissues such as transplanted organs.

Q What are the steps in a B-cell lymphocyte (humoral) immune response?

A The steps in a B-cell lymphocyte immune response are as follows:

- Step One. A macrophage engulfs and processes the antigen, pushing the antigen to its cell surface. Here, the antigen interacts with the B cell and helper T cell. The helper T cell's involvement is essential. In acquired immunodeficiency syndrome (AIDS), the helper T cells are destroyed. This is part of the reason why the immune system does not respond in the AIDS patient.

- Step Two. The antigens bind to both the B cell and the helper T cells, activating both.

- Step Three. The activated helper T cells secrete a lymphokine that stimulates the B cells to produce a clone (a group of identical cells formed from the same parent cell). Included in the clone subgroups are plasma cells and memory B cells. The memory cells do not participate in the attack but they do remember the initial encounter with the antigen and are helpful in future encounters with the same antigen. The plasma cells produce large amounts of antibodies to travel through the blood to the antigen.

Q What is an immunoglobulin?

A The antibodies secreted by the B cells are proteins called immunoglobulins. There are five classes produced in humans: immunoglobulin G, M, A, D, and E. They are abbreviated as "IgG," "IgM," and so forth. The first three are the most abundant. Specifics about each type are as follows:

- IgG—the most common, accounting for 75 percent of the antibodies in the blood. Not only is IgG abundant in the blood, but it is also found in the lymph, synovial fluid, peritoneal fluid, cerebrospinal fluid, and breast milk. IgG is the only immunoglobulin that crosses the placenta to provide temporary immunity in neonates.

- IgM—accounts for 5–10 percent of the antibodies in the blood and is the dominant antibody in ABO incompatibilities. It triggers the increased production of IgG in acute infections and complement fixation required for an effective antibody response.

- IgA—accounts for 15 percent of the antibodies in the blood. Also found in tears, saliva, the respiratory tract secretions, the stomach, and accessory organs. It combines with a protein in the mucosa and defends body surfaces against invading microorganisms.

- IgD—accounts for less than 1 percent of the antibodies in the blood. Its biological function is unknown.

- IgE—accounts for less than 1 percent of the antibodies in the blood. It is found in some tissues and on the surface membranes of basophils and mast cells. IgE is responsible for immediate (type I) hypersensitivity reactions.

Q What are the steps in a cell-mediated (T cell) immune response?

A The steps in a cell-mediated immune response are as follows:

- Step One. The antigen on the surface of the pathogen is engulfed by a macrophage. After digesting the pathogen, the macrophage pushes the antigen to its surface.

- Step Two. Specific T cells bind to the antigen and become activated. Activation of the T cell always requires an antigen-presenting cell such as a macrophage.

- Step Three. The activated T cell divides repeatedly creating a large number of clone T cells. There are four subgroups of clones: the killer T cells (destroy the antigen), the helper T cells (stimulate both T and B cells), the suppressor T cells (inhibit or stop the immune response), and the memory T cells (remember the reaction for the next time it is needed).

Q What are examples of cellular interactions in the immune response?

A Examples of cellular interactions in the immune response include the involvement of cytokines (e.g., lymphokines and monokines), antigen processing, antigen presentation and antigen recognition, T cell and B cell differentiation.

Q What is the status of the immune system in the fetus or neonate?

A Fetal immunity is derived primarily from maternal IgG and IgM antibodies. Following delivery, these persist until the neonate's own B cells take over. A substantial number of antibodies is also transferred via the breast milk, one of many reasons experts favor breast-feeding.

Q What is the status of the immune system in the elderly?

A T cell and B cell function is deficient in the elderly. Depressed lymphocyte function is accompanied by a decrease in macrophage activity. Therefore, the elderly are more prone to develop infections and recover slowly. In addition, the elderly have increased levels of autoantibodies (antibodies directed against the patient). This is one of the reasons why the elderly are prone to develop an autoimmune disease.

Q What are the triggers of the body's typical response to inflammation?

A Typical triggers of the acute inflammatory response include lethal cellular injury, nonlethal cellular injury, and other microorganisms.

Q Does stress affect the immune response?

A People who are stressed secrete excessive amounts of steroids such as cortisol. Cortisol suppresses the immune system and that is why stressed people experience a larger number of upper respiratory infections.

Studies have shown that many facets of the immune system are inhibited by stress. Steroid production is one mechanism, but others are likely responsible (e.g., endorphin production in the central nervous system).

Q What is the role of mast cells in inflammation?

A Mast cells release histamine and other chemicals involved with inflammation. They are produced in almost all organs and tissues, especially the liver and lungs.

Q What is the role of the synthesis of leukotrienes and prostaglandins in the inflammation response?

A Both leukotrienes and prostaglandins are inflammatory mediators. They serve multiple roles, the most important of which is attracting WBCs to the site of infection or foreign body "invasion."

Mediators, when produced in excess, may also be harmful to a person. Both leukotrienes and prostaglandins play a role in the pathogenesis of shock.

Q What is the role of plasma protein systems in the inflammation response?

A Plasma protein systems include the complement system, the clotting system, and the kinin system. Each separate system consists of a cascade of biochemical reactions such that as one compound is produced, it catalyzes the formation of the next one.

- The complement system plays a vital role in attracting WBCs to the site of the infection (chemotaxis), as well as initially attacking bacteria. The activation of the complement system during a severe illness, though, may lead to "self-destruction" by activated components.
- The clotting system is vital to the formation of blood clots in the body as well as facilitating repairs to the vascular tree.

In some cases, the clotting cascade is inappropriately activated, causing the thrombotic occlusion of small vessels (microangiopathy) and multiple organ system dysfunction. This clotting process uses up clotting factors, resulting in bleeding in the larger vessels. The combination of microvascular clotting and macrovascular bleeding is termed diffuse intravascular coagulation, or DIC.

- The bradykinin cascade releases vasodilators, which are important in the regulation of blood flow.

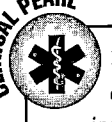

The release of bradykins in disease states, however, may also contribute to the development of shock by worsening vasodilation.

Q What are the cellular components of inflammation?

A The cellular components of inflammation include phagocytes, polymorphonuclear neutrophils, monocytes, macrophages, and eosinophils. The role of each of these components is as follows:

- Phagocytes—engulf foreign matter and bacteria.
- Polymorphonuclear neutrophils—destroy invading organisms, primarily bacteria, through the production of lysosomal enzymes.

- Monocytes—are produced in the bone marrow and through the process of phagocytosis (cellular eating), they enter tissues and are transformed into macrophages.
- Macrophages—are produced in almost all organs and tissues and through the process of phagocytosis (cellular eating), they present antigens to the helper T cells and polymorphonuclear neutrophils.
- Eosinophils—are produced in the bone marrow and destroy parasites. Eosinophils also play a major role in the pathogenesis of allergic reactions and asthma.

What cellular products are involved in the inflammation response?

The cellular products that are involved in the inflammation response include interleukin-1, interleukin-2, and lymphokines (e.g., migration inhibitory factor, macrophage activator factor). The roles of each of these cellular products are as follows:

- Interleukin-1, interleukin-2—attract WBCs to the sites of injury and bacterial invasion.
- Lymphokines—stimulate lymphocytes. Macrophage activator factor stimulates macrophages to help engulf and destroy foreign substances. Migration inhibitory factor keeps WBCs at the site of infection or injury until they can perform their "mission."

What are systemic responses to acute inflammation?

The systemic responses to an acute inflammation include fever, leukocytosis, and an increase in the circulating plasma proteins or acute phase reactants. The fever results from the production of pyrogens by WBCs that are attracted to the site of inflammation by acute phase reactants.

What are the characteristics of a chronic inflammation response?

Chronic inflammation responses are usually caused by an unsuccessful acute inflammatory response due to a foreign body or persistent infection or antigen. Their characteristics include:

- Persistent acute inflammation response.
- Neutrophil degranulation and death.
- Lymphocyte activation.
- Fibroblast activation.
- Infiltration or the development of pus.
- Tissue repair or scar development.

What are the local effects of an inflammation response?

The local effects of an inflammation response are vasodilation, increased capillary permeability, and the development of exudate. Exudate is fluid, cells, or other substances that have been slowly discharged through small pores or breaks in cell membranes.

What are the normal phases of the resolution and repair of wounds?

Normal wound healing involves four steps: repair of damaged tissue, removal of inflammatory debris, restoration of tissues to a normal state, and regeneration of cells.

What are examples of problems leading to dysfunctional wound healing?

Both local and systemic factors may influence normal wound healing. Local factors include:

- Infection—wound infection almost always slows the rate of wound healing.
- Blood supply—inadequate blood supply, as in diabetes, produces tissue hypoxia, which slows wound healing. It may also promote infection.
- Foreign bodies—the presence of a foreign body in a wound stimulates acute and chronic inflammation, which interferes with wound healing.

  Systemic factors that influence wound healing are:
- Nutrition—data have repeatedly demonstrated that poor nutritional intake leads to poor scar formation and suppression of the immune system.
- Hematologic abnormalities—proper wound healing requires the presence of adequate numbers of WBCs. Patients who have impaired bone marrow stores or WBC production may not only be susceptible to infection, but often heal slower.
- Systemic disease (e.g., diabetes, AIDS)—both diabetes and AIDS directly affect the cells of the immune system that play a direct role in wound healing. In addition, there is an increased tendency for wound infection, which also interferes with normal healing. As mentioned previously, diabetic patients often have circulatory impairment, especially to the lower extremities, that significantly retards the rate of healing and increases the likelihood of wound infection.
- Steroid use—steroids decrease the initial inflammatory response required for the proper formation of scar tissue. They also increase the risk of wound infection by suppressing the immune system.

Q **What is meant by the terms hypersensitivity, allergy, autoimmunity, and isoimmunity?**

A The definitions are as follows:

- Hypersensitivity—any bodily response to any substance that a patient is abnormally sensitive to. This is a generic term for a variety of reactions.
- Allergy—an overreaction to an antigen causing a variety of symptoms ranging from mild to severe and life threatening.
- Autoimmunity—when a person's T cells or antibodies attacks them, causing tissue damage and organ dysfunction.
- Isoimmunity—formation of antibodies or T cells directed against antigens on another person's cells.

CLINICAL PEARL

The destruction of cells by antibodies may be either an autoimmune or an isoimmune reaction. A blood transfusion reaction is an isoimmune reaction to another's red blood cells (RBCs). Systemic lupus occurs as a result of our body forming antibodies against our own tissues, an autoimmune reaction.

Q **Explain the mechanisms of hypersensitivity?**

A There are four types of hypersensitivity reactions. They are:

1. Type I hypersensitivity reaction—an immediate reaction allergy that occurs rapidly and in response to a stimulus (e.g., bee sting, penicillin, shell fish, or iodine). This hypersensitivity reaction involves IgE antibodies. The most severe form of a hypersensitivity reaction is called anaphylaxis, which involves bronchoconstriction and cardiovascular collapse.
2. Type II hypersensitivity reaction—antibodies (not IgE) combine with antigens in normal locations, such as normal cells. Cells are then destroyed, either by complement (an inflammatory mediator) or other antibodies. Examples include transfusion reactions, newborn hemolytic jaundice, and Goodpasture's disease of the lungs and kidneys (causes kidney failure and hemoptysis).
3. Type III hypersensitivity reaction—involves the formation of immune complexes by the reaction of antibodies with antigens. The deposit of immune complexes in tissues forms the underlying abnormality. Reactions may be systemic or localized. The systemic form is called serum sickness and results from a large, single exposure to an antigen, such as horse antibody serum. The localized form is called an arthus reaction, consisting of a circumscribed area of vascular inflammation (vasculitis). An example of this is farmer's lung, a local hypersensitivity reaction in the lung from molds that grow on hay.

CLINICAL PEARL

Complement is usually activated in both type II and type III hypersensitivity reactions. In type II reactions, the immune complexes are formed where the antigens should be located. In type III reactions, they form where antigens are not normally found (e.g., circulating in the blood, deposited in the skin).

4. Type IV hypersensitivity reaction—is mediated by T cells, rather than by antibodies. There are two subtypes. The first type, delayed hypersensitivity, involves lymphocytes and macrophages. T cells respond to an antigen and activate CD4 lymphocytes. These release mediators that destroy the foreign substance. The other type, cell-mediated cytotoxicity, involves only sensitized T cells (CD8 lymphocytes). These kill antigen-bearing target cells rather than activating the CD4 lymphocyte to do so.

Q **What are some examples of autoimmune and isoimmune diseases?**

A Autoimmune and isoimmune diseases include the following:
- Graves' disease—a disease involving hyperthyroidism.
- Rheumatoid arthritis—a chronic, systemic, degenerative disease involving inflammation of the connective tissue in the joints.
- Myasthenia gravis—a neuromuscular disease of the lower motor neurons causing muscle weakness and fatigue.
- Immune thrombocytopenic purpura—a platelet disorder causing bleeding into the skin, mucous membranes, internal cavities, and organs.
- Isoimmune neutropenia—the presence of an unusually small number of neutrophil cells in the blood.
- Systemic lupus erythematosus—a chronic autoimmune inflammatory disease involving multiple systems that has periods of remission and exacerbation.
- Rh and ABO isoimmunization.

Q **What are some examples of immunity and inflammation deficiencies?**

A Immunity and inflammation deficiencies include the following:
- Nutritional deficiencies—any nutritional deficiency can hamper normal immune function and the inflammatory response. A lack of protein in the diet decreases the ability of the liver to manufacture inflammatory mediators and plasma proteins.

Poor nutrition also results in bone marrow depression, decreasing the formation of WBCs.

- Iatrogenic deficiencies—the most common iatrogenic immune deficiency is caused by drugs. Steroids, taken orally or inhaled, comprise the largest percentage of offenders. Idiosyncratic reactions to antibiotics may result in bone marrow suppression, as may reactions to chemotherapeutic drugs for cancer.

- Deficiencies caused by trauma—the stress of trauma by itself may cause immunodeficiency. Organ damage, shock, mediator production, and decreased nutrition may also contribute.

- Deficiencies caused by stress—physical or mental stress can result in decreased WBC and lymphocyte function, as well as a decreased production of various antibodies.

- AIDS—HIV infection results in a loss of normal CD4 helper T lymphocytes. This leads to a decreased ability of the body to fight many types of infection that are normally eradicated by type IV delayed hypersensitivity reactions.

Pharmacology

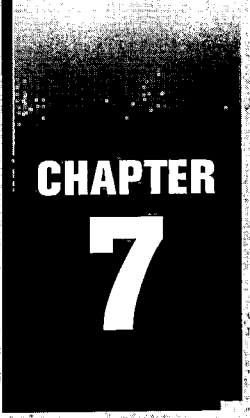

EMS providers have a responsibility to understand the principles and concepts of pharmacology, including such things as indications, contraindications, drug actions and interactions, side effects, and doses. They must also know how a drug works, why it is given, and when is it given. This chapter covers the aspects of pharmacology specific to the out-of-hospital patient. Please see Chapter 8 for all content related to medication administration.

Basic Pharmacology

❓ Is there a difference between a medication and a drug?

🅰 Yes. Although the two terms are used interchangeably, there is a difference. A medication is a medicinal substance used as a treatment or remedy, whereas a drug is any chemical substance that, when taken into a living organism, produces a biological response affecting one or more of that organism's processes or functions. For the remainder of this chapter, we use these terms interchangeably.

❓ What are the phases of drug activity?

🅰 Basically there are three phases of drug activity: pharmacodynamic, pharmaceutical, and pharmacokinetic.

❓ What is pharmacodynamics?

🅰 Pharmacodynamics is the study of how a drug works and why it works. Specifically, it looks at the biochemical and physiological effects on or interactions with the target organ(s) or tissue(s).

❓ What is pharmaceutics?

🅰 Pharmaceutics is the study of the various drug preparations and how they affect pharmacokinetic and pharmacodynamic processes. For example, a drug in liquid form given orally is absorbed quicker than a drug given in a solid form because the latter has to be dissolved before it can be absorbed. A drug administered IV is absorbed quicker than a drug taken orally because it is placed directly into the bloodstream.

❓ What is pharmacokinetics?

🅰 Pharmacokinetics is the study of how a drug is altered as it travels through the body. Once a drug has been introduced into the body it goes through five distinct stages:

- Stage one. When a drug enters the body, by any method, and reaches the bloodstream, this is the *absorption* stage.
- Stage two. The drug moves through the bloodstream to the target organ and this is the *distribution* stage.
- Stage three. If administered properly, the drug produces the desired effect.
- Stage four. A chemical breakdown of the drug occurs, and this is the metabolism or biotransformation stage.

- Stage five. The drug is removed from the body, and this is the elimination or excretion stage.

What are the general properties of drugs?

Medications are administered to achieve a therapeutic (healing) effect, a prophylactic (preventative) effect, or a diagnostic (attempting to identify) effect. The interaction between a drug and a body organ or tissue is only a physiologic modification of that organ or tissue because drugs do not produce new functions. Drug-induced physiologic changes to a body function or process are known as a drug action. A drug usually affects more than one organ or tissue and varies in degree of desired or undesired effects. There are several ways by which a drug affects a body organ or tissue; this is referred to as the drug's "mechanism of action." The major mechanism by which a drug affects the body is by joining with receptors located on the target organs or tissues.

What is a drug receptor?

A drug receptor is any part of a cell with which a drug molecule interacts to trigger its desired effect. Drugs that affect the autonomic nervous system (ANS) are commonly used in emergency and out-of-hospital settings. There are two general types of receptors, *cholinergic* and *adreneric,* that respond to various drugs that either influence or block the ANS.

How do drugs affect or block the ANS?

The ANS is the division of the nervous system that is responsible for maintaining control of the involuntary vital functions of the body such as blood pressure, respiratory status, and cardiac rhythm. Autonomic drugs in general affect the entire body rather than a target organ. The ANS is subdivided into sympathetic and parasympathetic systems. Drugs that affect the ANS are categorized according to the part of the ANS they stimulate or inhibit. When a drug stimulates a receptor, it is called an *agonist,* which means "to act or to activate." When a drug inhibits a receptor, it is called *antagonist,* which means "to block."

What is an adrenergic receptor?

Adrenergic receptors respond to neurotransmitters epinephrine and norepinephrine acting on the sympathetic response. Dopamine, an antecedent in the formation of epinephrine, can also act as a neurotransmitter in the sympathetic nervous system. Drugs that mimic the functions of the sympathetic nervous system are called *sympathomimetic* drugs. This group of drugs is commonly used in out-of-hospital emergency care, par-

ticularly within ACLS. These are a few of the drugs used in the out-of-hospital setting:

- Dobutamine.
- Dopamine.
- Epinephrine.
- Isporeterenol.
- Norepinephrine.

Antiadrenergic is a group of drugs that block the function of the sympathetic nervous system and are called *sympatholytic* drugs. Some examples include:

- Atenolol.
- Esmolol.
- Labetolo.
- Metoprolol.
- Propranolol.
- Timolol.

What is a cholinergic receptor?

Cholinergic receptors respond to the neurotransmitter acetylcholine. Drugs that perform similarly to acetylcholine and mimic the parasympathetic response are referred to as cholinergic or *parasympathomimetic.* This group of drugs is not utilized in out-of-hospital care. Drugs that block the cholinergic receptors and parasympathetic response are called *parasympatholytic.* In this group of drugs, atropine is probably the most commonly used drug in out-of-hospital care. Primarily, atropine blocks parasympathetic stimulation of the heart causing the rate to decrease, but it also affects other body systems.

What are alpha 1 and 2 and beta 1 and 2 receptors?

There are two types of sympathetic receptors, adrenergic receptors and dopaminergic receptors. Adrenergic receptors are subdivided into four types: alpha 1 and 2, beta 1 and 2. When stimulated, the receptors effect certain responses:

- Alpha 1 receptors cause contraction (vasoconstriction) of smooth muscle.
- Alpha 2 receptors are inhibitory and stop the release of norepinephrine.
- Beta 1 receptors cause an increase in the rate, contraction, automaticity, and conduction of the heart.
- Beta 2 receptors cause bronchodilation and vasodilation.

Dopaminergic receptors affect the dilation of cerebral, coronary, and renal arteries. Many drugs are selective to affect any one of the four receptors, and some are nonselective and affect one or more of these receptors. For example, the sympathetic beta-blocker Timolol is nonselective and affects both beta 1 and 2 receptors.

Q How does a drug join with a receptor site?

A The joining of a drug and a receptor site is called affinity and is often compared to the connection of a lock and a key. The drug is the key and the lock is the receptor. Certain drugs have keys that fit perfectly into the lock and create a reaction; these drugs are called agonists. Some drugs fit partially into the receptor and do not create a reaction; these are called antagonists. There are drugs that fit and create a small reaction, but they block other responses; these are called partial agonists.

Q What are the other ways a drug affects a body organ or tissue?

A Two other drug mechanisms of action are drug–enzyme interaction and nonspecific drug interaction. Some drugs work by influencing the enzyme system of a cell, while other drugs alter the chemical composition of body fluid.

Q How does a drug get inside a cell or body part?

A All of the stages of drug processing through the body—absorption, distribution, metabolism, and excretion—are carried out by active transport or passive transport. To review these two types of transport, see Chapter 6, General Principles of Pathophysiology.

Q What is the difference between a drug action and an interaction?

A The expectation in the administration of a drug is to produce a desired, or therapeutic, effect on a target organ or tissue. A drug action is the effect of a drug on a specific body organ or tissue; this is called a local effect. Entire body systems may be affected; this is called a systemic effect. A drug interaction is the combined effect of drugs taken at the same time that alters the expected therapeutic effect.

The combined effect of two drugs may be *synergistic* or *antagonistic*. Two types of synergism are *additive effect* (two agreeable drugs produce an effect that neither could alone) and *potentiation* (the combined effects of two drugs are better than either could have produced alone). Three types of antagonism are *chemical, competitive,* and *physiologic.* A drug can block another chemically or compete with another for a receptor. Physiologic antagonism is when the biologic responses of two drugs are opposite each other.

- Synergism examples:
  1. Additive—The use of a combination of antihypertensives to produce a greater decrease in blood pressure than either drug could produce alone.
  2. Potentiation—Drinking alcohol while taking barbiturates results in one drug enhancing the effects of the other.
- Antagonism examples:
  1. Chemical—Giving activated charcoal to inactivate poisons. The charcoal binds with and adsorbs the toxins present in the GI tract to inactivate them.
  2. Competitive—Narcan has a greater affinity for a cell receptor than narcotic analgesics, so it binds to the cell and prevents it from responding. Competitive inhibition responses are usually reversible.
  3. Physiologic—When taking barbiturates and amphetamines at the same time, the biologic responses to the two drugs are opposite.

Q There are a number of other terms commonly associated with pharmacology, how are they defined?

A Other common terms specific to this area include:

- An *adverse reaction* is an unintended or undesirable response to a drug. The reaction may be sudden or take several days. For example, a patient taking lasix, a diuretic, develops ECG changes due to the loss of specific electrolytes that occurred with the increased urine output.
- *Cumulative effect* is the effect that develops when a dose is repeated before the prior dose has been metabolized. Unmonitored, this condition may lead to toxicity. Digitalis is a drug that can become toxic quickly and has to be monitored very closely. The patient with renal or hepatic failure is at a high risk for a cumulative effect because digitalis is metabolized by the liver and excreted through urine.
- *Habituation* is the psychological or emotional dependence on a drug after a repeated use. Analgesics are a good example of a class of drugs that a patient can become accustomed to from frequent use.
- *Half-life* refers to the amount of time that a drug remains at a therapeutic level to produce a desired effect and the time it takes the body to metabolize or inactivate a drug's concentration by 50 percent. This information about a drug is important when determining dosage and how often a drug is to be administered.
- *Hypersensitivity* is an exaggerated response to a drug, usually idiosyncratic in origin. This is an allergic reaction as might be seen when antibiotics are given and a patient develops itching, a rash, or shortness of breath.

- *Idiosyncrasy* is an abnormal or unpredictable response to a drug that is peculiar to an individual rather than a general group. For example, you administer the same drug in the same dose to three individuals having chest pain. One of the patients develops the reaction of shortness of breath instead of the intended reaction of relieving the chest pain. That one patient is said to have had an idiosyncratic reaction.

- *Side effect* is a response to a drug that is not the principal intent for giving that drug. A side effect may be considered desirable or undesirable depending on the effect it produces. Some of the most common undesirable side effects include headache, nausea, or dizziness. A desirable side effect might be administering nitro to a patient who is dangerously hypertensive to decrease the blood pressure.

- *Tolerance* to a drug is the decrease in the expected response with repeated doses. Patients taking analgesics are prone to this condition; consequently, the dose has to be increased. This can become a problem for the patient and the physician. With increased doses of painkillers, which are often narcotic in part, the patient cannot tolerate the side effects of the drug (e.g., increased respiratory depression). The solution is a change of medication rather than increasing the dose.

How long does a drug stay at a receptor site causing an effect?

How long a drug remains at a receptor site varies with each drug's receptor interaction, the drug response relationship, and the biological half-life of the drug.

What is a loading dose and a maintenance dose of a drug?

A loading dose is considered to be a single dose or the accumulation of several closely repeated single doses (boluses) used to obtain the therapeutic level to achieve a desired effect. As a drug loses its therapeutic level during its half-life, any additional administration given either as a single dose or an IV drip to maintain the desired effect is called a maintenance dose. For out-of-hospital patients, lidocaine is an example of a drug that is given initially as a loading dose or single bolus of 1 mg/kg followed by an IV drip of 2 mg/min as a maintenance dose.

What is the blood–brain barrier?

The blood–brain barrier is a physiologic barrier that exists between circulating blood and the brain. This barrier protects brain tissue and cerebral spinal fluid from exposure to certain substances. It is very particular about allowing the movement of many drugs into the brain. This barrier ensures that most drugs are absorbed more slowly by the brain than by other tissues.

How are drugs metabolized?

The liver metabolizes most drugs. Drug effects are temporary because the body works to detoxify and eliminate foreign chemicals such as drugs. One of the major functions of the liver is to detoxify and metabolize chemicals and drugs so the kidneys can easily eliminate them. The kidneys also metabolize quite a few drugs. Other tissues such as plasma, lungs, and intestinal mucosa may be involved in this process.

What does iatrogenic mean?

An iatrogenic disorder is an adverse mental or physical condition induced inadvertently in a patient by a physician, medical treatment, or diagnostic procedures. For example, a paramedic starts an IV on a patient without using aseptic technique; the patient develops an infection leading to septic shock.

Drug Nomenclature

What is the difference between the chemical, generic, trade, and official names of a drug?

The chemical name is the first name given to a drug and is usually a description of the chemical makeup of the drug. The generic name is often an abbreviated form of the drug's chemical name. It is the official name of a drug in the United States and is assigned by the U.S. Adopted Name Council. The trade or brand name is a name assigned by the manufacturers and is usually registered to protect it. One drug may have several trade names. A registered trade name is capitalized and followed with the symbol®.

The official name is the same as the generic name and is followed by the initials USP (U.S. Pharmacopoeia) or NF (National Formulary) denoting its listing in one of these official publications. The following is an example of the four names of a drug:

- Chemical name: N-(4-hydroxypheny) acetamide.

- Generic name: acetaminophen.

- Official name: acetaminophen USP.

- Trade or brand name: Tylenol®, Tempra®, and Datril®.

The EMS provider is primarily responsible for knowing the generic and brand names of a drug. However, some drugs are a combination of two or more drugs and will have the name of one drug listed as its chemical abbreviation. For example, hydrochloride, abbreviated as HCK, may follow a generic or trade name (e.g., trazodone HCK), making a new drug from a combination of two. Therefore, the EMS provider is also responsible for knowing these types of chemical suffixes.

What are the main derivatives of drug products?

Drugs and drug products are developed from several sources:

- Plants (e.g., atropine and digitalis).
- Animals and humans (e.g., epinephrine and insulin).
- Minerals (e.g., iron and iodine).
- Synthetic or chemical (e.g., Heptavax).
- Microorganisms (e.g., penicillin).

How are drugs classified?

Drugs may be classified in many ways and many drugs fit into more than one classification. The categories and an example of each are:

- Chemical class—barbiturate or opiate.
- Mechanism of action or functional classification—ACE inhibitor, beta-blocker, or bronchodilator.
- Therapeutic classification—acetylcholine or analgesic.

What is an ACE inhibitor?

Angiotensin converting enzyme (ACE) inhibitors work by affecting the renin-angiotensin-aldosterone system. This system supports the sodium and fluid balance of the body and maintains blood pressure. Renin, an enzyme produced in the kidney, separates angiotensinogen to form angiotensin I, which is then converted to angiotensin II. The angiotensin II is a powerful vasoconstrictor that can raise blood pressure, but it also causes the release of aldosterone, which contributes to sodium and water retention.

When this system is disrupted by kidney damage or some other mechanism, hypertension can result. By inhibiting the angiotensin I from converting to the angiotensin II with ACE, the system is suppressed and the blood pressure is lowered.

ACE inhibitors are mild antihypertensives used to treat young to middle-aged adults. Some of the most common ACE inhibitors are Capoten®, Vasotec®, and Prinivil®. Anti-inflammatory drugs, such as Advil® or Motrin®, can slow the actions of ACE inhibitors. Be sure to check for any over-the-counter medications a patient is taking to get the full picture.

How is classification different from standardization?

Recall that the classification of a drug is a categorization based on how it works or what it is made of. Standardization is the method for making sure a drug's dosage and reliability are accurate. Because many drugs are made from plants, the strength from plant to plant may be different based on a number of variables such as where it was grown and how it was processed.

The method by which the strength and purity of a drug (chemical or biologic) is determined is known as an assay. A chemical assay is a test that determines the ingredients and their exact amounts. The bioassay is another test that is used on drugs that have an unknown active ingredient or cannot be tested by other means. Bioassay tests determine how much of a drug is needed to produce a specific effect. This test process is done on laboratory animals under specific standard conditions.

What are some resources available for obtaining drug information?

Fortunately there are many resources for getting information on drugs. In the United States, all drug manufacturers include drug inserts in the drug packages. Additional resources include:

- Drug information centers.
- Poison control centers.
- Pharmacists.
- Internet Web sites (e.g., Yahoo! Health–Medication or Drug).
- Professional journals.
- Physician's Desk Reference (PDR).
- American Medical Association (AMA).
- Hospital Formulary.
- U.S. Pharmacopoeia—A U.S. government publication and the only official book of drug standards in the United States since 1980. All drugs listed in the book have met high standards of quality, purity, and strength.

What are the key legislative acts controlling drug use and abuse in the United States?

Prior to the early 1900s, many people were injured by, became addicted to, or died because of certain ingredients contained in medications and remedies. In 1906, the U.S. government passed the first law to protect the public from impure or mislabeled drugs. The Pure Food and Drug Act of 1906 required drug manufacturers to label certain dangerous ingredients on the packages. However, it did not provide for the safety or effectiveness of drugs. This Act also designated the U.S. Pharmacopoeia and the National Formulary as official standards and empowered the federal government to enforce them.

The Sherley Amendment of 1912 prohibited the use of fraudulent therapeutic claims. Soon after came the Harrison Narcotic Act of 1914, which was the first Act passed by a nation that controlled the sale of narcotics and drugs that cause dependence.

The Federal Food, Drug, and Cosmetic Act of 1938 was enacted to ensure that drugs are tested for safety and that the labels accurately list all ingredients used to prepare the drug and the directions for its use.

The Kefauver–Harris Amendment in 1962 required proof of both safety and efficacy before a new drug could be approved for use. The Comprehensive Drug Abuse Prevention and Control Act (Controlled Substance Act of 1970) superseded the Harrison Narcotic Act. This Act sets forth the rules for the manufacture and distribution of drugs that have the potential for abuse. Because of this Act, a new classification system was established that classifies this specific class of drugs into five categories or schedules.

Q **What are the five addictive drug schedules of the Controlled Substance Act of 1970 (Table 7–1)?**

A Controlled substances are divided into five schedules depending on their potential for abuse.

- Schedule I—High abuse potential with no accepted medical uses. Used for research, analysis, or instruction only (e.g., heroin, LSD).
- Schedule II—Strictly regulated due to high abuse potential (e.g., morphine, codeine).
- Schedules III and IV—Moderate abuse potential (e.g., codeine with aspirin [ASA]).
- Schedule V—Low abuse potential (e.g., cough syrups, diarrhea medications).

TABLE 7–1

Drug Schedules		
Schedule	Specifics	Examples
I	High abuse potential. No accepted medical use. For research or teaching only.	Opioids, psychedelics
II	High abuse potential. Strictly regulated with accepted medical use.	Barbiturates, opioids, and stimulants
III	Less abuse potential than I or II. Prescription with accepted medical use.	Barbiturates, opioids, steroids, and stimulants
IV	Less abuse potential than III. Prescription with accepted medical use.	Barbiturates, benzodiazepines, opioids, steroids, stimulants, and others
V	Lower abuse potential than IV. Accepted medical use with or without prescription.	Cough preparations and anti-diarrheal medications containing limited quantities of opioids

Q **What are the roles of the Food and Drug Administration (FDA) and the Drug Enforcement Agency (DEA)?**

A The FDA controls the testing and marketing of prescription drugs, as well as the availability of drugs, either by prescription or over the counter. The DEA in the Department of Justice became the nation's sole drug enforcement agency in 1973.

Q **Are drug manufacturers liable for injuries caused by their products?**

A Certainly, drug manufacturers are legally responsible for knowing the effects of their products and anyone who has been harmed by a defective product can sue the manufacturer. The U.S. Pharmacopoeia Convention, Inc. manages a drug product problem-reporting program that informs the product manufacturer, the labeler, and the FDA of potential health hazards and defective drug products. Defects in drug products may be reported by any health professional. The report is submitted in writing to the FDA in Maryland.

For drug product liability to exist, the following three criteria must be met:

- The defect caused harm.
- The defect occurred before it left the manufacturer.
- The product is defective or not fit for its intended reasonable uses.

Q **Why does it take so long to get new drugs on the market?**

A Before a new drug enters the market, it has to go through a lengthy and costly process to determine if it is safe and effective. This process has been developed primarily by the FDA in order to protect the consumer. The process has multiple steps, which include the following:

- Investigational drugs—discovery of the drug, standardization, animal and human testing.
- FDA approval—the drug has to complete four phases to ensure its safety and efficacy.

These phases include testing, approval, and marketing requirements before new drugs can reach the consumer.

1. Phase I. Involves human trials of an investigational drug, usually on 20 to 80 healthy volunteer subjects. These studies are designed to determine the metabolic and pharmacological actions of the drug in humans.
2. Phase II. Involves several hundred people and is designed to obtain preliminary data on the effectiveness of the drug for a particular indication(s) in patients with the disease or condition. Also, it is designed to determine the side effects and risks associated with the drug.

3. Phase III. Involves several hundred to several thousand people and is intended to obtain data about overall effectiveness and safety to evaluate the benefit–risk of the drug.

4. Phase IV. Involves the drug's post-marketing surveillance. This phase is designed to monitor the new drug through voluntary information reported by health care professionals.

On average, it takes approximately 12 years and $10 million to get a new drug on the market. This makes it very difficult for drug manufacturers to research drugs to treat rare or chronic diseases. In 1983, the FDA established the Orphan Drug Act to provide grants to encourage research for diseases such as AIDS and cystic fibrosis. Approximately 500 new drugs have been discovered since this Act was implemented.

What are different forms of drugs?

There are many preparations of drugs and typically, they are subdivided into solids and liquids. Each form has benefits and drawbacks.

1. **Solids:**
   - Capsule—a container made of gelatin that holds a single dose and is designed to eliminate the taste of the drug (e.g., Contact® cold capsules).
   - Pills—a single dose that is shaped like a pellet and can be chewed, swallowed whole, or dissolved sublingually. A pill, tablet, or capsule may be coated (enteric-coated) with a substance that keeps the drug from dissolving until it reaches the small intestines (e.g., ASA).
   - Powders—a collection of fine granules that is usually mixed with a liquid before administration (e.g., glucagon or Alka-Seltzer®).
   - Suppositories—single doses that are contained in an oblique-shaped capsule made of soap, gelatin, or cocoa butter and are designed to be placed in the rectum, vagina, or urethra to be dissolved (e.g., ASA for children or Valium).
   - Tablets—single dose that is shaped like a disc and can be chewed or swallowed whole (e.g., baby aspirin).
   - Troches (lozenges)—a single dose combined with sugar and mucilage and designed to be placed in the mouth to be dissolved (e.g., a cough drop).

2. **Liquids:**
   - Douches—a spray or stream of solution pointed at a body part and designed as a treatment for a local condition (e.g., vinegar and water vaginal douche).
   - Solutions—liquids that contain dissolved drugs (e.g., eye drops).
   - Suspensions—liquids with solid particles mixed within but not dissolved (e.g., activated charcoal).

   - Syrups—concentrated sugar with small amounts of medicine that cover the taste and smell of the medicine (e.g., cough syrup).
   - Tinctures—drug preparations made using alcohol to extract the medicinal substance from a vegetable or animal (e.g., tincture of belladonna).
   - Topical creams—medicinal creams designed to be placed on the skin for slow absorption to a local area (e.g., cortisone cream or Bengay®).
   - Transdermal patches—similar to topical creams, but the medication has a gel-like texture and comes on a patch similar to a Band-Aid®. They are placed on the skin for absorption at a fixed rate to attain a systemic effect (e.g., nitro patch, MS patch, or nicotine patch).

How can the medications a person is taking give us clues about their medical history?

Because drugs are classified by their chemical class, mechanism of action, or therapeutic effect, examining a patient's medications can provide useful information quickly, especially if the patient has an altered mental status (AMS), is in distress, or just doesn't know what they are taking. It is easy to identify a hypertensive, cardiac, or respiratory medical condition by looking at a patient's medications. By looking at the dates of the prescriptions and how much is in the container, you may also be able to ascertain if they are compliant with their medication schedules.

What are the factors that influence the action of a drug?

There are many factors that can influence the action of a drug. Some of these include:

- Age. Geriatric and pediatric patients have a higher risk of adverse reaction. Because neonates, infants, and toddlers have immature liver and kidney functions, they cannot metabolize and excrete drugs like adults. The elderly may have a poor response to drug therapy due to a decline of their liver and kidney functions; this often occurs with a coexisting disease process.

- Body weight. Total body weight and the amount of a drug given has a direct association over the distribution and concentration of a drug. The average adult dose is based on the drug amount that will produce a particular effect in 50 percent of persons who are between the ages of 18 and 65 and weigh about 150 pounds. Very lean and very obese people may need doses adjusted to their body mass. Most medications have no pediatric recommended doses, so they are administered according to body weight and physician direction.

- Gender. Differences in weight, body fat, and water weight can vary the effects of a drug. Females are usually smaller than men. Because many drugs are fat-soluble, they bind to proteins and concentrate in the fatty tissues of the body, which results in a prolonged drug effect. Other places that drugs can accumulate are muscle tissue, bone, and plasma. When this occurs, these areas act as drug reservoirs and have the tendency to delay the drug's onset of action and prolong the duration of its effect.

- Pathological state. Geriatric patients have an increased incidence of illness and disease. With age comes a decrease in circulation as well as renal and liver functions, which in turn causes a decrease in the metabolic rate and results in more drugs in their system. The increased amount of drugs in the system can reach lethal levels, commonly referred to as drug toxicity. Some of the most common drugs that produce drug toxicity are digitalis, lidocaine, and various beta-blockers. When a person is injured, the amount of a drug needed to produce a desired effect will vary based on the severity of the injury.

- Genetic factors. Pharmacogenetic abnormalities, such as metabolic deficiencies or abnormal receptor sites, can affect a drug response.

- Psychological factors. The way a person thinks about how a drug will work can actually alter the drug's effects. This is one reason why double-blind testing with placebos (an inactive substance) is used in the controlled testing of drugs.

- Pregnancy. In the pregnant patient, many drugs can rapidly cross the placental barrier to reach and affect the fetus. Protein binding is decreased during pregnancy and hepatic metabolism is delayed.

- Drug storage. Many drugs become ineffective or unsafe due to age, the temperature at which they are stored, or exposure to light. All drugs have a limited viable time, called shelf life, during which their potency and safety can be ensured. Any drug with a shelf life of less than one year has to be labeled with a warning that displays the date of expiration. Some drugs require refrigeration or they become ineffective or dangerous, while most other drugs just need to be stored away from extreme hot or cold temperatures. Nitro tablets are an example of a drug that can quickly become ineffective shortly after the package has been opened or when exposed to light. Usually these drugs are packaged in dark containers.

Q **What are the factors that slow or enhance the absorption of drugs?**

A There are a great number of factors that can affect the absorption rate of a drug. The following list contains the most predominant factors:

- Disease and illness. Disease and illness are two major factors that can slow the absorption of a medication. Patients that have an illness or disease that decreases their cardiac function, circulation, or renal and liver functions will have a decrease in the metabolic rate. When this is unrecognized or unchecked, it can lead to increased drugs in the system. The increased amount of drugs in the system can eventually reach lethal levels.

- Injury. When a person is injured, the amount of a drug needed to produce a desired effect varies based on the severity of the injury. The hemodynamic state of the body is a significant factor in the absorption of medications. For example, when the body is in a state of shock, it has decreased peripheral perfusion. A medication administered intramuscularly will have a slow absorption rate and a subcutaneous administration will be even slower. The decreased motility in a shock state also slows absorption.

- Route of administration. The parenteral routes of drug administration have a quicker absorption rate than the enteral routes.

- Dosage. Drugs administered in higher doses often have a quicker absorption rate than lower doses.

- Solubility. The form of the drug affects the absorption rate. Drugs in liquid preparations have a quicker absorption rate than drugs in solid form.

- pH. The pH of a drug, how acidic or alkalinic it is, can affect the rate at which it diffuses across a cell membrane. Because this membrane has an affinity for uncharged chemicals, it allows for the rapid passage of uncharged chemicals while slowing the passage of charged chemicals. The pH of the body changes a drug's chemical reaction from charged or uncharged depending on the pH of the environment. The chemical acidity of the climate through which a drug must pass will vary with the route of administration. The mouth has a pH of 7.0, which is neutral; the stomach is approximately 1.4, the small intestine is 5.3, and the colon is 7.3. Drugs that enter these different climates are affected in various ways. Drugs that have a weak acidity, such as barbiturates, are absorbed better in the stomach than in the intestine. Drugs that have a weaker base, such as morphine sulfate, have a better reaction if given by a route other than orally so as to avoid the high acidity of the stomach.

- Body temperature. When a drug is administered peripherally, cold ambient temperature can slow the absorption rate.

Medication Administration

EMT-Bs (basic) are trained to assist patients to take a limited number of their own prescribed medications. EMT-Is (intermediate) and EMT-Ps (paramedic) not only assist patients, but also are permitted to administer a variety of drugs. EMS providers must have an excellent knowledge of the drugs they use to treat their patients. In addition, they should be familiar with the most commonly prescribed medications and general principles of pharmacology. The administration of medications is a great responsibility that carries with it accountability, liability, obligation, and duty. This chapter discusses these responsibilities and the principles of medication administration in the out-of-hospital setting.

Accountability and Obligation

What are the legal implications of medication administration?

The basic principle of medication administration is the same as that of medicine, which is, "First do no harm." Administration of medications is an area that can help or harm a patient significantly. Only a licensed physician can prescribe the drugs administered by EMS providers. Medications are administered by the orders of medical direction, either on-line (direct) or off-line (indirect). If EMS providers administer a medication without an order, they are "practicing medicine without a license." Although the medical director is ultimately responsible for the EMS provider's field practice in general, the individual provider is legally responsible for her actions.

Direct orders for medication administration are received over the radio, telephone, or in person from a physician. Confirm direct medication orders twice, including the specific drug, dose, and route of administration.

Indirect orders for medication administration are commonly used with specific circumstances such as an asthma attack or a cardiac arrest. These orders are written as standing orders and referred to as protocols. These protocols, although similar, vary somewhat from one region to another.

Document all medications administered on a prehospital care report (PCR). Include the drug, dose, route of administration, time, initials of the person administering the drug, and the patient's response.

This report is a legal document and can be used in court. If the report is not complete or is carelessly completed, the EMS provider may encounter problems if testimony based on the report is needed in court. At the very least, most documentation goes through a quality review process within the EMS provider's own department.

When working with controlled substances, the procedures are more stringent. There are many protocols in place to safeguard the use of these drugs. EMS providers must keep precise records of drug inventory, management, and administration.

Further, the EMS provider has an obligation to understand the patient's rights regarding medication administration. A patient must give informed consent before receiving any medication. Always respect patient confidentiality regarding medical treatment. This is discussed in Chapter 4, Medicolegal Issues.

ⓠ What are the "six rights" of medication administration?

ⓐ This phrase refers to some of the universal principles of medication administration. In an effort to avoid making an error when giving a patient a medication, the person administering the drug checks and rechecks to ensure that the *right* patient is getting the *right* drug in the *right* dose through the *right* route at the *right* time and that the *right* documentation is completed.

In the past, the "five rights of drug administration" has been used to describe these principles of medication administration. In the 1998 EMS provider curriculum and in the texts that support it, you will see the "six rights of drug administration" with the sixth right referring to the proper documentation of medication administration on an out-of-hospital care report. Following is an explanation of each of the six rights:

1. *Right Patient*
   - For assisted medication administration, check that the medication on hand is in fact the prescribed medication for that patient.

2. *Right Drug*
   - Check for the name of the drug on the container label; check the expiration date, color, and clarity; and look for leakage and the absence of foreign substances.

3. *Right Dose*
   - Compare the concentration and amount of drug on hand to the dose ordered.

4. *Right Route*
   - Check that the form supplied is for the route you expect to use.

5. *Right Time*
   - Record the time of administration.

6. *Right Documentation*
   - Document the order for the drug administration as either a direct order or a standing order, the dose, the route, the time of administration, any repeated doses, the initials of the person who administered the drug, and the patient's response or lack of response to the drug.

ⓠ Is there a standard procedure to document medication administration?

ⓐ Yes, there are accepted practices for documenting or charting medication administrations. For example, to avoid errors when recording doses that are less than a whole number, place a zero before the decimal and always list the unit of measurement (e.g., record a half milligram as 0.5 mg). When documenting medication administration, *do not:*

- Erase. Erasing or deleting information gives the appearance of hiding information. Instead, mark a single line through the error, write your initials next to it, and then write the correction.
- Add. Once written, do not add information at a later time or date. If additional information is needed, document the change clearly, and date and initial it on all copies. Many legal advisors recommend clearly identifying a subsequent entry as "late entry."
- Change. It is not acceptable to change or write over a notation to fix an error such as changing a one to a four. This creates confusion as to which is the correct notation and gives the appearance of hiding an error. If a change is required, document the change clearly and initial it on all copies.

CLINICAL PEARL

Standard procedure in many locales is to use a single line to mark out the error (e.g., ~~four~~) followed by the word "error," the correction, your initials, and the date and time changed.

General Precautions

ⓠ What do the terms universal precautions, BSI, standard precautions, and PPE mean?

ⓐ *Universal precautions* is a term for the precautions used by health care providers in the care of every patient. In out-of-hospital settings, gloves should be worn for all patient contacts. Masks, goggles, and gowns should be worn whenever there is the potential to be exposed to blood or body fluids. Body substance isolation *(BSI)* is a term for a process used by health care providers to isolate themselves from potentially dangerous body substances (e.g., blood, urine, or vomitus), especially in situations where it is difficult to distinguish exactly what body fluid is present. Established in 1996, *standard precautions* are the Centers for Disease Control's (CDC) revised guidelines regarding isolation precautions and replaces BSI and universal precautions. *PPE* is personal protective equipment such as gloves, goggles, and gowns used by health care providers to isolate or protect themselves from potentially dangerous body substances. Throughout this book, we use the terms *BSI* and *standard precautions* interchangeably.

During the administration of medications to a patient, there is always a potential risk for exposure and infection. Because most of the out-of-hospital drugs are given parenterally, the risk for exposure is higher for out-of-hospital care providers. Presently, exposure to and transmission of the hepatitis C virus (HCV) is occurring in alarming numbers in health care providers. The CDC predicts that the death rate from HCV will exceed that of AIDS within the next 10 years.

In studies that assessed risk factors for infection, accidental needle sticks or cuts with sharp instruments have been associated with the transmission of HCV and one study reported the transmission of HCV through a blood splash to the conjunctiva. The message here is to always use PPE and be very careful when working with sharps, especially in the uncontrolled environment of the field.

> *Studies show that the greater the risk of body fluid exposure, the less likely health care providers use appropriate PPE. Remember that your first responsibility is to ensure your own safety!*

❓ What is the difference between clean and sterile techniques? When would each be used?

🅰 Sterile or aseptic technique is a method used during a procedure to prevent contamination to the body using instruments that are sterilized and by wearing sterile gloves, masks, and gowns. Usually, persons performing the procedure have washed their hands and arms using special disinfectants following protocols. The word *asepsis* means a condition free from germs, infection, and any form of life. Surgery is performed with aseptic technique.

In out-of-hospital care, no procedure can be performed with total aseptic technique. However, certain procedures do require the highest aseptic technique possible. For example, deep suctioning through an endotracheal (ET) tube is a procedure that is performed with sterilized equipment, including sterile solution, catheter, and gloves. The goggles and mask are usually not sterile, gowns are rarely worn for this procedure, and of course, the environment is not sterile.

Most of the remaining procedures are performed with a very clean technique using sterile and clean equipment. Starting an IV, medication administration, and inserting an ET tube are all pro-

> *The term "sterile technique" refers to the use of sterile gloves, sterilized instruments, and antiseptic skin preparations under ideal conditions. Virtually no medical procedure is 100 percent "aseptic" or "sterile," though the operating room environment comes close. The out-of-hospital setting, despite all provider efforts, is no exception. When we use the term "sterile technique," the implication is that the EMS provider did everything under the circumstances to maintain as much sterility as possible.*

cedures that are performed with both sterile and nonsterile equipment.

❓ What are sharps and why are they dangerous?

🅰 Sharps are any medical product that can cause a puncture or cut to anyone that handles them. This can include any broken medical glassware, syringes, needles, scalpel blades, suture needles, and disposable razors. The CDC recommends that, in addition to PPE, standard precautions include the appropriate disposal of needles and other sharps and hand washing immediately following patient contact.

The danger with sharps is more than just being cut or punctured. The risk is being exposed to a contaminated sharp and contracting a disease. To prevent accidental sticks, needles should *never* be recapped. Studies have shown that recapping needles significantly increases the chance of injury and exposure. Because the potential risk for exposure is present, dispose of all sharps in sharps containers, a special puncture-resistant container usually made of thick plastic and colored red. Using this special container for the disposal of sharps is the only proper way to dispose of a sharp. Therefore, a sharps container must be at the patient's side when procedures are done. When a sharps container is full, it is considered medical waste and has specific disposal requirements.

Medication Administration Principles and Procedures

❓ When should EMS providers draw blood samples?

🅰 In the out-of-hospital setting, blood drawing is usually guided by local protocol. Any patient receiving medication or fluid should have a blood sample drawn beforehand in accordance with local protocols. However, in a true emergency, such as anaphylaxis or cardiac arrest, there may not be time. A great deal of information may be obtained by testing blood samples. Though additional in-hospital tests may be required, blood samples drawn in the out-of-hospital setting are helpful in detecting:

- Possible acute myocardial infarction (AMI)—samples are used for cardiac enzyme testing and possible fibrinolytic therapy.
- Possible cerebrovascular accident (CVA)—samples are used for possible fibrinolytic therapy.
- Hypovolemia—samples are used for blood type and cross, and hemoglobin and hematocrit levels.
- Diabetic emergency—samples are used for glucose levels.
- Possible overdose—samples are used to determine substance levels for possible toxicity.

- Altered mental status (AMS)—samples are used to determine the cause of the AMS.

- Allergic reaction—samples are used to check for poisoning and the level of allergens.

Although there is more than one way to obtain a blood sample, the preferred method is to obtain the sample while starting the IV. Collect samples in vacuum-sealed blood tubes with a rubber cap. The vacuum creates negative pressure inside the tube, helping to draw blood in. Some of the tubes contain small amounts of chemicals to keep the blood from clotting or to otherwise prepare it for testing. The color of the rubber stopper indicates the contents of the tube. A "red top" has no chemicals, "purple tops" and "blue tops" contain different anticoagulants. Check the expiration date on each tube before use. Though in-hospital specimens may be kept on ice, this is rarely done in the out-of-hospital setting.

The most popular device used to take blood samples is a Vacutainer®. This is a plastic barrel-shaped syringe with an opening at one end that slips over the tube and a small opening at the other end that a covered needle is threaded into (Figure 8–1).

- The needle has a port at the end outside the Vacutainer® holder that plugs into an angiocatheter that has been cannulated (placed in a vein). The needle draws (pulls) the blood from the cannulated vein into the tube. The Vacutainer® stays in place while tubes are switched after filling. After drawing the samples, the holder is removed and the IV line is inserted into the angiocatheter.

- Another method to draw blood using the Vacutainer® is to use an adapter needle with needles on both ends. One of the needles has a long hollow shaft that is used to pierce a vein directly without having to start an IV first.

Other equipment needed includes a tourniquet, alcohol preps (when taking blood alcohol samples, use iodine instead), a small gauze, and tape or a Band-Aid®.

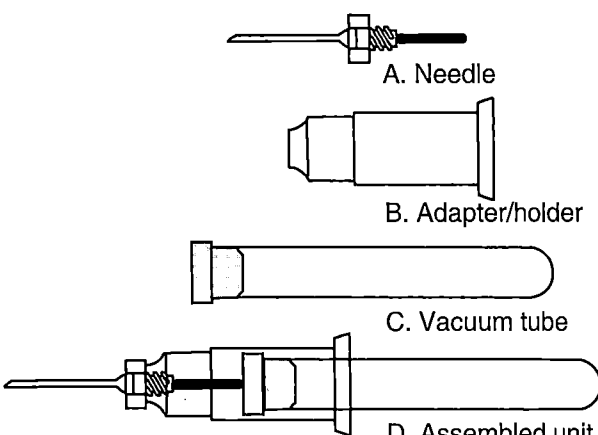

A. Needle

B. Adapter/holder

C. Vacuum tube

D. Assembled unit

FIGURE 8–1 Vacutainer® with needles.

Before Vacutainers® became popular, the method used to obtain blood samples was to draw the blood into a large syringe and then transfer the blood into the blood tubes. This is done by threading a cannulated needle onto a syringe and directly inserting it into the vein. When the syringe is full, the blood is transferred into the blood tubes by placing the needle into the rubber top of the tube. If an IV was started first, a syringe with a Luer-Lok™ tip could be screwed directly on to the angiocatheter and filled. When the syringe is filled, it is unscrewed from the angiocatheter and a needle is attached to the syringe. The tubes are filled by placing the needle into the rubber top.

Whatever method is used, the preparation procedure is the same:

- Place a tourniquet above the vein to be cannulated or drawn from (usually on the back of the hand or on the arm) to create a back up of venous blood that will make the veins stand out.

CLINICAL PEARL

A tourniquet should only occlude venous blood flow. When a tourniquet is placed too tight, it occludes the arterial flow and the veins will not stand out. Often a BP cuff is used as a tourniquet. To occlude only venous blood flow, do not inflate the cuff more than 70–80 mmhg.
- *Clean and prep the skin at the site of injection with an alcohol prep or iodine to minimize the risk of infection.*
- *Puncture the vein and obtain the appropriate blood sample.*

Q **Why are there different colored tops on blood sample tubes?**

A The different "colors" of the tops indicate the contents of the tube. Table 8–1 summarizes the most common tubes.

Q **In what order are the tubes filled?**

A Generally, dry tubes are filled first to prevent cross contamination with tubes containing fluid. However, local protocol, which is often driven by local hospital preference, will guide the answer to the order of filling blood tubes.

Q **What are the complications associated with drawing blood samples?**

A There is a potential for exposure to infectious disease if the patient's blood enters your body through a break in the skin (e.g., puncture or cut). The most common complication is that the patient develops a local infection at the site of injection. This is directly associated with poor (dirty) technique by the person who performed the skill. Other risks include secondary or systemic infections that originated from the local infection, soft tis-

TABLE 8-1

Colored Blood Tubes			
Color Top	Contents	Use	Pseudonyms
Light blue top	Sodium citrate (anticoagulant)	Clotting function tests (PT, INR, PTT)	Blue top, citrate tube, coag tube
Red/gray (speckled) top	Polymer gel and silica activator to separate serum and cells	Any test where serum is required	Tiger top, serum separator tube (SST), separator tube, speckled top, camouflaged tube
Plain red top	None (silicone-coating)	Must be used for blood banking; may be used whenever serum is required for testing	Clot tube, plain red
Green top	Freeze-dried sodium heparin (anticoagulant)	Ammonia, ionized calcium, tissue typing	Green top
Lavender top	EDTA (anticoagulant)	Complete blood count (CBC), platelet count, sed rate	Purple top
Yellow top	Acid-citrate-dextrose (anticoagulant, sugar mixture)	Blood banking, DNA, paternity testing	Yellow top

sue hematoma, muscle or nerve damage, and miscannulation of an artery instead of the vein.

Q **If a police officer wants the EMS provider to draw a blood sample for blood alcohol testing, can the EMS provider refuse?**

A This is a sensitive area—state, system, and local protocols provide guidance. Basically, your agency and medical director should answer this question before it arises! Be sure you understand what your system's requirements are and what the procedure entails. If the EMS provider does take a sample, in most cases the drawing has to be witnessed by the officer requesting the sample to maintain a chain of evidence. No alcohol preps are used to prepare for the needle stick as it may skew the sample. Document the procedure and the entire call well and be prepared to go to court later.

CLINICAL PEARL

Though rare, health care providers have been arrested for refusing to comply with police requests. Convictions have been few, but the expense and embarrassment of litigation takes a significant toll. Have written protocols in place before this situation ever occurs!

Q **What are the ways to administer medications?**

A The following is a list of many but not all of the routes for drug administration. The EMS provider may be trained to perform any of these and more, but local protocol will dictate which of these they can actually perform in the out-of-hospital setting.

- ET (parenteral)—injection into an endotracheal tube.
- Epidural (parenteral)—injection into the spinal canal on or outside the dura mater that surrounds the spinal column.
- Inhalation (parenteral)—inhaled as a gas or aerosol.
- Intraaticular (parenteral)—injection into the synovial cavity of a joint to relieve joint pain and reduce inflammation.
- Intracardiac (parenteral)—injection into the chambers of the heart.
- Intraosseous (IO) (parenteral)—injection into the bone marrow.
- Intraperitoneal (parenteral)—injection into the peritoneal cavity.
- Intraplueral (parenteral)—injection into the pleura.
- Intrathecal (parenteral)—injection into the spinal column.
- Intramuscular (IM) (parenteral)—injection into skeletal muscle.
- Intravenous (IV) (parenteral)—injection directly into the bloodstream.
- Lingual/buccal (enteral)—dissolved between the cheek and gum.
- Nasogastric (enteral)—injection directly into the stomach through a tube inserted into a nostril, down the esophagus, and into the stomach.
- Oral/ingestion (enteral)—swallowed and absorbed in the stomach or small intestine.
- Oral spray (enteral)—absorbed across the mucous membrane of the mouth.
- Pulmonary route—aerosolized through metered dose inhaler (MDI) or small volume nebulizer (SVN).
- Rectal (enteral)—suppositories placed per rectum.
- Subcutaneous (SC or SQ) (parenteral)—injection under the dermis into connective tissue or fat.
- Sublingual (enteral)—dissolved under the tongue and absorbed across the mucous membrane of the mouth.
- Transdermal/topical (parenteral)—absorbed through the skin.

- Umbilical (parenteral)—injection directly into the bloodstream through a special angiocatheter placed in the umbilical stump of a neonate.

❓ What is the difference between enteral and parenteral routes of administration?

🅰 Enteral drug administration is through the GI tract either orally or per rectum. The parenteral routes of administration include any route other than the alimentary canal and are for injected drugs.

❓ What are the advantages and disadvantages of enteral versus parenteral medication administration?

🅰 The enteral drug route advantages are that it is considered the most convenient and the most economical. The disadvantages are that it is the slowest and least reliable route. The parenteral routes work well for emergencies because of the faster and more predictable absorption effects. For example, in the case of a severe allergic reaction, diphenahydramine (Benadryl) administered IV will have a much faster effect than IM or PO (oral intake). PO would have to travel through the gastrointestinal (GI) tract before it becomes effective. IM is quicker than PO, but when shock is present as in an allergic reaction, absorption will be too slow. Therefore, IV administration is the best choice if IV access is quickly available.

❓ How are parenteral drugs administered?

🅰 Parenteral drug routes include any route that is not enteral (oral or per rectum). Most medications administered by the EMS provider are parenteral because the effects from absorption are faster and more predictable than enteral. The most common parenteral routes for drug administration used by the paramedic include:

- IV—intravenous injection directly into the bloodstream using a catheter over the needle or butterfly needle. Alternate IV access routes include two types of central venous catheters (CVC). These types of catheters are positioned in the inferior vena cava, superior vena cava, or the right atrium of the heart. The first type of catheter is a surgically placed indwelling catheter used for long-term care. Hickman®, Brovia, and Groshong catheters are examples of this type of catheter, which has a distal port (access point) outside of the chest. The second type of CVC is also surgically placed. The Port-A-Cath®, Medi-Port®, and INFUSAPORT® require a special type of catheter (Huber needle) to access the port that lies under the skin, usually on the upper chest or arm of the patient. This is an area where there should be a local protocol and training to orient EMS providers in the use of these devices (Figure 8–2).

- IM—intramuscular injection into skeletal muscle using a 19- or 21-gauge, 1½- to 2-inch needle.
- SC—subcutaneous injection under the dermis into connective tissue or fat using a 23- or 25-gauge, ½- to ⅝-inch needle or tuberculin (TB) syringe.
- IO—intraosseous injection into the bone marrow using a commercial I/O or bone marrow biopsy needle.
- Percutaneous—transderm or topical that is absorbed through the skin or mucous membranes.
- ET—endotracheal, nasal tracheal, or transtracheal injection into an endotracheal tube.
- SLI—sublingual injection directly into the bottom portion of the base of the tongue. Though aesthetically unpleasant, this route provides rapid central circulatory access. Drugs given in less than 1 cc of volume are absorbed in all nonarrested patients as rapidly as in a central IV line. Follow your local protocols.

❓ In which sizes do needles and syringes come?

🅰 Needles vary in length from ⅜ inch to 3 or more inches. The gauge can vary from 12 gauge (very large lumen) to 28 gauge

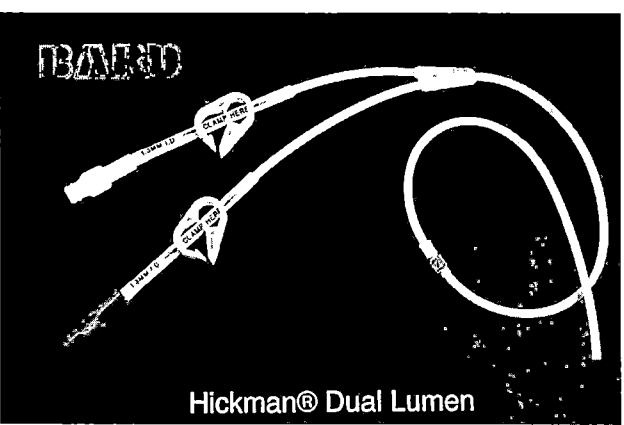

Hickman® Dual Lumen

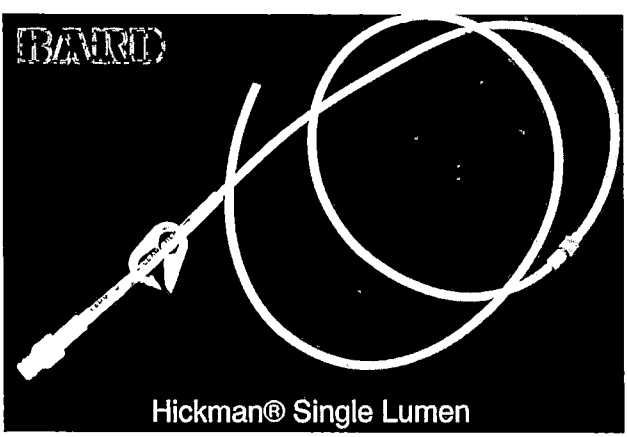

Hickman® Single Lumen

FIGURE 8–2 Hickman® central venous catheter.

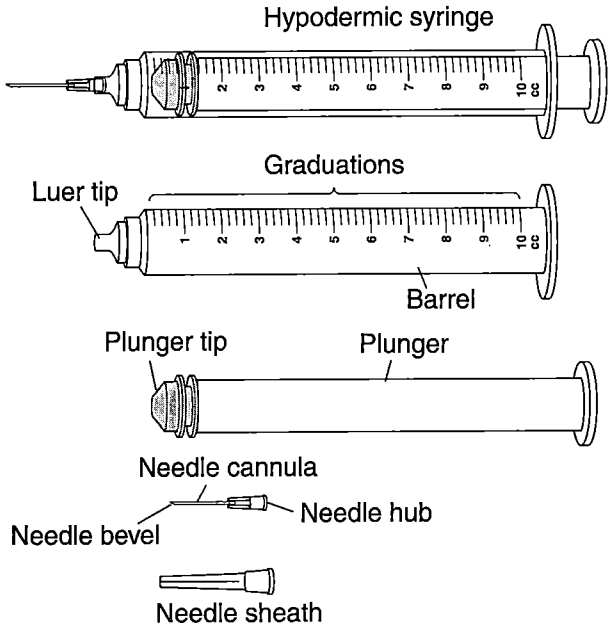

Hypodermic syringe

Graduations

Luer tip

Barrel

Plunger tip   Plunger

Needle cannula

Needle hub

Needle bevel

Needle sheath

FIGURE 8-3 Syringe.

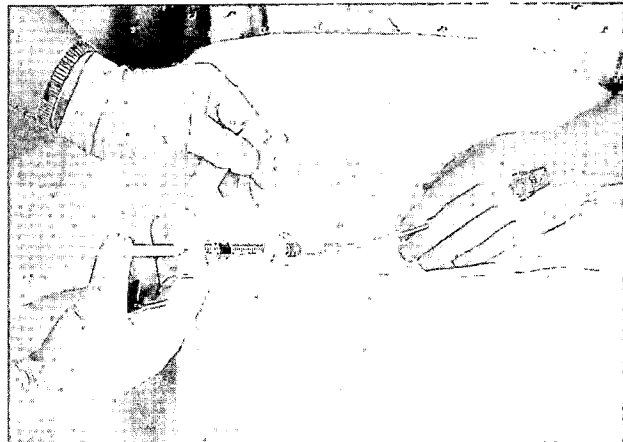

FIGURE 8-4 Needle injection port/saline/heparin lock.

(very small lumen). Commonly used syringes range in size from 1-ml TB and insulin syringes to 60-ml. Syringes have markings to accurately measure liquids and liquid medications (Figure 8–3).

🅠 Where are the locations for administering medications with needles?

🅐 The size and length of a needle to be used is determined by the location of the injection. Larger needles are used for IM sites, while smaller needles are used for SC sites. The anatomical locations for each type of injection are:

- IM. The deltoid muscle of the shoulder and upper arm, the upper outside quadrant of the gluteus muscle, or the vastus lateralis and the rectus femoris muscles located in the thigh are commonly used.

- SC. For these injections, the total volume to be injected is usually less then 0.5 ml. The deltoid muscle of the shoulder, the anterior thigh muscles, or the lateral abdominal muscles are common sites.

- IO. This method of cannulation is used most often in the emergent pediatric patient with no immediate vascular access. The preferred site for cannulation is usually the proximal tibia, 2 cm below the tibial tuberosity. Another site is the distal tibia, just above the medial malleolus.

- IV. Use the injection or access port closest to the patient, and clamp the IV line above the injection port during administration to prevent the medication from back flowing in the line (Figure 8–4). After the injection is complete, unclamp the line and flush the medication through.

🅠 What is the difference between IM, SC, and intradermal medication administration?

🅐 IM is a route of drug administration directly into body muscle for slow absorption (Figure 8–5). The total volume of medication given via this route is no more than 5 cc's, but is usually less (as in 1–3 cc's). Outside the hospital, the most common drugs administered IM are glucagon, Narcan, morphine, and Valium®.

SC or SQ is a route of drug administration directly into the subcutaneous or fatty tissue under the skin and overlying the muscle so that the medications are absorbed into the systemic circulation (Figure 8–6). The rate of absorption is slower than with the IM and IV routes. The total volume of medication given via this route is small, usually no more than 1 cc. The most

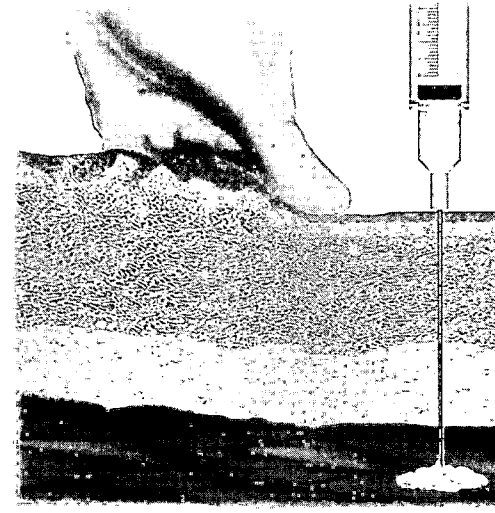

FIGURE 8-5 IM injection is a common route for administration of epinephrine in the field.

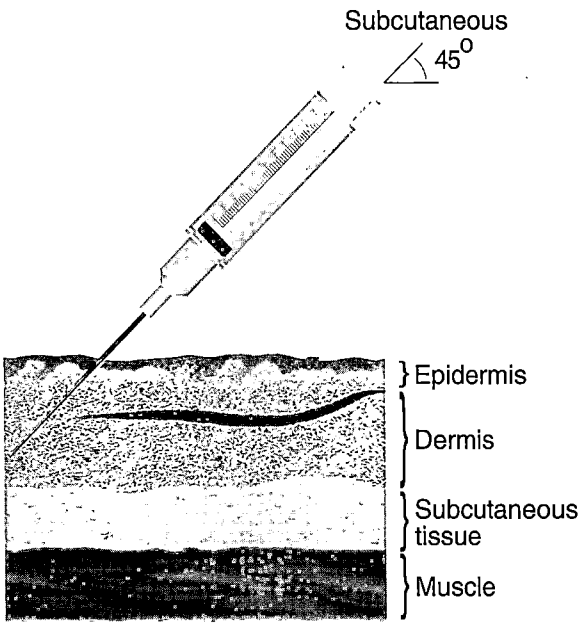

Subcutaneous

45°

} Epidermis

} Dermis

} Subcutaneous
tissue

} Muscle

FIGURE 8-6 SC injection technique.

common site for an SC injection is the deltoid muscle of the shoulder. The out-of-hospital drug most commonly given SC is epinephrine. Intradermal injection is a route of drug administration directly below the epidermis as seen with the Mantoux test for tuberculosis.

Poor perfusion and a cold ambient temperature can cause delayed absorption in any of the routes of drug administration. IM drug administration should be avoided in patients suspected of having an AMI (acute myocardial infarction), as it may elevate enzyme levels (lactic dehydrogenase or LDH) and delay or prevent a speedy diagnosis of AMI.

When is IV medication administration indicated?

Out-of-hospital IV drug administration is the fastest route for drug absorption and is ideal for emergencies.

Why is it necessary to flush the IV line after administering a drug or between administering different drugs?

The primary reason to flush an IV line after administering a drug is to get the drug out of the sometimes lengthy IV line and into the bloodstream. Adenosine is a drug with an extremely short half-life, so a large and rapid flush is required to get the drug into the bloodstream before it becomes inactive.

It is necessary to flush an IV line between the administration of different drugs because some drugs, such as sodium bicarbonate combined with calcium, can cause precipitates

(deposits) to form and clog the line. Bicarbonate can also interact with other drugs and inactivate them; for example, when combined with catecholamines and vasopressors such as epinephrine and dopamine.

When is IO medication administration indicated?

IO infusion is a quick access route for drugs and fluids. Access is gained by placing a hollow needle with a stylet into the medullary cavity of a bone. The proximal tibia is the preferred site, but the distal tibia and the distal femur may be used.

Is IO access better than IV access?

When vascular access is not immediately available, IO is fast and reliable; however, it is used only as a temporary access. IV access is better for long-term vascular access. IO access is generally used with a pediatric patient; however, it is not restricted to pediatric use.

What are the special considerations when using inhaled medications?

Inhaled drugs work directly on the lung tissue with little systemic effects. When administering aerosolized medications, be sure not to inhale the drug yourself. Wearing a mask can reduce this risk.

What exactly is the EMS provider's responsibility when administrating medications?

All health care professions who prescribe, dispense, or administer medication are legally responsible for their actions. EMS providers are required to document the time, dose, and route of medications administered on a PCR, as well as the patient's response to the medication. When a narcotic has been administered to a patient, most systems require additional documentation from both the person administering the drug and the physician who gave the order.

What do the abbreviations p.o., n.p.o., p.r.n., q.i.d., and b.i.d. mean?

The following is a list of abbreviations used in medication administration.

- b.i.d. = twice a day.
- b.i.n. = twice a night.
- /d = per day.
- n.p.o. = nothing by mouth.

- p.o. = by mouth.
- p.r.n. = as needed.
- q.h. = every hour.
- q.i.d. = four times a day.
- q.d. = per day.
- t.i.d. = three times a day.
- t.i.n. = three times a night.

What are the general principles for administration of parenteral drugs?

EMS providers *are* responsible for knowing the indications and contraindications for any drug they administer. In addition, they must understand and be prepared to manage any adverse reactions and potential side effects that develop as a result of that drug. The "six rights" of drug administration must be practiced each time.

Adhere to local protocols, using direct or indirect medical control when necessary. Each agency should have written procedures for storing, stocking, and restocking of all medications.

What are the complications associated with parenteral drug administration?

The complications are the same as for drawing blood samples. Additional complications, such as unexpected adverse reactions and side effects, may result from the following medication administration errors:

- Incorrect route of administration.
- Incorrect dose as prescribed by the physician.

How are enteral drugs administered?

Because enteral routes are through the alimentary canal, which begins at the mouth and ends at the rectum, enteral drugs are taken orally (PO) or rectally (PR). Oral drugs are easy to take, making them the most popular form of home medication. Oral medications can be prescription or over-the-counter (OTC). As discussed in Chapter 7, Pharmacology, they are available in many forms.

Nausea and vomiting are common in a variety of illnesses. For this reason, patients are given nothing by mouth (n.p.o.), including oral medications. Once at the hospital, many procedures (e.g., anesthesia) require an empty stomach and few people can swallow pills without drinking something. One of the few medications that is given orally by the EMS provider is baby aspirin. Baby aspirin is very useful in the presence of an AMI, tastes good, and can be chewed easily without drinking anything. Other examples include activated charcoal, oral glucose, and ipecac.

What is the difference between oral, lingual, sublingual, and buccal medication administration?

Oral drug administration is when a drug is placed in the mouth, chewed, and swallowed for digestion by the GI system. Lingual refers to the tongue. An example of a drug given lingually is nitro spray; it is sprayed directly on the tongue. Sublingual medications are placed under the tongue as in the administration of nitro pills. A buccal tablet is designed to be placed in the mouth between the cheek and gum. It is dissolved there through the buccal mucosa. Generally speaking, the mucosa in the mouth is highly vascular and absorbs drugs quickly.

When would a drug be administered rectally?

Rectal drugs are given to pediatric patients who cannot take oral medications easily or at all, unconscious or altered mental status patients, vomiting patients, and patients with upper GI ailments. This route is also an alternate route for the seizure patient with difficult IV access. The rectum is vascular, allowing for a rapid absorption that does not go through biotransformation in the liver before reaching target organs.

Some medications come in the form of suppositories—a single dose of a drug in an oblique-shaped capsule made of soap, gelatin, or cocoa butter. Suppositories are placed into the rectum where they dissolve. Others are given in liquid form. Drugs that may be useful rectally in the out-of-hospital setting include Phenergan®, aspirin, or Valium®.

Is any special equipment required for rectal drug administration?

Adult suppositories may have a commercial injector to facilitate placement in the rectum. A common method for pediatrics is to draw up the appropriate dose in a syringe and attach a #10 French suction catheter. Lubricate the catheter and carefully place it into the rectum approximately 3–5 cm and insert the medication. A small flush, 5 ml, with normal saline to clear the catheter is recommended. This method works in adults as well.

What special considerations apply when administering medication through an ET tube?

The choice of drug administration via the ET tube is usually chosen when vascular access is unavailable. The drugs given via this route are emergency medications and are administered at 2 to 2.5 times the recommended vascular dose diluted in a total of 10 ml of normal saline. Not all drugs can be administered by this route. The emergency drugs that can be so administered are represented by the acronyms LEAN or LANE.

L—lidocaine.

A—atropine.

N—Narcan.

E—epinephrine.

The acronym NAVEL was taught for many years and included the drug Valium® (diazepam); however, this is no longer recommended. A few other drugs that have been effective through the ET route are the nebulized medications such as Albuterol and atrovent.

When is a drug administered through a gastric tube?

A gastric tube may be in place through the nose (nasogastric tube, Levin's tube®) or through the mouth (orogastric tube). The gastric tube is not a primary route for medication administration; however, it is an available route when a patient will not swallow, has an altered mental state (AMS), is unconscious, or unable to swallow. Activated charcoal is an example of a medication that may be given by nasogastric tube.

Are there any possible complications with gastric tube medication administration?

The primary concern with this procedure is to ensure that the airway is protected. The reason a gastric tube is placed is either to evacuate the gastric contents by lavage or to relieve distension of the stomach.

How are medications given through a gastric tube?

Before placing anything down the gastric tube, confirm its correct placement by aspirating with a syringe or listening with a stethoscope over the epigastrium while injecting 20 cc of air. Check the "six rights" of medication administration. Once correct tube placement is confirmed, measure the dose of medication into a syringe, attach the syringe to the tube, and inject the medication. Observe for vomiting, possible aspiration, adverse reactions, and side effects.

When would an IV drip be used for medication administration?

An IV piggyback (IVPB) drip is used to maintain the desired therapeutic effect of a drug over a longer period of time, usually at a lower concentration than a bolus. Blood is often infused via a piggyback setup with an IV of normal saline. Watch for the backup of blood into the primary IV (usually normal saline) bag, indicating an obstruction of the IV flow.

Basics of Drug Dosages and Calculations

What are the three systems of measure used for drug administration?

The metric system is the standard system used internationally. The apothecary system is the old system used before the metric system. The household method is a system commonly used in the home, also called the United States system, and is based on the traditional English system.

What are the major units of measure in the metric system?

The metric system uses the decimal system, which is based on the number 10. The basic unit of mass (weight) is the gram; the basic unit of volume is the liter; and the basic unit of length is the meter. Adding prefixes to the basic unit name produces all of the other units of measure and these prefixes indicate how many times smaller or larger than the basic unit the new unit is (Table 8–2).

What are the major units of measure in the apothecary system?

Although the apothecary system is rarely used for ordering drugs anymore, there are some drugs that are available only in grains (1 grain = 64.7989 mg or 0.0648 gram). This is why the EMS provider should be able to use this system. The major units of measure for liquids and solids are as follows:

Liquids:

- Minims.
- Fluidrams.
- Fluidounces.
- Pints.
- Gallons.

TABLE 8–2

Metric Prefixes and Their Meanings	
Mega-	x 1,000,000
Kilo-	x 1,000
Hecto-	x 100
Deka-	x 10
Basic unit	1 (gram, liter, meter)
Deci-	1/10
Centi-	1/100
Milli-	1/1000
Micro-	1/1,000,000

Solids:

- Grains.
- Drams.
- Ounces.
- Pounds.

🅠 What are the major units of measure in the household system?

🅐 The major units of measure are:

- Drop.
- Teaspoon.
- Tablespoon.
- Cup.
- Glass.
- Pint.
- Quart.
- Gallon.

🅠 Is one milligram (mg) the same as one cubic centimeter (cc) for medications?

🅐 Not always, cc is the physical measurement of a liquid, while mg is the concentration of the drug. For example, epinephrine may be packaged as 1 mg in 1 cc or as 10 mg in 1 cc. The latter is 10 times the concentration of the first, but both are in the same amount of fluid.

🅠 Is there a difference between cc and ml?

🅐 Cubic centimeter (cc) is a volume and milliliter (ml) is a capacity, but the U.S. equivalent for both is 0.061 cubic inch.

🅠 What is the difference between KVO and TKO?

🅐 There is no difference. KVO, *keep vein open,* and TKO, *to keep open,* both refer to the drip rate of an IV. This rate is approximately one drop every two seconds. This is the standard rate used when an IV is kept in place for purposes other than replacing fluids.

🅠 What is the difference between a macro and micro drip set?

🅐 The number of drops needed to equal 1 ml by a drip set is called the gtt (drops) of the set. A micro drip set is fixed to drip

60 gtt or 60 drops to equal 1 ml. The macro drip set is fixed to allow larger drops in 1 ml to get fluids through faster. The three common macro drip sets are 10 gtt, 15 gtt, and 20 gtt.

🅠 What mathematical principles should the EMS provider understand in order to administer drugs?

🅐 The EMS provider must have a reasonable understanding of several mathematical concepts to understand the units of drug measurement:

- Percentages—a part of a whole expressed in hundredths.
- Proportions or ratios—the relation of one part to another or to a whole.
- Fractions and decimal fractions—a numerical representation such as 1/2 or 3.323 indicating the quotient of two numbers.
- Roman numerals—a numeral in a system of characters that is based on the ancient Roman system.
- Multiplication.
- Division.
- Calculation methods for drug dosages.
- Fahrenheit—a scale for measuring temperature with the boiling point of water at 212 degrees and the freezing point at 32 degrees above zero.
- Celsius—also called centigrade, a scale for measuring temperature with the boiling point of water at 100 degrees and the freezing point at 0 degrees.

🅠 Does an EMS provider have to know any conversion ratios?

🅐 Yes, the EMS provider should know or at least be familiar with the mathematical equivalents used in pharmacology. One does not have to commit them all to memory, but should be able to locate and understand them from a reference source. The four conversions listed here are the most common used in out-of-hospital care.

1. Conversion within the same system:
   - First, review Table 8–2. Given this information, how many grams are there in 1,500 mg? (Answer: 1.5 grams)
   - How many centimeters are in 2 meters? (Answer: 200)
2. Conversion between the metric and household systems:
   - Given the following example, how many tablespoons should the patient receive if the order is for 30 ml of a specific medication? (Answer: 2) One tablespoon = 15 ml, so divide 30 ml by 15 ml = 2 tbl.

     Example: 30 ml = 1 ounce
                 15 ml = 1 tbl.
                  5 ml = 1 tsp.

3. Conversion between pounds (lbs) and kilograms (kgs):

- The formula is to divide the pounds by 2.2 to arrive at the approximate equivalent in kilograms. (220 lbs ÷ 2.2 = 100 kg)

- For a quick conversion, take half of the patient's body weight, in pounds, and subtract 10 percent.

4. Conversion between Fahrenheit and Celsius:

- The formula to convert Fahrenheit to Celsius is to subtract 32 and multiply by 5/9. $(101°F - 32) \times 5/9 = 38.3°C$

- To convert Celsius to Fahrenheit, multiply by 9/5 and add 32. $35°C \times 9/5 + 32 = 95°F$

Q What drug calculations must the EMS provider be able to perform in order to administer medications in the field?

A The following formula calculations are the most frequently used in the field:

- The formula for dose of drug is:

    dose ordered × unit of measure ÷ amount on hand

    Example: The order is to administer 200 mg of aminophyline. You have a 10-ml vial that contains 500 mg of the drug. How many ml will you give? Using the formula, calculate the dose to be given.

$$200 \text{ mg} \times 10 \text{ ml} \div 500 \text{ mg}$$
$$4 \times 1 \text{ ml} = X$$

Answer: X = 4 ml

Using the formula, calculate the following problem:

The order is to administer 0.5 mg epinephrine of 1:1000 subcutaneously (SC) and the drug comes in a preloaded cartridge containing 1 mg in 1 ml of 1:1000. How much epinephrine is administered? (Answer: 0.5 ml)

- The formula for drug per kg:

    Step 1. Convert lb to kg (lbs ÷ 2.2 = kg).

    Step 2. Amount of drug × number of kg = amount to be given.

    Example: The order is to administer 0.01 mg per kg of epinephrine.

The patient weighs 24 lbs. Using the formula above, calculate the dose to be given.

Step 1. 24 lbs ÷ 2.2 = 10.91 kg (round up to 11 kg)
Step 2. 0.01 mg × 11 kg = 0.11 mg
Answer: 0.11 mg

Using the formula, calculate the following problem:

The order is to administer 5 mg per kg of Bretylium®, and the patient weighs 175 lbs. How much Bretylium® is administered? (Answer: 400 mg) To get the answer, the patient's weight must be converted to kg, and then multiplied by 5: 175 ÷ 2.2 = 79.55 (round to 80) × 5 = 400.

- The formula for drug or solution bolus over time:

    IV rate (gtt/min) = (volume to be given *in ml × gtt/ml* ÷ time for infusion *in min*

    Example: The order is to administer a 100-ml bolus over 30 minutes using a 15-gtt drip set. How many drops per minute will infuse the bolus?

Example: rate = (100 ml)(15 gtt/ml) ÷ 30 min
Answer: 50 gtt/min

Using the formula, calculate the following problem:

The order is to administer a 250-ml bolus of normal saline in 10 minutes, using a 10-gtt drip set. How many drops per minute will infuse the bolus?

rate = (250 cc)(10 gtt/ml) ÷ 10 min.
Answer: 25 gtt/min

Q What does percent mean to a pharmacist?

A Mathematically, percent means that portion of 100. For example, 10 percent is 10/100 or 1/10, a tenth. Percent has a much more specific definition to a pharmacist. Basically, the percentage number is the number of grams of a substance (solute) placed in every 100 cc of solvent (usually distilled water) to make up the drug. This mixture is constant whether making up 100 cc of the drug or a 55-gallon drum. Therefore, D5W is really D5%W, meaning every 100 cc of water has 5 grams of dextrose in it.

With this in mind, complete this exercise. Which one has more sugar in it, a Bristoget™ of D50 (packaged in a 50 cc preloaded syringe) or infusing 500 ml of D5W in a drip? The answer is that they both have the same amount of sugar, although there is much more water in the drip. Compare the following:

D50:

- Contains 50 grams per 100 cc of solvent.

- Each vial (amp) is 50 cc.

- So, if there are 50 grams in 100 cc, there are 25 grams in 50 cc.

- An amp of D50 (50 cc) contains 25 grams of sugar.

D5W:

- Contains 5 grams of sugar per 100 cc of solvent.

- Because every 100 cc of D5W contains 5 grams sugar, 500 cc contains five times as much or 25 grams of sugar.

Q How are the most common emergency drugs packaged?

A Many emergency drugs come in pre-loaded syringes (e.g., Abboject™, BristoJect™) that are fast and easy to use. The following is a list of the most common drug packaging devices currently used in the field:

- Pre-loaded cartridges—a prefilled cartridge that resembles a very small syringe, but does not include a barrel or plunger. The commercial injector (Tubex®) is reusable plastic (older Tubex® injectors were made of steel) that holds the prefilled cartridge and serves as the barrel and plunger.
- Pre-loaded syringes—include the barrel, the plunger (holds the drug), and the needle tip. The caps are removed from the barrel and plunger, and the two are threaded together.
- Vials—small glass containers with a rubber top containing the drug. The drug is extracted from the vial with a needle and syringe. Because many of the vials are very small, a volume of air equivalent in volume to the amount of drug to be withdrawn must first be injected into the vial to prevent a vacuum from forming.
- Ampules—small glass containers with an elongated top or neck that must be snapped off to access the drug. The top is scored to assist with opening; however, because the ampule is made entirely of glass, the potential for injury from a sharp edge is present. The drug is withdrawn with a needle and syringe. Be sure to check that the ampule is scored; otherwise, it will not break properly and may cause an injury. Hold a gauze pad over the top while snapping the ampule open to minimize the risk of injury.
- Needles and syringes—includes the barrel, which has markings for measuring the volume of product, and a plunger to push out the drug. A needle may come attached to a syringe or one can be threaded to the tip of the barrel.
- Transdermal patches—are small patches that resemble Band-Aids® and contain medication that is absorbed through the skin. Care must be taken when applying or removing these topical patches because anyone handling it can absorb the drug on the patch.
- Sprays—metered dose inhalers and small volume nebulizers dispense aerosolized medication. The inhaler is the classic "puffer" or inhaler that asthmatics use to self-administer their bronchodilator medication. The nebulizers produce an aerosolized mist that the patient inhales through a tube or mask.
- High dose for IV drip use only—high concentration medications that typically come in vials and have a warning (often a red label) that indicates the drug is to be mixed (diluted) prior to administration.

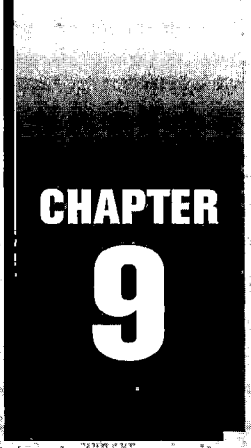

CHAPTER 9

Basic Cardiac Life Support

This chapter discusses the International Guidelines 2000 for basic life support (BLS). The focus is on the latest BLS changes and updates as well as *why* the changes have been made.

What are BLS and BCLS?

Basic life support (BLS) is the care provided in the first few minutes of a life-threatening emergency. Together with advanced cardiac life support (ACLS), it is part of the emergency cardiac care provided to patients experiencing symptoms of a heart attack. BLS is used interchangeably with basic cardiac life support (BCLS) when discussing cardiac care. Finally, BLS is often used to refer to the technique of cardiopulmonary resuscitation (CPR) when managing a cardiac arrest. For purposes of this chapter, we use the acronym BCLS to mean the resuscitative care of a patient with an acute coronary syndrome.

> **CLINICAL PEARL**
>
> *An acute coronary syndrome ranges from acute angina to myocardial infarction. It is a "catch all" term devised to emphasize that many times it is impossible to tell the difference between unstable angina and infarction. Your first task is to recognize that the patient may have an acute coronary syndrome.*

Where did the International Guidelines 2000 come from?

A series of discussions and debates have been conducted since March 1999 by internationally recognized experts in resuscitation. In September 1999, there was an evidence evaluation conference attended by more than 250 people. In February 2000, more than 500 people continued to review, debate, and discuss the proposals, and ultimately came to a consensus on the guidelines. During the following months, the guidelines were finalized through the use of a restricted-access Web site where drafts were posted and revised. In September 2000, the finalized guidelines began to be disseminated to the American Heart Association (AHA) National Faculty and the resuscitation community at the Emergency Cardiac Care Conference and Exposition in San Diego, CA.

Where can the unabridged version of the International Guidelines 2000 be found?

These were published in American Heart Association publication, *Circulation*, Vol. 102, No. 8, August 22, 2000.

What was the goal of the International Guidelines 2000 committee?

The goal was to develop valid, widely accepted international resuscitation guidelines that were based on scientific evidence and accepted by the international resuscitation community. Clearly, International Guidelines 2000 is not merely an AHA document because 40 percent of the participants at the conference were not from the United States. At least one U.S. scientist and one non-U.S. scientist evaluated each guideline topic.

What is meant by "new guidelines?"

New guidelines include a reappraisal of existing recommendations as well as new recommendations for medical devices, drugs, and interventions.

What were the levels of evidence used to develop the Guidelines?

The Guidelines were developed using an evidence-based, rigorous review of the published scientific evidence and studies on resuscitation. The principles of evidence-based medicine classifies interventions into one of five categories: Class I, IIa, IIb, Indeterminate, and III.

What is a Class I designation?

According to the Guidelines, "Class I guidelines are supported by excellent, definitive evidence of effectiveness in humans; must have at least one prospective randomized, controlled, positive clinical trial." Examples of Class I BLS interventions (the ALS interventions are listed in Chapter 52, Advanced Cardiac Life Support) include:

- Early defibrillation within five minutes of the EMS call.
- First responders should provide defibrillation, when appropriate, in less than three minutes in all areas of hospital and ambulatory care facilities.

What is a Class IIa designation?

According to the Guidelines, "Class IIa guidelines are supported by very good evidence of effectiveness and safety in humans." Examples of Class IIa BLS interventions and recommendations include:

- During rescue breathing, a ventilation tidal volume of 10 ml/kg (700 to 1,000 ml) delivered over two seconds until a well-defined chest rise is observed when using mouth-to-mouth or mouth-to-mask without supplemental oxygen.

- Chest-compression-only CPR when the rescuer is unwilling or unable to perform mouth-to-mouth rescue breathing.
- Chest-compression-only CPR for use with dispatcher-assisted CPR instructions to simplify the technique so bystanders can intervene rapidly.
- Lay rescuers will no longer be taught to check for a carotid pulse. Instead, they will be taught to look and examine for "signs of circulation," which include normal breathing, coughing, or movement.
- Health care providers with a duty to perform CPR should be trained, equipped, and authorized to perform defibrillation.
- Early defibrillation capability, including equipment and trained first responders, should be available throughout hospitals and affiliated outpatient facilities.
- Response time intervals for in-hospital resuscitation events are often inaccurate and must be corrected before documented defibrillation can be considered reliable.
- BLS responders such as police, firefighters, security personnel, ski patrol members, ferryboat crews, and airline flight attendants should be trained in CPR and the use of an automated external defibrillator (AED).
- Biphasic waveform defibrillation with shocks of less than 200 joules is safe and has the equivalent or higher efficacy for the termination of ventricular fibrillation as the higher-energy escalating, monophasic waveform shocks.
- Leaving the nontraumatic cardiac arrest victim, after an adequate trial of BLS and ALS has been done, and supporting the survivors.
- Having a medical director available for real-time consultation and able to authorize cessation of the resuscitation when an adequate trial of BLS and ALS has been unsuccessful. This is the time to change the focus to supporting the survivors.

What is a Class IIb designation?

According to the Guidelines, "Class IIb guidelines are supported by fair to good evidence of effectiveness and safety in humans; no evidence of harm." Examples of Class IIb BLS interventions and recommendations include:

- Hospital-based intra-arterial fibrinolytic agents may be beneficial within three to six hours of symptom onset in stroke patients with middle cerebral occlusions.
- Patients with suspected stroke and airway compromise or altered level of consciousness (LOC) merit the same high priority for dispatch, treatment, and transport as patients with AMI or major trauma.

- EMS providers should transport stroke patients, and provide prearrival notification, to an emergency facility with the proven capability to initiate fibrinolytic therapy within one hour of arrival unless such a facility is more than 30 minutes away by ground ambulance.

- A tidal volume of 6 to 7 ml/kg (approximately 400 to 600 ml) is delivered over one to two seconds until a chest rise is observed when a bag-valve mask (BVM) or mouth-to-mask device with supplemental oxygen is used.

- Alternative airway devices, such as the laryngeal mask airway (LMA) or Combitube®, may be better than BVM ventilation when used by trained health care providers who are able to maintain their knowledge and skills through practice.

- The compression rate for one and two rescuer adult CPR is increased to 100 per minute.

- The ratio of 15 compressions to 2 ventilations is recommended for both one and two rescuer adult CPR for the adult victim with an unprotected (nonintubated) airway.

- For teaching and performing CPR, audio timing prompts may help the rescuer achieve the required rate of performing chest compressions.

- Emphasis for the foreign body airway obstruction (FBAO) of an unresponsive adult should be placed on opening the airway, providing ventilation, and delivering chest compressions.

- Use of AEDs in children over eight years of age is recommended.

- The two-thumb-encircling-hands chest compression technique is the preferred method for two health care providers to use on newborns and infants of appropriate size.

What is a Class Indeterminate designation?

According to the Guidelines, "Class Indeterminate interventions or actions are proposed guidelines with insufficient evidence to support a final recommendation for clinical use. Often these are ideas at a preliminary research stage, promising but in need of more research at a higher level." Examples of Class Indeterminate BLS interventions and recommendations include:

- A "special situations" section should be added to all BLS lay rescuer training materials to identify exceptions to the phone-first and phone-fast rules.

- Victims who are unresponsive and breathing and have signs of circulation should be placed in a recovery position. The recovery position is lying the patient on his side with the head and neck extended so fluid can drain from the mouth.

- Citizens at work sites or in public places should have CPR and AED training.

- Use of AEDs in infants and children under eight years of age.

What is a Class III designation?

According to the Guidelines, "Class III interventions or actions are almost always existing guidelines that continue to be reviewed and researched. New evidence or review of old evidence strongly suggests or confirms the probability of harm. These interventions are not useful, may be harmful, and thus are unacceptable." Examples of Class III BLS interventions include:

- Abdominal thrusts in infants.

- Transportation of nontraumatic cardiac arrest victims to an ED after an adequate trial of BLS and ALS has been provided. Pulselessness should be documented and continuous during the trial of therapy.

Is it true that the American Heart Association is planning to offer first aid courses?

Actually they already do. The Heart Facts course is a collaborative effort of both the American Heart Association and the National Safety Council. Critics of that course have said that there simply is too much material covered in a very short amount of time. Following the evidence-based process, work is ongoing to issue several evidence-based first aid guidelines. The necessity of CPR and AED training in the workplace is evident in most cases of workplace cardiovascular emergencies. By adding evidence-based first aid training, instructors will be able to provide a complete package to meet most regulatory requirements for training in the workplace.

Is it true that the "Do Not Resuscitate" designation has been replaced?

The terminology has been changed to "Do Not Attempt Resuscitation" or DNAR.

Should the EMS provider, the ED personnel, and hospital personnel be responsible for locating and honoring a DNAR order?

The Guidelines reaffirmed that many individuals are executing their right of self-determination and declaring that they do not want attempts at resuscitation if they are unresponsive, not breathing, and pulseless. These wishes take the form of living wills, advance directives, or other documents. Some states allow bracelets and anklets to be worn by the patient to announce the patient's DNAR wishes. It is the responsibility of the health care provider to search for and honor a DNAR that is deemed valid.

Must a patient's DNAR be honored if it is deemed valid?

Yes, it must be honored. The DNAR is an expression of self-determination that must be honored when valid. To do otherwise is unethical and prohibited by law in many jurisdictions.

> **CLINICAL PEARL**
> *Remember that the guidelines are not intended to be legal standards of care despite the fact that some courts have recognized them as such.*

What do the Guidelines say about death pronouncement in the field?

The Guidelines reaffirmed that there are very few instances that require transporting a nontraumatic cardiac arrest patient who has failed a successfully executed out-of-hospital ACLS resuscitation effort to an ED to continue the resuscitation attempt. Rare exceptions may include profound hypothermia and toxin or drug overdose. A successfully executed out-of-hospital resuscitation includes an "adequate trial" of BLS and ALS including the following:

- Airway control with tracheal intubation or advanced airway device, confirmed proper tube placement, and secured tube to prevent dislodging.
- Oxygenation and ventilation are effective.
- Ventricular fibrillation has been shocked when present.
- The patient has been given epinephrine or vasopressin, atropine, and antiarrhythmics as appropriate for their ECG rhythm.
- Special resuscitation circumstances have been considered, located, and corrected if reversible.
- The patient has continued to be in continuous documented pulseless arrest after all of the preceding has been accomplished.

What is the position of the Guidelines 2000 with respect to the pronouncement of death?

The Guidelines reaffirm that EMS systems should develop criteria for stopping resuscitation attempts in the out-of-hospital setting. The ALS providers, in collaboration with the on-line medical control physician, can gather clinical data to allow the medical control physician to declare the patient dead. This must comply with state law that requires a licensed physician to certify death.

> **CLINICAL PEARL**
> *Follow your local protocols; field pronouncement protocols should include a relatively foolproof way to detect hypothermia (e.g., a rectal thermometer that reads well into the low 80 degrees F).*

What are necessary components of a survivor support plan?

According to the Guidelines, EMS providers acting as on-scene family advocates should know:

- Advanced plans for leaving a body at the scene.
- How to perform death certifications and complete the certificate.
- How to transfer the body to a funeral home.
- How to help the family accept nontransport of the dead person.
- Calling a chaplain or family minister for grief counseling.

What is the position of the Guidelines with respect to early defibrillation?

For a decade now, early defibrillation has been proven to be the intervention that saves the lives of adult patients. Evidence accumulated over the last 10 years continues to reaffirm all guidelines on defibrillation. The Guidelines reaffirm the need for timely defibrillation in public places, in the homes of high-risk patients, and in commercial aircraft, airports, hospitals, doctors' offices, and outpatient clinics.

Are there any changes in defibrillation concerning pediatrics?

The use of the AED is encouraged for all patients over the age of eight (or about 25kg/55lbs). The reason why this is a IIb recommendation is merely due to the fact that the data are limited. Regardless of the weight, a biphasic defibrillator provides non-escalating defibrillation energy doses of 150 joules (6 J/kg) for the 25-kg child. A monophasic defibrillator with escalating dose will provide approximately 200 joules (8 J/kg) initially for the 25-kg child and then higher doses.

> **CLINICAL PEARL**
>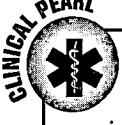
> *Despite promising data on biphasic defibrillation, either form of defibrillator promptly and properly used is better than no defibrillator at all!*

Q Has the emphasis on early defibrillation been expanded?

A Yes! The Guidelines highly recommend that authorization to use a defibrillator be expanded to nontraditional responders such as police, firefighters, and security personnel in casinos, on the ground, and in airports.

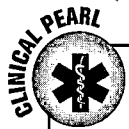

> *The guidelines merely lend "official" credence to a practice that is already underway in some areas. Hopefully, this support will encourage further development of early AED programs.*

Q What has the evidence shown to be the most economically efficient method for saving cardiac arrest patients?

A The research has questioned the value of medications, advanced airways, oxygenation, and ventilations, while continuing to amass evidence that early defibrillation is key. Limited funds are better spent on removing the barriers to training the lay public in CPR and public access defibrillation. Clearly, all the medications do not save as many patients as getting the defibrillator operator there faster!

> *Early defibrillation is the single acute intervention that really makes a difference in saving lives.*

Q What can each community do to improve cardiac arrest survival?

A Train the lay public and all levels of responders in CPR and public access defibrillation. The relative value of early defibrillation to reduce the interval from arrest to the first defibrillation by one to two minutes does more to improve the probability of survival for a patient than all of the medications, airway interventions, and newly designed defibrillation waveforms combined.

Q What is the difference between the phone-first and phone-fast rules?

A Phone first is used with adults and children over the age of eight who most likely need the defibrillator to help manage their arrest. Phone fast is used with children under the age of eight who are in cardiac arrest, which may be secondary to a primary respiratory event.

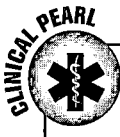

> *Remember that respiratory events are the most common cause of cardiac arrest in children under eight years of age.*

To keep the sequence for lay-rescuer CPR simple, the Guidelines emphasize that consistent, simple educational messages should be given. However, to maximize survival from cardiac arrest, rescuers should tailor rescue sequences to best meet the needs of the collapsed victim. Thus, the Guidelines recommend that the simple message be continued, but that information in the texts address exceptions to the rule. When appropriate, such as the pediatric with preexisting cardiac problems, health care providers can suggest that family members learn a different sequence.

Q Is there an exception to the phone-fast rule when phone first would be more sensible for children?

A The major exception to the phone-fast rule is those children under eight years old known to be at risk for ventricular fibrillation (VF)/ventricular tachycardia (VT) (e.g., known cardiac dysrhythmias, congenital heart disease) who experience sudden witnessed collapse.

Q Is there an exception to the phone-first rule for adults?

A The adult guidelines list five special resuscitation situations where airway compromise, rather than sudden VF/VT, is the cause of the arrest. The new BLS guideline for these people is phone fast, but provide one minute of CPR prior to phoning. The situations are: submersion/near-drowning, poisoning, drug overdose, trauma, respiratory arrest.

Q Is it true that the Guidelines are reemphasizing the use of the bag-valve-mask resuscitator (BVM) for health care providers?

A Yes, it is true and the health care providers must master the skill of using the BVM on adults as well as infants and children. The Guidelines make this class IIa recommendation the primary method of ventilatory support, especially when the transport time is short.

Q In the past decade the BVM has been de-emphasized in light of the studies showing that it was difficult for single rescuers to achieve effective ventilation

volumes with a one-handed mask seal. Why is this device back again?

[A] With the de-emphasis of the BVM, emphasis was placed on using either a pocket mask with a two-handed mask seal or trying to place an ET tube in the patient. In a recent study, conducted with pediatric patients in Los Angeles, the BVM was compared to the ET tube. The EMS system has short transport times and the providers are trained, but inexperienced, in pediatric intubation. The study results showed that children who received BVM ventilation had survival rates equivalent to those who received tracheal intubation.

CLINICAL PEARL

The reason why some training programs may back off on the "four hands" approach, especially without ET tube, is the fact that the required tidal volume seems to be less than thought and that two-handed BVM (one hold, one squeeze) ventilation can now deliver adequate volumes.

[Q] So, is the BVM an effective device to use in resuscitation?

[A] Yes. The BVM provides effective ventilation when used by properly trained providers who practice the skill. So, the responsibility is on the EMS educators to ensure that all EMS providers are properly trained in the technique. It is also necessary for EMS providers to practice the technique on a mannequin frequently to ensure that they will be adept at using the BVM. This is especially true if the EMS provider is not confronted with clinical situations requiring the BVM on a regular basis. According to the Guidelines, the bottom line here is that the BVM is a fundamental skill that should be mastered by all health care providers.

[Q] When using the BVM, what should be mastered?

[A] The best practice is to use the device with two rescuers. In that way, there can be a two-handed mask seal/hyperextension done by one rescuer and the other rescuer can squeeze the bag. In circumstances involving only one rescuer, the EMS provider should practice a one-handed mask seal (the "C" / "E" clamp) while hyperextending the patient's neck (assuming there is no neck trauma). Squeeze the bag slowly to avoid an explosive ventilation that might end up in the esophagus.

[Q] How can the EMS provider's technique of BVM use be best evaluated by the team leader?

[A] Watch the chest rise, mask seal, and hyperextension. This may be best seen by looking at the profile (side view) of the patient being ventilated. One thing to watch out for is EMS providers who get too close to the patient and move the airway into a neutral position. This closing of the airway is often enough to make it difficult to squeeze in an adequate volume of gas. The ventilator should be positioned approximately 18 inches above the head of the patient, hyperextend the airway, and use the weight of the left arm, which is sealing the mask, to hold the airway in the hyperextended position. The other hand can be used to squeeze the bag against itself. If you are having difficulty squeezing the bag, you can gently squeeze it against the patient's head. We do not recommend techniques that squeeze the bag against the rescuer's leg because the rescuer is then positioned too close to the patient and often loses sight of how well the airway is being hyperextended.

[Q] What technique should be used if you suspect the patient has a neck injury?

[A] The BVM should not be used by a single rescuer if the patient has a suspected neck injury. Because the neck must remain in a neutral position and in-line stabilization applied, the technique for opening the airway must be the jaw thrust maneuver. It is not possible to do a jaw thrust, jutting both sides of the jaw anterior, with only one hand. This technique involves one rescuer on the airway doing the jaw thrust and sealing the mask, while a second rescuer squeezes the bag. If only one rescuer is available and the patient is not intubated, a positive pressure ventilator with a trigger that can be depressed while two hands are sealing the mask is an effective device.

[Q] What is an effective tidal volume when using a BVM?

[A] The latest studies have shown that smaller BVM ventilation volumes than previously taught (800 to 1,200 ml) with supplemental oxygen can support adequate oxygen saturation, while also reducing the risk of gastric inflation. Ventilations delivered by mouth-to-mouth or a mouth-to-barrier device should average 700 to 1,000 ml delivered over two seconds. If supplementary oxygen is available, the EMS provider should provide smaller tidal volumes (400 to 600 ml over one second) during mouth-to-mask and BVM ventilation. However, if the smallest tidal volumes are used, the chest should rise visibly and the oxygen saturation should be maintained at greater than 90 percent.

CLINICAL PEARL

When larger tidal volumes were mandated, even well-trained rescuers were unable to deliver these using just two hands and a BVM. Now that we realize that lower volumes are adequate, single-rescuer operation (with the exception of a patient with a potential cervical-spine injury) is practical.

Q What technique should the rescuer use if the patient has clenched teeth and jaws (trismus) or is unable to cover an infant's nose and mouth?

A Studies have shown that some rescuers have difficulty covering both the mouth and nose of an infant with the rescuer's mouth. Mouth-to-nose breathing is an acceptable alternative to the mouth-to-nose-and-mouth breathing if the rescuer is unable to cover the infant's nose and mouth. It is also acceptable to do mouth-to-nose if the patient's mouth cannot be opened for any reason.

Q Are there any advanced airway devices recommended for use by EMS providers and other health care providers who are not advanced providers?

A Yes, the Combitube® and LMA are considerations for health care providers. They are discussed in Chapter 11, Airway Management and Ventilation, and Chapter 52, Advanced Cardiac Life Support.

Q Is it true that the pulse check has been removed from the CPR sequence?

A In the CPR technique for the lay rescuer, the pulse check has been replaced with an assessment of circulation. The circulation assessment includes three things: looking for signs of normal breathing, listening for a cough, and doing a quick body scan for signs of patient movement. In the absence of these three signs, the patient is said to be absent signs of circulation, and CPR and the AED should be employed.

Q Why was the pulse check dropped for the lay rescuer?

A Considerable studies have looked at the ability of the lay responder to take a pulse. The studies have demonstrated three things: lay rescuers have trouble locating the correct place for palpation of the carotid, they take more than the recommended 5 to 10 seconds, and when palpating the correct location for as long as needed to find the pulse, they are still often inaccurate. A type II (false-negative) error is committed by the lay rescuer 10 percent of the time. This means that 1 out of 10 cardiac arrest patients do not receive either chest compressions or defibrillation attachment.

The decision was made to drop the pulse check by the lay rescuer. The feeling is that dropping the pulse check does not result in as much potential harm as would keeping the pulse check.

Q Will health care providers still be checking a pulse in the CPR sequence?

A Yes, they will. The actual procedure for circulation assessment includes four things: looking for signs of abnormal breathing, listening for a cough, doing a quick body scan for signs of patient movement, and palpating for a carotid pulse. In the absence of these four signs, the patient is said to be absent signs of circulation and CPR and the AED should be employed.

Q Why is the health care provider told to check for abnormal breathing and the lay person told to check for normal breathing during the circulation check?

A The health care provider understands what agonal breaths are, which are clearly abnormal. The course for the lay person does not spend the time trying to explain agonal breaths. The lay person is just told to look for normal breaths.

Q Is it true that the lay rescuer will no longer be taught FBAO for the unconscious or unresponsive patient?

A Yes. According to the Guidelines, the FBAO maneuver for the unconscious patient will no longer be taught to the lay rescuer. Instead, they will begin standard CPR when an unrelieved, responsive choking patient becomes unresponsive, or an unresponsive person suspected of an FBAO is encountered, evaluated, and treated. The only difference from regular CPR is that the rescuer should open the airway widely whenever ventilations are attempted to look for a foreign object and remove it. Blind finger sweeps should not be used by lay rescuers on any patient. The FBAO for the unconscious patient will still be taught to the health care provider.

Q How many people die from a foreign body airway obstruction?

A In the United States, approximately 3,000 people a year die from choking. Compare this number to the more than 20,000 children a year who die from trauma and more than 225,000 adults who die from sudden cardiac arrest.

Q So, why was the FBAO sequence for the unconscious patient eliminated for the lay rescuer?

A Management of FBAO in the responsive infant, child, and adult is very important in preventing choking deaths. However, management of FBAO in the unresponsive patient is a complex skill that requires too much time and practice to master in a CPR course, thus, detracting from the practice time for more essential skills.

Q Are chest compressions effective in relieving a foreign body?

A Yes, in fact, a recent study conducted on adult cadavers found that chest compressions generated at least as high or higher intrathoracic pressures than abdominal thrusts. Therefore, the chest compressions used in CPR are helpful in dislodging a FBAO in the unresponsive patient. In fact, for many years rescuers have been taught to use chest compressions on adult pregnant patients as well as obese patients.

> *The bottom line is that chest compressions have the same effect on intrathoracic pressure as abdominal thrusts (the "Heimlich maneuver").*

Has the location of the rescuer's hand for CPR compressions been changed?

No. Actually, the method of describing the location has been simplified. When training lay rescuers in CPR, the phrase "in the center of the chest, right between the nipples" will be used to teach how to locate the point on the adult chest for chest compressions. The old technique of locating this site was difficult to explain and visualize.

What is the new chest compression rate for adult patients?

The new chest compression rate for the adult is 100 compressions per minute.

Why was the compression rate changed to a faster rate?

Studies support the need for the faster compression rate. This rate is better for blood flow and pressure. Evidence showed that frequent interruptions in compressions significantly reduces blood flow. Also, rescuers compressing at the slower rate slow even more as they fatigue. It is expected that eliminating a rate range and mandating a specific higher rate will influence rescuers to use a faster and more effective rate.

Has the compression to ventilation ratio changed?

Yes. In adults, two rescuers should be using a compression–ventilation ratio of 15:2. Once the airway is secured with an ET tube, it is acceptable to ventilate after the fifth compression.

Why has the adult compression–ventilation ratio been changed to 15:2 from the old 5:1?

The ratio of 5:1 produces too many chest compression interruptions while one ventilation is being given. This leads to

marked reduction in the blood flow and pressure. With a 5:1 ratio, the single ventilation sandwiched between short periods of rapid compressions leads to faster and more forceful ventilations. This type of ventilation often leads to greater risks for gastric inflation, regurgitation, and aspiration.

Has the ratio been changed for pediatrics?

The Guidelines have reaffirmed that the 5:1 ratio should be used in pediatric arrest by professional responders regardless whether one or two rescuers are involved. At this time, there is no evidence to justify a change. Emphasis on oxygenation and ventilation is justified in infants and children because the causes of cardiac arrest are primarily respiratory in origin.

Has the technique for doing compressions on an infant changed?

For many years, the two-thumb-encircling-hands chest compression technique was an acceptable alternative in the neonate. The Guidelines recommend this as the primary method for compressions for the neonate. The data show that the technique can provide better blood flow than the former two-finger technique. Because it may be difficult to perform with a single rescuer, this technique is only taught to the health care provider doing two-person CPR.

Is it true that it is now acceptable to teach CPR to the public without the mouth-to-mouth component?

The Guidelines have reaffirmed that CPR with compressions and ventilations remains the ideal method of maintaining blood flow until the arrival of the AED. However, if unwilling to perform mouth-to-mouth breathing on an adult patient, the rescuer should at least do the following:

- Access the EMS system.
- Open the airway.
- Assess for signs of circulation.
- Perform chest compressions at the rate of approximately 100 compressions per minute.

> *In a witnessed arrest, a significant amount of oxygenated air remains in the lungs for at least a minute. Thus, compressions without ventilations may still be effective. Compressions with or without ventilations are better than no compressions at all.*

Is CPR without ventilation a new skill?

Not really, because CPR without ventilation has been taught by some emergency medical dispatchers over the phone to bystanders who were not willing to ventilate.

Which area of the Guidelines contains the most new recommendations?

Actually, the airway management and ventilation section contains the greatest new changes that apply to health care providers at both the BLS and ALS levels. This is due to the volume of information, new products, and new insights since the last guidelines. Because these Guidelines are international, they now consider devices, such as the LMA, that previously have been unknown to many of the AHA training faculty.

What fact has the resuscitation community learned from conducting airway and ventilation quality assessments?

A number of national and international research centers conducting research on airway and ventilation have given the resuscitation community valuable information on the merit of different devices and approaches. Some of these studies have shocked the resuscitation community with unequivocal demonstrations that health care providers, in their best intentioned efforts to save lives, have the capacity to severely harm their patients.

What do the Guidelines say about the harm that has been done to some patients by the inappropriate use of airway and ventilation devices?

By adhering to the key principle of medicine, "first, do no harm," the resuscitation experts came to a consensus on a number of quality improvement initiatives that look at patient outcomes. The following Guidelines were identified as items requiring medical director involvement:

- Both ALS and BLS airway support techniques used in clinical settings.
- Reviews should be more than just descriptive statistics (e.g., how many medics per population) and process descriptions (e.g., average number of tracheal intubations per medic per year). The focus should be on measuring health status outcome (e.g., survival to hospital discharge of patients intubated versus not intubated in the field).

- Weigh outcome evaluations against the training, skill level, and experience of ALS providers in a given ALS system or code responders in a given hospital. All patient and system characteristics that can affect the evaluation outcome must be considered (e.g., witnessed versus unwitnessed arrests, bystander CPR versus none, short versus long transport times to hospitals, field use versus prohibited use of paralytic agents, and high versus low annual case frequency).
- Determine whether the outcomes are satisfactory. If not, question whether the sophistication and training requirements for use of the airway devices match the skill levels and experience of the EMS providers.
- Consider alternate action steps that might begin the improvement process.
- Develop action plans addressing problems identified in the quality improvement process.
- Observe the outcome from the action plans.
- Adjust training, programs, protocols, and equipment as necessary.
- Continue to monitor to determine whether the system interventions have been effective.

What do the Guidelines say about the laws in many states prohibiting EMT-Basics from doing advanced airway management?

The two new airway devices, LMA and Combitube®, are strongly recommended for use by BLS personnel; however, the Guidelines also recognize that this may not be legal in a number of states. Understanding that changing state law may take time, the resuscitation community did want to go on record with the evidence from a number of studies supporting their recommendations.

The evidence shows that, under certain clinical conditions, both the LMA and Combitube® are clinically superior to the BVM and clinically equivalent to the ET tube. For more information on these devices, review Chapter 52, Advanced Cardiac Life Support.

Does this mean that the paramedics who currently use ET intubation should switch over to the LMA or Combitube®?

Not necessarily. Prior to making this decision, many factors must be considered by the medical director using the quality improvement process outlined earlier.

CHAPTER 10

Life Span Development

This chapter discusses physiological, psychological, and sociological changes throughout human development, from infancy to late adulthood. The focus is on *why* patients present in a certain manner and *why* you need to respond in a certain way to their presenting problems. An understanding of and an ability to integrate the physiological, psychological, and sociological changes with assessment and communication strategies for patients of all ages is essential for proper patient care.

General Principles and Concepts

Q What is meant by "human life span development?"

A Human life span development refers collectively to all physiological, psychological, and sociological changes that a person normally undergoes from infancy to late adulthood. Though each category is listed separately, it is essential that health care providers view each patient as a "complete person."

Q What does the term "complete person" refer to from a health care point of view?

A Medically, a "complete person" refers to the combination of physiological, psychological, and sociological factors present at any point in a person's life. It is essential that health care providers be able to integrate all aspects of their patients to provide the best possible care.

Q What physiological parameters change during life span development?

A Though there are differences between stages, the following parameters are relatively predictable at different stages of life span development:

- Vital signs.
- Weight.
- Cardiovascular system.
- Pulmonary system.
- Renal system.
- Immune system.
- Nervous system.
- Musculoskeletal system.
- Dental system.
- Sensory system.
- Endocrine system.

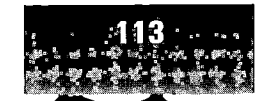

[Q] What psychosocial parameters change during life span development?

[A] Though there are differences between stages, the following parameters are relatively predictable at different stages of life span development:

- Family.
- Self-concept.
- Temperament.
- Trust.
- Ability to deal with stress.

[Q] What are the stages of human life span development?

[A] The most commonly used terms to describe human life span development are:

- Infancy—birth to one year old.
- Toddler—1 year to 3 years old.
- Preschool—3 to 5 years old.
- School age—6 to 12 years old.
- Adolescence—13 to 18 years of age.
- Early adulthood—19 to 40 years old.
- Middle adulthood—41 to 60 years old.
- Late adulthood—61 years of age and older.

Infancy—Birth to One Year Old

[Q] What are the typical changes in vital signs during infancy?

[A] Changes differ somewhat, depending on the particular parameter measured:

- Heart rate—During the first 30 minutes after birth, the heart rate ranges from 100 to 160 beats per minute. It gradually slows to an average of 120 beats per minute during the first year of life.

CLINICAL PEARL

Remember that a heart rate less than 100 bpm in a newborn is abnormal. Rates below 80 bpm usually require CPR.

- Respiratory rate—At birth, the respiratory rate is normally between 40–60 breaths per minute. It drops rapidly after the first few minutes of life (30–40 breaths per minute), and slows

to 20–30 breaths per minute by the time the infant reaches his first birthday. The tidal volume gradually increases during the first year of life. At birth, it is 6–8 ml/kg, and gradually increases to 10–15 ml/kg by one year.

- Blood pressure—The average systolic blood pressure increases from 70 mmHg at birth to 90 mmHg at one year of age.
- Temperature—Once stabilized after birth, the infant's normal temperature remains between 98 and 100 degrees Fahrenheit.

[Q] What types of weight changes are expected during the first year of life?

[A] The average newborn weighs 3.0–3.5 kg at birth. There is a normal weight loss of five to ten percent during the first week of life due to the excretion of extracellular fluid present at birth. Typically, infants exceed their birth weight by the end of the second week of life. During the first month, the infant grows by approximately 30 grams per day. As a result, the infant's weight should double by 4–6 months and triple by 9–12 months. The head circumference (in centimeters) should equal 25 percent of the infant's total body weight in the first year.

[Q] What changes take place in the infant's cardiovascular system shortly after birth?

[A] Exposure to atmospheric pressure leads rapidly to an increase in systemic vascular resistance. Pulmonary vascular resistance decreases at the same time. These circulatory changes lead to:

- Closing of the ductus arteriosus—the channel of communication between the main pulmonary artery and the aorta of a fetus.
- Closing of the ductus venosus—the smaller and shorter of the two branches into which the umbilical vein divides after entering the abdomen.
- Closing of the foramen ovale—the opening between the two atria in the fetal heart.

When these changes are complete, the infant has made the shift from fetal circulation to normal infant circulation.

[Q] What happens to the heart during the first year?

[A] The left ventricle strengthens and enlarges slightly during the first year of life.

[Q] How is the infant's pulmonary system unique?

[A] Compared to children and adults, the infant pulmonary system has several unique features:

- The airway is shorter, narrower, less stable, and thus, more easily obstructed due to the smaller diameter.
- Infants breathe only through their nose until they are four weeks old.

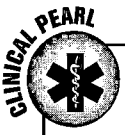

The fact that infants are obligate nose breathers during the first four weeks of life has important implications. Any occlusion of the nares is the functional equivalent of an upper airway obstruction.

- The lung tissue is fragile and more prone to barotrauma.

The fragility of infantile lung tissue mandates extreme care during any form of artificial ventilation.

- There are fewer alveoli with decreased collateral ventilation.
- Accessory muscles of respiration are immature and susceptible to early fatigue.
- The chest wall is less rigid.
- The ribs are positioned horizontally, causing diaphragmatic breathing.

How does an infant's metabolic and oxygen consumption rate compare to that of an adult?

Infants have higher metabolic and oxygen consumption rates than adults. Thus, they have higher respiratory rates that may lead to rapid heat and fluid loss through exhaling condensation and warm air.

How well do the infant's kidneys concentrate urine?

During infancy, the kidneys are unable to concentrate the urine, resulting in a specific gravity usually no greater than that of distilled water (1.000). Combined with an increased insensible fluid loss due to a rapid respiratory rate, the infant is more predisposed than an older patient to hypovolemia. Specific gravity is

Fluid balance in the infant is precarious. Seemingly simple factors, such as minor temperature changes, may lead to significant fluid imbalance. Carefully evaluate infants for signs of dehydration. In addition to the usual signs found in adults, be alert for the child who is not making tears, has a depressed fontanelle, and a furrowed tongue.

the weight of a substance compared to the weight of an equal volume of water.

What protects the infant against diseases?

At birth, the infant immune system is relatively undeveloped. Antibodies transferred from the mother maintain passive immunity throughout the first six months of life. By then, the infant's own immune system has begun to provide protection, at least to some extent.

What are normal movements in the first year of life?

The normal infant has a strong, coordinated suck and an intact gag reflex. The extremities should move equally when the infant is stimulated. At rest, an infant's extremities are in a semi-flexed position.

What are normal reflexes in the first year of life?

Normal reflexes include:
- Moro reflex—the "startle" reflex consisting of rapid abduction and extension of the arms, followed by adduction of the arms, such as in an embrace. The reflex is elicited by striking the surface near the infant's head. This reflex is usually not obtainable after three months of age.
- Palmar grasp reflex—light pressure on the palm leads to reflex grabbing of the examiner's finger by the infant. This reflex is usually not obtainable after six months of age.
- Sucking reflex—stroking the lips leads to a normal sucking motion by the infant. This reflex is usually not obtainable after four months of age while awake, seven months while asleep.
- Rooting reflex—stroking the cheek of an infant produces the rooting reflex, which consists of turning the mouth toward the stimulus. This reflex is usually not obtainable after four months of age while awake, seven months while asleep.

At what ages do the posterior and anterior fontanelle close?

The posterior fontanelle closes by three months of age. The anterior fontanelle closes between nine and eighteen months of age. Remember that depressed fontanelles may indicate dehydration.

Depressed fontanelles suggest hypovolemia but bulging fontanelles are less specific. Straining or crying may cause bulging in the absence of intracranial pathology.

What is the normal infant sleep pattern?

Initially, the infant sleeps 16–18 hours per day; sleep and wakefulness is evenly distributed over a 24-hour period. Gradually, sleep time decreases to 14–16 hours per day with most (9–10 hours) occurring at night. Most infants sleep through the night at two to four months of age. Whether sleeping or not, a normal infant is easily arousable.

How do bones grow?

Bones increase in length by growth at the epiphyseal or growth plate, near the ends of the bone. Bony thickness increases by the deposit of new bone on top of old bone (in concentric circles, like tree rings).

What factors influence bone growth?

Many things play a role in bone growth. These include:

- Growth hormone—deficits lead to retarded bone growth and short stature. Excess growth hormone levels lead to abnormal bone growth and acromegaly.

- Genetic factors—though the exact pattern of inheritance is yet unclear, height is transmitted (at least to some extent) genetically.

- Thyroid hormone—abnormal levels of thyroid hormones lead either to rapid (hyperthyroidism) or retarded (hypothyroidism) bone growth.

- Parathyroid hormone—the parathyroid glands are contained within the thyroid gland and produce parathyroid hormone, essential for normal bone metabolism.

- General health—a patient in poor general health is less likely to have normal bone development, especially in infancy, than a healthy person.

What percentage of body weight in an infant is muscle tissue?

Muscle comprises roughly 25 percent of body weight in normal infants.

At what age do the teeth start to develop?

This is actually a trick question because *all* of the infant's teeth (baby and adult) are present and fully developed at birth! They are simply below the gum line. The first baby teeth begin to erupt at five to seven months of age.

What are the major "milestones" of development during infancy?

Growth and development occurs rapidly during the first year of life. Table 10–1 summarizes major "milestones" during the first year that many infants are able to accomplish.

What is meant by reciprocal socialization?

Reciprocal socialization describes the concept that children should socialize their parents as opposed to the current pattern of parents socializing their children. Psychologists theorize that adults have a bad habit of telling children how to think, feel, and act. Parent–child relationships are based on intimidation, which, more often than not, results in the suppression of the child's own intuitive sensitivity.

What is "scaffolding" in terms of psychosocial development?

Scaffolding means doing some of the work for the infant who isn't quite ready to accomplish a task independently. Like

TABLE 10–1

Milestones of Infancy	
Age in Months	Milestone(s)
2	• Tracks objects with eyes
	• Recognizes familiar faces
3	• Moves objects to mouth with hands
	• Displays primary emotions with distinct facial expressions
4	• Drools without swallowing
	• Reaches out to people
5	• Sleeps throughout the night without food
	• Discriminates between family and strangers
6	• Sits upright in a highchair
	• Makes one syllable sounds (e.g., ma, mu, da, di)
7	• Exhibits fear of strangers (stranger anxiety)
	• Quickly changes from crying to laughing
8	• Responds to "no"
	• Sits alone
	• Plays "peek-a-boo"
9	• Responds to adult anger
	• Pulls self to a standing position
	• Explores objects by mouthing, sucking, chewing, and biting
10	• Pays attention to her own name
	• Crawls well
11	• Attempts to walk without assistance
	• Shows frustration to restrictions
12	• Walks with help
	• Knows own name

the supports that construction workers use on buildings, scaffolding is intended to be temporary. It is there to aid the completion of a task and it is eventually removed.

Q **What is meant by "attachment theory?"**

A *Attachment theory* is the description of relationships between children and parents. Many theorists suggest that the attachments formed during the first two years of life determine much of the remaining socialization process, and that the mother is the most important attachment object. Other theorists suggest that the early years for attachment are important, but no more so than the later years, and that mothers are no more important than any other interested adults. Current research indicates that more securely attached children are more likely to trust people and to exhibit normal psychosocial function as an adult.

Q **So, how does all this fancy psychological theory apply to clinical practice?**

A Due to the complex interactions between infant and parents (or caregivers), we are always dealing with both the patient *and* the family. With few exceptions (e.g., evidence of child abuse), this bond and interaction must be respected and used to the patient's advantage. Try to involve the parent in the care of the child as much as is possible.

Q **What are the terms used to describe an infant's temperament?**

A Typical terms are:

- Easy child—pleasant, likes everyone, rarely fusses.
- Difficult child—very discerning, selective about who he likes, fussy, temperamental.
- Slow to warm-up child—a shy child who is easy once she develops a relationship with another person.

Q **Why do infants cry?**

A Crying is an expression of many potential needs or feelings:

- Basic cry—a response to many situations that would be met with verbal responses at an older age.
- Anger cry—the infantile version of screaming or yelling in response to displeasure and anger.
- Pain cry—a response to pain; this cry is usually different from the basic or anger cry. Even adults sometimes cry in response to pain.

Q **What is the primary determinant of trust development in an infant?**

A Most psychologists believe that the development of trust is based on consistent parental care. Once this trust is established, the infant is more susceptible to parental separation reactions when the parent leaves the child's side. Reactions differ between children. They may include cries of protest, despair, or merely taking on a withdrawn appearance. Normally, the infant's behavior normalizes rapidly when the parent reappears.

Q **What is the role of pediatric growth charts?**

A Pediatric growth charts are useful for comparing a particular infant's physical development to the norm for age. Consistent deviations above or below normal may indicate disease states. These charts are of limited use in the out-of-hospital setting.

Toddlers and Preschool Children

Q **What are the normal vital signs in toddlers and preschool children?**

A Normal toddler and preschooler vital signs are summarized in Table 10–2.

Q **How does weight gain in toddlers and preschoolers compare to that of infants?**

A The rate of weight gain slows dramatically as the infant becomes a toddler. The average child gains only two kilograms per year during this period.

Q **What changes take place in the following body systems from age 12 months to 5 years: cardiovascular system, pulmonary system, renal system, immune system, nervous system, musculoskeletal system, and dental system?**

A The changes during years one to five are summarized in Table 10–3.

TABLE 10–2

Normal Toddler and Preschooler Vital Signs		
Parameter	Toddler	Preschool
Heart rate	80–130 BPM	80–120 BPM
Respiratory rate	20–30/MIN	20–30/MIN
Systolic BP	70–100 MMHG	80–110 MMHG
Temperature	96.8 DEG F	96.8 DEG F

TABLE 10-3

Changes in Body Systems of Toddlers and Preschoolers	
System	Change(s) from 12 Months to 5 Years
Cardiovascular	• Capillary beds develop to better assist in thermoregulation • Hemoglobin levels approach normal adult levels
Pulmonary	• Terminal airways continue to branch • Alveoli increase in number
Renal	• Kidneys are fully developed in toddler years • Specific gravity (ability to concentrate) and other urine findings similar to adults
Immune	• Passive immunity from maternal antibodies is lost • Increased susceptibility to minor respiratory and gastro-intestinal infections • Develops immunity to common pathogens as exposure occurs
Nervous	• Brain grows to 90 percent of adult weight • Myelination increases, leading to greater cognitive development • Development allows effortless walking and other basic motor skills • Fine motor skills begin to develop
Musculoskeletal	• Muscle mass increases • Bone density increases
Dental	• All primary teeth have erupted by 36 months

Isn't this the time when parents start thinking about toilet training? When is the toddler really ready and how long should it take?

Most children are physiologically capable of toilet training by 12 to 15 months of age. Psychologically, however, they are not ready until between 18 and 30 months. The average age for completion of toilet training is 28 months.

What about sensory system development?

Visual acuity averages 20/30 during the toddler years. Hearing reaches peak (maturity) levels at three to four years of age.

What cognitive milestones does the child normally reach during the toddler and preschooler period?

The following are major cognitive milestones in normal children:

• The basics of language are usually mastered by 36 months, with continued refinement throughout childhood.

• Understands cause and effect between 18–24 months.

• Develops separation anxiety (fear and crying when separated from parents or primary caregiver) at approximately 18 months.

• Develops "magical thinking" (e.g., fantasy, imagined play-mates) between 24 and 36 months.

How do play patterns change during the toddler and preschooler phase?

As a rule, exploratory behavior accelerates (making toddlers more susceptible to injury and accidental poisoning). They are able to play simple games and follow basic rules. Early displays of competitiveness are commonly seen at this age.

CLINICAL PEARL

Observation of play by trained therapists may uncover frustrations or other psychological conditions that are otherwise unexpressed or unnoticed. Similarly, "play therapy" is used commonly in child psychology. In out-of-hospital care, the use of dolls or stuffed animals (new for each patient) may help a child to express symptoms or emotions. For example, "Show me on Mr. Teddy bear where you hurt . . ."

What is sibling rivalry?

Sibling rivalry is competition between children for affection from others, particularly their parents. Toddlers and preschoolers often develop sibling rivalry shortly after a new baby enters the family. Initially, there is a period of excitement that is followed by jealousy because the infant is suddenly getting too much attention (at least in the mind of the toddler). Many times, toddlers and preschoolers respond to "new additions" by regressing—behaving like they were months or years younger. Though first-born children usually maintain a special relationship with their parents, they must be expected to exercise self-control and show responsibility when interacting with their younger siblings.

What role do peer groups play at this age?

Peer groups tend to form among children of similar age and maturity levels. From the child's point of view, these provide information about the outside world and other families. Developmentally, a child's peers become more important as he progresses through childhood.

What are different theories on parenting? Do their effects on children differ from style to style?

Child psychologists describe four styles of parenting: authoritarian, authoritative, permissive-indulgent, permissive-indifferent. Whether or not each individual style has a given effect on any given child is still unclear.

• Authoritarian parenting—this style is one that uses strict discipline, and children must follow rules. Obedience is often enforced through harsh punishment, and parents attempt to control their children to make them conform to an absolute set of standards. Emphasis is placed on obedience, respect for authority, and respect for tradition. Verbal give-and-take between parent and child is discouraged, as authoritarian parents expect the rules to be followed without any further explanation. Children who are subject to this type of parenting are habitually discontented, withdrawn, and distrustful.

- Authoritative parenting—parents that practice the authoritative style maintain a good middle ground; they are clearly in control while encouraging the child to strive for personal autonomy in certain areas. There is an expectation of mature behavior, and clear standards are set using nonpunitive discipline only when necessary. The child's individuality is accepted and communication between parent and child is encouraged.

- Permissive parenting—is characterized by more warmth and tolerance toward the child's impulses. Parents use a minimal amount of punishment and make few demands on the child to act maturely. Usually, the children are left to regulate their own behavior. Children of permissive parents have been found to be immature, lacking in impulse control, social responsibility, and independence. Permissive parenting has been further subdivided into two types based on two levels of responsiveness (e.g., warmth, acceptance, involvement) in permissive families. Parents that were low in authority and high in responsiveness were typified as engaging in an indulgent style of parenting *(permissive-indulgent parenting)*. These parents are committed to their children and are tolerant, warm, and accepting, but they do not exercise much authority and make few demands for mature behavior on the part of the child. On the other hand, parents who display no signs of responsiveness are described as indifferent parents *(permissive-indifferent parenting)*. These parents show no attempt to keep track of their children or get involved in their interests. Indifferent parents are often too preoccupied with their own problems to worry about their responsibilities as parents.

CLINICAL PEARL

Parenting styles may be apparent when caring for a child. Regardless of your personal feelings, refrain from comment. Conflict may arise when a parent suddenly shifts her style in response to the stress of a situation. For example, a normally controlling authoritative parent may become withdrawn and difficult to communicate with.

Q What factors mediate the effects of divorce on toddlers and preschoolers?

A Each child is different. Effects are mediated by:

- Age.
- Cognitive and social competency of the child.

- The degree of dependency of the child on the parents.
- The type of day care given to the child.
- The parents' ability to respond to the child's needs.

Q Does television affect children at this age?

A Though there is still some controversy, many experts believe that viewing violence on television causes increased aggression in toddlers and preschoolers. Limited data suggest that careful screening of television exposure may be effective in reducing levels of violent behavior in later years.

Q What is modeling?

A Modeling is imitation of another's behavior, dress, mannerisms, or attitudes. Toddlers and preschool children soon recognize differences between males and females. They may begin to model themselves based on a person's sex. For example, little girls may want to put on makeup and fancy dresses. On the other hand, modeling after a person of the opposite sex is not generally considered abnormal at this age (e.g., a little boy wants to wear his sister's dresses).

School-Age Children

Q What are the normal vital signs for school-age children?

A Normal vital signs are:

- Heart rate—70 to 110 beats per minute.
- Respiratory rate—20 to 30 breaths per minute.
- Systolic blood pressure—80–120 mmHg.
- Temperature—98.6 degrees Fahrenheit.

Q How fast does the average school-age child grow?

A The average child gains 3 kg per year in weight and grows 6 cm per year in height.

Q What are the usual changes in bodily functions during this period of development?

A Most bodily functions reach adult levels during this period. Common features include:

- Lymph tissues in school-age children are proportionately larger than the adult. The thymus gland is present until late adolescence.

- Brain function increases in both hemispheres.
- Primary teeth are lost; replacement with permanent teeth begins.

What are the usual trends in the parent–child relationship during this period of time?

As a rule, children are allowed more self-regulation, though parents still provide general supervision. In families with both parents working or divorced, parents tend to spend less time with children in this age group than when the child was younger.

How do interactions with adults and children lead to the development of a self-concept at this age?

With each interaction, school-age children compare themselves with others. This leads to the development of self-esteem, either positive or negative. Self-esteem tends to be higher during the early years of school than the later years and is often based on external characteristics (e.g., appearance, weight). Negative self-esteem can be damaging to further normal development and may be promoted by:

- Peer popularity (or lack thereof).
- Rejection.
- Emotional support (or lack thereof).
- Neglect (e.g., by parents, friends, and teachers, whether perceived or real).

When do children start to develop morals?

Moral development varies considerably from child to child and depends on many factors (e.g., family status, religious beliefs, peer groups). Though many psychological theories have been advanced, it is clear that individuals move through this development throughout school age and young adulthood at very different paces.

What are the psychological reasoning processes that may underlie moral development?

There are three types of reasoning processes described by child psychologists and sociologists:

- Preconventional reasoning—the "old school" where guilt, emphasis on obedience because "rules are rules," and punishment for a failure to abide were common. Nonconformers are often highly individualistic and driven by a specific purpose.
- Conventional reasoning—the "typical" method of moral development where there are acceptable norms for interpersonal behavior. If people are moral as individuals, then so is the social system as a whole.
- Postconventional reasoning—"futuristic" or "liberal" development of morals. Emphasis is more on community rights rather than on individual rights. Supporters condone a set of "universal ethical principles."

Realistically speaking, most of our morals derive from a combination of these types of reasoning. For example, we practice good patient care because:

- Failure to do so may result in job loss or a lawsuit (preconventional reasoning).
- We believe in the Hippocratic principle "First do no harm . . ." (conventional reasoning).
- Our society, as a whole, deserves the best health care possible (postconventional reasoning).

Adolescence

What are the normal vital signs for adolescents?

Normal vital signs are:

- Heart rate—55 to 105 beats per minute.
- Respiratory rate—12 to 20 breaths per minute.
- Systolic blood pressure—100 to 120 mmHg.
- Temperature—98.6 degrees Fahrenheit.

Don't most adolescents experience a "growth spurt?" What really happens and when does it stop?

Most adolescents experience a rapid growth spurt lasting two to three years. It begins distally with an enlargement of the feet and hands. Enlargement of the arms and legs follows. These changes may lead to a temporary lack of coordination or clumsiness. During the final stage of the growth spurt, the chest and trunk enlarge. Though some adolescents continue growing into their early 20s, girls are mostly done growing by age 16, boys by age 18.

What are the typical stages of secondary sexual development in adolescents?

In both genders, there is a noticeable development of the external sexual organs with development of pubic and axillary hair. Voice quality changes occur, though they are usually more prominent in males. Females undergo menarche (onset of menstruation).

Q What endocrine changes take place in females during adolescence?

A Gonadotropins, such as follicle stimulating hormone and luteinizing hormone, are released by the pituitary gland. These promote the production of estrogen and progesterone by the ovaries, which contributes to further development of secondary sexual characteristics and to sexual maturity.

Q What is meant by secondary sexual characteristics?

A The secondary sexual characteristics are the external physical characteristics of sexual maturity resulting from the action of sex hormones. These include male and female patterns of body hair, fat distribution, and development of external genitals.

Q What endocrine changes take place in males during adolescence?

A Gonadotropins, such as interstitial cell-stimulating hormone, are released by the pituitary gland. These promote the production of testosterone by the testes, which contributes to further development of secondary sexual characteristics and to sexual maturity.

Q What other significant body changes take place during adolescence?

A Many changes occur—those of major interest are:

- Muscle mass and bone growth are nearly complete by age 20.
- Body fat decreases early in adolescence, but begins to increase later. Females require that 18–20 percent body fat be present for menarche to occur.
- Blood chemistry values are nearly identical to adult levels.
- The skin toughens due to activity of the sebaceous glands. This often leads to skin problems, such as acne vulgaris ("zits" or pimples).

Q What are some common reasons that conflicts often arise between adolescents and other family members?

A Four major reasons are:

1. Adolescents strive for autonomy—adolescence is a midpoint between childhood and adulthood. At times, the adolescent thinks and acts like a child (requiring much parenting). Other times (usually unpredictable), she rejects any parental influence.
2. Biological changes associated with puberty—adolescents are often overwhelmed by sudden changes in their bodies over

which they have no control. They "rebel" by attempting to regain control over whatever they possibly can, including suggestions or instructions from other family members.
3. Increased idealism—adolescents often imagine a better world than the one they live in. To them, the "grass is always greener …" regardless of "the lawn's true condition." This idealism is healthy in many cases and leads to the development of many novel ideas and products. On the other hand, the failure of an adolescent to realize his "dreams" may lead to severe depression, even suicide.
4. Independence and identity changes—a major struggle for adolescents is answering the question, "Who am I?" This quest for a personal identity and independence follows many years of dependency on others (e.g., parents, siblings, other caregivers).

Q What takes place as adolescents develop their own identity?

A Several events typically occur; some are potentially dangerous. Adolescents progress through various stages depending on their ability to handle crisis. They include:

- Increased self-consciousness.
- Increased peer pressure.
- Increased interest in the opposite sex.
- Desire to be treated like adults.

CLINICAL PEARL

In our modern day society, peer pressure and risky behavior often takes place in school-age children before they reach adolescence. Don't assume that these problems and challenges are unique to adolescents!

Q When does "antisocial behavior" peak?

A Typically, antisocial behavior peaks around eighth or ninth grade. Minority adolescents tend to have more identity crises than nonminority adolescents.

Q What are the effects of body image in adolescents?

A Body image is of great concern. Adolescents continually compare themselves to their peers. As a result, eating disorders are common, especially in females. To gain acceptance, some adolescents turn to self-destructive behaviors such as tobacco, alcohol, or illicit drugs. Depression and suicide are more common during adolescence than in any other age group.

Q What about ethical development?

A Development of a personal "code of ethics" varies widely among adolescents. Most have the intellectual capability for logical, analytical, and abstract thinking. Whether or not a particular adolescent translates this innate ability into lifestyle changes depends on many variables.

Early Adulthood

Q What are the normal vital signs for early adults?

A Normal vital signs are:

- Heart rate—averages 70 beats per minute.
- Respiratory rate—16 to 20 breaths per minute.
- Blood pressure—averages 120/80 mmHg.
- Temperature—98.6 degrees Fahrenheit.

Q Typically, what is the status of body systems during this period?

A As a rule, all body systems are at optimal performance. Persons reach a peak in physical conditioning between 19 and 26 years of age. In addition, adults develop lifelong habits and routines during this time.

Q What is the leading cause of death among early adults?

A Accidents are the leading cause of death in this age group.

Q What are the usual psychosocial milestones during this period?

A Early adulthood is less associated with psychological problems related to well-being than other periods of human development. Major stressors involve jobs and family relationships:

- People tend to experience the highest levels of job stress during early adulthood.
- Serious "love interests" are most likely to develop at this age, leading to a combination of romance and affection. Marriage is common.
- Along with love and marriage, having children is most common during this period. New family units provide new challenges and stress for early adults.

Middle Adulthood

Q What are the normal vital signs for middle adults?

A Normal vital signs are:

- Heart rate—average 70 beats per minute.
- Respiratory rate—16 to 20 breaths per minute.
- Blood pressure—average 120/80 mmHg.
- Temperature—98.6 degrees Fahrenheit.

Q What are the common trends in vision and hearing during this period?

A Generally, the body is still functioning at a high level with varying degrees of degradation. Vision predictably changes—near vision (reading) becomes more and more difficult without reading glasses. Hearing decreases, but to a variable degree among people.

Q What other medical considerations are common during this period of development?

A Common and important considerations include:

- Cardiovascular disease—cardiovascular health becomes a major concern. The cardiac output decreases throughout this period and cholesterol levels tend to increase.
- Cancer is more common in this age group.
- Weight control is more difficult.
- Menopause begins in women—usually in the late 40s and early 50s.

Q What are an individual's concerns with the "social clock" versus the "biological clock?"

A During this period, adults are more concerned with the "social clock" than the "biological clock" (growing old). Though aging is a real concern, many people become extremely task oriented as if feeling pressed for time to accomplish lifelong goals. Though this tendency engenders stress, a beneficial side effect is that middle-age adults tend to approach problems more as challenges rather than as threats. This leads to less stress and a greater sense of accomplishment when goals are achieved. The "biological clock" is also a term used to mean the time when a woman is approaching the end of her child-bearing years. This too can be stressful in some cases.

What is the "empty-nest syndrome?"

The empty-nest syndrome occurs when all of a parent's children become old enough to leave home (e.g., college, marriage, employment). The home situation returns, in a sense, to the way it was prior to the birth of children. Often, this is very exciting for couples because they are able to spend previously unavailable time together. On the other hand, couples that have "grown apart" while raising their children are now alone with each other. This may present serious challenges to the integrity of a marriage—divorce is common during this stage, even after long years of marriage.

CLINICAL PEARL

A common cause of stress in middle adulthood is marital discord in a previously "happy" marriage. This may aggravate physical complaints as well as lead to antisocial behavior (e.g., alcohol, drugs, sexual promiscuity).

What specific financial concerns arise during middle adulthood?

Middle-age adults are often burdened by financial commitments for elderly parents as well as young adult children. This further increases the potential stress of the "empty-nest syndrome."

Late Adulthood

What are the normal vital signs for late adults?

Heart rate, respiratory rate, and blood pressure depend on the patient's physical and health status. The normal temperature remains 98.6 degrees Fahrenheit.

What are the differences between "life span" and "life expectancy"?

Life span is the total duration of one's life from birth to death. Although the maximum human life span is thought to be approximately 120 years, the seventh decade is more common. *Life expectancy* is the amount of time remaining before a person is expected to die. The average life expectancy depends on many factors including the year of birth. Older individuals typically have a shorter life expectancy than younger persons.

CLINICAL PEARL

Life span is a retrospective measurement—it measures how long a person actually lived. Life expectancy, on the other hand, is a prospective measure. It indicates the likelihood of remaining alive for any given period of time. For example, a person with a terminal illness may have a life expectancy of only months.

What are the major changes in cardiovascular function during this period?

Aging affects the blood vessels, the heart, and the blood cells:

- Blood vessels—vessel walls thicken, often due to arteriosclerosis. The result is an increase in peripheral vascular resistance with variable reductions in organ blood flow. By 80 years of age, there is a 50 percent decrease in blood vessel elasticity. Baroreceptors within blood vessels lose their sensitivity. As a result, late adults are more sensitive to orthostatic (positional) changes. Postural hypotension becomes more common because of inadequate compensatory mechanisms.

CLINICAL PEARL

Many late adults have a high blood pressure when taken by BP cuff but it is relatively normal when direct intra-arterial measurements are taken. This is due to their "stiffer" vessels as late adults.

- Heart—the myocardium is less able to respond to exercise because the muscle is less elastic. This leads to an increased workload on the aging heart. Increased heart size (cardiomegaly) may occur for any of a number of reasons including mitral or atrial valve disease. Cardiomegaly further increases the workload of the heart. Because cardiac reserves become limited, stress (e.g., tachycardia) is not well tolerated. Finally, the conduction system develops fibrous (scar) tissue, particularly in the sinoatrial node. Combined with a loss of normal cardiac pacemaker cells, arrhythmias are more common.

CLINICAL PEARL

Degeneration of the cardiac conduction system may lead to a combination of brady- and tachydysrhythmias. This is often termed the "tachy-brady" syndrome or "sick-sinus syndrome." Patients alternate from normal sinus rhythm to supraventricular tachycardias to bradycardia and AV-block without apparent logic. Either too fast or too slow rates may lead to symptoms, though bradydysrhythmias are typically more likely to cause syncope in these patients.

- Blood cells—with aging, the bone marrow produces fewer red blood cells (RBCs) and platelets. There is also a decrease in a person's functional blood volume. Decreased iron levels from poor nutrition or malabsorption further decrease the levels of RBCs, making low-grade anemia relatively common (though *not* normal) in late adulthood.

> **CLINICAL PEARL**
>
> *Remember that anemia decreases the oxygen-carrying capacity of the blood. This worsens oxygen delivery to tissues, including the myocardium. Thus, anemia in late adulthood may worsen already tenuous cardiac function.*

What changes take place during late adulthood in the respiratory system?

Changes occur in the mouth, nose, and lungs. Tissues atrophy and lose normal mucous membrane linings. As a result, inhaled air is less humidified. Metabolic changes also have potential effects on gas exchange. Years of exposure to pollutants inevitably lead to decreased diffusion of gases through the alveoli and a generalized decrease in lung capacity. Decreased muscle mass leads to relative chest wall weakness. This, combined with decreased elasticity of the diaphragm, leads to decreased respiratory function. Older persons often have an ineffective cough reflex due not only to the weakened chest wall and diaphragm, but also due to weakened bone structure in the ribs, vertebrae, and sternum.

What are the major changes in endocrine system function during late adulthood?

Insulin production decreases, leading to abnormalities in glucose metabolism. Other endocrine organs are also affected:

- The thyroid gland shows diminished T3 (thyroid hormone) production. Patients are more likely to show clinical evidence of hypothyroidism during this period.

> **CLINICAL PEARL**
>
> *New onset atrial fibrillation in the late adult period is more likely due to either ischemic heart disease or* hyperthyroidism *even if the patient has no obvious symptoms. So-called "occult hyperthyroidism" in the elderly presents clinically with lethargy and weakness. As such, beta-blocker treatment may be lifesaving.*

- Cortisol production by the adrenal glands is diminished by 25 percent. Because cortisol is produced during stress, the late adult is less equipped to handle bodily stresses (e.g., severe infection).

> **CLINICAL PEARL**
>
> *Relative hypoadrenalism is common in shock, even in previously normal persons. This is the basis for consideration of replacement dose corticosteroids in sick individuals. This is* not *considered routine care, in or out of hospital, at this time.*

- The pituitary gland is 20 percent less effective. The result is a generalized decrease in all endocrine function because the pituitary or "master gland" is responsible for regulating the entire system.
- Reproductive organs atrophy—this occurs in both sexes, though changes may be more obvious in women.

What are the major changes in the gastrointestinal system during late adulthood?

The mouth, teeth, and saliva are all affected by aging. Teeth weaken and may be missing. Salivary enzymes decrease in volume and potency, leading to digestive difficulty. Other GI secretions, such as stomach acid, are also decreased. This leads to poor absorption of nutrients—vitamin and mineral deficiencies are common during this period. Peristalsis throughout the entire GI tract is decreased. The result is a tendency toward bowel slowdown (ileus) and blockage (obstruction). Muscular sphincters (e.g., esophageal, rectal) become less effective, resulting in acid reflux and stool incontinence.

What are the major changes in the renal system during late adulthood?

Nearly 50 percent of functioning nephrons are lost during this time. Glomerular abnormalities (for a variety of reasons) are more common. As a result, decreased excretion of fluid, salts, and waste products (e.g., urea, creatinine) may occur.

> **CLINICAL PEARL**
>
> *Changes in renal function have a major effect on the metabolism of many drugs in the older patient. Always check to determine whether the dose of a drug must be decreased in late adulthood. A common example is lidocaine—"standard" loading doses may result in toxicity in the small, late adulthood patient.*

What are the major changes in the sensory system during late adulthood?

Virtually all sensory systems exhibit decreased responsiveness during this period:

- Taste and smell sensations are decreased.
- Pain perception is decreased—this may result in development of a serious disease (e.g., appendicitis) with very few clinical signs or symptoms.

CLINICAL PEARL

Nondescript abdominal pain in an older patient may be due to a serious disease (e.g., appendicitis, cholecystitis, myocardial infarction) and they may be unable to sense the pain appropriately.

- Kinesthetic (body position) sense is decreased—the result is a loss of balance and falling, often with devastating consequences (e.g., hip fracture or central nervous system [CNS] bleed).

CLINICAL PEARL

A hip fracture, regardless of the type, results in a significantly increased mortality rate over the next year. If the patient already had an underlying disease before falling, the mortality rate goes even higher. This is why the prevention of fractures (e.g., treatment of osteoporosis, attention to safety issues) is extremely important.

- Visual acuity is diminished—the result, combined with decreased kinesthestic sensation, is falling. In addition, decreased vision (and hearing) make driving potentially dangerous.
- Reaction time is decreased.
- Hearing is decreased; presbycusis refers to the "normal" hearing loss due to aging.

CLINICAL PEARL

All of these sensory changes present significant challenges to the late adult, especially in the operation of machinery and motor vehicles.

What are the major changes in the nervous system during late adulthood?

Normal aging results in a loss of neurons and neurotransmitters. The clinical effects are variable. Generally, the sleep–wake cycle is disturbed. People in late adulthood typically go to sleep early and arise early in the morning.

What is the terminal drop hypothesis?

The terminal drop hypothesis is a *theory* suggesting that death is preceded by a decrease in cognitive function over a five-year period prior to death. The relevance of this theory to clinical practice is uncertain.

What are the major psychosocial challenges of late adulthood?

Aging leads to numerous concerns. These are discussed further in Chapter 45, Geriatrics: Abuse and Assault. In summary, challenges include:

- Decreased self-worth—previously productive persons are no longer able to work.
- Declining well-being—aging is often accompanied by health problems.
- Financial burdens—with retirement comes a fixed income. Increased medical costs and poor insurance coverage pose a real concern to all patients, especially in late adulthood. Sometimes people refuse necessary medications or medical care because they feel unable to pay for it.
- Death or dying of friends and companions—the reality shock of our limited life span becomes clear as one's friends and companions start to die. For many people, this realization takes place in early or middle adulthood with the death of a parent. The loss of a close friend or spouse further solidifies the fact that we are not immortal.

Comparison Between Various Life Span Stages of Development

NOTE: As it is impossible to compare and contrast every potential difference between each stage in life span development, the authors have chosen specific areas to summarize in tabular form.

How do normal vital signs vary during different stages of life span development?

The differences in vital signs across age groups are summarized in Table 10–4.

How do weight and growth vary during different stages of life span development?

The differences in weight and growth from group to group are summarized in Table 10–5.

TABLE 10-4

Differences in Vital Signs				
Vital Sign Stage	Heart Rate	Respiratory Rate	Blood Pressure	Temp
Infancy	100-160 bpm first 30 min; then 120 bpm	Initially 40-60; drops to 30-40 after a few minutes; slows to 20-30 by 1 year	Average systolic BP at birth = 70 mmHg; increases to 90 mmHg at 1 year	98-100 Deg F
Toddler	80-130 bpm	20-30/min	70-100 mmHg	98.6 Deg F
Preschool	80-120 bpm	20-30/min	80-110 mmHg	98.6 Deg F
School age	70-110 bpm	20-30/min	80-120 mmHg	98.6 Deg F
Adolescence	55-105 bpm	12-20/min	100-120 mmHg	98.6 Deg F
Early adulthood	70 bpm	12-20/min	120/80 mmHg	98.6 Deg F
Middle adulthood	70 bpm	12-20/min	120/80 mmHg	98.6 Deg F
Late adulthood	Depends on patient's health	Depends on patient's health	Depends on patient's health	98.6 Deg F

TABLE 10-5

Weight and Growth Differences	
Stage	Weight and Growth
Infancy	• Normally 3.0-3.5 kg at birth • Normally drops 5-10 percent in first week (loss of ECF) • Exceeds birth weight by second week • Grows at 30 gm/day during first month • Should double weight by 4-6 months • Should triple weight at 9-12 months • Head in cm = 25 percent of total body weight
Toddler	• Rate of weight gain slows dramatically • Average child gains 2 kg per year
Preschool	• Rate of weight gain slows dramatically • Average child gains 2 kg per year
School age	• Average child gains 3 kg per year • Average child grows 6 cm in height per year
Adolescence	• Rapid 2-3 year growth spurt • Begins with enlargement of feet and hands • Enlargement of arms and legs follows • Chest and trunk enlarge during final stage • Most girls done by age 16; most boys by age 18
Early adulthood	• Peak physical conditioning between 19 and 26 years of age • All body systems at optimal performance • Little, if any, growth during this period
Middle adulthood	• Body functioning at high level with varying degrees of degradation • Weight control more difficult
Late adulthood	• No new growth takes place • Height may decrease due to osteoporosis of spine

Q **How does the cardiovascular system change during different stages of life span development?**

A The changes in the cardiovascular system from age group to age group are summarized in Table 10-6.

TABLE 10-6

Cardiovascular System Changes	
Stage	Cardiovascular Changes
Infancy	• Increased systemic vascular resistance • Decrease in pulmonary vascular resistance • Closing of the ductus arteriosus • Closing of the ductus venosus • Closing of the foramen ovale • Left ventricle strengthens throughout the first year
Preschool	• Capillary beds better developed to help thermo-regulation • Hemoglobin levels approach normal adult levels
School age	• Adult levels reached
Adolescence	• Adult levels reached
Early adulthood	• Adult levels reached
Middle adulthood	• Cardiovascular health becomes a concern • Cardiac output decreases • Cholesterol levels increase
Late adulthood	• Blood vessels thicken with increased peripheral resistance, reduced blood flow to organs • Decreased baroreceptor sensitivity • Increased cardiac workload • Fibrous tissue in conduction system • Decreased RBC and platelet count • Blood volume and iron levels decreased

How does the respiratory system change during different stages of life span development?

The changes in the respiratory system from age group to age group are summarized in Table 10-7.

How does the renal system change during different stages of life span development?

The changes in the renal system from age group to age group are summarized in Table 10-8.

TABLE 10-7

Respiratory System Changes	
Stage	Changes in the Respiratory System
Infancy	• The airways are shorter, narrower, less stable, and thus, more easily obstructed • Infants breathe only through their nose until they are four weeks old • The lung tissue is fragile and more prone to barotrauma • There are fewer alveoli with decreased collateral ventilation • Accessory muscles of respiration are immature and susceptible to early fatigue • The chest wall is less rigid • The ribs are positioned horizontally, causing diaphragmatic breathing • Infants have higher metabolic and oxygen consumption rates than adults • Infants have higher respiratory rates that may lead to rapid heat and fluid loss
Preschool	• Terminal airways continue to branch • Alveoli increase in number
School age	• Adult levels reached
Adolescence	• Adult levels reached
Early adulthood	• Adult levels reached
Middle adulthood	• Adult levels reached
Late adulthood	• Changes occur in the mouth, nose, and lungs; tissues atrophy and lose normal mucous membrane linings • Decreased diffusion of gases through the alveoli • Generalized decrease in lung capacity • Decreased muscle mass leads to relative chest wall weakness • Decreased elasticity of the diaphragm leads to decreased respiratory function • Ineffective cough reflex

How do the endocrine and reproductive systems change during different stages of life span development?

The changes in the endocrine and reproductive systems from age group to age group are summarized in Table 10-9.

TABLE 10-8

Renal System Changes	
Stage	Changes in the Renal System
Infancy	• Kidneys are unable to concentrate the urine • Specific gravity usually no greater than 1.000
Preschool	• Kidneys well developed • Specific gravity and other urine findings similar to adults
School age	• Kidneys well developed • Specific gravity and other urine findings similar to adults
Adolescence	• Kidneys well developed • Specific gravity and other urine findings similar to adults
Early adulthood	• Adult levels reached
Middle adulthood	• Adult levels reached
Late adulthood	• 50 percent of functioning nephrons are lost during this time • Glomerular abnormalities (for a variety of reasons) are more common • Decreased excretion of fluid, salts, and waste products (e.g., urea, creatinine) may occur

TABLE 10-9

Endocrine and Reproductive System Changes	
Stage	Changes in the Endocrine and Reproductive Systems
Infancy	• No significant changes
Preschool	• No significant changes
School age	• No significant changes
Adolescence	• Secondary sexual development occurs • Gonadotropin promotes release of estrogen and progesterone (female), and testosterone (male)
Early adulthood	• Adult levels reached
Middle adulthood	• Menopause in women
Late adulthood	• Insulin production decreases, leading to abnormalities in glucose metabolism • The thyroid gland shows diminished T3 (thyroid hormone) production • Cortisol production by the adrenal glands is diminished by 25 percent • The pituitary gland is 20 percent less effective • Reproductive organs atrophy—this occurs in both sexes, though changes may be more obvious in women

[Q] **How do the nervous and sensory systems change during different stages of life span development?**

[A] The changes in the nervous and sensory systems from age group to age group are summarized in Table 10–10.

[Q] **What are the behavioral norms, "milestones," and typical mental focus during different stages of life span development?**

[A] The behavioral norms, milestones, and typical mental focus from age group to age group are summarized in Table 10–11.

TABLE 10–10

Nervous and Sensory System Changes	
Stage	Changes in the Nervous and Sensory Systems
Infancy	• Strong, coordinated suck • Intact gag reflex • Extremities should move equally when the infant is stimulated • At rest, an infant's extremities are in a semi-flexed position
Preschool	• Brain grows to 90 percent of adult weight • Myelination increases, leading to greater cognitive development • Development allows effortless walking and other basic motor skills • Fine motor skills begin to develop • Visual acuity averages 20/30 • Hearing reaches peak (maturity) levels at three to four years of age
School age	• Brain function increases in both hemispheres
Adolescence	• Adult levels reached
Early adulthood	• Adult levels reached
Middle adulthood	• Reading vision gets worse • Hearing less effective
Late adulthood	• Taste and smell sensations are decreased • Pain perception is decreased • Kinesthetic (body position) sense is decreased • Visual acuity is diminished • Reaction time is decreased • Hearing is decreased • Loss of neurons and neurotransmitters • Disturbance of sleep-wake cycle

TABLE 10–11

Behavioral Norms and Milestones	
Stage	Behavioral Norms, Milestones, and Focus

Infancy	• By one year:
	  – Responds to "no"
	  – Sits alone
	  – Explores objects
	  – Recognizes own name
	  – Crawls
	  – Walks with help
	• Temperament developed (easy, difficult, slow to warm up)
	• Specific cries developed
	• Trust based on consistent parental care
	• Demonstrates parental separation reactions

Preschool	• Basics of language by 36 months • Understands cause and effect at 18–24 months • Separation anxiety at 18 months • Magical thinking at 24–36 months • Play behavior possible • Sibling rivalry may develop • Peer group interactions begin • Television may affect behavior • Children may exhibit modeling
School age	• Develop self-concept • Develop self-esteem • Develop morals
Adolescence	• Familial conflicts likely • Develop self-identity • Body image of great concern • Self-destructive behaviors may begin • Depression and suicide more common than any other age group
Early adulthood	• Job stress common • Love interests develop • Child bearing common
Middle adulthood	• Concern with "social clock" and completion of life goals • Approach problems more as challenges than as threats • Empty-nest syndrome common • Financial burdens of adult children and aging parents common
Late adulthood	• Decreased self-worth • Declining sense of well-being • Financial burdens • Death or dying of companions and friends

Airway Management and Ventilation

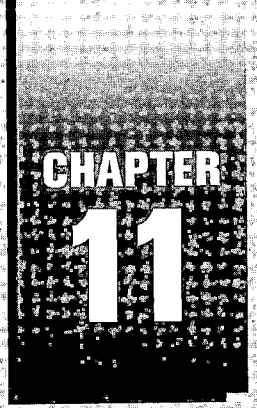

CHAPTER

11

This chapter discusses basic and advanced airway management and ventilation. The focus is on *why* patients present in a certain manner and *why* you must respond in a certain way to their presenting problems. Management of the airway is paramount to successful patient care. Without an adequate airway, all patients ultimately die.

Physiology

Q **What is the relation between the pulmonary circulation, oxygenation, and ventilation?**

A Ventilation refers to the movement of carbon dioxide out of the lungs during breathing. This process differs from oxygenation, the movement of oxygen into the lungs, though they are often interrelated. Normally, each alveolus is surrounded by a functioning pulmonary capillary and carbon dioxide passes from the blood and is eliminated by breathing (Figure 11–1). Simultaneously, oxygen is absorbed from the alveolus into the capillary. It is then transported to the cells via the RBCs. If either the pulmonary circulation or the alveoli are disrupted, a mismatch of blood flow (perfusion) to alveolar gas flow (ventilation) occurs. This is called a "ventilation-perfusion" defect and is common in many abnormal conditions, such as pulmonary embolus.

Q **What is meant by the partial pressure of a specific gas?**

A The combined pressure of all atmospheric gases is the total pressure. At sea level, the pressure, measured in torr, should add up to 760 torr and the percentage should equal 100 percent.

CLINICAL PEARL

Ventilation is the movement of carbon dioxide out of the lungs; oxygenation is the movement of oxygen into the lungs. Ventilation and oxygenation are not always interrelated. When a patient hypoventilates (e.g., narcotic overdose), hypoxia occurs due to the slow respiratory rate. On the other hand, patients with pulmonary emboli commonly hyperventilate, but their partial pressure of oxygen (PO_2) is usually low. People with diabetic ketoacidosis also hyperventilate to compensate; most have normal PO_2 levels.

The partial pressure is the pressure exerted by a specific atmospheric gas. The normal concentration of gases in the atmosphere at sea level is: nitrogen 597.0 torr (78.62 percent), oxygen 159.0 torr (20.84 percent), carbon dioxide 0.3 torr (0.04 percent), and water 3.7 torr (0.50 percent). Note that torr and mmHg are interchangeable terms.

Q **How does the alveolar gas concentration differ from the atmosphere?**

A There is less nitrogen and oxygen, and more carbon dioxide and water in the alveolar gas. Specifically, the concentrations are:

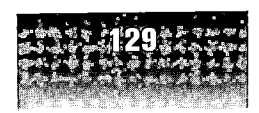

129

Nose—mouth

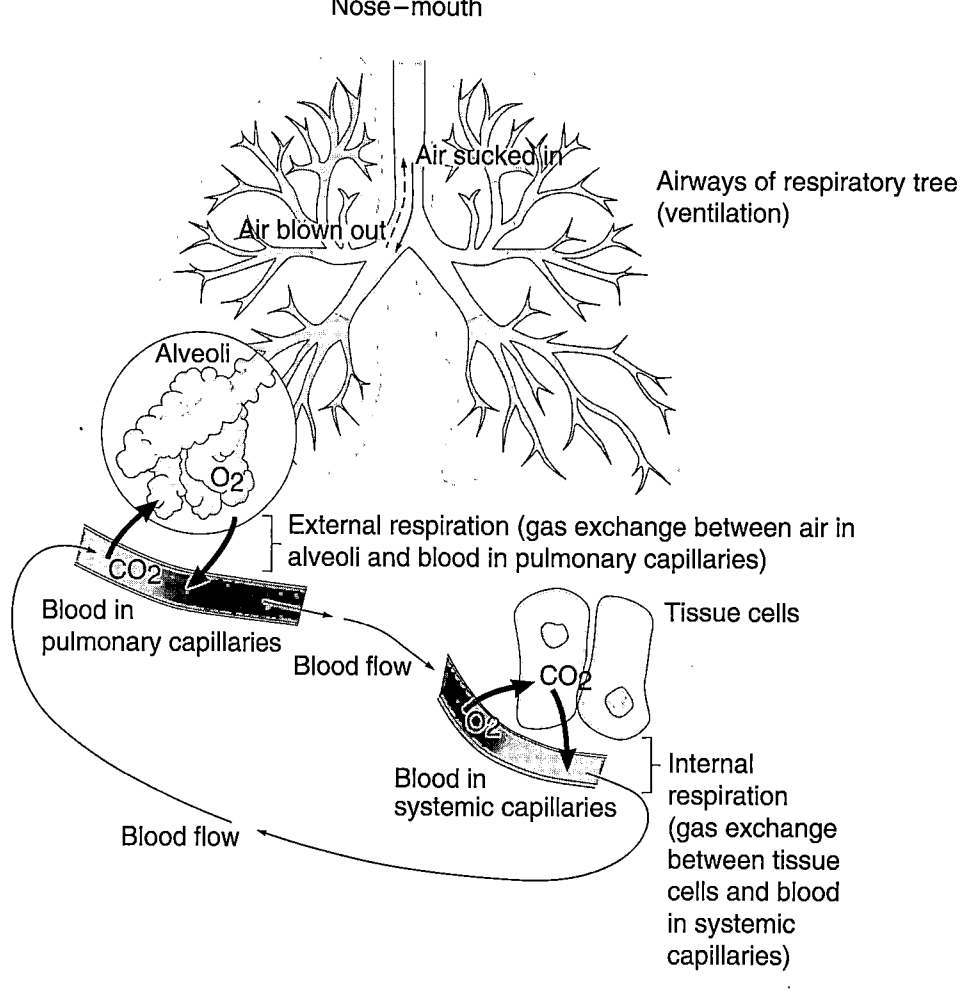

FIGURE 11–1 Respiration.

nitrogen 569.0 torr (74.9 percent), oxygen 104.0 torr (13.7 percent), carbon dioxide 40.0 torr (5.2 percent), and water 47.0 torr (6.2 percent).

What are the factors that affect the respiratory rate?

The respiratory rate is the number of times per minute that a person breathes. Overall, the major controlling factors of respiratory rate are the central nervous system and the patient's metabolic status, especially acid–base balance. These are often closely linked.

The rate of respiration is controlled by the medulla and pons in the brain. The medulla is the primary involuntary respiratory center. It is connected to the respiratory muscles by the vagus nerve. The pons has the secondary control center of respirations called the apneustic center. It takes over if the medulla fails to initiate breathing. The pneumotaxic center is responsible for the control of expirations.

Chemoreceptors control respiration by measuring the Ph of the blood and cerebral spinal fluid. This analysis sends messages to the brain to increase or decrease the respiratory rate. Chemoreceptors are most plentiful in the carotid sinus and the aortic arch.

Finally, the rate of respiration can also be increased by other factors such as fever, drugs and medications, pain, emotion, hypoxia, and acidosis. Respirations can be decreased by sleep and medications or drugs.

What is hypoxia and hypoxemia?

Hypoxia is a lack of oxygen in the tissues of the body (e.g., temporary decreased blood flow to a portion of the heart due to a coronary vessel spasm). Hypoxemia is a lack of oxygen in the blood (e.g., carbon monoxide taking up all of the oxygen receptor sites on the hemoglobin). There are conditions where there is adequate oxygen in the blood, but it cannot get to the tissues (e.g., tissue swelling). Anoxia is the total absence of oxygen (e.g., a complete coronary vessel blockage or a patient trapped in an environment that has no oxygen). This causes anaerobic metabolism, which is very inefficient and produces lactic acid.

Q What is the voluntary versus involuntary regulation of respiration?

A The involuntary regulation of respiration involves nervous system controls and monitoring of oxygenation at the cellular level by the brain. Voluntary regulation involves changing the respiration rate due to anxiety, a stress reaction, a psychological reaction, or pain (e.g., rib fracture).

Airway Control

Q Besides the tongue, what are the most common forms of airway obstruction, and what are other causes of airway obstruction?

A Common causes of airway obstruction include foreign bodies, laryngeal spasm, edema, a fractured larynx, and aspiration. Less common causes are muscle diseases (e.g., myasthenia gravis), in which the supporting muscles lose tone and cause an obstruction.

CLINICAL PEARL

Patients with neurological problems (e.g., stroke, transient ischemic attack [TIA], coma), tend to hypoventilate even though they may look fine. Assume that any patient with a neurological emergency is hypoventilating and hypoxemic until proven otherwise.

Q What are the signs and symptoms of a foreign body airway obstruction (FBAO)?

A The patient may present with choking, gagging, stridor, dyspnea, aphonia (the inability to speak), or dysphonia (difficulty speaking).

Q What causes laryngeal spasm?

A Laryngeal spasm is a closure of the vocal cords and surrounding muscles. A frequent cause is trauma from an overly aggressive intubation attempt. It may also occur following extubation, in drowning (especially cold water exposure), and in allergy shock (anaphylaxis).

Q What causes laryngeal edema?

A The glottic opening may become extremely narrow or totally obstructed due to a bacterial infection in the epiglottis called epiglottitis or a severe allergic reaction. This can also occur due to swelling from the trauma of inhaling smoke, superheated gases, or caustic toxic substances.

Q How can a fractured larynx cause an airway obstruction?

A The patency of the airway is dependent on the intact muscular and skeletal structures of the jaw, hyoid bone, and larynx. When a patient receives blunt trauma to the neck, the larynx may be fractured. The result is a decreased diameter from swelling, a lack of muscular tone, and an increased ventilatory effort. This increases the airway resistance, much like breathing through a straw.

Q What effect can aspiration have in obstructing the airway?

A Besides the obvious effect of a mouth or airway full of foreign materials, such as blood, secretions, beer and peanuts, or the last meal, aspiration significantly increases mortality by obstructing the airway and decreasing the ability to ventilate. Regurgitated or vomited stomach acids can easily destroy delicate lung tissue and introduce pathogens into the lungs. The resulting chemical aspiration pneumonia may be fatal. The EMS provider's ability to clear the airway properly and prevent aspiration is paramount.

Q What are some signs to identify a patient with an airway problem?

A Signs to identify a patient with an airway problem include:
- Observation of the rise and fall of the chest.
- Observation of gasping and nasal flaring.
- Observation of the color of the skin—red or pink usually suggests good oxygenation; blue, grey, or pale skin is an indicator of poor oxygenation.
- Observation of pursed lips that allows patients to let the air out of their lungs slowly.
- Observation of muscle retractions in the intercostal spaces, suprasternal notch, supraclavicular fossa, and subcostal areas.

Q How is a complete airway obstruction handled in the field?

A Basic life support (BLS) techniques range from using proper airway positioning, finger sweeps with adult patients (when something is seen in the mouth), abdominal thrusts (formerly called Heimlich maneuver), and chest thrusts with small children and pregnant and obese patients. Advanced life support

(ALS) techniques include using Magill forceps, attempting to visualize the obstruction, attempting to push it down the right mainstem bronchus, and surgical airway procedures. The technique of choice depends upon the provider's training, scope of practice, and protocols. More specifics on the latest guidelines for health care providers in the management of foreign body airway obstruction are found in Chapter 9, Basic Life Support.

Q **What is the purpose of suctioning the upper airway?**

A The upper airway is suctioned to remove fluid, blood, or secretions so the patient does not aspirate foreign substances into the lungs.

Q **What are the different types of suction devices?**

A There are many different types of suction units: vacuum-powered devices onboard the ambulance; manual units such as a "turkey baster," bulb syringe, V-Vac®, or foot pump unit; oxygen-powered units; battery-powered units; and electrical units that are either AC or DC powered.

Q **What are the advantages and disadvantages of the different suction units?**

A Manual units usually work, but often have very small collection bottles. They are lightweight, portable, usually inexpensive, and mechanically simple. They take one or two hands or even your foot to operate, reducing the number of other things that you can do. It may be helpful to have a bystander pump the foot suction device. The "turkey baster" or V-Vac® unit is easy to employ and small enough to carry in a "first-in" bag. No matter which suction unit you choose, it does little good sitting out in the truck if the patient is vomiting in the house! Select one that you can easily carry in and *always* carry it when you conduct an initial assessment of the patient.

Oxygen-powered units work well, but they deplete your oxygen source rapidly. Some of the older units have very small collection bottles that do not stand upright easily. That is usually not a concern, but if the unit is on its side sometimes the fluid that has collected will interrupt the suction. Oxygen-powered units work off the venturi principle: gas flows through a small pin hole at high pressure and creates a draft of the room air behind. This produces a very accurate mixture of oxygen and room air with large volumes of gas, mostly the room air. When used in a suction unit, the flow of the room air is channeled through the top of the collection bottle so there is suction at the end of the tubing. This unit works well provided there is an adequate source of oxygen and the bottle is not tipped over, disrupting the venturi flow.

Mounted vacuum-powered suction devices have an extremely strong vacuum that is adjustable. The fluid contact components are usually disposable for ease of cleaning. These are not portable and fixing them in the field is not possible if they break down. Always have a backup unit available in the ambulance.

Battery-powered units are most commonly used in the field because they are lightweight and portable. They have been improved over the years so that they have large collection bottles similar to those used in the hospital. Disposable components reduce any potential contact with the biohazards in the tubing and collection bottle. The biggest problem with any battery-powered device, such as a portable radio or suction unit, is the regular charging schedule of the batteries. All batteries must be charged, maintained, deep discharged (depending on the type), and replaced regularly. Check your suction units every shift to make sure they are ready for service.

Q **When is it necessary to use sterile technique to suction a patient?**

A Whenever any catheter or tube is placed in a patient's mouth, it should be clean. If the catheter is going to be passed into the tracheobronchial region, it must be sterile and you should use sterile gloves and technique. This is because the introduction of foreign materials or germs on a non-sterile catheter can cause a serious infection in the lungs. Always hyperoxygenate before and after suctioning and limit the time of suctioning to 10 to 15 seconds. When suctioning down an ET tube, injecting three to five cc's of sterile water may be necessary to loosen the secretions.

Q **Why do most textbooks say to limit the time for suctioning to 10 to 15 seconds?**

A The principle here is that time spent suctioning is time *not* oxygenating. This has always been confusing to the new EMS providers because they would like exact numbers and the textbooks often do not agree. You should also remember that while the suction unit is on, it is "sucking out" air and fluid, thus emptying the patient's respiratory tree of oxygen. That is why the time the unit is on has to be limited. Enter the oropharynx first, *then* turn on the suction as you evacuate the pool of fluid on your way out. Never just leave the suction unit tubing, catheter, or rigid tip inside the patient. Once it finishes sucking out the liquid, it will also suck out gas from the lungs, removing the patient's oxygen.

Q **What is vagus nerve stimulation and why is this important to understand when suctioning a patient?**

A The vagus nerve is a cranial nerve that affects much of the body. There are many ways to stimulate it. Examples of vagal stimuli include applying pressure to the eyes, tickling the back of the throat, carotid sinus stimulation, or changes in the intrathoracic pressure (e.g., bearing down). When the vagus nerve is stimulated, the heart rate slows. This can be quite a problem for the patient who is having a myocardial infarction (MI), has a dysrhythmia, or has a very fragile medical condition. In some circumstances, a vagal stimulus can be the precursor to ventricular fibrillation and death. When you suction patients, limit your time to 10 to 15 seconds, then reoxygenate. If the patient is on a heart monitor, watch the monitor or listen for the beeps that indicate a slowing of the patient's heart rate. If the patient's heart rate begins to slow, finish suctioning quickly and reoxygenate the patient with the bag-valve-mask (BVM).

When is it inappropriate to insert a flexible suction catheter into the nasopharynx?

When suctioning the pharynx in adults, a rigid-tip device is preferred because you can direct where the tip is going and handling it is easier. Rigid suction tips are uncomfortable if placed through the nose. A flexible catheter is designed to be passed down a tube such as the ET tube or a nasal airway. If you suspect that the patient may have a basilar skull fracture, do not pass a catheter into the nose blindly. The catheter could actually enter the fracture site and possibly pass into brain tissue.

How do I know when I should suction the patient?

When patients make gurgling sounds or have visible secretions or blood in their airway, they should be suctioned. Most patients begin to collect secretions in the back of their throat and mouth when lying down. The situation is worse in those without a gag reflex. Medical patients should be placed in the recovery position so their airway can drain. Apply suction as necessary. In a trauma patient, maintain manual in-line stabilization of the neck and have another rescuer apply suction. If you cannot keep up with the fluid, it may be necessary to log roll the patient on the side to clear the airway while maintaining manual in-line stabilization of the neck.

Remember, suction units are designed for blood, fluid, and secretions. They are not designed for big chunks of food or other substances. Sweep out the big stuff with your gloved finger.

What are the advantages of and indications for oral airways?

Oral airways or oropharyngeal airways are hard plastic tubes designed to prevent the tongue from obstructing the glottis. They are indicated for unconscious patients or any patient who does not have a gag reflex. Oropharyngeal airways are noninvasive, are easily placed as shown in Figure 11–2, and help to prevent blockage of the glottis by the tongue. They do not guarantee that the airway will remain patent. That is your responsibility and may involve manual positioning and suctioning to maintain the airway.

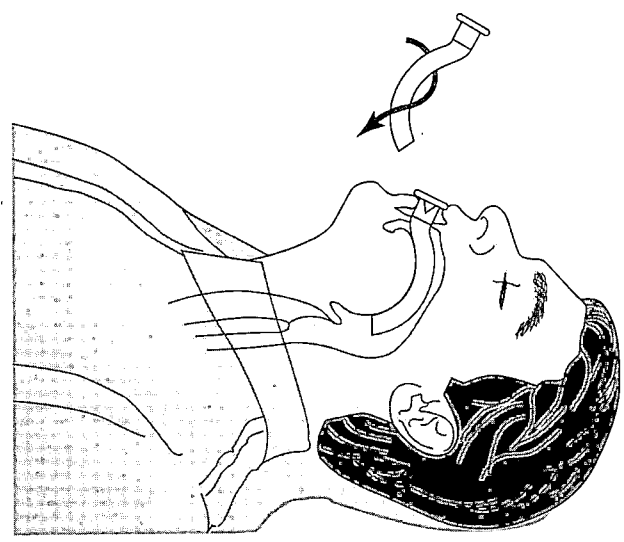

FIGURE 11–2 OPA insertion.

What are the advantages of and indications for nasal airways?

Nasal airways are indicated for unconscious patients and patients with an altered level of consciousness. Because they do not go down into the throat, a suppressed gag reflex is helpful but not essential (Figure 11–3). Using one in each nostril can also be useful. Nasal airways can be suctioned through, provide a patent airway, and can be tolerated by conscious patients. Nasal airways can be safely placed blindly and do not require the mouth to be opened during insertion.

Why are nasal airways curved with a bevel on the end?

The airway is curved to follow the natural curvature of the nasopharynx. The bevel on the end is designed to face the nasal

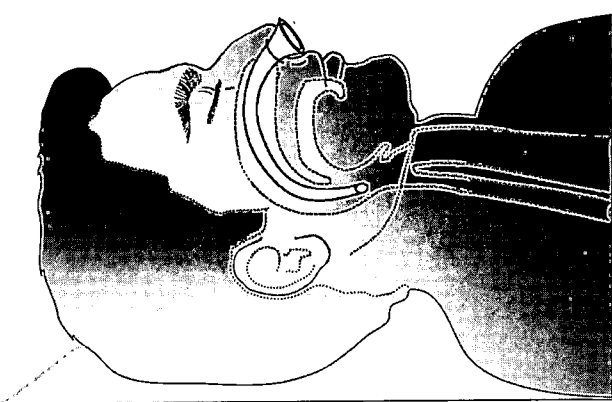

FIGURE 11–3 In this model, the NPA is clearly behind the tongue in a position where it can help to protect the airway, yet it does not often stimulate a gag reflex.

septum. For that reason, nasal airways are usually designed to be inserted in the right nostril. That does not mean they cannot be used in the left if there is difficulty inserting one in the right.

Q What is the rule of thumb for sizing a nasal airway?

A Use an airway that is the same diameter as the patient's "pinky" (fifth or "little") finger.

Q Why should only a water-soluble jelly be used when lubricating a nasal airway and what are some examples of these products?

A Petroleum jelly, such as Vaseline®, and other hydrocarbon-based products are not biodegradable and can collect in the lung tissue causing a chemical aspiration pneumonia. Water-soluble products, such as KY®, Lubifax®, and Surgilube®, are less irritating to the tissue if a small amount should get into the lungs. Also, hydrocarbon-based products may break down the plastic, latex, or rubber of the airway itself.

Respiratory Distress

Q What are the general causes of respiratory distress?

A Causes of respiratory distress may include upper and lower airway obstruction, inadequate ventilation, impairment of the respiratory muscles, and impairment of the nervous system. Many factors can contribute to any of these general categories.

Q How does the EMS provider assess a patient's breathing?

A Observe the patient. At rest, an adult normally breathes between 12 and 24 times per minute. Each breath should be regular, steady, and effortless. The patient should have no difficulty speaking in full sentences and no obvious use of positioning (e.g., sitting up to breathe better) and accessory muscles (e.g., supraclavicular or intercostal retractions).

Q What is pulsus paradoxus and when does it occur?

A Pulsus paradoxus is present when the systolic BP drops more than 10 mmHg with inspiration. A change in the pulse quality may also be detected during inspiration. This is seen in chronic obstructive pulmonary disease (COPD) patients and patients with pericardial tamponade. It may also occur during an asthma attack. The cause is felt to be increased intrathoracic and pericardial pressures that decrease the venous return to the heart.

Q What protective reflexes are used by patients to modify their respirations?

A Patients may modify their respiration with any of the following protective reflexes:

- Cough—forceful exhalation that aids in clearing the bronchi and bronchioles.
- Sneeze—clears the nasopharynx of mucous and foreign material.
- Gag reflex—also called a swallow reflex, a spastic pharyngeal and esophageal reflex due to a stimulus of the posterior pharynx.
- Sighing—involuntary deep breath that increases the opening of alveoli to prevent atelectasis (localized collapsed areas of nonaerated lung), which occurs an average of once every hour.
- Hiccup—intermittent spastic closure of the glottis.

Q What are examples of respiratory patterns other than normal breathing?

A Normal breathing is referred to as eupnea. There are many different respiratory patterns as shown in Figure 11–4. Five of the most common respiratory patterns are:

- Cheyne-Stokes—gradually increasing rate and tidal volume, which increases to a maximum, then gradually decreases. This pattern occurs when the brain stem has been injured.

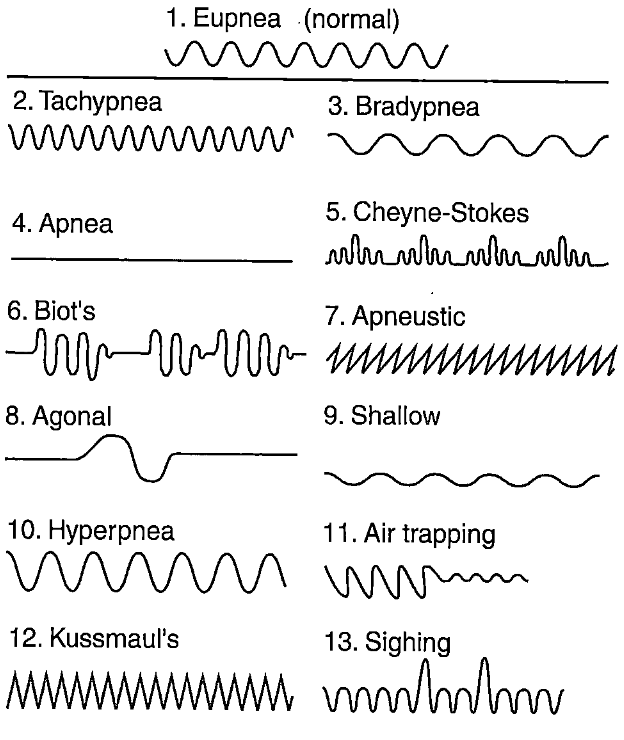

FIGURE 11–4 Respiratory patterns.

- Kussmaul's—deep gasping respirations, representing hyperventilation, "blow off" (breath out) excess CO_2 and compensate for an abnormal accumulation of metabolic acids in the blood (metabolic acidosis). Though possible in any patient with metabolic acidosis (e.g., aspirin poisoning, alcoholic ketoacidosis, methanol poisoning, kidney failure, sepsis), this respiratory pattern is best known with diabetic ketoacidosis.
- Biot's—irregular pattern and volume with intermittent periods of apnea found in patients with increased intracranial pressure.
- Central neurogenic hyperventilation—deep, rapid, regular respiration found in a patient who has increased intracranial pressure.
- Agonal—slow, shallow, irregular respiration that results from brain anoxia.

What is meant by modified forms of respiration?

Patients may modify their respirations by positioning themselves to make it easier to breathe (e.g., sniffing position, Fowler's position, or tripod position).

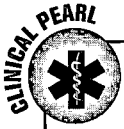

> *Patients are not usually consciously aware that they took on a "special breathing position."*

What is gastric distension and how is it caused?

Gastric distension is an expansion of the stomach usually due to an excess of trapped air. When the rescuer is giving too much ventilatory volume (usually too fast) or the airway is not properly opened, excess air enters the esophagus and, ultimately, the stomach. This causes two major problems. First, a rapidly enlarging stomach places pressure on the diaphragm and limits the lung expansion. This creates resistance to bag-valve-mask (BVM) ventilation. Second, if there is food in the stomach, the introduction of air increases the chances of regurgitation and the potential for aspiration. This is discussed in more detail in Chapter 9, Basic Cardiac Life Support.

How can gastric distension be managed in a noninvasive manner in the field?

The noninvasive method of managing gastric distension is to increase the BVM ventilation time in adults to 2 seconds per inspiration and in pediatric patients to 1 to 1.5 seconds per breath. It can be relieved by *being prepared* to suction potentially large volumes, placing the patient in the left lateral position, and then *slowly* applying pressure to the epigastric region, suctioning as necessary to ensure that the patient does not aspirate.

What are the indications for and advantages of using a gastric tube?

A gastric tube is a tube placed in the stomach for gastric decompression and emesis control. Nasogastric decompression is indicated when there is a threat of aspiration or the need to lavage the patient. It is tolerated by conscious patients, does not interfere with intubation, permits the patient to talk, and mitigates recurrent gastric distension and nausea.

What are the contraindications for and disadvantages of using a gastric tube?

Nasogastric decompression should be used with extreme caution in patients with esophageal disease or trauma, facial trauma, or esophageal obstruction. These patients may have weaknesses in the wall of their esophagus that could be damaged by the tube. It is uncomfortable for the patient, may cause the patient to vomit during placement even if the gag reflex is suppressed, and interferes with a mask seal.

> *Naso- or orogastric intubation causes vagus nerve stimulation and may lead to bradycardia, heart block, or asystole. The risk is greatest in persons with inferior myocardial infarction. Though it may occur in anyone, in most cases, patients respond promptly to atropine and termination of the procedure.*

Where did the old 800 cc minimum standard ventilation come from?

The 800 cc standard is an average minimum for the typical 150-pound patient. The 150-pound patient is an average of the male and female normal weights. When ventilating, the patient needs 10 to 12 cc's of ventilation volume per kilogram of body weight. Because there are 2.2 pounds in each kilogram, the 150-pound patient should require approximately 680 to 818 cc's as a minimum. This is only a minimum, especially for heavier patients such as the 220-pound patient (100 Kg) who requires between 1,000 and 1,200 cc's. As discussed in Chapter 9, Basic Cardiac Life Support, the Guidelines 2000 have decreased the required ventilation volume, especially in cases where 100 percent oxygen is being administered.

> *The myth of the ideal "70 kg (150 pound)" patient is just that. The formula is a "cookbook." Make sure you are a "thinking cook!"*

🅀 What is the risk of infection to the EMS provider associated with ventilation?

🅰 Managing the airway can be a serious hazard due to the exposure to body fluids. Protect yourself from body fluids that could spread diseases such as hepatitis, tuberculosis (TB), meningitis, or influenza. Always use disposable gloves, an eye shield, and mask when suctioning and ventilating a patient. This helps to prevent spurting materials from getting into your mouth or eyes. In addition, consider the contents of the suction unit tubing, catheter, and canister to be a biohazard and dispose of them properly. If you do not have a completely disposable system, always wear personal protective equipment (PPE) when cleaning the suction unit.

🅀 What are the safety considerations to keep in mind when handling oxygen tanks and regulators?

🅰 Oxygen tanks are pressurized vessels and, as such, they can be very dangerous if not handled safely. If a tank is accidentally dropped, the weakest point is the valve stem or regulator if one is attached to the tank. The regulator can be easily damaged. If the valve stem broke, it could send the pressurized vessel flying like a missile, injuring everything and everyone in its path.

Add to this the oxygen stored in the tank that supports combustion and will cause a fire to burn rapidly. Here are some simple rules to follow:

- Only use tubing, pressure gauges, and regulators that are designed for oxygen use.
- Use nonferrous metal oxygen wrenches for changing gauges and regulators and adjusting flow rates to avoid sparks.
- Make sure the valve seal inserts and gaskets are in good condition and there are no leaks at the tanks or gauge.
- Cylinders have to be hydrostatically tested every five years. If a tank has a star after the test date, it is good for a 10-year period.
- Use medical grade oxygen because industrial grade oxygen contains impurities.
- Do not use adhesive tape on oxygen tanks or to mark or label tanks or delivery devices. The oxygen could react with the adhesive and debris and cause a fire.
- Open the valve of an oxygen cylinder fully, then close it a quarter turn.
- Store spare oxygen tanks in a vented, cool room, properly secured in place.
- Be careful not to drop a cylinder or let it fall against an object. When transporting a patient with an oxygen tank, be sure to strap it in or secure it to the litter.
- Oxygen cylinders in a standing position must be secured.

- Clearly mark the area of oxygen use with signs that say "OXYGEN—NO SMOKING."
- Do not use oil, grease, or fat-based soaps on devices that will be attached to an oxygen tank. Do not handle these devices with greasy hands. Use greaseless tools for connections.
- Do not drag or roll an oxygen cylinder on its side or bottom.

CLINICAL PEARL

Many newer providers think that the "flying oxygen tank" is a myth. I thought so too until I saw a flying tank take out a brick wall!

🅀 What is the normal maximum tank pressure and how does it get reduced down to the liters per minute that is administered to the patient?

🅰 The pressure of the tank (tank pressure) is usually around 2,200 PSI when the tank is full. High-pressure regulators are designed to be attached to the cylinder stem and deliver the cylinder gas under high pressure. High-pressure regulators are also used to transfer cylinder gas from tank to tank, as in a cascade system. The high pressure must be first reduced down to a lower pressure so that it can be delivered to the patient in the normal range of 10 to 15 liters per minute. A therapy regulator is designed to be attached to the cylinder stem, or wall of the ambulance, and is generally set at 50 PSI. The actual delivery to the patient is adjustable on the flowmeter to liters per minute.

🅀 What is the maximum pressure recommended for positive-pressure ventilation?

🅰 The pressure of a positive-pressure ventilator should not exceed 30 cm of water pressure.

🅀 Which oxygen delivery devices are potentially useful in out-of-hospital care for breathing patients?

🅰 The following oxygen delivery devices may be helpful:
- Nasal cannula.
- Non-rebreather mask.
- Small volume nebulizer.
- Simple face mask.
- Partial-rebreather mask.
- Venturi mask.

We also use "blow-by" oxygen or can poke oxygen tubing through the bottom of a plastic or paper cup for pediatric patients. The oxygen is blown by the face of the child in this manner. Do not use a styrofoam cup because the child may inhale the fluorocarbons.

When is a nasal cannula used and what are its advantages and contraindications?

Nasal cannulas are usually used on patients receiving low to moderate oxygen enrichment for long periods. In the field, it is common to use a nasal cannula to continue the therapy of a patient on a nasal cannula who is not in respiratory distress. It is contraindicated in patients who are mouth breathers and patients with a poor respiratory effort, severe hypoxia, or apnea. Nasal cannula oxygen is tolerated well. It offers, even if inadequate, an alternative for hypoxic patients who simply will not tolerate a mask.

When is a non-rebreather mask used and what are its advantages and contraindications?

The non-rebreather mask delivers from 80 to 95 percent oxygen at 15 liters per minute. It is indicated whenever a patient needs oxygen, has a good respiratory effort, and is not apneic. An advantage is that it provides the highest oxygen concentration enrichment with a high volume. When patients inhale, they receive oxygen-enriched gas from the reservoir bag rather than residual air from a partial-rebreather bag.

How should the liter flow for a non-rebreather mask be set?

Before placing the mask on the patient's face, set the flow at 15 liters per minute and close the valve inside the mask. This allows oxygen to fill the reservoir bag. After watching the patient breathe, make sure the liter flow is adjusted so the bag is at least ¾ full before each breath.

Why do some non-rebreather masks have a port without a valve?

A true non-rebreather mask has three valves. Two are on the outside of the mask. These close when the patient inhales so the inspired air comes directly out of the bag and does not leak in through the mask from the environment. The third valve is inside the mask on the top of the bag and opens when the patient inspires so the patient receives only oxygen from the bag. Some non-rebreather masks are provided with only one valve on the outside of the mask. This is done by the manufacturer as a safeguard in case the patient was not closely watched and the caregiver allowed the reservoir bag to completely empty. Should that situation occur, the patient is able to obtain room air from the open, uncapped valve. In the out-of-hospital setting, it makes the most sense to use the non-rebreather with three valves and pay attention to the reservoir bag. If the patient is overbreathing the bag, turn up the liter flow.

What is a small volume nebulizer?

A small volume nebulizer is another form of administering oxygen combined with a medication, such as albuterol. The medication is delivered to the patient in an aerosolized form. Pressurized oxygen enters the aerosol (medication) chamber, which contains 3–5 cc's of fluid. The result is a mist of oxygen and medication (an aerosol) that is inhaled easily.

What is a laryngectomy and how is a patient altered?

When a patient has the larynx removed, usually due to cancer, the airway may be attached to the end of a stoma in the neck. This is called a complete laryngectomy. When doing rescue breathing, you ventilate into the stoma as shown in Figure 11–5. If the patient has a partial laryngectomy, there may still be an open pathway through the mouth as well as a stoma. In this case, when ventilating through the stoma, you have to cover the mouth so the air does not exit there.

Why is the two-person (or even three person) BVM technique preferable to the one-person technique?

Much evidence supports the notion that one rescuer using a BVM on a medical patient is less than optimal. The key is that there should always be two hands on the mask to seal it to the face. Thus, an additional person has to squeeze the bag. If the patient is being ventilated and has an ET tube in place, the need for a rescuer to hold the mask is eliminated. Still, studies have suggested that two hands squeezing the bag are better than one!

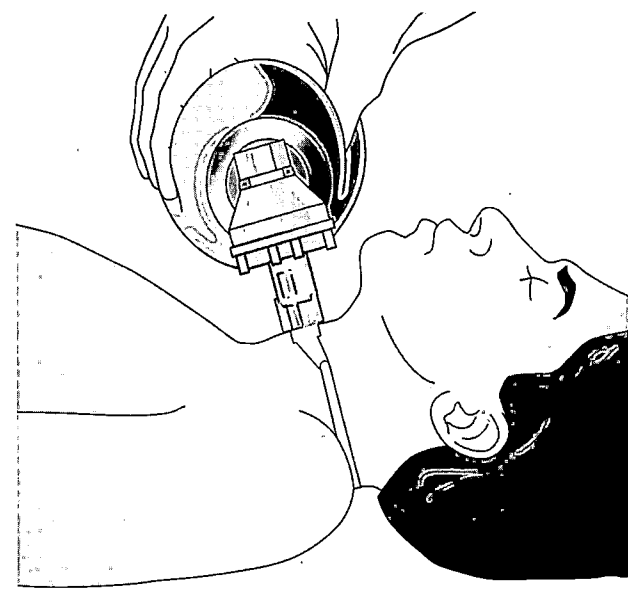

FIGURE 11–5 Ventilating a stoma.

Why is the use of a BVM with one rescuer less than optimal?

Research has shown that a one-handed mask seal on a medical patient is difficult to master, even for short periods. The tidal volume delivered is dependent on the mask seal's integrity. In a trauma patient, doing a one-handed mask seal and a jaw thrust with only one rescuer is impossible.

Then why is BVM ventilation tested on practical exams?

That's a good question! Practice and evaluation often lag behind research findings. Also, there may not be two rescuers to dedicate to the airway, so all health care providers should be capable of using a BVM by themselves, even if for a short period of time.

CLINICAL PEARL

Studies on BVM and the required "number of hands" have shown repeatedly that the one-handed technique delivers less than 800 cc. Fortunately, the research used in the Guidelines 2000 has "lowered the bar." It is now acceptable to ventilate with lower volumes provided the BVM is attached to 100 percent oxygen. Remember that tidal volume estimates are based on the "average" patient and larger patients require more volume. Thus, the one-handed technique is likely to be even more ineffective in a larger patient.

What is the best technique to achieve a good mask seal?

For the best mask seal, position yourself approximately 18 inches above the head of the patient. Seal the mask on the face using a jaw thrust, with the thumbs on the mask and the index or middle fingers jutting the jaw. With a medical patient, tilt the head back as if you were trying to "stand the patient on his head." With a trauma patient, do not tilt the head, simply jut the jaw as shown in Figure 11–6. If you hear or feel air leaking around the mask, reposition it. *Any* air leak reduces the volume that the patient receives dramatically.

Can I use my leg to help squeeze the BVM?

Some instructors have allowed their students to squeeze the BVM bag against their leg as they kneel directly at the head of the patient. Usually, this is done because the instructor has concluded that, due to small hands, the student is unable to squeeze an adequate volume of air out of the bag. However, with the com-

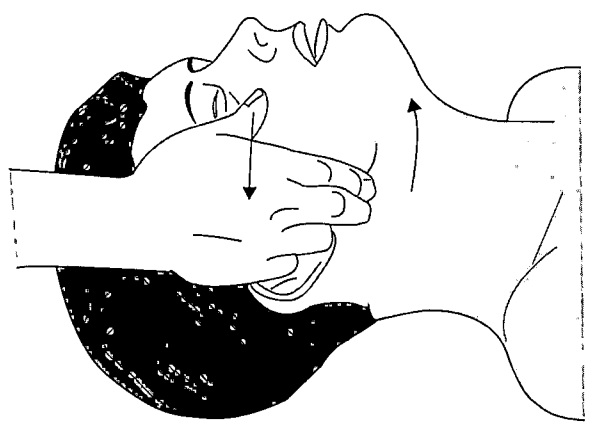

FIGURE 11–6 Jaw thrust maneuver.

bination of a proper seal, proper rescuer positioning, and rescuers using the weight of their arms to hold the airway open, this situation is unlikely. Placing the patient's head between one's legs in order to squeeze the bag, makes visually evaluating the airway very difficult for the rescuer.

If there are two rescuers on the BVM, how should they be used?

One rescuer seals the mask and juts the jaw using the jaw thrust, while the second rescuer squeezes the BVM bag. If trauma is suspected, an untrained assistant is best used to squeeze the bag.

Why are pediatric pop-off valves not recommended on the adult BVM?

If you are going to ventilate an adult, use an adult BVM. If you are going to ventilate an infant or child, use the infant or child size BVM. A pop-off valve should not be used or engaged on any size BVM during resuscitation. Some EMS providers have been sold adult BVMs with pop-off valves and led to believe that the pop-off valve will avoid overinflation if it is used on a child. Actually, when the valve senses pressure, it opens and the excess air is expelled, rather than being administered to the patient. There have been cases when an adult BVM was used to ventilate a pediatric patient and the EMS provider did not realize that all of the volume was exiting through the pop-off valve and no air was going to the patient. Thus, the patient received no oxygen during the entire resuscitation!

If you have a BVM with a pop-off valve, replace it because it may be a serious problem. If you do not have the proper size for children, then get them. Do not improvise because the danger of ineffective equipment can be fatal. Airway management and resuscitation equipment has to fit the patient; it can't be adjusted like splinting.

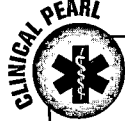

Using pop-off valves is a surefire invitation to the courtroom.

Once a cervical collar is applied to a patient, can it be removed for intubation or if there is a problem opening the airway?

The priority is *always* the airway. If the patient has a potential spine injury, "adjust" your technique to avoid moving the head or neck by using the jaw thrust without a head tilt. This can usually be accomplished with the proper size collar. Occasionally, it may be necessary to remove the collar if there is difficulty keeping the airway open. Most anesthesiologists prefer removing the anterior portion of a cervical collar if a Philadelphia® collar is used because this allows for easier movement of the jaw. Of course, whenever the patient's head and neck is not taped down to the long board, there must always be two hands providing manual in-line stabilization until the neck is cleared in the ED.

What are the indications and contraindications for intermittent positive-pressure breathing (IPPB)?

IPPB is indicated when a conscious or unconscious adult patient needs a high volume of high concentration oxygen. It is not indicated in noncompliant patients (breathing patients that fight the device), patients with poor tidal volume, and small children.

What are the advantages of IPPB?

IPPB can be self-administered, and it delivers a high volume and a high oxygen concentration. There is no oxygen wasted because it is delivered in response to the inspiratory effort. This also helps to reduce the risk of overinflation when the pressure delivered is less than 30 cm of water.

What are the disadvantages and complications of IPPB?

With IPPB, you cannot monitor lung compliance. To operate, an oxygen source is required. Complications include gastric distension if the airway is not properly opened and overinflation often occurs. The patient can also experience barotrauma with IPPB that is not properly administered.

Why can't a "demand-valve" be used on a nonbreathing patient?

The patient has to be breathing to create negative pressure on the valve. The device then administers oxygen to the patient throughout inspiration. Nonbreathing patients do not create this negative pressure. What caused the confusion in the past was a manufacturer's product called "Demand Valve," which actually was a multifunction device, involving both the demand feature and a positive-pressure ventilator.

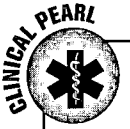

Automatic transport ventilators eliminate problems intrinsic to BVM ventilation.

What are the indications and advantages of an automatic transport ventilator (ATV)?

ATVs are used in some field applications that involve extended ventilation of intubated patients such as critical care transports. ATVs allow for control of the ventilation volume and rate. They are lightweight, portable, durable, and mechanically simple, and adaptable to portable oxygen tanks. By setting the ATV properly, the ventilation can actually be delivered over two seconds, minimizing airway pressure and the risk of gastric distension. To do this manually using a BVM over a period of time is difficult at best.

What are the contraindications and disadvantages of an ATV?

The ATV is contraindicated in awake patients who might fight the device, and with obstructed airways or increased airway resistance due to pneumothorax, asthma, or pulmonary edema. Disadvantages include: tube displacement is not detectable, it does not detect increasing airway resistance, securing it is difficult, and it is dependent on the oxygen tank pressure.

What is meant by "noninvasive ventilation" and what is its use in the field?

"Noninvasive ventilation" refers to positive-pressure ventilation using a tight-fitting nasal or face mask, but without ET intubation. The first use of this technique originated in-hospital when continuous positive airway pressure (CPAP) was applied by mask to respiratory and cardiac patients. It was so successful that portable units were devised and used at home, especially by people with sleep apnea. The principle is that the patient constantly breathes against a small amount of positive pressure. The pressure causes previously collapsed (atelectatic) airways to open, improving oxygenation.

The next step was the development of biphasic positive airway pressure (BiPAP) devices. They were similar to CPAP masks, but could vary the degree of positive pressure during inspiration and expiration separately. The ability to vary the pressure made the system more comfortable and was effective in most patients. In-hospital and ED work with these devices has been very promising. It has been used with many diseases including COPD, asthma, and acute cardiogenic pulmonary edema. A few small field trials have had excellent results.

The major advantage of noninvasive ventilation is that intubation is avoided by some patients who might previously have required it. This "middle-of-the-road" population avoids the risks of "traditional" mechanical ventilation and improves much quicker than with simple ventilatory adjuncts alone. Be alert to the increased use of BiPAP systems in out-of-hospital care in the future.

What is atelectasis and how is it caused?

The collapse of the smaller airways and alveoli due to hypoventilation or obstruction is called atelectasis. Literally, the term means collapse due to inadequate aeration. Atelectasis is sometimes a complication of abdominal surgery or rib fractures because taking a deep breath is very painful for patients. As a result, they decrease their tidal volume. When we sigh or take a larger breath, it helps to open the smaller airways that are not always well ventilated and prevents atelectasis. Patients in pain fail to sigh as deeply or as often as is normal.

Why is the ET tube more likely to inadvertently slide into the right mainstem bronchus than the left?

This occurs because it's a "straight shot" from the trachea to the right mainstem bronchus. The angle to enter the right mainstem is much less acute than on the left side. To enter the left mainstem bronchus, the ET tube has to make a sharp turn.

What is the "sniffing position" and when is it used?

The "sniffing position" is used to help visualize the vocal cords during intubation. Envision sitting upright holding a rose six inches from your nose. The "sniffing position" is when you move your nose and head forward to try to take a sniff without moving your entire torso. We try to use this position to intubate supine medical patients by placing a folded hand towel behind the head to approximate the sniff position.

When is it appropriate to extubate a patient?

Generally, it is *rarely* appropriate to extubate a patient in the out-of-hospital setting unless the patient has died and the coro-

ner (or medical examiner) has granted permission. Once you intubate a patient in the out-of-hospital setting, the best policy is to leave the tube in until the patient is turned over to the ED.

At times, patients may extubate themselves. This is not a safe practice as they may injure themselves if the tube's cuff is still inflated or they may aspirate on vomitus. If a patient does seem like she is trying to pull the tube, consider physical and chemical restraint after consulting with medical control. Should the decision be made to extubate the patient, always be prepared to turn them on their side and suction their airway immediately following removal of the tube. If a patient does extubate herself, the EMS provider should reevaluate the need for intubation. If the patient's condition has stabilized (e.g., looks good, good oxygen saturation, etc.), administering oxygen and observation is reasonable. Be certain to follow local protocols and always inform medical control of any changes, including self-extubation by a patient.

> **CLINICAL PEARL**
> *Though still controversial, the appropriate use of paralytic agents (e.g., succinylcholine) prior to intubation is a safe and useful field procedure.*

What are the visual landmarks for direct laryngoscopy?

Whether using a straight or a curved blade, the object is to expose the glottis by upward traction on the handle. You should be able to see the vocal cords on either side of the glottic opening and the epiglottis anteriorly. Depending on the lighting and the patient's anatomy, the arytenoid cartilages may or may not be easily visible.

What is the Sellick's maneuver and when is it used?

The Sellick's maneuver is also known as "cricoid pressure." It is used to ease intubation and to decrease the chances of regurgitation. A second rescuer (or properly coached bystander) places firm, downward pressure on the anterolateral aspects of the cricoid cartilage with the thumb and index finger, as shown in Figure 11–7. The pressure must be maintained until after the ET tube is inserted *and* the cuff is inflated. It is important that this pressure be on the lateral edge of the cartilage, rather than the middle, otherwise visualization of the glottic opening may actually be more difficult.

> **CLINICAL PEARL**
> *The Sellick's maneuver has been called the "sore luck maneuver"—if the EMS provider applies pressure improperly, airway obstruction results.*

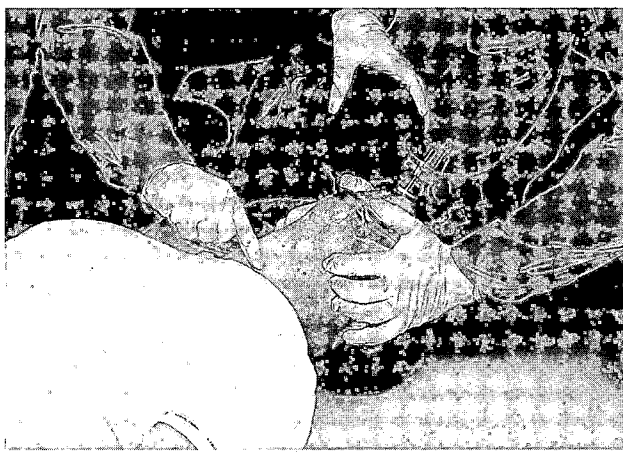

FIGURE 11-7 The Sellick maneuver.

[Q] **Why are airway adjuncts such as the esophageal obtu-rator airway (EOA), esophageal-gastric tube airway (EGTA), Combitube®, or pharyngeotracheal lumen air-way (PTL) considered indirect methods and not the "gold standard" of airway control?**

[A] The definitive "gold standard" of airway control is the ET tube. Most other "advanced" airway adjuncts are inserted blindly and indirectly provide ventilation and oxygenation by attempting to seal the esophagus. The EOA and EGTA have both fallen into disfavor over recent years and are rarely used in the field. Both the Combitube® and the PTL® offer rescuers an alternative when ET intubation is not readily available or is difficult to achieve. The Combitube® is probably easier to use because there is no need to maintain a mask seal with the device. Both devices have been shown to provide adequate airway control in the field. Given the choice, however, you should opt for ET intu-bation when it is available and the EMS providers are experi-enced in the technique. The introduction of the laryngeal mask airway (LMA) to field use in the Guidelines 2000 has caused many EMS Service medical directors to begin to ask the question, "Is there a better device for field use if my EMS providers are not experienced in ET intubation?" For more information on this topic, review Chapter 9, Basic Cardiac Life Support, and Chapter 52, Advanced Cardiac Life Support.

[Q] **What is an LMA and when should it be used?**

[A] The laryngeal mask airway or LMA, as shown in Figure 11-8, is an airway that has been used in the operating room for many years. In the Guidelines 2000, the LMA and Combitube® have been recommended as secondary airway adjuncts when ET intu-bation is difficult or not available.

This device is easy to insert into the airway because, like the Combitube®, it is inserted blindly. However, it does not protect the airway from gastric contents, vomitus, or other secretions. The criteria for its insertion include:

• The patient must have an absence of a gag reflex.

• The patient should have an empty stomach. This is difficult to ensure in the out-of-hospital setting, but studies have shown the risk of regurgitation is low.

• The device cannot be used under high-pressure airway condi-tions (e.g., chest trauma, airway trauma, or restrictive COPD.)

The LMA comes in a number of sizes for use on newly born patients to over-100 kg adults. Initial training and competency retraining is necessary; however, this takes far less time than ET tube placement training and retraining. The manufacturer has a number of versions of the product available. Versions vary from the disposable single-use model used in the field (the Unique LMA®) to the reusable LMA Classic® model.

[Q] **What is tactile or digital intubation and when is it used?**

[A] Digital or tactile intubation involves placing the first two digits into the mouth to push the tongue down. The ET tube is placed between the fingers, which guide the tube beneath the

CLINICAL PEARL

Currently, the EOA and EGTA are of historical interest only. Their use may now be grounds for a medical neg-ligence suit. If ET intubation is not available, either the Combitube® or the PTL offer an alternative. The LMA has been used in anesthesia for many years. Euroasian work has shown it to be an effective adjunct in the out-of-hospital set-ting. Field use of the LMA in the United States has not caught on due to the risk of gastric aspiration. The risk is low accord-ing to the studies and this may all change very quickly as the Guidelines 2000 are implemented across the country.

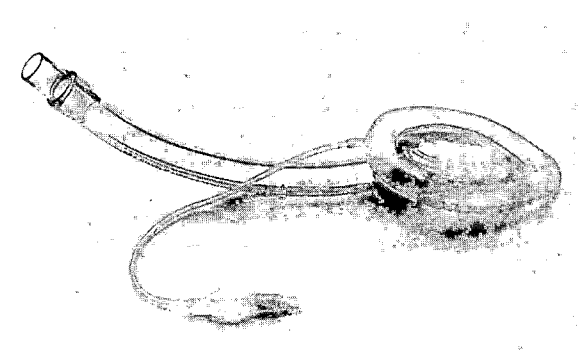

FIGURE 11-8 The laryngeal mask airway. *(Courtesy of LMA)*

epiglottis and anteriorly toward the larynx. This technique is most helpful in an unconscious patient when either the larynx cannot be seen on direct laryngoscopy (e.g., difficult anatomy, hemorrhage) or there is suspected cervical spine injury.

What is retrograde intubation and when is it used?

Retrograde intubation involves placing a needle through the cricothyroid membrane. A guide-wire is then threaded upward toward the oropharynx. The ET tube is placed over the guide-wire into the trachea. The wire is removed when the tube is in place. This technique, though effective, involves an invasive procedure beyond intubation. It should be reserved as a last resort and performed only by properly trained providers.

What is pulse oximetry and when is it used?

Pulse oximetry is a noninvasive technique that involves an electrode placed on the patient's fingertip and an infrared light beam to measure the oxygen saturation of the blood. The normal reading is 95 percent or greater. Patients whose saturation values are below 90 percent usually need supplemental oxygen.

CLINICAL PEARL

Though often called "the fifth vital sign," EMS providers must be aware that, like any test, pulse oximetry is only one parameter. If the patient looks sick and the pulse oximetry reading is normal, the patient is still sick!

Why does a pulse oximeter sometimes give false readings?

The principle of pulse oximetry assumes normal capillary blood flow, normal hemoglobin concentration, and a normal hemoglobin molecule. Any conditions that alter these "assumptions" may lead to false values. Thus, pulse oximetry may not be reliable during cardiac arrest, hypovolemia, hypothermia, in patients wearing nail polish, carbon monoxide poisoning (or any other disease with an altered hemoglobin molecule), shock, and severe anemia.

What is an end-tidal CO_2 (colormetric) device and how is it used?

Colormetric devices attach to the ET tube and detect exhaled CO_2 via color changes in the center of the device. Normally, intra-tracheal tube placement results in the exhalation of CO_2. If the tube is in the esophagus, CO_2 is absent. These devices do not work well for continuous monitoring because the mois-

ture in expired air ruins the paper filter in the device. Capnography is the preferred method for continuous monitoring.

What is capnography?

Capnography is an assessment of the level of carbon dioxide exhaled by the patient. End-tidal CO_2 ($EtCO_2$) is the concentration of carbon dioxide (CO_2) in the exhaled gas at the end of exhalation. The normal range of $EtCO_2$ is 36–44 mmHg. The readings obtained can help to determine whether a patient is breathing effectively or if an airway adjunct is properly inserted. The Guidelines 2000 have placed a strong emphasis on the use of end-tidal CO_2 monitoring as a secondary confirmation method of ET tube placement. (Review Chapter 9, Basic Cardiac Life Support, and Chapter 52, Advanced Cardiac Life Support for more information on these topics.)

When used for the evaluation of proper tracheal tube placement, capnography can confirm placement within seconds after an intubation attempt. Capnography also provides for continuous monitoring, which is the recommendation in the Guidelines 2000.

The presence of exhaled CO_2 indicates that tube placement is correct. The lack of $EtCO_2$ usually indicates that the tube is misplaced in the esophagus. Before an accurate reading is obtained, the patient should be ventilated 5–6 times to wash out any residual $EtCO_2$ that may be present in the esophagus, especially in non-perfusing patients.

False readings do occur. The most common scenarios for false readings are in non-perfusing patients, premature neonates < 2kg, the presence of a pulmonary embolism, and patients that had ingested carbonated liquids before a cardiac arrest.

What is the difference between a capnograph and a capnometer?

A capnograph provides $EtCO_2$ readings in two forms, one is a number and the other is a wave form or graph. The capnometer provides the reading in a number form only.

Besides listening to the lungs, how else can the proper placement of an ET tube be assessed?

The proper placement of an ET tube can be determined by a combination of the following:

- Always observe the tube go through the cords.
- Hold the tube at the teeth and take note of the number at the teeth. Once the tube is in the correct position, keeping track of the number is an easy way without an X-ray to monitor intra-tracheal tube position.
- Apply an esophageal intubation detector and withdraw air into the syringe.

- Listen over each lung field as well as the epigastrium.
- Consider applying an end-tidal CO_2 monitoring device as well as a pulse oximeter.
- Document what you did to ensure the tube was properly placed and recheck it frequently.

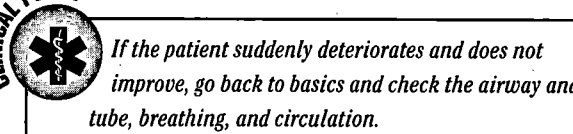

If the patient suddenly deteriorates and does not improve, go back to basics and check the airway and tube, breathing, and circulation.

🔲 What is an esophageal intubation detector and how is it used?

🅰 An esophageal intubation detector, as shown in Figure 11–9, is a syringe-like device that is helpful in verifying tracheal, versus esophageal, intubation. Attach the device when the patient is intubated and draw back on the syringe. If there is fluid in the syringe, the tube is probably in the esophagus. If pulling back the syringe is easy or there is some condensation, the tube is most likely in the lungs. If there is some difficulty withdrawing air into the syringe, it is probably because the tube is in the esophagus, a flat tube that collapses when suction is applied through the syringe. On the other hand, the trachea does not collapse due to the cartilaginous rings that maintain its shape. A few studies have questioned the reliability of this device. Always combine your clinical intuition with other methods of verification (e.g., breath sounds, patient response, visualization of the cords) to decide proper ET tube placement.

🔲 How often should I check the ET tube placement?

🅰 Placement is checked after intubation, after taping the tube, if the patient becomes difficult to ventilate, every few minutes, and after each patient move. Also, you should document that the tube placement was checked. Never leave the BVM attached when defibrillating the patient. The weight of the BVM tends to pull the tube out.

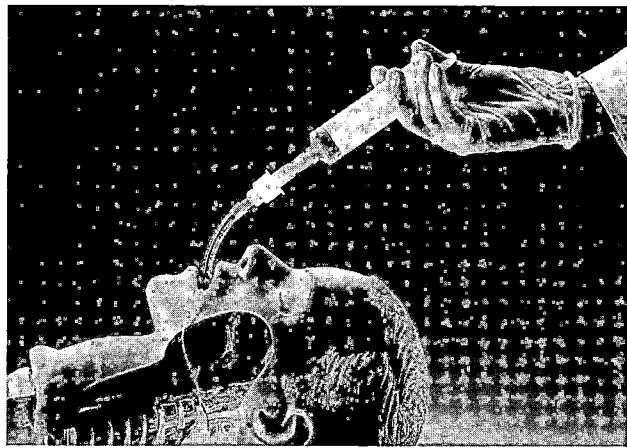

FIGURE 11–9 The esophageal intubation detector device (EID). *(Courtesy of Ambu, Inc., Linthicum, Maryland)*

🔲 Why are some ET tubes uncuffed?

🅰 Non-cuffed ET tubes are used for pediatric patients less than eight years old because the cricoid cartilage narrows the trachea and serves as a functional cuff.

🔲 What are the indications for and advantages of nasotracheal intubation?

🅰 Nasotracheal intubation is used in breathing patients only. Nasotracheal intubation does not require a laryngoscope, the sniffing position is not needed, and the tube is more easily secured. In addition, the patient cannot bite the tube.

🔲 What are the contraindications for and disadvantages of nasotracheal intubation?

🅰 Nasotracheal intubation is contraindicated or should be used with caution in patients with facial trauma or a deviated nasal septum. The major disadvantage is that this is a "blind" technique and may be used only in breathing patients.

🔲 Why is apnea a contraindication for nasal intubation?

🅰 Apnea is a contraindication because the tube is passed blindly and advanced as you hear the sounds of air moving through the glottic opening and vocal cords. If the patient is in respiratory arrest, there is no air movement.

🔲 What is a BAAM® adapter and how is it used?

🅰 A BAAM® (Beck Airway Airflow Monitor) adapter is used in nasal intubations because it makes a noise when air flows through it. Often, hearing the air flow past the cords without a device such as the BAAM® is difficult.

🔲 What is an Endotrol® tube?

🅰 An Endotrol® is an ET tube that has a plastic ring handle that, when pulled, bends the tip of the tube. This is especially helpful for nasal intubation because it allows the rescuer to flex the tube end to reach the vocal cords and glottic opening.

What are the indications for a needle cricothyrotomy?

Needle cricothyrotomy is a last-resort technique in a patient with a complete airway obstruction or in whom tracheal intubation is otherwise impossible. It may be done as a prelude to translaryngeal cannula ventilation as well.

What is translaryngeal cannula ventilation (TLCV) and when is it used?

It is a means of providing ventilation through a large-bore needle that is directly inserted through the cricothyroid membrane. TLCV is useful when there is complete airway obstruction or in a patient who urgently requires an airway and all other alternatives have failed.

What is transtracheal jet insufflation?

This is the same technique as TLCV. The catheter is connected to a pressure-controlled oxygen outlet incorporating a one-way valve.

What is rapid sequence induction (RSI) and when is it used?

RSI involves the administration of a neuromuscular blocker (paralyzing) drug, such as succinylcholine (SUX), usually with some type of sedative (e.g., benzodiazepine or narcotic) to simplify ET intubation. Though far from universal, many EMS systems are using paralytic drugs for RSI. Data have shown that, used appropriately, RSI is safe and may actually reduce morbidity by improving airway access. Patients who are conscious, uncooperative, and in severe respiratory distress are ideal candidates. RSI in combative, head-injured patients may be life saving. The sedative component is also very important, so that the patient's anxiety level is not raised during the short period of neuromuscular paralysis.

What neuromuscular blocking agents are used for RSI?

There are many agents available. The most commonly used paralytic is succinylcholine (SUX). It is safe and short-lasting (less than one hour). It can produce muscular tremors (fasciculations) that are generally of no consequence in most patients. Rarely, these tremors lead to hyperkalemia (elevation of serum potassium). SUX is contraindicated in patients with massive tissue damage (e.g., burns or severe crush injuries) due to the risk of hyperkalemia.

History Taking and Therapeutic Communication

E stablishing a rapport with a patient and taking a health history are a significant portion of the patient interview. It begins from the time the call is dispatched and lasts until the patient is turned over to the emergency department. Obtaining a good history is often difficult or impossible for many reasons. The patient may be a poor historian, have an altered mental status, be unconscious, be overwhelmed, or be nonverbal. Even when the patient is cared for by relatives, health care facilities, or resides in an adult residence home, pertinent patient information often is not available.

This chapter discusses why obtaining a patient history can be challenging and the techniques to obtain a patient history, including the history of the present illness or injury, and past medical history. Some tips on how therapeutic communication can help find the information when the patient is unable or unwilling to provide it are also discussed.

Health History

Q What forms of communication does the EMS provider use during patient care?

A As with most professions, communication is an integral component of the EMS profession. The communication process used by the EMS provider focuses around a message (information). The message moves through various forms:

- Written—messages placed on a report, document, letter, PCR, or e-mail.
- Verbal—exactly what is said and the tone and volume used.
- Nonverbal—posture, position, and facial expressions.
- Encoding—interpreting what message to send.
- Message—what points you were trying to convey subject to encoding and decoding perceptions.

- Decoding—interpreting what message was received.
- Receiver—the person for whom the message is intended.
- Feedback—a response to a message that was sent based on the receiver's interpretation of the original message.

Q How can the EMS provider assess a patient's mental status using interview techniques?

A Speaking with the patient is the best way to assess the mental status. Determine the AVPU (alert, verbal, painful, unresponsive) during the initial assessment and follow up using the Glasgow Coma Scale (GCS). During the patient interview, you should be able to determine whether the patient is conversing normally, is responding reasonably to questions, and is oriented. It is important to keep in mind that many factors can alter the assessment and interview: alcohol, drugs, and posttraumatic complications such as hypotension (BP < 80 systolic), and hypoxia.

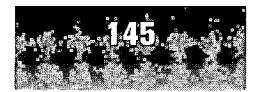

What is a health history?

A complete health history is all of the medical events and conditions that have ever occurred to the patient. This means every surgery, hospital visit, illness (adult and childhood), injury, immunization, and psychiatric problem. It also includes all medications, allergies, family history, and activities, including exercise, diet, career, smoking, drug and alcohol use, religious beliefs, daily routines, patient outlook, relationships, sleep patterns, and other personal stress factors. Not all of this information will be of use to the EMS provider, nor will it be pertinent to the current event. Sometimes, it is easy to determine what parts of a patient's health history may be relevant to today's chief complaint (e.g., previous scars on chest, taking lasix and nitro are relevant to a possible acute myocardial infarction (AMI), but the old inguinal hernia from 20 years ago may not be).

> **CLINICAL PEARL**
>
> *The EMS provider rarely needs to obtain a truly "complete" medical history. In fact, the time required to do this may actually hamper patient care. The "focused" history and physical is appropriate in many circumstances.*

What is the purpose of obtaining a health history?

For most people, the purpose of obtaining a health history is to provide the physician with necessary information about that patient before treatment can be provided. These patients are seeking care for symptoms of a current illness or injury. Another reason health care providers obtain a health history is as a requirement for new employee baseline information. This baseline information should be updated on a regular basis, the frequency depending on the type of employment. Many health care providers are required to file annual "self-assessment" forms as well as undergo TB testing. In addition to baseline information and annual updates, the current health status, past history, and the status of any ongoing, recurrent, or present illness, should be updated after any visits to the patient's physician.

What is a focused history?

A focused history is the chronological history of the present illness. It is the information obtained from the patient or bystanders about the current event, including what led up to it, why EMS was called, and what has been done thus far and its positive, negative, or lack of effect. If this is a recurring event for the patient, obtain additional information if possible:

- Is this similar to a previous event?
- When was the last event?
- How many times has this happened?
- What treatment was received at the last event?

What additional information should be obtained about the present illness or injury?

In the field, the acronym OPQRST is used to remember the set of questions to be asked to obtain information about the present illness or injury. Get the patient to elaborate on the chief complaint.

    O—onset of pain or discomfort (e.g., came on suddenly).

    P—provocation or what brought this on (e.g., shoveling heavy snow).

    Q—quality of the pain or discomfort (e.g., vague pressure sensation).

    R—radiation, relief, recurrence. Does it hurt anywhere else (e.g., jaw also hurts); did you do anything to relieve yourself of the pain (e.g., took an aspirin); has this ever happened before, and if so, when and what did you do then (e.g., took a nitro previously and it went away).

    S—severity; compare this event to a similar event or use a scale to rate the severity (e.g., on a scale of 1 to 10, this is a five).

    T—time; when did this begin or how long has it been like this. Frequency, how often does this happen (e.g., pain began about 15 minutes ago).

What questions should be routinely asked about a patient's health history?

Just as OPQRST is used to remember questions about the current or present event, SAMPLE is used to remember the set of questions about the patient's past medical history.

    S—signs and symptoms, similar events.

    A—allergies, especially to medications.

    M—medications, including over-the-counter (OTC) (e.g., aspirin and antacids), herbal, homeopathic, home remedies, and prescribed (e.g., diuretics or birth control).

    P—previously diagnosed conditions or diseases, surgeries, prior hospitalizations, trauma, and pregnancy.

    L—last oral intake, last menses, medication administration, similar event.

    E—events that led up to what the patient was doing when the episode began.

What is or is not relevant about the past medical history (PMH)?

For the EMS provider, the PMH of relevant and recent events will be most important. Patients who state that they had their tonsils removed 25 years ago likely are not supplying information that is relevant to the EMS provider. Examples of relevant PMH are:

- Recent surgery.
- Recent illness.
- Recent trauma.
- Recent period of immobilization (e.g., long bone cast).
- Any hospitalization.
- Change in mental status.
- Change in physical ability.
- Change in medications.
- Change in daily routine or activities.
- Family history similar to the current event.
- Disabilities or handicaps.
- Blood transfusions.

CLINICAL PEARL

The medication history is extremely important. Always ask if the patient is taking any OTC medications, including birth control pills, vitamins, or herbal medications. Also ask if the patient has changed medications (started, stopped, or modified doses with or without a physician's knowledge) in the past month.

Interviewing

[Q] Why is it important for the EMS provider to be empathetic when obtaining a health history?

[A] Showing empathy is a therapeutic communication technique to help the patient with their feelings and to obtain more information.

[Q] How should the patient be addressed during history taking?

[A] Using a patient's proper name, Mr., Mrs., or Ms. Jones shows respect. If the patient gives permission to use another name, such as a first name or nickname, then it is okay to use that name. However, it is disrespectful to use terms such as dear or honey.

[Q] What is an open-ended question?

[A] An open-ended question is one that requires more than a simple "yes or no" answer, and does not lead the patient to any particular conclusion. Open-ended questions are useful to obtain descriptive information in a narrative form. For example, ask the patient to describe the last episode of chest pain.

[Q] When are open-ended questions effective?

[A] EMS providers are taught to avoid the use of open-ended questions. It is better to use direct questions when interviewing a patient. However, they do have a place, such as being a good introduction, "Why did you call us here today?" or "How is the pain different today?" They are also appropriate when there is less urgency in the patient's condition and there is more time to spend with the patient.

[Q] When is it better to ask direct questions?

[A] Due to the limited time the EMS provider spends with a patient and the level of distress the patient may be in, the need to get to the point quickly becomes significant. Therefore, direct questions are asked when you require specific information or facts. When a patient is in severe distress, ask questions that require a one- or two-word answer. "Are you having chest pain now?" requires a "yes or no" answer. "When did the pain begin? 10 minutes or two hours ago?" Be careful not to lead the patient to an answer or put words in the patient's mouth by the way you phrase your question. It is better to ask the patient, "Is your pain sharp like a stabbing or dull?" instead of asking, "Do you have a crushing chest pain under your breastbone?"

CLINICAL PEARL

Open-ended questions encourage patients to talk freely. In some situations, time requirements may discourage verbal exchanges, but should not prevent proper communication. Many patients get "turned off" by rapid "yes or no" questions and simply blurt out an answer to get the process done quickly. Be specific if you have to, but not at the risk of causing the patient to "clam up" and refuse to give you an accurate history.

[Q] What should be avoided during the interview?

[A] One of the most important aspects of an interview is to maintain privacy for the patient. Avoid asking personal questions in front of coworkers or even certain family members. When you are not getting an appropriate answer, consider that the patient may be embarrassed or does not want other people to know. Examples of questions to avoid in public are: "Are you pregnant?" and "Do you have psychiatric history?"

- Avoid the use of complicated medical terminology. Stick to lay terms as much as possible. If you are caring for a health care professional who understands medical jargon, it should become apparent quickly and the use of medical jargon may be appropriate.

- Avoid leading questions that put words into the patient's mouth (e.g., Do you have sharp chest pain?). Some patients may tell you what you want to hear rather than how they really feel. For example, you might ask, "What does the pain feel like?" Follow this with a list of choices, including *none of the above,* if the more open-ended question doesn't work first.

- Avoid condescending or judgmental questions (e.g., "You don't smoke, do you?"). The patient may not be comfortable with this and may probably lie about this or other things.

- Avoid negative nonverbal communications. The look on your face, body language (e.g., standing over a patient, arms crossed), or inattentiveness can also make a patient feel uncomfortable and lead to information being withheld.

- Do not provide false reassurance when the situation is serious. It is better to explain what is happening and what is going to happen next. If the patient perceives that you are lying, you may not get the cooperation you need.

- The amount of physical *space* between you and the patient is important and can vary with different people, especially different cultures. Not everyone can tolerate you up close in their face. Some cultures, such as Arabian, Asian, Indochinese, and Native American, may consider direct eye contact impolite or aggressive and may avoid eye contact during an interview.

What other techniques are useful during the interview?

The way we respond to a patient's answers should encourage expression. This is accomplished using several techniques:

- *Facilitation* is the way you speak, how your posture and your actions encourage the patient to say more. Positive examples include sitting close to the patient and making eye contact, while you nod or say, "I'm listening," "Please tell me more," or "Continue." Negative examples include standing over a patient, barking out questions without waiting for responses, or not making eye contact while interviewing.

- *Reflection* is to repeat or echo the patient's own words as a way of encouraging the flow of conversation without interrupting the patient's concentration. An example of reflection is to say, "You say the chest pain woke you up this morning at 5 A.M." Reflection helps the patient feel that you are listening and can confirm information that is pertinent to the event.

- *Clarification* is used when the patient's responses are confusing or ambiguous. For example, ask the patient to clarify by saying, "Using your finger, please point to where the pain is."

- *Explanation* is necessary to help put a patient at ease and can make the interview, assessment, and entire call go better. Explaining procedures or the steps of a procedure to a patient beforehand lets the patient anticipate and feel informed (e.g., "I am going to lift your shirt to listen to your breathing now").

- *Confrontation* is used when you have observed a response, either verbal or physical, that conflicts with other information you have been given. For example, "You say that you are not having any pain, but when you move you are guarding and protecting your stomach."

- Interpretation is reasoning based not on what you observed about the patient, but what you have concluded from the information you have compiled. For example, "It seems that whenever you exert yourself physically, you develop a shortness of breath."

- *Empathy* is used to recognize and state a feeling openly. It allows patients to feel accepted and can help them to deal with the feeling. For example, just hold a patient's hand when you can see they are scared.

- *Silence* has a useful purpose at the right times. You can use silence to give patients time to organize their thoughts and to observe nonverbal clues while you perform essential tasks.

Challenges to Getting Information

Where can I look for information about patients when they are unable to tell me themselves?

There are a number of information sources found on patients in the field. Some wear necklaces or bracelets, while others use smart cards, computer chips, or wallet cards. When examining the patient, these devices are usually found during the initial assessment. Take a quick look at the medical identification device to see whether it offers any pertinent information about today's problem.

Of all the devices available, the most common ones are the necklaces and bracelets available from the MedicAlert® Foundation (www.medicalert.org), which maintains a 24-hour Emergency Response Center. The toll-free EMS phone number (1-800-629-3780) is answered by a trained representative who can fax copies of the patient's medical data and can assist with language translation services via AT&T Translation Service. Conditions noted on these devices include allergies, diabetes, hypertension, clotting disorders, seizure disorders, Alzheimer's, and implanted devices (e.g., automatic internal cardiac defibrillator [AICD] and pacemakers).

Another service is the Global MED-NET® to which patients may subscribe. The patient wears a symbol that is supplied as a sticker to put on a key chain or wallet. On calling the toll-free phone number (1-800-650-0409) with the patient's membership identification number, EMS providers can receive the patient's complete medical profile.

Look for medication containers because they can tell you a lot about a patient. For example, you can learn if patients have a cardiac or respiratory history, or if they have hypertension. You can determine whether they are compliant with their medications by checking the date and amount of prescription fill and then counting the remaining amount. If you do not have a medication reference handy to tell you what type of medication you have found, be sure to bring all of the medications, or a list of all medications and the doses, with you to the hospital.

If the medication is not in plain view, look in the medicine cabinet, bedrooms, and kitchen. Be sure to look in the refrigerator. Here you may find insulin for the diabetic, other medications requiring refrigeration, and possibly a Vial of Life®. The Vial of Life® is a rolled piece of paper with pertinent medical information about the patient that is kept in a plastic jar.

CLINICAL PEARL

Law enforcement personnel are experts at performing safe and legal searches, and can find patient medications that the rest of the crew missed.

Many people use Lifeline MedCom, a service that centralizes personal health data, emergency contacts, and insurance information for emergency retrieval 24 hours a day via the Internet (http://info@lifelinemed.com) or live call center. The EMS provider who has access to the Internet may consider accessing this service for information on the patient.

What obstacles may be encountered during the interview?

There are numerous challenges that are encountered during the interview that cannot be simulated in the classroom or in a book. Some EMS providers are more comfortable with these special challenges than others. Therefore, let the person who is most experienced or most comfortable do the interview for that particular patient. This allows other crew members to observe and learn.

- Language barriers—ideally the best solution is to find a translator. Otherwise, use positive body language, such as friendly facial expressions and slow movements to assess, take vital signs, and provide treatment.

- Hearing impaired—speak facing the patient or write out communications. If the patient owns a hearing aid, be sure they are using it. If the patient can sign, attempt to provide a translator. Once at the hospital, the ADA requires that the hospital provide a sign interpreter within 30 minutes of the patient's arrival.

- Blind—announce who you are, why you are there, and explain as much as possible. Ask permission before touching the patient.

- Developmentally disabled—give the patient the opportunity to provide you with information. If the condition is severe or information is omitted, family or caregivers may be able to provide information.

- Intoxicated—be careful not to escalate an event by challenging or aggravating this patient. Do not hesitate to get additional backup from the police before it is actually needed.

- Hostile—anger and hostility is often misdirected at the caregiver. Do not get angry in return. As with the intoxicated patient, do not escalate the event. Many EMS providers do a "pat-down" during the patient evaluation and act with caution, assuming that a weapon could always be present. Technically, EMS providers are not allowed to search a patient. Remember that anything can be used as a weapon, so be very careful with hostile patients.

- Anxious—be sensitive and alert to nonverbal clues. Reassurance, an explanation, or a distraction often help reduce anxiety.

- Depressed—be alert for signs of depression such as sleep disorders, appetite disturbances, an inability to concentrate, or lack of energy. Do not hesitate to ask a patient about their feelings. Depression is associated with some psychological illnesses.

- Confused—when the patient is displaying an acute confusing behavior or the history is confusing, be alert for medical or trauma causes. When the confusion is known to be part of the history, be alert for a mental illness or dementia. Look to family or caregivers for information.

- Abused—abuse comes in many forms, so let the most experienced crew member do the interview. Sometimes the patient will decide whom they want to talk to, if they talk at all. This is okay too. For example, an abused female may only want to talk to another female.

- Overtalkative—this patient can be a challenge when faced with limited time for interview and care. It is easy to become impatient with this type of patient. Use direct questions requiring yes or no answers, summarize frequently, and do not expect to obtain too much relevant information.

- Multiple symptoms—this is a patient that requires an experienced interviewer. The task of sorting through the multiple symptoms to discover and prioritize the complaints takes practice.

- Asymptomatic—use the experienced crew member (your best detective) to ask questions after the initial interviewer has finished.

CHAPTER 13

Techniques of Physical Examination

Each patient is unique with respect to physical attributes, psychological demeanor, and current emergency or crisis. Therefore, your approach to each patient will be distinctive. Although your approach to the physical exam (PE) should be logical, there should be flexibility to modify and adjust to the dynamic environment of the out-of-hospital setting. This chapter discusses the techniques used to perform a PE and specific assessment skills.

The chief complaint and the initial assessment guide the focused PE and any subsequent reassessments. The PE is performed predominantly by inspecting, listening, and feeling (palpation) with and without the use of additional equipment. The PE provides the information needed to make clinical decisions. Learning the components of the PE takes time and becoming proficient takes practice.

Assessment Skills

[Q] **Which skills are used during the PE?**

[A] Cognitive skills include assessing the patient's mental status, taking a history, and priority decision making. Physical skills include examining the patient through observation, palpation, auscultation, and percussion and taking vital signs. Taking standard precautions (formerly called universal precautions) to prevent the exchange of body fluids and hand washing after each patient contact are included as a skill in patient assessment.

The list of components of the PE are found in Table 13–1 and additional EMS provider skills are found in Table 13–2. The list of skills used based on findings made during the PE are listed in Table 13–3.

TABLE 13-1
Cognitive and Physical Skills

1. Don appropriate personal protective equipment (PPE)
2. Evaluate mental status
3. Interview
    - Focused history
    - SAMPLE
    - OPQRST
4. Vital signs
5. Respiratory
    - Rate
    - Effort
    - Depth
    - Speech
    - Lung sounds
6. Pulse
    - Presence or absence

- Rate
- Regularity
- Quality
- Location
7. Blood pressure (palpation, auscultation)
    - Adult
    - Child
    - Infant
8. Skin:
    - Color: normal, pale, flushed, cyanotic.
    - Temperature: oral, rectal, axillary, forehead, tympanic, electronic.
    - Condition: dry, diaphoretic, turgor, edema.

TABLE 13-2
Additional EMS Provider Skills

1. Assessing pupils
    - PEARLA
2. Motor and neurological functions (traumatic brain injury or spinal cord injury)
    - Pulses Motor Sensation (PMS) + 4 with or without deficit
    - Blood glucose
3. ECG monitoring and diagnostic 12 lead
4. Pulse oximetry monitoring
5. End tidal CO_2 monitoring
6. Doppler (may be used in some locations)
7. Otoscope (used in some regions)
8. Opthalmoscope (used in some regions)

TABLE 13-3
Skills Used Based on Findings Made During the PE

- Treatment decisions.
- Reassessment.
- Transportation decisions.
- Record keeping.

What equipment is used in the field to perform a PE?

PPE, including gloves, mask, eyeshield, and gown (as needed), stethoscope, BP cuff, Doppler, paper, pen, flashlight, tongue depressor, watch, thermometer, ECG monitor, pulse oximeter, glucometer, and capnograph.

What are the techniques of the PE?

Inspection, or looking at the patient, is the first component of the PE and is quickly used in conjunction with the skills of palpation and auscultation. Inspection, both visual and using the sense of smell, is used immediately as the EMS provider begins to form a general impression of the patient. Look for signs of distress and begin to differentiate normal from abnormal findings. By looking closely at the patient's symmetry, body size, weight, grooming, and personal hygiene, the overall state of health becomes apparent. When focusing on a specific body system in the detailed PE, observe for specific characteristics.

Auscultation, or examining by listening to the body, may be performed using the ear alone or with the use of a stethoscope. Listening to the body is first used during the initial assessment, but may be a part of forming a general impression of the patient, such as the patient presenting with audible wheezing from a few feet away. Listening skills become honed as you learn how to auscultate lung sounds, heart sounds, bruits, bowel sounds, and blood pressures in places with loud ambient noises.

Palpation is examining through touch or feel. Using light touch or deep touch and feeling for symmetry, compare one side of the body to the other.

Prior to palpation, reduce the patient's anxiety, fear, and muscle tensing by explaining where and how you are going to touch and warm your hands prior to touching.

Percussion is a skill that is occasionally used in the PE, but not regularly in the field. This skill combines touching (tapping the fingertips on various body parts) and listening to determine the size, position, and consistency of underlying structures of the body. Various areas of the body have what is called "normal percussion tone." Think of this as the normal sound when "tapped." Diseases, such as the accumulation of fluid in the lungs, dull (hyporesonant) or flatten the tone. Abnormal collections of air, such as in a pneumothorax, make the percussion tone louder (hyperresonant).

What do we look for in the general appearance of the patient?

Look for the presence (or absence) of distress and its level; the patient's behavior, age, gender, and skin color, temperature, and condition (CTC); and whether the patient's dress is appropriate for the surroundings. Consider the location of the call. Is the patient at home, work, store, health-care facility, or nursing home? Then, consider who else is present: family, friends, coworkers, strangers, or caregivers.

What should be recognized and evaluated during the PE using the techniques of observation, palpation, and auscultation?

Signs of distress can be obvious or quite subtle. The more practiced one becomes with the PE and what normal findings are, the easier it becomes to recognize the less obvious signs of distress. Following are findings that should be evaluated during the patient PE:

Observation:

- Poor skin color, temperature, and condition.
- Labored breathing.
- Positions of comfort and discomfort.
- Obvious deformity.
- Patient looks sick.

Auscultation:

- Labored or irregular breathing.
- Moaning, grunting, crying, or silence.
- Unilateral, diminished, or no breath sounds.
- Absent bowel sounds.
- Muffled or murmured heart sounds.

Palpation:

- Asymmetry—compare one side of the body to the other.
- DCAP-BTLS:
  a. Deformity—fractures, dislocations, depressions.
  b. Contusions—new, old, or indicative of abuse.
  c. Abrasions—active bleeding, presence of debris.
  d. Punctures—entrance or exit.
  e. Burns—degree and body surface area.
  f. Tenderness—light versus deep palpation, rebound.
  g. Lacerations—length and depth.
  h. Swelling—edema or hemorrhagic.
- Irregular body textures:
  a. Edema—local or generalized abnormal accumulation of fluids in body tissues.
  b. Tenting—indication of poor skin turgor; tent-like shape remains when skin is pinched.
  c. Crepitis—grating bone pieces.
  d. Subcutaneous emphysema—air trapped under skin creating "bubble wrap" feel when palpated.
  e. Bloating, distention, ascites (fluid in abdominal tissues).

CLINICAL PEARL

If you know what normal looks like, abnormal is often not subtle. An abnormal finding supports your assessment. Negative findings are less likely to rule out a condition. Remember—a normal exam does not mean a normal patient. Take advantage of the body's natural symmetry. If something is asymmetrical, it is more likely to be abnormal. Remember also, though, that a patient may be symmetrically abnormal.

Why is the PE performed in a head-to-toe fashion?

The head-to-toe method of performing a PE is a systematic approach used to keep in sequence and to avoid overlooking any body parts.

Is the head-to-toe exam used on all patients?

No, a complete head-to-toe exam is primarily used on trauma patients to avoid overlooking any injuries. After the initial assessment, the focused PE centers on the chief complaint and the source of the illness or injury discovered in the initial assessment. The pediatric PE is often performed in the opposite direction, from toe to head.

Why is the PE performed differently on children?

In children, the PE is performed in a toe-to-head fashion so as not to frighten the child. For infants and small children the ears and throat are the most uncomfortable to examine and the child may become upset.

What does the EMS provider look for when examining the head?

HEENT is an acronym used to describe the areas examined: hearing, eyes, ears, nose, and throat.

- Hearing—acute changes.
- Eyes—pupil response, six cardinal fields of gaze. (Described in Chapter 24, Neurology.)
- Ears—otorrhea (ear infection with a purulent discharge).
- Nose—rhinorrhea (a watery discharge from the nose).
- Throat—airway patency, edema.

Common abnormal findings of the head and face include muscle tics and twitching, decreased skin turgor, facial drooping, and irregular speech. Facial asymmetry is an abnormal finding; however, minor facial asymmetry is normal, especially below the nose.

What abnormal findings can be located when examining the neck?

Abnormal findings in the area of the neck include the presence of jugular venous distension at 45 degrees, the presence of bruits in the carotid arteries, a restricted range of motion, and the presence of swollen glands or nodes.

Q What is a bruit and where does the EMS provider auscultate for them?

A A bruit is a swishing noise heard over arteries that indicates turbulent blood flow. The most common location the out-of-hospital provider assesses for bruits is the carotid arteries. A carotid bruit can be heard when the lumen becomes occluded by one-half to two-thirds; for example, in atherosclerosis.

To auscultate for carotid bruits, place the patient's neck in a neutral position. Lightly place the bell of the stethoscope over the carotid artery. Listen first at the base of the neck, then halfway up the neck, and then at the angle of the jaw.

Perform this procedure with extreme care so as not to compress the artery. Doing so may dislodge plaque or stimulate a vagal nerve response.

CLINICAL PEARL

> *Though bruits may be caused by the partial occlusion of an artery, complete occlusion results in silence, not a bruit.*

Q What is examined in the chest and back?

A Chest wall symmetry (similarity from right to left sides) and integrity (no holes or flail segments), respiratory effort, and lung and heart sounds.

Q What is the difference between the bell and diaphragm of a stethoscope?

A The bell has a shape like a cup and is used to listen for deep and low-pitched sounds such as abnormal heart sounds. It is placed very lightly on the skin, enough to form a seal. Not all stethoscopes have a bell. The diaphragm has a flat shape and is used to listen for high-pitched sounds such as breath, bowel, and normal heart sounds. Unlike the bell, the diaphragm is placed firmly against the skin.

Q Where are lung sounds most frequently auscultated?

A Although it is possible to listen to breath sounds on the back or posterior surface, it is most common to listen on the chest or anterior surface, especially in cases involving trauma. In trauma, patients are often managed in the supine position to maintain the integrity of the spine. To listen for bronchial breath sounds, place the diaphragm of the stethoscope on the chest over the intercostal space at the mid-clavicular line on one side of the chest. Then, compare to the other side. To listen for vesicular breath sounds, place the diaphragm over the fifth anterior axillary line and mid-axillary line and repeat bilaterally.

Q Where are heart sounds ascultated?

A To auscultate heart sounds, place the bell of the stethoscope at the fifth intercostal space at the mid-clavicular line. Listen to determine whether the heart sounds are normal or abnormal. Normal heart sounds have two clear distinct sounds, "lub-dub." Muffled or distant heart sounds may indicate the presence of fluid as with a pericardial tamponade or hemothorax.

Q What are examples of what is found on examination of the abdomen?

A The abdomen should normally be soft and not tender. There should be nothing abnormal such as tenderness, masses, ascites, bloating, distention, rigidity, absent bowel sounds, or signs of incontinence.

Q When and how does the EMS provider assess for the presence of bowel sounds?

A Changes in bowel sounds are most helpful in evaluating patients with possible peritoneal irritation, regardless of the cause. Listen for bowel sounds in any person with acute abdominal distress or trauma. Part of the reason that bowel sounds are not routinely assessed in the field is that it takes a few minutes and there can be very little background noise.

CLINICAL PEARL

> *Many words have been used to describe bowel sounds. The most helpful finding is the complete absence of bowel sounds. This almost always indicates serious intra-abdominal pathology. Other changes in the bowel sounds (e.g., hyperactive, hypoactive) are less sensitive and have very poor reliability.*

Q What is the difference between light and deep palpation?

A Light palpation may be used to assess most body parts, while deep palpation is usually reserved for the abdomen. Light palpation is used to assess for softness, tenderness, large masses or deformities, and abnormal body temperature. To palpate the four quadrants of the abdomen using light palpation, use the pads of your fingers and gently depress each abdominal quadrant one at a time, about one centimeter. Palpate the area of complaint last.

Deep palpation is not frequently used in the out-of-hospital setting. To assess the abdomen by deep palpation, one or both hands may be used to depress two to three inches in each abdominal quadrant. Often two hands are used with an obese or muscle tense abdomen. Deep palpation is used to appreciate the size of the liver, tenderness of the gallbladder (Murphy's sign), and to further evaluate any masses or enlarged organs. Remember to warm your hands first to prevent muscle tensing and never palpate over bruits (may rupture plaque).

CLINICAL PEARL

A common fear among less experienced examiners is that they will worsen a patient's condition by palpation. Done properly, the examination should never cause harm. Deep palpation requires practice and knowing when to stop.

What is examined on the extremities?

The presence of distal pulses, symmetry, BP, restricted range of motion, shortening, abnormal rotation, and DCAP-BTLS are checked. If injury is present, check for pulses, and motor and sensory function.

Why is it important to use the proper size BP cuff on a patient?

There are many factors that cause inaccurate readings when taking a BP. Using the wrong size BP cuff is one of them. A properly sized cuff should be centered on the upper arm and cover about two-thirds. If the cuff is too big, the reading will be inaccurately low; if the cuff is too small, the reading may be too high.

Other common errors made while taking a BP that can cause false readings are:

- Releasing the air too fast from the cuff.
- Immediately reinflating the cuff on the same side.
- Positioning the patient's arm above the level of their heart.
- Taking the BP while the patient's bladder is distended.
- Taking the BP on the side with a mastectomy, shunts, or old cerebrovascular accidents (CVAs).
- Taking the BP while the patient is smoking.
- Loud ambient noises (e.g., sirens).
- Any source of patient anxiety (e.g., pain).

CLINICAL PEARL

Recent studies have shown that many people exhibit an elevated BP due to anxiety and the stress of an acute injury or illness. Look at the patient as well as at trends in vital signs before concluding that the BP is truly abnormal.

What are Korotkoff's sounds?

Korotkoff's sounds are the sounds heard with a stethoscope while taking a BP that, when combined with readings on the gauge, indicate the systolic and diastolic readings.

When and how is a BP taken by palpation?

Taking a BP by palpation means not using a stethoscope to listen for Korotkoff's sounds. A BP by palpation is performed by placing a BP cuff on the upper arm and before inflating the cuff, palpating for a distal pulse (usually a radial pulse). While continually palpating the pulse, inflate the cuff until the distal pulse is no longer felt. Then inflate the cuff to 10 mmHg above the point where the pulse was felt. While still feeling for a pulse, slowly release the cuff's pressure until a pulse returns and note the number. This is the systolic pressure. No diastolic pressure can be obtained using this method.

This method is often performed when no stethoscope is immediately available or the ambient noise is too loud to hear while using a stethoscope.

What is an apical pulse and how is it taken?

An apical pulse is the pulse felt or heard directly over the apex of the heart. It is used frequently to assess the pediatric patient, as well as assessing irregular pulses, acute thoracic injury, and patients with cardiac or pulmonary diseases.

The apical pulse is heard by placing the diaphragm of a stethoscope on the chest in the midaxillary line (MAL) between the fourth, fifth, or sixth intercostal spaces. It may be palpated by placing your fingers over the same area.

Can a BP be taken anywhere else?

The thigh is another site used by placing the BP cuff on the upper leg similar to placing it on the upper arm. Use the popliteal pulse behind the knee either by palpation or with a stethoscope.

Taking a BP by using a Doppler is another method of obtaining a systolic blood pressure on pediatric patients, obese patients, and patients who are hypoperfused.

How does a Doppler work and how is it used?

The Doppler principle states that the intensity of sound waves changes as the source changes distance from the listener. For example, when an ambulance approaches, the siren gets louder, reaches a peak as it passes, and then decreases in intensity. Doppler ultrasound devices take advantage of this principle by using fixed sound waves (the probe) to measure a moving target (flowing blood). Occasionally, the Doppler may be used to detect blood flow in the extremities where a pulse is difficult to obtain.

Where shouldn't a BP be taken?

Whenever possible, avoid taking a BP on an extremity that is painful or injured. Taking a BP on patients with arteriovenous shunts or fistulas, or on the postmastectomy side should be avoided because it can cause pain as well as inaccurate readings.

How is edema assessed?

Edema is an abnormal accumulation of fluid that settles within the intracellular space of the body. With the help of gravity, the spaces where edema settles are closest to the ground. For example, many people have edema in their feet, ankles, lower legs, arms, and hands because they are usually standing or sitting. When a patient is non-ambulatory or bedridden, edema tends to settle in the sacral area and lungs, although it may be present in the extremities.

Edema is rated as none present, mild, moderate, or severe using a four-point scale. First, observe if there is edema, then note if it is pitting. Assess for pitting by pressing your thumb or finger firmly into an area that appears to be edemous and then release. Note the depth of the indentation (pitting) on the skin and how long it takes the skin to return to normal. The deeper the indentation and the longer the skin takes to return to normal, the more severe the edema. Note if pitting edema is absent. The four-point scale is listed in Table 13–4.

TABLE 13–4

Pitting Edema 4-Point Scale		
+1 = 0″–1/4″		
+2 = 1/4″–1/2″		
+3 = 1/2″–1″		
+4 => 1″		

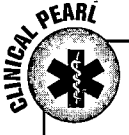

The presence of edema, whether pitting or not, is significant. Pitting edema, however, is more likely to represent a significant heart, lung, or kidney problem.

How is skin turgor assessed?

Assessing the elasticity of the skin (turgor) indicates the patient's state of hydration. To assess the skin, gently pinch a small section such as the forearm, back of the hand, anterior chest, or abdomen. When the skin is released, it should return to its original shape quickly. If the skin remains pinched or the natu-

ral contour returns slowly, this is decreased skin turgor and indicates dehydration. It is possible to have increased skin turgor due to increased tension or a connective tissue disease.

Aging also affects turgor; elderly people commonly have poor skin turgor due to a loss of connective tissue.

How is jugular vein distention (JVD) assessed?

The jugular veins are like a dipstick to the heart and give a measure of central venous pressure (CVP). Distention indicates increased CVP. To accurately assess for the presence of JVD, it is important to place the patient in a semi-Fowler's position with the heart at a 30–45 degree angle. The semi-Fowler's position is sitting up halfway. Position is important (Figure 13–1) because JVD is a normal finding in a patient who is lying supine. In a patient at a 45 degree angle, it is abnormal. At a 90 degree angle, JVD may indicate serious pathology such as severe right heart failure, pericardial tamponade, or tension pneumothorax. Unilateral JVD is abnormal and may indicate a local vein blockage or restriction.

How is the hepatojugular reflex assessed?

Begin by placing the patient in a semi-Fowler's position with the head at a 30 degree angle. Observe the jugular veins to determine whether they are normal or distended. Then, observe the jugular veins while simultaneously performing a deep palpation on the upper-right quadrant of the abdomen for approximately 30 to 60 seconds. If an increase of more than 1 cm in JVD is noted, this finding may indicate right heart failure or fluid overload.

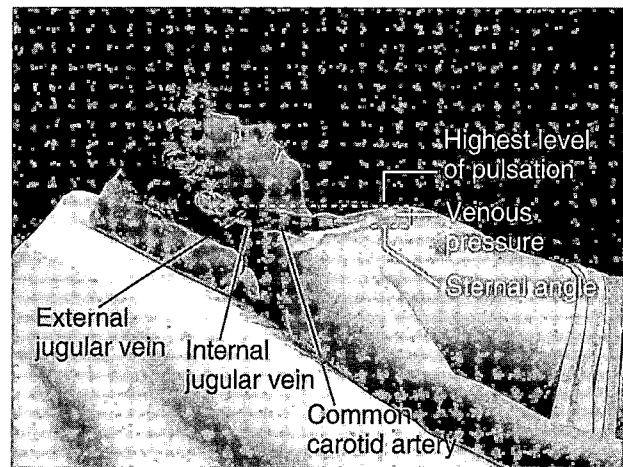

FIGURE 13–1 Inspection of the jugular vein for distension.

How is an otoscope used?

The otoscope consists of a light source projected through a cone-shaped device that is placed into an orifice, either the nose or ear. This allows the examiner to inspect the inner structures, such as the eardrum, for redness, purulence, and foreign bodies. (Figure 13–2).

What is the otoscope used to find that may be relevant to out-of-hospital care?

The most common helpful findings made with an otoscope include:

- Inflammation of the eardrum (suggesting middle ear infection).
- Inflammation of the ear canal (external ear infection such as swimmer's ear).
- Rupture of the eardrum.
- Foreign bodies.

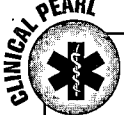

When looking for a foreign body, don't advance the scope tip blindly. You may inadvertently push the foreign body in further.

How is an ophthalmoscope used?

The ophthalmoscope is a combination of several lenses and a light source. The examiner looks through the ophthalmoscope at the patient's eye by focusing the scope with the lenses.

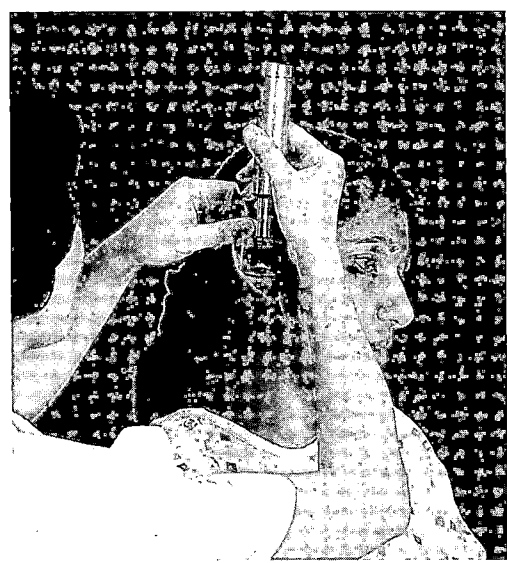

FIGURE 13–2 The otoscope.

What is the opthalmoscope used for that is relevant to out-of-hospital care?

The opthalmoscope may be used to identify foreign bodies, some corneal abrasions, other external eye injuries, and numerous conditions within the globe. These include:

- Papilledema (swelling of the optic disk due to increased intracranial pressure).
- Diabetic retinopathy (changes in the blood vessels due to diabetes).
- Hypertensive retinopathy (changes in the blood vessels due to high BP).
- Bleeding within the globe.

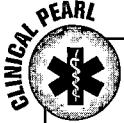

Use of the opthalmoscope requires practice. It is not used routinely in out-of-hospital care.

When would an EtCO$_2$ detector be used?

An end-tidal CO$_2$ monitor is a device that measures the amount of carbon dioxide during each breath at the end of exhalation. It is used to determine whether ET tube placement is correct and to trend CO$_2$ levels once the patient has been intubated. This skill is discussed further in Chapter 52, Advanced Cardiac Life Support.

EtCO$_2$ monitoring has been used to follow resuscitation during cardiac arrest. As blood flow to the lungs increases, EtCO$_2$ goes up. The failure of EtCO$_2$ to rise during a resuscitation effort portends a poor prognosis and has been used by some EMS systems as an indication to stop resuscitation.

When is pulse oximetry used?

Pulse oximetry is used to assess the oxygen saturation of hemoglobin (SpO$_2$). The technique is used routinely on patients that present with a chief complaint of shortness of breath, evident tachypnea, dyspnea, cyanosis, altered mental status, smoke inhalation, or post-bronchodilator therapy, during manual ventilation and post-intubation.

Are there any special considerations with the use of pulse oximetry?

Yes. Pulse oximetry may give false high or low readings under certain conditions. Readings may be falsely high in the presence of carbon monoxide. Chronic smokers have elevated carbon monoxide levels secondary to smoking. Therefore, these patients have higher than normal pulse oximeter readings. Hypothermia and shock alter peripheral circulation and, therefore, affect readings. Patients may also have inaccurate indicators if they are in an anemic state.

Never withhold oxygen from a patient to obtain a pulse oximetry reading when the clinical condition indicates oxygen is needed!

CLINICAL PEARL

Look at the patient, not the number! If the patient looks sick and the pulse oximetry reading looks good, then the patient is still sick.

What are the various ways to take a temperature in the field?

The antiquated mercury in the glass thermometer found in a patient's home may be the only instrument available to some EMS providers to measure a temperature. However, the patient must be able to follow instructions. The two and a half minutes it takes to get a reading makes it untimely in emergent situations.

* Rectal route—used when other routes are not practical. There is also a hazard with accidental perforation of the rectum.

* Tympanic—probe is placed in the ear. This method is safe, fast, and uses one patient disposable probe cover.

* Electronic—many types are available for use in various places (e.g., oral, rectal, or continuous). These are safe and fast and designed for single-patient use. The device must be calibrated and charged on a regular basis. To assess the temperature of a patient that you suspect is hypothermic, a special thermometer must be used that covers lower temperatures than most normal thermometers.

CLINICAL PEARL

Tympanic membrane temperatures are easy to obtain. Some data, however, has called their accuracy into question, especially in persons with severe infections. If the patient looks sick, feels warm, and the tympanic membrane temperature is normal, consider using a different type thermometer.

How is blood glucose obtained in the field?

There are two general methods for obtaining blood glucose in the field.

* Glucometers are fast and easy to use, and are reliable when calibrated to the manufacturer's specifications. The meters provide an LCD readout very quickly after placing a drop of venous blood on the test strip and inserting the strip into the meter.

* Chemstrips, BGS, Dextrostix®, and others are reagent strips and are not as accurate as glucometers, but are still used in the field. Testing with these strips requires placing a drop of venous blood on a test strip and waiting a specific number of seconds for a color change, and then comparing the color on the strip to a chart. Because there are several variables that can affect the reading, it is always more accurate when combined with a meter.

CLINICAL PEARL

Reagent strips by themselves are not as accurate as when combined with a meter; however, the results still provide sufficient information to determine whether blood sugar is low or high.

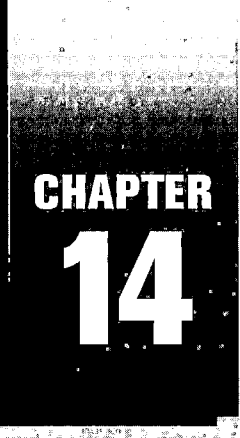

CHAPTER 14

Patient Assessment Overview

Patient assessment in the field is unique because the out-of-hospital care provider incorporates many aspects that are not found in the controlled environment of a clinical setting such as an ED or physician's office. These aspects include incomplete and often erroneous dispatch information, scene size-up, patient handling, and various transportation considerations.

This chapter discusses the overview of patient assessment. There are very specific steps in the assessment process; however, the unique aspects of each call make the out-of-hospital patient assessment a highly dynamic process. The EMS provider is expected to manage any possible emergency or crisis when they arrive at a scene and to provide meaningful emergency care. This level of responsibility represents the complex decision making the EMS provider must be able to carry out. The focus is on *why* patients present in a certain manner and *why* you must respond in a certain way to their presenting problems.

Components of Assessment

Q What are the components of the out-of-hospital patient assessment?

A The list of patient assessment components for the EMS provider begins with the *scene size-up* and ends when the patient is *transferred* to the ED. In between, are the other components.

1. Scene size-up—medical, trauma, or a combination of both.
2. Initial assessment—mental status (MS), ABCs, physical appearance, and psychological (emotional) presence.

- General impression—the absence of or the level of distress from physical, emotional, or psychological causes.
3. Focused history and physical exam (PE)—based on chief complaint and initial assessment (medical vs. trauma).
4. Baseline vital signs.
5. Transportation.
6. Detailed PE.
7. Ongoing assessment.

- Documentation.
- Legal component.
- Ethical component.

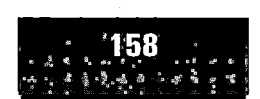
158

Many times the patient's chief complaint is urgent or critical. The patient's mental status, emotional state, physical condition, and the location of the call may change the usual progression of the assessment. Considering the dynamics of out-of-hospital patient assessment, clinical judgment and experience dictate when specific steps should be omitted, deferred, or repeated.

What are the components of scene size-up?

The components of scene size-up include:

- Assessing the scene and surroundings for obvious and potential hazards.
- Assessing the need for additional resources.
- Assessing the need for the appropriate body substance isolation (BSI).
- Determining the mechanism of injury (MOI) or nature of illness.

The scene size-up is discussed in detail in Chapter 15, Scene Size-Up and Initial Assessment.

What are the components of the general impression?

The components of the general impression of the patient include determining from your first impression the following:

- Gender.
- Age or approximate age.
- Severity or level of distress.
- Observation of environment.

Getting the general impression of a patient is discussed in detail in Chapter 15, Scene Size-Up and Initial Assessment.

What are the steps of the patient assessment?

To help remember the sequence of the steps in a patient assessment, use Figure 14–1.

What does the initial assessment tell us about the patient?

The initial assessment guides the decision-making process for the remaining steps in evaluating, treating, and transporting the patient. The purpose of the initial assessment is to determine the patient's mental status, to find and manage any life-threatening conditions, and to make appropriate transportation arrangements.

What is a focused exam?

A focused exam hones in on a specific area of complaint. When a patient has a chief complaint of abdominal pain, after performing the initial assessment, the progressive direction of the exam is to focus or vector in on the abdominal assessment. The head to toe sequence is altered to adapt to the presenting episode. Vectored (focused) exams combine body systems when examining most body parts. For example, when assessing the abdomen, you include components of the skin, musculoskeletal, circulatory, and GI systems for a complete physical exam (PE). Detailed vectored exams for respiratory, cardiac, neurological, behavioral, abdominal, trauma, geriatric, and pediatric patients are discussed elsewhere in this text.

What are the components of the detailed PE?

The detailed PE is the standard head to toe exam all out-of-hospital providers perform on all patients. In practice, it is not actually performed on all patients because it is really not necessary. The latest curriculum has been modified so that the detailed PE is performed on the trauma patient with significant MOI enroute to the hospital. The detailed PE is performed in a logical sequence so as to avoid missing any body parts. However, it does take time to perform, and time may not be available due to the patient's condition or short transport time. The components are as follows:

Assess:

- General appearance.
- Neurological status.
- Vital signs.

Examine:

- Skin.
- Head, scalp, cranium.
- Face, eyes, ears, nose, mouth, tongue, throat.
- Neck, jugular vein distention (JVD).
- Back.
- Upper extremities.
- Anterior chest.
- Abdomen.
- Pelvis.
- Lower extremities.

When appropriate, consider the following diagnostic information: ECG, SpO_2, $EtCO_2$, blood glucose, and temperature.

Explain how to determine whether to take spinal precautions?

When a patient has an obvious deformity, or swelling or bruising to the neck or spine, the decision to immobilize the spine is simple. A common scenario for spinal precautions is the patient who has a chief complaint of pain in the neck or back

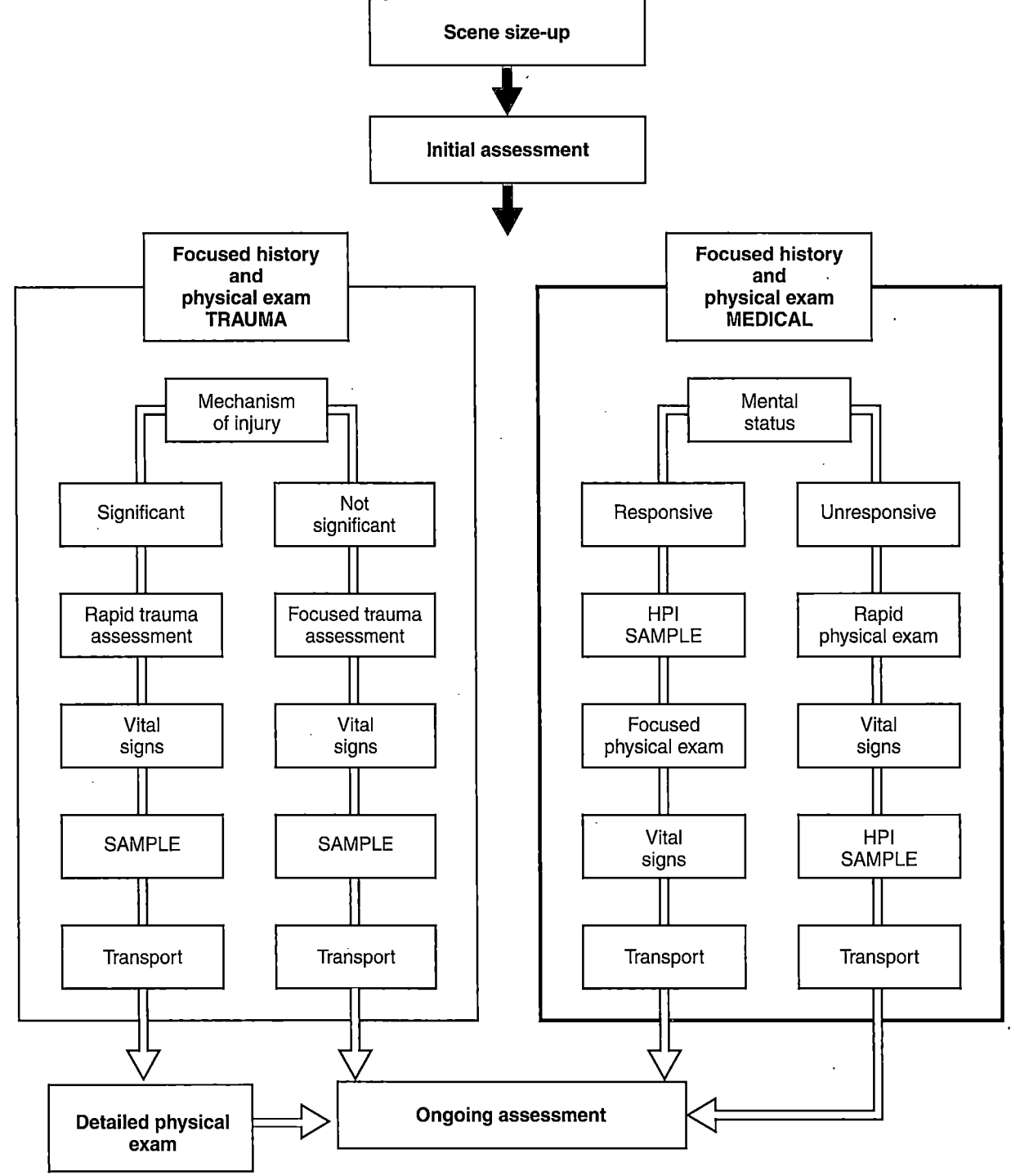

FIGURE 14-1 The patient assessment algorithm

after a traumatic event such as a car collision or a fall. These cases are easy to recognize as requiring immobilization measures. The patient who does not have signs or symptoms of injury after sustaining a significant MOI is more complicated. These are the cases where you must visualize the probable trauma the body

sustained and consider the potential for injury. Therefore, the decision to take spinal precautions should be based primarily on the MOI, rather than the absent signs or symptoms of pain and injury. Significant MOI are listed in Table 14–1.

TABLE 14-1

Significant MOI

- Falls from significant height (greater than 20 feet).
- An event producing a sudden acceleration, deceleration, or lateral movement of the spine.
- An event that impacts violently on the head, neck, torso, or pelvis.
- A head injury with an altered mental status.
- The presence of significant helmet damage.
- An explosion.
- Shallow water diving accidents.
- Motor vehicle rollover.
- Ejection from a motor vehicle.
- Struck by a vehicle moving over 20 mph.
- Major damage to the patient compartment of a vehicle.
- Patient was a survivor of car accident where a death occurred in the same vehicle.

What is "trending" and why is it important?

Trending is an important tool in patient care. *Trending* is the process of obtaining a baseline assessment, repeating the assessment multiple times, and using the information to determine whether the patient is getting better, worse, or shows no change. An example of trending performed on each patient is obtaining baseline vital signs, repeating the vital signs, then modifying treatment using the information recorded.

What are the components of the rapid trauma exam?

The components of the rapid trauma exam are directed at a quick and gross head to toe assessment of the body. It is similar to the detailed PE, but not as thorough.
Assess:

- General appearance.
- Neurological status.
- Vital signs.

Grossly assess:

- Head, face, and neck.
- Anterior chest.
- Abdomen and pelvis.
- Posterior.
- Extremities.

What are the differences when performing a PE on an unresponsive patient?

With the unresponsive patient you have to omit the components of the assessment that require patient communication. Depending on where the patient is found, it may be possible that the patient's family, coworkers, friends, or bystanders can provide essential information about the patient.

Like the conscious patient, the ABCs are the highest priority; however, managing the ABCs in an unconscious patient may take all available manpower. The patient's positioning becomes a higher priority due to airway maintenance. Mental status (MS) is evaluated using deep pain response, reflexes such as Babinski's and doll's eye (only if no spinal injury), pupillary reactions, and the Glasgow Coma Scale. Diagnostic information, such as ECG, SpO_2, $EtCO_2$, and blood glucose, becomes even more essential when caring for the unresponsive patient.

What are the components of the ongoing assessment?

The components of the ongoing assessment are to repeat assessments, repeat vital signs, trend the findings, and modify treatment decisions accordingly. Each patient requires a different level of ongoing assessment based on the severity of her specific event. For example, the ongoing assessment of a patient with an isolated extremity injury includes reassessing distal pulses, motor, and sensation of the injury, while a patient with a traumatic head injury requires reassessment of the MS, ABCs, and neurological system.

Why is documentation part of the patient assessment?

Documentation of the assessment is a tool used by health care professionals and is the legal record of the patient contact.

What are the legal and ethical components of patient assessment?

The medicolegal and ethical components of patient assessment include:

- Respecting the patient's autonomy in the decision-making process.
- Being accountable to the patient.
- Respecting patient confidentiality and privacy.
- Obtaining consent.
- Recognizing assault and battery.
- Understanding and respecting advanced directives.
- Accurate, factual, and nonjudgmental documentation.

These topics are discussed in detail in Chapter 4, Medicolegal Issues, and Chapter 5, Ethical Issues for the EMS Provider.

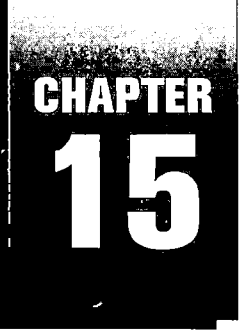

CHAPTER 15

Scene Size-Up and Initial Assessment

T his chapter discusses the first assessment of the scene as well as the first assessment of the patient. The focus is on *why* patients present in a certain manner and *why* you must respond in a certain way to their presenting problems. Proper assessment of the scene can prevent the EMS provider from being seriously injured or killed. Proper initial assessment of the patient is paramount to successful care of the patient.

Scene Size-Up

What is meant by scene size-up?

The scene size-up is the EMS provider's first assessment of the scene and surroundings to obtain valuable information about the safety of the scene, the need for body substance isolation (BSI) precautions, and the mechanism of injury (MOI) or nature of illness.

Why do EMS providers assess for scene safety?

It is not uncommon for the scene of an EMS incident to be potentially hazardous to the EMS provider and crew, the bystanders, and the patient.

What are some examples of actual or potential hazards to the EMS provider at the scene of a call?

Some examples of actual or potential hazards to the EMS provider include:

- Domestic disputes.
- Patient's pets.
- Traffic at the scene of a collision.
- Hazardous materials.
- Below grade (i.e., under the street or in confined spaces), low-oxygen level environments.
- Extreme weather conditions.
- Falling debris.
- Electrical lines or underground transformers.
- A fire at the scene.
- Unstable footing.
- Ice or snow.
- Weapons at the scene.
- Perpetrator who is still at the scene.
- Street gangs.
- One of the biggest hazards, getting to the scene in your emergency vehicle, is discussed in more detail in Chapter 48, Ambulance Operations and Multiple Casualty Incidents.

Why is it so important for the EMS provider to recognize hazards?

The first and foremost priority is safety. We may tell the public that the patient comes first, but in reality we can't take care of the patient if we haven't taken care of ourselves first! If you look for hazards, you will find many that can be easily controlled. At a minimum, notify the proper authorities as soon as possible so they can control or secure the scene.

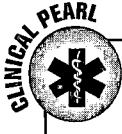

> *It's always better to call out the "troops" and not need them, than not calling in the first place.*

What makes a scene unsafe?

Any potential hazard that can injure the EMS providers, the bystanders, or further injure the patient makes a scene unsafe (e.g., fire, broken glass, dangerous crowds, downed power lines, etc.).

What clues indicate there may be hazardous materials involved in the incident?

Always be suspicious if there is a tanker collision or multiple patients at the scene with medical complaints (e.g., shortness of breath [SOB], nausea, headaches). This usually means there is something in the air.

What is an example of a subtle hazard to the EMS provider?

That cute little family dog can very quickly become a threat to you once it perceives you as a threat or as inflicting pain on its owner. Just ask postal carriers why many of them carry pepper spray in their bag! When an EMS provider conducts a PE or does a painful procedure, like starting an IV, the family pet can quickly turn vicious. Always insist on having someone secure the pet in another room to protect yourself and your crew from injury.

How can the EMS provider make a scene safe?

The EMS provider can best make a scene safe by looking for the hazards. At the scene of a collision, consider doing a quick walk around the entire vehicle prior to rushing in to assess the patient.

Why are BSI precautions a part of the scene size-up?

As one of the first things the EMS provider does on arrival at the scene, taking BSI precautions is an essential step in protecting yourself from contracting a disease that could easily be life threatening. Don your gloves prior to touching the patient or any objects their body substances have contacted. If there is spraying or spurting blood or body fluids, consider the use of a disposable mask, goggles or eyeshield, and a gown. The safest rule is: "If it is wet and it is not yours, don't touch it without BSI precautions."

What are examples of unsafe scenes that the EMS provider should not enter?

Examples of unsafe scenes include:
- A vehicle that is hanging precariously on the side of a cliff or embankment or an unstable vehicle.
- A low-oxygen environment such as a confined space, a water treatment facility holding tank, or a silo.
- An electrified vehicle either with downed wires on top of it or sitting on top of a transformer box.
- A bar fight or scene where there are street gangs involved.
- A crime scene with the perpetrator still present.
- A domestic dispute with the family members still arguing.

What does the term "secure scene" mean?

The term "secure scene" is a police term. It is used by the police once they have attempted to make a potentially violent scene as safe as possible so EMS providers can enter. It is a safe practice for EMS providers to stage a block away when the dispatch information indicates there may be a threat of violence. Police should be dispatched to secure the scene prior to EMS leaving the staging area to enter the scene.

What is an example of a scene in a residential area that could be a threat to the EMS provider?

Examples of potential threats to the EMS provider in a typical residential area include:
- A night response to a house that has no lights on.
- Walking up to the front door of a house and hearing screaming.
- Walking up to the front door and seeing a broken window.

Q **Once you arrive at the scene of a call in a private residence, what things can you do to help keep it a safe scene for you and your partners?**

A As you knock on the door, be sure to stand to the side of the doorway. Always bring a portable radio and do not get separated from your partner until you are reasonably comfortable that it is a safe scene. Watch each other's back all the time. Look around the room for real and potential weapons. Real weapons include guns, ice picks, and knives. Potential weapons include sharp objects such as letter openers, scissors, glass bottles, or one of those swords hung up on the wall! Look for blunt objects that could be used as weapons such as hammers, statues, or a baseball bat. If for any reason you suspect any threat to your life, cautiously exit and call for the police to come to the scene. Always have a clear exit and leave a crew member to guard the exit. For additional information on this topic, review Chapter 51, Crime Scene Awareness.

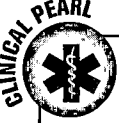
CLINICAL PEARL

> *Remember, just about any object can be used as a weapon (e.g., pen, flashlight, ashtray, beer bottles, paper clip) by just about anyone. Never assume you are totally safe, especially if your gut feelings indicate otherwise.*

Q **What is a subtle example of an infectious process at a scene that could involve a hazard to the EMS provider's well-being?**

A The EMS provider should always be suspect of more subtle signs such as a sickly looking patient who has shortness of breath, a fever, and a bad cough. He may have an airborne disease as minor as a cold or as major as tuberculosis (TB). Consider donning a protective mask and eyeshield in addition to gloves.

CLINICAL PEARL

> *In a nonjudgmental fashion, always assume the patient has something you don't want, and that you have something she doesn't want.*

Q **What is an example of an unstable scene that can easily be stabilized?**

A An unstable scene that can easily be stabilized is a vehicle that was involved in a collision and is found on all four wheels. The driver may have forgotten to put the vehicle in park or neutral with the emergency brake engaged. You can easily resolve this situation provided you look for it first.

Q **What are examples of incidents where EMS providers have been purposely injured either by the patients or by the people who called for help?**

A There have been instances where angry crowds have hurt public safety personnel. EMS providers have been shot at and trapped in deliberately set fires. In some cities, the EMS providers wear bulletproof vests. This is a somewhat controversial issue, but one thing is clear, wearing a vest should never give the EMS provider a "false sense of security" such that they go places or do things they ordinarily would not do.

Q **What is an example of an incident where an EMS provider was seriously injured by mistake?**

A As a responding EMS provider, you should always be careful when at the scene of a call, especially when attempting to enter a residence without actually being let in by the patient or bystanders. In most communities, EMS providers wait for police to respond if it becomes necessary to force a door or window to enter the residence.

One interesting incident occurred in early 2000 when an EMS provider was trying to assist a disabled woman who had called 911 for help. Apparently the patient's door was locked, so the EMS provider went around the back and found a bathroom window ajar. As he climbed into the neighbor's window, the neighbor was startled by an intruder breaking into his home at midnight and shot the EMS provider with a 9mm pistol.

Fortunately, after five hours of surgery to remove bullet fragments, he did live to tell the story. You can be sure he will not be so quick to climb in someone's window the next time!

Q **What is one of the greatest hazards to EMS providers?**

A Traffic at the scene of a collision. Never take the passing motorist lightly. Always wear bright reflective clothing at night and always be careful when working in or around traffic. Drunk drivers and rubberneckers have been known to drive right into the emergency personnel. Many police, fire, and EMS providers have been seriously injured or killed by this type of incident. Be aware that the ambulance lights may be blocked from the oncoming motorist when the doors are open to load the stretcher. Always call for the police to help take control of the traffic flow to minimize the potential dangers to you and your partners.

CLINICAL PEARL

> *Always assume that oncoming traffic is unaware of your presence. For your own protection, also assume that drivers will not be able to avoid you if you wait for them to make the first move.*

The Initial Assessment of the Patient

[Q] What are some examples of common MOIs?

[A] Common MOIs include collisions, gunshot wounds (GSW), stabbings, assaults, abuse, falls, sports-related injuries, burns, water-related accidents, and environmental injuries (e.g., too hot or too cold).

[Q] What are some of the common "nature of illness" complaints for medical problems?

[A] Common examples of the nature of illness include, SOB, dizziness, syncope, chest pain, seizure, altered mental status (AMS), obstetrical emergencies, poisoning or overdose (OD), stroke, hemorrhage (e.g., GI bleed), and general body weakness.

[Q] What are some examples of how an understanding of the MOI can help the EMS provider predict patterns of injury?

[A] When an EMS provider takes the time to learn about common MOIs, he can make some predictions or be more attuned to specific injury patterns. Examples of predictable fall injuries, motor vehicle collision (MVC) impacts, and blunt and penetrating trauma are included in Table 15–1.

TABLE 15-1

Common MOIs	
Feet first impact	The initial injuries are to the heel, fractures to ankles, legs, and hips. If the patient fell from more than three times her own height or there is an open ankle fracture, also suspect spine fracture (Fx).
Head first impact	Injuries to the cranium and cervical spine. Also consider thoracic aortic disruption if rapid deceleration was involved.
Fall on out-stretched arm	Wrist, elbow, or Colles' fracture (silver fork deformity) are common
Fall or twisting of the knee	These injuries are from physical activities that involve planting the foot as the body is still twisting (e.g., basketball, skiing, racketball). These often injure the supporting structures of the knee.
Up and over the steering column or dash	These injuries occur to unrestrained passengers in the front seat of a vehicle. Suspect facial lacerations and head and cervical spine injuries. The secondary injuries are to the chest and abdomen.
Down and under the steering column or dash	These injuries occur to unrestrained passengers in the front seat of a vehicle. Suspect knee, femur, hip, pelvis, and spine injuries.
Lateral impact (broadside)	The injury on side of impact is more serious if 12 inches or more of vehicular intrusion. This usually involves fractures of

the humerus, ribs, pelvis, and femur on same side, and may involve a head injury.

Coup-contra-coup head injury	Striking one side of the head often causes blunt trauma to the brain in the area that was struck as well as the opposite area of the brain.
Penetration from high velocity projectile (>200ft/ second). Severity is determined by what was hit (e.g., the heart, the lung, soft tissue) and tumble, fragmentation, profile, and cavitation.	*Tumble*—the bullet tumbles or rolls through space with the potential that the side of the bullet, rather than the point, may enter the patient's skin. *Fragmentation*—the projectile bursts into many smaller pieces or fragments and each causes its own injury path. *Profile*—the shape of the bullet. Does it have a solid or soft hollow nose to it? The solid ones penetrate further. The soft-nose bullets mushroom out causing very large temporary spaces (20 times diameter of bullet) and a large permanent injury tract. *Cavitation*—the momentary acceleration of tissue laterally away from the projectile tract. This is like the ripple effect of a rock dropped into a pond. These waves of tissue can cause damage and explain why a bullet near the spine can actually injure the spine. It also explains why the exit wound is usually larger than the entrance wound.
Injury that leads you to suspect other underlying injuries	Examples include a contusion over the left side of the ribs with a possible underlying liver or spleen injury and a steering wheel imprint on the chest with underlying lung contusion.
Physical signs on the vehicle that lead you to suspect underlying injuries	Examples include a starred or cracked windshield, a broken steering wheel, a broken dash, intrusion into the side of the passenger compartment.
Abuse injuries	Injuries in areas that are not usually injured (e.g., upper arms, upper back) or unusual injury patterns (e.g., dipping burn lines, cigarette burns, or rope burns from being restrained).
Waddell's triad	When struck by a vehicle, an injury pattern in children involving the legs, chest, and head: the legs from a direct blow, the chest from being thrown onto the car hood, and the head from being thrown clear of the vehicle when the vehicle comes to a stop. Children have large heads (proportionately) so they "fly" like a javelin head first.
Blow to the side of the head	Striking the temples of the cranium with a blunt object causes the middle meningeal artery to bleed and an epidural hematoma to develop. That is why baseball players wear batter's helmets.
Ejections from a vehicle	It is estimated that the chances of a spinal injury increase up to 1,300 times when not wearing a seat belt and being thrown clear of the vehicle. Of course, that is assuming you are not run over by another vehicle.
Partial ejections	Often the patient's arms and legs are severely crushed when the vehicle rolls when extremities flop outside the vehicle.
Motorcycle injuries	Road rash (serious abrasions) from laying the bike down. Two fractured femurs from being ejected over the handlebars. Crushing injuries to the leg from sideswiping a vehicle.

Why is it so important to identify the total number of patients at an EMS call as soon as possible?

On arrival at the scene, as you ensure that the scene is safe and size it up, be sure to count the number of patients. In some communities, the multiple casualty incident (MCI) plan is put in place for more than three patients. At a minimum, if you need another ambulance or other rescue assistance, you should call right away because it takes time to respond. Some communities have an automatic response to collisions with one engine, two ambulances, and the police because the patients often do not go to the same hospital and are often immobilized on long back-boards. Optimal care is to have no more than one immobilized patient or one critical or unstable patient per ambulance.

Imagine being on the scene of a collision and just as you are about to transport your patient, a police officer asks you to check out the other driver who is now complaining of back pain. If you had counted potential patients on arrival and asked for the proper number of ambulances to be assigned, there should be a unit at the scene by now to care for the other patient rather than you having to wait for its arrival.

Why is it necessary to "choreograph" a scene following size-up?

Scene choreography can make the difference between a well-managed call and a chaotic scene. This requires one person on each unit to be in command and it requires teamwork. The team must work well together, be coordinated, be practiced, and clearly understand each other's roles. Otherwise, an uncoordinated "EMS mob" tends to look like the 20 clowns piling out of a small car at the circus!

Even if there is only one unit responding with two EMS providers, someone should be in charge. If your unit arrives first on the scene of an incident involving multiple units, assess the scene and think about issues like vehicle placement, access and egress, and safety concerns. If you are not the first to arrive, report to the incident commander to obtain a quick report and an assignment for your crew. Once assigned a job, do it, and don't question it unless it could be unsafe. When the assignment is completed, report back to the incident commander for another task. Do not freelance or go off on your own looking for things to do. Freelancing leads to a confusing duplication of efforts and losing track of crew members.

What is a general impression and why is it important for each patient?

The general impression is your first impression of the patient as you approach. This has been referred to as the "look test," a "gut reaction," or your "assessment from the doorway."

It includes the patient's gender, approximate age, your impression of the degree or severity of the patient's distress, and the environment. Examples of general impressions include a male, middle aged, in mild distress, sitting in a chair or a teenage female, unconscious at the bottom of the stairs.

What is an initial assessment of the patient and what general steps does this include?

The initial assessment (IA) is the EMS provider's first assessment of the patient. It is designed to find and begin to deal with life threats as well as prioritize the patient for care and transport. The general steps are:

- BSI precautions.
- Mental status evaluation.
- Airway.
- Breathing.
- Circulation assessment.
- Determining patient priority and the need for additional assistance (e.g., helicopter, critical care transport unit).

What BSI or standard precautions are needed during the initial assessment of the patient?

As you approach the patient, you should have donned disposable gloves and should consider whether goggles or eye-shields and a mask, or even a gown, are needed to protect you from body substances.

What are the methods of assessing the patient's mental status during the initial assessment?

The mental status (MS) is assessed first by introducing yourself to the patient. Start off your assessment by saying, "Hi, I'm (your name) and I am a/an (your level of training). What is your name and how can I assist you?" To determine the patient's level of consciousness (LOC) or MS, we use AVPU: alert, verbally responsive, pain response, or unresponsive. To assess "A," you ask the patient three questions to determine orientation to person, place, and day. Ask, "What's your name?," "Do you know where you are?," and "What day of the week is it today?" Don't bother asking the date because most people have to look at their watch for that answer. A patient correctly answering one or two questions may be considered verbally responsive. A patient answering all three correctly may be considered alert. Verbal responses (not how he speaks, but how he responds to your voice) can be appropriate or inappropriate. You might ask him to show you two fingers.

To assess for a painful response (how the patient responds to some painful stimuli), you have to apply a little pain to the patient. Carefully explain what you are doing so the family members or bystanders do not misinterpret this activity. You can pinch the axillary or squeeze a fingernail. If this does not work, pinching the sternocleidomastoid muscle above the clavicle often works. The response to pain is either appropriate (withdraw from the pain or try to push the pain source away), inappropriate (push into the pain source or elicit a neurological posture), or no response at all. Neurological posturing is either decorticate (flexing the arm to the core of the body) or decerebrate (extending the arm).

What are the differences between the primary survey, the expanded primary survey, and the initial assessment?

Assessment has evolved over the past 30 years of EMS training. First, we learned to do the primary survey, which involved checking ABCs. Then, the survey was expanded to include the management of the life threats identified by the primary survey and referred to as the expanded primary or "ABCDE." Today, we do the initial assessment, which is "MS-ABC," involving assessing and managing life threats to the mental status, ABCs, and prioritizing the patient for transport.

CLINICAL PEARL

When "push comes to shove," regardless what we call the steps, the essence of what we do is unchanged:

- *Make sure the scene is safe.*
- *Immediately evaluate MS.*
- *Immediately evaluate the ABCs.*
- *Maintain the integrity of the cervical spine.*
- *Call for help early, rather than later.*
- *Consider what may be going on.*
- *Consider what you are going to do about it.*

What are the LOCs for patients of different ages (adult, child, infant)?

The LOCs or mental status of all ages is recorded as AVPU. There are subtle changes for the infant or small child (toddler) who has not yet developed language skills. Incorporate the assistance of the parent or caregiver to determine whether the reaction to verbal stimuli is normal for the child.

What is the difference between LOC and MS?

Though these terms are often used interchangeably, they have different meanings:

- Level of consciousness (LOC)—the degree of the patient's alertness, wakefulness, or arousability.
- Mental status (MS)—the appropriateness of the patient's thinking. A psychiatric patient may, for example, have a normal LOC but markedly altered affect or response.

Why don't we use terms like "semi-conscious," "lethargic," "stuporous," "obtunded?"

These terms are inexact, confusing, and difficult to define in such a way that all health care providers can use them the same way. When comparing changes in the patient's LOC or MS, it is important to use the same yardstick!

What is different when assessing the LOC of patients of different ages (adult, child, infant)?

It is more difficult to assess the mental status of a small child or infant. You can't ask an infant to identify the day of the week and expect a correct answer! In these cases, the EMS provider must rely heavily on the caregiver or parent. Try asking questions like, "Would this be a normal reaction for your child to a stranger?" or "Would this be a normal reaction to flicking the soles of the feet?" or "Is he acting different today and if so, explain how?" This same approach may be taken with a psychiatric patient or an Alzheimer's patient.

CLINICAL PEARL

Sometimes we see the term "A&Ox3," meaning "alert and oriented times three" (person, place, and day). Don't get into the dangerous habit of writing this. How do you determine that a two-month-old child is "A&Ox3?" For children, descriptive terms of their behavior better communicate the point:
- *Three-month old infant who looks awake and follows me as I move around the room.*
- *Five-month old infant who looks awake and follows me as I move around the room.*
The described movement also helps to rule out significant neck stiffness.

What is neurological posturing?

An unconscious patient who exhibits (decorticate or decerebrate) posturing is exhibiting neurological posturing. This may occur all the time or only when pain is applied. It is illustrative of low-level brain functioning. Most commonly, this is due to herniation and compression of the brain stem or from metabolic causes (e.g., severe diabetic ketoacidosis, sedative overdose).

Q Why is it important to assess the airway in all patients, and what should the EMS provider look for?

A The pediatricians say that, for children, the initial assessment should be renamed from "MS-ABC" to "AAA" because assessing the airway is so important in younger patients. In an unresponsive patient, there is usually little control of the airway, gag reflex, or swallow reflex, so they are apt to aspirate without close attention to the airway. It is the responsibility of one EMS provider to manually position the airway and ensure that it stays open and clear. This can become a great deal of work if the patient is heavily secreting, is vomiting, or has a suspected spinal injury.

Assessing the airway status may be easier on the responsive patient, but do not be lulled into a false sense of security. A crying baby is usually a good sign that the airway is open, but that does not mean it will stay that way. Even if patients are responsive to verbal stimuli or are alert, they may still have serious airway compromise problems (e.g., broken jaw and nose). The EMS provider should ask three questions when assessing the airway:

- Is it open?
- Will it stay open?
- Does anything endanger the airway?

If the airway is not open, the EMS provider must immediately use the head tilt–chin lift technique. If injury is suspected, use the jaw thrust technique.

Q Why is it so important to treat for a cervical spine injury when opening the airway and assessing the mental status of a patient?

A If the airway of a spinal injured patient is excessively manipulated using a head tilt maneuver instead of the jaw thrust maneuver, it is possible to cause further damage to the patient, including severing or compressing the spinal cord and rendering the patient paralyzed for life.

Q What are some examples of situations that would lead you to treat for a spine injury?

A Any time a patient has received a high-energy impact to the clavicles or superior to the clavicles, the EMS provider must consider the possibility of neck injury and use the jaw thrust, rather than the head tilt, maneuver to open the airway. Always consider that MOIs, such as falls and motor vehicle collisions, are indicators for spinal management. In addition, manual stabilization and spinal immobilization are appropriate for these patients.

Q What questions should the EMS provider ask when assessing breathing?

A There are six questions the EMS provider should ask about the patient's breathing:

- Is the patient breathing?
- What's the respiratory rate?
- Is the rate adequate?
- Does anything endanger breathing?
- Can the patient take a deep breath?
- Is the patient having trouble breathing (dyspnea)?

Q What should the EMS provider do if unsure whether the patient is breathing?

A If you find that it is difficult to determine whether the patient is actually breathing, perhaps because the respirations are very shallow or absent, begin to assist ventilations with a pocket mask or bag-valve-mask (BVM). If the patient is breathing on his own, there will be no harm done by a ventilation or two. If the patient is not breathing on his own, waiting and staring at the chest and abdomen just allows a bad situation to get worse!

Q What is the difference between "adequate" and "inadequate" minute volume?

A Minute volume is the amount of gas inspired or expired in a minute. An inadequate minute volume exists if the respirations are shallow and the rate is too slow (hypoventilation).

Q What are some problems that may cause inadequate breathing?

A Evaluate whether there is a trauma or medical condition that may endanger breathing efforts. Some conditions are obvious, such as a patient pinned under a concrete slab who is having difficulty expanding the chest. Other conditions are more subtle, such as a few broken ribs sustained in a motor vehicle crash that limit the patient's ability to expand the chest due to the pain.

The patient with a penetrating injury to the chest may have worsening dyspnea unless managed appropriately with an occlusive dressing and ventilation. The asthmatic patient with bronchoconstriction and thick mucous in the lower airways may exhibit life-threatening breathing difficulty. A person may have been in an enclosed room during a fire or explosion or in a poorly ventilated area working with paint or chemicals.

ⓠ Are the methods different for assessing the breathing status of an adult, a child, or an infant?

ⓐ The focus on looking, listening, and feeling for air exchange is still the same. Infants are nose breathers, so the impact of a stuffy nose from a cold or upper respiratory infection (URI) is more significant. Basically, "mucous is potentially deadly" in the first four months of life! You can watch the abdomen of a small child to count the respirations.

ⓠ What are the differences between the methods of providing airway care to an adult, a child, or an infant?

ⓐ The neck of the infant should not be hyperextended when opening the airway because this can close off the airway. The small child may have heavy secretions, and they tend to suck more air into their abdomen, which can make ventilations difficult. When inserting the oral airway in a child, place it straight in with the assistance of a tongue blade. Do not flip it over 180 degrees, as in an adult. When intubating an infant, the landmarks are also different (see Chapter 44, Pediatrics).

ⓠ What is the method used to obtain a pulse during the initial assessment of an adult, a child, or an infant?

ⓐ During the initial assessment, the pulse is taken at the carotid for the "quick check" to determine whether the adult or child patient has a pulse. In infants, this is done at the brachial artery in the upper arm. Assessing the radial pulse is more useful in the initial assessment than a carotid pulse because it gives information about the effectiveness of the distal circulation. In certain shock states, a patient may have a palpable carotid pulse, but the distal circulation is so poor the radial pulse cannot be palpated. This helps with estimating the systolic blood pressure without actually applying a BP cuff. In an adult, it takes approximately 80 mmHg of pressure to be able to palpate a radial pulse. A femoral pulse takes about 70 mmHg and a carotid takes approximately 60 mmHg.

ⓠ Why is it so important to assess the patient for external bleeding during the initial assessment?

ⓐ If the patient has serious life-threatening external bleeding, it should be located and controlled during the initial assessment because death could otherwise result. An artery that is severed and spurting must be dealt with immediately.

ⓠ What is assessed in the patient's skin?

ⓐ When assessing the skin, the EMS provider should look at the skin color and feel for the temperature and condition (CTC).

Regardless of the underlying skin pigmentation, the normal skin of the palms and soles is similar in most persons. It should be pink, dry, and warm (depending on the surrounding weather conditions).

ⓠ How is the color of the patient's skin assessed, and what do the different colors mean?

ⓐ Skin color is assessed by looking at the nail beds, lips, and eyes. Abnormal skin color includes:

- Pale—indicates constricted blood vessels, possibly resulting from blood loss, shock, hypotension, or emotional distress.
- Blue (cyanotic)—indicates a lack of oxygen resulting from inadequate breathing or heart function.
- Red (flushed)—indicates heat exposure, hypertension, or emotional excitement.
- Yellow or jaundiced—indicates abnormalities of the liver (e.g., hepatitis, renal failure).

ⓠ Why has capillary refill time been downplayed in adults over the past few years?

ⓐ Recent training curricula have downplayed the use of capillary refill time because there are many unreliable factors that can interfere with the capillary refill time, such as heavy smoking history, skin color, normal poor distal circulation, and cool or cold skin or ambient temperature.

ⓠ How is the capillary refill time assessed in an infant or child?

ⓐ To assess the capillary refill time in an infant or child, press on the nail bed. It should blanch or turn white. Normal capillary refill time after the release of pressure is two seconds or less. (The amount of time it takes to say "capillary refill.") Longer time periods are abnormal, suggesting decreased peripheral perfusion.

ⓠ How is the patient's skin temperature and condition assessed, and what do the findings mean?

ⓐ Place the back of your hand on the patient's forehead and then on the patient's forearm. Normally, the skin should be warm and dry, although the temperature may vary a little with the surrounding environment. Abnormal skin temperature and conditions include:

- Cool and clammy—suggests shock or that the body is losing heat.

- Cold and dry—suggests exposure to cold, hypothermia, or poor peripheral circulation.

- Hot and dry—suggests high fever or heat exposure.

- Hot and moist—suggests high fever or heat exposure.

- Piloerection or "goose pimples" with shivering, chattering teeth, blue lips, and pale skin—suggests chills, exposure to cold, communicable disease, pain, or fever.

- Tenting of the skin—after gently squeezing and pulling the skin, it should quickly drop back to its original position. In a dehydrated patient, the skin stays up in this "tented" position.

Q Why is it so important to prioritize the patient for care and transport as the last step in the initial assessment?

A The last part of the initial assessment is an important decision because it sets the tone for the rest of the patient contact. There are various formats used to classify patients into different priorities.

Q What are some examples of systems used to prioritize patients in the initial assessment?

A Examples of systems to prioritize patients include the high-low classification; the critical, unstable, potentially unstable, or stable (CUPS); and a priority 1,2,3 system. The use of the CUPS format to prioritize is shown in Table 15–2.

TABLE 15–2

The CUPS Format
Critical Actual or impending cardiorespiratory arrest, respiratory failure, decompensated shock (hypoperfusion), rising intracranial pressure, severe upper airway difficulties. Management should include circulatory and ventilatory assistance, CPR, BVM, oxygen administration, and volume resuscitation. Priority is high for all patients.
Unstable Cardiorespiratory instability; respiratory distress; compensated shock (hypoperfusion); two or more bone fractures; trauma with associated burns; amputation proximal to wrist or ankle; penetrating injury to the head, neck, chest, abdomen, or pelvis; uncontrollable external bleeding; chest pain with BP < 100/p; severe pain; general poor impression; unresponsive patients or responsive but not following commands. Management should include supplemental oxygen. Priority is high for all patients.
Potentially Unstable High potential for cardiorespiratory instability, MOI is a "hidden injury," major isolated injury, general medical illness, uncomplicated childbirth. Management should include careful monitoring. Priority is low for the adult and high for the infant or child.

Stable
Low potential for cardiorespiratory instability, low-grade fever, minor illness, minor isolated injury, uncomplicated extremity injury.
Management should include continued observation.
Priority is low for all patients.

Q Why isn't trauma stabilized at the scene?

A It usually requires the "bright lights and cold steel" of a surgical suite to stop internal bleeding. This is not something that can be done in the field. The basic rule is that the internal bleeding is stopped by the surgeon within the first hour after the injury (the golden hour).

Q What are some examples of steps that an experienced EMS provider can skip or expedite when caring for a trauma patient on the scene?

A If the patient is critical, it is acceptable to abbreviate a few steps, such as using the minimum adequate bandaging required, or using the long backboard as a "full body splint" instead of taking the time to splint every fracture the patient may have.

PEARL

There is a major difference between sufficient bandaging and splinting and "sloppy" work. It's all right to minimize on scene time as long as the care given is proper.

Q What are some examples of steps that should not be skipped or expedited when caring for a trauma patient on the scene?

A If the patient is critical, it is not acceptable to skip airway control, bleeding control of life-threatening external bleeding, or full spinal immobilization. You can consider using the rapid extrication technique to get the patient out of the car if necessary. Airway control and cervical spine immobilization should be done simultaneously.

PEARL

Remember the most important steps, once you've ensured your own safety: airway, breathing, circulation (with attention to cervical spine control).

Q Once the initial assessment has been completed, what are the two general categories of patient classification?

A After the initial assessment, patients are assessed as either medical or trauma.

Q Does every patient fit neatly into these two categories?

A No! Consider the patient who has a syncopal episode (passes out) at the top of the stairwell or in the driver's seat of a moving car. Initially, the patient may have a medical problem, but often the reason the EMS system is activated is the trauma from falling to the bottom of the stairwell or crashing the vehicle into the bridge abutment. The trauma may be the obvious part for the EMS provider to assess, but the medical aspects that caused the incident in the first place also need to be investigated. Could it have been a dysrhythmia, a seizure, hypoglycemia, or any number of other medical problems?

CLINICAL PEARL

Many patients "don't read a medical textbook" before getting sick or hurt! Always suspect the unusual and the unexpected.

Q Why has there been a shift from "diagnosis-based curricula" to "assessment-based curricula"?

A It is often difficult, if not impossible, to make a definitive field diagnosis. The same is true in the ED. The EMS provider's major responsibility is not to make a "final diagnosis." Rather, it is to form an "initial impression" based on priorities:

- Identify and treat immediate life threats.
- Determine whether transportation (admission) is necessary.
- Initiate necessary evaluation steps (e.g., ECG, blood glucose, pulse oximetry).
- Stabilize the patient until definitive care is available.

For more information on this topic, review Chapter 18, Assessment-Based Management.

Q What is the rapid trauma assessment?

A The rapid trauma assessment is a quick assessment of the head, neck, chest, abdomen, pelvis, extremities, and posterior of the body to detect signs and symptoms of injury. This is discussed in detail in Chapter 17, Focused History and Physical Examination: Trauma Patient.

Q What is the ongoing assessment?

A The ongoing assessment describes what is done in the ambulance enroute to the hospital. It includes reassessing vital signs, checking on interventions such as medications, and redoing the initial assessment as needed. This is discussed in detail in Chapter 19, Ongoing Assessment and Clinical Decision Making.

Q Why is it necessary to reconsider the MOI when assessing the patient?

A The MOI is very important and might be initially overlooked. It should be reconsidered throughout the patient assessment, especially when sorting trauma patients by "significant MOI" and "nonsignificant MOI." Take a mental snapshot of the MOI and try to imagine what forces the patient's body experienced. When possible, get a Polaroid® photo to show the physician in the ED.

Q Why is the initial assessment a part of the ongoing assessment?

A The initial assessment is repeated in the ongoing assessment in cases where the patient's condition may be rapidly changing and life-threatening problems have developed that must be managed.

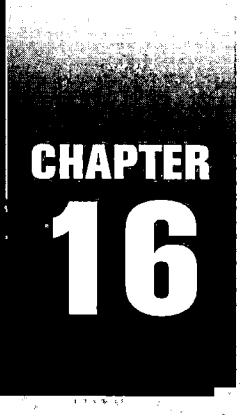

CHAPTER 16

Focused History and Physical Examination: Medical Patient

This chapter discusses the focused history and physical examination (PE) of the medical patient who is either responsive or unresponsive. The emphasis is on conditions that can be managed in the field.

Medical Patient Assessment

Q When is the focused history and PE of the medical patient performed?

A After the initial assessment has been completed, the next step in the assessment is to focus on the patient's chief complaint. In the absence of trauma and mechanism of injury (MOI), the patient most often will have a medical complaint, which was usually the reason why EMS was called.

Q What are the components of the focused history and PE for the medical patient?

A The focused history often begins concurrently with the assessment. When the patient is unresponsive, a rapid PE follows the initial assessment and management of the ABCs. The components of the medical patient assessment are listed in Figure 16–1.

Q What information is collected in the focused history?

A Gather a SAMPLE history and the history of the present illness (HPI). Collect the positive findings or the information that is clearly relevant to the chief complaint. Also collect the pertinent negatives, those symptoms the patient does not have that

may be relevant to the case (e.g., there was no loss of consciousness, patient denies any shortness of breath). The acronyms in Table 16–1, Table 16–2, and 16–3 should be helpful.

TABLE 16-1
Acronym for Patients with Pain
O–Onset.
P–Provocation.
Q–Quality.
R–Radiation, Relief, Recurrence.
S–Severity.
T–Time.

TABLE 16-2
Acronym for Patients with Altered Mental Status (AMS)
A–Alcohol (acute or chronic).
E–Epilepsy, endocrine, exocrine, electrolytes.
I–Infection (local or systemic).
O–Overdose (intentional or accidental).
U–Uremia (traumatic or renal causes, including hypertension).
T–Trauma (old or new), temperature.
I–Insulin (hypo- or hyperglycemic).
P–Psychoses (many possibilities).
S–Stroke (hemorrhage or ischemic), shock, space occupying lesion, subarachnoid bleed.

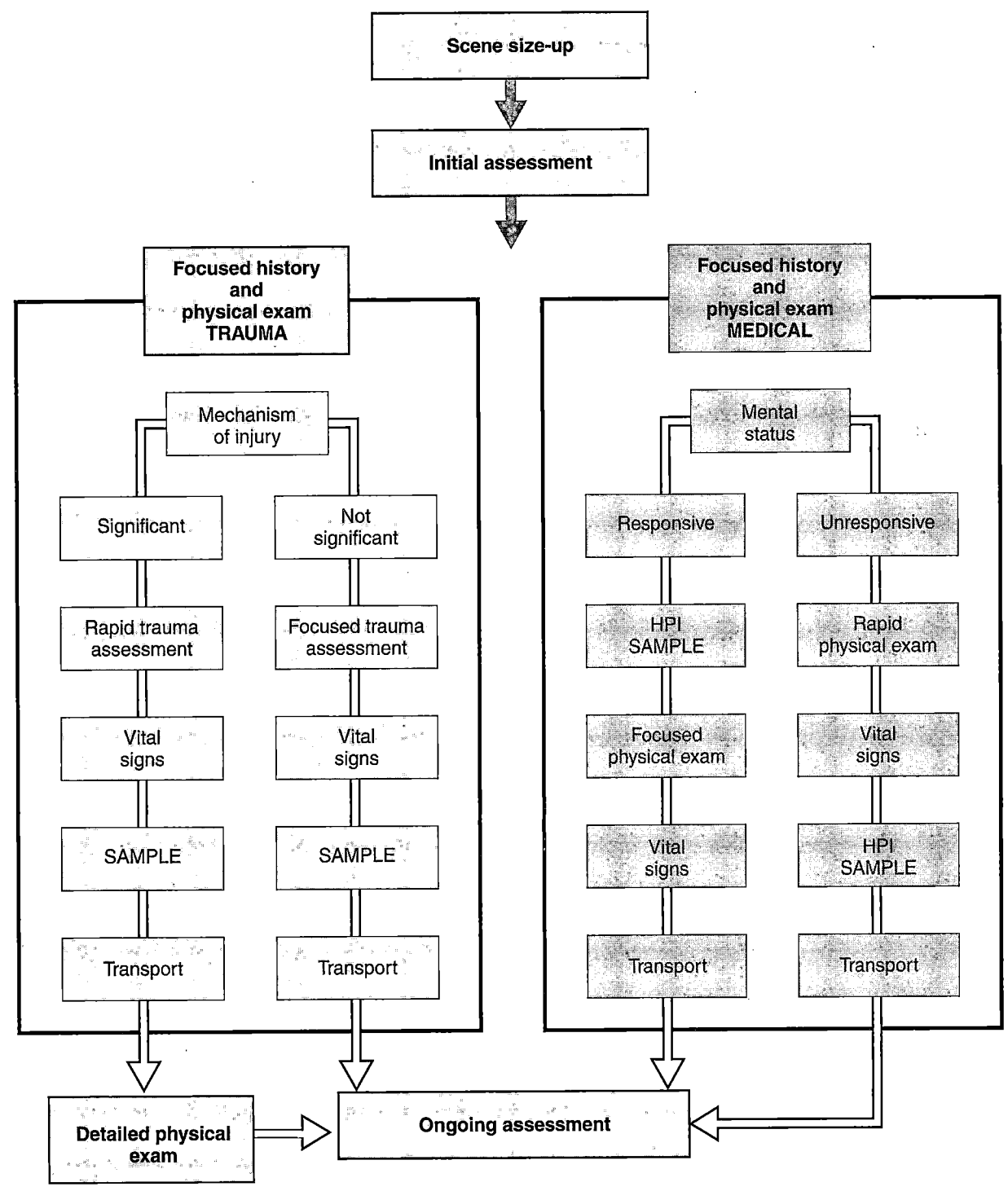

FIGURE 16-1 The patient assessment algorithm.

TABLE 16-3

Acronym for Patients With Shortness of Breath (SOB)
C—Chest pain with breathing.
A—Activity at onset.
P—Prolonged bed rest or limited mobility.
E—Exposure to toxin or pollution; smoker (packs per day and number of years).
C—Cough; productive—color, amount, blood.
H—History of lung disease and intubation history.
O—Orthopnea (unable to breathe unless in an upright position).

Q Why do we talk to a medical patient before touching them?

A In most cases, it is necessary to establish a rapport and get consent for treatment before touching a patient. To gain a patient's trust and cooperation, it is necessary to demonstrate professionalism and to show respect. Not only is it the right thing to do, it is the legal thing to do.

Q How is the focused history (FH) and PE of a medical patient different for responsive and unresponsive patients?

A When a patient is responsive, the interview process begins concurrently with or just before performing the initial assessment. When the patient is unresponsive, the initial assessment and management of the ABCs is started immediately. Because the patient is not able to provide a history, the rapid PE follows. Information about the patient's history may or may not be available depending on whether anyone is present at the scene that can provide additional information.

Q Why was patient "responsiveness" used to differentiate medical patients into two categories?

A In the revised curriculums, which are assessment based, the patients are separated into two categories of "severity." Using the earlier diagnosis-based curricula, the EMS provider would have attempted to make a presumptive field diagnosis on medical patients (e.g., trying to separate patients with angina from those with suspected acute myocardial infarction [AMI]). Today, when using assessment findings, the level of responsiveness is used to separate patients into the two categories of severity.

Q Why don't we just make a field diagnosis to differentiate medical patients?

A Many of the presenting medical problems involve the same field management in the first 30–60 minutes, so it is not always necessary or practical to make a diagnosis in the field (e.g.,

angina vs. AMI, transient ischemic attack [TIA] vs. cerebrovascular accident [CVA], fracture vs. dislocation).

CLINICAL PEARL

Strive to assess emergent signs and symptoms, stabilize patients to the best of your ability, and transport them to the nearest appropriate facility.

Q What is DCAP-BTLS?

A This acronym is used to remember what is assessed about the patient's skin.

D—Deformity.	B—Burn.
C—Contusion.	T—Tenderness.
A—Abrasion.	L—Laceration.
P—Puncture/penetration.	S—Swelling.

Q What are the components of the rapid PE?

A Even if trauma has been ruled out in the unresponsive patient (e.g., a witness saw the patient pass out, caught the patient, and laid the patient on the floor without injury), this does not mean that the patient has not very recently sustained some other form of trauma. Therefore, do not overlook DCAP-BTLS during the rapid PE. The components of the rapid PE are:

- Head—assess the head and face for skin color, temperature, and condition (CTC); asymmetry; neurological deficits (e.g., facial droop); pupillary response; and DCAP-BTLS.

- Neck—assess the skin CTC, JVD, and DCAP-BTLS.

- Chest—assess the skin CTC, breath sounds, heart sounds, and DCAP-BTLS.

- Abdomen—assess the skin CTC, softness, rigidity, masses, distention, and DCAP-BTLS.

- Pelvis—assess skin CTC, distention, and DCAP-BTLS.

- Posterior—assess for DCAP-BTLS.

- Extremities—assess skin CTC, distal pulse, motor function, sensation, and DCAP-BTLS.

- Mental status (MS) is further evaluated using deep pain response reflexes such as Babinski's, doll's eye (only if no spinal injury), pupillary reactions, and the Glasgow Coma Scale.

Q What are the components of the focused PE?

A The components of the focused PE are guided by the chief complaint, the findings of the initial assessment, and the findings during the focused PE. For example, when a patient has a chief complaint of shortness of breath, after performing the initial assessment, the progressive direction of the exam will be to focus on the respiratory system. While listening to breath sounds you hear an abnormal heart sound, so now you adapt the focused PE to include the cardiac system as well. Focused PEs often combine multiple body systems. For example, when assessing the abdomen, you include components of the skin, musculoskeletal, circulatory, and GI systems for a complete PE.

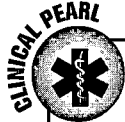

CLINICAL PEARL

The answer to one question may open new "doors."
However, don't lose track of the original complaint.

Q **What are the different focused PEs used by the EMS provider?**

A Detailed focused exams for respiratory (Chapter 22), cardiac (Chapter 23), neurological (Chapter 24), behavioral (Chapter 31), abdominal (Chapter 27), geriatric (Chapter 45), and pediatric (Chapter 44) patients are discussed in other chapters. A summary of the key components of these exams is in Table 16–4.

TABLE 16-4

Key Components of Focused Exams for Medical Patients

RESPIRATORY
- Skin CTC.
- Position.
- Abnormal respirations.
- Use of accessory muscles to breathe.
- Lung sounds.
- Abnormal chest contour.
- Medic Alert® tag.
- Clubbing of finger tips or nails.

CARDIAC
- Skin CTC.
- Jugular vein distention (JVD).
- Medic Alert® tag.
- Transdermal patches.
- Pacemaker or automatic internal cardiac defibrillator (AICD).
- Midsternal scars.
- Midline pulsations and aortic aneurysms.
- Lung sounds.
- Heart sounds.
- Point of maximal impulse (PMI).
- Pulses.

- Liver distention.
- Peripheral edema.

NEUROLOGICAL
- MS exam, including the AVPU (alert, verbal, pain, unresponsive) trauma alertness scale, the Glasgow Coma Scale (GCS), and memory loss.
- Motor symptoms (e.g., paresis, paralysis, weakness, inability to move a part of the body, impaired coordination).
- Sensory symptoms (e.g., decreased sensation, hypersensitivity, "pins and needles" feelings, and pain).
- Seizures.
- Headache.
- Stiff neck.
- Neck or back pain.
- Loss of bowel or bladder control.
- Abnormal respirations.
- Vision disturbances.
- Speech disturbances.
- Vertigo.
- Syncope.
- Coma.

BEHAVIORAL
- Presentation
- Position
- Behavior
- Affect
- Speech (e.g., clarity, intonation, speed, content, word choice).
- Dress (e.g., hygiene, appropriate clothing).
- Judgment.
- Memory.

ABDOMINAL
- Skin CTC.
- Position.
- Orthostatics (e.g., hypotension in the standing position).
- Presence of blood in vomitus, urine, or feces.
- Color of stool.
- Tenderness.
- Masses.
- Ascites (accumulation of fluid between the tissues and organs of the abdomen).
- Abdominal scars.
- Bowel sounds.

GERIATRIC INDEPENDENT ASSESSMENT
- Physical or mental inability to perform daily living activities, including living environment, support systems, and hazards.
- Considerations of aging process (e.g., anatomical changes, mental status, and emotional well-being).
- Past medical history (e.g., concurrent illnesses, complete medication list, and surgeries).

PEDIATRIC
- Toe to head exam in small children.
- Age appropriate inference.
- Consideration of anatomical differences.
- Consideration of emotional differences.

Associated Symptoms

What is the difference between vertigo and dizziness?

Vertigo is often used as a synonym for dizziness or light-headedness. True vertigo is a vestibular disorder that includes motion sickness. The patient experiences a false sensation of motion. Dizziness encompasses a variety of complaints: hazy, light-headed, faint, giddy. Making a differential diagnosis is not quick or easy. It involves getting a good history and completing a thorough exam with diagnostic procedures. Common causes of vertigo include:

- Traumatic brain injury (TBI).
- Stroke.
- Medications, especially antibiotics.
- Ear infections.
- Viruses.
- Stress.
- Advanced old age.

CLINICAL PEARL

It is sometimes helpful to ask the patient if he felt like the room was spinning (favors vertigo) or if he felt like passing out or was wobbly (favors dizziness).

What causes dizziness?

There are many possible causes including:
- TBI.
- Stroke.
- Medications.
- Narcotics or alcohol.

Dizziness may be associated with:
- Standing up. This may indicate low blood pressure.
- Moving the head. This may indicate an inner ear problem.
- Nausea, vomiting, headache, or hearing loss. This may also indicate an inner ear problem (e.g., vertigo, Meneire's disease).

What causes nausea and vomiting?

Nausea or vomiting is associated with many disorders. Frequently, but not always, vomiting is preceded by nausea. When brought on by injury, or accompanied by severe abdominal pain or headache, nausea or vomiting may indicate a serious condition. The vomiting reflex is located in the vomiting centers in the medulla. The reflex can be stimulated by several mechanisms:

- Sensory receptors in the stomach and intestines may stimulate the reflex due to infection, food irritation, or injury.
- Chemoreceptor trigger zones in the vestibular system are stimulated by:
    a. Inner ear disorders (e.g., dizziness, vertigo, motion sickness).
    b. Various drugs (e.g., morphine, digitalis, and various anesthetics).
    c. Endogenous toxins.
- Increased intracranial pressure can stimulate the vomiting reflex as seen with brain disorders (e.g., TBI, infections, tumors, migraine).
- Stimulation of the cerebral cortex and limbic system by noxious stimuli or stress.
- Voluntary stimulation of the gag reflex.

What is the difference between vomiting and regurgitation?

Vomiting is an active process in a conscious patient; regurgitation is a passive process in an unconscious patient.

Can vomiting alone lead to potential complications?

Yes, a patient with an AMS or unprotected airway may aspirate while vomiting. Dehydration can become a severe problem especially in infants, children, and older patients. Vomiting can also be a sign of more serious conditions. Prolonged or frequent vomiting may produce GI bleeding as a result of the reflux of acid and bile. It can also cause Mallory-Weiss tears.

Why are some patients medicated to prevent vomiting?

Some patients are medicated to prevent the complications from dehydration and gastrointestinal (GI) distress. Cardiac patients are medicated to prevent the vagus stimulation that occurs with vomiting. In many cardiac conditions, the patient cannot tolerate the slower heartbeat and its accompanying decrease in cardiac output as well as the potential for myocardial irritability causing extrasystoles. Patients with serious conditions (e.g., brain disorders, GI blockage) that produce nausea and vomiting are medicated to prevent further discomfort from and complications of the preexisting condition.

Medications commonly used are antihistamines (e.g., meclizine, cyclizine, and phenegan) and posphorylated carbohydrate solution (e.g., Emetrol®).

Why do so many people die in the bathroom?

The bathroom is a very likely location for a syncopal event to occur. The patient usually slips and falls, or passes out first and then falls, and strikes the porcelain (tub, sink, or commode) and sustains trauma. They may not be found immediately and die of a cardiac event, drowning, head injury, or hemorrhage. One of the common causes of syncope in the bathroom is a parasympathetic response from stimulation of the vagus (e.g., bearing down on the commode, shaving the neck stimulating the carotid artery, pressing on the eye while manipulating contact lens). The patient having an AMI usually has an ischemic heart that is irritable and does not tolerate the sudden drop in pulse rate from vagal stimulation. Often the irritable heart throws more extrasystoles setting up the potential for ventricular fibrillation to occur.

What are some of the causes of syncope?

The causes of syncope are numerous and are listed as cardiac or noncardiac in Table 16–5.

TABLE 16–5

Causes of Syncope

CARDIAC CAUSES
- Heart block and bradycardias.
- Dysrhythmias (e.g., supraventricular tachycardia [SVT], Stokes-Adams syndrome, Sick Sinus syndrome).
- Aortic stenosis.
- AMI.
- Angina.

NONCARDIAC CAUSES
- Neurologic.
- Hemorrhagic.
- Vasovagal.
- Micturition (urination).
- Dehydration.
- Respiratory.
- Pharmacologic.
- Emotional (e.g., stress, anxiety, fright).

Many drugs can cause a syncopal event. Following are drug classifications for common medications that may cause syncope:

- Beta-blockers.
- Diuretics.
- Antihypertensives.
- Narcotic analgesics.
- Antiarrhythmics.
- Nitrates.
- Digitalis.

- ACE inhibitors.
- Psychiatric medications, especially tricyclics.

Should every patient that has experienced a syncopal event be transported?

Yes, especially pregnant patients and any patients over the age of 50. Unless the patient has a clear cut vasovagal faint, most experts recommend in-hospital evaluation at the ED.

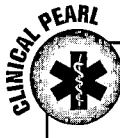

CLINICAL PEARL

Numerous diseases, ranging from pulmonary emboli to cardiac dysrhythmias, may cause syncope. Always assume the worst and treat the patient accordingly.

What is the value of orthostatic vital sign changes?

They are helpful if positive and the patient is symptomatic. They are not always significant or reliable because most people normally have subtle vital sign changes when going from a supine or sitting position to a standing position. Orthostatic hypotension occurs due to a sudden peripheral vasodilation with a compensatory increase in cardiac output. This is common in aging people, from prolonged bed rest, from certain medications, and from hypovolemia with a blood loss greater than 1,000 cc.

CLINICAL PEARL

There are wide variances in "normal ranges" for orthostatic vital signs. More significant are positional symptoms, especially if associated with significant pulse or BP changes.

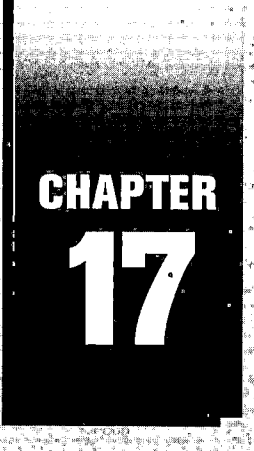

CHAPTER 17

Focused History and Physical Examination: Trauma Patient

This chapter discusses four essentials of trauma patient management: (1) classifying trauma patients into one of two categories by the mechanism of injury (MOI), (2) the rapid trauma exam, (3) the focused history and physical examination (PE) of the trauma patient, and (4) the detailed PE. The focus is on *why* trauma patients are different from medical patients and *why* EMS providers must respond differently to their presenting problems. In one word, "time" is not on your side with the trauma patient and most of your effort is to fight against the clock to ensure appropriate assessment and management in as little time as possible.

Trauma Patient Assessment

Q Why are safety, scene size-up, and MOI important when assessing the trauma patient?

A For the assessment to progress quickly and effectively, these three steps are vital. Safety and the correction of hazards are the top priorities before any other steps. Next, a scene size-up is done to determine how many patients are involved and what additional personnel and equipment are needed to provide care. Evaluating the MOI to understand the pathology of what happened combined with the first two steps forms the foundation of excellent trauma patient care. Examples of common MOIs are listed in Table 15–1 in Chapter 15.

Q What are life-threatening conditions that require immediate intervention?

A Life-threatening conditions include any injury that interferes with the ABCs. The factor involved most often in traumatic injuries is shock.

> **CLINICAL PEARL**
>
> *The most important aspect of trauma assessment is the MOI. Know this, maintain an airway, breathing, and circulation (with cervical spine control), and proceed accordingly.*

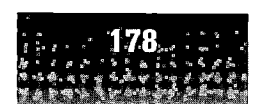

Q What are the primary concerns during the assessment and treatment of the trauma patient?

A When managing the trauma patient, you must consider what the patient needs and what you can provide. For the critical trauma patient, definitive treatment is in the OR. Critical patients have the best chance for survival if they can reach definitive care within one hour of the onset of injury. This is called the golden hour. The maximum time the EMS provider should spend on scene, barring any extrication, is no more than 10 minutes. This is an instance when less is better. This 10-minute field time is called the "platinum 10 minutes" when it is referenced with the "golden hour." The primary concerns for the critical trauma patient are:

- A—assess for a patent airway. Use the jaw thrust and suction as needed to maintain an open airway.
- B—assess breathing and ventilation, provide high-flow oxygen, and assist ventilations if needed.
- C—assess perfusion and control hemorrhage.
- Rapid transport and notification to definitive care.

For the noncritical patient, the concerns are similar; however, the priorities are changed. There is time for a thorough focused history (FH) and PE. A detailed PE and rapid transportation may not be required in the noncritical patient.

Q What are the components of the trauma assessment?

A During the scene size-up, it is crucial to quickly, but carefully, evaluate and understand the MOI because this is the starting point of the trauma assessment. The focused history often begins concurrently with the assessment. The components of the trauma patient assessment are shown in Figure 17–1.

Q Why is the MOI used to classify trauma patients into significant and nonsignificant categories?

A The general impression of the patient often provides information about the overall condition, but not always. Patients can sustain a significant MOI without an apparent major injury or any injury at all. This does not mean they should be managed lightly or not at all. Because unrecognized traumatic injury is how so many patients have died, the Committee on Trauma of the American College of Surgeons, together with other national groups, have developed courses such as prehospital trauma life support (PHTLS), critical trauma care (CTC), basic trauma life support (BTLS) and advanced trauma life support (ATLS). These trauma courses teach the principles of appreciating the MOI, when to suspect possible injuries associated with various MOIs, as well as the management of the trauma patient.

Proper evaluations of the MOI can help the EMS provider predict injuries that may or may not be readily apparent. Based on this information, the responder can better provide the appropriate assessment and management.

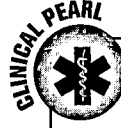

CLINICAL PEARL

If the MOI suggests a potentially life-threatening injury, treat the patient as such, regardless of how stable he looks.

Q Why don't we use the field diagnosis to classify trauma patients into two categories?

A Experts agree that assessment-based patient care, not diagnostic-based care, provides the best chance for the survival of critical trauma patients. This is because it takes time to make a diagnosis. When you consider the golden hour, there is not enough time to diagnose injuries in the field, and often not even in the ED.

Q What are the steps of the *rapid trauma exam*?

A The steps of the rapid trauma exam are performed using the assessment techniques of observation, listening, and palpation to rapidly examine each of the following areas of the body. Begin by taking body substance isolation (BSI) precautions.

- Head—assess for deformity, contusion, abrasion, puncture/penetration, burn, tenderness, laceration, and swelling (DCAP-BTLS), crepitation on the head and face, and pupillary response.
- Neck—assess for DCAP-BTLS, crepitation, and jugular vein distention (JVD).
- Chest—assess for DCAP-BTLS, crepitation, symmetry, paradoxical motion, and breath sounds.
- Abdomen—assess for DCAP-BTLS, softness, rigidity, masses, and distention.
- Pelvis—assess for DCAP-BTLS, crepitation, and stability.
- Posterior—assess the back and buttocks for DCAP-BTLS.
- Extremities—assess for DCAP-BTLS, distal pulse, motor function, and sensation.
- Glasgow Coma Score (GCS).

Q What is the detailed physical examination (DPE)?

A The DPE is a complete head-to-toe exam for nonlife- or limb-threatening injuries.

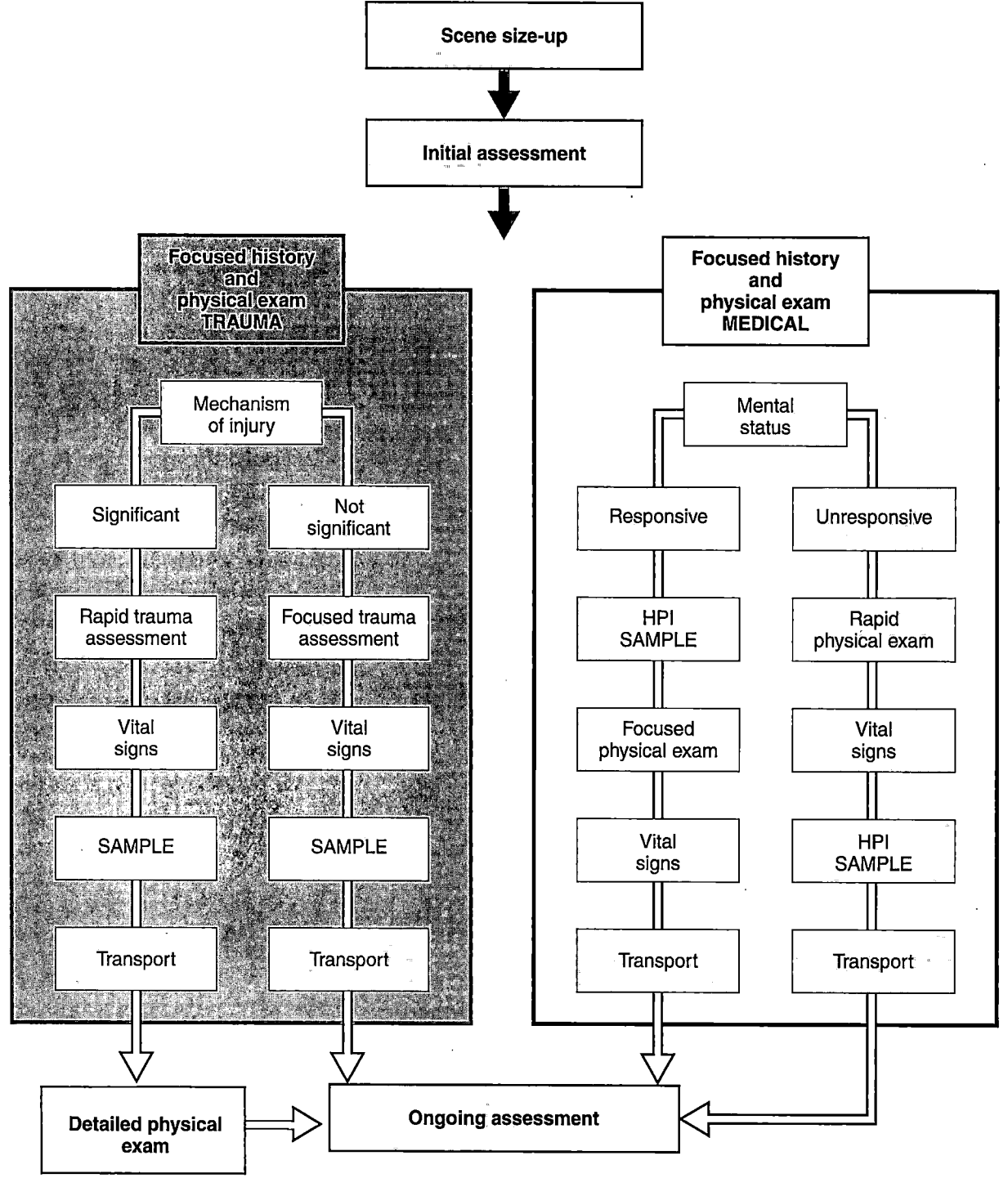

FIGURE 17-1 The patient assessment algorithm.

What are the steps in the DPE?

The steps are similar to, but more thorough than, the rapid trauma exam. Begin by taking BSI precautions.

- Head—assess for DCAP-BTLS and crepitation on the head and scalp.

- Face—assess for DCAP-BTLS, crepitation, and symmetry.
- Eyes—assess for DCAP-BTLS, pupillary response and eye movement, and discoloration.
- Nose—assess for DCAP-BTLS and drainage.
- Ears—assess for DCAP-BTLS and drainage.

- Mouth—assess for DCAP-BTLS, crepitation in mouth and jaw, loose or broken teeth, swelling or laceration of tongue or throat, unusual odors, discoloration, and drainage.
- Neck—assess for DCAP-BTLS, crepitation, and JVD.
- Chest—assess for DCAP-BTLS, crepitation, symmetry, paradoxical motion, and breath sounds.
- Abdomen—assess for DCAP-BTLS, softness, rigidity, masses, and distention.
- Pelvis—assess for DCAP-BTLS, crepitation, and stability.
- Posterior—assess the back and buttocks for DCAP-BTLS.
- Extremities—assess for DCAP-BTLS, distal pulse, motor function, and sensation.

Is it acceptable not to do a DPE on a trauma patient? What if I don't have enough time?

The DPE is conducted only if time permits, usually enroute to the hospital. When a patient is critical, necessary interventions, serial initial assessments, trending vitals signs, and transport time often do not allow enough time to perform the DPE. These steps have priority over the DPE; however, very few patients (approximately 10 percent of trauma patients) are so critical that omitting the DPE is rare.

If the patient deteriorates rapidly, where is it acceptable to save time in the field management of the trauma patient?

It is never acceptable to skip the scene size-up, safety, initial assessment, or intervention for ABCs. However, there are areas that may be "downplayed" to minimize scene time.

- Perform a rapid extrication rather than using a short spine immobilization device.
- Use a long board device rather than immobilizing individual extremities.
- Use BLS skills for the ABCs and perform invasive skills, such as intubation and IV access, enroute to the hospital.
- Delay bandaging until you have time enroute, unless it is an arterial bleed needing a pressure bandage.

When should ALS be called to the scene and what can they offer to the trauma patient that BLS can not?

Determining whether ALS should be called depends on what they have to offer the patient. Airway management above BLS measures, such as ET, Combitube®, laryngeal mask airway (LMA), rapid sequence induction (RSI), chest decompression, and IV volume replacement for hemorrhagic shock, may be bene-

ficial for some trauma patients. The call for ALS can be made at any point during the call. However, if there is even a remote possibility that ALS may be needed, call early. Sometimes the extra set of hands and advanced assessment skills can be valuable. You can always cancel the call if you do not need them or you have arrived at the hospital.

Transportation should not be delayed while waiting for ALS to arrive. Make the call and begin transport. Have ALS meet you enroute (intercept) to the hospital.

> **CLINICAL PEARL**
>
> *As a rule, don't wait for ALS to arrive; begin transport and meet enroute. If you are awaiting the arrival of an aeromedical helicopter, go promptly to the chosen landing zone.*

When should rapid transport be considered for the trauma patient?

The transportation decision is usually made after the assessment for the MOI and the initial assessment have been completed. The information obtained at this point is enough to determine the patient's condition and to make the decision to "load and go" or "stay and play."

Why should we examine first before obtaining the history of a trauma patient?

The out-of-hospital provider must quickly identify the patient's condition, provide essential intervention, and make a meaningful management and transportation decision. Every additional minute spent on scene could be valuable time taken away from the golden hour, reducing the patient's chance for survival. In most cases, the focused history is obtained during the assessment in the interest of time.

> **CLINICAL PEARL**
>
> *In trauma, simultaneous assessment and history taking are often the rule rather than the exception. The time saved may make the difference between life and death.*

When should a cervical collar be applied?

The decision to apply a cervical collar is made by considering the following:

- The MOI (e.g., major vehicular deformity).
- The presence of an obvious deformity of the neck or spine.

- A conscious patient complains of pain or tenderness with or without palpation.
- An unconscious patient with unknown MOI or unknown cause of loss of consciousness (LOC).

Maintain manual stabilization of the patient's cervical spine until after the initial assessment and critical interventions have been completed. Then, apply the cervical collar. Continue to maintain stabilization until the patient is fully immobilized.

Trauma Centers

Who established the criteria for trauma center designation?

Under the Federal 1204 series grants and the direction of Doctor David Boyd, trauma center designation was started using criteria set forth by The American College of Surgeons (ACS) Committee on Trauma (COT).

What are the levels of trauma centers and their differences?

Trauma centers are classified into four levels based on the resources and programs available at each facility.

- *Level I* is a regional center that serves as a leader in trauma care for a specific geographical area. Most Level I trauma centers have a full range of resources, services, and programs.
- *Level II* has the capability of definitive patient care, but may not have all of the resources of a Level I.
- *Level III* is designated in communities without Level I or II trauma centers. They have the capability for stabilization, but, when necessary, transfer patients to a Level I or II for further intervention and ongoing care.
- *Level IV* is established for rural and remote communities. A Level IV may be a clinic rather than a hospital. The goal is to provide initial stabilization and then transfer to a Level I, II, or III.

What are the criteria for transport to a Level I trauma center?

The needs of the patient and the capabilities of the trauma center determine the criteria for transportation to any level trauma center. These criteria are based on the regional structure of a trauma care system and often can be found in local protocols.

Examples of criteria for transport to a Level I trauma center are severe burns or major trauma to a pediatric, geriatric, or pregnant patient. A traumatic cardiac arrest is most often transported to the nearest hospital even if it is not a Level I trauma center. The reason for this is that the survival rate of a traumatic cardiac arrest is so low that the closest facility that can provide stabilization may be the patient's best chance.

What are the criteria and procedure for aeromedical transport?

The criteria and specific procedures for aeromedical transport vary with geographical locations; however, there are advantages to established guidelines in each county. The following is a list of advantages of aeromedical evacuation.

- Situations where the time required for ground transport poses a threat to the patient's survival or recovery.
- Access to remote areas.
- Access to specialized critical care personnel or specialty units in certain hospitals (e.g., neonatal intensive care unit, re-implementation, transplant center, burn center).
- Access to personnel with specialty skills (e.g., surgical airway, thoracotomy, rapid sequence intubation).
- Access to specialty supplies and equipment (e.g., aortic balloon pump).

What is the trauma score?

The trauma score was developed in 1980 as a scale to be used for triage and to predict patient outcome. Howard Champion, MD is the physician responsible for the latest version of the trauma score referred to as the Revised Trauma Score. This is a numerical grading system that combines the Glasgow Coma Scale (GCS) (Table 17-1) and measurements of cardiopulmonary function as a gauge of the severity of injury and a predictor of survival after blunt injury to the head. Each parameter is given a number with high being normal and low being impaired or absent function. The severity of injury is determined by summing the numbers for the following categories: respiratory rate, respiratory expansion, systolic BP, pulse, capillary refill, and a conversion scale for the GCS, as shown in Table 17–2. The trauma score has a value from 1 to 16 with 1 being a patient with virtually no percentage of survival, 8 having a 26 percent chance of survival, 12 having an 87 percent chance of survival, and 16 having a 99 percent chance of survival.

TABLE 17-1

Glasgow Coma Scale (GCS)		
Eye opening response:	Spontaneous	4
	To voice	3
	To pain	2
	None	1
Best verbal response:	Oriented	5
	Confused	4
	Inappropriate words	3
	Incomprehensible sounds	2
	None	1
Best motor response:	Obeys commands	6
	Localizes pain	5
	Withdraws from pain	4
	Flexion to pain	3
	Extension to pain	2
	None	1

TABLE 17-2

Glasgow Coma Score (GCS) Conversion for Trauma Score	
GCS Total Points	Apply to Trauma Score
14 to 15	5
1 to 13	4
8 to 10	3
5 to 7	2
3 to 4	1

Special Considerations in Trauma Assessment

Q What are the unique aspects of the pediatric trauma patient?

A Trauma is the number one killer of children in the United States. The following is a list of MOIs unique to pediatric trauma.

- The most common MOI is falls.
- Head injury is the most common cause of death.
- Trauma in children, as compared to adults, more often involves multisystem trauma, rather than an isolated injury.
- Common patterns of injury are prevalent.
- Children have unique physiological responses to trauma, such as the ability to compensate for blood loss longer than adults. However, when they reach the point that they can no longer compensate, unlike adults, they deteriorate quickly and severely.

Q What are the special considerations in the assessment of the pediatric trauma patient?

A Because children are continuously growing and most body organs, systems, and structures have not matured, special consideration must be given to the assessment of the pediatric patient.

Incomplete calcification of bones makes them softer and less likely to fracture than adult bones. Therefore, when a deformity of a bone is apparent, you must suspect that a significant amount of energy was involved in the injury and that there may also be accompanying internal injury as well. Missed orthopedic injuries can leave a child with a permanent deformity or long-term disability.

- Airway—large tongues and anterior airway structures make the pediatric airway prone to obstruction.
- Neck—spinal cord injury without radiological abnormality (SCIWORA) means that children can sustain spinal cord injuries without having the same injuries visible on X-ray studies. The same injuries are much easier to observe on X-ray studies in an adult patient.
- Chest—rib fractures are rare due to soft bones. When present, the risk of mortality is increased.
- Abdomen—large and exposed with little protection from the ribs or spine, the abdomen is at increased risk for injury (especially the liver and spleen).
- Pelvis—check for stability and crepitus.
- Extremities—growth plate injuries must be ruled out in the ED.

Q What are the special considerations for assessing the elderly trauma patient?

A Preexisting medical conditions may precipitate a traumatic injury, such as a syncopal event leading to broken bones from a fall. Chronic and degenerative disease processes can make an injury, even a minor one, worse. As the body ages, body systems begin to deteriorate. The key is to attempt to learn what the patient's baseline condition was so you can assess for acute changes.

- The thermoregulatory system makes the body susceptible to cold and heat, as well as electrolyte imbalances.
- As the immune system fails, the body's response to infection falls short and puts the patient at risk of system infections from open wounds.
- Cardiac stroke volume and respiratory capacities decrease.
- Body fat decreases minimizing the body's padding against traumatic injury.

- Brain mass decreases leaving voids in the skull that the brain can strike with acceleration and deceleration forces.

- Increased calcification of cartilage and developing osteoporosis make bones fragile and increase the risk of bone fractures significantly. This is especially true of the ribs, hips, thighs, and pelvis.

- Sensory deficits, such as hearing and vision, can make the patient interview and management a challenge.

- Mental capacities may make it difficult to establish a baseline. Does the patient have memory loss due to Alzheimer's, dementia, or a concussion?

- Many factors can mask signs of deterioration. The use of beta-blockers, for example, slows the heart rate and lowers the BP. When a patient is in compensated shock, you expect to see tachycardia, but not when a beta-blocker is used.

- Symptoms, such as pain or tenderness, may take longer to develop due to an increased pain tolerance and a loss of sensory function that develops with age.

- Ventilating a patient with a bag-valve mask (BVM) is a challenge to manage when the patient has no teeth.

▐Q▌ What are the special considerations for assessing the pregnant trauma patient?

▐A▌ When dealing with this trauma patient, you now have two or more patients. Pregnancy causes many changes to a woman's body that the EMS provider must be aware of for proper assessment and management.

- If the fetus is to survive, the mother must survive.

- A pregnant woman's blood volume increases by nearly 50 percent; however, oxygen-carrying blood cells do not increase.

- A blood loss of 30 percent can occur before any signs of shock develop (e.g., tachycardia, obvious vasoconstriction, or hypotension). Therefore, the MOI must be taken very seriously.

- Vitals signs change during pregnancy. The heart rate increases 10 to 15 bpm over the term of the pregnancy. The BP decreases in the first trimester and returns to normal by the second and third trimesters. The respiratory rate does not change; however, due to the large size of the fetus and decreased lung expansion in the third trimester, taking a deep breath is difficult, especially when lying down.

- Slowed peristalsis creates a full stomach, increasing the risk of nausea and vomiting and the possibility of aspiration.

- Abruptio placenta (placenta detaches from uterine wall) is life threatening to the mother due to blood loss and is often fatal to the fetus.

- Vena cava compression syndrome occurs when a woman lies on her back causing the weight of the fetus to clamp down on her vena cava, thereby decreasing the return of blood flow to the heart. This condition can be quickly remedied by turning the woman on her side, left lateral preferably. If she is immobilized on a long board, just tilt the board up 15 degrees to the left side.

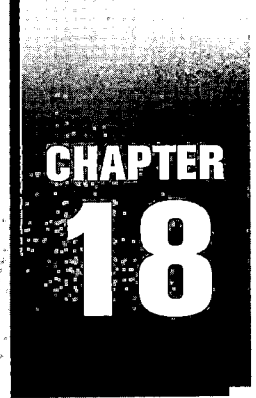

CHAPTER 18

Assessment-Based Management

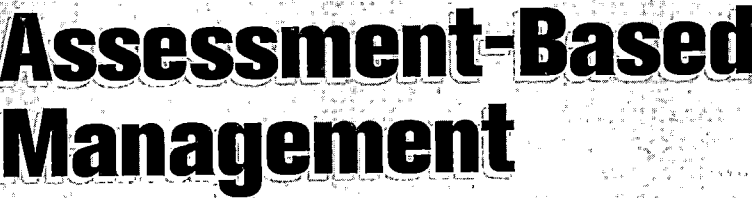

This chapter discusses assessment-based management. Although the term "assessment based" was new to the latest editions of the EMT-B, First Responder, and EMS provider curriculums, as you read through the questions and answers in this chapter you will see that the concepts are not new at all. The focus is on *what* an assessment-based approach to patient care is and *why* you should respond in a certain way to their presenting problems.

Importance of Assessment

Q How important is the assessment?

A An assessment is the foundation of care. It is difficult to report or manage a problem that you did not find! The EMS provider must gather, evaluate, and synthesize information in order to make appropriate decisions.

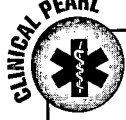

Decisions are only as good as the information they are based on.

Q What accurate information is critical to decision making?

A Decision making involves a combination of the following sources of information: the history, the physical exam (PE), recognition of patterns, a field impression, and existing BLS or ALS treatment protocols.

Q What is the importance of history?

A It is estimated that approximately 80 percent of a medical diagnosis is based on the history. One's knowledge of a disease and its assessment findings, as well as maintaining a degree of suspicion about a particular problem, affects the quality of a history taken from the patient. The history should be focused toward the organ systems that are associated with the complaint.

Q What is the value of a complete PE of the patient?

A The PE is an important step in the assessment of the patient. You cannot benefit from the information obtained from the PE if you overlook some part or just do a cursory PE. The PE must be focused on organ systems associated with the complaint.

Q What is the usefulness of pattern recognition?

A The EMS provider should continually expand their knowledge base of diseases and disorders. As this occurs, it becomes easier to compare patterns found during the field assessment to one's knowledge base. This comparison and recognition of patterns can help the EMS provider begin to accurately determine the patient's presenting problem.

Q What part do protocols have in the critical decision-making process?

A First, the EMS provider must arrive at the right field impression in order to follow the right protocol. This is especially true in regions where the protocols are still diagnosis based as opposed to assessment based. It is also important to understand that protocols are "guidelines for care" and dictate when and how an EMS provider may deviate from a protocol if the patient's condition warrants.

Q What are some of the factors that affect assessment and decision making?

A Factors that may impede decision making or making a proper field assessment include:

- EMS provider attitude (e.g., a bias against people who do not have a similar background to that of the EMS provider).
- Uncooperative patients (e.g., the argumentative patient or patient unwilling to share important medical history information).
- Obvious distracting injuries (e.g., a severely crushed extremity or a degloving injury).
- Tunnel vision (e.g., going right to the crashed car without first assessing the overall vehicular damage).
- Labeling patients (e.g., drunks or system abusers, not listening to their medical complaints).
- The environment (e.g., in very noisy, rainy, snowy, hot, or cold conditions).
- Patient compliance (e.g., a patient who argues and doesn't want the oxygen, immobilization, or other needed treatment).
- Manpower considerations (e.g., there is a limited number in the crew and a critical or very heavy patient).

Q How can EMS providers obstruct the assessment process?

A It is important that the EMS provider be nonjudgmental and objective. Having a biased or prejudicial "attitude" or attempting to classify patients by a social status can cause the EMS provider to miss vital pieces of information, often short circuiting the information-gathering process.

Q How can the perception of a patient being uncooperative obstruct the field assessment process?

A Sometimes uncooperative and belligerent patients are perceived as intoxicated. This can alter the course of the EMS provider's assessment plan. Remember, restless or uncooperative behavior can also be caused by hypoxia, hypovolemia, hypoglycemia, or a head injury.

Q How can an obvious distracting injury obstruct the field assessment process?

A Often when a patient presents with an obvious distracting injury, such as a severely angulated compound fracture of the leg, the EMS provider may ignore the initial assessment priorities (MS-ABC) and focus on the injury. Although difficult to do, it is important to focus on the priorities first.

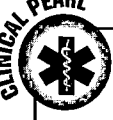

CLINICAL PEARL

Don't let impressive, but not dangerous (i.e., no immediate threat to the ABCs) injuries distract you from more serious life threats.

Q What is the problem with labeling patients?

A Labeling patients is unfair to the patient because they may not be afforded the full attention that all patients deserve. Labels, such as "just another drunk" or this guy is a "frequent flyer," can be very destructive to the assessment process. Remember, even the intoxicated patient or people who you feel abuse your services get sick and injured once in a while.

Q How can tunnel vision impede the assessment process?

A Making a decision too early or before all of the facts are gathered can lead to poor decision making by the EMS provider. Beware of "gut instincts" that may cause you to rush and make a judgment too early in the assessment process. For example, seeing a patient who is a local drug abuser and immediately blaming his disorientation on drugs rather than considering that it could be some other medical problem today.

Q How can the environment obstruct the assessment process?

A Chaos at the scene or violent or dangerous situations can make it difficult to conduct a proper assessment. In this case, deal with the scene safety issues first and remove the patient to your "office," the ambulance, for further assessment. Crowds of bystanders or EMS providers can sometimes be very noisy and interfere with the assessment process. If there are too many rescuers present, move the patient to a quiet place. Extra rescuers holding side conversations can be very distracting and send the wrong message to the patient. Tell them to move the socializing out of view of the patient!

How can the number and level of training of the EMS providers affect the way an assessment is obtained?

With one EMS provider there is sequential information gathering and treatment. With two, there can be simultaneous information gathering and treatment, which is more efficient. In situations with multiple responders, it is suggested that one person be responsible for the assessment and establishing a rapport with the patient and delegate the management skills to others. Do not try to assess by committee because it is too confusing to the patient to be asked questions by different responders and no one ever gets the entire story.

How can scene choreography be improved?

Preplanning, practice, and communication are always a good starting point. Some agencies assign critical roles or positions based on the equipment an EMS provider carries into the call. For example, the person who carries the drug box and defibrillator may be the team leader, and the person carrying the oxygen and intubation kit may go right to the patient's head for airway control.

What is the team leader–patient care provider concept?

This is a plan of the responsibility division based on two positions the EMS providers may take on a scene. It is useful in situations where both EMS providers have similar training. One EMS provider fills the role of the team leader and the other fills the role of the patient care provider.

What are some of the responsibilities of the team leader?

The team leader is usually the EMS provider who will accompany the patient through definitive care. The team leader takes on many of the following responsibilities:

- Has a concerned dialogue with the patient.
- Obtains the history.
- Does the PE.

- Gives the radio report and ED patient presentation.
- Completes the documentation.
- Maintains overall patient perspective and designates tasks.
- Coordinates transport.
- Acts as the initial EMS command at a mass casualty incident (MCI).
- Interprets ECG, talks on the radio, gives drug orders, controls the drug box, and keeps notes on all interventions during an ACLS code.

What is the role of the patient care provider?

The patient care provider is responsible for providing scene "cover" to make sure no one gets hurt. In addition, the patient care provider handles the following responsibilities:

- Gathers scene information, talks to the family and bystanders.
- Obtains the vital signs.
- Performs skills as requested by the team leader (e.g., attaches ECG monitor leads, administers oxygen, performs venous access, administers medication, obtains transport equipment).
- Acts as the triage group leader at an MCI.
- Administers drugs, monitors tube placement, and monitors BCLS during an ACLS code.

What is the essential equipment that should be brought to the side of every patient?

The essential equipment is that needed to conduct the initial assessment of the patient's priorities. Specifically, the first-in kit(s) should contain the following items:

- To expose the patient—scissors and a space blanket.
- Airway control—oropharyngeal airways (OPAs), nasopharyngeal airways (NPAs), suction, rigid Yankauer nozzles and flexible suction catheters, laryngoscope and blades, ET tubes, esophageal detector device, stylette, MaGill forceps, 10 cc syringe, tape, and tube restraint device.
- Breathing control—pocket mask, bag-valve mask (BVM) and spare masks, oxygen tank, flowmeter, non-rebreather, cannula, oxygen tubing, occlusive dressings, and large bore IV catheters for thoracic decompression.
- Circulation control—dressings, bandages, and tape; BP cuff; and stethoscope.
- Disability or dysrhythmia—rigid collars, flashlight or penlight, ECG monitor, and automated external defibrillator (AED).
- Pad and pen for notes.

Q **What are helpful aspects of the general approach to a patient?**

A Your general approach to a patient should be made with a calm orderly demeanor. You should have a preplan to avoid the appearance of confusion, and be carrying all of the essential equipment. Obtain a good initial scene size-up and proceed with the initial assessment.

Q **What is meant by a calm and orderly demeanor?**

A The EMS provider should look and act the part as a health care professional. Bedside manner is very important if you want the patient to trust you with their medical history. Patients may not be able to rate medical performance, but they can rate your people skills and customer service.

Q **How important is an EMS provider's ability to effectively communicate patient information?**

A The EMS provider's ability to effectively communicate patient information is an essential part of the job. This is done routinely with every patient encounter: face-to-face, over the telephone or radio, and on the prehospital care report (PCR).

Q **Why are effective oral presentation skills important?**

A These skills are important because they help establish trust and credibility. A good assessment and effective oral presentation go hand in hand. Basically, you cannot report anything that was not found and you cannot treat things that were not found. A good oral presentation suggests effective patient assessment and care; a poor presentation suggests poor assessment and care.

Practice your radio presentation. Other health care providers are usually not interested in listening to a rambling or disjointed presentation that omits vital information.

Ongoing Assessment and Clinical Decision Making

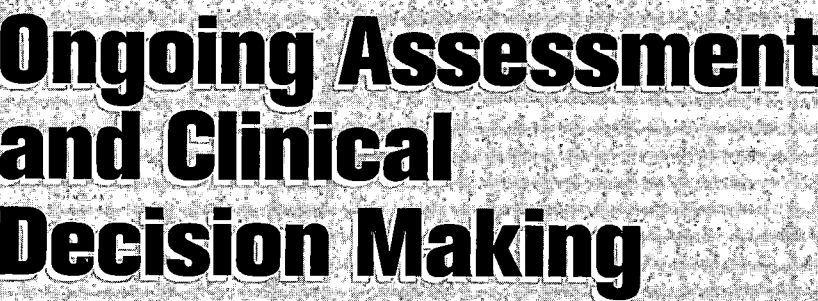

This chapter discusses ongoing assessment and the elements of clinical decision making. The focus is on *why* patients present in a certain manner and *why* you should respond in a certain way to their presenting problems.

Ongoing Assessment

What are the key aspects of ongoing assessment?

The key aspects of ongoing assessment are:

- Trending—mental status, vital signs, level of distress.
- Modifying—treatment interventions after reassessment.
- Time constraints—limited amount of time if the facility the patient is being transported to is nearby.
- Manpower limitations—may be limited based on the configuration of the crew (e.g., two or three people, two EMT-Basic, or two medics).
- Anticipating—changes and possible deterioration patterns or responses to interventions such as side effects and adverse reactions.
- Altering—changes based on medical versus trauma complaints, predictable patterns of injury, or illness from specific mechanisms of injury (MOI) or disease processes.

How often is an ongoing assessment repeated on a patient?

The ongoing assessment of the critical patient, either trauma or medical, is repeated every five minutes. For the non-critical patient, it can be repeated every 15 minutes.

Why is trending an essential part of patient care?

Trending is an important tool in patient care. It is the process of obtaining a baseline assessment, repeating the assessment multiple times, and using the information to determine if the patient is getting better or worse or has experienced no change. Treatment is then continued or modified using the information obtained from trending. This is especially important with the head-injured patient whose condition may be deteriorating very quickly. The earliest indicators are often subtle changes in the patient's mental status (MS).

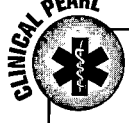

CLINICAL PEARL

Isolated measurements or observations are generally far less helpful than are changes *or* trends *measured over a period of time.*

What are the essential concepts of clinical decision making for the EMS provider?

The cornerstone of being an effective EMS provider is having the ability to think and work effectively under pressure. This consists of gathering, evaluating, and processing information while developing and implementing appropriate patient management.

The entire plan of care is based on patient assessment; therefore, adequate assessment skills are a must. Based on the ongoing assessment and evaluation, a new plan may be formulated and additional interventions may be required.

Verify assessment data that is significantly out of the normal range. For example, if you find an abnormal BP reading, 280/180, double check it or ask a partner to check it. If you do not remember a treatment parameter or protocol, look it up or ask for the information. Remember, many doctors carry pocket references. It is unprofessional and unethical to guess. Do not be embarrassed to get a second opinion.

The EMS provider should possess a sense of self-awareness to guide his actions. Follow your judgment. Critical thinking integrates objective and subjective data. Always ask, "Why?" Encourage the patient to actively participate in the process (e.g. provide information, ask questions, use teaching moments).

What are the major patient care differences in the out-of-hospital setting versus the traditional hospital or clinic setting?

The most obvious difference is that the traditional clinical setting is a relatively controlled environment. Care in the field is heavily influenced by environmental factors such as weather, hazards, time constraints, limited personnel and resources, extrication, and access. Other differences, such as getting a general impression of the patient in their home or seeing the MOI, are significant components that affect patient care. In the hospital setting, consultation with experts is often easier.

CLINICAL PEARL

Though there are similarities between out-of-hospital care and in-hospital care, the out-of-hospital setting requires ongoing adaptability and "thinking on the fly."

How diverse is the range of patient care in the field?

The EMS provider is expected to respond to and appropriately manage any possible emergency or crisis that arises. The range spans nonlife-threatening to potentially life-threatening to critical life-threatening situations.

What are examples of nonlife-threatening, potentially life-threatening, and critical life-threatening situations?

Examples for each situation include:

- Nonlife-threatening—an isolated extremity injury without neurovascular compromise, or a call for assistance in lifting or moving a patient.
- Potentially life-threatening—multisystem injuries or concurrent disease presentations.
- Critical life-threatening—acute myocardial infarction (AMI), end-stage chronic disease process, major multisystem trauma, or major single-system trauma.

What are the fundamental elements of critical thinking for the EMS provider?

The fundamental elements of critical thinking for the EMS provider include:

- Achieving and maintaining an adequate body of knowledge (training). As with any health care provider, this is an ongoing process because the medical field is dynamic and continually improving.
- Focusing on specific, as well as multiple, elements of data.
- Gathering and organizing data and forming concepts.
- Identifying and managing medical ambiguity.
- Differentiating between relevant and nonrelevant data.
- Analyzing and comparing similar situations.
- Recalling contrary situations.
- Articulating and documenting decision-making reasoning and constructing valid arguments.

What are the components and sequences of critical thinking for the EMS provider?

The framework and flow of the critical-thinking process should follow a logical plan that resembles the following format:

1. Collecting information and formulating concepts using:
   - Scene size-up, general impression, MOI.
   - Initial assessment, chief complaint.
   - Focused history and physical exam (PE).
2. Interpretation and processing information varies with:
   - Knowledge base and experience.
   - Information gathered.
3. Application of treatment and management using:
   - Field impression.
   - Differential assessment.
   - Protocols, standing orders, and medical control.

4. Reevaluation:
  - Continue or modify treatment.
5. Reflection:
  - What was learned from the call.

How does the "fight-or-flight" response affect the EMS provider's critical decision making?

The hormonal fight-or-flight response to stress can affect the EMS provider's decision-making ability both positively and negatively. The natural hormonal responses include:

- Improved reflexes and muscular strength.
- Enhanced visual and auditory acuity.
- Diminished concentration and assessment abilities.
- Impaired critical-thinking skills.

What are some of the stimulants of the fight-or-flight response for EMS providers?

There are many stimulants and variants for the individual. The most common stimulants are alarms, pagers, dispatch information, lights and sirens, traffic, and other hazards. A seasoned EMS provider can become desensitized to some of these stimuli to a certain degree, but may then develop other stimulants of the fight-or-flight response, such as appreciating the risks for exposure and the potential for unknown hazards.

PEARL

Though the thrill of lights and sirens often attracts individuals into EMS, the "epinephrine high" can also lead to reckless driving and a dangerous feeling of immortality.

What are some things the EMS provider can do to keep the fight-or-flight response in check?

Experience is the best teacher. For most, the more an individual is exposed to an experience, the better able they are to manage similar experiences. However, we all have bad days and can backslide no matter how experienced we become. The following is a list of mental preparation tricks to fall back on when critical thinking becomes clouded:

- Stay calm—scan the situation, stop and think before acting. This will help to avoid panicking.
- Anticipate—plan for the worst. This will help you maintain a systematic, controlled plan of action.

- Reassess—frequently reevaluate, facilitate a dynamic course of management using a systematic approach.
- Pause—take a deep breath when experiencing a sensory overload and fall back on the priority MS-ABC plan.

What are the benefits of protocols, standing orders, and patient-care flow charts?

The benefits of using protocols, standing orders, and patient-care flow charts include promoting a standard approach to patient care, defining performance parameters, and speeding the application of critical-care interventions. They also provide some structure for the EMS provider.

What are the disadvantages of protocols, standing orders, and patient-care flow charts?

Disadvantages of protocols, standing orders, and patient-care flow charts include only fitting the "textbook" patient injury or illness, and failing to cover multisystem failures, nonspecific complaints, and concurrent disease processes.

What are the "six *R*s" of putting it all together?

The DOT National Standard Curriculum for the Paramedic describes the six *R*s as the following:

- Read the patient—
a. Observe for loss of consciousness (LOC), skin color, position, location, and obvious injury.
b. Interview for chief complaint (e.g., acute or chronic).
c. Assess the ABCs, color, temperature, and condition of the skin (CTC), pulse, and lung sounds; rule out life threats; obtain baseline vital signs; and triage.
- Read the scene—MOI, environmental conditions, and immediate surroundings.
- React—treat as you go, correcting life threats first.
- Reevaluate—reassess initial focused history and detailed PE, responses to treatment interventions, and secondary problems.
- Revise—dynamic intervention based on focused history and ongoing assessment.
- Review—discuss and analyze after the call.

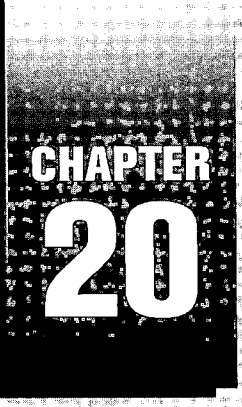

CHAPTER 20

Communication

This chapter discusses one of the most basic, yet essential, skills of the EMS provider: the ability to communicate. Inadequate communication places people at a disadvantage when obtaining important information. Although communication can be verbal and nonverbal, the focus of this chapter is on the verbal modes of communication.

Exchange of Information

Q How is communication important when providing emergency medical services?

A Communication is an essential component of emergency medical services. The EMS provider is an extension of the in-hospital team and must effectively communicate patient assessment and management to the ED physician. This way, the receiving hospital can prepare for the patient's arrival and assist the EMS providers with treatment orders.

In some EMS systems, ambulances routinely notify the hospital of the patient's condition on all calls. In other EMS systems, field-to-hospital communication is limited to contacting medical control for consultation, orders, and to notify the receiving hospital.

Q What are the steps involved in the communication of information between two individuals?

A The basic model of communication has six steps:

- The sender has a message (e.g., you perceive additional help is needed on the scene).

- The sender encodes the message (e.g., you think of the right way to ask for additional help over the radio so the dispatcher will understand what you want).

- The sender sends the message (e.g., you make a radio transmission).

- The receiver receives the message (e.g., dispatcher hears the transmission).

- The receiver decodes the message (e.g., dispatcher interprets exactly what to send to the scene).

- The receiver gives feedback to the sender (e.g., dispatcher acknowledges that medic 620 will be dispatched).

Q What are the phases of communication necessary to complete a typical EMS call?

A The phases of communication on a typical EMS call are shown in Table 20–1.

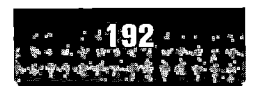

TABLE 20-1
Phases of Communication

Name	Example
Occurrence	An elderly man feels sick. He pulls his vehicle over to rest and passes out.
Detection	A citizen driving by notices the patient and calls 911.
Notification	On receipt of the information, the dispatcher sends EMS.
Response	The ambulance and police respond to the incident.
Treatment	The EMS providers may confer with medical control over the patient's field treatment.
Preparation for transport	Notify the dispatcher where the ambulance is transporting to and notify the hospital of what they are bringing in.
Preparation for the next call	Notify the dispatcher that the ambulance is back in service, clearing the hospital.

What is the role of verbal communication in EMS?

It is virtually impossible to receive, respond, assess, manage, transport, and turnover a patient to the ED without verbal communication. The best EMS providers are usually excellent at verbal communication because this is such an important interpersonal skill. Verbal communication can be face-to-face or over a radio or telephone. On a typical EMS run, verbal communication is necessary for the following segments of the call:

- Receiving the call information from the emergency medical dispatcher (EMD).
- Communication with the EMD to let her know you have arrived on the scene and to request additional resources.
- Interacting with other emergency services personnel on arrival at the scene.
- Interacting with other crew members and bystanders or family members on arrival at the scene.
- Interacting with the patient to introduce yourself and your crew, obtain permission to treat, obtain a history, do an assessment, and explain all of the needed treatment.
- Interacting with family and bystanders to obtain assistance as necessary (e.g., moving furniture, obtaining the patient's medications and medical insurance cards).
- Communicating with the EMD to inform her of the destination for transportation.
- Communication with medical control or the receiving hospital for medical orders and notification of a patient report.
- Communication with the EMD to inform her of your arrival at the destination hospital's ED.
- Communication with the triage nurse on arrival at the hospital to determine which room the patient is to be taken to.

- Communication with the ED staff who will be taking over the management of the patient.
- Communication with the pharmacy or stock room personnel to obtain replacement supplies.
- Communication with the EMD to inform her of your availability for another assignment.

CLINICAL PEARL

Remember that "body language" comprises nearly 97 percent of nonverbal communication. Be sure to make eye contact, smile appropriately, and treat the patient with respect.

What is the role of written communication in EMS?

Documentation is an essential skill that the EMS provider must acquire. It is not sufficient to merely tell the ED what the assessment findings are and how you have managed the patient. The EMS provider must leave a complete and accurate prehospital care report (PCR) with the ED staff. Additional information on what should be included in the PCR is found in Chapter 21, Documentation.

What is the role of electronic communication in EMS?

Electronic communication is expanding at a rapid pace in EMS. One example is the "code summary" on a monitor–defibrillator unit that prints out all ECG changes and the time of occurrence, pulse oximeter reading, end-tidal CO_2 readings, and BP readings on one record. Another example is the use of handheld computers (e.g., Palm Pilots®) for protocols and drug calculation charts. Electronic devices offer events or information in real time. Electronic technology can be integrated with diagnostic technology. Today, it is not uncommon to obtain a printout from the end-tidal CO_2 monitor or pulse oximeter, the Glucometer®, and an interpretation of the 12-lead ECG taken from the patient.

Electronic communication helps to reduce dependence on traditional means of documentation such as written reports. A "pen based" PCR can prompt the EMS provider with relevant suggestions for documenting various patient assessment and management conditions. A good example of advanced technology being used to improve patient management is the cellularly transmitted 12-lead ECG. Patients who have a 12-lead taken and transmitted to the ED, in addition to a thrombolytic checklist done in the field, often receive "clot-busters" faster on arrival in the ED. Some actually bypass the ED and go straight to the coronary catheterization laboratory.

Why is it so important to use the proper terminology in EMS communication?

EMS communication must be very exact to prevent confusion or the possibility of multiple interpretations. Do not make up your own phrases. Use the common language of your EMS system. Many of the services that previously used the 10-codes have changed to plain English. Other services have eliminated "special codes or radio identifiers" used only during mass casualty incident (MCI) operations and replaced them with plain English. Using these special codes, like EMS 900 instead of EMS Command, adds an unnecessary level of complexity during a MCI.

> *Fancy jargon sounds "cool" on television, but is potentially harmful to both providers and patients in real life. Use plain English as much as possible to communicate.*

Why is it important to use proper verbal communication during an EMS call?

Proper verbal communication helps to prevent confusion. Pronounce each word and letter clearly. Mumbling into the microphone makes the radio transmission difficult to hear and understand.

What are some examples of factors that impede verbal communication?

There are two factors that tend to impede verbal communication—semantics and technical terminology. Semantics is actually the study of the meanings in language, whereas technical terminology relates more to the specific "buzzwords" of our profession. We should select our words and phrases with the audience in mind. When talking to our peers or other health care professionals, more technical terms can be used.

When talking to a patient or child, minimize the technical terms. Some examples to consider when selecting your words are:

- Say, "I would like to touch your wrist to feel your pulse" instead of "I would like to take your pulse." A child might wonder where you are going to take it and if are you going to give it back.
- Ask the patient if he has had problems with his heart or lungs rather than, "Is this your first heart attack?"
- When inserting an IV say, "It will just hurt for a second" rather than, "It's just a little prick."
- Don't refer to a patient's pulse rates as irregular in front of them.

- Don't use terms like "bottomed out" or "crashing" in front of the patient.
- Don't refer to pacing as "shocking the patient" in front of them.
- Don't say, "Did your water break?" Say, "Has there been a fluid discharge from your vagina?"

What are some examples of factors that enhance verbal communication?

Speaking clearly can enhance verbal communication. Open your mouth, don't mumble words, and use terms that are easy to understand. When speaking into a radio microphone, depress the microphone key for a moment before you begin speaking so you do not cut off your first word or two.

> *Regardless of assigned channels, the airways are public. Assume that radio transmissions are open for all to hear. Never say anything over the radio, including divulging patient names, that you would be uncomfortable saying on public television. Follow your local protocols.*

What are the components of an EMS communication system?

The components of a local communication system include the public safety access point, the emergency medical dispatcher, pre-arrival instructions, and the system dispatcher.

What are the functions of each component of a local communication system?

The functions of the components of the local communication system are as follows:

- Public safety access point (PSAP)—is the means of alerting police, fire, and EMS agencies in each community. It has been estimated that 78 percent of the communities in the United States have switched from a seven digit phone number to the three digit standardized access number 911. Dialing the operator or "O" is not advisable in most communities because it is possible that you can be switched to an operator thousands of miles away who is not familiar with your local community. This can add unnecessary delays to the dispatch and arrival of the proper emergency services. Other means of accessing the public safety access point may include highway call boxes, citizen band radio, and amateur radio.
- The emergency medical dispatcher—is a professional who has been trained in each of the following aspects of dispatch: telephone interrogation, triage, radio dispatch, logistics

coordination, resource networking, and phone pre-arrival instruction.

- Pre-arrival instructions—are instructions given by a trained EMD to the caller telling the caller specific skills to perform (e.g., how to position the airway so vomit can drain, how to perform rescue breathing, how to control bleeding).
- The system dispatcher—depending on the size of the system and the frequency of calls, it may range from one person who answers the phones and dispatches emergency service agencies to a room full of call receiving operators and another group of dispatchers, one or more for each of the emergency services (police, fire, and EMS).

What are the "four cardinal rules of priority dispatching?"

The EMD is trained to determine the answer to the following four key questions before proceeding with specific questions focused on the potential patient complaint:

- What is the patient's chief complaint or the type of incident?
- Is the patient conscious?
- Is the patient breathing?
- What is the patient's approximate age?

What are the dispatch and field time intervals in an EMS call?

Dispatch and field time milestones include the following:

- Response time—the interval from the time the call is received by medical dispatch to the time the unit (ambulance) arrives on the scene. In some instances, true arrival is when the EMS personnel arrive at the side of the patient, which is different than arrival in front of the building.
- Scene time—the time that the EMS crew spends assessing and managing the patient on the scene prior to transport.
- Transport time—the time from when the ambulance leaves the scene to arrival at the hospital.
- Hospital time—the period of time from the ambulance's arrival at the hospital until the crew calls in service. This usually includes transferring patient care to the ED personnel, completing the PCR, and cleaning and restocking the vehicle.

What is the "queue" time?

This is the time between the receipt of the call and the time the call is given to the unit to respond. During this time, the dispatcher determines the type of call, the most appropriate units to dispatch, and their response mode.

How is the scene time lengthened artificially?

Scene time begins when the unit arrives in front of the building. If it takes a few minutes to actually get to the patient's side, this extra time appears to be scene time. Also, the time to transport patients from where they were found to the ambulance is included in the scene time. On calls where the patient is on the street, the scene time is usually accurate. On calls where it takes a while to find the patient, the scene time can be extended. This extra scene time should be explained on the PCR.

> **CLINICAL PEARL**
>
> *On-scene times are used in research studies to determine the risk–benefit ratio of out-of-hospital interventions (e.g., 12-lead ECG). Artificially lengthened scene times lead to inaccurate scientific conclusions. Always document factors that prolong scene time (e.g., extrication, 10 flights of stairs). Unless these factors are accounted for, studies carry an incorrect bias that on-scene interventions lengthen scene time.*

What is the difference between 911 and enhanced 911?

The 911 system has been available since the late 1960s. An enhancement to this system, called E911, was added later to include computer displays of the caller's telephone number and location as well as instant callback capabilities in case the caller hangs up too fast. In areas where 911 service is in place, there is a direct link between locations with multiple phone lines, such as a hotel, and the emergency center. A number of states are reviewing this policy because switching to enhanced 911 gives the dispatcher direct access to the actual room where the call was made instead of the address of the hotel property.

> **CLINICAL PEARL**
>
> *Proper planning and public education can avoid delays when responding to large hotels or motels. Some facilities encourage patrons to call the front desk or an internal "emergency" number. In some cases, a hotel employee responds first. If the employee is untrained in emergency care, this response only lengthens the time prior to calling 911. A few larger complexes have security staff trained in CPR and basic first aid skills, and are equipped to operate an automated external defibrillator (AED). In this case, simultaneous notification of EMS and in-house rescuers is appropriate.*

What is meant by a first-party caller?

A first-party caller is the patient calling for herself.

Q What is meant by a second-party caller?

A A second-party caller is someone who is in direct contact with the patient but is not actually the patient.

Q What is meant by a third-party caller?

A A third-party caller is someone who is calling for the patient that is not in direct contact with the patient.

Q EMS providers use radio communication on every call. What is the role of the Federal Communications Commission (FCC)?

A The FCC is responsible for regulating all aspects of the communication industry. Its primary goals include promoting competition in communication, protecting consumers, and supporting access by every American to existing and advanced telecommunication services.

The plan for the evolution of the FCC involves a transition from an industry regulator to a market facilitator. In the past, the FCC served as the regulator of large communication monopolies. It is expected that in the early part of the twenty-first century, the U.S. communications markets will be characterized by vigorous competition. In this changing market, the FCC will have to address issues that will not be solved by the market. The "new FCC" will have to do the following:

- Create a model agency for the digital age.
- Promote competition in all communication markets.
- Promote opportunities for all Americans to benefit from the communication revolution.
- Manage the electromagnetic spectrum (the nation's airwaves) in the public interest.

Q How does the EMD function as an integral part of the EMS team?

A The EMD is an integral part of the EMS team by being the true "first" responder to the patient through interrogation and providing pre-arrival instructions that may, in some cases, be lifesaving.

Q What is the Clawson's Medical Priority Dispatch® system?

A Jeff Clawson is the physician from Salt Lake City, Utah, who is credited with changing the way dispatchers were trained, and developing the Medical Priority Dispatch® system. Clawson's visionary system has been recognized as an appropriate intervention by the American College of Emergency Physicians, the National Association of EMS Physicians, and the National Institutes of Health. The emergency medical dispatchers trained using Clawson's system provide pre-arrival instructions that effectively create a "zero-minute" professional response time. The pre-arrival instruction cards (Figure 20–1) are designed for life-threatening conditions like arrest, choking, and childbirth. This new level of care was defined in 1989 as dispatch life support. Most modern dispatch centers use this system.

Q What is a CAD system?

A A computer aided dispatch (CAD) system uses a computer to assist the EMD in determining which units to send to which calls. More specialized versions of these systems use devices placed in each emergency vehicle that constantly send messages to the dispatcher's computer screen giving the EMD the exact location of the vehicle. This helps the computer determine which unit is actually the closest to the incident location. It may also be programmed to incorporate a system status management designed to deploy units from dynamic locations rather than static locations.

Hospital Radio Reports

Q What is the purpose of the verbal communication of patient information to the hospital?

A A verbal report over the radio or telephone helps prepare the ED for the arrival of the patient. In some instances, they may need to clear a bed, locate a specialty surgeon, prepare the transplant team, or complete other time-consuming activities.

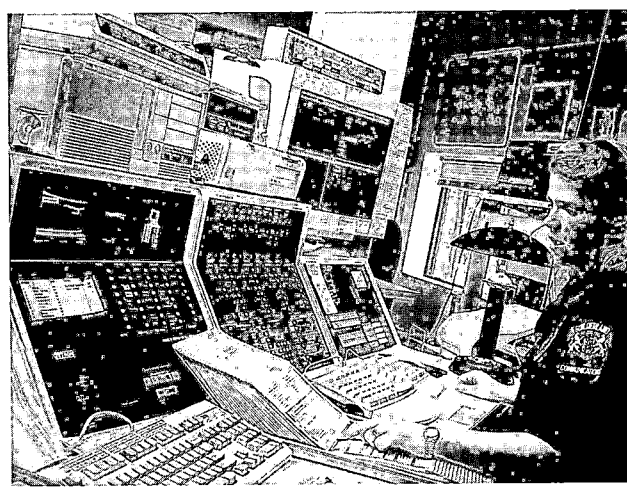

FIGURE 20–1 The EMD is using medical dispatch cards to offer pre-arrival instructions.

What information should be included in a report over the radio or phone?

The typical radio report is given in the following format. There may be some local variances based on your hospital's needs and your medical director's wishes.

- Unit identification (ambulance #____).
- Level of provider.
- Estimated time of arrival (ETA).
- Patient's age and gender.
- Chief complaint.
- Brief, pertinent history of present illness or injury.
- Major past illnesses.
- Mental status (MS).
- Baseline vital signs.
- Pertinent findings of the PE.
- Emergency medical care given.
- Response to emergency medical care.
- Does medical direction have any questions or orders?

What information should be included in a report to medical control?

The same information as listed previously plus ALS modalities and drugs administered and requests for additional orders from medical control. In some areas of the country, a 12-lead ECG is also transmitted.

Why are codes discouraged when communicating over the radio?

Codes are being replaced with plain English because often the receiver is unfamiliar with the codes used and they actually create confusion.

What is a 10-code?

The 10-code is a system used primarily by police agencies to reduce the length of radio transmissions and convey a precise meaning. The number 10 before the code number is designed to alert the listener mentally that a code is about to be spoken. There are many local versions of these codes that make them confusing if you are not familiar with their use. The Association of Public Safety Communications Officials (APCO) has an official list of 10-codes that is used by many police departments and other emergency service agencies. The list of these 10-codes is shown in Table 20–2.

TABLE 20–2

APCO 10-Codes

- 10-1 signal weak
- 10-2 signal good
- 10-3 stop transmitting
- 10-4 affirmative (OK)
- 10-5 relay (to)
- 10-6 busy
- 10-7 out of service
- 10-8 in service
- 10-9 repeat (say again)
- 10-10 negative
- 10-11 ____ on duty
- 10-12 stand by (stop)
- 10-13 existing conditions
- 10-14 message/information
- 10-15 message delivered
- 10-16 reply to message
- 10-17 enroute
- 10-18 urgent
- 10-19 (in) contact
- 10-20 location
- 10-21 call (____) by phone
- 10-22 disregard
- 10-23 arrived on scene
- 10-24 assignment completed
- 10-25 report to (meet)
- 10-26 estimated time of arrival
- 10-27 license/permit information
- 10-28 ownership information (vehicle)
- 10-29 records check
- 10-30 danger/caution
- 10-31 pick up
- 10-32 ____ units needed (specify)
- 10-33 help me quickly
- 10-34 time

CLINICAL PEARL

With the widespread availability of citizen's band radio, 10-codes became very popular. Unfortunately, different groups and areas often use different codes. Unless mandated by local protocol, avoid these; use plain English instead.

What are some of the principles of proper radio system usage?

When using a radio to communicate, keep these principles in mind:

- Make sure the radio is turned on, is on the correct frequency, and the volume is properly adjusted.
- Reduce background noise by closing the window if transmitting from the front cab of the vehicle.

- Listen first to ensure the frequency is clear prior to beginning your transmission.
- Depress the talk button, then wait a second prior to talking so you do not cut off your first few words.
- Speak slowly and clearly with your lips about two to three inches from the microphone.
- Keep transmissions brief; use plain English; and avoid codes, slang, and phrases that serve no purpose.
- When calling another unit or base station, use their unit number or name followed by yours (e.g., "Dispatcher, this is Medic 641.")
- When transmitting a number, say each digit for clarity (e.g., not 15, rather one five).
- Do not use the patient's name over the radio. Remember, there are numerous people in your community with scanners who may be listening in.
- Use "affirmative" and "negative" instead of "yes" or "no."
- Courtesy is assumed, so do not waste time saying "thank you," "please," or "you are welcome."
- Use the EMS frequencies only for authorized EMS communications and use only official codes and abbreviations.

Q **Why is it necessary to repeat back medical orders?**

A This is referred to as "echoing." It should always be done when confirming a medication order to ensure that you received and interpreted the message correctly.

Equipment Issues: Low Tech and High Tech

Q **What is the cause of radio interference?**

A Radio interference is caused by many things. Interference is any undesired radio signal on a frequency that comes from other radio transmitters or sources of electromagnetic radiation. Nuisance interference can be heard but does not override system signals. Destructive interference overrides system signals. Sometimes a buzzing or 60-cycle interference can occur when the radio is too close to a computer, fluorescent light fixture, or electronic motor.

Q **What are some basic definitions that apply to radio transmissions?**

A The following definitions apply:

- Amplitude modulation—a transmitting radio frequency carrier fixed in frequency, but increasing or decreasing in amplitude in accordance with the strength of the applied audio.
- Frequency—the number of repetitive cycles per second completed by a radio wave.
- Repeater—In some EMS systems, the radio power (watts) of the portable unit is not strong enough to reach the base station. Instead, it is transmitted to the ambulance, which has a higher-powered transmitter. The ambulance radio repeats the message so it can reach the base station or other mobile units. Repeaters are also used on radio towers to send the message along to the next tower and ultimately on to the end point.
- Frequency modulation—deviation of carrier frequency in accordance with the strength of the applied audio. Because this band is less susceptible to interference than amplitude modulation, it is more frequently used in EMS communication.
- Very high frequency—the radio frequencies between 30 and 300 MHz. This spectrum is further divided into high and low bands.
- Ultra high frequency—the radio frequencies between 300 and 3,000 MHz. The 460 MHz range is most commonly used for EMS communication.
- Telemetry—the ability to transmit biological patient information over the airwaves or cellular band. The best example of this is the transmission of a patient's ECG to the ED by the EMS provider in the field.
- Call simplex—when a radio transmits and receives on the same frequency. It is not possible to do both simultaneously. After your transmission, you must listen for the receiver's response. Frequently, users of a simplex device say something like "over" or "kay" at the end of their message to signal the listener that they are done talking and ready to listen.

Q **What is a duplex communication device?**

A When a radio transmits and receives at the same time, it is called a duplex. There are two frequencies involved, both of which have the capability to transmit and receive. The telephone is a good example of a duplex system, whereas a voice-activated telephone or speaker system is an example of a simplex system. Duplex systems also allow the transmission of ECG, but not speaking and transmitting ECG at the same time.

Q **What is a multiplex communication device?**

A A multiplex system is similar to a duplex system; however, it is also possible to transmit data, such as an ECG, at the same time you are having a two-way conversation. This is not really recommended because it downgrades the quality of the ECG transmission.

What is a trunked communication device?

Many of the communication systems that operate in the 800-MHz range use trunking. A trunked system uses a pool of frequencies and a computer to route the transmission to the next available clear frequency in the "trunk." The "trunk" is like a cable with hundreds of smaller strands of cable inside it. In this way, each transmission could literally be on a different frequency depending on the number of users and the volume of transmissions in the pool of frequencies.

What is an analog transmission?

Analog is a voice transmission. Most systems are switching over to digital communication because analog is time consuming and often difficult to understand. There is also a limited number of radio frequencies that can be used for analog technology. In the cellular phone communication network of many of the busier markets, analog cellular systems are fast approaching system capacity, so digital technology will become essential.

What is digital communication?

All common forms of communication (e.g., TV, telephone, CD player, camera, radio station, and cable company) are in the process of switching over to digital communication. In a digital system, the message is translated or encoded into a condensed digital code that is transmitted faster, taking up less airtime. When received, it is decoded or translated back to the voice or photo message that was originally sent. This technology makes it difficult for people with scanners to listen in on transmissions and helps to minimize transmission time. Some EMS systems have mobile data terminals that can receive a call from a dispatcher and print it out. They may have a button for the EMS provider to depress that signals they have received the call location, and that the unit is enroute or is at the scene of the call. Because these transmissions are digital, they do not require voice transmission time over the radio.

What is a cellular communication device?

Because everyone seems to own a cellular phone, it is difficult to believe this is a fairly new form of communication. In 1981, the FCC created a commercial cellular radio–telephone service using 50 MHz of the 800 MHz frequency band. A cellular system operates by dividing a large geographical service area into cells and assigning the same channels to multiple, nonadjacent cells. This allows channels to be reused, increasing spectrum efficiency. As you travel across a service area, your message is handed off from one cell to another without noticeable interruption. Because unique radio–telephone and control equipment service each cell, there is an allocation of a set of voice channels and a control channel for each. The FCC estimates that there are over 30 million portable cellular units and more than 20,000 cell sites operating in the United States.

The latest ECG monitors often have the ability to transmit a 12-lead ECG by use of a digital cellular device to the ED. This is a more accurate means of transmission than the previously used method.

Are telephones still used for EMS communication?

Absolutely! In some areas, it may be more practical, especially when in the patient's home standing right next to a telephone, to call directly to medical control or the poison control center for advice. Telephone conversations are less formal than radio transmissions. One disadvantage of telephone calls is that some EMS systems routinely tape record all radio transmissions for quality improvement and medicolegal issues. Phone conversations, unless connected through the dispatch center, are not recorded.

How are pagers used for EMS communication?

Many EMS systems use pagers to alert personnel that there is a call. When the dispatcher sets off the pager, it sounds a tone or actually transmits the dispatcher's voice announcement. Some systems use the digital pagers to receive the actual address of the assignment. Paging systems have come down in price as the general public ran out to buy cell phones. It is now possible, even for a small EMS agency, to purchase a paging system and encode their own messages to be sent to all or certain pagers in their system. This enables the system to send specific digital messages.

What is a facsimile (fax)?

A facsimile (fax) machine is a quick way to send printed information to another fax machine or computer. The message is digitalized line-by-line and transmitted over the telephone line to another fax machine or computer. On the other end, it is decoded and printed out. Some hospitals use a fax as a means of sending information about patients from one office to another. Another use is by a physician's office to provide additional history information to the ED on arrival of the patient. The disadvantage of the fax is that telephone lines limit available service. In addition, the message must be received by a device with fax capabilities.

What other forms of communication are being used in EMS?

The laptop computer and palm computer are used on a limited basis by many EMS agencies. They are useful for storing tremendous amounts of reference material, writing reports, storing protocols, storing contact information, storing calendars and task lists, and many more applications.

The computer has changed the way we live, work, play, shop, and communicate. Most EMS providers have a computer and use an Internet service provider (ISP) to gain access to the World Wide Web.

Most EMS providers also use e-mail communication, and many EMS educators use the computer to develop lectures and notes. These can be easily shared with other students or instructors across the country by attaching the file to an e-mail note or posting it to a site on the Internet. We are not far from the time when each EMS provider will arrive at the station and

- Sign on to the computer to get their messages and assignments for the shift (if they have not already read them at home on their own computer).
- Do continuing medical education at their own pace on the computer.
- Transmit their vacation requests on the computer.
- Transmit their vehicle check list and supply order list on the computer so the supervisor or quartermaster can deliver the supplies later in the day.

What are some uses of technology to collect and exchange patient and/or scene information electronically?

Since the first days when NASA transmitted live broadcasts of astronauts walking in space and transmitted all of their biological data to the control center physicians on Earth, many have wondered how this technology could be applied to routine medical care. In some areas where physicians are not immediately available, a caregiver has the ability to transmit live video and audio to a physician in an ED. This can be helpful in determining whether the patient should be transported to the ED or can be managed off-site. A number of prison clinics are incorporating systems of this type. In the digital age, the potential of communication is often a mere function of the ideas that we can come up with!

What is the legal status of medical information exchanged electronically?

This is not intended to be legal advice. Recent court decisions have upheld the right of law enforcement officials to access electronic transmissions, either stored or during actual transmission. To do so, however, requires either a search warrant or a court order, depending on the circumstances and type of information desired. Also, court decisions have held that computer disks and hard drives are not "closed containers" that require separate search warrants. If a computer is searched or seized, disks and drives become "fair game."

Documentation

This chapter discusses the importance of properly documenting your actions as an EMS provider. The focus is on *why* it is neccessary to document patient assessment and management as well as *what* to document. Some say the paperwork is almost as important as the care itself! The proper documentation of patient care is one more step toward keeping clear of legal entanglements.

Why Document?

Q What is the general principle regarding the importance of EMS documentation?

A In medicine, there is a saying, "If you didn't write it down, you didn't do it!" That is how important documentation is to patient care. Poor documentation is usually an indication of a poor assessment.

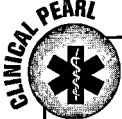

> *Whether or not your care was optimal, poor documentation is a difficult hurdle to overcome.*

Q How are documents used in out-of-hospital care?

A The documentation that is done for out-of-hospital care is important. It is the written and legal record of the incident. The paperwork also provides a professional link between the field assessment and management and in-hospital care.

Q What is meant by the minimum data set?

A The National Highway Traffic Safety Administration (NHTSA) has standardized a minimum data set to be included in all out-of-hospital care reports. This standardization helps make it easier to compare data from different agencies and systems. Most forms contain administrative data as well as patient data.

The run data includes the date, times, service name, unit, and the names and level of training of the crew members. The patient data includes patient name, address, date of birth, gender, and age. The patient data also includes the nature of the call, mechanism of injury (MOI), location of the patient, SAMPLE history, signs and symptoms, treatment administered prior to the arrival of the EMS provider, baseline vital signs, patient management, changes in the patient condition, and the disposition of the call.

Q What is a PCR?

A The prehospital care report (PCR) is the out-of-hospital care report used by EMS providers in the field. Some services refer to this document as a trip ticket, run sheet, or ambulance call report.

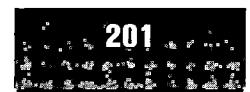

Q **What administrative information is pertinent to record on the PCR?**

A The PCR should contain patient demographic information (e.g., address, date of birth, phone number) and the pertinent times (e.g., dispatch, enroute, onscene, enroute to facility, arrival at facility, and in-service times).

Q **What are some of the other uses of the PCR?**

A PCRs are used for medical audits, run reviews, quality improvement, conferences, or other educational forums. The patient's name must be removed or completely covered if the forms will be used for discussion with providers other than those who were present on the specific call.

Q **How are PCRs used in quality improvement?**

A The PCR may be used to tally an EMS provider's number of patient care procedures (e.g., traction splint applications, oral airway insertions, and successful IV sticks) and to review individual performance (e.g., calls with patients who presented with chest pain and received high-flow oxygen and nitroglycerin if not hypotensive).

CLINICAL PEARL

Copies of PCRs may be used to document ongoing skill maintenance. For example, many EMS services mandate that a provider perform a certain number of IV starts or ET tube placements per year to maintain a skill level.

Q **What is the importance of documentation for agency reimbursement?**

A In many EMS agencies, the costs of the system are paid for by a combination of a tax subsidy and direct billing. Many patients have some form of insurance (third-party payer) that requires very specific information about the patient and the call before paying the bill (e.g., age, birth date, address, social security number, presumptive field diagnosis, procedures and medications administered). A failure to obtain necessary billing information could ultimately jeopardize the ability of the EMS agency to continue to provide services to the community. Many EMS agencies have a separate billing form for insurance because most insurers require a patient or physician signature.

What to Document

Q **What is meant by the documentation "standing on its own"?**

A A PCR should, by itself, provide a complete and accurate portrait of the patient's needs and the care given.

CLINICAL PEARL

By "stand on its own," we mean that a record contains everything it should in a clear, legible, and concise fashion. That way, you or anyone else should be able to refer to it in the future and be perfectly clear about what happened.

Q **What is meant by being objective, specific, and concrete on a PCR?**

A When documenting, always try to use objective language and not make judgments. Instead of writing that "the patient's home was dirty and disorganized," write that "there were cobwebs and piles of papers all over the bedroom." Rather than writing that "the patient vomited a lot of times last night," be specific and write that "the patient stated he vomited three to four times last night."

Be concrete by documenting exactly what you see, hear, feel, or smell. Avoid adding your interpretation of the reasons why the patient exhibited specific behavior. For example, do not write that "the patient was crying from his depression;" instead, write that "the patient was crying during the initial assessment."

Q **Why is it necessary to document multiple sets of vital signs on the PCR?**

A It is difficult to make decisions based solely on one set of vital signs. Multiple sets are taken and documented to show trends in the patient's condition. Take vital signs every five minutes for critical or unstable patients and every 15 minutes for stable patients. Also, take vital signs after interventions, such as medication administrations, to determine the effect (positive, negative, or no change).

Q **Why is it necessary to document the presence of distal pulses, motor, and sensation (PMS) before and after the immobilization of a suspected fracture or dislocation of a long bone or after spinal immobilization?**

A The presence or absence of PMS function is very important in instances where an extremity or the spine has to be immobilized. This is especially true if the extremity must be manipulated prior to splinting. Be sure to document on the PCR that you checked these functions before and after splinting because this is essential information to pass on to other health care providers.

> *Failure to document the adequacy of the neurovascular supply both before and after immobilization is unfortunately common. Excellent documentation of pre- and post-splinting (or immobilization) findings may be vital when defending your care.*

How should the EMS provider document a patient's words?

If the patient makes statements to questions that do not appear in a check box on the PCR (e.g., a dying statement, admission of guilt in a criminal activity, or a threat of suicide), the EMS provider should document the statement using quotes on the PCR. For example, "I drank two six-packs," "I was trying to kill myself," or "I only shook the infant a little bit before he stopped crying."

What are examples of standard abbreviations used in EMS documentation?

A list of standard abbreviations can be found in Table 21–1. For a more comprehensive listing of abbreviations, see p. vii.

What are examples of standard terms and planes referred to on EMS documentation?

A list of standard terms and planes appears in Table 21–2.

What are examples of word parts, such as prefixes and suffixes, that are used to make up the standardized medical terminology used in medical documentation?

A list of standard word parts used to make up medical terms appears in Table 21–3. The prefix comes at the beginning of the word and the suffix comes at the end.

What is the importance of preparing complete and accurate documentation?

Often, decisions about the patient's care are made based on PCR documentation. The PCR must be an accurate reflection of

TABLE 21–1
Standarized Abbreviations

=—equal.	D5W—5 percent Dextrose.	oz—ounce.
+—positive.	d/c—discontinue.	p̄—after.
—negative.	DC—direct current.	prn—as needed.
>—greater than.	Dr.—doctor.	q—every.
<—less than.	h—hour.	qd—every day.
R—right.	h/o—history of.	qh—every hour.
L—left.	hz—hertz.	qid—four times a day.
x—times or multiply.	kg—kilogram.	qod—every other day.
@—at.	l—liter.	r/o—rule out.
ā—before.	mA—milliamps.	s̄—without.
AC—alternating current.	mg—milligram.	tid—three times a day.
Bid—twice a day.	ml—milliliter.	w/—with.
c̄—with.	mm—millimeter.	WNL—within normal limits.
c/c—chief complaint.	mmHg—millimeters of mercury.	w/o—without.
cc—cubic centimeters.	n/a—not applicable.	y/o—year old.
cm—centimeters.	Ohm—electrical resistance.	
c/o—complained of.	PSI—pounds per square inch.	

TABLE 21-2

Standard Terms and Planes

Abduction—movement away from the body's midline.

Adduction—movement toward the body's midline.

Afferent—conducting impulse toward a structure.

Anterior—the front surface of the body.

Anterior to—in front of.

Caudad—toward the tail.

Cephalad—toward the head.

Circumduction—circular movement of a part.

Coronal plane—an imaginary plane that passes through the body from side to side and divides it into front and back sections.

Craniad—toward the cranium.

Deep—situated remote from surface.

Distal—situated away from the point of origin.

Dorsal—pertaining to the back surface of body.

Dorsiflexion—bending backward.

Efferent—conducting impulse away from a structure.

Elevation—raising a body part.

Extension—stretching or moving jointed parts into or toward a straight condition.

External—situated outside.

Flexion—bending or moving jointed parts closer together.

Frontal plane—an imaginary plane parallel to the long axis of the body and at right angles to the median sagittal plane.

Inferior—situated below.

Internal—situated inside.

Lateral—situated away from the body's midline.

Lateral rotation—rotating outward away from the body's midline.

Left lateral recumbent—lying horizontal on the left side.

Mediad—toward the midline of body.

Medial—situated toward body's midline.

Medial rotation—rotating inward toward body's midline.

Median sagittal plane—an imaginary plane that passes through the body from front to back and divides it into right and left halves.

Palmar—concerning the inner surface of the hand.

Peripheral—away from a central structure.

Plantar—concerning the sole of the foot.

Posterior—pertaining to the back surface of the body.

Posterior to—situated behind.

Pronation—lying face down or turning a hand so the palm faces down or back.

Prone—lying horizontal, face down and flat.

Protraction—a pushing forward.

Proximal—situated nearest the point of origin.

Recumbent—lying horizontal.

Retraction—a drawing back.

Right lateral recumbent—lying horizontal on the right side.

Rotation—turning around an axis.

Superficial—situated near the surface.

Superior—situated above.

Supination—lying face up or turning the hand so the palm faces forward or up.

Supine—lying horizontal, flat on the back and face up.

Transverse plane—an imaginary plane that passes through body and divides it into upper and lower sections.

Ventral—front surface of the body.

TABLE 21-3

Standard Medical Word Parts

A—not, without, lacking, deficient.
Ab—away from.
-Able—capable of.
Abdomin/o—abdomen.
Ac—pertaining to.
Acou—hear.
Acr/o—extremity, top, peak.
Acu—needle.
Ad—to, toward.
Aden/o—gland.
Adip/o—fat.
Aer/o—air.
Af—to.
-Algesia—painful.
-Algia—suffering pain.
Algi—pain.
All—other.
Ambi—both sides.
Ambl/y—dim, dull, lazy.
Amphi—on both sides, around both.
Ampho—on both sides, around both.
Amyl/o—starch.
An—without, negative.
Ana—upward, again, backward, excess.
Andr/o—man, male.
Anemia—blood.
-Anesthesia—sensation.
Angi/o—blood vessel, duct.
Anis—unequal.
Ankyl/o—stiff.
Ant—against, opposed to, preventing.
Ante—before, forward.
Antero—front.
Anti—against, opposed to, preventing.
Ap—to.
Apo—separation, derivation from.
-Arium—place for something.
Arteri/o—artery.
Arthrio—joint, articulation.
Articul/o—joint.
As—to.

-Ase—enzyme.
At—to.
Audi/o—hearing.
Aut—self.
Aur/o—ear.
Aut/o—self.
Bi—two, twice, double, both.
Bis—twice, double.
Bi/o—life.
Blephario—eyelid.
Brachi/o—upper arm.
Brady—slow.
Bronch/o—larger air passages of lungs.
Bucc/o—cheek.
Cac/o—bad, evil.
Calc/o—stone.
Calcane/o—heel.
Calor/o—heat.
Cancr/o—cancer.
Capit/o—head.
Caps/o—container.
Carcin/o—cancer.
Cardi/o—heart.
Carp/o—wrist bone.
Cat—down, lower, under, against, along with.
Cata—down, lower, under, against, along with.
-Cele—tumor, a cyst, hernia.
Celi/o—abdomen.
Cent—hundred.
-Centesis—perforation or tapping with a needle.
Cephal/o—head.
Cerebr/o—cerebrum.
Cervic/o—neck, cervix.
Cheil/o—lip.
Chil/o—lip.
Cheirio—hand.
Chir/o—hand.
Chlor/o—green.
Chol/e—bile, gall.
Chondr/o—cartilage.
Chrom/o—color.

Chromat/o—color.
Chron/o—time.
-Cid—cut, kill, fall.
-Cide—causing death.
Circum—around.
-Cis—cut, kill, fall.
-Clysis—irrigation.
Co—with.
Col—with.
Col/o—colon, large intestine.
Colp/o—vagina.
Com—with, together.
Con—together.
Contra—against, opposite.
Cor/e—pupil.
Core/o—pupil.
Cost/o—rib.
Crani/o—skull.
Cry/o—cold.
Crypt/o—hide, cover, conceal.
Cyan/o—blue.
Cyst/o—urinary bladder, cyst, sac of fluid.
-Cyte—cell.
Cyt/o—cell.
Dacry/o—tear.
Dactyl/o—finger, toe.
De—down, from, not.
Deca—ten.
Deci—tenth.
Demi—half.
Dent/o—tooth.
Derm/o—skin.
Dermat/o—skin.
Dextr/o—right.
Di—twice, double.
Dia—through, across, apart.
Dipl/o—double, twin, twice.
Dips/o—thirst.
Dis—to free, to undo.
Dors/o—back.
-Dynia—painful condition.

(continued)

TABLE 21-3 *(continued)*

Standard Medical Word Parts

Dys—bad, difficult, abnormal, incomplete.

-Ectasia—dilation or enlargement of organ or part.

Ecto—outer, outside of.

-Ectomy—the surgical removal of an organ or part.

Ef—out.

Electr/o—electric.

-Emesis—vomiting.

-Emia—condition of the blood.

En—in, into, within.

Encephal/o—brain.

End—within.

Endo—within.

Ent—within, inner.

Ento—within, inner.

Enter/o—small intestine.

Ep—over, on, upon.

Epi—over, on, upon.

Erythr/o—red.

-Esthesia—feeling, sensation.

Eu—good, well, normal, healthy.

Ex—out of, away from.

Exo—outside, outward.

Extra—on the outside, beyond, in addition to.

Faci/o—face, surface.

Febr/i—fever.

-Ferent—bear, carry.

Fibr/o—fiber, filament.

Fore—before, in front of.

-Form—shape.

-Fufal—moving away.

-Fuge—to drive away.

Galact/o—milk.

Gangli/o—knot.

Gaster—the stomach, the belly.

Gastr/o—stomach.

Gen/o—come into being, originate.

-Genesis—production or origin.

-Genic—giving rise to, originating in.

Gloss/o—tongue.

Glyc/o—sweet.

Gnath/o—jaw.

-Gog—to make flow.

-Gogue—to make flow.

-Gram—drawing, written record.

-Graph—an instrument for recording the activity of an organ.

-Graphy—the recording of the activity of an organ.

Gynec/o—woman.

Gnos/o—knowledge.

Hem/a—blood.

Hem/o—blood.

Hemat/o—blood.

Hemi—one-half.

Hepat/o—liver.

Heter/o—other, dissimilarity.

Hidr/o—sweat.

Hidrot/o—sweat.

Hist/o—tissue.

Holo—all.

Hom/o—same, similar, unchanging constant.

Home/o—same, similar, unchanging constant.

Hydr/o—water, fluid.

Hyp—under.

Hypn/o—sleep.

Hyal/o—glass.

Hyper—beyond, normal, excessive.

Hypo—below normal, deficient, under, beneath.

Hyster/o—uterus, womb.

-Iasis—condition, pathological state.

Iatr/o—healer, physician.

-Ible—capable of.

-Id—in a state, condition of.

Idio—peculiar, separate, distinct.

Il—negative, prefix.

Ile/o—ileum.

Ili/o—ilium.

Im—negative, prefix.

In—in, into, within.

Infra—beneath, below.

Inter—between.

Intra—within.

Intro—within, into.

Ir/o—iris.

Irid/o—iris.

Ischi/o—ischium.

-Ism—condition, theory.

-Ismus—abnormal condition.

Iso—same, equal, alike.

-Itis—inflammation.

-Ize—to treat by special method.

Juxta—near.

Karyo—nucleus, nut.

Kata—down.

Kera—horn, indicates hardness.

Kerat/o—cornea.

Kinesi/o—movement.

-Kinesis—motion.

Labi/o—lip.

Lact/o—milk.

Lal/o—talk.

Lapar/o—flank, abdomen, abdominal wall.

Laryng/o—larynx.

Latero—side.

Lept/o—thin, small, soft.

Leuc/o—white.

Leuk/o—white.

Lingu/o—tongue.

Lip/o—fat.

Lith/o—stone.

-Logist—a person who studies.

Log/o—speak.

-Logy—study of.

Lumb/o—loin.

Lymph/o—lymph.

-Lysis—destruction.

Macr/o—large, long.

Mal—bad, poor, evil.

Malac/o—a softening.

Mamm/o—breast.

-Mania—mental aberration.

Mast/o—breast.

Medi/o—middle.

Mega—large.

Megal/o—large.

-Megaly—an enlargement.

Melan/o—dark, black.

Men/o—month.

Mes/o—middle.

Meta—change, transformation, exchange.

-Meter—measure.

Metr/o—uterus.

Micr/o—small.

Mio—less, smaller.

Mon/o—single, only, sole.

Morph/o—form.

Multi—many, much.

Myc/o—fungus.

Mycet/o—fungus.

My/o—muscle.

Myel/o—marrow, also refers to spinal cord.

Myx/o—mucous, slime-like.

Narc/o—stupor, numbness.

Nas/o—nose.

Ne/o—new.

Necr/o—corpse.

Nephr/o—kidney.

Neur/o—nerve.

Niter—nitrogen.

Noct/I—night.

Non—no.

Norm/o—rule, order, normal.

Nucleo—nucleus.

Null/I—none.

Nyct/o—night.

Ob—against, in front of, toward.

Oc—against, in front of, toward.

Ocul/o—eye.

Odont/o—tooth.

-Oid—shape, form, resemblance.

Olig/o—few, deficient, scanty.

-Oma—tumor, swelling.

Omo—shoulder.

O/o—egg.

Onych/o—nail.

Oophor/o—ovary.

Opisth—backward.

-Opsy—a viewing.

Opthalm/o—eye.

Opt/o—sight, vision.

Optic/o—sight, vision.

Or/o—mouth.

Orch/o—testicle.

Orchid/o—testicle.

-Orium—place for something.

Orth/o—straight, upright.

Os—a mouth, a bone.

-Osis—process, an abnormal condition.

Oste/o—bone.

-Ostomosis—to furnish with a mouth or outlet.

-Otomy—cutting.

Ot/o—ear.

Ovari/o—ovary.

Oxy—sharp, acid.

Ov/I—egg.

Ov/o—egg.

Pachy—thicken.

Palat/o—palate.

Pan—all, entire, every.

Para—beside, beyond, accessory to, apart from, against.

Path/o—disease.

-Pathy—disease of a part.

-Penia—an abnormal reduction.

Peps/o—digestion.

Pept/o—digestion.

Per—throughout, completely, extremely.

Peri—around, surrounding.

-Pexy—fixation.

Phag/o—ear.

Pharyng/o—throat.

Phas/o—speech.

Phil/o—like, have an affinity for.

Phileb/o—vein.

-Phobia—fear, dread.

Phon/o—sound.

Phor/o—bear, carry.

Phot/o—light.

Phren/o—diaphragm.

-Phylaxis—protection.

Physi/o—nature.

Pil/o—hair.

-Plasia—development, formation.

-Plasm—to mold.

-Plasty—surgical repair.

-Plegia—paralysis, a stroke.

Pleur/o—rib, side, pleura.

Plur—more.

Pnea—breath, breathing.

Pneum/o—lung, air, breath.

Pneumat/o—air, breath.

Pneumon/o—lung.

Pod/o—foot.

-Poiesis—formation.

Poly—much, many.

Post—after, behind.

Pre—before.

Pro—before, in front of.

Proto—first.

Proct/o—anus.

Pseud/o—false.

Psych/o—mind, soul.

-Ptosis—abnormal dropping/sagging of part.

Pulmon/o—lung.

Py/o—pus.

Pyel/o—renal pelvis.

Pyr/o—fire, fever.

Quadri—four.

Rach/I—spine.

Radio—ray, radiation.

Re—back, against, contrary.

Rect/o—rectum.

Ren/o—the kidneys.

Retro—located behind, backward.

-Rhage—hemorrhage, flow.

-Rhaphy—a suturing or stitching.

-Rhea—to flow, indicates discharge.

Rhin/o—nose.

-Rrhage—abnormal discharge.

-Rrhagia—hemorrhage from an organ or body part.

-Rrhea—flowing or discharge.

Sacchar—sugar.

Sacro—sacrum.

Salping—a tube, relating to a fallopian tube.

Sanguin/o—blood.

Sarc/o—flesh.

Schiz/o—split.

Scler/o—hardening.

-Sclerosis—hardening condition.

Scoli/o—twisted, crooked.

-Scope—an instrument for observing.

-Scopy—to see.

-Sect—cut.

Semi—one-half, partly.

(continued)

TABLE 21-3   *(continued)*
Standard Medical Word Parts

Sept/o—infection.	Syn—joined together, with.	-Tripsy—surgical crushing.
Seps/o—infection.	Tachy—fast.	Troph/o—nourish.
Somat/o—body.	Tele—distant, far.	Ultra—beyond, excess.
Son/o—sound.	Tetra—four.	Uni—one.
Spermat/o—sperm, semen.	-Therapy—treatment.	Ur/o—urine.
Sphygm/o—pulse.	Therm/o—heat.	Ureter/o—ureter.
Splen/o—spleen.	Thio—sulfur.	Urethr/o—urethra.
-Stasis—stopping, controlling.	Thorac/o—chest cavity.	-Uria—relating to urine.
Sten/o—narrow.	Thromb/o—clot, lump.	Vas/o—vessel, duct.
Stere/o—solid, three-dimensional.	Thyro—thyroid gland.	Ven/o—vein.
Steth/o—chest.	-Tome—surgical instrument for cutting.	Ventr/o—belly, cavity.
Sthen/o—strength.	-Tomy—surgical operation on an organ or body part.	Vesic/o—blister, bladder.
-Stomy—surgically creating a new opening.	Top/o—place.	Viscer/o—internal organ.
Sub—under, near, almost, moderately.	Trache/o—trachea.	Xanth/o—yellow.
Super—above, excess.	Trans—through, across, beyond.	Xen/o—stranger.
Supra—above, over.	Tri—three.	Xer/o—dry.
Sym—joined together, with.	Trich/o—hair.	Zo/o—animal life.

what the EMS provider found and what was done for the patient because the EMS provider will not be present to explain her findings to all who ultimately read the PCR. The form should be so complete that it "speaks for itself!"

The existence of a complete and accurate record may help avert further legal action during the discovery phase of a lawsuit. The presumption is that a well-documented PCR equals a well-conducted assessment that, in turn, equals a well-managed patient.

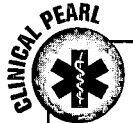

Like it or not, the public's perception determines the standard of care to at least some extent.

[Q] What are examples of extraneous or nonprofessional information on a PCR?

[A] The PCR is a legal document and the EMS provider should be careful to ensure that the expressions and terms used on the PCR are standardized and professional. Examples of extraneous or nonprofessional statements include:

- Judgmental biases (e.g., "patient was asking for a beating," "patient acts like he rarely bathes").
- Stereotyping (e.g., "These people are usually dirty," "These people have a high threshold for pain").

- Derogatory terms (e.g., "skell," "bum," "gomer," "woodchuck").
- Reference to an EMS system abuse call (e.g., "frequent flyer," "taxi ride").

[Q] What is the difference between subjective and objective findings on the PCR?

[A] Subjective findings are things the patient or bystanders tell the EMS provider. This information consists of symptoms or answers to questions. Objective findings are things the EMS provider can measure such as vital signs, pulse oximeter, or the patient's color.

[Q] What is the importance of confidentiality to an EMS document?

[A] Patients have a right to have their medical conditions held in confidence and breaching that right may cause harm or embarrassment to the patient and their family. For this reason, any discussion for quality improvement or educational purposes that relates to a PCR should not include the patient's name or specific identifying information.

What are the potential consequences of poor documentation?

An incomplete, inaccurate or illegible PCR can create problems where none really exist. This is because the presumption might be that the EMS provider either did not give the proper care or had something to hide.

Documentation of Procedures

What should be documented when an ET tube is inserted?

There has been considerable attention to the issue of misplaced tubes in both the hospital setting and the field. Checking a box that says ET is simply not enough today. When an ET tube is placed, the EMS provider should document at least the following information:

- The size of the tube.
- Who placed the tube.
- When the tube was placed.
- At least three methods of ensuring that the tube was properly placed (e.g., visualization, auscultation over both lungs and epigastrium, use of a pulse oximeter, use of an esophageal intubation detector device [EIDD], use of a colo-metric CO_2 device, or the use of an end-tidal CO_2 device).
- The depth of the tube (e.g., 22 cm at the teeth) and the method of securing.
- That the tube was reassessed periodically and after patient movement.
- The correction of misplaced tubes.

What should be documented when an IV is administered?

When an IV is started in the field, the following things should be documented on the PCR:

- The type of fluid administered, the drip rate, and how much was administered prior to leaving the patient at the ED.
- The size of the needle used.
- Who started the IV.
- The site of the IV.
- The number of attempts if the first was not successful.

What should be documented on the PCR when narcotics are administered to the patient?

Often, there is other additional paperwork associated with narcotic administration. When the patient receives a narcotic, such as morphine, in out-of-hospital care, the EMS provider should document the following on the PCR:

- The patient's name.
- The drug name, route, dose, and time administered.
- The physician authorizing administration of the narcotic.
- What effect the medication had on the patient.
- Reassessment of the patient's vital signs.
- Exactly how any left-over medication was disposed of and the observing witness's name.

Documenting Special Situations

What are the special considerations for documentation when a patient refuses care or transportation?

The proper documentation of a refusal of care or transportation is very important. The procedure for doing this is described in Chapter 4, Medicolegal Issues.

What are the special considerations for documentation at a mass casualty incident (MCI)?

Triage tags are often used as the first line of documentation at an MCI. Once the patient is transported, most EMS agencies require a PCR for each patient treated. It is a good practice to reference the same incident somewhere on the PCR (e.g., patient 4 of 6 from Main St. incident). Sometimes, this may not be practical because you do not know the total number of patients until completion of the incident. To clear the hospital quickly and return to the scene, try to abbreviate the PCR without eliminating any essential assessment or management information. Some of the demographics can always be added in at a later time (as an amended PCR, not just on the agency copy) because most understand that a call with many patients is not the regular course of business.

CLINICAL PEARL

If you minimize the information contained in the initial PCR, remember you must go back and finish the report properly. Don't wait until the entire incident is past history.

Q What is a pertinent negative and how are these documented?

A A pertinent negative is a negative response, such as the answer to a question, that adds to the assessment. For example, "patient was involved in a collision, struck his head, and denies any loss of consciousness" is an important pertinent negative finding.

Q What is the most appropriate way to correct errors on the PCR?

A The proper way to correct an error on the PCR is thoroughly discussed in Chapter 4, Medicolegal Issues.

Q What are some examples of unusual situations that should be documented on the PCR?

A Each service should have a standard operating procedure that clearly lists unusual circumstances that must be documented on the PCR. In some cases, services also use a special incident report. Examples of situations that should be documented on the PCR include the following:

- An injury occurred to the patient (e.g., dropping the stretcher) or EMS provider (e.g., lifting a patient who was too heavy).

- A blood borne exposure occurred.
- There was a delay in response time (e.g., inclement weather, wrong initial dispatch address, vehicle malfunction).
- Equipment failure that may have impacted on patient care.
- An emergency vehicle collision occurred.
- Radio failure or out of range delaying direct medical control.
- Police request to draw blood (if this is done by EMS providers in your system).
- Patient needing restraint.
- Hostile and abusive patients.

CLINICAL PEARL

Some services document provider injuries, ambulance accidents, etc., separately on an incident report alone, and not in the PCR. Follow your local protocols. Incident reports or other tools used for quality improvement purposes are potentially accessible for legal purposes. In-hospital quality control documents are somewhat more protected, but never assume that just because a document is done under the guise of quality improvement, it is completely safe from others.

Special Thanks

Bob Elling, MPA, REMT-P, for the abbreviations, standard medical word parts, and terms and planes from his book *Pocket Reference For The EMT-B and First Responder,* 2nd Ed., 2001, Prentice-Hall.

(1) W. J. Ginsburgh. (1998 May). Prepare to be shocked: the evolving standard of care in treating sudden cardiac arrest. *American Journal of Emergency Medicine, 16,* 315–319.

Pulmonary and Respiratory

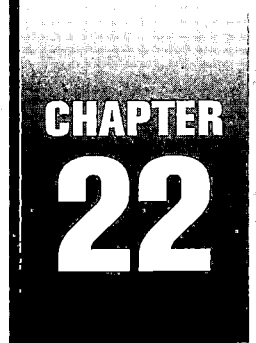

This chapter discusses basic and advanced pulmonary and respiratory problems. The focus is on *why* patients present in a certain manner and *why* you need to respond in a certain way to their presenting problems. Respiratory complaints are among the most common medical complaints in the field. With a thorough knowledge of pulmonary and respiratory disorders, the EMS provider will be able to understand the importance of recognition and management in these patients.

Chronic Versus Acute Disorders

Q **If respiratory problems are divided into "acute" and "chronic," why would it be true to say that nearly all persons with respiratory problems who come to the attention of EMS providers will have an acute condition?**

A Many persons are completely healthy before developing a breathing problem. Patients with chronic respiratory problems, such as chronic obstructive pulmonary disease (COPD), however, usually present with an *acute exacerbation* of their *chronic* condition. In this sense, nearly all persons with respiratory problems who come to the attention of EMS providers will have an acute condition.

Q **What is the significance of the oxyhemoglobin saturation curve?**

A This curve plots the percentage saturation of hemoglobin by oxygen on the vertical axis and the partial pressure of oxygen (PO_2) in arterial blood on the horizontal axis. The result is a sigmoid-shaped curve as shown in Figure 22–1. Normally, hemo-globin saturation is greater than 90 percent once the PO_2 exceeds approximately 70 mmHg.

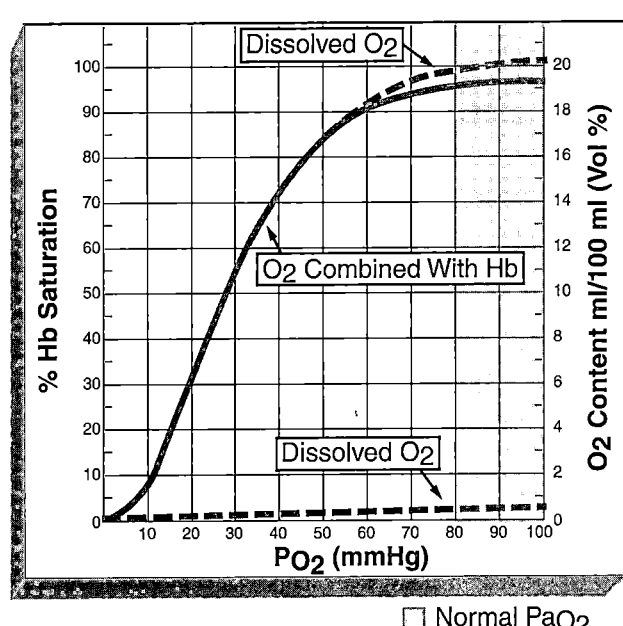

□ Normal PaO_2

FIGURE 22-1 The Oxyhemoglobin Dissociation Curve.

Shifts of the curve to the right or to the left affect the affinity of hemoglobin for oxygen. Look at the curve. If it moves to the right, the PO_2 must be *higher* to maintain 90 percent saturation. If the curve moves to the left, the PO_2 can be *lower*. This means that shifts in the curve indicate a change in the *affinity of hemoglobin for oxygen*. A rightward shift *decreases* it, while a leftward shift *increases* the binding (affinity) of oxygen to hemoglobin. Remember, as the affinity of hemoglobin for oxygen *increases* (leftward shift of the curve), the tissue oxygen delivery *decreases*, and vice versa (rightward shift of the curve *increases* tissue oxygen delivery).

Q Which factors shift the oxyhemoglobin saturation curve to the right, thus increasing tissue oxygen delivery?

A Increased body temperature and acidosis are the most common causes. Increased levels of the blood protein 2,3-diphosphoglycerate (2,3-DPG) have the same effect, but we have little control over this in the field. When fever develops, the cells' metabolic rate increases and so does their oxygen need. Because it is a law of nature that this rightward shift of the curve occurs with increased body temperature, the body automatically tries to provide more oxygen to the tissues.

Q Which factors shift the oxyhemoglobin saturation curve to the left, decreasing the tissue oxygen delivery?

A Decreased body temperature and alkalosis are the most common causes. Low levels of 2,3-DPG have the same effect, but are of little significance in most aspects of emergency care. The leftward shift of the curve with decreased body temperature helps explain why cells may survive prolonged periods of hypothermia.

CLINICAL PEARL

Alkalosis affects tissue oxygen delivery. This is the reason sodium bicarbonate has lost favor in the treatment of cardiac arrest and metabolic acidosis. Shifting the oxyhemoglobin saturation curve to the left may increase *the pH (make the patient more alkalotic), but* decreases *tissue oxygen delivery by* increasing *the affinity of hemoglobin for oxygen.*

Q What do I need to know to understand a blood gas report?

A To understand arterial blood gases, you have to look at four things:

- The patient's name.
- The pH (normally 7.35–7.45) indicates acid–base balance. Too high means the patient is alkalotic (basic), while too low indicates the patient is acidotic (acidic).

- The pCO_2 measures ventilation (exchange of carbon dioxide); normal levels are 35–40 mmHg. pCO_2 is a respiratory acid—increased levels cause an *increase* in the blood acid level and a *decrease* in the pH, or acidosis. Decreased levels result in a *decreased* blood acid level and an *increased* pH or alkalosis. Every 10 mmHg change of the pCO_2, up or down, results in a 0.1 change in the pH in the *opposite* direction. For example, by hyperventilating and "blowing off" 10 mmHg of pCO_2, the pH is *raised* by 0.1—say, from 7.40 to 7.50.

- The PO_2 measures oxygenation at sea level and should normally run greater than 80 mmHg.

CLINICAL PEARL

Other than the patient's name, pCO_2, pH, and PO_2, all other parameters on the blood gas report are calculated, not measured. They offer little more to interpretation than potential confusion.

Q Do changes in PO_2 always occur when there are changes in the pCO_2 level, and vice versa?

A Definitely not! Sometimes changes in the pCO_2, such as hypoventilation due to narcotic intoxication, leads to severe hypoxia (decreased PO_2) and elevated pCO_2 due to CO_2 retention. Other times, a patient may hyperventilate (lower the pCO_2) yet the PO_2 may be high, low, or normal. The only predictable and reproducible relationship in blood gases is between the pH and the pCO_2.

Q What is the difference between a respiratory and a metabolic acidosis or alkalosis?

A For a review of these conditions, see Chapter 6, General Principles of Pathophysiology.

Q How quickly does respiratory compensation for a metabolic alkalosis or acidosis occur?

A Respiratory compensation occurs within minutes. On the other hand, metabolic compensation for a respiratory process (e.g., CO_2 retention in COPD or asthma) takes hours to days to occur. Consequently, you are most likely to see patients with *uncompensated* primary respiratory processes, while many with primary metabolic processes will have *respiratory compensation*.

Q Is there an easy way to figure out the primary "instigating" process from a set of blood gases?

A Yes. The answers to three simple questions usually identify the primary cause: respiratory acidosis, respiratory alkalosis, metabolic acidosis, or metabolic alkalosis.

1. Is the PO_2 low (below 80 mmHg)? If so, fix it. Otherwise, move onto the second question. Other than recognizing and treating hypoxia, the PO_2 value contributes no additional information to the proper interpretation of a blood gas result.

2. Which way did the pH go, up (too high) or down (too low)? In most acute situations, the pH will have moved one way or the other.

3. Did the pCO_2 move in the *opposite* direction from the pH? If so, the primary problem is *respiratory*. If not (it did not move or moved in the same direction as the pH), the primary problem is *metabolic*.

These rules are all you need to make sense out of just about any set of blood gas data. They are based on the fixed and predictable relationship between the pH and the pCO_2. If the pCO_2 and pH move in opposite directions, the primary problem is respiratory. If not, the primary problem has to be metabolic!

CLINICAL PEARL

Most EMS providers are scared to death of blood gas interpretation. This fear is a total waste of worry time! Blood gases are very straightforward if you follow the rules. They are based on a sound law of nature—the "happy marriage" between pH and pCO_2—they always move in opposite directions by a 10 to 0.1 ratio.

Pathophysiology

Q What respiratory abnormalities commonly affect ventilation?

A Those primarily affecting ventilation (exchange of oxygen and carbon dioxide) include:

- Upper airway obstruction (e.g., trauma, epiglottitis, foreign body obstruction, tonsillitis).
- Lower airway obstruction (e.g., trauma, obstructive lung disease, mucous accumulation, smooth muscle spasm or bronchospasm, airway edema).
- Impairment of chest wall movement (e.g., trauma, hemothorax, pneumothorax, empyema, pleural inflammation, neuromuscular diseases such as multiple sclerosis or muscular dystrophy).
- Problems with neurologic control involving either the central nervous system (e.g., CNS depressant drugs, stroke, other medical condition, or trauma) or the peripheral nervous system (phrenic or spinal nerve dysfunction due to trauma or neuromuscular diseases).

Q What respiratory abnormalities commonly affect diffusion?

A Diffusion-related (movement of gases across membranes) conditions include:

- Inadequate oxygen concentration in the ambient air.
- Alveolar pathology (e.g., asbestosis, blebs from COPD, inhalation injuries).
- Interstitial space pathology either due to elevations of hydrostatic pressure ("water pressure") in the pulmonary circulation (e.g., pulmonary edema, pulmonary hypertension) or secondary to abnormal permeability of the pulmonary vessels (e.g., adult respiratory distress syndrome [ARDS], environmental lung diseases, near-drowning, hypoxia, inhalation injuries).

Q What respiratory abnormalities commonly affect perfusion?

A Perfusion-related (pumping of blood from the heart to the tissues) factors may also impair gas exchange. These include:

- Inadequate blood volume or hemoglobin levels (e.g., hypovolemia, anemia).
- Impaired circulatory blood flow (e.g., pulmonary embolus, cardiac tamponade).
- Chest wall pathology (trauma).

General Assessment

Q What should your priority in any respiratory emergency be?

A *Scene size-up always comes first!* Pulmonary complaints may be associated with a variety of toxin exposures including carbon monoxide, products of combustion, or oxygen-deficient environments (e.g., silos, enclosed storage spaces, below grade). Assure a safe environment for all EMS providers before initiating patient contact. If necessary, use individuals with specialized training and equipment to remove the patient from a hazardous environment.

CLINICAL PEARL

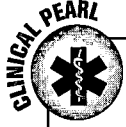

Your own safety always comes first regardless of the situation.

What is the major focus of your initial patient assessment in a person with a respiratory problem?

Many pulmonary diseases present a very real risk for patient death. Recognition of immediate life-threatening conditions and prompt initiation of resuscitation takes priority over a detailed assessment.

What findings suggest that an immediate life threat is present in a patient with respiratory problems? Why are these particular findings "red flags?"

The following are signs of potential life-threatening respiratory distress in adults:

- Alterations in mental status (MS)—suggestive of hypoxia, carbon dioxide retention, or both.

- Severe cyanosis—usually a late stage, and indicates significant hypoxia.

- Absent breath sounds—the inability to hear breath sounds in patients who are obviously struggling to breathe means poor air movement. Often, they are "too tight to wheeze." Sometimes COPD patients have quiet breath sounds. This differs from absent lung sounds in a person with obvious clinical distress. A quiet chest in an acute asthmatic indicates impending respiratory failure.

- Audible stridor—stridor is an uncommon finding, but should alert you to the possibility of an upper airway obstruction (e.g., croup, epiglottitis, foreign body obstruction).

- One or two word dyspnea—the fewer words a person can speak before stopping to take a breath, the worse the disease is. Patients who are only able to say one or two words without pausing to breathe are in severe respiratory distress.

- Tachycardia of greater than 130 beats/minute—though nonspecific, tachycardia often indicates stress. Combined with the clinical picture of a person who is short of breath, significant tachycardia is worrisome. In addition, hypoxia and carbon dioxide retention can lead to cardiac dysrhythmias, which may also cause a rapid pulse rate (e.g., atrial fibrillation, supraventricular tachycardia, ventricular tachycardia).

- Pallor and diaphoresis—these are nonspecific findings, but are worrisome when they accompany a shortness of breath.

- The presence of retractions or the use of accessory muscles of respiration—both retractions and the use of accessory muscles show that the patient is working harder than normal to breathe.

- Grunting—a sound that occurs primarily in infants and small toddlers when the child breathes out against a partially closed epiglottis, grunting is usually a sign of respiratory distress.

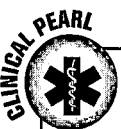

A quiet-sounding chest in a patient who appears to be markedly short of breath is a bad sign!

What chief complaint may a patient with a respiratory problem present with?

The patient may present with a chief complaint such as:

- Dyspnea—"I can't breathe," "I can't catch my breath."
- Chest pain—"My chest hurts," "My chest is tight."
- Cough—"I have a bad cough." Or, "I have been coughing up red/green/pink/black stuff." It is important to note if it is a productive or nonproductive cough.
- Wheezing—"I am starting to wheeze." Sometimes the EMS provider can actually hear the wheezing without the assistance of a stethoscope.
- Signs of infection—"I have been running a fever," "I have the chills."

What are specific areas in the patient's focused history (FH) that should always be explored in detail?

Especially relevant areas to explore in the patient's *history* are:

- Has the patient had experiences with similar or identical symptoms? If the current problem represents an exacerbation of a chronic condition, the patient's subjective description of the acuity may be helpful. Ask the patient what happened the last time he had an attack this bad. Perhaps he had to be tubed in the hospital the last time.

- Does the patient have a known pulmonary diagnosis?

- Has the patient ever required intubation? A history of previous intubation is an accurate indicator of severe pulmonary disease and suggests that intubation may be required again.

- What medications does the patient take? Be certain to ask not only how the medications were prescribed (i.e., *supposed* to be taken by the patient), but when the patient *actually* takes them. Also determine if the patient has any medication allergies. People who are on oral corticosteroids typically have a severe, chronic disease. Inhaled steroid use is now common for both asthma and COPD, even in patients with mild disease.

- Determine the details of the present episode.

- Determine any possible toxic exposures, especially cigarette smoke or toxic gases.

Focusing on these specific questions is paramount in a respiratory distressed patient. Be aware that the patient may deteriorate quickly, soon being unable to answer any questions.

What factors should be assessed when forming the general impression of a patient during the physical exam (PE)?

Form a general impression of the patient's condition based on your assessment of the following:

- Position—the patient's position often indicates the degree of respiratory difficulty. Dyspneic persons often sit, leaning forward on their hands, with the feet dangling. This is known as the *tripod position,* and suggests moderate to severe respiratory distress is present.
- Mentation—confusion suggests hypoxemia or hypercarbia (carbon dioxide retention) until proven otherwise; both fear and hypoxemia can cause restlessness and irritability. Severe lethargy or coma is a sign of severe hypoxia or hypercarbia.
- Ability to speak—a good indicator of breathing difficulty is a patient's ability to speak freely without having to stop and breathe. Rapid, rambling speech often indicates anxiety and fear, though many other conditions may be responsible (e.g., pulmonary embolus, drug intoxication).
- Respiratory effort—patients who look as if they are working to breathe usually are!
- Skin color and appearance—Cyanosis, either peripherally or centrally, is always worrisome.

What potential value are vital sign measurements in persons with respiratory emergencies?

Obtain baseline vital signs; use these in combination with your other findings to evaluate the severity of the patient's condition:

- Pulse—tachycardia is a sign of hypoxemia and fear. It may also occur because of sympathomimetic medication use such as inhaled bronchodilators. In the face of a respiratory problem, bradycardia is an *ominous* sign of severe hypoxemia and suggests imminent cardiac arrest.
- Blood pressure—hypertension may be associated with fear, anxiety, dyspnea, use of sympathomimetic medications, or a combination of factors.
- Respiratory rate—isolated measurement of a patient's respiratory rate is an inaccurate measurement of respiratory status unless it is very slow (less than 8–10 breaths per minute in an adult). More helpful are changes in the measured respiratory rate. Trends are essential in evaluating any patient. A slowing

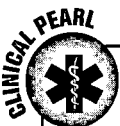

Trends are usually more helpful than the measurement or observation of any single parameter.

respiratory rate in the face of an unimproved condition suggests patient exhaustion and impending respiratory failure.

Why is pursed-lip breathing often present in exacerbations of COPD and asthma?

The common denominator in both conditions is decreased expiratory air flow. Pursed-lip breathing causes resistance to exhalation at the mouth. This leads to a "backup" of airway pressure into the lungs. The pressure forces previously atelectatic (collapsed) airways to open and improves oxygenation. Many patients with chronic lung disease have taught themselves to feel better using pursed-lip breathing. In others, it may be a subconscious defense mechanism.

What are the signs and symptoms of right-sided heart failure?

Distended neck veins, peripheral edema, and ascites are the most common manifestations of right-sided congestive heart failure (CHF), whatever the underlying cause.

How does lung disease cause right-sided heart failure?

Many forms of lung disease cause increased resistance to blood flow in the lungs (pulmonary hypertension). To compensate, the right heart must work harder. Even after enlarging to compensate (hypertrophy), the right ventricle has such little mass (compared with the left) that it is soon unable to counteract completely the pulmonary resistance to flow. Blood backs up into the venous system. The result—venous distention (especially the neck veins), peripheral edema, and sometimes ascites. The liver and spleen are also engorged with blood backup through the portal circulation, though this may not be easy to detect in the field.

What causes the "barrel chest" deformity in COPD and sometimes in asthma?

Increased expiratory resistance to flow and air-trapping underlie the pathogenesis of both. Trapped air leads to hyperinflation of the lungs, resulting in a widening of the anterior-posterior diameter of a person's chest. In most individuals, this looks (from the side) like a barrel as shown in Figure 22–2.

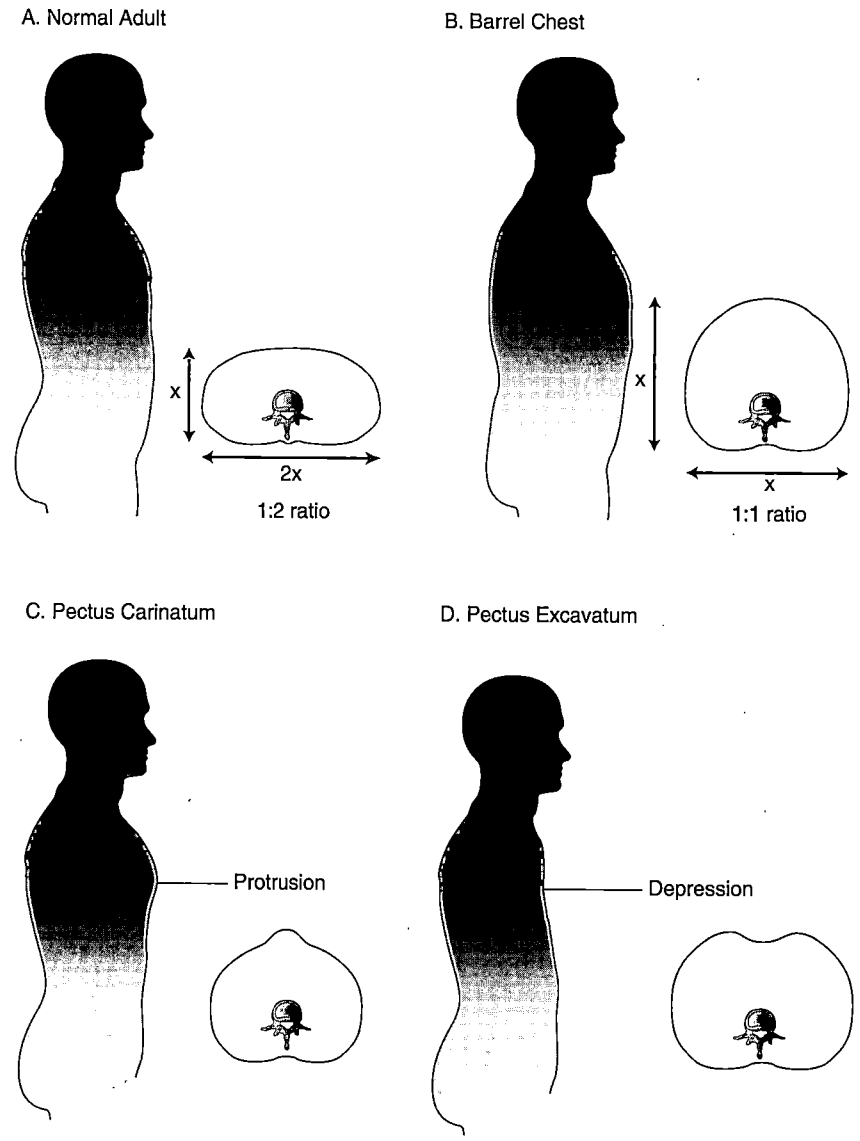

A. Normal Adult

B. Barrel Chest

x
2x
1:2 ratio

x
x
1:1 ratio

C. Pectus Carinatum

D. Pectus Excavatum

— Protrusion

— Depression

FIGURE 22-2 Chest configurations.

Q What generates breath sounds?

A Air movement through airways of different sizes, as transmitted through the chest wall to the stethoscope, leads to both normal and abnormal breath sounds.

- Wheezes result when small airways constrict; the transmitted sound becomes high pitched and somewhat squeaky. The sound of wheezes may be "drawn-out" or longer than normal breath sounds, reflecting resistance to expiratory air flow.

- Crackles usually result from fluid in the airways, in the interstitial tissue, or in both.

Q Why do many experts now avoid the use of the term "rales" when describing breath sounds?

A Many studies proved that there was little, if any, agreement between listeners as to exactly which sound constitutes a rale. Various groups (e.g., physicians, nurses, respiratory therapists, paramedics) failed to agree with each other when asked to listen to recorded lung sounds. Even more interesting was the fact that people did not even agree with themselves—when asked to listen to the same sounds two weeks later, over half the listeners classified them differently than they did their first attempt.

Descriptive terms, such as "crackles," "wheezes," and even "wet lungs," more effectively communicate the message.

CLINICAL PEARL

Some instructors still emphasize apparent differences between "wheezes," "rales," and "rhonchi." True, each has a "dictionary definition," but repeated studies have shown that groups of health care providers are unable to reliably identify the differences. Therefore, it's often better to use descriptive terms to improve communication.

Q What is carpopedal spasm and why does it occur?

A Carpopedal spasm is a spasmodic contraction of the hands, wrists, feet, and ankles. This condition is associated with decreased carbon dioxide levels (hypocapnia) resulting from periods of rapid, deep respirations (whatever the cause). Low pCO_2 levels lead to a respiratory alkalosis—the change in pH increases the binding of calcium to albumin. This leads to a decreased level of unbound (ionized) calcium in the blood. Because calcium participates in nerve transmission and muscle contraction, both are affected, leading to spasm.

Q Why is carpopedal spasm not just a sign of "anxiety-hyperventilation?"

A Anxiety is only one of many causes of hyperventilation. Any condition that leads to a respiratory alkalosis may cause carpopedal spasm. The safest approach is to assume that the patient has something seriously wrong (e.g., pulmonary embolism, diabetic ketoacidosis, myocardial infarction) until proven otherwise.

CLINICAL PEARL

Assuming a hyperventilating patient only has anxiety-hyperventilation is dangerous. Give the patient the benefit of the doubt—assume something bad is happening and treat accordingly with oxygen and appropriate monitoring.

Q What is the best way to use peak flow readings clinically?

A Peak flow meters are easy to use and provide a baseline assessment to follow therapy. Isolated readings on their own are potentially misleading—follow trends instead.

Obstructive Airway Disease

Q Why is obstructive airway disease a spectrum?

A *Obstructive airway disease* is a generic term for a spectrum of diseases that affect many individuals worldwide. The most common diseases include asthma and COPD. COPD is sometimes subdivided into emphysema and chronic bronchitis, though many patients have clinical features of both.

Q What factors may exacerbate underlying respiratory conditions?

A Factors that may exacerbate underlying conditions include:

- Stress—a significant exacerbating factor, particularly in adults.
- Infection—upper respiratory infection is a common precipitant of acute exacerbations of both asthma and COPD.
- Exercise—though exercise may exacerbate any respiratory condition, exercise-induced wheezing and asthma are especially common.
- Tobacco smoke—increases the chances of developing COPD and heart disease. The exposure of others to second-hand smoke affects them similarly. Children with asthma who are surrounded by cigarette smoke have an increased frequency of asthmatic attacks.
- Allergens—various substances (e.g., foods, animal dander, dusts, molds, pollens) in one's environment may precipitate or worsen obstructive lung disease. One purported reason for the increased incidence of asthma in inner-city children is exposure to cockroaches.
- Drugs—allergic reactions to any medication may lead to wheezing. Certain drugs (e.g., beta-blockers) affect the ability of the sympathetic nervous system to cause bronchodilation and may provoke or worsen obstructive lung disease.
- Occupational hazards—many occupational exposures have been shown to cause or worsen obstructive lung disease. One of the most significant to health care providers is latex allergy. Many health care workers have developed a latex allergy because of our widespread use of latex-containing products, especially gloves. Patients may also be latex sensitive—the failure to have equipment that is latex-free may place you in a serious medicolegal situation.

CLINICAL PEARL

Exercise-induced wheezing or cough is a common manifestation of obstructive lung disease, especially in children and teenagers. It may be precipitated by an upper respiratory infection (URI).

How can the pathophysiology of obstructive airway disease be summarized?

The underlying pathophysiology of all forms of obstructive lung disease is decreased expiratory airflow and air trapping, primarily due to obstruction in the small bronchioles.

What pathological factors lead to airway obstruction in obstructive lung disease?

Obstruction is usually a result of several factors including:

- Smooth muscle spasm—various irritants cause the bronchiolar wall smooth muscle to contract, resulting in bronchospasm, obstruction, and wheezing. These muscles contain beta-receptors that respond to sympathetic stimulation, resulting in bronchodilation. Bronchoconstrictors have the opposite effect (e.g., beta-blockers).

- Mucous—goblet cells line the respiratory tract and normally produce a layer of mucous that is continuously swept out of the lungs by cilia, moving hairs. Anything that disrupts the movement of the cilia leads to an accumulation of excess mucous in the airways. Abnormal ciliary movement occurs in obstructive lung disease and in many other conditions, such as cystic fibrosis. Sometimes, the disruption is temporary, but the damage might be permanent (e.g., chronic bronchitis, cystic fibrosis).

- Inflammation—obstructive lung disease occurs in the face of both acute and chronic inflammation. This finding has completely changed our approach to the treatment of asthma in recent years. Data also suggest that chronic inflammation underlies COPD. Acutely, infection leads to inflammation that may exacerbate any form of obstructive lung disease.

Why does air trapping develop in obstructive lung disease?

No matter the mechanism, an obstruction may be reversible or irreversible. Typically, asthmatics improve between attacks, though some never achieve normal pulmonary function. On the other hand, at least part of the damage in COPD is irreversible, leading to continuous air trapping:

- Bronchioles dilate naturally on inspiration as they fill with air.

- Dilation enables air to enter the alveoli even if the lumen (opening) of the bronchiole is narrowed due to obstruction.

- Bronchioles naturally constrict on expiration.

- Air becomes trapped distal to the site of the obstruction during exhalation.

What is asthma?

Acute asthma is a recurring condition of completely or partially reversible acute airflow obstruction in the lower airway. Asthma is exhibited by constriction of the bronchi, wheezing, and dyspnea. Asthma is the leading cause of chronic illness in children.

What is the series of events that happens when asthmatic airways are irritated?

People with asthma have extra-sensitive bronchial airways that are easily irritated. When the airways become irritated, a series of events occurs:

- Bronchospasm—tiny muscle layers surrounding the bronchioles go into spasm and narrow the lumen of the airways. Bronchospasm is similar to pinching a drinking straw; it limits the movement of air. The result is wheezing as air is forced through the narrowed airways. Shortness of breath follows because not enough air reaches the alveoli.

- Increased mucus production—because of the irritation, the bronchial airways produce an abnormal amount of mucus. This secreted mucus is particularly thick, making it difficult to remove with coughing. Because mucus is no longer being removed through normal processes, it clogs the smaller bronchioles further decreasing the airway diameter. This makes breathing even more difficult.

- Swelling and edema—fluid collects in the lining of the irritated airways, causing them to swell, which further blocks the flow of air.

- Inflammatory cell proliferation—white blood cells (WBCs) accumulate in the airway. These cells secrete substances that worsen the muscle spasm and increase mucus production.

Is asthma always "completely reversible" between attacks?

No—a severe asthma patient may have ongoing inflammation in the lungs despite appearing clinically normal. The patient may depend on daily medication to prevent attacks.

What are the most common triggers of asthma attacks?

Common asthma triggers include:

- Respiratory infections—the most common asthma triggers, they include colds, the flu, and sinus infections. These illnesses

CLINICAL PEARL

Recent evidence clearly documents that asthma is a chronic inflammatory condition despite presenting in clinical paroxysms. These findings underlie the basis for chronic anti-inflammatory therapy for asthma, such as inhaled steroids. One reason that the death rate from asthma continues to rise, despite our increased knowledge, is the undermedication *of many patients (not enough use of anti-inflammatory drugs). Inhaled steroids were originally thought to result in less side effects than the oral preparations. Unfortunately, this is not absolutely true—dose-dependent side effects can still occur (e.g., cataracts, osteoporosis, adrenal suppression). As a consequence, the pharmacy profession has invented other anti-inflammation drugs, such as the leukotriene blockers.*

trigger asthma attacks because they temporarily inflame and damage the lining of the air tubes causing bronchospasm, increased mucus production, and swelling. Asthma attacks that occur with a respiratory infection are usually worse than those that occur at other times.

- Allergens—are substances that can trigger an allergic reaction that irritates the bronchial airways. Children are more likely to have allergies that trigger attacks than are adults who develop asthma later in life. The most common allergens are pollen, dust, animal dander, lint, insecticides, food, mold, and drugs (e.g., aspirin, penicillin, local anesthetics, anti-inflammatory drugs such as ibuprofen). Street drugs may cause acute asthmatic attacks in sensitive individuals. Contrary to popular belief, food allergies are very rare. Nuts and seafood are the most common causes of food allergies that trigger asthma attacks.

- Irritants—these triggers are substances that can irritate anyone's bronchi, but in persons who have asthma, they can trigger an attack. Examples include odors, cigarette smoke, air pollution, and fumes. Work place irritants are particularly common among people who work in factories where dust or fumes are present.

- Exercise—fast breathing, especially during cold weather, irritates the bronchial airways. They become more sensitive and produce more mucus that can lead to an asthma attack. Another common trigger among children is exercise. It is natural for children to run and exercise outdoors, especially in the spring and fall when pollen fills the air.

- Emotions—any strong, subjective feeling or reaction may cause an asthma attack. Although there has been less research conducted in this area than on other asthma triggers, examples of emotions that might trigger an attack include crying,

yelling, or even laughing. Stress from personal or work-related worry is a particularly powerful trigger.

- Chemicals—many people have severe asthma reactions to specific chemicals. Common examples include: red and yellow dye (not only in food, but also in colored pills), sulfur dioxide in red wine, aspirin (and other anti-inflammatory drugs), and sulfites that are often used to preserve fruits and vegetables and are found at food and salad bars.

- Changes in environmental conditions—sun, cold, wind, or humidity.

CLINICAL PEARL

Sulfites are sometimes used as preservatives in prescription nebulized bronchodilators, such as isoethrane. If given to a sulfite-sensitive patient, the situation is worsened rather than aided. Always look at the packaging, if possible, of any nebulized solutions used at home by the patient.

Q What is status asthmaticus and why is it so worrisome?

A *Status asthmaticus* is a severe prolonged asthma attack that does not respond to standard medications. Its onset may be sudden or insidious and is frequently caused by a viral respiratory infection. Status asthmaticus requires immediate transport because the patient is in imminent danger of respiratory failure. Out-of-hospital treatment is the same as for acute asthma; however, rapid transport is more important. Patients should be closely monitored. Anticipate the need for intubation and aggressive ventilatory support.

Q Why is the death rate from asthma still climbing?

A Despite leaps and bounds in our level of knowledge, the asthma death rate continues to soar. Once thought to be the result of too many inhaled sympathomimetic drugs ("puffers"), this is no longer felt to be the case. Two factors underlie the fatal trend:

- Inadequate use of anti-inflammatory medications, such as steroids or leukotriene blockers.

- Decreased airway sensitivity in severe asthmatics. Many severe asthmatics lose their awareness of dyspnea until it is too late. Studies have shown that there is a genetic defect in some asthmatic patients that makes their lungs *less* sensitive to stretch. Normally, resistance to breathing (as in asthma) distends (stretches) the lungs. This triggers "stretch receptors" and leads to the sensation of dyspnea, even before physical findings (e.g., wheezes, decreased peak expiratory flow) are present. Asthmatic patients who lack this sensitivity will not feel short of breath until their attack has progressed to near death—a point at which even the most sophisticated specialists and facilities often make no difference!

Can we identify the patients who are at high risk for fatal asthma attacks?

We cannot identify them, at least in time to make a difference for most. The "typical" clinical picture is a female between 20 and 40 years of age with a history of near-fatal asthma attacks. Any asthmatic patient meeting these criteria is a "priority" patient. Any asthma attack can turn fatal rapidly.

There is some promising news on the horizon—genetic studies may be able to identify asthmatic patients with a chromosomal abnormality. In addition, routine home monitoring of peak expiratory flow by computer has been shown to identify early downward trends. Be certain to ask patients if they do home monitoring—bring a copy of the record (if one exists) to the hospital with the patient.

CLINICAL PEARL

A genetic defect has been found in some asthmatic patients with a history of near-fatal attacks. The defect can be passed from generation to generation. Current investigations are directed at the early identification of people with this defect. In addition, some type of gene transplant will likely be tried in the near future to restore the normal system.

What is COPD?

COPD is a progressive and irreversible disease of the airway marked by a decreased inspiratory and expiratory capacity of the lungs. COPD may result from chronic bronchitis (excess mucus production) or emphysema (lung tissue damage with a loss of the elastic recoil of the lungs). COPD patients usually suffer from a combination of chronic bronchitis and emphysema.

What typically happens when a COPD patient seeks EMS assistance?

Patients with COPD function at a certain baseline level until an event occurs that causes decompensation. This is known as an

acute COPD episode (exacerbation) and is usually when EMS is called for help.

Anatomically, how does the pathology of chronic bronchitis differ from that of emphysema?

Chronic bronchitis results from overgrowth of the airway mucus glands and an excess secretion of mucus that blocks the airway. These patients have a productive cough for at least three months per year for two or more consecutive years. *Emphysema* results from a destruction of the walls of the alveoli as shown in Figure 22–3. Normally, exhalation is a passive process resulting from the elastic recoil of the lungs after they have expanded, similar to air coming out of a balloon after it has been blown up. The loss of normal alveolar structure leads to a decrease in the elastic recoil, which creates resistance to expiratory airflow. Air is trapped within the lungs, resulting in poor air exchange.

CLINICAL PEARL

It's difficult to discriminate between emphysema and chronic bronchitis in early emergency care (out-of-hospital or ED). The good news is: it doesn't really matter. The clinical approach is identical for nearly all patients with COPD.

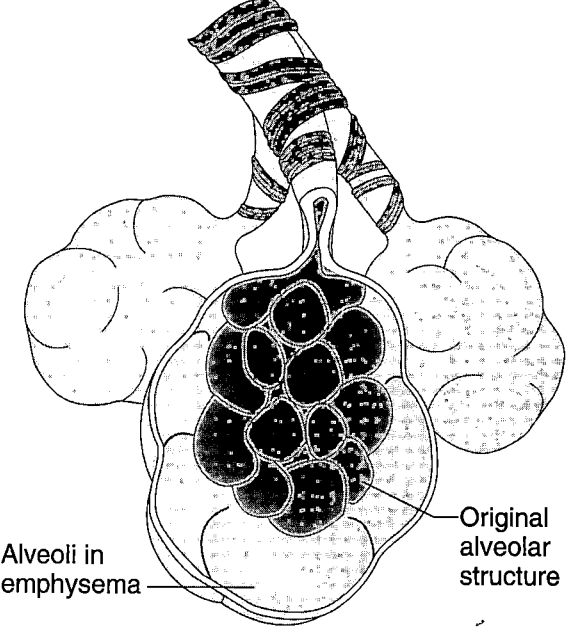

Alveoli in emphysema

Original alveolar structure

FIGURE 22–3 The alveoli of the emphysema patient.

Most patients with COPD have a combination of the features of both chronic bronchitis and emphysema. They have marked resistance within their airways to air movement. The work required to breathe is considerable.

Q What causes COPD?

A The major cause of COPD is cigarette smoking. Industrial inhalants (e.g., asbestos and coal dust), air pollution, and tuberculosis also contribute to the condition.

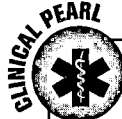

Very few individuals develop COPD without a smoking history. Nonsmokers who develop COPD often have a congenital deficiency of a lung enzyme, such as alpha-1-antitrypsin.

Q What are the differences, if any, between the typical onset of an asthmatic attack versus an acute exacerbation of COPD?

A Many asthmatic patients keep medications at home for attacks. Usually, they try these remedies before calling EMS. Victims will often report a recent upper-respiratory infection, often with a cough. Their symptoms often come on relatively quickly, as compared with persons with COPD. The patient with an acute COPD episode complains of a shortness of breath with symptoms gradually increasing over a period of days.

Be certain to ask about the recent use of over-the-counter asthma medications (e.g., Primatine Mist®). Though these agents are helpful, some patients react adversely to the inactive "filler" ingredients.

Q What is meant by the statement "all that wheezes is not asthma?"

A Wheezing may also be present with other diseases that cause dyspnea, such as COPD, heart failure, pulmonary embolism, pneumothorax, toxic inhalation, foreign body aspiration, and other pathological states. Always consider the possibility of a foreign body in the airway, especially in young children with wheezing and no history of asthma. A complete history and thorough patient examination are necessary for appropriate emergency care decisions.

Remember, "all that wheezes is not asthma." Isolated inspiratory wheezing suggests foreign body obstruction, especially in a child.

Q Why are the following medications potentially useful in the treatment of obstructive lung disease: epinephrine (e.g., terbutaline), aminophylline, inhaled sympathomimetic agents (e.g., albuterol), parasympatholytic drugs (e.g., ipratropium, atropine), steroids, and leukotriene antagonists?

A Many medications have bronchodilating effects. Nebulized bronchodilators, such as albuterol, are the most commonly used field agents.

- Epinephrine—once the treatment of choice for an acute asthma attack, epinephrine remains an option in severe cases. In these individuals, intravenous epinephrine (1:10,000) 1–5 cc (0.1 mg to 0.5 mg) may be lifesaving. A continuous infusion (1 mg in 250 cc D5W or NaCl titrated to effect) is another option.

- Terbutaline—has a beta-stimulating effect similar to that of epinephrine, but lasts 6–8 hours and may result in fewer side effects. Terbutaline may be given either subcutaneously (.25 mg) or via nebulizer.

Though there are only a few out-of-hospital studies, terbutaline is an effective and underused alternative treatment for obstructive lung disease.

- Aminophylline—once a drug of choice for both asthma and COPD, aminophylline (theophylline) derivatives are used far less commonly now. Though the data surrounding their use are controversial, studies still show that a group of patients will benefit. The clinical challenge is that is it difficult to predict, *in advance*, who will benefit. Aminophylline remains an option, generally for in-hospital use, because it is rarely carried by EMS providers in the field anymore.

- Inhaled sympathomimetic agents—a variety of drugs are available, though albuterol is used most commonly in the United States. Stimulation of the sympathetic nervous system, predominantly via beta-1 receptors, causes bronchodilation. Though you should always follow your local protocols when administering any drug, data suggest that nebulized treatments need *not* be given 20 minutes apart. The effect of up to three consecutive treatments, waiting only to re-evaluate the patient, is well established as safe and effective in most cases.

- Parasympatholytic drugs—because the parasympathetic nervous system effects tend to be the *opposite* of those of the sympathetic nervous system, it should come as no surprise that parasympathetic stimulation causes *bronchoconstriction*. Though this has been known for many years, atropine was not widely used in the treatment of obstructive airway disease. An atropine analogue, ipratropium bromide (Atrovent®), is now available in aerosol ("puffer") and nebulized form.

> **PEARL**
>
> *Some EMS systems are currently evaluating a combination of albuterol and ipratropium for routine use, but the verdict is not yet in.*

- Steroids—the anti-inflammatory effects cover many abnormal chemical mediators and cells present in acute asthma attacks. Some evidence also suggests that inflammation underlies many exacerbations of COPD. Steroids are beneficial in the chronic treatment of nearly all asthmatic patients and many COPD patients. As such, inhaled steroids have been first-line drugs in many patients. The inhaled form results in fewer side effects than the oral preparations, though inhaled steroids are not free of side effects. Additional steroids, either oral or parenteral, underlie the successful treatment of acute obstructive airway disease (e.g., asthma and COPD). Because these drugs require at least one to two hours to have an effect, the earlier they are given, the better. Though far from a field "standard of care," some EMS systems are routinely administering steroids along with nebulized bronchodilator agents.

> **PEARL**
>
> *Some EMS systems carry steroids. Because these drugs take at least one or two hours to work, initiating therapy in the field has a sound scientific basis. Follow your local protocols.*

- Leukotriene blockers—one of the major inflammation-causing compounds ("inflammatory mediators") produced in asthma are leukotrienes. They are blocked, to some extent, by steroids. Specific agents that directly attack leukotriene production or action have emerged in the past few years. These drugs either block the leukotriene receptor or block an enzyme (5-lipoxygenase) that synthesizes leukotrienes. Leukotriene blockers are not indicated as acute therapy at this time. Their success in chronic therapy has been somewhat disappointing, though approximately 35 percent of patients show some benefit.

Q **Which leukotriene blockers are currently available?**

A Three agents are commercially available in the United States. All are oral preparations and are *not* indicated for emergency ("rescue") use:

- Zafirlukast (Accolate®), montelukast (Singulair®)—block the leukotriene receptor, thus exerting an anti-inflammation effect.
- Zileuton (Zyflo®)—blocks the enzyme 5-lipoxygenase that catalyzes the synthesis of leukotrienes. The net effect is anti-inflammatory.

Q **Does magnesium offer any benefit to asthmatic patients?**

A Several studies have shown minimal additional effects of magnesium sulfate infusions in asthma. The magnesium acts as a smooth muscle relaxer. No data have shown magnesium to be harmful. It may be of benefit in selected patients, but data do not support routine emergency use, in- or out-of-hospital.

Q **Do all patients with obstructive lung disease require IV fluids?**

A There are really two different issues here—the first involves IV access overall. Few would disagree that having an IV lifeline available before things "hit the fan" is better. The real issue is whether or not IV or oral hydration allows people with obstructive lung disease to clear their secretions better. This approach was routine for asthma, and for some COPD patients, for years. The pendulum has swung. Currently, the approach is to reduce fluids unless the patient is dehydrated clinically. There are two reasons for this change:

- Studies showed that IV fluids really did not affect a person's ability to cough and clear secretions unless the person was clinically dehydrated to begin with.
- Steroids are used commonly in the treatment of both asthma and COPD. It is possible that chronic steroid use could predispose a patient to fluid retention problems, possibly even pulmonary edema, if excessive fluids were routinely used.

Q **How much oxygen should be administered to a patient in respiratory distress? Does a history of COPD influence the decision?**

A Unfortunately, there is still some disagreement in EMS about giving oxygen to patients with COPD. The basis for this argument is the fact that there are two separate respiratory drives:

- The carbon dioxide drive. When you hold your breath, CO_2 accumulates in the blood. After a period, the level of CO_2 gets high enough to stimulate breathing centers in the brain. The reflex response is to take a breath. The accumulation of carbon dioxide in our blood is the major stimulus that normally causes us to breathe.

- The hypoxic drive. A secondary mechanism that stimulates breathing is a lack of oxygen in the blood. If the level of oxygen in the blood goes very low, brain breathing centers are stimulated, leading to the reflex response of breathing.

A small number of patients with COPD do not effectively excrete carbon dioxide from their lungs. Carbon dioxide is always elevated in their bloodstream. These patients are called carbon dioxide retainers. These patients have lost their carbon dioxide drive to breathe. The only thing that stimulates breathing is the low level of oxygen in their blood (the hypoxic drive).

If a high level of oxygen is given to a CO_2 retainer, hypoxia, the only remaining stimulus for breathing, is eliminated. The patient could develop hypoventilation and eventually respiratory arrest. Based on this logic, some EMS protocols limit the use of oxygen to a low concentration. Others recommend the field use of Venturi masks to give precise O_2 concentrations.

Only a few COPD patients are at risk for developing respiratory arrest from a high oxygen concentration. Unfortunately, determining in the field who these patients are is impossible. A reasonable approach to take is as follows:

- Unless the patient is in marked respiratory distress, give 1–3 lpm via nasal cannula. If the patient is on home oxygen, use the prescribed setting. This is not enough oxygen to harm patients in the field even if they are CO_2 retainers.

- If the patient is in severe distress and appears to require higher oxygen concentrations, use what you decide to be appropriate. Observe the patient carefully for changes in the respiratory rate and MS. If the patient begins to deteriorate, the O_2 concentration may be decreased. Bear in mind that problems other than excessive oxygen can cause these patients to deteriorate. Assist their breathing as necessary.

- As a rule, give the patient the amount of oxygen you consider necessary for his condition; do not withhold high-concentration oxygen, when required, just because the patient might be a CO_2 retainer. In reality, this is quite unusual.

Pneumonia

Q What is pneumonia?

A *Pneumonia* is an acute inflammatory condition of the lungs, usually caused by either bacterial or viral infection.

Q What factors predispose patients to pneumonia?

A Several risk factors make people more likely to get pneumonia:

- Cigarette smoking—the smoke directly inhibits the normal movement of mucus via bronchial cilia out of the lung. As a result, the lung is unable to clear pathogens (e.g., bacteria, viruses) as effectively. Allowed to remain, these infectious agents multiply, resulting in pneumonia.

- Alcoholism—drinkers are especially likely to get aspiration pneumonia (inhaling their vomit) during passing-out spells. Even without aspiration, chronic alcoholics have an increased risk of acquiring infections because of a weakened immune system due to the ethanol.

- Cold exposure—though it is a myth that mild cold exposure causes pneumonia, prolonged acute or chronic hypothermia exerts a severe toll on the body's immune system. Pneumonia is especially common in elderly patients who are chronically hypothermic, often under less than ideal living conditions.

- Extremes of age—both the very young and the elderly are more susceptible to pneumonia than other groups of people.

- Abnormal immune system—diseases such as acquired immunodeficiency syndrome (AIDS) predispose victims to severe infections, including pneumonia. Other potential high-risk patients include those on chronic steroid therapy (especially oral), cancer chemotherapy, or antirejection drugs following a transplant.

Q What types of infectious agents cause pneumonia?

A Pneumonia is most commonly bacterial, though viruses and fungi may also cause it. Community-acquired pneumonia is often caused by *Diplococci* or *Mycoplasma pneumoniae* organisms. These infections do not tend to be as severe as hospital-acquired ones that are more commonly due to gram-negative bacteria such as *Pseudomonas*.

CLINICAL PEARL

On balance, the risks of hypoxia by failing to give an appropriate concentration of oxygen to a patient are far greater than any theoretical risk of suppressing the respiratory drive in a COPD patient with CO_2 retention. Clinical data have shown that even if oxygen administration results in an increase in the pCO_2, the minute volume (amount of air exchanged in a minute) remains unchanged.

> *It is impossible to tell in the out-of-hospital setting whether a person has bacterial versus viral pneumonia. Fortunately, the clinical approach is identical.*

Q | What clinical findings are present in the "typical" patient with pneumonia?

A | The "typical" picture of bacterial pneumonia is heralded by an acute onset of fever and chills. Cough productive of purulent (rust-colored or green) sputum soon follows. Depending on the location of the infection, the patient may have pleuritic chest pain—pain that worsens with deep breathing or moving due to inflammation near the external lung surface. Physical findings vary widely, though crackles and signs of pulmonary consolidation (e.g., bronchial breath sounds, decreased breath sounds) are often present.

> *Pneumonia in older patients is a common precipitant of congestive heart failure or pulmonary edema (Figure 22–4). Pneumonia may also coexist with exacerbations of chronic lung disease.*

Q | How do patients with "atypical" pneumonia differ from those with the "typical" disease?

A | "Atypical" symptoms are more common in viral pneumonia, and in the very young or very old. These include:

- Nonproductive cough.
- Headache.
- Myalgias (muscle aches).
- Fatigue.
- Sore throat.
- Nausea, vomiting, diarrhea.
- Fever and chills (continuous versus the dramatic onset that occurs in "typical" pneumonia).

Q | What should be your first consideration when dealing with a patient who may have pneumonia?

A | Consider any patient with possible pneumonia to be contagious and act accordingly.

Q | What is the role of drug therapy in the field treatment of pneumonia? Do antibiotics play a role?

A | At times, inhaled beta-2 agonists (e.g., albuterol) may be helpful, especially if the patient has accompanying obstructive

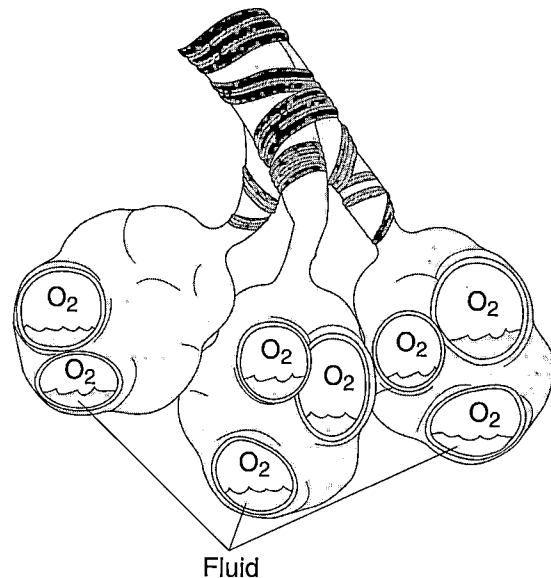

Fluid

FIGURE 22–4 Pneumonia often is accompanied by pulmonary congestion.

lung disease—follow your local protocols. Generally, antibiotics are not given in the field. Use aspirin or acetaminophen for pain and fever if permitted by your local protocols.

Upper-Respiratory Infection (URI)

Q | What is an upper-respiratory infection (URI)?

A | URI is an acute, usually self-limited infection of any part of the upper-respiratory tract. Most commonly, the mouth, throat, and ears are affected.

Q | How does a URI differ from the "common cold?"

A | The terms are nearly interchangeable provided the URI is caused by a virus, as is the "common cold." Sometimes either the throat (pharyngitis) or the ears (otitis) are selectively affected. Still, either a virus or a bacterium may be responsible. Because it is impossible to tell the cause in the out-of-hospital setting, the generic term "URI" is preferable.

Q | How does a URI differ from influenza (the "flu")?

A | Influenza or "the flu" is a specific type of viral infection that may affect both the upper (e.g., dry, hacking cough with diffuse muscle aches) and lower respiratory tracts (pneumonia). There are some drugs that may alleviate flu symptoms, but they must be given within the first 48 hours of symptom onset. No drug has yet been shown to specifically improve a viral URI, except influenza. Influenza pneumonia is rare, but results in severe hypoxia (see "atypical pneumonia").

How common is URI?

Most people have a URI once or twice a year. Patients with an underlying disease, such as COPD or cancer, may have them more frequently. People with more than six URIs in a year should be evaluated by a physician for possible immune deficiency diseases.

What are the causes of URI?

Viruses are the most common cause. Some bacteria, such as *Streptococcus pneumoniae* or *Haemophilus influenzae* are also common causes. It is impossible to differentiate viral from bacterial causes without cultures. There is too much overlap in the clinical features of both to be helpful, in- or out-of-hospital.

What is the pathophysiology of URI?

Typically, the organism invades the lining (mucosa) of the upper-respiratory tract. This results in localized inflammation and swelling. Lymph nodes usually trap the organisms and prevent further spread.

What are the signs and symptoms of URI?

The clinical presentation varies depending on the organism and the location(s) infected. Typically, most patients have a combination of:

- Fever, chills.
- Muscle and joint aches (myalgias, arthralgias).
- Diaphoresis.
- Sore throat.

Some viral URIs cause bronchospasm, even in people without a history of obstructive lung disease. They may present with wheezing. The clinical treatment is similar to that for asthma. Once the URI resolves, the bronchospasm usually (but not always) disappears. A few patients develop a chronic obstructive lung disease, especially asthma, from early viral URI. The rapidity of treatment does not seem to influence this outcome.

- Cough (usually nonproductive).
- Earache.
- Swollen lymph glands in the neck and under the jaw.

What complications can occur from a URI?

Most patients with a URI have a spontaneous resolution of symptoms within seven days, with or without antibiotics. People who have an underlying disease (e.g., immune suppression, COPD, congestive heart failure) may develop more severe infections, such as pneumonia or sepsis. In addition, viral URI is a common precipitant of acute exacerbations of asthma and COPD.

What is the out-of-hospital management of patients with a URI?

Other than the maintenance of the ABCs, there is little specific care to provide for a URI in the field. Remember, most URIs are contagious, so act accordingly. Rarely, people develop an airway obstruction or respiratory failure. Fever may lead to dehydration and hypotension, but rarely causes shock unless a systemic infection is also present. Follow your local protocols regarding alternative transportation routes and sources of health care for stable people with an acute URI.

What about patients who have had their spleen removed (splenectomy)? Doesn't this increase the danger of a "simple" URI?

YES! Patients who have undergone a splenectomy, regardless of when the surgery was performed, lose resistance to common organisms that often cause a bacterial URI (*Streptococcus pneumoniae*). Remember, the spleen is responsible for the production of lymphocytes. Without prompt parenteral antibiotic treatment, their "mild cold symptoms" may progress to full-blown septic shock. This rapid demise often occurs in less than 24 hours. Assume that any person who has had the spleen removed and presents with a URI to have a life-threatening illness! They require prompt transport to an appropriate hospital. These patients are *not* appropriate candidates for any type of "treat and release" or "alternative transportation" plan that may exist for minor illness.

Neoplasm of the Lung

As EMS providers we often transport patients who have neoplasms. What does the term "neoplasm" mean?

"Neoplasm" literally means "new growth." In modern medical terms, it refers to some type of tumor, either benign (non-cancerous) or malignant (cancerous). Benign neoplasms are relatively common and rarely require emergency care. Malignant lung neoplasms ("lung cancers") are far more worrisome.

> *Some patients have had benign nodules removed from their lungs. These are not cancerous, though the patient may refer to them as "tumors." Try to ascertain whether or not the patient was told the lesion was "cancerous," and what type, if any, of treatment was used after removal of the lesion.*

What are the types of lung cancer?

Malignant neoplasms (referred to as "lung cancer") may be either primary or metastatic:

- Primary tumors arise from lung tissue (including the bronchi).
- Metastatic tumors spead to the lung from another site by direct invasion, via the blood, or through the lymphatic system.

What are the causes of lung cancer?

The most common cause of primary lung tumors is cigarette smoking. Other diseases, such as coal miner's lung and asbestosis, also predispose people to lung cancer, but cigarettes often still play a role. There are no specific factors that determine whether or not a tumor in another part of the body will spread to the lungs.

What are the signs and symptoms of lung cancer?

Many lung cancers are asymptomatic and discovered on routine chest x-ray examination. Some patients present with weakness, weight loss, or cough. Others have pneumonia that does not resolve in the normal period of time. Sometimes patients discover swelling in the axilla (armpit) or supraclavicular fossa (above the clavicle) due to lymph node metastases. Rarely, patients present with shortness of breath or hemoptysis due to the rupture of a previously unknown tumor into a large pulmonary blood vessel.

Where does primary lung cancer tend to metastasize?

Primary lung tumors commonly spread:
- Within the lung itself.
- To the opposite lung.
- To the pleura.
- To the ribs.
- To the lymphatic system.
- To the liver and spleen.

Which tumors commonly metastasize to the lung?

Any tumor can metastasize to the lung. The most common are:

- Breast.
- Colon.
- Liver.
- Prostate.

What types of treatment modalities are employed by cancer specialists (oncologists) for lung cancer?

Usual treatment includes chemotherapy, radiation therapy, or a combination of both. Often, EMS providers get involved in the transport of patients who are going for their treatments or who have experienced the side effects of the treatments.

What are the side effects of chemotherapy for lung cancer? How might these come to the attention of the out-of-hospital provider?

The most common side effects from chemotherapy are nausea, vomiting, diarrhea, and hair loss. Some patients become significantly dehydrated following therapy. Many drugs also lead to bone marrow suppression. This may result in decreased numbers of red blood cells (anemia, weakness), white blood cells (increased susceptibility to infection), and platelets (increased risk of bleeding). Some forms of chemotherapy cause peripheral nerve problems, resulting in severe pain (usually in the legs and feet).

What are the side effects of radiotherapy for lung cancer? How might these come to the attention of the out-of-hospital provider?

A number of side effects may occur, though most rarely come to the attention of the out-of-hospital care provider. Sometimes irradiation leads to bone marrow depression and severe infection. More commonly, patients have a dry cough or are asymptomatic. Scar tissue from radiation treatment may restrict lung expansion, leading to a shortness of breath or pneumonia.

What is an implanted IV port? Can I use this to give out-of-hospital fluids and medications?

Though there are many varieties and names, all have a long IV catheter either attached to a reservoir port (usually implanted in the subcutaneous tissue) or an IV cap (e.g., a long-line heparin lock or Hickman catheter®). Avoid using these as "quick and easy" IV routes.

What complications of lung cancer are likely to come to the attention of out-of-hospital providers?

Cancer is a chronic disease and may lead to a number of problems including malnutrition, and fluid–electrolyte imbalance. Both chemotherapy and radiotherapy may also result in serious side effects. Specific problems directly related to primary or metastatic lung cancer include:

- Loss of normal lung tissue and a shortness of breath.
- Cavitating disease (air filled cavities due to the destruction of normal tissue); these may rupture, leading to a spontaneous pneumothorax.
- Invasion of a pulmonary or bronchial blood vessel. A rare, but dramatic, event is the erosion of a lung tumor into a large artery. The result is severe hemoptysis (coughing up blood). Unstopped, death often results. Sometimes deliberately placing a large ET tube down the affected bronchus allows the patient to be selectively ventilated through the other lung. This is relatively easy if the lesion is on the patient's right side. Special blades and tubes are often required to obtain selective left mainstem intubation.
- Some lung tumors lead to the abnormal production of parathormone (parathyroid hormone), which causes bone breakdown, raising serum calcium levels (hypercalcemia). Weakness, depression, abdominal pain, and hypotonic muscles may result.

What is the out-of-hospital treatment for patients with lung neoplasms?

Most often, out-of-hospital treatment is directed toward breathing problems, respiratory infections, or the side effects of either chemotherapy or radiation, rather than the cancer itself. The fact that a patient has cancer does not mean that she cannot have other medical problems. Always do a complete patient survey.

CLINICAL PEARL

Avoid the temptation of developing "cancer vision"— assuming that any problem in a cancer patient is always related to the cancer. Just like any other patient, there may be a different and treatable cause. Also remember, you cannot "catch" cancer from a patient. Use the same body substance isolation (BSI) procedures you would on any patient. There is no need to act differently.

Pulmonary Edema

What is pulmonary edema?

Pulmonary edema refers to the filling of the lungs with fluid in the interstitial spaces, the alveoli, or both. It is not a disease in itself, but rather a pathophysiological condition resulting from many causes.

What are the classifications of pulmonary edema based on mechanism?

Mechanistically, pulmonary edema is classified as either *high pressure* or *high permeability*. The origin of this differentiation is based on a law described early last century by the physiologist, Starling. He noted that two factors determine the flow into or out of a fluid-filled biological tube, such as a pulmonary capillary:

- The permeability of the tube's walls.
- The hydrostatic pressure ("water pressure") of the fluid inside.

Thus, we classify pulmonary edema based on whether the pressure is elevated (high pressure) or whether the permeability is abnormal (high permeability). Though the physiology is fascinating, it is often difficult to distinguish clinically (especially in the field) one form from the other.

CLINICAL PEARL

The most common form of pulmonary edema we see in the out-of-hospital setting is cardiogenic hydrostatic due to myocardial ischemia. Sometimes it's difficult to differentiate this from COPD—some EMS systems routinely use both inhaled bronchodilators and furosemide in this situation.

Why are the terms "high-pressure" and "high-permeability" pulmonary edema more accurate than "cardiogenic" and "noncardiogenic?"

The most common causes of high-pressure pulmonary edema are cardiac, though other diseases (e.g., scorpion bites, brain injury, diving accidents) may also raise the hydrostatic pressure in the lungs. Consequently, many people often, though incorrectly, refer to high-pressure pulmonary edema as "cardiogenic." Similarly, the term "noncardiogenic pulmonary edema" is often used for high-permeability edema when, in reality, noncardiac factors can also raise the hydrostatic pressure.

Sometimes health care providers incorrectly classify *all* noncardiogenic pulmonary edema as adult respiratory distress syndrome (ARDS). ARDS is a highly specific diagnosis consisting of high-permeability pulmonary edema, due to any of several causes, *and* the inability to adequately oxygenate the blood despite 100 percent FiO_2. Administering 100 percent oxygen often requires a ventilator in a hospital setting, and arterial blood gas measurements are needed to confirm the diagnosis. Even when these are both available, the diagnosis of ARDS is often erroneously applied! The proper classification of acute pulmonary edema is based purely on mechanism, that is high pressure or high permeability.

How is gas exchange impaired in high-pressure pulmonary edema?

In high-pressure pulmonary edema:

- Ischemia leads to acute failure of the left ventricle.
- The inability of the ventricle to pump blood adequately results in an increase in ventricular pressure.
- Increased ventricular pressure is back-transmitted to the left atrium, then the pulmonary vessels, causing an increase in the pulmonary venous pressure.
- Elevated pulmonary venous pressure results in increased pulmonary capillary hydrostatic pressure.
- The engorged vessels leak fluid into the interstitial space due to the elevated hydrostatic pressure (Starling's mechanism).
- As coughing and lymphatic drainage fail to drain the excess fluid, it accumulates in the interstitial space.
- Fluid accumulation causes expansion of the interstitial space, which impairs the diffusion of gases.
- If the amount of interstitial fluid is significant, alveoli fill with fluid and may also rupture from the pressure.

How is gas exchange impaired in high-permeability pulmonary edema?

During high-permeability pulmonary edema, the alveolar–capillary membrane is disrupted by any of several causes:

- Severe hypotension.
- Severe hypoxemia (e.g., post drowning, post-cardiac arrest, severe seizure, prolonged hypoventilation).
- High altitude.
- Environmental toxins (e.g., chlorine gas inhalation).
- Septic shock.

Because of the membrane disruption, fluid leaks into the interstitial space. The widening of the interstitial space by fluid impairs diffusion. Though possible, alveolar filling with fluid in high-permeability pulmonary edema is less frequent than in high-pressure pulmonary edema.

What are common similarities and differences between high-pressure and high-permeability pulmonary edema?

The most common presentation of pulmonary edema, whatever the cause, is an acute onset of shortness of breath. In high-permeability cases, symptoms may develop over a longer period, but an acute onset is still common.

CLINICAL PEARL

The "classic" presentation of cardiogenic hydrostatic pulmonary edema is a rapid onset (over minutes) of severe shortness of breath. Exacerbations of asthma or COPD typically develop over hours to days.

Why are the terms "congestive heart failure" and pulmonary edema often confused?

Pulmonary edema is a general term for fluid in the lung, for any of several reasons. Congestive heart failure (CHF) is a spectrum ranging from mild to severe decreases in cardiac function. Sometimes people with severe CHF develop pulmonary edema—typically, they do not. People with acute pulmonary edema due to cardiac ischemia have severe CHF, but not all patients with severe CHF have pulmonary edema.

Why do patients with either CHF or pulmonary edema have an increased shortness of breath while lying down (orthopnea)?

The recumbent position *increases* venous return to the heart. The result is an increase in the preload or amount of blood that the heart must pump out. The normal heart compensates for this by dilating slightly, pumping harder, and pumping faster. In CHF or pulmonary edema, this "defense mechanism" is ineffective. Pressure backs up into the lungs, causing increased fluid flow from the pulmonary capillaries into the interstitial spaces. This fluid is then absorbed into lymphatic channels, causing distention of lung tissue. Stretch receptors in the lung parenchyma (tissue) fire, resulting in the sensation of dyspnea. When the patient sits or stands, the preload decreases, and the process reverses.

What percentage of patients with high-pressure pulmonary edema have an acute myocardial infarction (MI)?

Less than 50 percent of patients with acute cardiogenic high-pressure pulmonary edema suffer a concomitant MI. Pulmonary edema, like MI, angina or sudden death, is just another manifestation of severe myocardial ischemia.

Why do patients with acute pulmonary edema often refuse to wear an oxygen mask?

High-flow oxygen is preferable, but people with acute pulmonary edema often refuse a mask. The reason is that they are already markedly short of breath—putting a mask over their face may make them feel like they are suffocating. This worsens patient anxiety and causes the release of epinephrine from the patient's adrenal gland. Epinephrine causes the heart to work harder, worsening myocardial function. So, unless you are easily able to convince the patient to wear the mask, use a nasal cannula initially. Of course, if a patient's condition is deteriorating, assisted ventilation and intubation as required must be performed.

What are the current roles for nitroglycerin, furosemide, and morphine sulphate in the treatment of acute high-pressure pulmonary edema due to myocardial ischemia?

General information and the most commonly used doses of each drug follow. Adhere to your specific local protocols.

- Nitroglycerin—dilates both the veins and the arteries. Vasodilation decreases the amount of blood returned to the heart (preload), thus decreasing the amount it must pump out with each stroke. Arterial dilation decreases the workload against which the heart must pump (afterload). Generally, if the patient's systolic BP is greater than 100 mmHG, then sublingual (one 1/150 grain [0.4 mg] tablet) or nitroglycerin (NTG) spray (one spray) is a first-line drug in cardiogenic pulmonary edema. The dose may be repeated every five minutes, to a limit of three, as needed.

- Furosemide (Lasix™)—has several effects in acute pulmonary edema. It vasodilates causing a decrease in the cardiac preload (venous return). In addition, furosemide increases lymphatic flow from the lungs back into the circulatory system, helping to drain the lungs of fluid. Finally, the diuretic effect causes the kidneys to eliminate the excess fluid from the body. Furosemide is usually given IV (initial dose is 40 mg; may be repeated in 10–20 minutes as needed) in acute pulmonary edema.

- Morphine sulfate—a narcotic analgesic (painkiller) that also has significant effects on the central nervous system, causing dilation of both veins and arteries. As with nitroglycerin, both cardiac preload and afterload are reduced, allowing the heart to work more efficiently. Morphine sulfate also allays patient anxiety. Morphine is usually given IV (2 mg every five minutes as needed) in acute pulmonary edema.

What other drugs are "on the horizon" for possible field use for pulmonary edema?

There are two types of drugs that we are likely to see as part of our routine therapy for pulmonary edema, referring specifically to high-pressure "cardiogenic" pulmonary edema:

- Angiotensin converting enzyme (ACE) inhibitors—block the conversion of angiotensin I to angiotensin II in the lungs. Angiotensin II is a powerful vasoconstrictor—by blocking it, vasodilation occurs, leading to a decrease in cardiac work. Other mechanisms are likely involved as well. ACE inhibitors have been used to treat hypertension and CHF for years. They are emerging into the forefront of therapy, both oral and IV, in both acute MI and pulmonary edema. The most studied of these is captopril (Capoten®)—limited data suggest that 12.5 mg either sublingual or IV leads to improvement beyond that already engendered by nitroglycerin, furosemide, and morphine.

- Spironolactone (Aldactone®)—blocks the action of the hormone aldosterone on the kidneys. Aldosterone, when active, causes the retention of sodium and water and the excretion of potassium. Spironolactone has been used in the treatment of mild hypertension for many years but because it was a relatively weak agent, others replaced it. Recent data show that simply adding oral spironolactone to the drug regimen of people with chronic CHF improves their two-year survival rate significantly. If this "pans out" for "acute CHF" (pulmonary edema), it will likely be used alongside ACE blockers as first-line therapy.

What about the role of positive pressure breathing in the treatment of pulmonary edema?

Positive pressure breathing is a generic term for several different types of both invasive and noninvasive ventilatory assistance. Increased airway pressure causes the expansion of previously atelectatic (collapsed) portions of the lung and improves overall ventilation. In addition, it may increase intrathoracic pressure and counteract increased pulmonary capillary hydrostatic pressure.

ET intubation is *not* always required to take advantage of positive pressure breathing. A demand-valve resuscitator (DVR) is a form of positive pressure ventilation. Studies have shown that by increasing intrathoracic pressure, positive pressure breathing with a simple DVR leads to significant improvement in pulmonary edema patients.

Various devices for external noninvasive ventilation have evolved. Continuous positive airway pressure (CPAP) face masks improve oxygenation in many diseases including asthma, COPD, and some cases of acute pulmonary edema. They also provide necessary oxygenation for people with sleep apnea, a condition that results in periodic cessation of breathing during sleep.

The most recent development is *biphasic positive airway pressure* (BiPAP)—positive pressure is delivered to the lungs throughout the respiratory cycle via a tight-fitting nasal mask. The provider can vary the inspiratory and expiratory pressures independently. BiPAP masks have been used successfully in intensive care units, hospital floors, and EDs. Limited data from the out-of-hospital setting look promising. Depending on the results of ongoing studies, BiPAP noninvasive ventilation may become routine for many patients with respiratory emergencies, not just for pulmonary edema.

CLINICAL PEARL

Sometimes the use of a simple positive-pressure mask (DVR) will, if tolerated initially, increase the intrathoracic pressure sufficiently to effect marked improvement in patients, even without drug therapy.

Pulmonary Thromboembolism

Define pulmonary embolism. What is the difference between pulmonary embolism and pulmonary thromboembolism?

Pulmonary embolism (PE) is the blockage of a pulmonary artery by foreign matter as in Figure 22–5. Usually, the obstruction is due to a piece of a blood clot that has broken away from a pelvic or deep leg vein. The term *thromboembolism* refers to a combination of two processes, the formation of a venous thrombus (clot) followed by a fragment breaking off into the venous circulation (embolus).

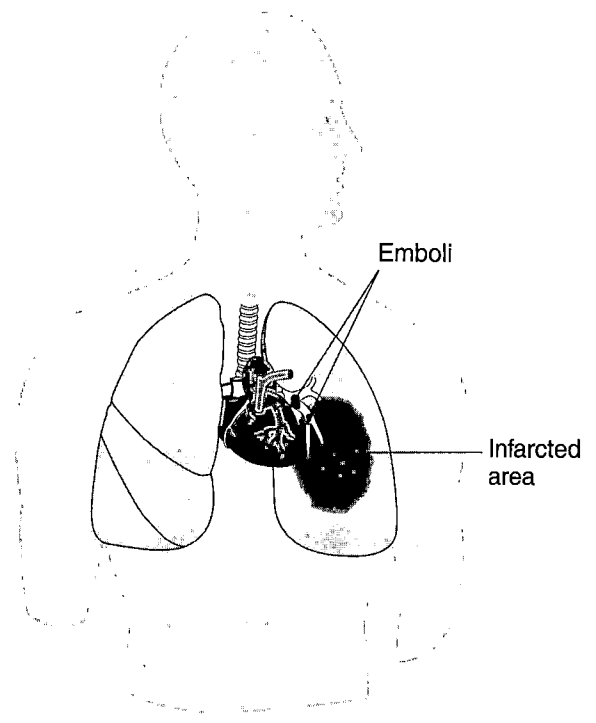

Emboli

Infarcted area

FIGURE 22–5 Pulmonary emboli.

What else, besides blood clots, causes pulmonary emboli?

Other causes of pulmonary emboli include fat, amniotic fluid, air, or tumor tissue.

What are common risk factors for PE? Why does each increase the patient's risk?

Risks for PE include:

- Sedentary lifestyle (prolonged inactivity or being bedridden)—normally venous blood is returned to the heart by the "milking action" of muscular contractions. Prolonged inactivity (e.g., long auto ride, flying) or being bedridden decreases much of this normal muscle movement. As a result, venous flow may become hampered, leading to localized activation of the blood clotting (coagulation) system and thrombosis formation. Pieces of thrombi break off becoming pulmonary emboli. PE is common in hospitalized patients and in those who have completed long auto or airplane trips.

- Obesity—decreased movement likely plays a role. In addition, obesity may have direct effects on the coagulation system.

- Infection—severe infection occurs in bedridden people. In some infections, particularly sepsis, abnormal activation of the coagulation system may lead to emboli.

- Cancer—certain tumors (e.g., kidney, lung) produce substances that make the blood more coagulable ("thicker") and increase the risk of embolism.

- Thrombophlebitis—an inflammation of the veins for any cause predisposes patients to localized thrombus formation.

- Oral contraceptives (birth control pills)—affect levels of natural anticoagulants in the blood resulting in a hypercoagulable state.

- Fracture of a long bone (e.g., femur, humerus)—the source of emboli is fat released from the bone marrow.

- Pregnancy—amniotic fluid embolism may occur during delivery. It is often fatal.

- Recent surgery—patients may remain in the same position on the operating table for several hours, leading to blood clot formation in the veins of the pelvis and legs.

- Blood diseases—rare blood disorders can make a patient's blood more likely to clot.

- Autoimmune (connective tissue) diseases—these (e.g., systemic lupus erythematosus) affect the body's level of intrinsic anticlotting proteins. The result is a hypercoagulable state in the blood.

PE is often an evasive diagnosis. Due to the variety of less common conditions that result in hypercoagulability (e.g., lupus), a good history may help diagnose a life-threatening condition.

What is the typical development of a PE?

Typical development of a PE follows this progression:

- Blood flow is altered in the peripheral vein due to injury to the vein wall, decreased movement of the patient, or other factors that increase the coagulability of the blood.
- Altered blood flow leads to platelet aggregation and activation of the body's coagulation system.
- A thrombosis or clot forms in the deep vein.
- For unknown reasons, pieces of the clot dislodge into the venous circulation and return to the heart as emboli.
- Emboli pass from the right atria through the tricuspid valve to the right ventricle. From there, they transverse the pulmonic valve and lodge in the pulmonary arterial circulation.
- As the clot passes through progressively smaller and smaller branches of the pulmonary circulation, it becomes lodged and a blockage occurs.
- Larger emboli occlude larger, more proximal branches of the pulmonary artery, while smaller ones travel to the smaller, more peripheral branches.
- The lung tissue supplied by the blocked artery becomes ischemic. If circulation to the lung is sufficiently compromised, the affected area dies (infarcts).
- If large pulmonary emboli occlude major branches of the pulmonary arteries, the heart is forced to pump blood against very high pressures. The result is often acute right-sided heart failure (acute cor pulmonale), syncope, shock, or cardiac arrest.
- Occlusion of the artery not only results in a decreased blood supply, but leads to the release of vasoactive substances (e.g., histamine) from white blood cells (WBCs). This causes a bronchospasm in the region of the clot and may be responsible for localized wheezing sometimes heard during the physical exam.

What findings may be present in a massive PE?

Patients with massive pulmonary emboli often suffer cardiac arrest or a syncopal spell as the first symptom of the illness. Altered MS, severe cyanosis, or profound hypotension also suggests the presence of a life-threatening embolus in a proximal location.

What are the typical findings for smaller pulmonary emboli?

Patients with smaller emboli may have the following signs and symptoms:

- Sudden, unexplained onset of chest pain that increases in intensity with a deep breath (pleuritic chest pain). The pain may be localized to the area of the chest overlying the involved lung tissue.
- Respiratory distress and shortness of breath. The patient's respiratory rate is usually increased. The patient may hyperventilate.
- Wheezing or coughing up of blood (hemoptysis).
- Anxiety.
- Shock (less common).
- Hypotension (less common).

What potentially serious diseases may mimic the symptoms and signs of a PE?

The signs and symptoms of a PE are often similar to MI or spontaneous pneumothorax.

Define pleuritic chest pain. What is its significance to people with respiratory problems?

Pleuritic chest pain is sharp discomfort felt when taking a deep breath. Pain clearly worsened by breathing is more likely to be due to a lung or chest wall problem than to myocardial ischemia. Of course, patients with acute MI may also have pleuritic pain, it is just less common. Pleuritic pain is common with small, peripheral pulmonary emboli because the pleural membranes next to the affected lung tissue become inflamed.

Though similar standards have not been published regarding out-of-hospital care, ED standards of care mandate that an important fact to determine in a patient with chest pain is whether or not it is pleuritic.

What are the common physical exam findings in patients with pulmonary emboli?

The most common physical findings are tachypnea and tachycardia. Breath sounds are usually normal, though localized wheezing is heard occasionally. After several hours, a grating sound (pleural friction rub) may be heard. Clinical evidence of deep vein thrombophlebitis is found in less than 50 percent of patients.

Q Why does a normal pulse oximetry reading *not* exclude the possibility of a pulmonary embolus?

A Though pulse oximetry often reveals low oxygen saturation, a normal value does *not* exclude PE. Like any test, it is most helpful when positive and confirmatory. A negative result rarely completely excludes the possibility of disease.

> **CLINICAL PEARL**
>
> *Unfortunately, the most common physical and diagnostic test findings in acute PE are "normal." Thus, we must always have a high clinical suspicion.*

Spontaneous Pneumothorax

Q What is spontaneous pneumothorax?

A Spontaneous pneumothorax is a sudden accumulation of air in the pleural space as shown in Figure 22–6. As the air enters the pleural space, the lung on the involved side collapses.

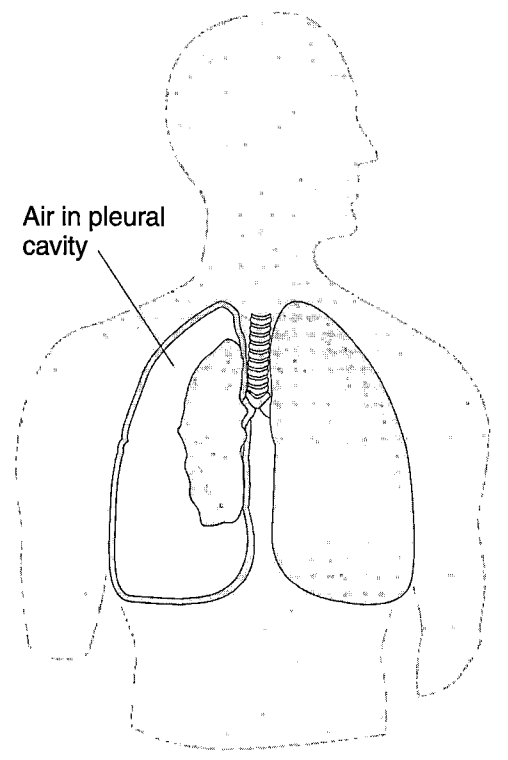

Air in pleural cavity

FIGURE 22–6 Pneumothorax.

Q Which patients are at highest risk for spontaneous pneumothorax and why?

A The most frequent cause of spontaneous pneumothorax is the rupture of a congenital defect (bleb) on the surface of the lung. A congenital bleb is an air-filled sac that has been present since birth. Young, tall, thin male smokers are most likely to develop pneumothorax from the rupture of a congenital bleb. The reasons for the association of smoking and bleb rupture are not clear.

Q Are there other potential causes of spontaneous pneumothorax besides congenital bleb rupture?

A Yes, less common causes of spontaneous pneumothorax include:

- Menstruation—spontaneous pneumothorax associated with menstruation is usually right-sided and occurs in women aged 20–30 years. It is thought to be secondary to the presence of endometrial tissue in the lung or a pleura that ruptures after swelling during the menstrual cycle.

- Lung disease involving the connective tissues of the lung.

- COPD—spontaneous pneumothorax associated with COPD is usually secondary to the rupture of defects that have formed from the destruction of normal lung tissue that results from COPD (bullae).

Q What is the typical clinical presentation of persons with spontaneous pneumothorax?

A Patients with spontaneous pneumothorax complain of the sudden onset of sharp chest pain accompanied by a shortness of breath. The pain is often localized to the side of the lung involved. Decreased breath sounds are present on the involved side and the patient's respiratory rate is increased. The patient may be coughing and be anxious or agitated.

Q What are the signs and symptoms of tension pneumothorax?

A The signs and symptoms of tension pneumothorax are:
- Increasing respiratory distress.
- Weak pulse.
- Cyanosis.
- Hypotension.
- Decreased breath sounds on the same side.
- Distended neck veins.

- Tracheal deviation away from the side of the pneumothorax—this is a late sign.
- Subcutaneous emphysema—crepitus may be felt in the skin of the chest wall overlying the collapsed lung.

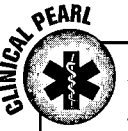

CLINICAL PEARL

Tension pneumothorax rarely occurs following spontaneous pneumothorax. However, always be alert to the possibility.

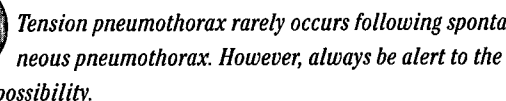

Hyperventilation

Q **What is hyperventilation?**

A *Hyperventilation* is a respiratory rate greater than that required for normal body function. It is the result of an increased frequency of breathing, an increased volume of air moved, or both. Hyperventilation causes an excessive intake of oxygen and the excessive elimination of carbon dioxide. Many disease states cause hyperventilation.

Q **What is anxiety-hyperventilation syndrome (also known as "hyperventilation syndrome")?**

A *Anxiety-hyperventilation syndrome* results in tachypnea without a physiologic demand for increased oxygen, leading to respiratory alkalosis.

Q **What is the pathophysiology of hyperventilation, whatever the cause?**

A Excessive excretion (blowing off) of carbon dioxide results in low blood levels (hypocapnia)—this disturbs the normal blood acid–base balance by increasing the pH. These pH changes can interfere with the normal function of other body systems.

Q **What conditions may result in hyperventilation?**

A Many conditions can result in hyperventilation. These include:
- Asthma attack.
- COPD.
- Myocardial infarction.
- PE.
- Spontaneous pneumothorax.

- CHF.
- Increased metabolism (e.g., exercise, fever, hyperthyroidism, infection).
- Central nervous system lesions (e.g., stroke, encephalitis, head injury, meningitis).
- Hypoxia.
- Accumulation of metabolic acids in the body (e.g., kidney failure, diabetic ketoacidosis, or alcohol poisoning).
- Drugs (e.g., cocaine, amphetamines, aspirin, epinephrine).
- Psychogenic factors (e.g., acute anxiety or pain).

Q **What is the major risk in caring for a patient with hyperventilation?**

A The major risk in caring for a patient with hyperventilation is to assume that anxiety is the basis of the symptoms. Many serious and life-threatening medical illnesses can cause hyperventilation. The patient can appear identical to someone with only a simple anxiety attack. A conservative approach demands that you assume the patient is seriously ill until it is proven otherwise.

CLINICAL PEARL

Assume that any hyperventilating patient has a serious problem until proven otherwise. Act accordingly.

Q **What is the current recommended role, if any, for "brown paper bag" treatment of hyperventilation?**

A Re-breathing is no longer an acceptable practice. Many patients who appear to have simple hyperventilation actually have a serious illness. Having the patient breathe into a paper bag causes a marked decrease in the available oxygen. Dangerous hypoxia can result. In addition, if the patient is hyperventilating as a compensatory mechanism against a metabolic acidosis (e.g., diabetic ketoacidosis), re-breathing expired air raises the pCO_2, *worsening* the acidosis!

CLINICAL PEARL

Research shows that the FiO_2 in a brown paper bag after only 30 seconds of re-breathing is significantly less than room air! Imagine a lawyer telling the jury: "By using this brown paper bag, these providers gave the deceased even less oxygen than he was getting before they arrived! He would have done better if they were never there in the first place!"

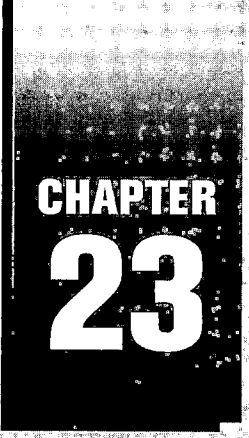

CHAPTER 23

Cardiology

This chapter reviews cardiac anatomy and physiology and discusses the pathophysiology of cardiac-related complaints. The focus is on the presentation and etiology of acute myocardial infarction and its management.

Physiology

Where is the location and what is the function of each cardiac valve?

There are two general types of valves: atrioventricular (AV) valves, which include the tricuspid (right) and mitral (left) and semilunar valves, which include the pulmonic (right) and aortic (left). These valves are shown in Figure 23–1. These valves are held in place by papillary muscles and chordae tendinea, which help to open and close the heart valves. The four valves of the heart normally open fully and close completely to promote the forward flow of blood. Any one or more of the four valves can become narrowed (stenotic) or leaky (regurgitant) through congenital damage or an acquired process such as hypertrophy, cardiomyopathy, or acute myocardial infarction (MI). The right heart pumps blood into the pulmonary circulation, while the left heart pumps blood into the systemic circulation.

What are pulse deficit, pulsus paradoxus, and pulsus alternans?

All of these conditions are a result of the irregular filling of the ventricles causing inconsistent cardiac output. *Pulse deficit* is present when the palpated distal pulse is less than the apical pulse. It occurs with dysrhythmias such as atrial fibrillation or ectopic beats. *Pulsus paradoxus* (paradoxical pulse) is when a pulse considerably decreases during inspiration. This can be associated with a number of conditions such as asthma, cardiac tamponade, pulmonary embolism (PE), tension pneumothorax, and hypovolemic shock. *Pulsus alternans* (alternate pulse) is present when a weak pulse alternates with a strong pulse in a regular cycle without changing the rate. This is present in cases of cardiac tamponade and left ventricular failure.

What are the normal heart sounds and what do these sounds represent?

The contraction and relaxation of the heart, combined with the flow of blood, generates characteristic sounds (heart sounds) when you listen with a stethoscope (auscultation of the heart). The normal pattern sounds much like "lub-DUB, lub-DUB, lub-DUB ..." The "lub" is referred to as the first heart sound (S1), and the "DUB" (emphasized because it's often louder) as the second heart sound (S2). S1 is caused by vibrations due to the sudden closure of the mitral and tricuspid valves at the start of ventricular systole. S2 results from the closure of both the aortic and pulmonic valves at the end of ventricular systole.

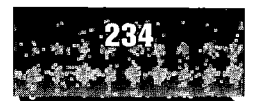

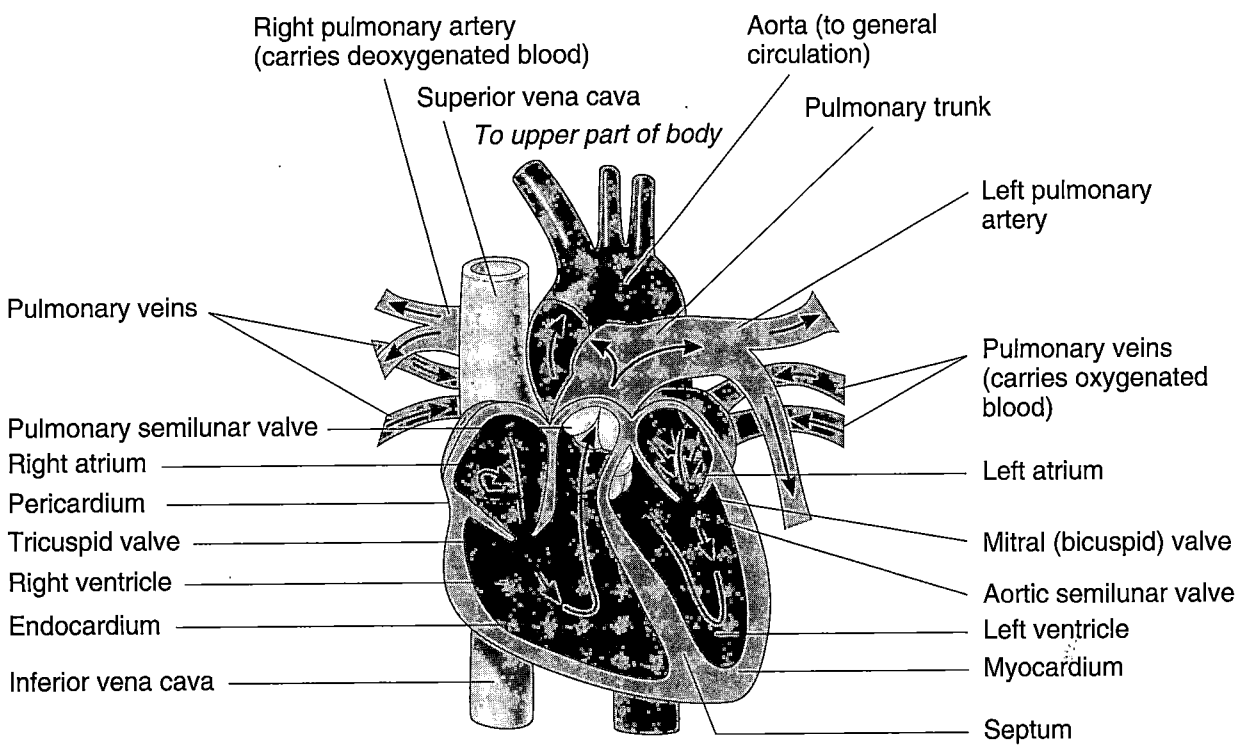

Right pulmonary artery
(carries deoxygenated blood)

Aorta (to general circulation)

Superior vena cava
To upper part of body

Pulmonary trunk

Left pulmonary artery

Pulmonary veins

Pulmonary veins
(carries oxygenated blood)

Pulmonary semilunar valve

Right atrium

Left atrium

Pericardium

Tricuspid valve

Mitral (bicuspid) valve

Right ventricle

Aortic semilunar valve

Endocardium

Left ventricle

Inferior vena cava

Myocardium

Septum

FIGURE 23-1 The heart and its valves.

What are the commonly heard abnormal heart sounds and what do the sounds represent?

A third heart sound (S3) is a soft, low-pitched sound heard about one-third of the way through diastole. Instead of hearing "lub-DUB," one hears "lub-DUB-*da*" with the "*da*" indicating the third heart sound. It is felt to represent the period of rapid ventricular filling due to vibrations set up by the in-rush of blood. Though sometimes present in healthy young persons, most commonly an S3 is associated with moderate to severe heart failure.

A fourth heart sound (S4) is a moderate-pitched sound occurring immediately prior to the normal S1. Instead of hearing "lub-DUB," one hears "*bla*'lub-DUB" with the "*bla*'" indicating the fourth heart sound. This represents either decreased stretching (compliance) of the left ventricle or increased pressure in the atria. An S4 is almost always abnormal.

A murmur is an abnormal heart sound usually caused when one or more valves fail to function properly. The "whooshing" noise is a result of turbulent blood flow. A pericardial friction rub sounds like a grating or scraping noise. It is sometimes mistaken for a cardiac-related sound. It occurs when inflammation is present in the parietal and visceral pericardium.

CLINICAL PEARL

If you know what the normal heart sounds like ("lub-DUB") then it is relatively easy to identify a sound that does not belong. Exactly what you call it is less important than noting the presence of an abnormal sound, describing its quality, and when it occurs (e.g., "whooshing sound" between the first and second heart sounds).

CLINICAL PEARL

Endocarditis is a potentially fatal bacterial infection of the endocardial layer of the heart, most commonly the heart valves. Myocarditis is a viral infection of the myocardium and may result in severe heart failure. Infection of the epicardium, by itself, is rare. Epicarditis more commonly occurs in the face of concomitant pericardial inflammation (pericarditis).

> **CLINICAL PEARL**
>
> *Abnormal collections of pericardial fluid are termed pericardial effusion. The rapid accumulation (e.g., following a steering wheel injury) of as little as 50 mls can result in pericardial tamponade and death. Pericarditis and effusion can also occur as a complication of acute MI, though pericardial tamponade is rare unless the myocardium ruptures.*

> **CLINICAL PEARL**
>
> *The Frank–Starling relationship denotes a normal physiologic mechanism. Think about it—the venous return to the heart (preload) varies constantly as we change position. The heart must be able to compensate on a second-to-second basis. It does this by pumping out the same percentage of blood (ejection fraction) with each contraction, despite changes in the venous return. Otherwise, when the preload increases, blood would back up into the venous system.*

Q What is meant by the terms positive and negative chronotropic effect, inotropic effect, and dromotropic effect as they relate to the heart?

A Chronotropism relates to influencing the rate of the heartbeat. Negative chronotrophy is the deceleration of the rate of the heartbeat. Positive chronotrophy is the acceleration of the rate of the heartbeat. Dromotropic is affecting the conductivity of nerve or muscle fibers. Positive dromotrophy is an increase in conductivity. Negative dromotrophy is a decrease in conductivity. Inotropic is influencing the force of muscular contractility. Positive ionotrophy is an increase in the force. Negative inotrophy is a decrease in the force. Table 23–1 summarizes these effects.

Q What is Starling's law of the heart?

A The relation between increased stroke volume and increased ventricular end-diastolic volume for a given intrinsic contractility is called Starling's law of the heart (or the Frank–Starling relationship). It is based on the fact that the greater the initial length or stretch of the cardiac muscle, the greater the degree of shortening will occur.

This relates to the preload of the heart. The larger the preload, the greater the stroke volume, until a point is reached when the muscle is so stretched, it can no longer contract. This is like stretching a rubber band, the greater you stretch the rubber band the greater the force of bouncing back to its original shape when you let go. Of course, there is a point when a rubber band will snap and the heart has a maximal point of stretch as well.

TABLE 23–1

Effects on the Heart			
Name of effect	Definition	Result of positive effect	Result of negative effect
Chronotropism	heart rate	increased heart rate	decreased heart rate
Dromotropism	state of conductivity	increased conductivity	decreased conductivity
Inotropism	force of cardiac contractility	increased force	decreased force

Q What are the special properties of cardiac muscle?

A Unlike other muscle tissue, cardiac muscle tissue has the ability to contract without neural stimulation, a property called automaticity. Specialized cardiac muscle cells, called pacemaker cells, normally determine the timing of contractions. Cardiac muscle tissue also has the ability to conduct (conductivity) these impulses rapidly throughout the heart; a property called self-excitation.

The most apparent structural difference in cardiac muscle cells is that they are branched, and each cardiac cell contacts several other cells at specialized sites called intercalated discs. These cellular connections contain gap junctions that provide a means for the movement of ions and small molecules and the rapid passage of action potentials from cell to cell, resulting in their simultaneous contraction.

Cardiac muscle cells are mechanically, chemically, and electrically connected in such a way with the intercalated discs that the entire tissue resembles a single, enormous muscle cell and has been called a functional syncytium.

Q What do the terms automaticity and conductivity mean?

A Automaticity refers to the pacemaker cells of the heart. These specialized cells have the distinct capability of self-repolarization. They "automatically" fire at a given rate under certain conditions, without external nerve stimulation. Conductivity refers to the special muscle cells of the heart designed to transmit the depolarization potential much quicker than regular myocardial cells.

Q How does the heart transmit the electrophysiologic impulse to contract?

A Cardiac muscle tissue uses three primary cation channels to bring about the changes in an action potential (the change in electrical potential of nerve or muscle fiber when it is stimulated; depolarization followed by repolarization). They are the potassium channels, the slow calcium–sodium channels, and the fast sodium channels. The three channels work in such a way as to time the action potentials to respond at slightly different times, allowing the atria to contract just before the ventricles.

Potassium, sodium, and calcium have important effects on cardiac function:

- Potassium—too much (hyperkalemia) or too little (hypokalemia) slows the heart rate.
- Sodium—too much (hypernatremia) slows the heart and too little (hyponatremia) causes fibrillation and death.
- Calcium—important to initiating muscle contractions, too much calcium (hypercalcemia) has the opposite effect of potassium causing spastic contractions. Too little (hypocalcemia) slows conduction, but by prolonging the Q-T interval may actually provoke dysrhythmias, such as torsade de pointes.

Why is the heart often referred to as a "self-starter?"

Because a cardiac muscle cell has the characteristics of automaticity, excitability, and conductivity, it is literally a self-starter. The pacemaker cells in the SA node normally initiate the electrical impulses that start the sequence of excitation and conduction through the heart. These discharge spontaneously at a rate of 60 to 100 times a minute.

If the SA node fails to discharge, the heart has backup or intrinsic pacemakers located in a pathway moving down through the heart. The AV node is the first backup and discharges at a rate of 40–60 times a minute. If the AV backup pacemaker should fail, the last backup is located in the ventricle, bundle branches, and Purkinje fibers—this pacemaker discharges at a rate of 20–40 times a minute.

CLINICAL PEARL

Backup cardiac pacemakers are often called "escape foci," meaning that if the normal pacemaker fails, the next one anatomically below it will take over stimulation of the entire sequence.

What is the refractory period?

During depolarization and repolarization of action potentials in the myocardium there are two distinctive periods of time when excitability of muscle tissue is resistant to stimulation of another action potential. Immediately after an action potential, the sodium channels close for a brief moment and will not permit any stimulus to set off another action potential—this is called the absolute refractory period. Following the absolute refractory period is a shorter relative refractory period. During

this time, repolarization is only partially complete. A stronger than normal stimulus can excite the muscle tissue and set off an action potential. This is a vulnerable period in the cardiac electrical cycle. A so-called "R on T phenomenon" occurs when a premature ventricular contraction (PVC) occurs during this vulnerable period and can easily lead to ventricular fibrillation.

What is the route of a stimulus through the conduction system?

Under normal conditions, pacemaker cells that are located in the SA node produce the stimulus for a contraction. From the SA node, the impulses flow through the atrial walls by way of internodal pathways to reach the AV node. After a brief delay, the impulses are conducted to the AV bundle (Bundle of His) and then continue on to the left and right bundle branches, through the Purkinje fibers, and out to the ventricular myocardial cells.

What determines the heart's pacemaker control, rate, and rhythm?

Specialized cells found only in the heart, called pacemaker cells, establish a regular rate of contraction. The fastest pacemaker sets the heart rate. Under normal condition, the fastest pacemakers are the ones located in the SA node of the heart. The autonomic nervous system (ANS) can alter the rate of pacemaker activity naturally or with the use of certain drugs. Irritable pacemakers located outside the SA node can overtake normal pacemakers when the heart experiences injury or insult. Backup or intrinsic pacemakers located in the AV node or the ventricles may take over when the SA node fails.

How does the ANS alter the heart rate, rhythm, and contractility of the heart?

Sympathetic nerves are located throughout the heart, while parasympathetic nerves are located primarily in the SA and AV nodes. These nerves affect the heart rate and the contractility of the heart by the use of the natural chemicals acetylcholine (Ach), epinephrine, and norepinephrine.

Ach, a neurotransmitter released by parasympathetic motor neurons, lowers the heart rate and stroke volume. Epinephrine and norepinephrine, catacholamines released by the adrenal medulla and sympathetic neurons during sympathetic activation, increase both heart rate and stroke volume.

What is reentry?

Reentry, aberration, and accessory pathways are related to the conduction pathway of the heart. Reentry refers to the alteration of a repolarization wave from its normal direction, which is blocked, to another pathway, which is not blocked. The wave then goes back up the original pathway to produce a contraction. This leads to a continuing series of premature beats.

Aberration is a deviation from the usual pathway. A bizarre and unusually wide-looking QRS complex characterizes aberrant conduction through the ventricles of an impulse generated in the supraventricular region. An accessory pathway is an irregular connection between the atria and ventricles that bypasses the AV node.

Q What is meant by the term electro-mechanical disassociation?

A Electro-mechanical disassociation (also referred to as pulseless electrical activity, PEA) is a pathologic state in which an action potential does not result in systole. Organized ECG activity is not accompanied by a cardiac contraction, therefore there is no pulse. It is paramount that one does not rely on the ECG to know whether the patient has a mechanical pulse. To be certain a pulse is actually present, you must feel it.

Q What should be anticipated in the care of a cardiac arrest victim?

A A cardiac arrest is a sudden stopping of circulatory function from the heart. There are many causes for cardiac arrest, half of which are directly related to coronary heart disease. Other causes include stroke, trauma, drowning, electrocution, suffocation, airway obstruction, drug intoxication, respiratory failure, congenital anomalies, and perinatal asphyxia at birth.

The arrhythmias that may be seen during cardiac arrest are ventricular fibrillation, asystole, and PEA.

The treatment for a person in cardiac arrest begins with BLS measures as soon as possible followed by ACLS as soon as possible. Critical actions in caring for a cardiac arrest patient are providing interventions such as CPR, early defibrillation of ventricular fibrillation, and clearing an obstructed airway immediately. As each minute after the arrest passes, the chance for survivability decreases. Post-resuscitation care begins with reassessing ABCs, if possible making a differential diagnosis, and continuing care as guided by medical control.

Etiology of Chest Pain

Q Why is the etiology of chest pain often difficult to determine in the out-of-hospital setting?

A Pains from the heart are vague because they are of a visceral origin. The nerve supply is less specific than pain of

somatic origin (e.g., a spot on the skin). There are many causes of chest pain that may arise from a variety of organs within the chest and abdominal cavities with many etiologies (e.g., cardiac, trauma, and infection). This is why all patients, particularly adults, with chest pain should be treated as having a cardiac problem until proven otherwise.

CLINICAL PEARL

Because so many different conditions, some life threatening, can cause chest pain, the EMS provider should consider that pain anywhere from the navel to the jaw is cardiac ischemia until proven otherwise!

Q What is the difference between visceral and somatic (parietal) pain?

A Patients who experience somatic pain most often are able to localize pain to a specific area. The pain is frequently characterized as sharp, constant, and aggravated by movement or coughing. Particular structures in the body that are innervated by sensory nerve fibers return to the spinal cord along specific nerve pathways located on the same side as the site of pain.

A patient with visceral pain feels pain that is usually intermittent, worsens with time, and may be described as dull, cramping, or even gaseous. Because visceral pain impulses are carried by nerve fibers that return to the spinal cord at several levels from both sides of the body, the pain is typically perceived by the patient as being poorly localized and ill-defined.

Q Then why does ischemia cause visceral pain in the heart?

A Generally speaking, a person cannot "feel" his heart, but ischemic cardiac muscle does exhibit a pain sensation. The most likely explanation is that ischemic muscle releases lactic acid, as well as other pain-producing substances such as histamine or kinins. The high concentrations of these abnormal products then stimulate pain endings in the cardiac muscle, and pain is felt. Because of the bilateral visceral nerve supply, the pain is poorly localized and usually dull or pressure-like in nature.

Q Is the location of the pain diagnostic of its etiology?

A No, the location of the pain often does not correspond to the actual source. For many patients, the severity or absence of pain is often unrelated to its life-threatening potential.

Altered pain sensation is more evident in elderly or diabetic patients. As a person ages and begins to lose various senses such as sight and hearing, another body function that deteriorates is the sense of pain. The elderly and the diabetic patient experiencing an acute myocardial infarction (AMI) often present with atypical symptoms. Any one or a combination of the following may indicate the presence of an AMI:

- Altered mental status (MS), confusion, or syncope.
- Weakness or fatigue.
- Dyspnea that is mild to severe.
- Epigastric, back, or neck pain.
- New-onset congestive heart failure (CHF).

Why do diabetic patients have silent AMIs?

Not all diabetic patients have silent AMIs, yet many do. The reason is altered pain perception due to chronic nerve damage (neuropathy) from diabetes. The loss of pain sensation in the feet is why diabetic patients often develop ulcers that are far advanced before they seek treatment. Similarly, a diabetic patient may suffer atypical symptoms from myocardial ischemia.

What are some of the medical life-threatening causes of acute chest pain that must be considered first when assessing a patient?

Some of the first life-threatening conditions to consider are myocardial infarction, unstable angina, pulmonary embolism, pneumothorax, aortic dissection, and esophageal rupture.

What are examples of some other conditions that present as chest pain and are not usually life threatening?

There is a long list of conditions that present as typical or atypical chest pain to include the following:

- Stable angina—chest pain that occurs with exertion, is often predictable, and usually is relieved with rest or nitroglycerin.
- Cholecystitis—an inflammation of the gallbladder that presents as upper-abdominal pain often with referred pain to the back or right shoulder.
- Acute viral pericarditis or other inflammatory cardiac disease—chest pain is usually worse while the patient is supine and often relieved when the patient leans forward.
- Aneurysm—sac formed by the dilatation of the wall of an artery, vein, or the heart, it is filled with fluid or clotted blood, often forming a pulsating tumor. Sometimes pain will result from pressure on contiguous parts.
- Hiatal hernia—protrusion of the stomach upward through the esophageal hiatus that presents with epigastric pain.
- Esophageal gastric reflux—backward or return flow of stomach contents into the esophagus causing pain and indigestion. This condition is often relieved with antacids or prescribed

medication. Beware—many patients confuse epigastric pain from MI with indigestion.

- Peptic ulcer disease—ulcer in the lower esophagus, stomach, or duodenum may present with upper-abdominal, epigastric, or chest pain that is often relieved with antacids.
- Pancreatitis—inflammation of the pancreas that presents with acute and intense epigastric pain, nausea, and vomiting.
- Costochondritis—inflammation of an area of the ribs or surrounding cartilage that causes pain with movement and breathing.
- Dyspepsia—painful digestion marked by abdominal pain, heartburn, nausea, and vomiting.
- Herpes zoster—virus infection, usually as a result of old chicken pox (varicella), that presents as a severe or stabbing neuralgic pain. Usually self-limited.
- Musculoskeletal—pain worsens with movement, sometimes with breathing.
- Chest wall tumors, pleural irritation, respiratory infections, and chest wall trauma.

So, what is all the "time is muscle" emphasis all about?

When there is an inadequate blood flow to an organ, such as the heart, ischemia (lack of oxygen) occurs. Infarction occurs when a portion of ischemic myocardium dies (necrosis). Following AMI, not all of the myocardium supplied by the affected coronary artery dies at once. The central "core" dies first, while the surrounding myocardium remains ischemic and potentially salvageable. Untreated, this ischemic muscle develops necrosis. However, reperfusion therapy (e.g., chemical thrombolysis, balloon angioplasty, coronary artery bypass) may restore flow, if begun early enough, minimizing the ultimate size of the infarction.

The sooner treatment is received, the better the chance for survival of a greater number of cardiac cells. The time when insult is occurring and has not yet resulted in permanent injury is the *window of opportunity*. Though most experts agree that "earlier is always better," the accepted "window" ranges from four to six hours in most institutions.

What does it mean when a patient has referred pain?

Referred pain is pain felt at a site that is different from that of the injured or diseased part of the body. For example, a patient having an angina attack usually feels pain beneath the upper sternum and often has pain in the left arm, shoulder, neck, or jaw. The reason for the distribution of pain is that the heart originates during embryonic life in the neck, as do the arms. Therefore, both of these structures receive pain nerve fibers from the same spinal cord segments.

Q Is radiating pain the same as referred pain?

A Yes, radiating pain is the term for a patient's subjective description of pain from the point of origin moving toward another location. Radiation of pain is the transmission of pain from a point of origin toward another anatomical location. The mechanism by which the pain is experienced is described medically as referred pain.

History

Q What are the acronyms OPQRST and SAMPLE used for regarding the cardiac patient?

A These are acronyms that pertain to the focused history (FH) of a patient. They represent a set of questions used to ask a patient about the chief complaint and past medical history. Each letter stands for the following:

OPQRST

- **O**nset—How did the symptom begin, suddenly or over a period of time? AMI is more often acute in nature, whereas CHF develops slower.

- **P**rovocation—What was the patient doing at the time of onset? Was the pain exertional (e.g., stable angina) or nonexertional (e.g., unstable angina, MI)?

- **Q**uality—What does the pain feel like? Encourage the patient to describe the pain or discomfort so you are able to distinguish one cause of pain from another. For example, if the pain is constant, it may be unstable angina, pleurisy, or an unstable dysrhythmia, whereas if the pain is intermittent, it may be stable angina, or progressive cardiac ischemia. You also should determine if there have been similar events. If there have been, ask the patient to compare these to the present event.

- **R**adiation, **R**egion, **R**elief—Determine if the pain is limited to one area or if it radiates from one point of origin to another. Cardiac chest pain is often described as a substernal chest pain with associated pain to the left arm, shoulder, neck, or jaw. Ask if the pain is worse when the area is palpated or when the patient coughs or takes a deep breath. This type of pain is usually associated with pleuritic or musculoskeletal rather than cardiac chest pain. Also ask the patient what was done before to resolve the episode (e.g., rest or take a nitroglycerin) because this may be the treatment you will use.

- **S**everity—Ask the patient to compare the pain now to the pain experienced from a previous occurrence or to use a rating system. A commonly used rating system is a scale of 1–10 with 0 being no pain and 10 being the worst pain imaginable. Ask patients, "Describe how you would rate the pain now." Use

this subjective information to compare how they felt at the initial onset of the pain, when it was the most intense, and after any interventions, by either you or them.

- **T**ime of onset—How long has the symptom been present? The onset may have been acute; however, a call for help is often delayed due to denial or atypical cardiac pain.

SAMPLE

- **S**ymptoms—When asking patients about their symptoms keep in mind the typical versus atypical symptoms of cardiac chest pain.

- **A**llergies—Look for allergies to medications that you might use to treat a cardiac problem (e.g., adenosine or lidocaine for dysrhythmias).

- **M**edications—Look for cardiac, respiratory, and hypertension medication, but look for all medications taken. Include prescription, over-the-counter (OTC), homeopathic, recreational, home oxygen, or someone else's medication (e.g., a spouse's).

- **P**ast medical history—Ask specific questions rather than general.

- **L**ast—Meal, oral intake, episode, treatment (e.g., last nitroglycerin taken).

- **E**vents—What led up to this episode? This question is similar to the **O**nset question.

Q Why is history significant with an AMI?

A In a significant number of cases, it is difficult to diagnose AMI based on any one component of an examination or test. An FH and physical exam together with clinical tests are all required for diagnosing an AMI. The three primary components used for diagnosis include a patient's history, abnormal ECG or ECG changes, and a cardiac enzyme analysis.

CLINICAL PEARL

Sometimes, even with in-hospital data, it is impossible to exclude or fully diagnose an AMI. The most important thing to consider is, "Could the patient's pain represent myocardial ischemia?" Even if the patient is not a candidate for acute reperfusion therapy of an AMI, ongoing ischemia is still potentially deadly.

Q How is Prinzmetal's angina different from stable or unstable angina?

A Angina pectoris is a severe pain caused by a lack of oxygen to the heart muscle. When the pain occurs with exercise or exertion and is predictable, it is referred to as stable angina. Usually relief is prompt with rest or nitroglycerin. Unstable angina pain results when patient's discomfort is more prolonged or severe than their usual stable angina. It may be an indication of an impending MI. It can occur anytime, even during rest, and should be treated as a medical emergency. Prinzmetal's angina is an atypical form of angina caused by the vasospasm of otherwise normal coronary arteries. Chest pain may be severe and can occur at rest similar to an unstable angina. Oxygen, nitroglycerin, and drugs that influence calcium metabolism by the myocardium are of benefit.

How do I know if a syncopal event was cardiac related?

There are many causes of syncope that are not cardiac in origin. It is significant to discern pre- and post-syncope information such as the position of the patient. Syncope in a supine patient is serious and most likely cardiac in nature. Syncope occurring after a patient stands up may be cardiac, but more often indicates orthostatic changes as seen with noncardiac syncope. Determine, if you can, if there has been any previous similar episodes. Ask about associated cardiac symptoms before the syncope (e.g., chest pain, shortness of breath, palpitations) and about post-syncope symptoms.

The duration of the loss of consciousness (LOC) is a helpful clue. Cardiac and neurologic syncope usually occur without warning and can last a few minutes in duration. Recovery is often slow with confusion, headache, dizziness, orthostatic changes, or local dysfunction. Noncardiac syncope often occurs in patients with no underlying disease, usually from a stressor such as pain, emotion, or medication and lasts only briefly with a quick recovery period. Despite these caveats, remember that the most common causes of syncopal spells are vasovagal faint, positional orthostatic hypotension, and cardiac dysrhythmias.

CLINICAL PEARL

Just because patients wake up quickly does not completely exclude the possibility of syncope due to cardiac dysrhythmia.

Are there any classical symptoms associated with ischemic chest pain?

Yes, the patient's chest pain may be associated with any of the following: dyspnea, diaphoresis, syncope, dizziness, nausea, vomiting, heartburn, indigestion, back-neck-jaw pain, tingling, or numbness.

What is the most common cause of AMI?

The most common cause of AMI (occurring about 90 percent of the time) is a coronary thrombosis (blood clot). Typically,

the coronary artery is already narrowed due to chronic atherosclerosis (hardening of the arteries) as shown in Figure 23–2. This area is called a "plaque." The acute event occurs because of plaque inflammation, rupture, and localized bleeding. The resulting blood completely blocks the already narrowed lumen (opening) of the artery, resulting in an AMI. Other precipitating causes include hypertension atherosclerosis, persistent angina, occlusion, trauma, and recreational drugs such as cocaine.

CLINICAL PEARL

Because an acute blood clot is responsible for the majority of AMIs, reperfusion therapy with either drugs, angioplasty balloons, or coronary artery bypass has become common. The mechanism that causes most heart attacks also causes nearly 70 percent of thrombotic strokes—a blood clot completely occludes a narrowed cerebral artery. This forms the basis for reperfusion therapy in stroke.

Often a person who is having a heart attack denies having chest pain. What other phrases do patients use to describe chest pain?

Patients often do not report that they are having chest pain for various reasons. Sometimes they are in denial, but other times the pain is atypical chest pain. The patient might use terms such as:

- I feel a pressure.
- My heart is racing.
- I feel palpitations.
- I just do not feel right.
- I feel tired.
- I feel weak.
- It is hard to take a breath.
- My chest feels tight.
- There is heaviness or squeezing in my chest.
- I cannot catch my breath.
- It feels like indigestion.
- Nothing is wrong.

The ECG

How does one interpret an ECG?

Electrical events occurring in the heart are powerful enough that they can be observed by the use of electrodes

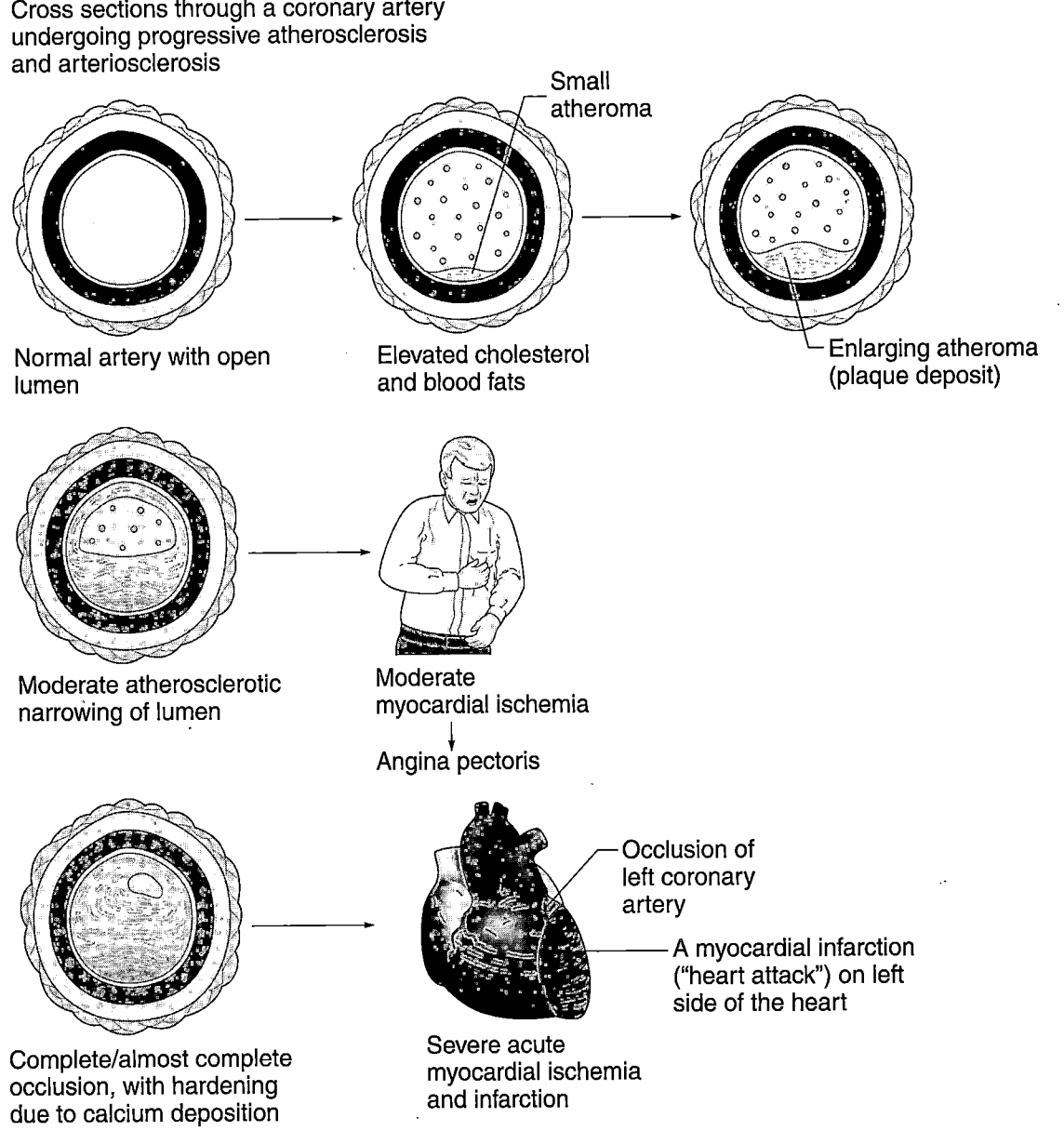

Cross sections through a coronary artery undergoing progressive atherosclerosis and arteriosclerosis

Small atheroma

Normal artery with open lumen

Elevated cholesterol and blood fats

Enlarging atheroma (plaque deposit)

Moderate atherosclerotic narrowing of lumen

Moderate myocardial ischemia

↓

Angina pectoris

Complete/almost complete occlusion, with hardening due to calcium deposition

Severe acute myocardial ischemia and infarction

Occlusion of left coronary artery

A myocardial infarction ("heart attack") on left side of the heart

FIGURE 23-2 The progression of atherosclerosis.

placed on the body. The electrical impulses are measured for duration and strength of amplitude on ECG recording paper as shown in Figure 23–3. On the paper, waveforms are marked from a baseline. The electrical activity is seen as waveforms and segments that are deflections away from or returning to the baseline. These may be positive (above the baseline) or negative (below the baseline) in direction.

The normal ECG is made up of a P wave, a QRS complex (group of wave forms), and a T wave. The QRS complex is usually composed of three separate waves.

- The P wave represents an electrical impulse generated as the atria depolarize before contraction.

- The P-R interval represents the beginning of the P wave to the beginning of the QRS complex, regardless of the deflection of the P wave or QRS complex on an ECG, and correlates to the impulse through the atria into the AV node and through the bundles to the ventricles.

- The QRS wave represents impulse generated as the ventricles depolarize before contraction.

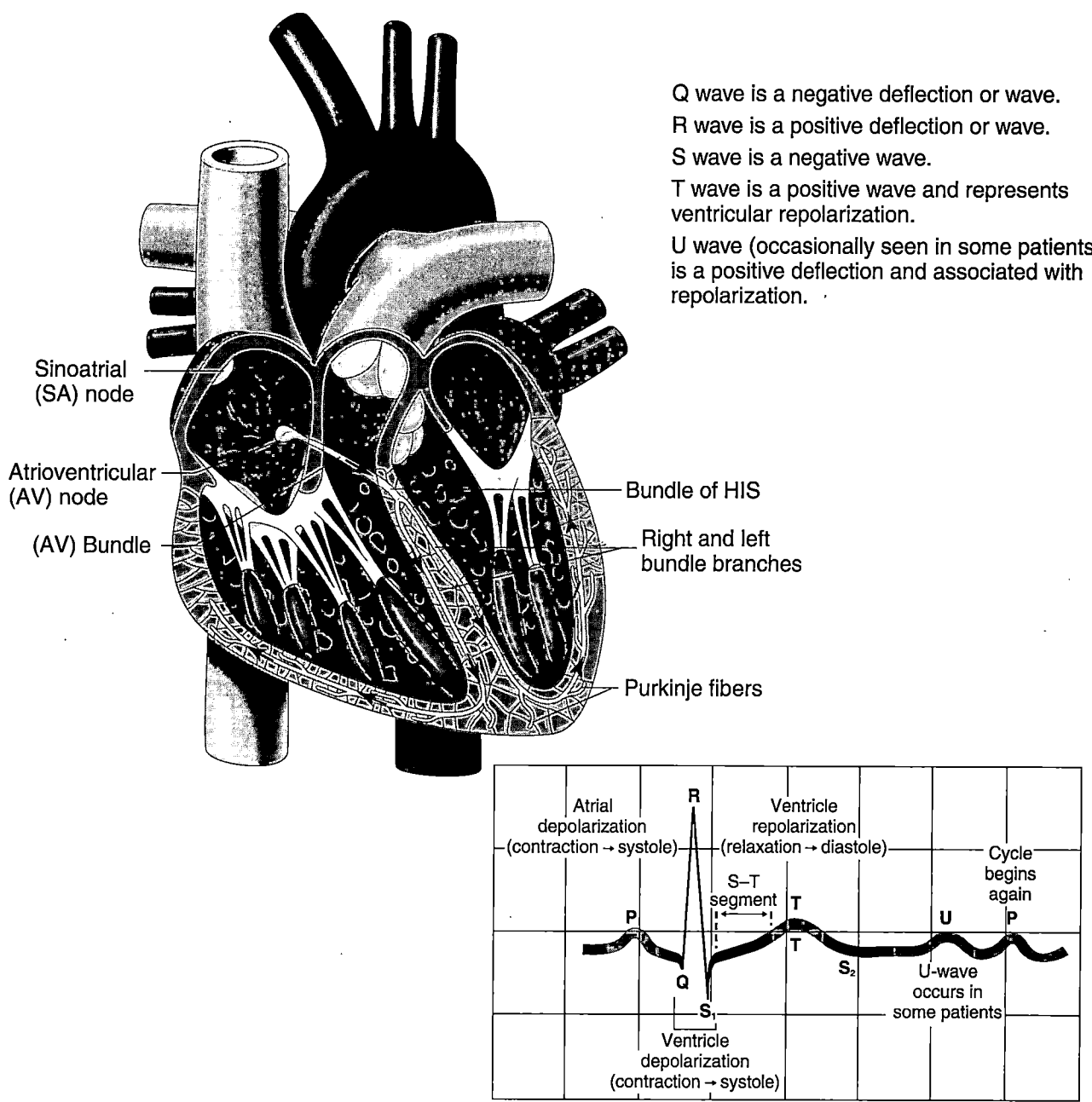

Q wave is a negative deflection or wave.

R wave is a positive deflection or wave.

S wave is a negative wave.

T wave is a positive wave and represents ventricular repolarization.

U wave (occasionally seen in some patients) is a positive deflection and associated with repolarization.

Sinoatrial (SA) node

Atrioventricular (AV) node

(AV) Bundle

Bundle of HIS

Right and left bundle branches

Purkinje fibers

| Atrial depolarization (contraction → systole) | R | Ventricle repolarization (relaxation → diastole) | Cycle begins again |

S-T segment | T

P

Q

S₁

S₂

U

P

U-wave occurs in some patients

Ventricle depolarization (contraction → systole)

FIGURE 23–3 Relationship between the heart's electrical conduction system and the ECG.

• The T wave represents repolarization of the ventricles. Repolarization of the atria cannot be seen on an ECG because the stronger impulses of the depolarization of the ventricles (QRS complex) cover it.

• The S-T segment represents the end of the QRS (J point) to the beginning of the T wave and correlates to the time between ventricular depolarization and repolarization.

• The Q-T interval represents the beginning of the Q wave to the end of the T wave and correlates as the total ventricular activ-

ity, both the depolarization (QRS) and the repolarization (S-T segment and the T wave).

Q How do you calculate the heart rate from an ECG recording?

A There is more than one way to do this. One popular method is to count the number of large squares between two consecutive QRS complexes and divide that number into 300. Another method is to count the number of small squares between two consecutive QRS complexes and divide that number into 1500. Another way is to count QRS complexes in a six-second strip and multiply by 10. These methods work well if the rhythm is regular. When the rhythm is irregular, obtain a longer strip to count and check for pulse deficits.

CLINICAL PEARL

Monitor readouts of heart rate are often unreliable, especially if the patient has large T waves or the rhythm is irregular. Whenever possible, print out a rhythm strip and estimate the rate yourself.

Q What is the difference in lead placements?

A The heart is a three dimensional structure that has to be viewed in the various dimensions. Placing electrodes in various positions on the body provides views at various angles. The way leads are placed also affects the appearance of the waves by altering the size and shapes of waves recorded.

By comparing the information obtained from electrodes placed at different locations on the body surface, you can check the performance of specific nodal, conducting, and contractile components. For example, when a portion of the heart has been damaged, the affected muscle cells no longer conduct action potentials, so an ECG reveals an abnormal pattern of impulse conduction. Physicians thus rely on ECGs to detect structural or functional problems in the heart.

Q What is Einthoven's triangle?

A Dr. Willem Einthoven invented the ECG machine in 1901. He described the placement of the first three standardized leads (lead I, II, and III) as a triangle over the body and around the heart (Figure 23–4). These leads provide three different views of the heart. To obtain the three standard limb leads, electrodes are placed on the two arms and the left leg to form the corners of the triangle.

- Lead I—positive electrode on left arm and negative on right arm.
- Lead II—positive electrode on left leg and negative on right arm.
- Lead III—positive electrode on left leg and negative on left arm.

Q Is there a difference between ECG and EKG?

A No, they are both abbreviations for electrocardiogram. However, for uniformity throughout this book we have chosen to use ECG.

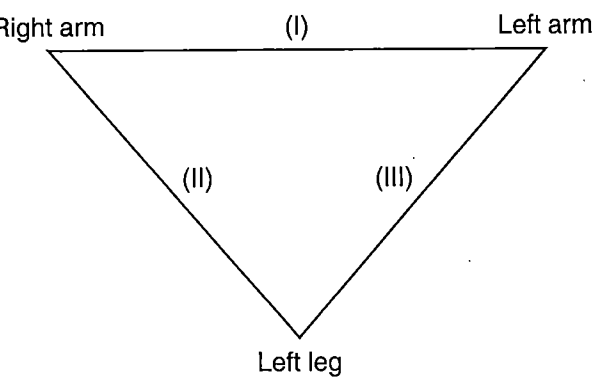

FIGURE 23–4 Einthoven's triangle.

CLINICAL PEARL

Dr. Einthoven was Dutch and spelled the name of his new invention "elektrokardiogram." Some purists prefer the term "EKG" in deference to him. It is also less likely to be confused with the term "EEG," representing electroencephalogram (brain wave test).

Q Which patients should have an ECG done?

A Certainly, an ECG should be obtained on any patient where the EMS provider feels she needs the data to confirm suspicions of cardiac irregularity. However, it is paramount that the ECG does not take priority over caring for life-threatening injuries such as a compromised airway or uncontrolled bleeding. The most likely candidates for ECG analysis would be those who:

- Complain of typical or atypical chest pain.
- Have experienced a syncopal or near syncopal event.
- Are unconscious or have an AMS.
- Have a complaint or symptom and an irregular pulse.
- Have possibly overdosed.
- Have experienced an electrical shock.
- May be experiencing hypoxia.
- May be experiencing an electrolyte imbalance.

CLINICAL PEARL

Remember "a normal test does not mean a normal patient!" Nearly 50 percent of people with proven AMIs have an initially normal ECG. The clinician (YOU!) is responsible for making or suspecting a given diagnosis, not a lab, ECG, or x-ray test.

What is the significance of S-T elevation or depression?

Many things can cause S-T segment elevation or depression (e.g., ischemia, infarction, normal variants, electrolyte disturbances). An elevation or depression of ≥1 mm (≥0.1 mV) above or below baseline, measured 0.08 seconds (2 small boxes) after the end of the QRS complex, is abnormal. Under many clinical circumstances, you *must* assume that these represent AMI until proven otherwise.

S-T elevation is usually a sign of severe myocardial injury. Other common causes of S-T elevation that may be confused with AMI are coronary vasospasm (e.g., Prinzmetal's angina) and acute pericarditis. S-T depression is also a common manifestation of myocardial ischemia. Other causes include left and right ventricular hypertrophy, left and right bundle branch block, and digitalis use.

Can an ECG alone rule out an AMI?

No, the three primary components that are utilized to diagnose an AMI include the patient's chief complaint or primary symptom, ECG changes or abnormalities, and a cardiac enzyme analysis. In a significant percentage of cases, it is still difficult to diagnose AMI. Studies have consistently shown that approximately 30 percent of out-of-hospital ECGs show ECG changes, such as S-T elevation or S-T depression, that are consistent with an AMI. The reason for this could be that there is only a short window of time when the S-T changes may occur, usually within the first hour of the event. Often a person with chest pain will wait to see if the pain resolves on its own before calling for help. By the time the out-of-hospital provider arrives, changes may have come and gone.

Is the 12-lead ECG really beneficial to guide treatment in the out-of-hospital setting?

Yes, the 12-lead ECG can help to identify the size and location of the infarction that is occurring. With this information, one can anticipate the most common complication associated with each type of infarct and thus, it helps to guide treatment. The Guidelines 2000 specify the use of an out-of-hospital 12-lead ECG as a Class IIa recommendation. For more on the Guidelines 2000, review Chapter 52, Advanced Cardiac Life Support.

For example, in the case of inferior infarction, the conduction system is often involved. This may result in an AV block (Type II, Mobitz II, or Type III), producing bradycardia that will not likely respond to atropine. Knowing this allows the EMS provider to choose pacing to treat the bradycardia or to anticipate that a heart block may develop.

Further, inferior infarction is often associated with right ventricular (RV) infarcts. Patients with RV infarcts often have problems with hypotension and decreased cardiac output, and are very sensitive to drugs that reduce preload such as nitroglycerin. This is because, with reduced RV function, the patient needs a high preload to maintain forward flow through the lungs. These patients often respond to fluid administration.

Conversely, anterior infarcts tend to be large, producing hypotension and decreased cardiac output due to left heart failure. This is treated with vasopressor agents more than fluids.

The following is a guide for the location of an infarct by lead placement:

- Inferior wall of left ventricle—look at leads II, III, and aVF.
- Anterior wall of left ventricle—look at leads V_3 and V_4.
- Lateral wall of left ventricle—look at leads I, aVL, V_5, and V_6.
- Septal wall—look at leads V_1 and V_2.
- Right ventricle—look at leads V_{4R}, V_{5R}, and V_{6R}.

CLINICAL PEARL

Numerous studies have proven that the field 12-lead ECG reduces the time required to administer thrombolytic therapy in the ED. The average increase in field time to perform the ECG is less than five minutes. Experts caution, however, that an EMS system should first allocate resources to providing early and rapid defibrillation before considering a field 12-lead program.

Dysrhythmias

What are the primary mechanisms that produce cardiac dysrhythmias?

The primary mechanism is heart disease, due to the effects of decreased blood flow to the heart. This in turn leads to the myocardium experiencing hypoxia and then ischemia. Any time the heart muscle experiences hypoxia and ischemia, it will become irritable and is prone to producing dysryhthmias. Other mechanisms that produce cardiac dysrhythmias include the use of drugs, electrolyte imbalances, electrical shock, and trauma.

Why is it recommended that asystole be confirmed in three leads?

Asystole has no discernable waves or complexes on an ECG. There are conditions that can mimic this tracing (e.g., loose or absent lead connection, placement, artifact). Asystole and fine ventricular fibrillation may be difficult to distinguish from one another on an ECG. To avoid incorrect interpretation, or delay of correct treatment, the presence of asystole should always be confirmed in two or three leads.

▣ What happens to a hypoxic heart?

▣ When heart muscle becomes hypoxic, the myocardium becomes irritable. This irritability may cause disturbances in the electrical conduction of the heart such as ectopy and dysrhythmias. Untreated, this could lead to myocardial ischemia, injury, and infarct. The classic pain of angina is usually accompanied by ectopy and dysrhythmias, followed by cardiac arrest and sudden death.

▣ What is Adams–Stokes Syndrome?

▣ Adams–Stokes syndrome, also called "Stokes Adams Attack," is a disorder found more commonly in the elderly and is characterized by a periodic loss of consciousness (syncope) due to a heart block.

▣ What is Wolff–Parkinson–White (WPW) syndrome?

▣ WPW syndrome refers to typical ECG changes indicating aberrant atrioventricular conduction in the presence of an extra conduction pathway. Also called pre-excitation syndrome, these changes may be asymptomatic or may be associated with paroxysmal supraventricular tachycardia (PSVT) or atrial fibrillation (AF). Typically, the ECG displays a short P-R interval and a wide QRS complex, which characteristically shows early QRS widening referred to as a delta wave.

Electrical Therapy

▣ What is the difference between synchronized cardioversion and defibrillation?

▣ Synchronized cardioversion is similar to defibrillation; however, in synchronized cardioversion, the shock is timed (synchronized) to the heart's existing electrical activity to avoid stimulation during the relative refractory phase (vulnerable) period. The shock is often delivered during the R wave. Synchronization, which is commonly used to treat patients with tachydysrhythmias who are symptomatic, reduces the energy required to convert and reduces the chance for post-shock dysrhythmias.

▣ What are the components of a pacemaker?

▣ A noninvasive transcutaneous pacer (TCP) is an electric, battery-operated device that may be either free standing or incorporated into a defibrillator monitor. Two large external pacer pads adhere to the chest wall. These are plugged into the pacing device and repetitive electrical impulses are sent to the

heart to regulate the heartbeat. The controls for setting heart rate and amplitude for pacing are located on the unit. The use of this device is a temporary measure until an invasive pacemaker can be placed in the patient.

Invasive pacers are surgically implanted under the skin and supply impulses to regulate the heartbeat as shown in Figure 23–5. This type of pacemaker has been placed in thousands of individuals. The site of implantation is usually in the left chest area. Electrode catheters attached to the pacemaker are then passed into the heart and anchored to the chest wall. This rather simple device has saved many people whose hearts cannot beat effectively alone.

> **CLINICAL PEARL**
>
> *Patients in cardiac arrest with implanted pacemakers will continue to have electrical activity, but without a pulse. Decisions to terminate resuscitation are sometimes difficult under these circumstances. Consult your local protocols and on-line medical direction for assistance.*

▣ What is the difference between anterior–posterior (AP) and anterior–left lateral (AL) pad placement when pacing a patient?

▣ TCP pacing pads are large pads that may be placed either AP or AL. The AP placement is more common and does not interfere with defibrillation if needed.

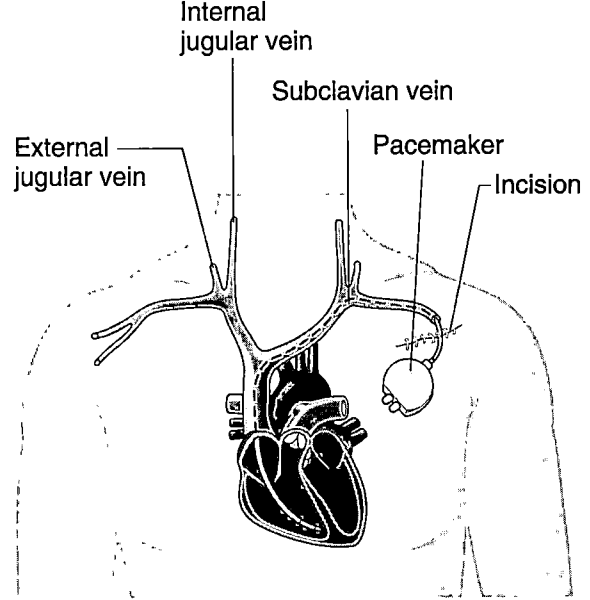

FIGURE 23–5 A pacemaker.

Why are there different types of pacemakers?

When injury to the myocardium affects the automaticity and the heart can no longer produce the normal pace or rhythm, an artificial pacemaker may be used. The location of the injury determines the type of pacemaker required. There are several types of pacemakers available and there is a five-letter pacemaker identification code developed by the Intersociety Committee on Heart Disease (ICHD) designed to explain how each works.

Diagnostic Tests

What test is the most accurate in the diagnosis of an AMI?

Cardiac enzyme testing is a reliable test performed in the hospital. When cardiac muscle dies, enzymes are released in the blood stream. The measurement of CK-MB (creatine kinase; M, muscle; B, brain) over a 12- to 24-hour period is currently the test of choice for the diagnosis of an AMI.

CLINICAL PEARL

CK-MB is still regarded as the "gold standard" by most experts, yet, other tests appear promising. Troponin is a component of the myocardium and is released into the blood during ischemia. Even in patients who turn out not to have suffered an AMI, elevated troponin levels may identify high-risk patients for life-threatening dysrhythmias.

Is there a field test for cardiac enzymes?

There are commercial kits available for the bedside determination of troponin levels. These have been tried experimentally in the field with good success. The problem lies less in a positive test *confirming* your clinical suspicions, but whether or not a negative test *excludes* AMI or myocardial ischemia. No tests to date, especially when performed early in the course of a patient's symptoms, reliably rule out ischemia.

Physical Examination

What is Kussmaul's sign and what does it suggest?

Kussmaul's sign is a paradoxical filling of the neck veins during inspiration and suggests a right ventricular infarction, massive pulmonary embolism, or pericarditis.

What is Levine's sign and when is it seen?

Levine's sign is the presentation of a sick-looking patient who places a clenched fist over the sternum to describe a chest pain. This sign is frequently associated with ischemic heart disease.

Reperfusion Therapy

What about clotbusters? Who should get them and why?

A clotbuster is a term for a drug classified as a thrombolytic or fibrinolytic. Blood thinners, such as aspirin or heparin, and thrombolytics are used to treat occlusions of coronary arteries due to thrombi after an AMI to restore blood flow. They are also used to treat deep vein thrombosis, pulmonary embolism, arterial thrombosis, arterial embolism, and arteriovenous cannula occlusion. Though several drugs are available, the most widely used is recombinant tissue plasminogen activator (RTPA). There may be severe complications with the use of these drugs such as cerebral hemorrhage, uncontrollable bleeding, and death. Therefore, some people are not candidates for this type of treatment.

What is a clotbuster checklist and when would it be used?

The checklist is used to determine whether a patient is a candidate to receive fibrinolytic therapy. The checklist includes reviewing the following conditions, which carry potential dangers from excessive bleeding, with the patient:

- Active bleeding.
- Severe hypertension.
- COPD.
- Renal disease.
- Hepatic disease.
- Cerebral embolism.
- Thrombosis or hemorrhage.
- Recent surgery.

If patients have any of these conditions, they will not be candidates for this type of therapy.

General Treatment

What is the safest initial approach to patients presenting with chest pain?

Assume that all patients with acute chest pain have a life-threatening event (e.g., AMI). Begin treatment with high-concentration oxygen, obtain IV access, and perform cardiac monitoring. Assist ventilations if respirations are inadequate. Continuous cardiac rhythm monitoring is essential for rhythm disturbances that require prompt treatment. IV access is necessary in case the patient's condition suddenly deteriorates necessitating fluid or medications. The goal is to reduce pain and provide oxygen to the heart. Nitrates are given to dilate coronary arteries to better perfuse the heart and analgesia is given to help reduce the pain. Aspirin is also given to help thin the blood in an effort to better restore perfusion. Transport the AMI patient quickly, but without increasing present anxiety.

Why is baby aspirin given in the field?

Most choose baby aspirin because it doesn't taste bad. As a result, it is easy to chew and swallow. Remember, people with myocardial ischemia often have nausea. Taking the aspirin in this form minimizes oral intake—the patient doesn't have to take a drink to swallow the medication.

Why is nitroglycerin used for patients with chest pain?

Nitroglycerin is an antianginal drug that relaxes vascular smooth muscle, resulting in peripheral vasodilation. This, in turn, decreases myocardial workload and myocardial oxygen demand and decreases the pain. It also helps to differentiate angina from AMI. Nitroglycerin tends to quickly relieve stable angina, Prinzmetal's angina, and esophageal spasm, whereas AMI and unstable angina may remain unrelieved.

CLINICAL PEARL

Though stable angina pain is typically relieved with sublingual nitroglycerin, don't assume that pain relief excludes a more serious condition. More importantly, if three sublingual nitroglycerin tablets (follow your local protocols) fail to alleviate the pain completely, the patient has an AMI until proven otherwise.

Pathophysiology of Vascular Disorders

What are the most common arteries affected by occlusive disease?

Coronary artery disease and cerebral vascular disease are the great causes of death and disability. Both are frequently associated with hypertension (HNT), or high blood pressure.

How does hypertension affect the cardiovascular system long term versus short term?

Hypertension is a devastating disease that affects the cardiovascular system in two ways. First, HTN places an increased workload on the heart. The left ventricle is more adversely affected by chronic HTN than the right. The left ventricle works harder to push the same volume of blood through arteries that are narrowed due to arteriosclerosis. The extra workload causes the left ventricle to hypertrophy. Myocardial geometry (shape) changes, causing the hypertrophied heart to work harder to maintain a given output. HTN also accelerates coronary arteriosclerosis. The combination of increased heart size and decreased blood supply often leads to ischemia and angina.

Secondly, just as coronary arteries develop arteriosclerosis, so do the blood vessels throughout the body. Arteries become damaged due to the excessive pressures and then become weakened. The weakened areas develop blood clots and thrombosis or they rupture and hemorrhage critically. Aneurysm, stroke, and renal failure are the primary types of damage that occur with chronic HTN. The small blood vessels in the back of the eye are also affected and may bleed.

What is a hypertensive emergency?

A hypertensive emergency is a life-threatening, sudden, and severe increase in BP that can lead to serious, irreversible end-organ damage within hours if left untreated. Currently it occurs in one percent or less of patients with hypertension. The organs most likely to be at risk are the brain, heart, and kidneys. Clinical features associated with this condition are headache, confusion, vision disturbance, nausea, and vomiting.

The treatment plan is to reduce the patient's BP within one or two hours to avoid permanent organ damage. Administer high-concentration oxygen, keep the patient calm, and medical direction decides what medication, if any, will be started in the field. Procardia may be given sublingually, but it has the adverse reaction of dropping the BP too fast and there is no way to quickly reverse its effects. For this reason, most experts strongly discourage its use in any hypertensive emergency.

The goal of drug treatment in a true hypertensive emergency is to give an agent that is easily titratable and that may be stopped rapidly if untoward side effects occur. The only two commercially available drugs meeting these criteria are IV drips of either nitroglycerin or sodium nitroprusside (Nipride®).

Hypertensive emergencies are related to other emergencies such as intracranial hemorrhage, pulmonary edema, myocardial ischemia, toxemia, and aortic dissection. When HTN is associated with these conditions, treatment should be directed to the primary problem.

What is cerebral autoregulation?

Cerebral autoregulation is a normal property of the brain that maintains cerebral perfusion within a fairly wide range of mean arterial BPs. This occurs with the opening and closing of sphincter muscles in the small arterioles of the brain. If autoregulation is lost, such as during a stroke or after head injury, the only way for the brain to maintain adequate perfusion is to elevate the arterial BP. So, it's expected to see a period of hypertension (24–48 hours maximum) as a direct response to the loss of cerebral autoregulation. In case of progressive patient deterioration or intracranial bleeding, the pressure still needs to be lowered rapidly. In many other patients, though, the period of hypertension is a *normal defense mechanism* designed to maintain cerebral perfusion. Lowering the blood pressure under these circumstances could be devastating.

CLINICAL PEARL

Treat the patient, not a number! Stroke patients commonly have a period of post-stroke hypertension. If the patient is normotensive or hypotensive, beware—this suggests either hypovolemia or septic shock from a central nervous system infection that caused the stroke in the first place. Trauma patients are usually not hypotensive from isolated head trauma—remember the normal response due to the loss of cerebral autoregulation is hypertension. *Look carefully for hypovolemia under these circumstances—pelvic fracture, internal bleeding.*

What is a "triple A" (AAA)?

Abdominal aortic aneurysm (AAA) is an aneurysm on the abdominal aorta. An aneurysm is a bulging sac in the wall of a blood vessel due to a localized weakness (Figure 23–6). The weakness in the wall may be caused by the effects of arteriosclerosis, infection, or a congenital condition. As the bulging of the sac continues to grow, the pressure it exerts on other structures often causes symptoms such as abdominal or back pain. Definitive treatment is surgical replacement of the damaged or weakened section of the wall with a synthetic graft. If the aneurysm goes unrecognized or untreated, it leaks, causing pain, or it grows and bursts like a balloon, usually resulting in sudden death.

Out-of-hospital management is limited to recognizing the possible life-threatening condition and initiating a rapid transport. Administer high-concentration oxygen, start an IV, keep the patient still, and advise the hospital early of your findings.

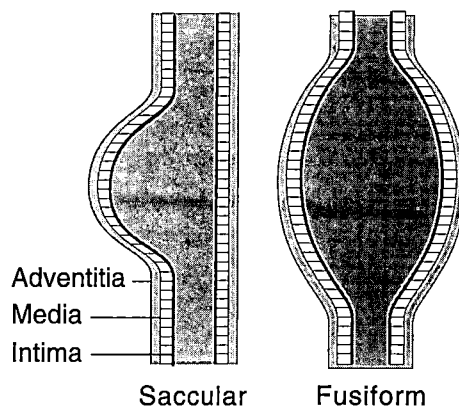

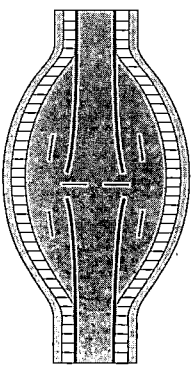

FIGURE 23–6 Types of aneurysm.

What is Marfan's syndrome?

It is a hereditary vascular disorder characterized by an abnormal length of the extremities, especially the fingers and toes; subluxation of the lens of the eyes; congenital anomalies of the heart; and other deformities such as aortic aneurysm. These patients develop aneurysms. Their aneurysms typically involve the aortic arch rather than the abdominal aorta, which would be more commonly caused by HTN.

What of significance happens to the Marfan's patients in out-of-hospital EMS?

Those affected with Marfan's may experience sudden death, usually from a spontaneous rupture of the aorta, often at an early age. Fortunately, some individuals have warning symptoms, such as shortness of breath or chest pain, prior to rupture. Having a general understanding of the possible consequences of the disease may help to prepare to manage this type of patient.

Q What is claudication?

A Claudication is a common manifestation of arteriosclerosis and presents with a severe pain in the lower extremity caused by inadequate blood supply. Similar to angina, it typically occurs with exertion and subsides with rest. The calf is most commonly affected.

Q What is phlebitis?

A Phlebitis is an inflammation of a vein causing pain in the affected part that is often accompanied by stiffness and edema. It can develop from intimal damage to the vein from catheters, injection of irritating substances, septic phlebitis, and the use of oral contraceptives. Thrombophlebitis refers to a thrombus developing in addition to the inflammation of the vein.

Congestive Heart Failure

Q How do preload, afterload, and left ventricular end-diastolic pressure correlate to the pathophysiology of heart failure?

A In a cardiac contraction, the degree of stretch of the contracting muscle is called the preload. This preload is also considered to be the volume of blood in the ventricles at the end of diastole, sometimes referred to as the end-diastolic volume. The load against which the heart exerts its contractile force is the afterload, or the pressure in the arteries leaving the ventricles. As the ventricles fill to higher atrial pressures, the strength of the cardiac contraction increases, causing the heart to pump increased quantities of blood into the arteries (Frank–Starling law of the heart).

When the heart muscle is injured and the ventricles can no longer pump effectively, the arterial pressures begin to change. The preload and afterload are directly affected. Therefore, the circulation of blood does not effectively reach all areas of the body and a backup of fluid develops in other areas.

Q What is heart failure?

A Heart failure occurs when the heart has been injured. The damage may be acute as a result of an AMI or dysrythmias, or progressive from disease such as HTN or another congenital disease. When cardiac pumping is insufficient to meet the circulatory demand of the body, it is called cardiac or heart failure. Two major problems that occur with failure are that cardiac output decreases and blood backs up in the venous system.

In the early stage of failure, the body senses the decrease in cardiac output. It attempts to compensate through sympathetic nervous system stimulation and fluid retention by the kidneys. The heart is stimulated to increase the rate and the force of contraction. The systemic circulation is stimulated to increase the tone in the blood vessels to provide better venous blood flow to the heart. The severity of damage to the heart will determine if the myocardium will recover or progress to cardiogenic shock.

The heart may fail in whole or part. Because the heart is literally two pumps, one or both of the pumps may fail initially. However, the stress of one injured pump will eventually lead to the entire pump failing. Left-heart failure is more common than right-heart failure because the left ventricle is more often affected by chronic HTN than the right. Often this is a "cumulative" problem resulting from multiple AMIs.

When the left ventricle fails to sufficiently pump blood, a backup of blood occurs in the lungs and pulmonary system because the heart is unable to push it out to the systemic circulation. This makes the right ventricle work harder, further elevating pulmonary arterial pressures and forcing blood through the lungs and into the weakened left ventricle. The increased BP in the pulmonary vessels leads to pulmonary edema, a buildup of fluids in the lungs. Consequently, pulmonary edema can occur so suddenly that death results after only 20 to 30 minutes from the onset of acute left-heart failure. If the left-heart failure is moderate, the patient may survive several days. In the case of a chronic failure, the lungs have built up delicate resistance and will not be as vulnerable to acute pulmonary edema (APE).

In right-heart failure, or *cor pulmonle,* blood is not pumped adequately from the systemic circulation into the lungs. The most common cause is left-heart failure, but other causes include HTN, COPD, and pulmonary embolism. The signs and symptoms of right-heart failure (Figure 23–7) may include tachycardia, venous congestion (e.g., peripheral edema, ascites, pericardial effusion), liver engorgement, and a history of AMI and the use of medications such as digitalis and furosemide (Lasix®). Right-heart failure is more often chronic than acute, and is usually not an emergency unless it is accompanied by left-heart failure and pulmonary edema. Rarely, acute right-heart failure can cause a great enough decrease in cardiac output that death may result. Patients do not generally call an ambulance for CHF, they call for weakness or shortness of breath due to acute pulmonary edema.

Q What is acute pulmonary edema (APE) and its relation to left ventricular failure?

A In the later stages of left-heart failure, the compensation mechanisms are stressed to the point that the left ventricle can no longer keep up with the right ventricle. Blood flow becomes congested, or backed up, in the pulmonary circuit and the patient suddenly develops severe pulmonary edema. Death may occur suddenly due to severe hypoxia and respiratory failure.

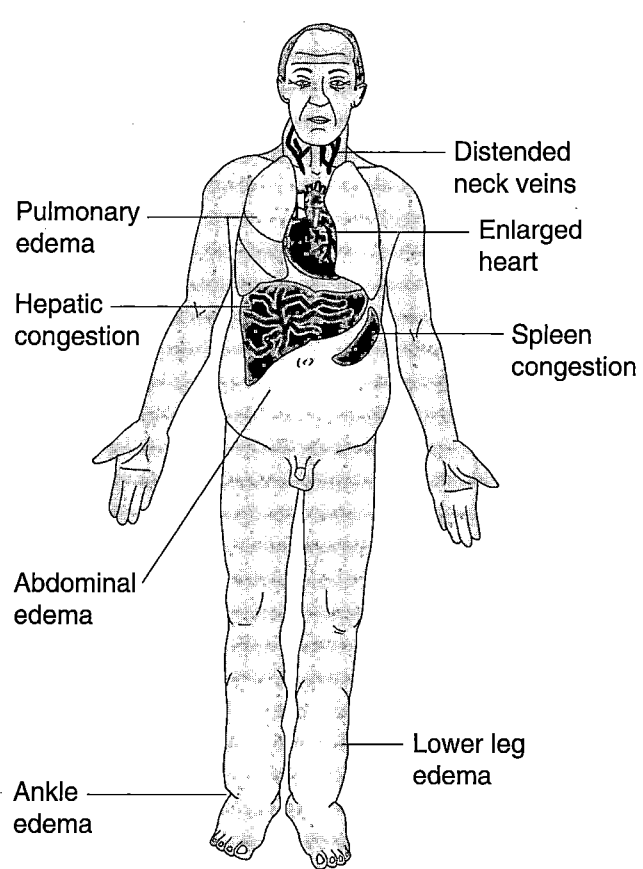

Pulmonary edema

Hepatic congestion

Abdominal edema

Ankle edema

Distended neck veins

Enlarged heart

Spleen congestion

Lower leg edema

FIGURE 23-7 Signs of heart failure.

The signs and symptoms of APE include the presence of shortness of breath with or without pink tinged sputum, presence of JVD, peripheral edema, chest discomfort, and cardiac dysrhythmia. Inspiratory rales or crackles in the base of the lungs are also associated findings for heart failure.

> **CLINICAL PEARL**
>
> *Pulmonary edema occurs both in chronic CHF, as late stage disease, and* de novo, *without warning. In the later case, APE usually develops as a response to acute myocardial ischemia. Less than half of patients with APE (not as progressive as CHF) have a concomitant MI. APE is their* sole *manifestation of ischemia.*

What is the clinical significance of paroxysmal nocturnal dyspnea (PND)?

PND refers to a shortness of breath that occurs during the night. Typically, the patient wakes suddenly from sleep and is extremely diaphoretic and short of breath. PND usually indicates significant CHF. Most people sleep in a prone or near-prone posi-

tion. Blood pools in the lungs leading to pulmonary congestion and difficulty breathing. Patients with a history of advanced heart failure will usually sleep with several pillows to keep them positioned upright (orthopnea) in order to prevent such attacks.

What is the clinical significance of edema of the extremity and sacral areas?

Edema is an accumulation of fluid most apparent in dependent portions of the body below the heart. Because gravity plays a large role in where edema settles, the legs will have more than the arms, and for bedridden or immobile patients, the sacral area is more prominently affected. Peripheral edema is more likely in chronic CHF because it takes several hours to develop. Stable patients who suddenly lapse into acute pulmonary edema often lack peripheral edema.

> **CLINICAL PEARL**
>
> *Peripheral edema and neck vein distension are far more common in* chronic CHF *than in acute pulmonary edema. Don't make the error of excluding the possibility of acute pulmonary edema simply because no peripheral edema is present!*

What are the interventions and most common drugs used to treat CHF?

The goal in the treatment is to improve oxygenation and ventilation by decreasing the preload, as well as the myocardial oxygen demand. Positioning the patient is paramount in this case. Sitting upright with legs dangling to assist in venous pooling aids in decreasing the preload. Though newer data will likely impact the acute treatment of APE, current therapy includes high-flow oxygen, nitroglycerin, furosemide, and morphine. Some EMS systems use inhaled bronchodilators and aminophylline as well. Pressor agents, such as dopamine, may be helpful in severe cases.

When a patient has progressed to a state of severe pulmonary edema, more aggressive and immediate treatment is required. Begin with assisting ventilations using a bag-valve-mask, followed by ET intubation if necessary. Though not widespread, noninvasive ventilation using nasal biphasic positive pressure breathing (nasal BiPAP) is being tried in the out-of-hospital setting. Preliminary data look promising.

What are the progressive stages of cardiogenic shock?

Cardiogenic shock is the most severe form of pump failure, resulting in inadequate cardiac output due to left ventricular malfunction. As a result of the greatly diminished blood flow throughout the body, tissues deteriorate rapidly and death ensues. The most common cause is a result of an extensive AMI.

Initially the signs and symptoms are the same as seen with AMI. As the body's compensating mechanism fails and shock progresses, severe hypotension develops and organ tissues die. Other signs and symptoms include altered mental status, tachycardia, dysrhythmias, diaphoresis, cyanosis, and tachypnea. Cardiogenic shock has a high mortality rate once shock has begun and hypotension remains.

Out-of-hospital management begins with treating for shock. Keep the patient supine, provide high-concentration oxygen and evaluate the need for assisted ventilation, establish an IV, and rapidly transport. The possible use of drugs might include dopamine or medications used to treat dysrhythmias.

Possible definitive treatment choices may include coronary artery bypass graft (CABG) or catheterization of the blocked coronary artery and the use of fibrinolytics (clot busters) such as tissue plasminogen activator (TPA).

Why is cardiogenic shock difficult to diagnose in the field?

The hypotension that is seen with cardiogenic shock can also be associated with other causes such as cardiac dysrhythmia, severe dehydration, hypovolemia, and infections, so making an out-of-hospital differential diagnosis is difficult.

How can you differentiate APE from COPD?

Sometimes it's really impossible to tell a difference. Patients with one condition often are at risk for the other. Both may present as a sudden shortness of breath with wet-sounding lungs. Past history may be helpful, though a person with a history of COPD is still prone to develop APE. To help differentiate between CHF and APE, look for a past medical history of heart disease because this is an important piece of information. A history of AMI is consistent with APE, while a history of COPD is consistent with CHF. However, a person may have both, making it

difficult to diagnose initially. Many providers, when in doubt, give both furosemide and an inhaled bronchodilator. This generally covers both conditions, as long as careful attention is paid to the basics of the ABCs.

What is cardiac tamponade and how is it produced?

Cardiac tamponade is an accumulation of fluids or a loss of blood into the pericardial sac. The pericardial sac is a fibrous sac that surrounds the heart and does not allow for expansion. The accumulation of fluids compresses the heart so that it cannot pump effectively and the patient dies of a sudden decrease in cardiac output.

This life-threatening condition quickly progresses from decreased cardiac output to cardiac failure and cardiogenic shock. This condition can develop from pericarditis, ventricular rupture following an MI, or a mechanical failure from a traumatic event such as a stabbing or compression in an automobile collision.

The major signs and symptoms are hypotension, dyspnea, tachycardia, and a weakening pulse. Look for the associated findings consistent with pericarditis and mechanism of injury from trauma. The treatment is pericardiocentesis, where a needle is inserted directly into the pericardial sac to remove the fluid. Out-of-hospital management is limited to recognizing the possible life-threatening condition and initiating a rapid transport. Administer high-flow oxygen, start an IV, keep the patient still, and advise the hospital early of your findings. Early hospital notification can be lifesaving. This will give the ED an opportunity to prepare to manage the patient immediately on your arrival.

What is Beck's triad?

Beck's triad is a combination of three symptoms characteristic of cardiac compression (tamponade) consisting of low arterial pressure (hypotension), high venous pressure (JVD), and quiet heart sounds. Beck's triad is named for the American surgeon, Claude Schaeffer Beck.

Neurology

The nervous system is clearly the most complex of the body systems. With all of the actions of a sophisticated computer working constantly, the nervous system acts as the control center of the body. Even today with our advanced medical research and knowledge, there are parts of the nervous system workings that are still not fully understood. Assessment and management of the patient experiencing a neurological emergency is a challenge. This chapter will explain the various components of the nervous system, review common and uncommon diseases and trauma-induced nervous system disorders, and lastly, discuss how to assess the patient with a neurological emergency.

Basic Terminology

What are common terms associated with the neurological system?

Common neurological terms include:

- Cognition—learning with understanding, reasoning, judgment, intuition and memory.
- Contralateral—pertaining to or affecting the opposite side of the body.
- Diplopia—double vision.
- Hemiplegia—paralysis of only one side of the body.
- Innervate—to stimulate, like a nerve stimulates an organ to respond.
- Ipsilateral—pertaining to the same side of the body; opposite of contralateral.
- Lateral—pertaining to a side, as to one side of the body.
- Neuralgia—pain in a nerve.

- Paralysis—temporary or permanent loss of function.
- Paresis—partial paralysis.
- Proprioception—perception of movement and position of the body.
- Ptosis—drooping eyelid.
- Sensorium—part of the brain that functions as a center of sensations.

Physiology

What are the different sections of the brain and their functions?

The brain is composed of the cerebrum, cerebellum, diencephalon, and brainstem. The components are shown in Figure 24-1.

- Cerebrum or telecephalon—the largest part of the brain; divided into right and left sides (hemispheres) that are connected by nerve tissue called the corpus callosum. Although certain areas of the brain have special purposes, no part of the brain works alone. Both sides of the brain communicate via the corpus callosum to carry out many complex functions. The cerebrum is the location of higher cognitive abilities such as learning, analysis, memory, and language. This area is also responsible for the control of specific sensory and motor functions. Each cerebral hemisphere is divided into five lobes; four of which are named for the bones that cover them. The five lobes of the cerebrum are:

   1. Frontal—each hemisphere controls voluntary motor functions on the opposite (contralateral) side of the body. The left hemisphere contains the speech sections called Broca's area and Wernicke's area, which control speech and the movement of the tongue, lips, and vocal cords; it basically "does the talking." The right side specializes in the perception of certain types of auditory stimuli such as coughing, crying, humming, and laughing, as well as the spatial perception of touch and sight.

   2. Parietal—receives and translates somatic sensations of pain, touch, pressure, heat and cold, and body position (proprioception). It also controls speech and memory.

   3. Temporal—primary auditory (hearing) and smell. It also controls speech and memory.

   4. Occipital—primary visual areas. It also controls memory.

   5. Insula—the central lobe of the cerebral hemisphere; it is triangular-shaped and lies in the floor of the lateral fissure. Also known as the Island of Reil, the insula is important in speech comprehension, expression, and recognition. It also modulates the autonomic response to irritative stimuli.

- Cerebellum—is located in the back of the skull beneath the cerebrum and surrounding the brain stem. It is responsible for maintaining posture, balance, and voluntary coordination of skilled movements.

- Diencephalon (between brain)—is located between the cerebrum and midbrain and contains the following five structures: the thalamus, hypothalamus, optic chiasma, limbic system, and the pineal body.

   1. Thalamus—responsible for sensation, emotion, alerting, and complex movement.

   2. Hypothalamus—responsible for many important functions for survival and pleasure such as eating, drinking, temperature regulation, and sex. It links the nervous and endocrine systems, as well as the mind (psyche) and body (soma).

   3. Optic chiasma—the area where the optic nerves cross before entering the brain.

   4. Limbic system—is a group of structures, such as the hypothalamus, hippocampus, and the amygdala, that are concerned with emotion and motivation.

   5. Pineal body—regulates the biological clock of the body.

- Brainstem—is located at the base of the brain; contains structures that are critical to the maintenance of vital functions. From top to bottom in the brain stem are the midbrain, pons, and medulla oblongata.

- Midbrain—controls reflexes for eye movement and pupillary reflexes (mediated by cranial nerves three and four). Also contains auditory, visual, and muscle control reflexes.

- Pons—contains reflexes mediated by the cranial nerves five to eight. Also contains the apneustic center, the stimulus to increase the length and depth of inspiration and the pneumotaxic center, the stimulus that affects the rate of respiration.

- Medulla—is located in the lower brain stem and attaches to the spinal cord. It is responsible for controlling vital reflex centers for breathing, heart rate, and vasomotor functions. The medulla also controls non-vital reflexes such as swallowing, vomiting, coughing, sneezing, and hiccupping.

Q What was the purpose of a frontal lobotomy in patients with severe behavioral problems?

A The lobotomy procedure was used previously on patients who did not respond to other treatments. The procedure was accomplished by an incision into the brain to disconnect certain pathways from the hypothalamic area to the prefrontal cortex. The lobotomy is no longer utilized.

Q How does the brain get its blood supply?

A Blood enters the brain from the two internal carotid arteries and the basilar artery, which connect into a cerebral arterial circle (Figure 24–2) called the "Circle of Willis." This structure forms a circle around the stalk of the pituitary gland and is a clever backup mechanism for complications that may arise with cerebral blood flow.

Normally, the internal carotid arteries supply the front half of the cerebrum. The basilar artery supplies the rest of the brain. If for any reason blood flow gets disrupted, the Circle of Willis may provide for collateral cerebral circulation, reducing the chances for serious complications.

Q What is CSF?

A Cerebrospinal fluid (CSF) is present in the subarachnoid space, cavities, and canals of the brain and spinal cord. CSF is produced in the ventricles of the brain and is completely replaced several times a day. There are three functions of CSF:

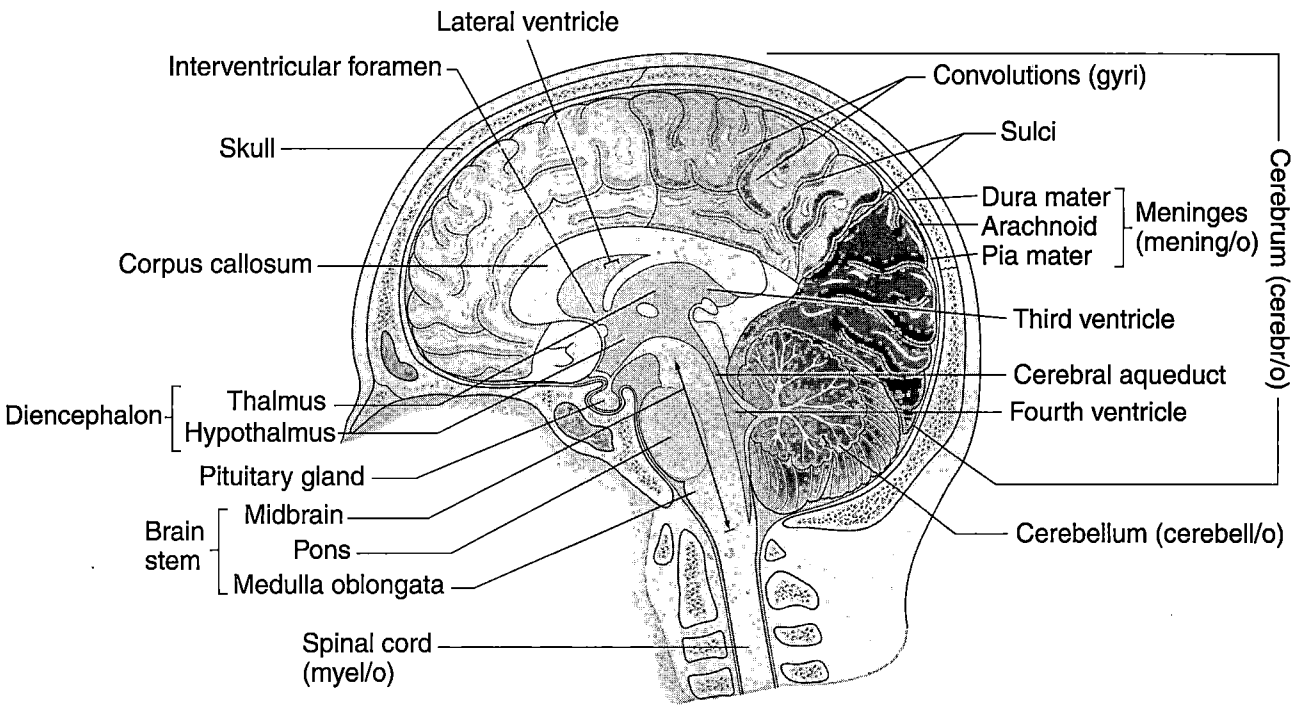

Lateral ventricle

Interventricular foramen

Skull

Corpus callosum

Diencephalon [Thalmus
Hypothalmus

Pituitary gland

Brain stem [Midbrain
Pons
Medulla oblongata

Spinal cord (myel/o)

Convolutions (gyri)

Sulci

Dura mater] Meninges
Arachnoid (mening/o)
Pia mater]

Third ventricle

Cerebral aqueduct

Fourth ventricle

Cerebellum (cerebell/o)

Cerebrum (cerebr/o)

FIGURE 24-1 The components of the brain on cross-section.

1. Protection as a cushion of fluid for the brain and spinal cord.
2. Supports the brain and spinal cord by diffusing nutrients, electrolytes, and metabolic end products between the extracellular fluid surrounding the CNS neurons and glia.
3. The brain monitors changes in the CSF CO_2 level and activates responses in the respiratory centers to regulate the CO_2 and pH of the body.

What is hydrocephalus?

Hydrocephalus is an increase in the amount of CSF due to either a blockage or decreased reabsorption. Sometimes this results in increased pressure within the skull (increased intracranial pressure). Treatment usually involves the placement of a shunt into the ventricles so that excess fluid can drain into the central systemic circulation.

What is the purpose of the meninges?

The meninges are three distinct layers of membranes that form a continuous sac surrounding the brain and spinal cord. These are called dura mater, arachnoid membrane, and pia mater.

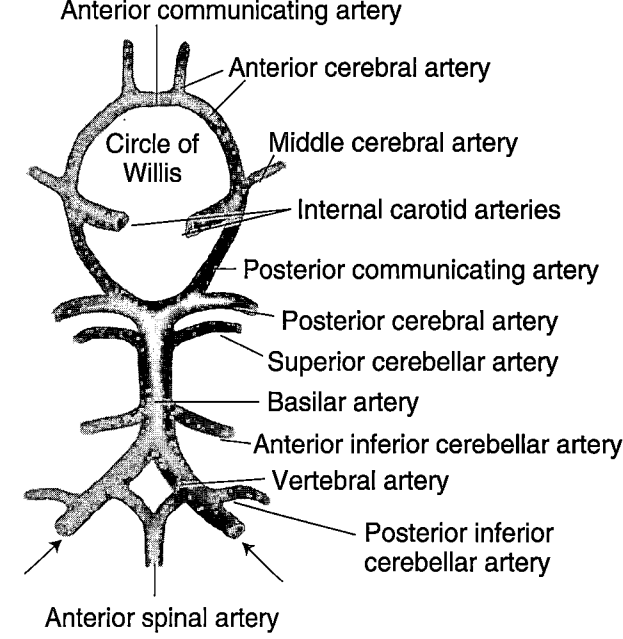

Anterior communicating artery

Anterior cerebral artery

Circle of Willis

Middle cerebral artery

Internal carotid arteries

Posterior communicating artery

Posterior cerebral artery

Superior cerebellar artery

Basilar artery

Anterior inferior cerebellar artery

Vertebral artery

Posterior inferior cerebellar artery

Anterior spinal artery

FIGURE 24-2 The major arteries of the brain.

- The dura mater is the outermost layer of the meninges. It is fibrous and inelastic. The Latin meaning of the word is "strong" or "tough." The space between the dura and the skull is the potential epidural space; it is here that meningeal arteries are located. When a bleed occurs in this potential space, it is called an epidural hematoma. The bleed is most often from the middle meningeal artery and can become life threatening very quickly.

  The dura mater has three significant inner extensions—the tentorium, falx cerebelli, and falx cerebri. The tentorium process of dura mater separates the cerebrum and cerebellum and supports the occipital lobes. The falx cerebelli separates the hemispheres of the cerebellum, while the falx cerebri partitions the two cerebral hemispheres.

- The arachnoid membrane is the middle layer of the meninges. The Latin meaning of the word is "web-like." This layer loosely covers the CNS. The subarachnoid space beneath the arachnoid is filled with CSF and has connections in certain areas with the pia mater. The space above the arachnoid membrane and between the dura mater is called the subdural (under the dura) space. When a bleed occurs in this potential space, it is called a subdural hematoma. The type of bleeding that occurs in this space is venous, unlike arterial bleeding in an epidural hematoma. The signs and symptoms of the subdural bleed usually do not appear acutely due to the slow venous bleed.

- Pia mater—is the innermost layer of meninges. It is highly vascular and covers the brain and spinal cord.

CLINICAL PEARL

Meningitis is an infection of both CSF and meninges that may be life threatening, especially when caused by bacteria. Encephalitis refers to the infection of the brain tissue itself and is usually viral in origin.

What is the gray and white matter?

Gray matter are the gray fibers of the CNS including the cerebral cortex, basal ganglia, and parts of the brain and spinal cord. This matter is nerve tissue comprised of cell bodies of neurons *not* covered with a protective myelin sheath (unmyelinated nerve fibers). White matter is the white fibers of the brain and spinal cord that is primarily composed of nerve fibers that are covered with myelin (myelinated).

What is a neuron?

A neuron, or nerve cell, is the fundamental component of the nervous system. The neurons are dependent on aerobic metabolism, meaning they require oxygen to function. When the hyper-

activity of a seizure depletes the neuron of oxygen, the neuron is injured. If this condition is prolonged, cell death occurs.

What are the parts of a nerve cell?

The nerve cell (neuron) has a surface that is sensitive to stimuli. The neuron communicates by means of initiating and transmitting nerve impulses from one part of the body to another. Neurons are classified as *functional,* labeled for the direction that they conduct impulses either to or from the CNS, or *structural,* labeled according to the number of processes projecting from the cell body.

There are three types of functional neurons: afferent (carry impulses from the tissues to the spinal cord and brain), efferent (carry impulses from the brain to the spinal cord, then to the tissues), and interneurons (located only in the brain and spinal cord) that connect afferent and efferent neurons.

There are three types of structural neurons: unipolar (two processes that form one axon), bipolar (one axon and one dendrite), and multipolar (one axon with several dendrites).

Each neuron (Figure 24–3) has three components—the cell body (soma), the dendrite, and the axon.

- The cell body contains DNA and RNA and is responsible for maintaining and renewing nerve fibers, as well as transmitting nerve signals.

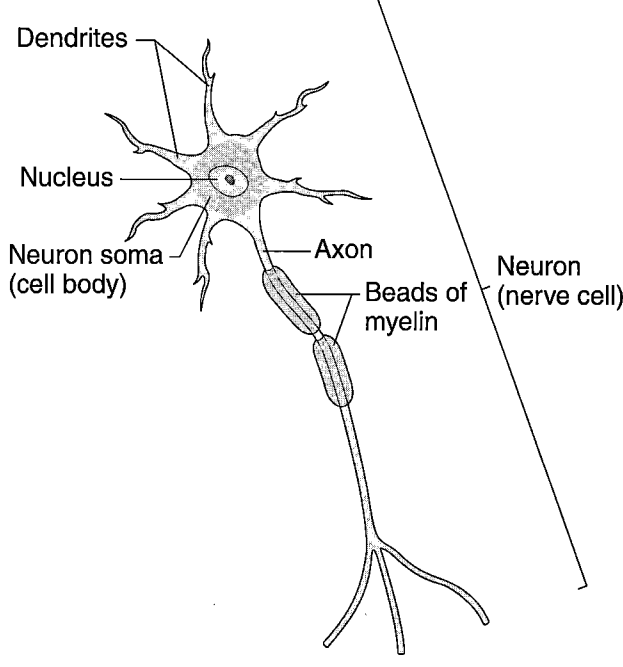

FIGURE 24–3 The neuron.

- Dendrites are extensions of the nerve cell body with branches that conduct impulses to the cell body, relaying information to the neuron.
- Axons are long efferent processes that project from the cell body and carry impulses away from it. Some axons are over a meter in length.

What are the supporting cells of the nervous system and what do they do?

The groups of supporting cells located in the CNS are called *glia;* in the peripheral nervous system (PNS) they are called Schwann and satellite cells. The supporting cells protect the neurons by forming sheaths creating the blood–brain barrier and the myelin sheath. They also provide metabolic support, which is imperative for normal neural function. Nervous tissue requires a tremendous amount of metabolic energy, specifically oxygen and glucose. The brain cannot create or store either of these, so it relies heavily on the supporting cells as a source of energy.

What is myelin?

Myelin is a layer or coating (sheath) around the axon that protects the axon process and increases the conduction of nerve impulses. Myelin has a high lipid content making it look white (white matter). Some disease processes, such as multiple sclerosis, interfere with the myelin sheath. The disease destroys the sheath and infects the nerve fibers, impairing nerve conduction.

How is an impulse transmitted from nerve to nerve?

The cell body and the dendrites are covered with thousands of synapses. The synapse (junction) is the place where impulses are transmitted to the axons and dendrites of other neurons. Nerve cells communicate with each other primarily via synapses. The signal may be propagated from cell to cell by either more synapses (synaptic transmission) or via the movement of ions (electrochemical transmission).

What is a reflex arc?

A reflex is an involuntary response to a stimulus. The reflex arc is the specific neural pathway used by the body in responding to a stimulus. A typical reflex arc includes a sensory receptor, an afferent neuron, a reflex center either in the brain or spinal cord, one or more efferent neurons, and an effector organ (usually a muscle or gland). The receptor senses a response and sends the information to the CNS. The CNS processes the information and sends out a signal to an effector organ to respond.

For example, a person's finger touches a sharp object and the sensation is forwarded to the brain through sensory pathways. The brain perceives the stimulus as pain and sends out a message as a motor response to the hand to pull away.

What is the limbic system?

Located within the diencephalon, the limbic system (emotional brain) is comprised of several brain structures that are involved with emotions—both the subjective experiencing and the objective expression of them. The limbic system also controls sense of smell and plays an essential role in coupling sensory inputs to short- and long-term memory.

What is the reticular activating system (RAS)?

High in the brain stem is the RAS that is responsible for maintaining the level of consciousness.

Which nerves are part of the PNS?

The PNS consists of 12 pairs of cranial nerves and 31 pairs of peripheral nerves exiting the spinal cord between each vertebra. Because the cranial nerves arise directly from the brain, they usually are affected by ipsilateral injuries. Before the peripheral nerves traverse the spinal cord, about three-fourths cross over (decussate) to the opposite side in the base of the brain within the medulla. Thus, the right hemisphere of the brain controls the left side of the body. This explains why a patient with a right-sided cerebral hematoma may exhibit an altered mental status, an enlarged right pupil (due to pressure on the third cranial nerve that controls pupil constriction), and *left*-sided weakness of the rest of the body.

What are the functions of the 12 cranial nerves?

The functions of the cranial nerves are summarized in Table 24–1.

Nervous System Disorders

What disorders of the central nervous system (CNS) should the out-of-hospital provider be familiar with?

The following list includes common diseases, uncommon diseases, and trauma-induced nervous system disorders that the EMS provider may find in patients in the field:

TABLE 24-1

Functions of the Cranial Nerves

Olfactory (I)	Smell
Optic (II)	Visual acuity, visual fields, funduscopic examination
Oculomotor (III)	Cardinal fields of gaze (EOM movement), eyelid elevation, pupil reaction, doll's eyes phenomenon
Trochlear (IV)	EOM movement
Trigeminal (V)	Motor: strength of temporalis and masseter muscles Sensory: light touch, superficial pain and temperature to face, corneal reflex
Abducens (VI)	EOM movement
Facial (VII)	Motor: facial movements Sensory: taste anterior two-thirds of tongue *Parasympathetic: tears and saliva secretion
Acoustic (VIII)	Cochlear: gross hearing, Weber and Rinne tests Vestibular: vertigo, equilibrium, nystagmus
Glossopharyngeal (IX)	Motor: soft palate and uvula movement, gag reflex, swallowing, guttural and palatal sounds Sensory: taste posterior one-third of tongue *Parasympathetic: carotid reflex, chemoreceptors
Vagus (X)	Motor and Sensory: same as CN IX *Parasympathetic: carotid reflex, stomach and intestinal secretions, peristalsis, involuntary control of bronchi, heart innervation
Spinal Accessory (XI)	Sternocleidomastoid and trapezius muscle movements
Hypoglossal (XII)	Tongue movement, lingual sounds

*Cannot be directly assessed.

EOM = extraocular muscle; CN = cranial nerve.

Functional Disorders

- Amyotrophic lateral sclerosis (ALS or Lou Gehrig's disease, named after the famous baseball player)—a rapidly progressive disorder leading to atrophy of all body muscles and death.

- Bell's palsy—unilateral facial paralysis due to the compression of cranial nerve VII (facial nerve).

- Cerebral palsy—blanket term for a nonprogressive group of disorders affecting the CNS. Associated with prenatal, perinatal, or postnatal CNS damage and classified by the extremities involved and the type of neurological dysfunction.

- Epilepsy—recurrent seizures of any form.

- Headache—a symptom rather than a disorder and is associated with many diseases and conditions, including emotional stress. There may be acute or chronic diffuse pain or ache any place in the head. A headache may also be associated with trauma or various intracranial or extracranial factors. Classified as tension (most common), vascular (migraine or cluster), and traction inflammatory (intracranial or cranial).

- Hydrocephalus—a condition of an increasing collection of CSF within the ventricles of the brain due to a blockage in the normal draining CSF.

- Multiple sclerosis—a chronic, progressive disease of the CNS characterized by exacerbation and remission of assorted multiple neurological symptoms.

- Parkinson's disease—a chronic and slowly progressive disorder characterized by low levels of the neurotransmitter dopamine in parts of the brain that control voluntary movement. The patient experiences weakness and muscle rigidity, irregular gait, and a fine resting tremor.

- Spina bifida—a malformation of the spinal column with an opening in the membrane that covers the vertebra. Spina bifida is the most common developmental defect of the CNS, occurring while in utero.

Infectious Diseases

- Brain abscess—intracranial infection; encapsulated collection of pus within the main portion of the brain. Signs and symptoms (listed with brain tumor) are similar to a brain tumor.

- Encephalitis—inflammation of the brain and spinal cord tissues that may temporarily or permanently affect neurological functions.

- Meningitis—inflammation of the tissues (meninges and CSF) that surround the brain and spinal cord. This condition may temporarily or permanently affect neurological function. Bacterial meningitis is most common, and is highly contagious. It may cause complications that include arthritis, blindness, cognitive deficit, deafness, hydrocephalus, myocarditis, and pericarditis. Viral meningitis is often short lived with benign recovery.

- Poliomyelitis (polio)—viral infection causing inflammation of the gray matter of the spinal cord that may temporarily or permanently affect neurological functions.

- Tetanus—bacterial infection of the CNS that is highly fatal. Characterized by painful muscle contractions.

- Shingles—acute viral infectious disease caused by *herpes zoster*, the same virus that causes chicken pox. Characterized by a painful, itching rash with blisters that follow the course of a sensory nerve. This is commonly found on the torso as shown in Figure 24-4. Rare complications include CNS infection, temporary paralysis, and muscle atrophy.

Tumors

- Brain tumor—intracranial lesion that may be benign or malignant. As the lesion expands within the main portion of the brain, signs and symptoms develop that vary with size and location and may include any of the following:

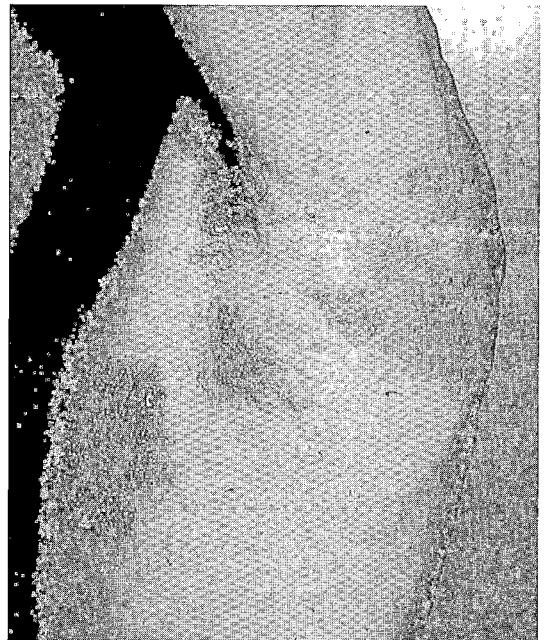

FIGURE 24-4 Shingles vesicles follow a nerve pathway.

a. Headache
b. Nausea and vomiting
c. Seizures
d. Memory loss
e. Impaired judgment
f. Depression
g. Psychotic behavior
h. Drowsiness

• Hematoma—a collection of blood caused by a ruptured blood vessel that is enclosed in an organ, tissue, or body space. The two most common hematomas that may develop within the brain are epidural hematoma and subdural hematoma, named by the location in relation to the meninges.

Vascular Disorders

• Cerebral aneurysm—congenital defect (weakness or bulge) on the wall of a cerebral artery. Usually not a problem until they rupture. Fourth leading cause of cerebrovascular disorder in the United States.

   Most ruptured aneurysms are classified as saccular (berry) aneurysms. These are small berry-like sacs that protrude outward in a pouch formation on cerebral arteries. The patient experiences a loud sound in the head when the rupture occurs, followed by severe headache. Altered level of consciousness and death may result.

• Cerebrovascular accident (CVA, stroke)—acute loss of blood supply to the brain.

• Transient ischemic attack (TIA)—acute temporary loss of blood supply to the brain.

Dementia (*often incorrectly* used synonymously with senility, is a general term for decreased mental intellect and cognitive function).

• Alzheimer's disease—chronic and progressive disorder leading to irreversible impairment of intellect and memory. AIDS dementia, Parkinson's disease, Huntington's disease, and Creutxfeldt-Jakob disease are additional classifications of dementia.

• Vascular dementia—caused by atrophy and death of brain cells due to decreased blood flow (e.g., atherosclerosis).

• Drug induced dementia—caused by chronic alcohol abuse, excessive use of drugs, or drugs that are toxic to the CNS.

• Head trauma dementia—caused by the death of brain cells from trauma, direct injury, or indirectly from edema caused by increased intracranial pressure (ICP).

What are the potentially reversible causes of dementia?

Some causes of dementia, if detected and treated in a timely manner, are completely or partially reversible. These include:

• Drugs, chemicals, or toxins.
• Emotional problems.
• Metabolic disorders.
• Vision or hearing deficits.
• Nutritional deficits.
• Tumors and trauma.
• Infections and fever.
• Stroke or vascular occlusion.

> **CLINICAL PEARL**
>
> *Always assume that a patient has a reversible cause for an altered level of consciousness (e.g., hypoxia, hypoglycemia) until proven otherwise!*

Traumatic Brain Injury

How common is brain injury?

Every 15 seconds, someone in the United States sustains a brain injury. This adds up to more than two million people each year. An estimated 5.3 million Americans currently live with disabilities resulting from brain injury. In addition, 80,000 Americans experience the onset of long-term disability following traumatic brain injury (TBI) annually.

What does secondary injury from TBI mean?

Medical research has demonstrated that all brain damage does not occur at the moment of impact; rather, it occurs over the next few hours and days. This is referred to as the secondary injury. Ischemia is the most common cause of secondary brain injury; the others are ICP, cerebral edema, and brain herniation.

What is a concussion?

A concussion is a mild closed-head injury that results in a transient loss of brain function with or without a loss of consciousness. Symptoms most commonly include headache, memory loss, and irritability that usually resolve in 24 hours, but may persist for months. Often patients demonstrate short-term memory loss after a temporal blow.

Anyone who has a concussion should be seen by a physician for an evaluation of the extent of injury. The doctor will have important instructions for the patient such as having someone wake them up every few hours within the first 24 hours of the injury and possible interactions with medications like blood thinners.

What is a contusion?

A contusion (brain tissue bruising) is a moderately severe closed-head injury with small bleeds and swelling (cerebral edema). Unlike a concussion, a contusion can be seen on a CT scan. Signs and symptoms can include a longer period of unconsciousness initially followed by amnesia, aphasia, and hemiparesis.

What is a contra-coup brain injury?

A contra-coup injury is one that occurs on the opposite side of the impact. The brain is bounced from one side of the cranium to the other, causing either a concussion or contusion (Figure 24–5). Because the cranium has sharp and protruding edges inside, the brain can be cut, torn, and bruised.

What is amnesia: retrograde versus anterograde?

Amnesia means loss of memory. There are different types of memory loss (e.g., short-term and long-term) and there are many causes of amnesia such as medication (i.e. benzodiazepines) or physical and emotional traumas.

- Anterograde—loss of memory for events after an adverse event. In this type of amnesia, the ability to establish new long-term memories is affected.
- Retrograde—loss of memory for events that occurred before an adverse event. This type of amnesia affects the ability to

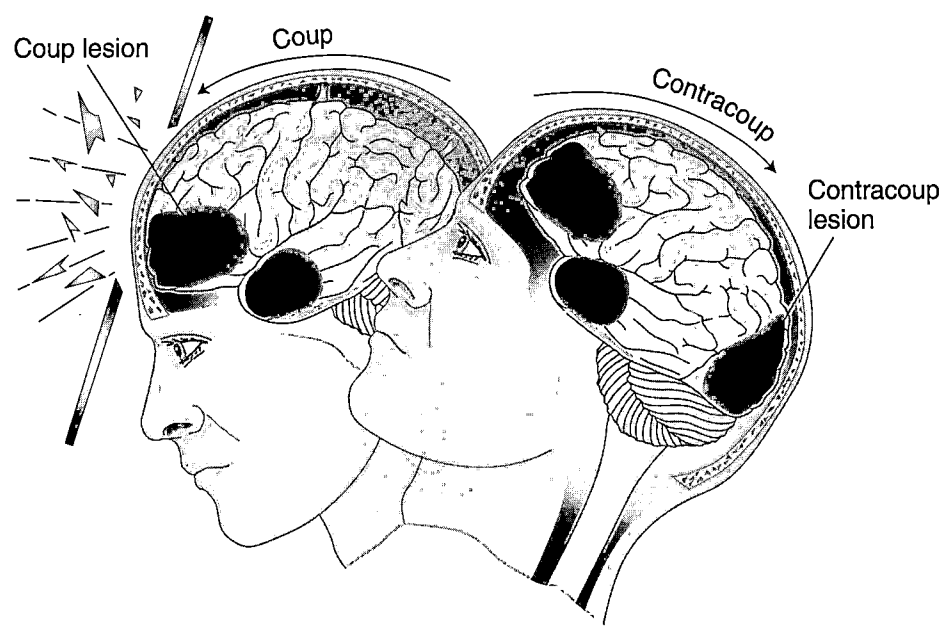

FIGURE 24–5 A coup-contracoup injury.

recall memories from the past; patients cannot access their long-term memory bank.

What is the significance of an open versus a closed skull fracture?

The main significance of *any* skull fracture is the degree of underlying brain damage and other associated injuries. In addition, an open fracture is associated with an increased risk of cerebral infection.

How does cerebrospinal fluid (CSF) leak out?

CSF leaks usually occur through fractures at the base of the skull. Fluid leaks through the nose. If the eardrum is ruptured, fluid may also leak out through the ears.

What steps by both the out-of-hospital and in-hospital caregivers provide significant reductions in mortality and morbidity of the head-injured patient?

The greatest reduction in mortality and morbidity are due to a combination of the following:

- Rapid transport to a trauma center.
- Prompt resuscitation.
- CT scanning.
- Prompt evacuation of significant intracranial hematomas.
- ICP monitoring and treatment.

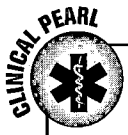

The best treatment for any patient is the maintenance of an airway, breathing, and circulation.

Is hyperventilation still used for patients with head trauma?

We used to teach hyperventilation as a treatment for head injury. Based on current research, the pendulum has swung in the opposite direction. Hyperventilation is no longer recommended for the head-trauma patient who does not have indications of rising ICP and brain herniation.

The guidelines of the Brain Trauma Foundation state that, "prophylactic hyperventilation (PaCO$_2$ <35 mmHg) therapy during the first 24 hours after severe traumatic brain injury should be avoided because it can compromise cerebral perfusion during a time when cerebral blood flow (CBF) is reduced." The guidelines do go on to state that hyperventilation therapy may be nec-

essary for brief periods when acute neurologic deterioration is present for longer periods or if there is intracranial hypertension that is refractory to sedation, paralysis, CSF drainage, and osmotic diuretics.

So when is hyperventilation recommended?

Consider hyperventilation in the field if traumatic brain injury (TBI) patients do not respond to verbal stimuli, and they do not respond appropriately (localizing) to axillary pinch or nail bed pressure and pupils are asymmetric or unreactive. The hyperventilation rates per minute are:

- 20 in adults.
- 30 in children.
- 35 in infants.

Should steroids be used for the TBI patient?

No, this is controversial, but current research shows that the use of steroids is not recommended for improving or reducing intracranial pressure in patients with severe head injury.

Neurologic Emergencies

What is a neurological emergency?

A neurological emergency is a sudden severe deficit in neurologic function. Causes may include trauma, infections, neoplasms, tumors, cerebrovascular disease, degenerative disease, and metabolic derangements.

What are the most common emergent neurologic conditions?

The most common neurological emergencies include:

- TIA.
- CVA.
- Seizure.
- Syncope.
- Headache.
- Expanding neoplasm, tumor, or abscess.

What is a TIA?

A TIA or mini-stroke is a temporary occlusion of an artery to the brain caused by a blood clot. TIAs are a strong predictor of stroke risk and may occur days, weeks, or months before a stroke. The major difference between a TIA and a stroke is that the TIA has no lasting effect.

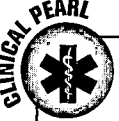

Even though patients with TIA may have no lasting neurological defects, consider TIA to be a "warning sign" of impending stroke within the next month. A physician should always evaluate these patients as soon as possible.

Who is at risk for TIA?

There are many risk factors for TIA and stroke, some that you can change or modify and some that cannot be changed. An undiagnosed TIA is a very high risk factor for a major stroke. Some of the risk factors include:

- Hypertension.
- Heart disease.
- Carotid artery disease.
- Arteriosclerosis.
- Diabetes.
- Family history.
- Overweight.
- Smoking.
- Unhealthy diet.
- Age.

What assessment findings would suggest the patient is having a TIA?

The following is a warning list, any one or more of the following acute changes may occur at the same time:

- Sudden confusion.
- Change in speech.
- Dizziness.
- Weakness.
- Numbness or paralysis.
- Headache with unknown cause.
- Nausea or vomiting.
- Incontinence of bowel or bladder.

The signs and symptoms are the same as for stroke; however, with TIA, they occur rapidly and last briefly, usually less than five minutes. Every TIA or stroke *must* be treated as a life-threatening

emergency! Just as "time is myocardium (heart muscle)," the same is true of brain cells. To receive "clot buster" (thrombolytic) therapy, the diagnosis of stroke must be made and treatment begun within three hours of the onset of symptoms.

If a stroke occurs during sleep, we must assume that the time of onset was shortly after the patient went to bed.

What is the management plan for the patient experiencing a TIA?

In the hospital ED, tests to rule out stroke or another medical problem will be performed. Out-of-hospital management includes:

- BLS, with the use of high-flow oxygen.
- Completion of a thrombolytic checklist.
- ALS, IV access with blood samples drawn.
- Supportive care and reassessment for changes.

What is a stroke?

A stroke or CVA has come to be known as a "brain attack." Stroke is a form of cardiovascular disease that affects the arteries leading to the brain. When an artery becomes blocked (thrombosis) or ruptures, blood and oxygen are cut off to the brain cells. The damage can be permanent or temporary depending on the location and size of the thrombosis, and how quickly treatment can begin.

What is the difference between a hemorrhagic and an ischemic stroke?

A hemorrhagic stroke occurs when a blood vessel to the brain ruptures. An ischemic stroke is the most common and is caused by a clot (thrombus) that blocks an artery. A smaller number of ischemic strokes are due to emboli that arise in other parts of the body, particularly the heart. Either way, part of the brain becomes ischemic due to the block. The out-of-hospital treatment is the same for both hemorrhagic and ischemic stroke. Definitive in-hospital therapy, however, varies.

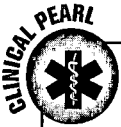

Stroke is a "heart attack of the brain." An "unstable angina of the brain" is a TIA.

What causes stroke?

The causes of stroke are the same as TIA.

What are the signs and symptoms of stroke?

The signs and symptoms of stroke are the same as for TIA, except that they do not resolve as quickly or at all. Signs and symptoms include:

- Acute onset may cause unconsciousness.
- Onset is more gradual if caused by thrombus.
- Numbness, weakness, and paralysis in face or extremity, more often unilateral.
- Sudden vision disturbances—blurred or decreased vision in one or both eyes.
- Change in speech—aphasia, dysphasia, and expressive aphasia.
- Ataxia—staggering, loss of balance or coordination, especially when combined with another symptom of stroke.
- Irregular breathing, expirational puffing of cheeks and mouth.

What are the effects of stroke?

Each year approximately 600,000 Americans will have a new or recurrent stroke. Stroke is the third leading cause of death in Americans (about 160,000) and a major cause of serious long-term disability.

Can stroke or TIA be prevented?

There are a number of risk factors that can be changed or modified to improve the chances of avoiding a stroke or TIA. Modifications to lifestyle made *slowly* can make a significant difference. Preventative steps include cessation of smoking, controlling hypertension or diabetes (decrease atherosclerosis), improved diet, and exercise. Risk factors such as family history, gender, and age cannot be changed; however, the ideal goal is to minimize the modifiable risk factors as the best preventive measures. This is probably the best reason for getting annual checkups.

How is stroke diagnosed?

A diagnosis for stroke by the physician includes the physical assessment, blood tests, ECG, CT scan, or MRI. Of all the tests, the physical assessment, combined with the patient's history, is usually the most informative.

What time of day do most strokes occur?

Thrombotic strokes typically occur during sleep. The patient falls asleep without any problems, then wakes up in the morning with a fixed neurologic deficit. Hemorrhagic or embolic strokes are more abrupt, occurring when the patient is awake.

CLINICAL PEARL

The natural history of thrombotic stroke is such that it often occurs during sleep. Because the time frame for thrombolytic therapy is short (three hours), most victims do not qualify because we must assume that the onset of the stroke was shortly after going to sleep.

What is the management plan for stroke?

Before any in-hospital treatment can begin, the diagnosis has to be made. All of the components of the diagnosis take time and this is where the out-of-hospital care provider can make a huge difference. Early recognition of the signs and symptoms of stroke can speed up the diagnosis, allowing for quicker and more effective treatment options and better patient outcomes. Perform the following steps in the out-of-hospital phase:

- Establish two IVs in different arms; one for "clot-buster" (thrombolytic drug) access and one for parenteral therapy. Avoid multiple needle punctures.
- Perform ECG, either 3, 4, or 12 lead, to help rule out cardiac conditions.
- Draw blood samples for the laboratory analysis (CBC, PT/PTT, platelets, fibrinogen, type and screen for packed cells, electrolytes, BUN, creatinine, CPK with isoenzymes).
- Rule out hypoglycemia with blood glucose; check all patients for altered mental status (AMS).
- Complete a thrombolytic checklist.
- Early notification of the ED.
- Transport to a facility with thrombolytic therapy ability.

Significant advancements have recently been made in the treatment of stroke, decreasing the death rate and reducing disability. Thrombolytic agents ("clot-busters"), such as tissue plasminogen activator (t-PA), are a major advance in treatment. However, not every patient is a candidate for clot-dissolving therapy. The primary reason is that the treatment has to begin within three hours of the onset of symptoms, and many do not seek care quickly enough.

What is a seizure?

A seizure is a sudden temporary change in behavior, sensory, or motor activity due to an excessive or chaotic electrical discharge of one or more groups of neurons in the brain.

What causes a seizure?

Causes of a seizure include stressors such as hypoxia, a sudden elevation in body temperature as seen with febrile seizures (pediatrics), or hypoglycemia. There are structural causes such as tumors, head trauma, eclampsia, and vascular disorders (e.g., CVA). Idiopathic epilepsy (chronic repetitive seizures) is the most common cause.

Seizures occur in patients of all ages, though the causes of seizures vary slightly in each age group. The most frequent causes of seizures by age group are:

Infant
- Trauma from childbirth.
- Infection.
- Electrolyte abnormalities.
- Congenital defects.
- Genetic disorders.

Toddler
- Trauma.
- Infection.
- Febrile seizure.

Child
- Trauma.
- Febrile seizure.
- Infections (meningitis).
- Idiopathic (epilepsy).

Adolescent
- Trauma.
- Drug or alcohol related.
- Idiopathic (epilepsy).

Young Adult
- Trauma.
- Alcohol (acute intoxication or withdrawal).

- Brain tumor.

Older Adult
- Stroke.
- Brain tumor.
- Intracerebral hemorrhage.
- Alcoholism.
- Metabolic disorders.

What are the different types of seizures?

Seizures are clinically referred to as generalized or partial. A generalized seizure has seizure activity that involves the entire body. Three types of generalized seizures are complete or full-motor seizure, absence seizure, and atonic seizure. Seizures can be broken down in the three phases: *preictal* (before), *ictal* (seizure attack), and *postictal* (after).

Generalized

- Complete motor seizure (also called tonic–clonic, formerly called grand mal) may include an aura, a distinctive sensation preceding seizure activity, in the preictal phase. This phase is followed by a loss of consciousness with muscle contractions (tonic) lasting 15–20 seconds and alternating muscle spasms (clonic) lasting up to 5 minutes. The tonic–clonic period disrupts the normal respiration causing hypoxia. Tongue biting and incontinence (more often urine) are common in this phase. The postictal phase follows the tonic–clonic phase. This is when consciousness slowly returns. The postictal phase will vary in length depending on which type of seizure was experienced. There will be disorientation, confusion, and often patient embarrassment. They may complain of a headache and usually experience extreme fatigue.

- Absence seizure (formerly called petit mal) is commonly seen in children. It appears similar to day dreaming or staring off into space. There is usually no aura or warning of any kind. The phase usually lasts for seconds to minutes and is followed by a relatively short postictal phase.

- Atonic seizure is a complete loss of postural control. The patient may have secondary injuries from falling. This type of seizure usually occurs in children.

Partial seizures affect a particular area of the brain and thus affect only a given area of the body, often without a loss of consciousness. Partial seizures include simple, complex, and partial with secondary generalization.

Partial

- Simple partial seizures were formerly called focal motor seizures. This type of seizure is characterized by the dysfunction of an isolated area of the body, such as a single arm shaking.

- Complex partial seizures, formerly called temporal lobe or complete psychomotor seizure, last approximately one to two minutes. They are characterized by an impairment of consciousness, including an aura. Aura with this type of seizure may include hallucinations of sounds, visuals, smells, and tastes (metallic taste). The patient may act confused or display personality changes that include outbursts and fits of rage.
- Partial seizure with secondary generalization, once referred to as Jacksonian march, initially involves one area of the brain, but then spreads to the entire brain. The seizure activity begins in one local area of the body, such as an arm, and then spreads (marches) throughout the entire body.

What information is important about the seizure activity?

Getting a good description of the seizure activity, including the duration of the tonic–clonic phase and postictal phase and evidence of incontinence can help determine what type of seizure the patient experienced. Also, determine if there was more than one seizure (status epilepticus) with this event.

> **CLINICAL PEARL**
>
> *Incontinence of urine, feces, or both is a well-described, though uncommon, finding in generalized seizures. Many people have seizures and are not incontinent. And, many incontinent persons have never had a seizure!*

What is status epilepticus?

Status epilepticus is a series of two or more seizures occurring in the same event without any intervening period of consciousness or a prolonged seizure lasting more than 10 minutes. Prolonged seizures tend to present with very little or no body movement (fixed gaze only). This does not mean the patient has stopped seizing. Their neurons are burning out, so treat for seizures (e.g., maintain their airway open and clear, administer oxygen, start an IV, and consider benzodiazepines). Brain damage can occur from a prolonged or repeated seizure, making *status epilepticus* a true emergency! If the EMS call was for a seizing patient and the patient is still seizing on your arrival, they probably are in status epilepticus!

> **CLINICAL PEARL**
>
> *A fixed gaze or disorientation may also be a sign of a prolonged postictal phase. Regardless of the cause, maintain the ABCs, consider treatable causes (e.g., hypoglycemia), and transport the patient appropriately.*

What other information should be obtained in the focused history (FH) of the seizure patient?

Determine, if possible, if this is a first-time seizure or if there is a history of seizures. If the patient has a history, inquire about compliance with medications, change of medication, and alcohol or substance abuse. If the seizure is the first one, ask about recent trauma, specifically head injury, illness, or infection. Always inquire about changes in medications or new medications. The first-time seizure patient should always be transported for further evaluation. Follow local protocols for the transportation of seizure patients and while caring for any seizure patient, be prepared for a repeat seizure.

> **CLINICAL PEARL**
>
> *In patients with known seizure disorders, always inquire if there was anything different about this particular event. Often families only call EMS when the patient's seizure differs from the usual pattern. This may be a clue to a new underlying problem, such as a tumor.*

What medications can cause syncope?

There are many drugs that may be the culprit of a syncopal event and the reason that EMS is called. Following are drug classifications for common home medications that may cause syncope:

- Beta-blockers.
- Diuretics.
- Antihypertensives.
- Narcotic analgesics.
- Antiarrhythmics.
- Nitrates.
- Digitalis.
- ACE blockers.
- Psychiatric meds (especially tricyclics).

What can a patient's medications tell me about their condition?

AMS is frequently associated with the patient's medications. Any changes in medications, such as starting on a new medication, stopping a medication, forgetting, or skipping a medication, can be the source of the problem. Once you become familiar with drug classifications, you can get a good idea of the patient's general medical condition.

> *If a patient is on a medication, with or without a prescription, assume it's part of the problem until proven otherwise.*

Q What is polymedication and polypharmacology?

A These are interchangeable terms. The dilemma occurs when a patient is prescribed multiple medications for concurrent diseases. This is seen commonly in the elderly for many reasons. When a patient sees multiple doctors and the doctors prescribe medications without being told by the patient about current medications they are on, medication errors occur.

- The multiple medications can create drug interactions.
- The patient becomes forgetful or confused and skips doses or takes too much.
- Financial challenges often play a role in not taking medications as prescribed.

> *Sometimes the patient is inadvertently taking both a trade preparation and a generic preparation of the same drug. They often look different, have different names on the labels, and are in different containers. With managed care and prescription drug regulations, this situation is likely to become even more common.*

Q Does the location of a headache indicate the cause?

A Not always; however, there are conditions that present with somewhat consistent localization of pain. For example, fever associated with the headache may indicate meningitis, brain abscess, or encephalitis, while hypertension with a headache may be seen with subarachnoid hemorrhage. The following are some additional findings associated with headaches:

- Cerebral aneurysm—localized to one side.
- Glaucoma—eye pain.
- Meningitis—back of head.
- Migraine—bilateral or unilateral.
- Stress—any area of the head.
- Subarachnoid—worst headache ever experienced.
- Temporal arteritis—pain or headache over temporal artery.
- Temporomandibular joint (TMJ) syndrome—pain with jaw movement.
- Trauma—any area of the head.

- Trigeminal neuralgia (also called tic douloureux)—pain in one or more of the three branches of the fifth cranial nerve (trigeminal nerve) that runs along the face.

Q What are the signs and symptoms of expanding cerebral neoplasms?

A Almost all signs and symptoms are slowly progressive. Cerebral neoplasms may present with a seizure, while a bleeding neoplasm will have signs and symptoms resembling a CVA. As cerebral edema develops, so does a slow onset of dulled mental status. Rarely, a neoplasm will affect the RAS causing an irreversible coma.

Brainstem tumors are slowly progressive with other localized neurological findings such as cranial nerve abnormalities appearing before a mental status change is apparent.

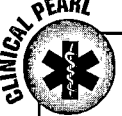

> *New onset seizures in patients over 21 years of age have a one in five likelihood of being due to a tumor.*

Q What are the various treatments and pharmacology available for the treatment of neoplasms?

A The treatments for cerebral neoplasms depend on the cause. For benign growth, surgical removal is often curative. For cancers, either primary or metastatic, a combination of surgery, radiation therapy, and chemotherapy is often required.

Q What are the signs and symptoms of a brain abscess?

A The signs and symptoms of a brain abscess may include headache, fever, and possibly sinusitis. Other findings are similar to that of space-occupying lesions such as seizures and focal neurologic deficits. The diagnosis is confirmed with a CT scan.

Q What is the treatment and pharmacology for abscesses?

A Treatment is aimed at the infections with the use of any of a number of antibiotics. Sometimes surgical drainage is also required.

Q What are the signs and symptoms of neurological diseases?

A Signs and symptoms of neurological diseases vary widely. Common presentations include:

- Motor symptoms (e.g., weakness, inability to move a part of the body, impaired coordination).
- Sensory symptoms (e.g., decreased sensation, hypersensitivity, "pins and needles" feelings, pain).
- AMS.
- Seizures.
- Headache.
- Stiff neck.
- Neck or back pain.
- Loss of bowel or bladder control.

What types of medications might a patient with a neurological disorder be taking?

Pharmalogical treatment will vary depending on the disorder. Listed are some examples of medications prescribed for Parkinson's, Alzheimer's, and seizure disorders.

Parkinson's disease:

- Drugs with central anticholinergic activity and anticholinergic agents (e.g., benxtropine, biperiden, prcyclidine, trihexyphenidyl).
- Drugs affecting brain dopamine (e.g., levadopa, amantadine, bromocriptine, pramipexole, ropinirole).
- MOAI (e.g., selegiline).

Alzheimer's Disease:

- Central-acting skeletal muscle relaxants (e.g., diazepam, carisoprodol, chlorphenesin carbamate, chlorzoxazone, cyclobenzaprine, metazalone, methocarbamol, orphenadrine).
- Direct-acting skeletal muscle relaxant (e.g., dantrolene).

Seizure disorders:

- Anti-seizure medications (e.g., diphenylhydantoin, phenobarbital, Tegretol®).

Focused Neurological Assessment

Why do a neurological assessment?

The neurological assessment is performed to either confirm or rule out a neurological disorder and to establish a baseline. Look for changes, either for better or worse, because everything is based on a comparison of repeated assessments. Isolated assessment findings have little value in the evaluation of the neurological patient. The neurological exam consists of six areas: mental status, cranial nerves, motor response, sensory response, coordination, and reflexes. A neurological exam should be performed for any patient with general neurologic complaints.

CLINICAL PEARL

The word "symmetry" makes neurological evaluation very straightforward. Though it is possible to be "symmetrically abnormal," any asymmetrical findings are abnormal until proven otherwise.

What are the signs and symptoms associated with a neurological emergency?

The following signs and symptoms could be associated with a neurological emergency and should be considered as such until they can be ruled out:

- Abnormal respirations.
- AMS.
- Memory loss.
- Headache.
- Weakness.
- Paresis.
- Paralysis.
- Vision disturbances.
- Speech disturbances.
- Motor disturbances.
- Vertigo.
- Syncope.
- Seizure.
- Coma.

How is the mnemonic AEIOU-TIPS used?

AEIOU-TIPS is used within the FH to help rule out conditions and begin to make a differential diagnosis of the patient with an AMS. Each letter is used as a reminder of the possible causes of AMS:

Alcohol (acute or chronic).
Epilepsy, Endocrine, Exocrine, Electrolytes.
Infection (local or systemic).
Overdose (intentional or accidental).
Uremia (trauma or renal causes, including hypertension).
Trauma (new or old), Temperature.
Insulin (hypo- or hyperglycemic).
Psychosis (numerous possibilities).
Stroke (hemorrhage or ischemic), Shock, Space-occupying lesion, Subarachnoid bleed.

Q What is significant about the acronym AVPU in the neurologic patient?

A Subtle changes in a patient's mental status are usually the earliest indicator of nervous system dysfunction. Out-of-hospital care providers utilize AVPU during the initial assessment of patients to obtain a rapid evaluation of their ability to respond to a voice and follow commands. The use of AVPU classifies the patient into one of four categories:

A—alert.
V—responds to verbal stimuli.
P—responds to painful stimuli.
U—unresponsive.

The significance of AVPU is that it can be performed quickly during the initial assessment to obtain a baseline of the patient's mental status. However, this method provides only a gross estimation of the neurological status of the patient and does not quantify the level of disability. Record information obtained from the AVPU on the prehospital care report (PCR). (For more information on AVPU see Chapter 15, Scene Size-Up and Initial Assessment).

Q How do I test for eye response?

A Look to see if the eyes are moving and watching you as you first move toward the patient. This is the best response (4 on the GCS). If the eyes are open and the patient does not focus on you until you give a verbal stimulus such as "Are you OK" or ask the patient to show you two fingers, the response is rated (3 on the GCS). To elicit a pain response, pinch a nail bed, (2 on the GCS). An example of no eye response is observing fixed pupils (1 on the GCS).

Q How should I adapt the GCS to an infant or toddler who does not have language skills yet?

A The American College of Emergency Physicians (ACEP) and American Academy of Pediatrics (AAP) in the APLS course (1998) recommend assigning a full verbal score (5 on the GCS) for crying or cooing without stimulation in children <2 years old. If it requires stimulation for crying, they get a score of (3 on the GCS).

Q How is the motor assessment for GCS performed?

A This is relatively easy on the unresponsive patient. However, to standardize the application of painful response, the Brain Trauma Foundation recommends placing the patient's arm in flexion and providing an axillary pinch. A localizing response by patients means they are attempting to pull your pinching hand away. If this test is not practical due to clothing, use pressure instead of pinching to see if the patient withdraws, flexes, extends, or is flaccid.

GCS motor assessment should be done on both sides. If the patient extends on one side and flexes on the other side, use the *best* response.

Q How can the GCS be helpful in the transportation decision?

A Some areas use the GCS as a triage mechanism. For example, the Brain Trauma Foundation guidelines suggest that patients with severe brain injury (GCS <9) should be transported directly to a facility with the capabilities for immediate CT scanning, prompt neurosurgical care, and the ability to monitor and treat intracranial hypertension.

Q What are the abnormal respiratory patterns associated with neurological emergencies?

A The following is a list of abnormal respiratory patterns associated with neurological dysfunction:

- Apneusis—extended inspiratory effort or gasping with a brief expiration due to pressure, damage, or surgical removal of part of the pons in the area of cranial nerve IV.
- Ataxic—breathing often precedes agonal breathing and apnea. There is no pattern or rhythm with depth or rate. Associated with lesions in the lower brain stem.
- Autisms—involuntary neurological activities such as yawning, hiccuping, coughing, and vomiting. When autisms are present together with AMS, this may indicate a lesion in the lower brain stem.
- Biot's respiration—pattern of repeated deep gasps and apnea due to increased ICP.
- Central neurogenic hyperventilation—pattern of extended hyperventilation with forced inspiration and expiration. Associated with respiratory alkalosis, or a lesion in the midbrain or upper pons. *This is not the same as an anxious hyperventilating patient.*
- Cheyne-Stokes respiration (CSR)—pattern of cycles of apnea and hyperventilation due to emergent conditions such as brain injury (cerebral) or drug overdose.
- Cluster breathing—pattern of breathing in short spurts and associated with lesions in the pons.
- Kussmal's breathing—pattern of very deep gasping respirations that is associated with coma and metabolic acidosis.

Q What do you look for with the eyes?

A The normal visual function of the eyes depends on the ability of both eyes to fix on the same object (binocular fusion) together with the retinal and CNS acuity mechanisms. Binocular fusion is controlled by the forebrain; if this reflex fails, double vision (diplopia) occurs. Three pairs of extraocular muscles, which are mediated by three cranial nerves, control binocular vision. Cranial nerve III innervates adduction, elevation, and lateral gaze; cranial nerve IV innervates medial gaze; and cranial nerve VI innervates lateral abduction. The reflexes in distance vision are called vergence reflexes. To see an object moving closer than 30 feet, the eyes move toward each other (convergence) and to see objects further away, the eyes move parallel (divergence) and return to conjugate gaze.

While examining the patient's eyes, assess for the following:

- Accommodation—refers to the adjustment of the eye to variations in distance.
- Acuity—sharpness of visual perception.
- Conjugate gaze—refers to the use of both eyes to look steadily in one direction. Deviation of both eyes to either side at rest indicates a structural lesion.
- Dysconjugate—one eye cannot move, may indicate intracranial trauma.
- Nystagmus—involuntary movement of the eyes that can be in any direction, but more often is either vertical or horizontal. May be induced by alcohol intoxication, irritation of the inner ear, blindness, and neurologic diseases.
- Doll's eye—the doll's eye maneuver test is used in comatose patients to assess for brain stem or oculomotor injury, *after neck injury has been ruled out*. With the patient's eyes opened, the head is turned quickly from side to side or up and down (Figure 24–6). The normal response is for both eyes to move

Normal (reflex present)

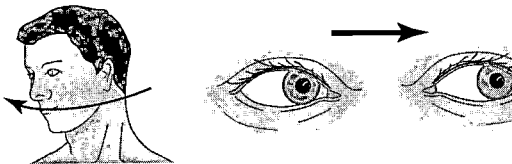

Head rotated to the right   Eyes move to the left

Abnormal (reflex absent)

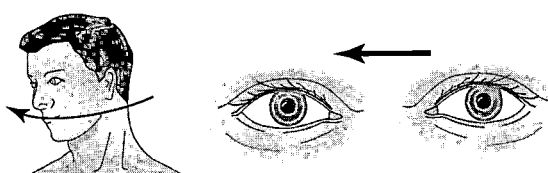

Head rotated to the right   Eyes follow

FIGURE 24–6 The doll's eye phenomenon.

in conjugate gaze to the opposite side of the head turning, similar to the doll with counterweighted eyes. The *abnormal response* is seen as the eyes staying in midposition (fixed) or turning in the same direction as the head is turned. This indicates severe forebrain or brain stem damage.

What can be learned from assessing the pupils?

Some say the pupils are the windows to the brain. Rods and cones are the photoreceptor cells located in the retina. The rods are stimulated by dim light and cones are stimulated by colors. Pupils are light sensitive—too much light they constrict, not enough light they dilate. Normal pupil size is 4 to 5 mm and pupil size can vary for a number of reasons. The ambient light is the first consideration in pupil size. If you are assessing the pupils in bright light, sunlight, or fluorescent lighting, the pupils should be constricted to a certain degree. In bright ambient lighting, instead of shining a light in the patient's eyes, cover or shade the eyes with your hand to see a change (dilation) in size. Head injury and many types of drugs can also change the pupil size.

- Constriction occurs naturally with age, other causes include photophobia, and the use of miotic drugs such as morphine sulfate, Eserine®, and physostigmine. Miosis is the abnormal constriction of the pupil due to certain types of infection. Miosis is seen in the early stage of meningitis, some types of drug overdose, brain lesion, and sunstroke. Pinpoint pupils are extremely small pupils due to excessive constriction, miotic drugs, and certain brain disorders.
- Dilation commonly occurs with blindness, intracranial trauma, fever, coma, glaucoma, ocular motor nerve paralysis, anoxia, and certain drugs such as atropine. Atropine is made from a plant called belladonna; some women actually use belladonna-like products to dilate their pupils because they believe it to be more "attractive." A fixed and dilated "blown" pupil is a very late sign of rising ICP. The mechanism for this occurrence is due to pressure on cranial nerve III due to herniation of the temporal lobe. This degree of herniation of the brain is severe and mental status will be significantly decreased; therefore, an alert patient with a blown pupil is not the classic picture of rising ICP.
- Fixed pupils do not respond to light. Lesions in the brain may cause pupils to look fixed; the size can vary from pinpoint to large depending on the location of the lesion.
- Accommodation of pupils is an expected mechanism that allows the normal eye to focus on objects closer than 20 feet.

CLINICAL PEARL

Remember, some opthalmic drops cause dilation or constriction of the pupils. Also, some patients have irregular pupils due to their corneal or cataract surgery.

What is considered a significant finding in assessing the pupils?

A difference of one mm or more in the size of the pupils is abnormal. A fixed pupil (<1 mm) to bright light is considered no response. A dilated pupil is greater than 4 mm.

CLINICAL PEARL

Nearly 10 percent of the population have congenital inequality of their pupil sizes, a condition known as anisocoria. Unless you are certain this finding is long standing, treat it as a major warning sign of a possible head injury.

What is glaucoma, what causes it, and why is peripheral vision testing important in these patients?

Glaucoma is a disease in which elevated pressure in the eye, due to an obstruction of the outflow of *aqueous humor,* damages the optic nerve and causes visual defects. Acute (angle-closure) glaucoma is a hereditary disorder with the iris blocking the flow of aqueous humor. Symptoms, which may occur suddenly, include dilated pupil, red eye, blurred vision, and severe eye pain, sometimes accompanied by nausea and vomiting. If untreated—by special eye drops or surgery—angle-closure glaucoma may result in permanent blindness within a few days. The much more common open-angle, or chronic, glaucoma, also hereditary, is one of the leading causes of blindness in the United States. Caused by a blockage of the canal of Schlemm, it produces symptoms very slowly with a gradual loss of peripheral vision over a period of years, sometimes with headache, dull pain, and blurred vision. Treatment involves the use of special eye drops. Glaucoma can also occur as a congenital defect or as a result of another eye disorder. Early glaucoma may be asymptomatic except for a loss of the peripheral visual fields.

What are muscle movement disorders?

Muscle coordination, balance, and gait are controlled through a complex system. Pyramidal and extrapyramidal tracts work together to control muscle movement and posture. Chemical mediators play an important role in neural transmission and include dopamine, the monoamines, seratonin, acetylcholine, GABA (gamma amine butyric acid), and possibly endorphins.

Pyramidal disorders cause weakness and spasticity, and also affect deep tendon reflexes and Babinski's sign. Extrapyramidal disorders affect involuntary movements and impair voluntary movements, causing changes in muscle tone. Examples of extrapyramidal disorders include:

- Akinesia—full or partial loss of muscle movement.
- Athetosis—condition of slow and irregular involuntary winding movement of the extremities, especially the fingers and hands. Some causes include drug toxicity or drug side effects, cerebral palsy, encephalitis, and Huntington's chorea.
- Ballism—intense, constant involuntary movement (jerking or twisting) of a proximal extremity caused by a lesion, infarct, or focal seizure.
- Chorea—brief involuntary movement of the distal extremities and face, which may blend with voluntary movements that can hide the involuntary motion. Chorea often occurs simultaneously with athetosis. Huntington's disease is the most prevalent cause; other causes include Parkinson's disease, thyrotoxicosis, and drugs such as antipsychotics.
- Dystonia—impairment of voluntary movement by sustained abnormal postures and disturbances of voluntary movement resulting in changes in muscle tone.
- Dyskinesia—involuntary movements of the extremities that are not repetitive, but may be stereotypical in nature.
- Myoclonus—rapid momentary contraction of a muscle or group of muscles. A hiccup is a normal form of myoclonus. Abnormal myoclonus can be caused by TBI and lesions, and is seen in degenerative neurologic diseases like Alzheimer's and Creutzfeldt-Jakob disease.
- Tics—rapid momentary involuntary movements that are repetitive and stereotypical, but not rhythmic, such as blinking.
  1. Tourette Syndrome—lack of muscle coordination; involuntary muscle movement; tics; and incoherent grunts, barks, and cursing. This disorder begins in childhood and is three times more prevalent in boys than girls.
  2. Tremors—a rapid quivering that may involve voluntary muscles as seen with shivering from being cold or involuntary muscles as seen in Parkinson's patients.

CLINICAL PEARL

Despite specific definitions for various types of movement disorders, many patients have an overlap of signs and symptoms. It is sometimes difficult to make a complete diagnosis even in the hospital setting, let alone in out-of-hospital care.

What are the six cardinal positions of gaze?

The six cardinal positions of gaze refer to the primary extraocular movements (EOMs), or movements of the eyeball due to the contraction of one or more of the attached extraocular muscles. An assessment of the six cardinal positions of gaze is used to evaluate cranial nerves III, IV, and VI to detect midbrain and pontine dysfunction. Checking EOMs is the best single method for measuring brain stem integrity.

Have patients hold their heads still while you direct them (using your finger) to move their eyes through six points of gaze—up and down laterally both left and right and side-to-side, in the shape of a large "H," like a stick-shift pattern. Observe for nystagmus, rapid oscillation of the eyeballs, simultaneously. An inability of one or both eyes to move as directed may indicate a neurological deficit. Paralysis of the upward gaze may also indicate an orbital fracture.

How can the location of a brain injury be determined from an assessment of cranial nerve function?

An assessment of the cranial nerves can help clue you in to the location of a brain injury or insult. Check EOMs in the conscious patient. An evaluation of the six cardinal gazes focuses on cranial nerves III, IV, and VI. Paralysis of the upward gaze may indicate an orbital fracture, while paralysis of a lateral gaze (either left or right) may suggest pathology in the brain. The loss of lateral eye movement is an early sign of rising ICP.

Assessment of the remaining cranial nerves:

- I—smell; not usually assessed in the field.

- II—optic; vision disturbances. Abnormalities may indicate problems anywhere in the visual pathway, including intrinsic eye injury or disease.

- V—speech; aphasia, dysphasia, dysarthria, difficulty swallowing or chewing (mastication), and blinking reflex. Instruct the patient to clench the teeth and ask the patient to move the jaw from side-to-side against resistance. Then have the patient bite down on the molars on each side.

- VII—facial asymmetry. Have the patient smile and "show me your teeth." Or ask the patient to purse the lips as if to whistle. Also have patients wrinkle the forehead and open their eyelids against slight resistance.

- VIII—lateralization of hearing loss; usually not assessed in the field.

- IX—symmetry of uvula and palate, ability to say "Ahhhh," gag reflex.

- X—vagus; slowed heart rate in the absence of beta-blockers. Also affects the swallowing reflex and voice.

- XI—shoulders shrugging and head turning left and right.

- XII—tongue midline and movement, listen for thick speech.

- Incontinence of urine or bowel may indicate spinal cord injury, seizure, or ethyl alcohol (ETOH).

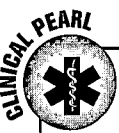

Remember that an evaluation of the cranial nerves is only one piece of information in the "puzzle" of diagnosis.

How can neurological problems affect speech?

In most people (including left-handed folks), the language function centers are located in the left hemisphere. Damage to any part of this specialized area of the cerebral cortex will interfere with language functions, including speech, writing, and sensory information.

Aphasia is the loss of an ability to speak due to a defect in or loss of language function. Expression (motor) or comprehension (sensory) of words may result. Aphasia is categorized as expressive or receptive:

- Expressive or nonfluent aphasia is associated with an injury of Broca's area and an abnormal processing of the motor function of language located in the frontal lobe. The speech is limited and unpredictable. The patient may be able to utter two or three words, may make up words, or exhibit involuntary cursing (involves the limbic system). Patients often know what they want to say, but are unable to speak their thoughts. There is no muscle impairment and patients understand what they hear or read. This often leads to frustration, anger, and depression for the patient.

- Receptive aphasia is the inability to understand words. In Wernicke's aphasia, patients are able to speak but unable to understand spoken or written words, impairing their ability to communicate effectively or socially.

Other common terms related to speech include:

- Ataxic—defective speech to muscular incoordination (expressive aphasia).

- Dysarthria—difficult or defective articulation of speech caused by disturbed motor control of the tongue or other muscles required for speech; there is no deficit in the ability to understand (patient is not aphasic).

- Dysphasia—impaired speech, word arrangement is mixed up (expressive aphasia).

- Dysphonia—difficulty speaking due to voice impairment, not due to aphasia (e.g., hoarseness or the changing of a boy's voice during puberty).

How do you test motor function?

The primary motor cortex located in the frontal lobe is connected with the association motor cortex in the basal ganglia and cerebellum. Assess patients for focal deficits of muscle strength, tone, and symmetry in all four extremities. If the patient has pain from injury or illness, the tests are unreliable and should not be performed.

Strength and movement:

- In the upper extremities, check for equal grip strength, hemiparesis, or hemiplegia.
- Assess pronator drift by having the patient close the eyes and hold out both arms with palms up. If one arm "drifts" lower or turns palm down, this may indicate motor deficit.
- In the lower extremities, check the dorsiflexors of the great toe.
- Flexing of the lower leg at the knee.

Cerebellar specific (fine motor movements):

- Have patients touch their index finger to your index finger.
- Have patients flip their hand palm up to palm down rapidly and repeat the movement. Faster is better.
- If not contraindicated, observe the patient walk to assess the balance and gait. Ataxia is an irregular gait caused by defective muscular coordination due to a variety of sources (e.g., alcohol, drugs, CVA, or inner ear infection). If patients can walk on their heels and then on the toes, they have intact muscular strength.

How is muscle tone described?

A patient's muscle tone is described using the following terms:

- Normal.
- Rigid.
- Spastic.
- Abnormal flexion.
- Abnormal extension.
- Limp or weak.

What are some examples of abnormal gaits?

Normal muscle tone, balance, coordination, and the pathways that connect these characterize the normal manner of walking (gait). When one, or more, of these components is disrupted or dysfunctional, a person's gait may become abnormal. The following is a short list of abnormal gaits:

- Ataxic—unsteady, uncoordinated, wide at base as seen with drunkenness, heavily medicated, or certain medical conditions.
- Festination—hurrying gait as seen in Parkinson's disease.
- Spastic hemiparesis—one-sided weakness with the toes of one foot dragging along.

- Steppage—steps appear to be going up steps due to a lesion in the spinal nerves.

How do you test sensory function?

This part of the neurological exam is the least exact and informative except in the case of spinal cord injury (SCI). The loss of sensory and motor function below certain levels in the spine defines an SCI. When this finding is present, mark the line of demarcation on the body during the baseline exam to compare with serial assessments.

For the non-SCI patient assess distal extremities for discriminative touch (sharp versus dull). There are at least six types of tactile receptors located in the skin and tissues below the skin. . There are several pathways for these receptors to transmit sensations, so it is uncommon to lose all sensations. Testing of the light touch determines the level and extent of damage in spinal cord lesions. Light touch is transmitted through pathways that are susceptible to insult and may be disrupted by a variety of causes. Dull touch can remain intact even with severe SCI:

- Meissner's corpuscles are located in the skin close to the surface and sense light touch.
- Merkel's disks are located in nonhairy areas of the skin and sense dull and continuous touch.
- Ruffini's corpuscles are located in the dermis of the skin and sense deep pressure and continuous touch.

Have patients close the eyes and, using a sharp-tipped object and a dull-tipped object, alternately touch the extremities. Ask if they can tell you where you are touching and which tip you are using.

Why is body temperature an important vital sign?

Extreme temperatures due to exposure or temperature regulation disorders are causes of AMS. Hypothermia below 32 degrees C or hyperthermia above 42 degrees C, by itself, can depress neurologic functioning enough to cause AMS. Often, this state is compounded by another condition, either medical or trauma, making diagnosis and treatment complex.

- Hypothermia—leads to hypoxia and dysrhythmias. This condition, by itself, can cause AMS. Hypothermia is not always obvious because exposure to profound cold is not necessary. For example, a drowning occurring in a backyard pool in 80 degree water during the month of August is often overlooked as being hypothermic in nature. However, if a person is impaired from performing normal behavioral responses, such as putting on clothing when cold, due to an AMS from intoxication, overdose, trauma, stroke, or tumor, the risk for hypothermia increases and the problem is compounded.

The elderly and the very young are especially at risk. The elderly often lose their ability to sense cold, while young children lose heat due to their large body surface area. Patients with altered sensorium, such as diabetic patients, are also at risk for hypothermia and may present with an AMS due to a single cause (hypo- or hyperglycemia) or compound causes such as hypo- or hyperglycemia and hypothermia.

- Hyperthermia—has many causes including exposure, insufficient acclimatization, infections, drugs, and metabolic disorders. Patients experiencing cerebral vascular accidents, including intracerebral or subarachnoid hemorrhage, can present with typical signs of heatstroke (e.g., AMS, neurological dysfunction, elevated temperature, hot and dry skin). There is often an overlap of conditions, making diagnosis and treatment complex. (For more information on hyper- and hypothermia, see Chapter 29.)

How are levels of consciousness described?

Because the cerebral hemispheres are the most susceptible to injury, the most common signs of brain dysfunction are AMS and behavioral changes. As other areas of the brain become affected, additional motor and pupillary changes occur. Respiratory and hemodynamic instability are the last signs to become apparent because the regulatory centers are located low within the brain stem in the medulla.

While assessing the patient's mental status, assess the patient's affect, behavior, cognition, and memory. When describing the patient's mental status avoid terms such as stupor, lethargic, obtunded. These terms are vague and have different meanings to different people. The following is a list of levels of consciousness:

- Conscious—alert and aware of self and surroundings. Oriented to surroundings, person, place, and time. The RAS is intact.
- Confusion—decreased concentration, agitation, and weariness.
- Delirium—fast onset.
- Dementia—slow onset.
- Hallucinations.
- Coma—profound depression of one's level of consciousness and awareness due to trauma or illness. Patients with a GCS of less than 8 have a high incidence (over 60 percent) of hypoventilation, regardless of their appearance, and often require ET intubation. There is also hypercarbia and a risk of aspiration.
- Progressive levels of deterioration:

1. Persistent vegetative state—loss of all cognitive functions, but reflex and vegetative functions remain.
2. Akinetic mutism—"open eye" syndrome where the patient cannot move or speak. Caused by a brain tumor or infarct in the brain stem, the patient is awake and aware, but can only respond with eye blinking.
3. Brain death—irreversibly damaged brain function including the brain stem.

What is neurological posturing?

Flexor-extensor posturing occurs progressively with other motor changes due to brain herniation and other severe brain damage. In the predictable pattern of central and lateral herniation, decorticate posturing may appear followed by decerebrate posturing (Figure 24–7).

Decorticate posturing, also referred to as flexion, is associated with a lesion at or above the upper brain stem. Characteristics include muscle rigidity with arms flexed and held tightly to the chest, fists are clenched, and legs extended and internally rotated. If the arms are flexed more to the "core" of the body, this is decorticate.

Decerebrate posturing, also referred to as extension, is associated with a lesion in the diencephalon, midbrain, or pons; severe hypoxia; and hypoglycemia. Characteristics include muscle rigidity with the jaws clenched and the neck and head extended. The arms are extended with the forearms turned out (pronated) and wrists and fingers are flexed. The legs are extended with the feet plantar flexed.

How is an unconscious patient assessed for neurological deficits?

Begin with the use of AVPU in the initial assessment followed by use of the GCS. Assess for the following in an unconscious or suspected unconscious patient:

- Irregular breathing pattern.
- Look for abnormal eye movement (e.g., doll's eye maneuver if no spinal trauma exists) and assess pupils for size, equality, and reactivity to light.
- Withdrawing from painful stimulus—pinching of nail beds.
- Babinski's reflex—elicited by stroking the lateral aspect of the foot. The normal reflex in anyone over six months of age is for the great toe to flex. If the great toe extends and the other toes spread out, this is abnormal in patients over six months of age, indicating spinal cord dysfunction.
- Muscle tone.
- Signs of rising ICP, early versus late.

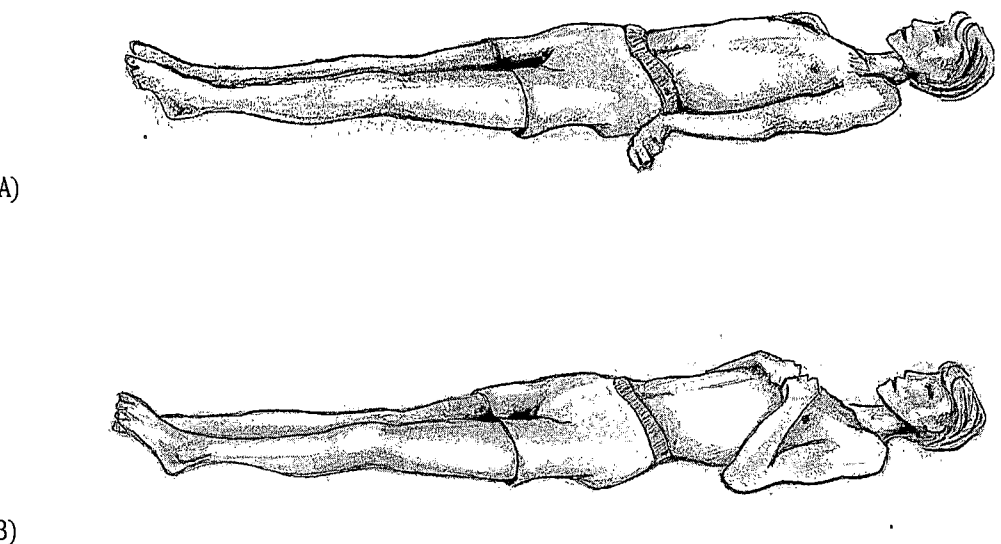

(A)

(B)

FIGURE 24-7 Neurological posturing exhibited in the GCS. (A) Decerebrate or extension and (B) Decorticate or flexion.

What are the signs of rising ICP?

The pattern of the syndrome of rising ICP is identified and described using early and late signs with progression to brain herniation.

Early signs of rising ICP:

- Increasing restlessness or confusion.
- Increasing severity of headache.
- Nausea and vomiting.
- Visual disturbances or deficits.
- Conjugate deviation.
- Sensory loss.
- Motor deficit; monoplegia, hemiplegia.

Late signs of rising ICP:

- Developing abnormal respiratory pattern.
- Decreasing level of consciousness.
- Pupillary changes.
- Cushing's triad.
- Muscle posturing (decorticate, decerebrate).
- Decrease or absence of reflexes or responses (e.g., gag, Babinski) and core temperature.

What is Cushing's triad?

The three signs of rising ICP are: rising BP, changing respiratory patterns, and a decreased pulse rate. Displayed together, they are called Cushing's triad and are a clear but late sign.

What is brain herniation?

Brain herniation means that parts of the brain are being displaced inferiorly due to pressure within the closed skull. The skull (cranium) is space restricted due to its shape. Brain tissue takes up approximately 1250 cc's; CSF, 250 cc's; blood vessels, 200 cc's; and the meninges, 50 cc's, leaving little room for anything else.

There is one large opening at the base (foramen magnum) through which the spinal cord leaves the brain. A bleed or increased ICP can increase the pressure either diffusely or focally. It is possible for the brain to herniate at more than one location. There are three primary patterns of herniation, each with distinguishing features:

1. Uncal herniation—occurs when one side (lateral) of the brain is displaced and pushed down on the temporal lobe, compressing the uncus (inferior portion of the limbic system), diencephalon, and midbrain to the opposite side. Cranial nerve III and the cerebral artery are compressed, causing ipsilateral pupil dilation. As herniation progresses, changes in consciousness occur due to the RAS being

affected. Late-stage changes are similar to central herniation with abnormal respiratory patterns (e.g., Cheyne-Stokes, ataxic) and bilateral positive Babinski responses, followed by flexor-extensor posturing, flaccidity, fixed pupils, and respiratory arrest.

2. Central herniation—occurs when the cerebral hemispheres are displaced downward on to the diencephalon and midbrain, pushing down through the foramen magnum. Early signs include AMS and bilateral pupil constriction due to pressure on the RAS and cranial nerve III, unlike lateral compression with uncal herniation. Central and uncal herniation may or may not occur together; however, as herniation progresses, the late signs are very similar as those described earlier.

3. Cingulate herniation—occurs when the cingulate gyrus (the more superior area of the limbic system that communicates with the prefrontal cerebral cortex) is displaced laterally and under the sharp edges of the falx cerebri. This causes a restricted blood flow leading to ischemia and increased ICP. There is limited information about signs and symptoms of this type of herniation.

What are the signs of brain herniation?

Brain herniation is a progressive order of deterioration following three phases.

Early phase of brain herniation:
- BP increases.
- Pulse slows.

- Abnormal respirations.
- Decorticate posturing.
- Pupil (on the injured side) reactive but sluggish.

Late phase of brain herniation:
- BP continues to increase.
- Pulse continues to decrease.
- Irregular respirations.
- Pupil (on injured side) midsize and fixed.

Terminal phase of brain herniation:
- BP falls.
- Pulse turns rapid and irregular.
- Absent or ataxic respirations.
- Flaccid and unresponsive.
- Pupil dilated and fixed "blown" on side of injury.
- Decerebrate posturing.

How important is psychological support in the care of the neurologic emergency?

Psychological support is paramount! Often, there will be confusion for the patient. Keep reorienting them as to what has happened, what is happening now, and what is going to happen. Other times, the patient may understand what has happened to them, but they are unable to communicate due to a new deficit, like when a stroke patient experiences aphasia.

Special Thanks

Gabriel, Ghajar, et al. *Guidelines for prehospital management of traumatic brain injury.* (2000). New York: Brain Trauma Foundation.

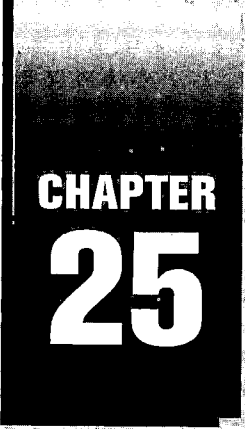

CHAPTER 25

Endocrinology

This chapter discusses various endocrine emergencies. Though the signs and symptoms vary widely, virtually all clinically significant conditions result in alterations of the ABCs, fluid balance, or sugar balance. The focus is on *why* patients present in a certain manner and *why* you need to respond in a certain way to their presenting problems.

General Concepts

Q What are the incidence, morbidity, and mortality of endocrinologic emergencies?

A The most common of the endocrinologic emergencies, diabetic problems, occurs more frequently than all of the rest put together. According to the American Diabetes Association, diabetes affects over 15.7 million people in the United States. Between 90 percent and 95 percent of those who have diabetes are classified as Type II diabetes (non-insulin-dependent) and the remainder have Type I diabetes (insulin-dependent). Diabetes and related complications affect approximately 5.9 percent of the U.S. population, but are responsible for nearly 16 percent of health care expenditures. Other endocrine diseases contribute to this burden, though far less significantly. Diabetes is also the leading cause of adult blindness, as well as the leading cause of nontraumatic lower extremity amputations and end-stage kidney failure.

Q What are the risk factors most predisposing to endocrinologic disease?

A Many endocrine diseases have a hereditary tendency, though specific genetic patterns are not always predictable. Rarely, toxic exposures cause endocrine disease (e.g., hypothyroidism, hypopituitarism).

Q What is the process of hormone secretion and what effect does it have on the regulation of homeostasis?

A The normal secretion of hormones is tightly regulated by a feedback mechanism involving the hypothalamus, the pituitary gland, the target gland, and the end-organ (the organ that the hormone affects). The steps in the process are:

1. Sensors in the body alert the hypothalamus of the need to change a condition.

2. The hypothalamus releases a protein (called a "releasing factor") that travels in closely attached blood vessels to the pituitary gland.

3. The pituitary gland is stimulated to manufacture a "stimulating factor" that travels in the systemic circulation to the target gland (e.g., thyroid, adrenal, pancreas).

4. Once the target gland is stimulated by the "stimulating factor," it produces the final hormone, which is released into the blood.

5. The hormone is carried to its "target organ" and carries out the necessary task.

6. Sensors in the body then alert the hypothalamus when the necessary hormone has been produced, released into the blood, and has exerted the needed effect.

7. In response to feedback from these sensors, the hypothalamus stops producing "releasing factor" until again "informed" by the sensor mechanism that more is needed.

This process is called negative feedback or feedback inhibition. The production of the final hormone "feeds back" to the hypothalamus, causing it to cease production of further stimulating factors. In some cases, the hypothalamus may also secrete inhibitory factors that terminate pituitary gland production of "stimulating factors."

What is the pathophysiology of endocrinologic emergencies?

Though the specific pathophysiology varies for each disease, endocrine emergencies typically arise due to one or more of the following:

- Failure of normal hormone production.
- Excessive hormone production.
- Failure of feedback inhibition systems involving the hypothalamus, pituitary gland, endocrine gland (e.g., pancreas, adrenals), and the target organ.

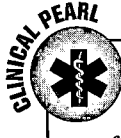

It is often impossible in the field to determine which of the potential causes is responsible for a patient's specific problem.

What general assessment findings are associated with endocrinologic emergencies?

Endocrine diseases may result in a variety of signs and symptoms. Determine the following information:

- Nausea, vomiting.
- Changes in energy level, alertness, sleep patterns, mood, affect, weight, skin texture, hair, sexual function, and personal appearance.
- History of hypopituitarism, hypothyroidism, polydipsia (frequent water intake), polyuria (frequent urination), polyphagia (frequent need to eat), diabetes, thyroid-associated eye problems (e.g., exophthalmus in hyperthyroidism).

How would the EMS provider identify the need for rapid intervention of the patient with endocrinologic emergencies?

As with any patient, any problem that interferes with airway, breathing, or circulation mandates immediate intervention. Significant alterations of vital signs (e.g., tachycardia, hypertension) or level of consciousness are also common in endocrinologic emergencies and mandate rapid assessment and intervention (e.g., hypoglycemia with unconsciousness).

Despite their intricate pathophysiology and biochemistry, most clinically significant endocrine problems result in alterations of the ABCs, fluid balance, level of consciousness, vital signs, and blood sugar level.

Diabetes Mellitus

What is diabetes and its underlying connection to insulin?

Diabetes mellitus is a chronic disease of the endocrine system caused by a decrease in the secretion activity of the hormone insulin. Insulin is released from the pancreas and, together with epinephrine and glucagon, regulates the blood sugar (BS) level. Insulin moves sugar molecules from the blood into the cells, where they are stored (Figure 25–1). In addition, insulin prevents the breakdown of fat tissue in the body. Glucagon and epinephrine have the opposite effects, raising the BS. They are often called counter-regulatory hormones.

Insulin is an anabolic ("builds up") hormone—it "feeds the tissues" causing an uptake of ingested glucose, amino acids, and free fatty acids from the GI tract. These are converted into glycogen, proteins, and triglycerides, respectively. Glucagon and epinephrine are catabolic ("breaks down") hormones. They tend to cause the breakdown of glycogen to glucose, stimulate new production of sugar by the liver (gluconeogenesis), protein breakdown to amino acids, and fat breakdown to free fatty acids and glycerol. Insulin tends to lower the BS, while glucagon and epinephrine tend to raise it.

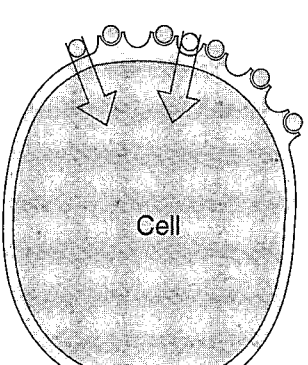

○ = Glucose
◎ = Insulin
ᴧᴧ = Insulin receptors

Insulin combines with insulin receptors on cell wall, allowing glucose to enter cell.

FIGURE 25–1 Insulin carries sugar from blood into the cells.

People with diabetes either do not produce enough insulin to regulate the BS level (Type I) or are relatively resistant to whatever insulin is produced (Type II). Because of a hormonal imbalance, the blood sugar level may become too high (hyperglycemia) or too low (hypoglycemia). Either condition can result in potentially life-threatening problems.

What is meant by Type I and Type II diabetes?

Diabetes is often classified based on whether or not exogenous insulin injections are required for life:

- Type I—insulin-dependent; patients typically have disease onset at a younger age, are prone to diabetic ketoacidosis (DKA), and require insulin injections to live. In the past, Type I diabetes was called "juvenile onset diabetes." Type I diabetes occurs as a result of an early viral infection of the pancreas leading to the formation of antibodies to pancreatic beta-cells that produce insulin. It is an "autoimmune" type of disease.

- Type II—non-insulin-dependent; usually, the onset of Type II diabetes is after the teenage years. Though DKA may develop in any diabetic patient, Type II diabetic patients are less prone. Though they may require insulin injections for optimal regulation of BS levels and the prevention of complications, exogenous insulin is not necessary for life. In the past, Type II diabetes was called "adult onset diabetes." Type II diabetes often develops in the face of obesity and is due to insulin receptor resistance, rather than an absolute deficiency of insulin. These patients have high insulin levels in their blood, but it is ineffective due to the receptor problem.

CLINICAL PEARL

The terms "juvenile onset" and "adult onset" diabetes have been replaced by "Type I" and "Type II" diabetes because these are more physiologically correct. The age of onset of a person's symptoms is less important than whether or not the patient requires insulin shots to live. Type I diabetic patients are absolutely dependent on exogenously administered insulin, while Type II diabetic patients typically are not.

What are the effects of decreased levels of insulin on the body?

When a person's insulin supply is insufficient, a state of cell starvation results. Though cells use glucose as their primary "food source," they will turn to secondary food sources like fat and then muscle if a lack of insulin is preventing the movement of glucose into the cells. When the body metabolizes fats, ketones and ketoacids result. This occurs in any malnourished

patient, not just with diabetes. The difference with diabetes is that the counter-regulatory hormones are also affected. Excess ketone accumulation upsets the acid–base balance in the body and acidosis develops.

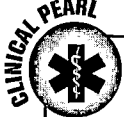

CLINICAL PEARL

Diabetic ketoacidosis is a homeostatic imbalance between the "yin-yang" of hormonal blood sugar regulation.

What are the effects of excess insulin levels on the body?

Glucose is the sole source of oxidative metabolism (nutrition) for the central nervous system (CNS). When the blood sugar level falls significantly (e.g., excessive insulin levels), altered states of consciousness or loss of consciousness may occur. Prolonged hypoglycemia (greater than 20 to 30 minutes) may lead to permanent brain cell damage.

CLINICAL PEARL

When a person loses consciousness from hypoglycemia, the longer the patient remains unconscious, the more likely there will be permanent damage to the brain!

Why do diabetic patients have "silent AMIs"?

Many diabetic patients, Type I or Type II, have an acquired dysfunction of the peripheral nervous system (neuropathy). In addition, increased insulin levels result in elevated blood lipid levels. The combination often leads to an earlier onset of coronary artery disease than in nondiabetic patients. Diabetic patients don't always have the "typical" clinical symptoms of myocardial ischemia (e.g., crushing substernal chest pain) due to altered sensation. They are more likely to simply present with general body weakness (e.g., the "blahs").

CLINICAL PEARL

New onset weakness ("blahs") in a diabetic patient is due to recent myocardial infarction (MI) until proven otherwise.

Why don't EMS providers give insulin in the field?

As a rule, EMS providers do not give insulin in the field. There are exceptions—critical care transport teams, areas where there are large numbers of known diabetic patients (e.g., the Pima Indian reservation in the Southwest). If uncertain of a patient's BS, it is always safer to err on the "low side," and assume that hypoglycemia is present. A period of hypoglycemia is far more dangerous to the patient than an equivalent period of hyperglycemia. Hypoglycemia of more than a 20–30-minute duration results in the production of toxic compounds (e.g., free radicals) in the brain that cause permanent neuronal damage. Even if the sugar is known, insulin administration (e.g., in diabetic ketoacidosis) requires continuous infusion and is not often done in the field.

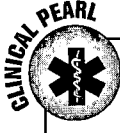

> *Always assume that the sugar is low and treat with D50, rather than assuming that it might be high and giving insulin. Symptomatic hypoglycemia is far more dangerous (at least for a few hours) to the patient than is an equivalent period of hyperglycemia.*

How would the EMS provider correlate abnormal findings in an assessment with the clinical significance in the patient with a diabetic emergency?

Many times it is difficult to tell whether a person's symptoms are more compatible with hypoglycemia, normal blood sugar levels, or hyperglycemia. The immediate problems with the brain not receiving an adequate amount of sugar can rapidly occur in hypoglycemia. As a result, when a diabetic emergency is present, assume that the problem involves hypoglycemia until proven otherwise, and care for the patient accordingly.

> *In a diabetic emergency, treat as though the patient is hypoglycemic until proven otherwise.*

What are BLS and ALS management of diabetic emergencies?

Certain aspects of management are universal for all patients with suspected diabetic emergencies:

- Ensure your own safety first.
- Maintain airway, breathing, and circulation.
- Monitor vital signs and the ECG.
- Determine the fingerstick blood sugar (according to local protocols).
- Treat specific findings (e.g., hypoglycemia) according to local protocols (usually considered ALS management); if you are unable to measure the blood sugar or are uncertain, assume that it is low (hypoglycemia).

- Consider whether the patient requires transport to the hospital (people with hypoglycemia are treated and released by protocol in some EMS systems).
- If necessary, transport the patient to the nearest appropriate medical facility.

How accurate are test strips for BS?

Without the concomitant use of a meter, some test strips may be inaccurate. Many of the older strips are unable to determine a specific BS numerical reading above 400 mg/dl or below 40 mg/dl. Regardless of their ability to "read" a specific sugar level, all *will* give a reliable subjective indication of "too high" (over 400 mg/dl) or "too low" (below 40 mg/dl).

> *A specific "number" for the BS is not terribly helpful in or out of the hospital. The general range, combined with the clinical presentation, is far better.*

How accurate is a glucose meter?

As long as it is calibrated and maintained properly, most hand-held glucose meters are relatively accurate. They provide sufficient information to determine the *range* of a person's glucose within 10–20 mg/dl.

What is a good cutoff of the BS level for treatment in the field with glucose or dextrose?

There is no specific level of low BS at which all people are symptomatic and require treatment. The usual average (follow your protocols) in a symptomatic patient is between 50–60 mg/dl.

> *The rate of decrease in the BS level also determines whether or not a patient is symptomatic. Some individuals with DKA who have their sugar levels lowered rapidly (e.g., from 350 to 200) have hypoglycemic symptoms, despite the fact that their sugar is far from what we normally consider "hypoglycemic" levels.*

Why is glucose (D50) no longer used in cardiac arrest?

Hypoglycemia is a rare cause for cardiac arrest, especially in adults. Most post-resuscitation survivors have hyperglycemia. Though documented hypoglycemia should be treated, the routine administration of glucose has been shown to increase the likelihood of post-resuscitation brain damage.

Q How can the EMS provider integrate the pathophysiological and the assessment findings to formulate a field impression and implement a treatment plan for the patient with a diabetic emergency?

A After ensuring your own safety, pay careful attention to airway, breathing, and circulation. Many patients with hyperglycemia are significantly dehydrated—fluid, not insulin, is the primary treatment. Always consider the possibility of hypoglycemia—prompt treatment is essential to avoid permanent brain damage.

Hyperglycemia

Q How can the EMS provider differentiate between the pathophysiology of normal glucose metabolism and diabetic glucose metabolism?

A Diabetic patients, whether Type I or Type II, lack (at least to some extent) the normal effects of insulin. As a result, sugar and other substances (e.g., free fatty acids, amino acids) fail to enter the cells properly. This results in two concurrent situations:

• "Hungry cells"—due to inadequate nutrient supply (insulin deficiency or resistance).

• Elevated blood sugar, and sometimes triglyceride levels.

Q What is the pathophysiology of hyperglycemia?

A *Hyperglycemia* is an elevation of the BS level above normal. The most common cause of hyperglycemia is diabetes. DKA is a metabolic condition consisting of hyperglycemia, dehydration, and the accumulation of abnormal compounds, called ketones and ketoacids, in the body. Another diabetic emergency, hyperosmolar hyperglycemic nonketotic coma (HHNC), occurs from a relative insulin deficiency that leads to marked hyperglycemia, but the absence of ketones and acidosis. It is summarized in Table 25–1.

Q What are the signs and symptoms of the patient with hyperglycemia?

A Hyperglycemia, by itself, may be asymptomatic. Even if symptomatic, not all people with symptomatic hyperglycemia have DKA or HHNC. By itself, hyperglycemia may lead to:

• Weakness.
• Lack of energy.
• Headache.
• Weight loss or gain.
• Frequent urination.
• Increased thirst.

> **CLINICAL PEARL**
>
> *Not all people with elevated BS levels have DKA or HHNC. Many people have glucose intolerance and hyperglycemia with absolutely no symptoms. Look at the patient, not at the number!*

Q What are BLS and ALS management of hyperglycemia?

A Maintenance of the ABCs is cardinal. Next, the most important decision is whether or not the elevated BS is the cause of a patient's symptoms. In the field, this is of less concern because insulin is not usually given. Always look for alternative sources of a patient's signs and symptoms besides the "obvious." If hyperglycemia is considered to be the main problem, consider fluid therapy according to local protocols.

Q How would the EMS provider assess the clinical significance of abnormal findings in the patient with hyperglycemia?

A The most important immediate problem in hyperglycemia is dehydration. Identify and correct it as soon as possible. Always

TABLE 25–1

Hyperosmolar Hyperglycemia Nonketotic Coma (HHNC)

Definition	Common Causes	History (Symptoms)	Physical Signs	Tests	Treatment
Syndrome of marked hyperglycemia, dehydration, and coma with markedly increased (>350) serum osmolality; minimal (if any) ketosis or acidosis	Severe underlying medical illnesses; often in elderly persons without history of significant diabetes (diet controlled Type II); usually precipitated by infection (pneumonia in women; urosepsis in men)	Progressive decrease in LOC over days; polyuria may occur	Decreased LOC; neurological findings (may mimic stroke); significant dehydration	BS markedly elevated; serum osmolality inc (normal ~ 290; pt often ~ 350); inc BUN/Cr due to hypovolemia; mild lactate elevations possible due to tissue hypoperfusion from massive hypovolemia	Critical Care unit: IV fluids, oxygen, potassium replenishment; insulin is a secondary treatment; treat underlying or precipitating cause

From Rothenberg, M. A., 2000. *Pathophysiology: Mechanisms of Disease.*

look for other sources of symptoms, especially if the patient has an altered mental status (AMS).

What is osmotic diuresis and its relation to diabetes?

Glucose is a big molecule and has a significant osmotic effect. When serum levels are elevated, it passes through the kidneys into the urine. The osmotic pressure of glucose causes fluids and electrolytes (particularly potassium) also to flow from the blood to the urine. Thus, diabetic patients have frequent urination and may be dehydrated. Depending on the severity of their condition, they may also be deficient in total body potassium, which may result in cardiac dysrhythmias.

How would the EMS provider integrate the pathophysiological principles and the assessment findings to formulate a field impression and implement a treatment plan for the patient with hyperglycemia?

Hyperglycemia leads to osmotic diuresis. Assume that symptomatic people are dehydrated and may be potassium deficient. Give IV fluids according to your local protocols and monitor the ECG carefully for signs of hypokalemia (U waves) and cardiac dysrhythmias.

Diabetic Ketoacidosis

What is DKA? What are the causes and the underlying pathophysiology?

DKA is a metabolic condition consisting of hyperglycemia, dehydration, and the accumulation of abnormal compounds, called ketones and ketoacids, in the body.

DKA occurs when a diabetic patient has inadequate insulin circulating in the blood to properly control the BS level. In addition, an excess of epinephrine and glucagon (counter-regulatory hormones) is present. The reasons for this excess are unknown.

The patient's BS rises significantly and the fatty tissue breaks down. The body forms compounds called ketones and ketoacids from the fat tissue. These substances change the acid–base balance in the body, harming the patient. The elevated BS level makes the patient urinate more frequently than usual, leading to dehydration and a loss of body chemicals (particularly potassium). (Figure 25–2)

The most common reason a diabetic patient develops DKA is an infection. This stress results in an increased insulin requirement in the body. Unless the diabetic patient recognizes the need to increase the daily dose of insulin when sick, metabolism and the regulation of BS level become abnormal.

CLINICAL PEARL

The term diabetic coma has been used in the past for diabetic ketoacidosis, but many patients with DKA are not in a coma. However, many patients with hypoglycemia or insulin shock are in a coma but are not in shock. Due to the confusing terms, the preferred terminology is hypoglycemia for low BS, and hyperglycemia for high BS. Some patients with hyperglycemia will have DKA, while many will not. Distinguishing between hyperglycemia alone and DKA in the field is difficult.

What is the mechanism of ketone formation and its relation to ketoacidosis?

During periods of insulin deficiency, stored fats are broken down to provide energy. Free fatty acids from stored triglycerides are released and metabolized in the liver to ketones. When ketones dissolve in the blood, they form ketoacids. If the level of ketones is high enough, the patient is not only ketotic, but develops an acidosis. The combination is called ketoacidosis.

What is the physiology of the excretion of potassium and ketone bodies by the kidneys?

Hyperglycemia leads to osmotic diuresis. Glucose and potassium travel together through the kidney into the urine. As a result, you should assume the following in patients with DKA:

- They are significantly dehydrated (average fluid loss over 24 hours in an adult is 6–9 liters).
- The total body potassium is depleted (regardless of the measured serum level because this only reflects a portion of the body's potassium stores; most is intracellular and not measured in the lab).

When ketone bodies accumulate in the serum, some are excreted in the urine. Urinary ketone excretion does not diagnose DKA nor correlate with the severity of a patient's condition.

CLINICAL PEARL

There is no predictable correlation between the elevation of a person's BS and the degree of ketoacidosis in the blood. Rely on patient appearance rather than a "number."

What are the clinical features of DKA?

These are summarized in Table 25–2.

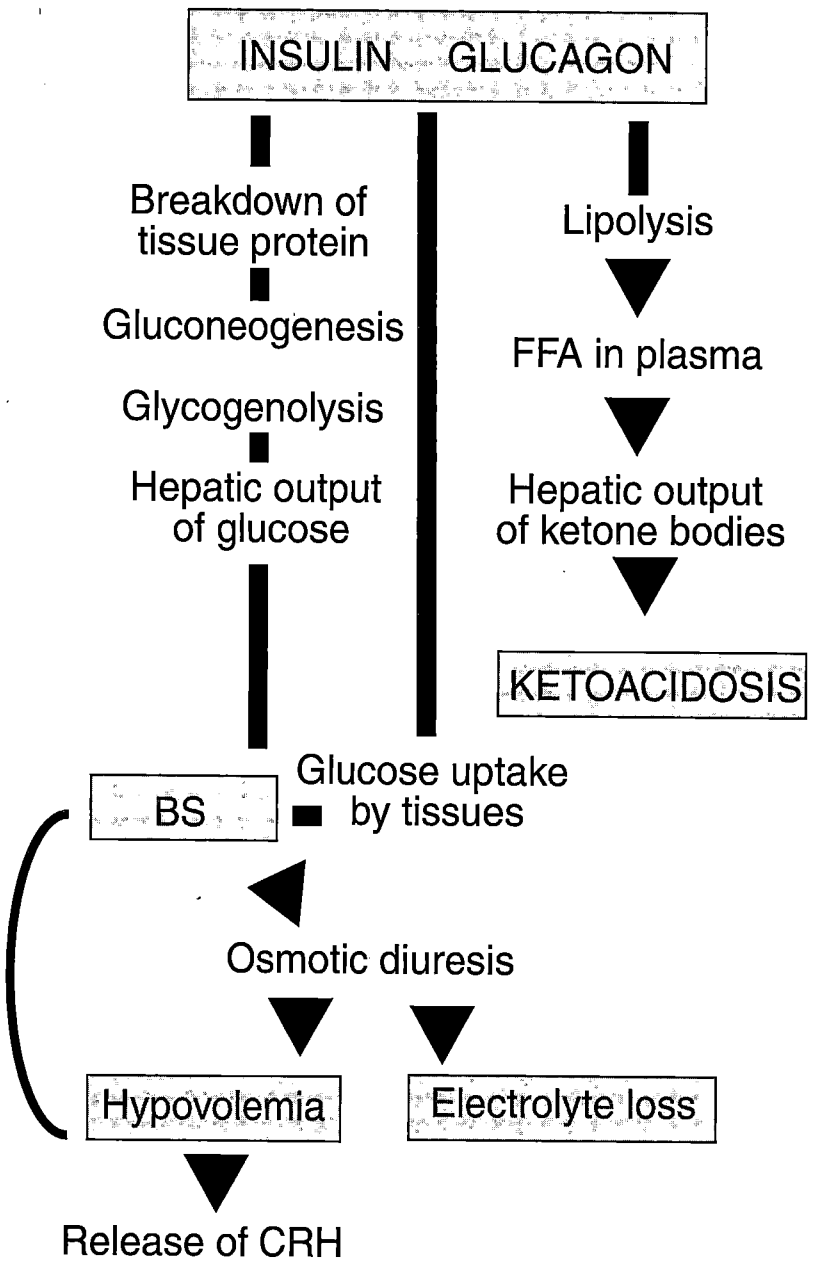

FIGURE 25-2 Insulin and glucagon breakdown. *(From Rothenberg, M. A., 2000.* Pathophysiology: Mechanisms of Disease.*)*

TABLE 25-2

Clinical Features of DKA					
Definition	Common Causes	History (Symptoms)	Physical Signs	Tests	Treatment
Metabolic disturbance caused by insulin depletion and counter-regulatory hormone excess resulting in hyperglycemia and the production of abnormal ketones and acids in the body	Underlying diabetes (usually Type I); precipitated by infection, usually viral gastroenteritis	12-48 hours of progressive weakness, nausea, vomiting; abdominal pain and coffee-ground emesis in 50 percent	Kussmaul respirations (hyperventilation); positive serum dehydration; mild alteration in LOC; acetone odor to breath (<50 percent of patients); normothermia; if hypo-thermic, this is associated with increased mortality	Increased BS, positive serum ketones; decreased HCO_3 on electrolytes; UA shows glucose and ketones; degree of acidosis does not correlate with degree of BS elevation or severity of DKA!	Fluids (mainstay of therapy); continuous insulin infusion, potassium. Avoid bicarb!

From Rothenberg, M. A., 2000. *Pathophysiology: Mechanisms of Disease.*

Hypoglycemia

[Q] What is the pathophysiology of hypoglycemia?

[A] The BS level decreases to the point where it results in symptoms. This level varies from person to person though the average range below which symptoms will occur is 50–60 mg/dl. Decreased BS levels result in the production of glucagon and epinephrine in the body's attempt to raise the sugar. Both counter-regulatory hormones also cause sympathetic-like symptoms (e.g., tachycardia, diaphoresis) that alert the patient to the need to take in sugar. Many longstanding diabetic patients lose this early warning system (production of glucagon and epinephrine) and remain asymptomatic until the sugar level drops low enough to result in loss of consciousness.

CLINICAL PEARL

Caffeine increases a person's sensitivity to hypoglycemia. A significant coffee intake, for example, may result in a person feeling hypoglycemic symptoms at a BS level not usually associated with causing problems (e.g., 75–80 mg/dl). Always elicit a history of caffeine intake by people with suspected BS abnormalities.

[Q] What is the utilization of glycogen by the human body as it relates to the pathophysiology of hypoglycemia?

[A] The production of counter-regulatory hormones (e.g., glucagon and epinephrine) stimulate enzymes that break down glycogen to glucose (glycogenolysis), as well as those that cause the liver to manufacture more glucose (gluconeogenesis). Together, these processes tend to raise the BS. Whether this increase is sufficient to overcome the patient's symptoms is another matter—often the response is inadequate and the symptoms persist or worsen.

[Q] What are the actions of epinephrine as it relates to the pathophysiology of hypoglycemia?

[A] Both glucagon and epinephrine stimulate enzymes that break down glycogen to glucose (glycogenolysis), as well as those that cause the liver to manufacture more glucose (gluconeogenesis). Together, these processes tend to raise the BS. These are known as counter-regulatory hormones because they attempt to counter the BS-lowering effects of insulin.

[Q] What are the signs and symptoms of the patient with hypoglycemia?

[A] Clinical features of hypoglycemia are summarized in Table 25–3.

CLINICAL PEARL

Hypoglycemia, by itself, does not usually result in hypotension. Look for another cause of the patient's symptoms if hypotension is present.

[Q] What are the compensatory mechanisms used by the body to promote glucose homeostasis?

[A] The release of glucagon and epinephrine constitutes the body's main compensatory mechanism to promote glucose homeostasis.

CLINICAL PEARL

Glucose homeostasis represents a "yin-yang" balance between insulin (lowers BS level) and glucagon/epinephrine (raises BS).

TABLE 25-3

Clinical Features of Hypoglycemia

Definition	Common Causes	History (Symptoms)	Physical Signs	Tests	Treatment
Decreased BS level that results in symptoms	Insulin, poor diet, oral diabetic drugs, alcohol	There is usually a rapid onset of anxiety, weakness, and altered LOC	Adrenergic signs early; altered LOC later; seizures uncommon in adults	BS low, though absolute value varies from patient to patient	ABCs, IV DW50; thiamine optional; glucagon is an alternative when no IV route possible; oral sugar in conscious patients

From Rothenberg, M. A., 2000. *Pathophysiology: Mechanisms of Disease.*

What are BLS and ALS management of a hypoglycemic patient?

To care for a patient with known or suspected hypoglycemia:

- Control the airway and assist breathing as necessary. Patients with an altered level of consciousness may have partial airway obstruction.

- Give oxygen by non-rebreather at a rate of 12–15 lpm.

- Monitor the ECG.

- If the patient is conscious, give orange juice with two packets of sugar dissolved in it. Alternatively, have the patient take a dose of oral glucose solution, corn syrup, or candy.

- Unless the symptoms are extremely mild, start an IV lifeline; draw blood before giving any fluid or sugar (D50).

- If permitted by your protocols, administer one amp D50 (25 grams of dextrose in 50 cc water) IV if the measured BS is less than 60 mg/dl. If you are unable to measure BS in the field, follow your local protocols regarding the administration of IV D50.

- Consider administration of glucagon, if necessary, according to your local protocols.

How much does an ampule of dextrose (D50) raise a person's BS level?

There is no predictable level to which an ampule of D50 raises any particular person's BS. Some people's BS actually *decreases* for unknown reasons. The only way to know for certain that the drug has made an impact is to observe the patient's clinical status and recheck the BS level in about five minutes.

Why is thiamine not given routinely with dextrose (D50)?

Thiamine is essential in the production of energy by the brain via glycolysis. The process involves the enzyme pyruvate dehydrogenase, of which thiamine is an integral component.

Because the brain usually obtains all of its energy from glycolysis, thiamine deficiency may result in severe brain damage by preventing the formation of adequate brain adenosine triphosphate (ATP).

The basis for empirically giving thiamine to hypoglycemic patients is that they may be nutritionally deficient, not only in glucose but in thiamine as well. Though "classically" thought necessary only in long-standing alcoholics with hypoglycemia, current thinking holds that thiamine may benefit *any* hypoglycemic patient who is also undernourished (e.g., due to cancer, AIDS, or other chronic disease).

Though academically sound, routine administration of thiamine is *not* considered a standard of care in most areas. Perhaps the more significant issue is that the *order* of administration is not crucial. Thiamine uptake is far slower than that of glucose. Even if thiamine is given first, glucose will exert its molecular effects first. The bottom line is simple—the emergent initial administration of thiamine is not absolutely necessary, though it may be beneficial in therapy once the patient is stabilized.

When should glucagon be used to raise the BS?

Exogenous glucagon will raise a person's BS level within 10 to 15 minutes of subcutaneous administration. It is indicated when you are unable to obtain intravenous access and significant hypoglycemia is present. Follow your local protocols and medical control directions.

How would the EMS provider assess the clinical significance of abnormal findings in the patient with hypoglycemia?

Always consider hypoglycemia as a potential cause of AMS. At the same time, don't forget that many other things (e.g., head injury, stroke, hypoxia) may result in similar symptoms. Whenever possible, perform a fingerstick BS prior to providing glucose therapy.

Q **How would the EMS provider integrate the pathophysiological principles and the assessment findings to formulate a field impression and implement a treatment plan for the patient with hypoglycemia?**

A The important steps here are the same as those that are key to the management of any potential diabetic emergency. Determining the exact nature of a diabetic emergency is difficult, even in the hospital. Your responsibility is to provide care based on your clinical assessment, rather than a specific diagnosis. Always pay close attention to the maintenance of airway, breathing, and circulation. Measurement of the fingerstick BS, if possible, provides valuable information. In addition, always determine the following:

1. History:
   - Has the patient's insulin dosage changed recently?
   - Has the patient had a recent infection?
   - Has the patient suffered any psychologic stress?
   - Has the patient had a change in the frequency of urination?
2. Physical:
   - AMS.
   - Abnormal respiratory pattern (Kussmaul's respirations).
   - Tachycardia.
   - Normotension (hypotension is rare).
   - Fruity breath odor (produced by ketones).
   - Skin color and temperature.
   - Hydration status.

Thyroid Disease

Q **What is the difference between thyrotoxicosis and thyroid storm?**

A Thyrotoxicosis is a general term for overactivity of the thyroid gland, or hyperthyroidism. Acute thyrotoxicosis, also known as thyroid storm, is a potentially life-threatening acute exacerbation of ongoing hyperthyroidism. For the purposes of this.text, the term thyrotoxicosis refers to thyroid storm, unless stated otherwise.

Q **What is the pathophysiology of thyrotoxicosis?**

A Thyrotoxicosis is an acute exacerbation of the hypermetabolism and excessive adrenergic symptoms of chronic thyrotoxicosis due to excess circulating levels of thyroid hormones (thyroxine and triiodothyronine). Normally, these regulate metabolism, growth, and development. In excess, they cause

massive sympathetic-like stimulation that may be life threatening, especially due to cardiac dysrhythmias. The most common causes are surgery, radioactive iodine therapy, or severe stress (e.g., uncontrolled diabetes, MI, acute infection).

Q **What are the signs and symptoms of the patient with thyrotoxicosis?**

A Signs and symptoms of thyrotoxicosis include:
- Fever.
- Flushing.
- Sweating.
- Marked tachycardia.
- Atrial fibrillation (especially new onset).
- Congestive heart failure (CHF).
- Agitation, restlessness.
- Delirium, coma.
- Nausea, vomiting, diarrhea.
- Fever out of proportion to other clinical findings.

CLINICAL PEARL

Protrusion of the eyeballs (exophthalmus) is common in chronic hyperthyroidism. If present during thyroid storm, the finding is helpful. Less than 50 percent of patients with acute thyrotoxicosis, however, have visible eye changes. Hyperglycemia is common in thyrotoxicosis due to insulin resistance and increased glycogenolysis.

Q **What is BLS and ALS management of thyrotoxicosis?**

A As usual, protect yourself and maintain airway, breathing, and circulation. If the diagnosis of thyroid storm is highly likely (on the basis of clinical criteria) and the patient is toxic, immediate therapy is indicated. Many of these necessary drug treatments are usually given in-hospital:

- Block the peripheral effects of the thyroid hormone—propranolol 1–2 mg IV every 15 minutes as needed. Dexamethasone, 2 mg orally, every six hours should also be considered in-hospital.
- Block the synthesis of further thyroid hormones (in-hospital therapy)—PTU (propylthiouracil).
- Block the release of thyroid hormones from the thyroid gland (in-hospital therapy—SSKI (supersaturated solution of potassium iodide).

Supportive care should also be given:
- Treat fever with Tylenol®.

- Treat heart failure with digitalis and diuretics.
- Identify and treat precipitating factors.
- Rehydrate.
- Consider the use of hydrocortisone, 100 mg IV, every eight hours.

Q How would the EMS provider assess the clinical significance of abnormal findings in the patient with thyrotoxicosis?

A Thyrotoxicosis presents as an acute hyperadrenergic state. Regardless of the cause, cardiac dysrhythmias may be life threatening. Careful attention to airway, breathing, and circulation is cardinal.

Q How would the EMS provider integrate the pathophysiological principles and the assessment findings to formulate a field impression and implement a treatment plan for the patient with thyrotoxicosis?

A Thyrotoxicosis presents as an acute hyperadrenergic state. Many other entities have similar presentations. Consider the following as well:

- Sympathomimetic toxidromes (e.g., amphetamines, caffeine).
- Anticholinergic toxidromes.
- Adrenal tumor (e.g., pheochromocytoma).
- Unusual drug reactions.

Q What is myxedema (hypothyroidism)?

A Hypothyroidism is a clinical syndrome due to a deficiency of thyroid hormones. Patients often have fatigue, lethargy, and gradual weight gain for years before the diagnosis is established. Characteristic symptoms include:

- Fatigue.
- Lethargy.
- Weakness.
- Cold intolerance.
- Dry skin.
- Coarse hair or hair loss.
- Weight gain.
- Constipation.
- Myalgias, arthralgias (pain in muscles and joints).
- Menstrual abnormalities.

Typical signs are:

- Cool dry skin.
- Coarse thin hair.
- Hoarse voice.
- Brittle nails.
- Hypertension.
- Slowed reflexes.

This constellation of hypothyroid symptoms is often referred to as myxedema. Originally, the terms referred to generalized nonpitting edema that was commonly present in hypothyroid patients. It has now become generalized to refer to the entire symptom and sign complex.

Q What is myxedema coma?

A Severe untreated hypothyroidism can result in myxedema coma, the ultimate state of long-standing hypothyroidism. Myxedema coma is characterized by:

- Hypothermia.
- Extreme weakness.
- AMS.
- Hypoventilation.
- Hypoglycemia.

Of all patients in full myxedema coma, 50 percent initially exhibit clinical shock (systolic pressure less than 100 mmHg), but perhaps another one-third of patients have a BP greater than 120/80 mmHg. Sinus bradycardia is the most common dysrhythmia seen in myxedema.

CLINICAL PEARL

Hypothyroid coma is rare and not well understood. In one series, it occurred in only 0.1 percent of all cases of hypothyroidism. It is extremely rare in the under-50 age group. Cold exposure, infection, or drugs often precipitate acute decompensation. Behavioral disturbances varying from confusion to frank psychosis are usually present before coma supervenes.

Q What is the pathophysiology of myxedema?

A Chronic hypothyroidism (myxedema) occurs due to a lack of sufficient thyroid hormones, for any of a number of causes. Normally, thyroid hormones contribute to normal metabolism. Their absence leads to decreased metabolism in most vital organs. Myxedema coma is an acute worsening of chronic symptoms due to an acute stress (e.g., cold exposure, infection, or drugs such as phenothiazines, phenobarbital, narcotics, benzodiazepines, anesthetics, lithium).

🅠 What is BLS and ALS management of myxedema?

🅐 Patients with myxedema (chronic hypothyroidism) may present with a number of complaints, whether related to the underlying thyroid condition or not. Symptom-based assessment and treatment, as well as careful attention to airway, breathing, and circulation, are essential. Myxedema coma may be life threatening and requires further steps (in-hospital treatment)—the single most important factor in survival is prompt, IV administration of significant doses of thyroid hormone.

🅠 How would the EMS provider assess the clinical significance of abnormal findings in the patient with myxedema?

🅐 Of prime importance are alterations in airway, breathing, and circulation. People with myxedema coma may have hemodynamically significant bradydysrhythmias and respiratory depression. Hypothermia may also be life threatening. Treatment of any of these findings takes high priority.

🅠 How would the EMS provider integrate the pathophysiological principles and the assessment findings to formulate a field impression and implement a treatment plan for the patient with myxedema?

🅐 In patients without myxedema coma, a wide variety of diseases may explain the signs and symptoms. If a patient has a history of thyroid disease and presents with acute hypothermia and an altered level of consciousness, suspect myxedema coma until proven otherwise. Prompt transportation to the nearest appropriate facility for further evaluation and empiric IV thyroid hormone replacement may be lifesaving.

Adrenal Gland Disease

🅠 What is Cushing's syndrome?

🅐 Cushing's syndrome is a metabolic syndrome resulting from hypersecretion of the glucocorticoid hormone, cortisol. The resultant excess affects carbohydrate, protein, and lipid metabolism.

🅠 What is the pathophysiology of Cushing's syndrome?

🅐 Eighty-five percent of cases result from excess production of adrenocarticotropic hormone (ACTH) by the pituitary gland or other sources (e.g., tumors). Other cases may result from adrenal gland disease (e.g., tumors, hyperplasia) or oral steroid replacement therapy. Steroid excess affects the metabolism of carbohydrates (raises BS), protein (breaks down to amino acids), and lipids (increases free fatty acid levels).

🅠 What are the signs and symptoms of the patient with Cushing's syndrome?

🅐 Typical signs and symptoms include:

- Abnormal pattern of fat distribution—centripetal obesity with wasting of the arms and legs; rounding of the face (moon facies), dorsocervical fat pad ("buffalo hump").
- Muscle weakness—usually affects proximal muscles (e.g., inability to stand up from a squatting position).
- Menstrual irregularities.
- Decreased libido.
- Adult-onset acne.
- Hirsuitism (excess growth of body hair).
- Skin striae—purple or dark "stretch marks."

🅠 What are BLS and ALS management of Cushing's syndrome?

🅐 The majority of persons with Cushing's syndrome present to EMS with problems that are not directly related to their underlying disease. Occasionally, a person suffers an acute complication (e.g., bleeding problem due to thinning of skin), but this is relatively uncommon.

🅠 How would the EMS provider assess the clinical significance of abnormal findings in the patient with Cushing's syndrome?

🅐 Any finding that impairs the integrity of airway, breathing, or circulation is clinically significant.

🅠 What are BLS and ALS management of the patient with Cushing's syndrome?

🅐 Because most people's acute complaint is not related directly to Cushing's syndrome, symptom-based assessment and management is the key to patient management.

Q How would the EMS provider integrate the pathophysiological principles and the assessment findings to formulate a field impression and implement a treatment plan for the patient with Cushing's syndrome?

A Because most people's acute complaint is not related directly to Cushing's syndrome, symptom-based assessment and management is the key to patient management.

Q What is adrenal insufficiency?

A Adrenal insufficiency is the inadequate production of adrenal hormones (primarily cortisol and aldosterone) for any of a number of reasons. Autoimmune destruction of the adrenal glands (Addison's disease) is the most common cause of adrenal insufficiency in the industrialized world. In the emergency setting, new adrenal insufficiency is rare. The most common cause of adrenal insufficiency in EMS is suppression of the hypothalamic-pituitary-adrenal axis as a result of long-term glucocorticoid therapy.

CLINICAL PEARL

> *Though oral steroid therapy is the most common cause of exogenous adrenal suppression, inhaled steriods (e.g., for asthma or COPD) may also have a similar effect.*

Q What is the pathophysiology of adrenal insufficiency?

A Exogenous glucocorticoid therapy (e.g., oral steroids) suppresses the normal feedback loop between the hypothalamus, pituitary gland, and adrenal glands. Both the hypothalamus and the pituitary gland "sense" sufficient circulating glucocorticoid (due to the exogenous medication). Thus, they suppress production of stimulating hormones. As long as the body is not stressed, no harm results.

When the patient is stressed and the body requires more steroids than those provided by the exogenous supply (e.g., the oral doses), the hypothalamus and pituitary gland are unable to respond because their ability to produce "stimulating hormones" is suppressed. The result is a lack of cortisol production by the adrenal gland and relative adrenal insufficiency. When the body lacks this normal stress response, life-threatening consequences may occur. Acute precipitating stresses include surgery, anesthesia, psychologic stresses, alcohol intoxication, hypothermia, myocardial infarction, diabetes mellitus, infection, asthma, and hypoglycemia.

Q What are the signs and symptoms of the patient with adrenal insufficiency?

A Chronic adrenal insufficiency presents with:
- Weight loss.
- Increasing fatigue.
- Vomiting, diarrhea.
- Anorexia.
- Salt craving.
- Muscle and joint pain.
- Abdominal pain.
- Postural dizziness.
- Increased pigmentation (e.g., extensor surfaces, creases of the palm, and oral mucosa).

Acute adrenal insufficiency (sometimes called Addisonian crisis) presents as hypotension, hypoglycemia, and severe hypovolemia.

Q What are BLS and ALS management of adrenal insufficiency?

A The acute life threats in adrenal insufficiency are hypotension and hypoglycemia. The former responds well to glucocorticoid replacement and IV hydration, and the latter to IV administration of dextrose.

- Addisonian crisis patients are often up to 20 percent volume depleted. Unless specifically contraindicated by the patient's cardiovascular status, correction of hypovolemia should be aggressive. One liter of normal saline may be infused over the first hour. Dextrose 5 percent is usually added to treat accompanying hypoglycemia. Up to a total of three liters may be required over the first eight hours. Optimal correction of hypotension will require both glucocorticoid and volume replacement.

- Treatment of hypoglycemia should be immediate. For symptomatic hypoglycemia or extremely low serum levels, IV glucose (50 to 100 ml of dextrose 50 percent in water) is preferable. If IV access is impossible, subcutaneous glucagon (1 to 2 mg) may be attempted, although a 10- to 20-minute period of latency should be anticipated.

Q How would the EMS provider assess the clinical significance of abnormal findings in the patient with adrenal insufficiency?

A Of prime importance are alterations in airway, breathing, and circulation. People with acute adrenal insufficiency have significant hypovolemia and often, hypoglycemia. Treatment of these findings takes high priority.

Q How would the EMS provider integrate the pathophysiological principles and the assessment findings to formulate a field impression and implement a treatment plan for the patient with adrenal insufficiency?

A Hypoglycemia, by itself, rarely causes hypotension. The combination, especially in a patient who has been on any form of steroids (oral or inhaled, such as for asthma), suggests acute adrenal insufficiency until proven otherwise.

Special Thanks

Tables 25–1, 25–2, 25–3, and Figure 25–4 are reproduced with permission from *Pathophysiology: Mechanisms of Disease,* by Mikel A. Rothenberg, M.D., © 2000.

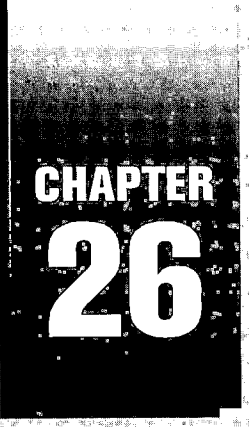

CHAPTER 26

Allergies and Anaphylaxis

This chapter discusses allergic reactions from the minor irritation to the life-threatening reaction. The focus is on *why* patients present in a certain manner and *why* you need to respond in a certain way to their presenting problem. The failure to rapidly recognize and rapidly manage a severe allergic reaction could cost a patient's life.

Definitions and Physiology

Q **What is an antigen?**

A An antigen is a foreign substance that when introduced to the body causes the production of antibodies.

Q **What is an antibody?**

A An antibody is a protein substance formed by the body in response to antigens that have entered the body.

Q **What is an immune response?**

A An immune response is a bodily response occurring when a foreign substance tries to invade the body. Protective cells are able to recognize infections or antigens as they enter the body and destroy them prior to them causing harm.

Q **What is immunity?**

A Immunity is a state of protection enabling the body to resist foreign substances. It can be natural or acquired. We are born with natural immunity. An acquired immunity develops in one's lifetime and is a reaction in the body occuring as a result of exposure to invaders.

Q **What is an allergy?**

A Allergies are an acquired hypersensitivity. First, the person is exposed or sensitized to the antigen. Repeated exposures cause a reaction by the immune system to the allergen. Signs and symptoms include redness, heat, swelling, and itching, as well as runny nose, coughing, sneezing, wheezing, and nasal congestion.

Q **What is an allergic reaction?**

A An allergic reaction is an overreaction by the body's immune system to normally harmless foreign substances that cause damage (e.g., swelling, cell wall breakdown) to body tissues.

Q **What is an anaphylactic reaction?**

A Anaphylaxis is an IgE (immunoglobulin) mediated hypersensitivity reaction leading to the most severe allergic reactions that involve respiratory distress and cardiovascular collapse.

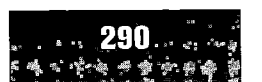

What is the pathophysiology of an allergic reaction?

When the antigen reacts with the IgE (antibody) on the basophils and mast cells, histamines, leukotrienes, and other mediators are released. Next, there is smooth muscle contraction (bronchoconstriction) and vascular dilation. Plasma escapes into the tissues, causing urticaria and angoiedema. This also decreases the plasma volume, ultimately causing shock. When fluid escapes from the alveoli, it causes pulmonary edema. When the reaction is prolonged, the patient may experience dysrhythmias and cardiogenic shock.

CLINICAL PEARL

Not every anaphylactic reaction results in all of the events described. The common step to all allergic reactions is the interaction of the IgE antibody with an antigen. The combination leads to the release of mediators from basophils and mast cells. Depending on many factors, the severity of the reaction (e.g., hives, wheezing, hypotension) varies significantly from patient to patient and exposure to exposure.

What is different with the reaction the body has from anaphylaxis compared to an allergic reaction?

Anaphylaxis involves IgE antigen interactions and includes the life-threatening cases involving progressive hives, lip and throat swelling, wheezing, respiratory distress, and hypotension as shown in Figure 26–1.

CLINICAL PEARL

The terminology of allergic reactions is somewhat confusing, as well as potentially deadly for the patient. IgE and other immunoglobulins are involved in many different types of allergic reactions. The term anaphylaxis refers to an immediate hypersensitivity reaction that occurs as a result of an antigen interacting with IgE, regardless of the symptoms. Progressive hives, wheezing, mouth or tongue swelling, and other symptoms are all considered anaphylaxis. Anaphylactic shock, however, involves any signs and symptoms of anaphylaxis and the presence of shock. All patients with any type of acute anaphylactic reaction need to be treated with epinephrine.

What are the potential routes of antigen entry into the body?

Allergens can enter the body by oral ingestion, injection (e.g., needles, stingers), inhalation, or topical exposure (through the skin).

What are examples of common allergens?

Common allergens include:

- Drugs—penicillin, sulfa, or codeine.
- Insects—bees and fire ants.
- Foods—shellfish, peanuts, chocolate.
- Animals—snakes and jellyfish.

What is urticaria?

Urticaria is the medical term for hives regardless of the size or number.

What is angioneurotic edema?

Swelling of the skin due to the leakage of fluid from the blood vessels into the interstitial and subcutaneous tissues. This may occur as a result of anaphylaxis or other types of reactions (e.g., cold or drugs).

What are the most common causes of anaphylaxis?

The most common causes of anaphylaxis are drugs, insect stings, blood products, and food.

What are the assessment findings in an allergic reaction?

Not all of the following signs and symptoms are present in every case; however, the following is a detailed listing:

- Mental status—the patient may be unable to speak, display restlessness, have a decreased level of consciousness (LOC), or be unresponsive.
- Upper airway—may be hoarse, have stridor, pharyngeal edema, or pharyngeal spasm.
- Lower airway—hypoventilation, labored accessory muscle use, abnormal retractions, prolonged expirations, wheezes, and diminished lung sounds.
- Skin—redness or rash, edema, moisture, itching, urticaria, pallor, and cyanosis.
- Vital signs—tachycardia, tachypnea, and hypotension.
- GI—abnormal cramping, nausea and vomiting, and diarrhea.

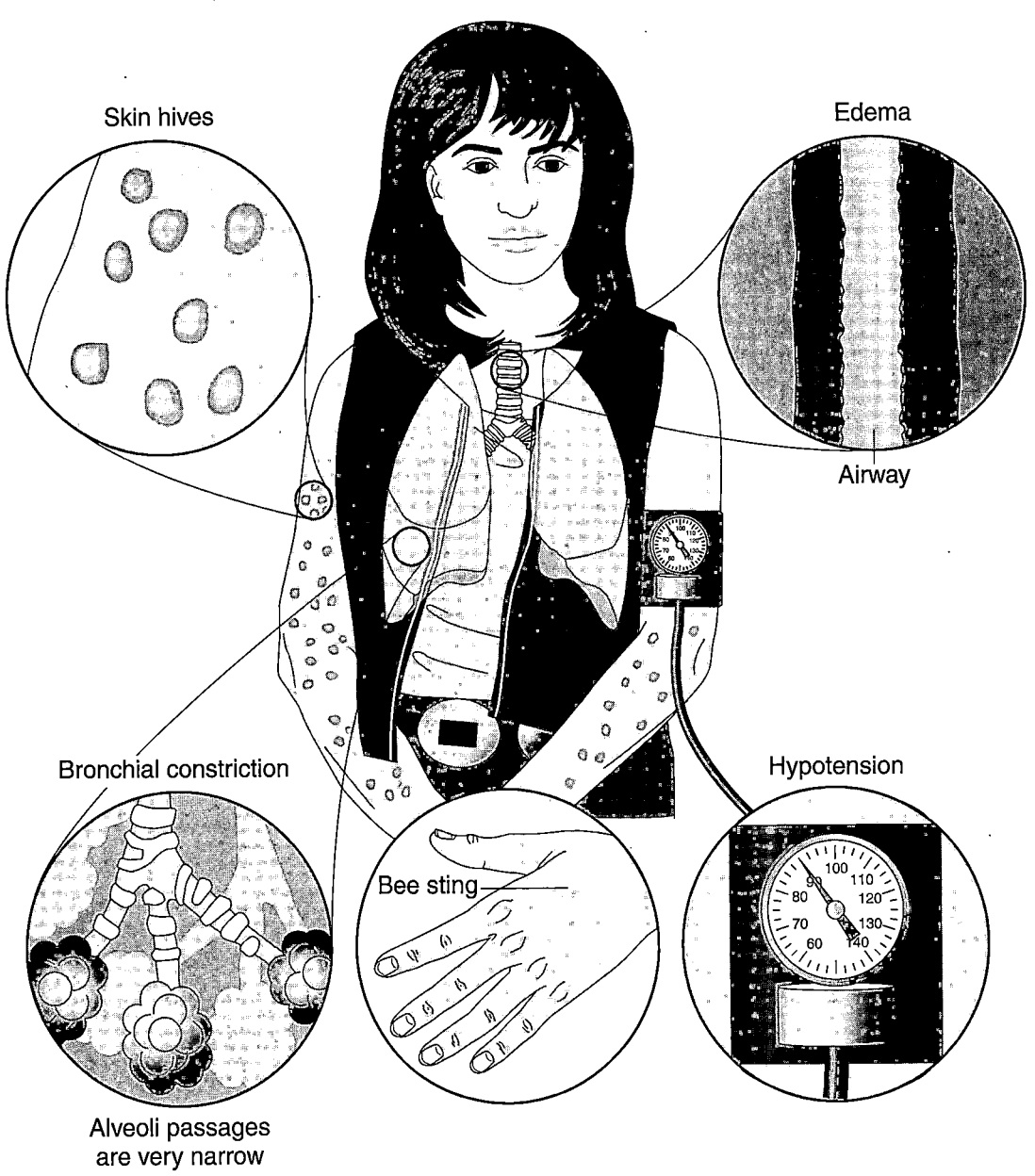

Skin hives

Edema

Airway

Bronchial constriction

Bee sting

Hypotension

Alveoli passages
are very narrow

FIGURE 26–1 A severe allergic reaction involves several body systems.

Anaphylaxis occurs as a result of the release of media-tors from mast cells. The majority of these cells "live" in the skin and the respiratory and GI tracts. Thus, the most common findings in anaphylaxis are urticaria (skin), wheezing (respiratory tract), and abdominal pain (GI tract).

Does an allergic reaction need to be managed in the field?

Allergies always need to be managed to rule out progressive hives or anaphylaxis because that should be treated with epinephrine. Provided the patient is only having mild local symptoms, it may be possible to treat and release advising of necessary follow-up should the condition worsen. This of course should only be done with the consultation and permission of medical control.

What is BLS management of anaphylaxis?

BLS management of anaphylaxis involves airway maintenance, position of comfort, oxygen administration, and assisting the patient with the administration of an epinephrine self-injector if they have one available. These patients should be transported to the nearest hospital.

What is an epinephrine auto-injector and when is it used?

An Epipen® is a prefilled syringe (0.3 to 0.5 mg epinephrine 1:1,000) that is designed to auto-inject when pressed firmly against the thigh. It is indicated when the following three criteria are met:

- The patient exhibits signs of a severe allergic reaction including respiratory distress, wheezing, progressive hives, throat or mouth swelling, or shock.
- A physician prescribes the medication for the patient.
- Medical direction authorizes (either direct or indirect protocols) use of the medication for the patient.

Are there contraindications for the use of the Epipen®?

Epinephrine is to be used with caution in patients over 50 years old and who have preexisting dysrhythmias. However, in a life-threatening situation, there is no real contraindication because the medication could be lifesaving.

What is the procedure for the use of an Epipen®?

After ensuring that the patient is a candidate for epinephrine, verify the medication is prescribed to the patient and medical direction authorizes (either on-line or off-line) the use of the drug, then do the following:

- Remove the cap from the auto-injector.
- Place the tip of the auto-injector against the patient's thigh (lateral portion, midway between the waist and knee).
- Push the injector firmly against the thigh until the injector activates.
- Hold the injector in place until the medication is injected (at least 10 seconds).
- Record the time of injection.
- Dispose of the injector in a sharps (biohazard) container.

Auto-injectors require a considerable amount of force to activate. This is a built-in safety precaution to prevent accidental activation. Empty training models are available for EMS provider and patient training. It is recommended that you try this yourself (with a test device), before using such a device on a patient.

Is there a different dose of epinephrine for adults as opposed to children?

Yes. The adult auto-injector contains 0.3 mg and the pediatric auto-injector contains 0.15 mg.

What other medications might be used by EMS providers in anaphylaxis?

Depending on your local protocols, patients may receive antihistamines, either oral or parenteral. The most common is diphenhydramine (Benadryl®). Antihistamines should *not* replace the administration of epinephrine when indicated.

The administration of antihistamines alone, such as Benadryl®, to a patient with ongoing anaphylactic reactions (e.g., progressive hives) is potentially fatal. Once the cascade of events is triggered, all anaphylactic reactions have the potential to progress to full-blown anaphylactic shock. Antihistamines do not block all of the released mediators, only histamine. The drug of choice is epinephrine. The supplemental administration of antihistamines is acceptable, but not absolutely necessary.

Q What is ALS management of anaphylaxis?

A The ALS management of anaphylaxis includes:

- Management of the airway—positioning, oxygen, assisting ventilations, ET tube placement as needed.
- Circulation—venous access and fluid resuscitation.
- Pharmacological—epinephrine is the main treatment as a bronchodilator and to decrease the vascular permeability. Antihistimines, such as Benadryl®, are useful.
- Steroids, such as solumedrol or hydrocortisone, may be helpful over the next few hours.
- Vasopressors may be helpful for hypotension not responsive to fluids alone.

Q Is it ever appropriate to use epinephrine 1:10,000 IV instead of 1:1,000 SQ?

A Yes, if the patient is in cardiovascular collapse and there is an IV started, the peripheral circulation may be so poor that a SQ injection will be ineffective.

Q What types of snakes and spiders usually cause an allergic reaction in most people?

A The pit viper snakes (e.g., water moccasin, copperhead, cottonmouth, and rattlesnake), coral snakes, the black widow spider, and brown recluse spider.

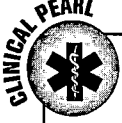

CLINICAL PEARL

True acute allergic reactions to spiders or snakes are unusual. Delayed reactions, especially to antivenin for snakebite, are far more common. Hypotension following an acute envenomation may be due to a direct effect of the venom. This is more common with neurotoxic venoms, such as in coral snakes.

Q How would the EMS provider distinguish the type of bite the patient has sustained?

A Distinguishing the type of bite may be difficult at best. A good history describing the markings of the animal is most helpful. Often spider bites are very small and the patient initially does not even realize she has been bitten. It has been reported that the sharp pain at the site of a brown recluse bite begins right away. The site of the recluse bite becomes edematous with an erythematous halo surrounding an irregular-shaped center of necrosed tissue. The black widow bite may be sharply painful or painless and initially only a tiny papule is visible.

Not all snakebites result in envenomation. Always observe the patient very closely for the development of signs and symptoms. It is common for the patient to have fang marks if bitten by a pit viper. There is a local burning pain immediately, leading to weakness, nausea, vomiting, paresthesia, and considerable swelling within the first five minutes. The coral snake bite may have little to no pain and no local edema or tissue necrosis because the damage is mostly neurotoxic.

Q What is latex?

A Latex is natural sap from the rubber tree used to make natural rubber products.

Q What does latex allergy result from?

A It has been shown that multiple skin contacts or inhalation exposures to the proteins found in natural rubber latex can cause a latex allergy.

Q How can an EMS provider be exposed to latex through inhalation?

A Gloves with powder contain the proteins responsible for latex allergies. When gloves are changed, the powder gets into the air and can be inhaled.

CLINICAL PEARL

Exposure to atmospheric powder from gloves is a common source of health care provider sensitization.

Q How many health care workers are sensitized to latex?

A Studies indicate that 8 to 12 percent of health care workers who are regularly exposed to latex become sensitized. That is they have a reaction, such as a rash, to the latex. More severe reactions may develop. It is impossible to determine ahead of time who will have a recurrent and more severe reaction with reexposure to latex.

CLINICAL PEARL

Some studies suggest that within a couple of years nearly 10 percent of health care providers will be unable to work in the profession due to an acquired latex allergy.

Q: Are health care workers more "at risk" than the general population?

A: Yes! Studies indicate that the general population has a one to six percent rate of being sensitized to latex.

Q: What are the symptoms of a latex allergy reaction?

A: The symptoms of a latex reaction include a skin rash and inflammation, respiratory irritation, asthma, and in rare cases, anaphylaxis. Death has been reported, even in people with a history of only one very mild reaction to latex in the past.

> **CLINICAL PEARL**
>
> *There are numerous cases reported in the United States over recent years of health care providers dying following reexposure to latex after having only relatively minor (e.g., wheezing, rash, hives) reactions in the past. Many had only one or two previous reactions. Assume that the possibility for a severe and life-threatening reaction is present in any person with a latex allergy.*

Q: Is latex allergy associated with other allergies?

A: Latex allergy is associated with allergies to foods such as potatoes, bananas, tomatoes, kiwi fruit, papaya, chestnuts, and apricots.

> **CLINICAL PEARL**
>
> *The reason for this association is that latex sap is chemically related to that of the listed fruits, vegetables, and nuts. This results in a "cross-reactivity" of antigens to IgE.*

Q: Why must the EMS provider beware of the significance of latex allergies in pediatric patients?

A: Though the "odds" are changing rapidly, children (especially those with a history of multiple surgeries, such as with spina bifida) are at a higher risk. Many of the "latex-free" products that are available do not include pediatric sizes.

> **CLINICAL PEARL**
>
> *Assume that any patient, regardless of sex or age, is potentially latex allergic and carry appropriate latex-free equipment. Remember, latex is in nearly every medical product we use (e.g., stethoscopes, gloves, ECG leads, tourniquets, syringe plungers, bandages).*

Q: When assessing a patient, what questions may indicate a potential risk for latex allergy?

A: Patients who are at risk include patients who:
- Have experienced swelling, wheezing, hives, or a rash after contact with latex.
- Have experienced an anaphylactic reaction during dental, rectal, or vaginal exams, surgery, bladder stimulation, and urinary catherization.
- Have history of allergic reactions to products containing latex or natural rubber.
- Have neural tube defect, such as spina bifida.
- Have genitourinary anomalies requiring chronic bladder catherization.
- Have a positive latex allergy test.
- Are on therapeutic protocols for neurogenic bowel or bladder.
- Have a history of multiple allergies.

Q: Why do spina bifida patients have latex sensitivity?

A: Though the specific reasons for this are unclear, most experts believe that a combination of frequent surgery and ongoing bladder catherization provide the chronic exposure to latex products. This results in the development of sensitivity.

Q: What are examples of supplies or equipment that EMS providers routinely carry that contain latex?

A: Examples of supplies and equipment that contain latex are:
- Airways, bite blocks, suction catheters, masks, and straps.
- BVMs and ET or NG tubes.
- BP cuffs, stethoscope tubing, electrodes, and IV sets.
- Hot water bottles and waterproof mattress covers.
- Dressings (Moleskin®, Colban®, Action wrap®) and Band-Aids®.
- Sterile or surgical gloves.
- IV sets and catheters (indwelling).
- Syringes, tourniquets.

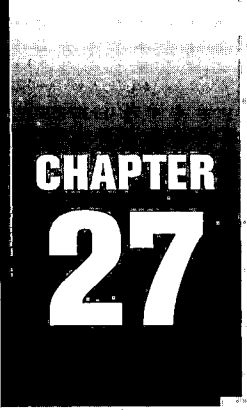

CHAPTER 27

Gastroenterology and Urology

This chapter discusses the problems patients may be having with their gastrointestinal (GI) and urinary systems. The focus is on *why* it is important for the EMS provider to understand the medical problems affecting these two body systems and how they affect our patients. It is important to distinguish between immediate life-threatening problems and acute problems that are managed in the ED setting. Trauma to the abdomen is covered in Chapter 41, Abdominal Trauma.

Gastroenterology Epidemiology

Q What are the common causes of acute abdominal distress?

A There are numerous mechanisms, both systemic and within the abdomen itself, that may result in acute abdominal pain. Common abdominal causes include:

- Bacterial contamination—usually caused by an infection in the bowel, the surrounding peritoneal cavity (peritonitis), or both.
- Chemical irritation—usually due to a leakage of bile or some other body substance (e.g., blood) into the wrong space, often the peritoneal cavity.
- Peritoneal inflammation—may be due to bacterial contamination, chemical irritation, or direct trauma.

(Bacterial contamination, chemical irritation, and peritoneal inflammation are all sometimes referred to as inflammatory abdominal pain because the basis for pain in all three is irritation of the abdominal contents.)

- Bleeding—bleeding anywhere in the GI tract may result in painful cramping; if blood seeps into the peritoneal cavity, peritoneal inflammation will result. This is sometimes called hemorrhagic abdominal pain.
- Obstruction—any factor that slows or blocks the movement of digestive contents through the bowel results in distention and pain. This is sometimes called nonhemorrhagic abdominal pain.

Numerous conditions that do not originate in the abdomen may also result in acute abdominal pain. These include:

- Thoracic conditions—pneumonia, spontaneous pneumothorax, myocardial infarction (MI).
- Spinal problems—nerve irritation from arthritis, herpes zoster, vertebral compression fracture.
- Metabolic problems—black widow spider bite, lead poisoning, kidney failure, diabetic ketoacidosis, anaphylaxis.
- Neurological problems—herpes zoster, herniated intervertebral disk.

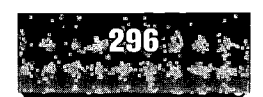

Q **What is the morbidity and mortality of GI emergencies?**

A GI emergencies account for a significant proportion of patients seen in EDs, outpatient clinics, and by EMS providers. There are many diseases that may cause acute abdominal pain and most are not life threatening. Common calls to EMS include complications of ulcers and potential ectopic pregnancy.

Q **Who is at risk for having a GI emergency?**

A Virtually anyone is at risk for suffering a GI emergency. Those at the greatest risk of suffering a bad outcome are the very young, the elderly, and pregnant women. The common denominator is that abdominal conditions tend to present atypically in all three patient groups. Unless the health care provider has a high index of suspicion, a potentially serious condition could be missed easily.

Q **What types of pain are associated with an acute abdomen?**

A There are three major types of acute abdominal pain: visceral, somatic, and referred.

- *Visceral pain* is caused by the sudden stretch or distention of a hollow organ (viscus). It is crampy, gaseous, and usually intermittent. Often, it is referred to the midline of the abdomen. It is diffuse and poorly localized. This type of pain is not well tolerated. Visceral pain is often accompanied by autonomic symptoms such as diaphoresis, nausea, vomiting, or dysrhythmias. Involuntary contraction of the abdominal muscles may also occur. Most acute intra-abdominal diseases requiring operations are preceded by obstruction (either functional or anatomical). The earliest clinical signs and symptoms are related to visceral pain. An example is the periumbilical crampy pain of early appendicitis.
- *Somatic pain* is caused by a stimulation of nerve fibers in the parietal peritoneum by chemical or bacterial inflammation. The patient usually lies quietly with the thighs flexed to relax the peritoneum. Any attempt at palpation is guarded by muscular contractions. This is referred to as involuntary guarding. Reflex cessation of bowel sounds commonly occurs. An example of this is the sharply localized lower-right quadrant pain of the later phase of appendicitis.
- *Referred pain* is pain from one area that is being sensed in another due to embryological nerve distribution patterns—the nerves for both areas originated from the same structure in early development. An example of this is diaphragmatic irritation being felt in the shoulder.

Q **What are some examples of pain referral patterns?**

A There are several characteristic patterns of referral of pain:
- Biliary pain commonly radiates around the right side to the back and angle of the scapula.
- Pain from the pancreas goes straight through to the back in the midline of the lower thoracic area. A posteriorly penetrating duodenal ulcer can present the same way.
- Blood or pus under the diaphragm presents as aching pain in the top of the shoulder.
- A leaking or ruptured aneurysm will cause pain in the lumbosacral area and occasionally in the upper thighs.
- Renal colic pain (kidney stones) will radiate to the groin and external genitalia.
- Uterine and rectal pain will often be felt in the lower back.

Q **Does the location of the pain correctly indicate the cause of distress?**

A Not necessarily, as certain disease processes typically cause pain in particular areas, though this may vary from patient to patient. The common causes of abdominal pain are summarized by their location in Table 27–1.

Note that there is fairly extensive overlap between the causes of pain and the quadrants of the abdomen that they may affect.

Q **Can acute abdominal pain be a symptom of an AMI also?**

A Yes, cardiac pain may radiate to or even originate in the abdomen. Abdominal pain of cardiac origin is often in the upper abdomen or epigastric area. Patients typically describe the pain as aching, though it may be sharp, "gassy," or indigestion-like.

TABLE 27–1

Common Causes of Abdominal Pain	
Location	Possible Conditions
Upper-left quadrant	Duodenal ulcer, pancreatitis, pyelonephritis, pneumonia
Lower-left quadrant	Ectopic pregnancy, ovarian cyst, kidney stone, pelvic inflammatory disease, diverticulitis
Upper-right quadrant	Cholecystitis, duodenal ulcer, pancreatitis, pneumonia with pleurisy, pyelonephritis
Lower-right quadrant	Appendicitis, diverticulitis, ovarian cyst, kidney stone, ectopic pregnancy, pelvic inflammatory disease
Epigastric	MI, duodenal ulcer, gastroenteritis
Periumbilical	Appendicitis, pancreatitis, abdominal aortic aneurysm
Unlocalized	Bowel obstruction, food poisoning, neurological lesion, metabolic problem (e.g., diabetic ketoacidosis)

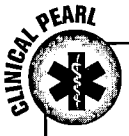

Pathophysiology

Q. What is a GI bleed?

A. GI bleeding is defined as the loss of blood from any portion of the GI tract due to a lesion of the mucosa (lining) itself. Swallowed blood (e.g., from a nosebleed) may mimic this.

Q. What is the difference between an upper and lower GI bleed?

A. An upper GI bleed is bleeding proximal to the duodenojejunal junction. A lower GI bleed involves bleeding located more distally. There are numerous causes for each. Common causes of upper GI bleeding include:

- Peptic ulcer disease.
- Acute gastritis.
- Esophageal varices.
- Esophagitis.
- Mallory–Weiss tear (torn esophagus from violent cough or retching).
- Angiodysplasia (arteriovenous malformations).
- Aortoenteric fistula.

Common causes of lower GI bleeding include:

- Diverticulosis.
- Angiodysplasia.
- Blunt abdominal trauma.
- Hemorrhoids.
- Fissures.
- Tumors.
- Polyps.

Q. How do you determine the cause of GI bleeding?

A. It is difficult, if not impossible, to determine accurately in the field the cause of either upper or lower GI bleeding. More importantly, initial out-of-hospital treatment is similar, regardless of the cause. Common symptoms include hematemesis (vomiting blood), hematochezia (bright red blood in the stool), and melena (tarry, sticky black stools). The patient may have vomited coffee ground-like material (suggestive of digested blood in the stomach). Pain may or may not be prominent. Estimates of the amount of blood lost from reports of stool and vomitus volume are likely to be unreliable. It takes only a drop of blood to turn the entire toilet bowl red.

Distinction of the bleeding location by history of bleeding depends on the amount and rapidity of bleeding, the source, and the transit time through the gut. Some guidelines to the clinical determination of the bleeding location are as follows:

- Hematemesis (vomiting of blood)—almost always an upper GI source.
- Hemoptysis—not from the GI tract, this is expectoration of blood from the respiratory tract.
- Hematochezia (bright red blood in the stool)—may be seen with upper GI bleeding and rapid transit or left colon or sigmoid colon bleeding.
- Dark red blood—usually bleeding from the ileum to the right colon.
- Black stool or blood (melena)—suggests at least 100 cc of rapidly lost blood. The source is usually duodenal or jejunal. It must be retained in the gut for eight hours to turn black.
- Silver stools—caused by biliary obstruction (e.g., cancer of the papilla of Vater) plus GI bleeding.

Remember that these are just guidelines. The determination of the precise bleeding spot is less important than stabilization of the patient.

Q. Can GI bleeding result in shock?

A. The physical examination may reveal signs of hypovolemic shock. Orthostatic BP and pulse changes ("tilt test") are useful to determine whether significant intravascular volume depletion has occurred. Orthostasis usually occurs with a 15–20 percent loss of circulating volume. Shock is almost invariably present when the patient loses more than 30 percent of the blood volume.

The color of the palmar crease, when the fingers are forcibly extended, is a useful bedside measurement for anemia. When the hemoglobin level is below 50 percent of normal levels, the creases do not turn red. The abdominal exam is usually nonspecific though tenderness, decreased bowel sounds, and surgical scars (possibly from graft placement) may be noted. The rectal examination will often reveal blood in the stool, either grossly or via special heme-testing solutions.

[Q] What is the field treatment for GI bleeding?

[A] Field treatment is the same, regardless of the cause. Initial treatment of any patient with GI bleeding, regardless of location, should progress as follows (always follow your local protocols):

- High-flow O_2—beware of continued vomiting and bleeding. In these cases, use oxygen via nasal cannula.
- Large-bore peripheral IV—fluid and rate as per your local protocols. The patient should have two lines if the BP is below 90 mmHg.
- Consider the use of military antishock trousers/pneumatic antishock garment (MAST/PASG). These may tamponade bleeding from a ruptured aortic aneurysm.

- Patients with hematemesis should be transported with the head and trunk elevated to prevent aspiration.
- Nasogastric (NG) tube placement, if permitted by local protocols, may be beneficial. The role of an iced saline lavage in controlling ongoing bleeding is somewhat controversial—the cold water not only vasoconstricts, decreasing bleeding, but may cause significant hypothermia. Studies have suggested that hypothermia in people with hemorrhagic shock markedly worsens their outcome.

[Q] What are the signs and symptoms, pathophysiology, and management of GI and genitourinary (GU) conditions seen in the field?

[A] The major GU and GI conditions seen in the field, as well as a summary of their diagnostic features and special treatment notes (where applicable), are summarized in Table 27–2.

TABLE 27-2

Major GI and GU Conditions	
Condition	Clinical Features
Appendicitis	Appendicitis is an inflammation of the appendix due to the occlusion of the lumen by a small piece of stool. As the obstructed appendix distends, its blood supply is cut off. Simple appendicitis then progresses to gangrenous appendicitis when tissue begins to die. Soon (usually within 24–48 hours from initial symptoms), the appendix ruptures, leading first to localized, then generalized peritonitis. The "classical" presentation is periumbilical crampy pain that then localizes in the lower-right quadrant. Nearly all persons with acute appendicitis have anorexia (markedly decreased appetite). Missed appendicitis is more common in young children, elderly patients, and pregnant women because the symptoms are often atypical.
Bowel obstruction	Blockage of any portion of the large or small bowel leads to a bowel obstruction. Potential causes are numerous. The most common include tumors (especially in obstruction of the lower colon) and scar tissue from previous abdominal inflammation or surgery ("adhesions"). The clinical picture usually evolves over 24–72 hours as the bowel gradually distends and "backs up." The result is abdominal distention, nausea, vomiting, and an inability to pass stool. A twisting of a loop of bowel on itself (volvulus) may also occur, resulting in rapid distention and progression of symptoms (including pain). In this case, urgent surgery is usually required.
Cholecystitis	Cholecystitis is an acute inflammation of the gallbladder, usually due to gallstones. These are particles of variable size that block the lumen, interfering with bile flow. Distention of the gallbladder causes upper-right quadrant pain that may radiate to the right shoulder area. Nausea and vomiting are common. Attacks may be accompanied by jaundice. The condition is not contagious, but clinical differentiation from acute hepatitis may be impossible.
Colitis	Colitis is a general term indicating inflammation of the colon for any of a number of reasons. The most common causes are infectious (viral), inflammatory disease (e.g., Crohn's disease, ulcerative colitis), and sexually transmitted disease (gonorrheal colitis).
Crohn's disease	Crohn's disease is a chronic condition resulting in bowel inflammation, usually of the small intestine. Patients have recurrent exacerbations consisting of pain, diarrhea, and sometimes lower GI bleeding. The initial presentation may mimic appendicitis, leading to emergency surgery and the correct diagnosis. Crohn's disease and ulcerative colitis, another inflammatory bowel disorder, are *not* contagious.
Diverticulitis	Diverticulosis is the presence of numerous small outpouchings in the colon called diverticula. Over 70 percent of lower GI bleeding is from this source, yet only 3–5 percent of patients with diverticula ever bleed from them. Diverticula may also become inflamed, resulting in diverticulitis and abdominal pain (usually in the lower-left quadrant).
Esophageal varices	Esophageal varices are dilations of the veins of the esophagus secondary to increased portal vein pressures. Alcoholic varices are secondary to cirrhosis caused by alcohol ingestion. Patients with alcoholic cirrhosis and varices may bleed from varices (40 percent of the time), but are as likely to have bleeding from gastritis, gastric ulcer (30 percent), or duodenal ulcer (20 percent). Patients with nonalcoholic cirrhosis and varices are four times as likely to bleed from varices than from peptic ulcer. Gastritis in these patients is rare.

(continued)

TABLE 27-2 *continued*

Major GI and GU Conditions

Condition	Clinical Features
Gastroenteritis	Gastroenteritis is a general term for the inflammation of any part or parts of the large or small bowel due to infection. The most common infection is due to viruses. These are usually self-limiting. Bacterial causes (e.g., salmonellosis) may be life threatening. Patients present with nausea, vomiting, diarrhea, general malaise, and variable degrees of dehydration. The maintenance of airway, breathing, and circulation (replenishment of fluid loss) is the best out-of-hospital approach, regardless of cause. Remember to observe body substance isolation (BSI) procedures—some of these agents are contagious.
Hemorrhoids	Hemorrhoids result from a dilation of veins in the lower portion of the colon (rectum). Though a common cause of lower GI bleeding, it is rarely hemodynamically significant. The most common symptoms are rectal itching and difficulty in defecation. Because hemorrhoids are nothing more than varicose veins of the rectum, they may occasionally clot (thrombosed hemorrhoid), leading to sudden and severe rectal pain. Though not life threatening, a thrombosed hemorrhoid requires prompt medical attention.
Hepatitis (acute)	Acute hepatitis refers to an inflammation of the liver for any reason. In common usage, we usually are referring to viral hepatitis, an infection. Patients present with malaise, nausea, and vomiting. Often jaundice and upper-right quadrant tenderness are present. Most forms of hepatitis are contagious.
Kidney stone	Kidney stones (urolithiasis) are small particles that form from a variety of substances. They are trapped in a portion of the kidney or ureter when the body attempts to pass them in the urine. The result is acute and severe pain, nausea, and often vomiting. The pain continues until the stone passes. Typically, patients have flank pain that radiates into the anterior lower quadrant on the involved side. People with kidney stones tend to writhe about in pain, unable to find any comfortable position. This fact may be helpful in diagnosis—people with inflammatory conditions (e.g., appendicitis) tend to lie quietly because movement usually aggravates their pain.
Reflux esophagitis	Esophagitis is caused by an erosion or irritation of the esophagus and may be a source of bleeding. The most common cause is acid reflux (backflow) from the stomach. The condition may be asymptomatic, may cause severe chest pain (mimicking AMI, thus the name "heartburn"), or any degree of symptoms in between. Even if a patient has a history of "heartburn," assume that chest pain is due to myocardial ischemia until proven otherwise.
Ulcers (peptic ulcer)	Peptic ulcer disease involves erosions of either the stomach or duodenum. Bleeding may occur, though pain and gastric distress are far more common. One out of six patients who bleed from a peptic ulcer have had no prior symptoms or history of ulcer disease. Gastritis presents in a similar fashion and is impossible to differentiate, in most cases, from peptic ulcer disease in the field. Acute gastritis results from erosions of the stomach lining, often caused by stress or a recent excessive ingestion of alcohol or salicylates.

[Q] Which causes of acute abdominal pain are immediate life threats?

[A] Four diseases are immediately life threatening:

- AMI—the pain of AMI may occur anywhere from the umbilicus upward.
- Ruptured abdominal aortic aneurysm—an outpouching of the abdominal portion of the aorta due to atherosclerosis. The aneurysm formation weakens the wall of the artery—if the aneurysm ruptures, severe abdominal and back pain, as well as shock, result. The patient may easily bleed to death.
- Ruptured ectopic pregnancy—occurs when the fertilized egg implants outside the uterus. Internal structures may rupture, causing severe internal bleeding. The patient has abdominal pain, vaginal bleeding, and shock.
- Ruptured viscus—viscus is a general term for any hollow organ. The most common viscus to rupture is the duodenum, usually due to a peptic ulcer. The patient develops the sudden onset of sharp epigastric pain and shock; the abdomen is rigid.

[Q] Which causes of acute abdominal pain require emergency surgery?

[A] Indications for surgery are more clinically based than cause based. In patients undergoing "emergency abdominal surgery," a cause other than that originally suspected is found in a significant percentage of patients (30–50 percent depending on the study). It is the clinical presence of a "surgical abdomen" that mandates emergency surgery. The most common nontraumatic causes are refractory GI bleeding, severe intestinal obstruction, severe acute inflammation with a high risk of rupture (e.g., appendicitis), and ruptured viscus (e.g., ruptured ulcer, ruptured appendix).

[Q] What additional diagnostic procedures may be used in the ED to locate abdominal bleeding?

[A] The return of bright red blood following placement of an NG tube may help differentiate upper- from lower-GI bleeding. However, over 30 percent of patients with ongoing upper-GI bleed have a negative NG aspirate. The reasons for this are unclear, but may include intragastric clots blocking the path of the tube. A negative NG return, thus, is not very helpful.

If the exact location must be known emergently, the "gold standard" is still GI angiography—placing a small catheter into the artery, injecting radiodense x-ray dye, and locating the bleeding vessel. Often, the angiographer can insert a thrombogenic (clot-forming) material into the artery to stop the bleeding once the exact site is identified. In recent years, therapeutic endoscopy has been used in both upper- and lower-GI bleeding. Both heated probes and lasers have been used, particularly in upper-GI bleeding, with success.

Why must ectopic pregnancy be ruled out in a female presenting with acute abdominal pain?

Any woman with an ectopic pregnancy is at risk for rupture. A ruptured ectopic pregnancy carries a high mortality due to hemorrhagic shock. In women of childbearing age, this is the most immediate life-threatening cause of abdominal pain and must be diagnosed or excluded promptly. Though pregnancy tests in the field are rarely performed, a woman with a sudden onset of abdominal pain, with or without vaginal discharge, has an ectopic pregnancy until proven otherwise. Assume it has already ruptured if she is in shock.

CLINICAL PEARL

Though not "officially recommended in protocols," the use of the MAST/PASG may be lifesaving in a woman with a ruptured ectopic pregnancy while transporting her to surgery. Always follow your local protocols and consult with medical control for direction.

What are the most common "missed diagnoses" in patients with abdominal pain?

Ectopic pregnancy, appendicitis, and AMI are the most frequently "missed diagnoses" of acute abdominal pain. Common errors (excluding misreading of 12-lead ECGs) include:

- The failure to perform a pregnancy test because a patient states she "cannot be pregnant." Ten to twenty percent of women with acute abdominal pain who have made this statement in EDs have positive pregnancy tests according to scientific evidence.
- Attributing symptoms of appendicitis to "the flu" or a urinary tract infection. Especially in the early stages, a patient's symptoms and signs may not point strongly to appendicitis, or even to an acute abdomen. If the patient has loose stools or urinary discomfort (both are common early in appendicitis), clinicians

may falsely reassure a patient. Adding to the potential confusion is the fact that when the distended appendix ruptures, the patient's pain often improves, at least transiently (due to the release of pressure). Peritonitis then develops over the ensuing hours.

- Deciding that epigastric pain and "indigestion" are due to gastritis or "heartburn" when they really indicate MI.

Assessment

Which questions should be asked in the focused history (FH) of the acute abdominal patient?

In general, use the "OPQRST" and "SAMPLE" acronyms to determine aspects of the following:

- The abdominal pain.
- Chest pain or shortness of breath (SOB).
- Recent change in diet.
- Food intolerance.
- Dysphagia (difficulty swallowing).
- Nausea and vomiting.
- Change in bowel habits.
- Past medical history.
- Medications—over-the-counter (OTC), antacids.

The history is the most important part of the diagnosis with acute abdominal pain. The *onset of pain* is very important. Was it sudden or gradual? Sudden, abrupt pain (if the patient can tell you the precise moment it started) suggests an acute perforation, strangulation, torsion, or vascular accident. Examples include ruptured ectopic pregnancy, perforated ulcer, mesenteric vascular occlusion, splenic, or renal infarction. Inflammatory lesions and obstructive phenomena are slower in their development. Examples include intestinal obstruction, appendicitis, and diverticulitis.

The *severity of the pain at onset* may be helpful. A good general rule is that the most severe entities cause the most intense pain and symptoms. Examples include perforated ulcer and dissecting or ruptured aneurysm. The exception to this rule is conditions where blood loss leads to shock; when this occurs, signs and symptoms of shock overshadow those of the pain.

Changes in the location of pain may be important in the diagnosis. Pain may become localized with abscess formation. On the other hand, the perforation of an abscess will lead to generalized pain. Periumbilical pain that moves to the lower-right quadrant suggests appendicitis. The sudden cessation of pain may signal perforation. Peritonitis may later develop. This, in fact, is what typically happens in an appendiceal abscess.

The *presence or absence of associated symptoms* may be helpful in refining one's impression:

- When prominent, nausea and vomiting suggest gastroenteritis, gastritis, acute pancreatitis, or obstruction.
- Pain precedes vomiting in acute appendicitis.
- Diarrhea is usually present with gastroenteritis.
- The failure to pass flatus (gas) suggests obstruction.
- Chills and fever are compatible with pyelonephritis or generalized bacteremia (of any cause).

Other associated events and diagnostic points include:

- GI distress in others sharing the same meal suggests food poisoning.
- A recent ingestion of fatty food preceding the pain suggests acute cholecystitis.
- A history of excessive alcohol consumption is compatible with pancreatitis.

The *age of the patient* is important to consider. Appendicitis usually occurs between ages 5 and 50. Cholecystitis is unusual in patients under age 20 and bowel obstruction is uncommon in patients less than age 35. One should also try to determine if there was a recent intake of drugs such as steroids, antibiotics, or antacids.

What are the major aspects in the focused physical examination of the acute abdominal pain patient?

Like the history, the physical examination of a patient with acute abdominal pain must be quite detailed. Note that the field evaluation may be limited by the patient's condition. Steps involved in the full abdominal exam include:

- General appearance of the patient—note first the patient's general appearance and obtain baseline vital signs. A patient with peritoneal inflammation lies still. A person suffering spasms or colic will usually be writhing in pain.
- Bowel sounds—are usually not checked in the field due to noise and time constraints. They may be difficult to characterize when present, but their absence is very significant and should be noted.
- Palpation—spasm of abdominal muscles, tenderness, masses. Spasm of the abdominal muscles can be tested by placing the hand on the abdomen, and depressing it slightly and gently. The patient is then asked to take in a long breath. During this maneuver, the muscle will relax if only voluntary spasm (guarding) is present. In true spasm (involuntary guarding), the muscle remains taut. This suggests peritoneal inflammation. Tenderness should be verified using one-finger palpation. It is best to start away from the stated area of pain. If pain is decreased with sitting (e.g., contraction of the abdominal muscles), it is likely intra-abdominal, and vice

versa. *Rebound tenderness* occurs when gentle pressure elicits less pain on the sudden release of that pressure. Keep in mind that the presence of rebound indicates peritoneal irritation. Any maneuver that jars the inflamed peritoneal cavity should result in rebound. This includes the direct release of palpation pressure, moving the cart sharply, or fist percussion of the soles of the feet. These alternative examination techniques may be especially helpful if the patient is hysterical or malingering. *Referred tenderness* occurs when pressure at a distance from an inflamed viscus causes pain over that viscus. An example of this is Rovsing's sign in acute appendicitis where lower-left quadrant palpation leads to lower-right quadrant tenderness. During palpation, note the presence of any masses in the abdomen.

- Genitorectal exam—although discussed in the National EMT-P curriculum, it probably is not done in the field. Check with your medical director for clarification on the field application of this examination in your region. During the genitorectal exam, the stool is examined for blood. Fullness, obstruction, and hernia are sought. If a hernia is present, it should be determined whether it is easily reducible or not.
- Pelvic exam—although discussed in the National EMT-P curriculum, it probably is not done in the field. Check with your medical director for clarification on the field application of this examination in your region. Tenderness on cervical motion ("chandelier sign") suggests pelvic inflammatory disease. A right-sided pelvic mass suggests an appendiceal abscess, and a left-sided one, tubo-ovarian abscess. Eight-five percent of those patients with an ectopic pregnancy have tenderness on direct cervical palpation.
- Special signs—although not usually considered field procedures, other signs may be present, further refining your impression:

  1. *Iliopsoas sign*—patients are first instructed to extend (straighten) their knee. They are then asked to attempt to flex (lift upward from a lying position) the thigh, keeping the knee straight, against the examiner's resistance (Figure 27–1). Alternatively, the examiner may extend the straightened leg backward with the patient on his side. If either maneuver causes pain, irritation of the underlying iliopsoas muscle is present, suggesting appendicitis or abscess.

  2. *Obturator sign*—the thigh is passively flexed to a 90-degree angle with the knee bent. The examiner internally, then externally, rotates the leg. Pain with this maneuver suggests pelvic appendicitis (right side) or diverticulitis (left side) (Figure 27–2).

- Pulmonary and cardiovascular exam—is crucial because abdominal pain may be due to disease above the diaphragm. Extraneous sounds in the lungs suggest pneumonia, heart failure, or MI. A left pleural effusion is common with pancreatitis.

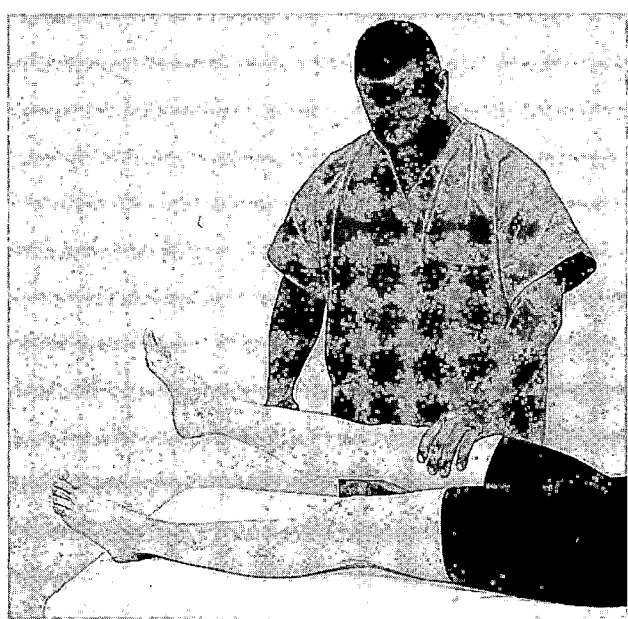

FIGURE 27-1 Iliopsoas muscle test.

The presence of atrial fibrillation or a prosthetic (artificial) heart valve suggests the possibility of emboli to the mesentery.

Q **What does a black stool indicate? What about other abnormalities in stool color?**

A "Colorful stools" may be due to a number of conditions, some benign and others potentially deadly:

- Dark, black, or tarry stool may indicate upper-GI bleeding or the ingestion of iron or bismuth preparations, such as antacids.

- Bright red discoloration of stool may be due to beets or other vegetables (red peppers) in the diet. Of course, the most immediate concern is GI bleeding. Bright red blood is usually due to lower-GI bleeding, but may also occur from upper-GI bleeding with rapid intestinal transit time.

- Gray (pale, clay-colored) stool may indicate obstructive jaundice. The gray color results from the loss of normal bile pigment (urobilinogen and stercobilin) in the stool.

- Yellow, fatty stools may be seen with a malabsorption syndrome of any cause.

Q **What test is used in the ED to detect nonvisible blood in the stool?**

A The guaiac test uses guaiac (a resin from a Guaiacum tree) on feces to detect occult blood in the intestinal and urinary tracts.

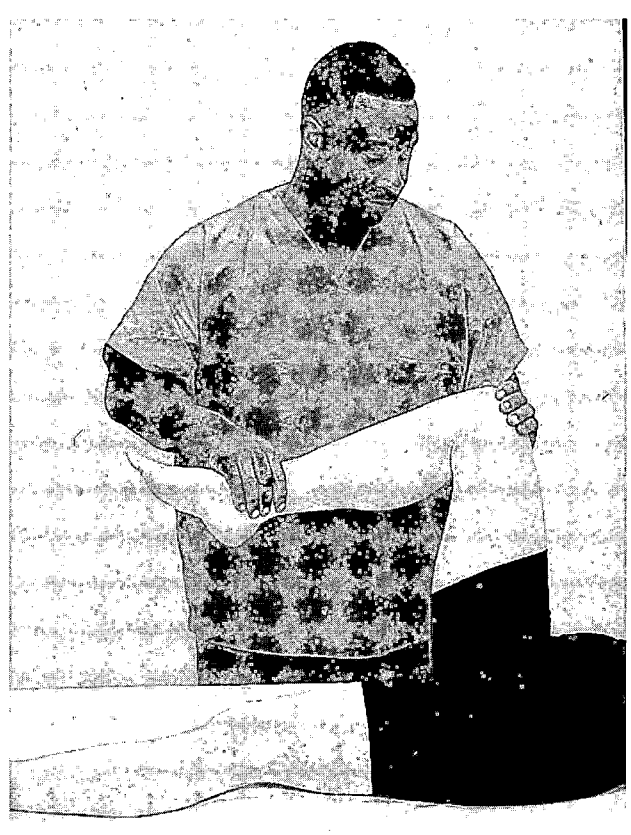

FIGURE 27-2 Obturator muscle test.

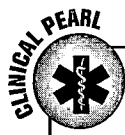 **PEARL**

Ingestion of red meat within the past three days causes a false positive test on the guaiac stool test.

Q **What is hepatojugular reflux?**

A Hepatojugular reflux refers to an increased venous pressure (distension) in the neck following gentle pressure on the liver. It is a sign of chronic congestive heart failure. This sign is not part of the routine physical assessment of people with abdominal pain.

Q **What is the tilt test and when is it used?**

A The tilt test measures orthostatic BP and pulse changes, and is useful in determining whether significant intravascular volume depletion has occurred. This means that the BP decreases, the pulse increases, or both, after changing from a supine to a sitting or from a sitting to a standing position. Many experts also consider the test positive if the patient has significant symptoms (e.g., dizziness, near syncope), regardless whether or not the vital signs change.

Orthostasis usually occurs with a 15–20 percent loss of circulating volume. Significant changes are an increase in the heart rate of 10–20 beats per minute or a decrease in the systolic blood pressure greater than 20 mmHg. The tilt test is more reliable in adults than children.

> **CLINICAL PEARL**
>
> *Normovolemic children, up to age 12, may show a heart rate increase of up to 30 or 40 beats per minute on standing. The BP may drop as much as 27 mmHg. Thus, these parameters are not helpful in patients under 13 years old. A review of adult data also suggests possible problems in interpreting adult values. The following changes occurred when going from lying to standing in normal adult patients:*
>
> *1. Heart rate increased up to 30 beats per minute.*
> *2. Systolic BP decreased 0 to 26 mmHg.*
> *3. Diastolic BP decreased 10 to 15 mmHg.*
>
> *Thus, it appears that orthostatic changes by themselves are difficult to interpret. Of course, when combined with an appropriate clinical picture, they mean far more.*

Why do certain foods cause abdominal pain?

Potential reasons for why a particular food causes abdominal pain in any given person are numerous. Foods that commonly cause GI distress include:

- Fatty foods—eating fat causes the gallbladder to contract, releasing bile. Bile contains special enzymes to digest fat so that it may be properly absorbed in the small bowel. If a person has a gallbladder disease (e.g., gallstones), contraction of the gallbladder may lead to distention and pain. Ingestion of fatty foods may also precipitate an attack of acute cholesystitis.
- Spicy foods—many spices (e.g., hot peppers) act as a direct irritant on the GI tract, especially the stomach. In sufficient amounts, they will cause pain in most people. Some people, however, are more sensitive than others and develop pain with smaller amounts. Though spicy foods may aggravate pain from gastritis or an ulcer, there is absolutely no scientific evidence that the ingestion of these foods *causes* either of these problems.
- Milk products—contain the sugar lactose. Lactose intolerance is probably the most common GI abnormality known to mankind. Some studies suggest that it affects more than half of the world's population. The symptoms include bloating, pain, and often violent diarrhea within minutes to hours of eating lactose-containing foods (e.g., milk, cheese). Acute gastroenteritis precipitates transient lactose deficiency even in people who are normally tolerant to lactose. There are several

low-lactose and lactose-free food preparations available commercially. In addition, patients may purchase (without a prescription) dropper bottles of the missing enzyme (lactase) to add to their food.

What do you listen for when listening for bowel sounds?

To auscultate bowel sounds, gently place the diaphragm (flat part) of your *warmed* stethoscope on each of the four quadrants of the abdomen. Allow it to remain in place for at least 15 seconds in each quadrant.

> **CLINICAL PEARL**
>
> *Some textbooks recommend listening for at least one minute in each of the four abdominal quadrants. In practice, this is rarely done. Follow your local protocols.*

Normally, you should hear intermittent gurgling sounds that are of a medium pitch. Bowel sounds (BS) are considered hyperactive if they occur more frequently than normal. Hypoactive BS are the opposite—they occur *less* frequently than normal. Realistically speaking, it is difficult to differentiate specific conditions by the presence of BS. More helpful is the total absence of BS in all four quadrants. This finding suggests serious intra-abdominal pathology, regardless of the reason.

> **CLINICAL PEARL**
>
> *Note whether BS are present or absent. Their absence is more important clinically (and easier to determine) than variations in sounds that are present.*

What is irritable bowel syndrome (IBS)?

IBS is a condition characterized by recurrent abdominal pain, usually crampy in nature, and diarrhea, often alternating with periods of constipation. It is most frequent in young adults and has no known cause. IBS is often associated with emotional stress and has also been called "spastic colon."

> **CLINICAL PEARL**
>
> *Unfortunately, some health care providers use IBS as a "wastebasket" diagnosis when they are not certain what is really wrong. This labeling of patients leads to complacency and the missed diagnosis of potentially serious conditions. Don't assume that just because a patient carries a diagnosis of IBS that something more serious can't be present!*

Do we need to save vomitus?

Unpleasant as it is, the answer is yes. An analysis of vomitus may provide significant diagnostic clues, especially in cases of unknown ingestions or an abdominal disease of unknown etiology.

What is the fluid wave test and how is it performed?

The fluid wave is a test for ascites (intraperitoneal, serous fluid). Sometimes tapping one side of the abdomen and feeling on the other may produce vibrations of fluid. Have the patient or an observer place the side of a hand along the midline to prevent the vibration of the anterior abdominal wall (and consequent misinterpretation). Gently tap one side of the abdomen with one or two fingers. At the same time, place your other hand (palm side toward the patient) on the opposite side to feel for the transmitted fluid wave. (Figure 27–3).

What are the pitfalls when evaluating elderly patients with acute abdominal pain?

Though not always, many older people have atypical signs and symptoms. This absence of "classic" findings is a dangerous trap for the unwary examiner. The list of possible "exceptions to the rule" is extensive. Some common ones include:

CLINICAL PEARL

The bottom line is simple: if the "classic findings" are there, they support your impression. It is far less likely that their absence *excludes a condition. If* you *think the patient is sick, she is sick until proven otherwise.*

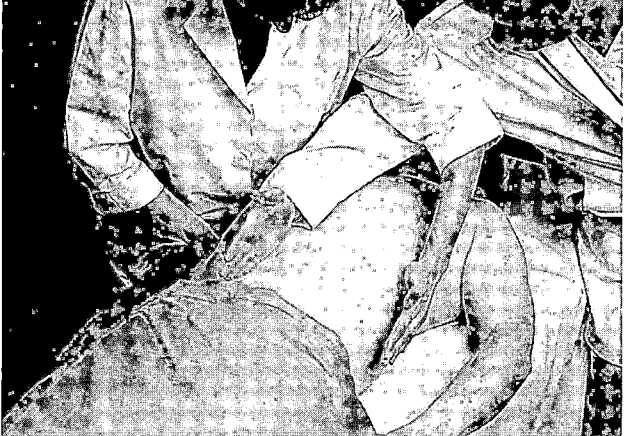

FIGURE 27-3 Palpation for ascites: fluid wave test.

- New onset diffuse weakness may be the only sign of peritonitis.
- The abdomen may not be rigid even in the presence of a perforated ulcer or ruptured bowel.
- Nausea or indigestion as the only signs of an MI.
- Back pain as a sign of a leaking abdominal aortic aneurysm.

What is the management plan for the patient with a GI emergency?

The approach to all patients with a GI emergency is similar regardless of the cause:

- Maintenance of airway, breathing, and circulation as per local protocols.
- Nothing by mouth.
- NG tube as per local protocols.
- Pain medicine as per local protocols.
- Transport by the most appropriate means to the appropriate health care facility.

When is the hematocrit level used in the ED for a patient with abdominal complaints?

The hematocrit measures the number of red blood cells (RBC) in the peripheral blood. It may be abnormal (e.g., too high, too low) due to a variety of conditions, including the patient's state of hydration. In abdominal trauma, alterations of the hematocrit are used to monitor blood loss. Similarly, trends are helpful in patients with GI bleeding.

When is diagnostic peritoneal lavage (DPL) used in the ED for a patient with abdominal complaints?

DPL has essentially no use in people with nontraumatic GI pain. DPL is reserved for patients with abdominal trauma and suspected internal organ injury (see Chapter 41, Abdominal Trauma).

Why do patients with acute GI emergencies get nothing by mouth (NPO)?

There are two major reasons why people with GI emergencies should be NPO:

- To rest the GI tract—food causes the release of digestive enzymes that often worsen most abdominal conditions.
- To minimize stomach contents in the event surgery is required—if a patient requires emergency surgery, the induction of general anesthesia may lead to the aspiration of stomach contents. Allowing the patient to eat or drink may delay necessary surgery.

🅠 What is the current thought on pain management for the acute abdominal patient?

🅐 There has been much debate regarding the role of pain medication with acute abdominal pain. Several studies have shown that small doses of narcotic medications (e.g., morphine) do *not* worsen diagnostic accuracy by "masking" signs and symptoms. On the contrary, investigators have shown that by making the patient more comfortable, the examiner is able to perform a more accurate physical exam. Despite these significant findings, many health care providers (especially surgeons) remain uncomfortable (as do the patients!) giving pain medications until definitive evaluation. Follow your local protocols.

🅠 Are MAST/PASG ever used on these patients when treating for shock?

🅐 "Official" recommendations on the use of MAST/PASG do not include abdominal conditions. However, many clinicians' experience dictates that they may be lifesaving, especially during prolonged transports, for patients with intra-abdominal bleeding (e.g., ectopic pregnancy, ruptured abdominal aortic aneurysm). Some reports also document efficacy in hemodynamically significant GI bleeding. Follow your local protocols.

Other Issues

🅠 What is dialysis?

🅐 Dialysis is a general term for a method, involving a semipermeable membrane, used to separate smaller particles from larger ones in a liquid mixture. Medically, this usually refers to *hemodialysis,* the procedure for filtering waste products from the blood of some kidney disease patients or for removing poisons or drugs. Another form of dialysis, *peritoneal dialysis,* is used on less sick individuals and involves fluid placement into the peritoneal cavity. In this case, the peritoneum itself serves as the dialysis membrane.

🅠 What types of emergencies can result from dialysis?

🅐 The most common emergency from peritoneal dialysis is an acute infection of the peritoneum. In this case, the patient presents with severe pain and often signs of early shock. Complications from hemodialysis may include:

- Vascular access problems—the most common problems are bleeding at the puncture site, thrombosis, and infection. Occluded grafts or fistulas (used for vascular access during hemodialysis) usually require surgery or the administration of a thrombolytic agent. Consider vascular access site infection whenever a dialysis patient has unexpected fever, malaise, or other signs of infection.

- Hemorrhage—renal failure patients have decreased platelet function. Thus, they are more likely to bleed significantly, whatever the inciting cause. Chronic renal failure also causes anemia, which limits the patient's RBC reserve. Control bleeding from an extremity with a fistula or graft in the normal function. Avoid obstructing circulation with the shunt.

- Hypotension—is common during hemodialysis and may result from a number of causes (e.g., reduction of intravascular volume, changes in electrolyte concentrations). Cautiously manage these patients with fluid expansion, taking care to avoid fluid overload.

- Chest pain—in addition to hypotension, mild hypoxia is common during hemodialysis. The combination may lead to myocardial ischemia and chest pain. Symptoms often respond to oxygen and nitroglycerin. Myocardial ischemia may also lead to cardiac dysrhythmias, especially when an electrolyte imbalance is present.

- Severe hyperkalemia—this is a life-threatening emergency that may occur in patients with chronic renal failure. It is rarely a complication of dialysis itself; rather, it is caused by the failure of the kidneys to excrete potassium adequately. ECG findings include peaked T waves, prolonged P-R interval, QRS widening, and eventually ventricular fibrillation. The presence of ECG changes or dysrhythmias in a hyperkalemic patient requires the immediate administration of calcium chloride or calcium gluconate to counteract cardiac membrane toxicity. Follow your local protocols.

- Disequilibrium syndrome—a group of symptoms that occur during or immediately after dialysis. Severity ranges from mild (e.g., headache, nausea) to severe (e.g., seizures, coma). The cause is unclear—some experts contend that it occurs as a result of an aluminum imbalance. Others believe that dialysis leads to an osmotic gradient between the brain and blood, leading to cerebral edema.

- Air embolism—though unusual, dialysis machine malfunction or loose tubing may lead to an accumulation of air in the right side of the heart. The patient may experience a number of different symptoms, including dyspnea, chest pain, or hypotension.

CLINICAL PEARL

Most hemodialysis centers were originally in-hospital. There are now a number of free-standing facilities resulting in a significant increase in EMS calls for hemodialysis-related emergencies. Dialysis technicians and nurses are highly trained and may offer valuable insight or suggestions.

What are the special considerations for the dialysis patient?

Special considerations for the dialysis patient include:

- Avoid the dialysis vascular access site for drawing blood or giving IV fluids; most experts recommend using the opposite arm if at all possible.
- Avoid performing BP measurements on any extremity with a graft or fistula in place.
- Under directions from medical control, dialysis access sites may be used. Pay careful attention to aseptic technique. Use caution to avoid puncturing the back wall of the vessel.

Urology Epidemiology

What are urological emergencies?

Urological emergencies are those that involve any portion or portions of the GU tract.

What are the common causes of urological emergencies?

The most common urological emergencies seen by the out-of-hospital care provider are:

- Kidney stones (renal calculi)—involve the formation of small rock-like concretions (stones), one to five mm in diameter. They are formed in the kidney and excreted with the urine. Most stones travel down the ureter to the bladder and eventually out the urethra. A small number become impacted and require surgical removal. The passage of a stone down the urinary tract tends to be accompanied by severe, intermittent crampy pain. This starts in the flank, but commonly radiates to the abdomen and groin. Nausea and vomiting are common.
- Urinary tract infection (UTI)—uncomplicated UTI is an infection that involves a structurally and functionally normal urinary tract. Next to respiratory infections, uncomplicated UTIs are the most common problem encountered in EDs. Between 10 percent to 20 percent of women will experience a UTI sometime in their lives. UTI in adult men is uncommon unless cystoscopy or catheterization has occurred. In institutionalized men and women, the incidence of UTI increases markedly. Nosocomial urinary infections are the most common hospital-acquired infections and account for significant morbidity and mortality. Clinically, a UTI is suspected on the basis of symptoms—dysuria (painful urination), frequency (frequent urination), urgency (immediate need to urinate), and suprapubic

(over the bladder area) pain. It is tentatively confirmed by the findings of pyuria (white blood cells in the urine) and bacteriuria (bacteria in the urine) on the microscopic examination of the urine.

- Pyelonephritis—one of the most common kidney conditions seen in out-of-hospital care is an acute bacterial infection of the kidneys. Usually the disease occurs as a complication of a bladder infection, although sexual transmission has been reported. The most common form affects young females and is due to the bacteria, *Escherichia coli*. As a rule, pyelonephritis is more serious than a simple UTI. Typically the patient will present with symptoms of flank pain, chills, and fever. Symptoms of lower UTI (e.g., urgency, nocturia, frequency, dysuria) may also be present.

The condition is diagnosed by the symptoms, physical findings of flank tenderness, and confirmed laboratory data in-hospital. Urinalysis will usually reveal white blood cells (leukocytes), hematuria (blood in the urine), bacteria, and casts. Often, the patient has a fever and an elevated white blood cell (WBC) count.

- Acute urinary retention—Acute inability to pass urine is referred to as acute urinary retention. The most common cause of this problem is prostatic enlargement (in males), urethral stricture (narrowing by scar tissue), or a blocked urinary catheter. Untreated, even brief (less than six hours) acute urinary retention can lead to a severe infection.

  In women, acute urinary retention is rare. Men commonly have acute urinary retention secondary to prostatic enlargement. Many disease processes may cause acute urinary retention in women. Postoperative and postpartum patients are most commonly afflicted. In one study, 13 of 45 female patients with urinary retention were found to have a pelvic mass as the cause of the retention.

  Acute urinary retention may be the initial presenting symptom of ectopic pregnancy. It is difficult to know if the urinary retention results from the mass effect of the ectopic pregnancy or from the inflammatory changes caused by peritoneal irritation. Either way, ectopic pregnancy *must* be ruled out in a woman capable of ovulating who presents with acute urinary retention.

  Common symptoms include discomfort and pain with attempted urination, as well as distention of the abdomen. Elderly people may present with an altered level of consciousness, but without complaints of discomfort or an awareness of their acute deterioration. Besides the markedly enlarged bladder, little may be found on the physical examination.

- Epididimitis—is an acute inflammation of the epididymis usually due to bacterial infection. The infection may or may not be sexually transmitted. The patient complains of a swollen, exquisitely tender, and enlarged scrotum. The pain develops suddenly in the scrotum and radiates along the spermatic cord, leading to discomfort in the lower abdomen, nausea, and vomiting. Often the patient will have a high fever in association with the disease.

- Prostatitis—is a bacterial infection of the prostate gland. Prostatitis is most often seen in males between the ages of 20 and 40 who present with the following findings: painful ejaculation, suprapubic pain, discharge from the penis, malaise and fever, and irritative symptoms of voiding—frequency, dysuria, and urgency. On physical examination, the physician discovers that the prostate gland is "boggy," warm, and swollen to the touch. The urinalysis, obtained following prostatic examination, contains WBCs and bacteria.

- Torsion of the testicle—is a condition when the testicle twists about the spermatic cord and epididymis, resulting in an occlusion of the blood supply. The condition is seen in about three to four patients per year in the ED of a large metropolitan hospital, most typically in a child or young adult (especially at the time of puberty). However, torsion has been described in older males as well. The condition is usually unilateral, although cases of bilateral torsion have been reported. Frequently the patient reports a sudden onset of pain in his testicle occurring during or after physical exertion, although the torsion is not necessarily associated with physical activity. The patient's symptoms include extreme testicular or scrotal pain and sometimes nausea, vomiting, and fever. The initial effect of testicular torsion is obstruction of the venous return. As the twisting of the spermatic cord persists, arterial thrombosis, edema, necrosis, and testicular atrophy develop. Even with timely treatment, some studies report a semen analysis to be abnormal after unilateral torsion. Testicular torsion is an acute urological emergency that threatens future reproductive capability in males.

- Renal failure—either acute or chronic, is less likely to come to your attention as the primary basis for a response. The major exception to this is problems during hemodialysis.

Q **What is the morbidity and mortality of urological emergencies?**

A Though very few urological emergencies are life threatening, they exact a significant toll in terms of morbidity. Dialysis treatment of chronic renal failure accounts for a significant percentage of the U.S. health care budget each year. UTI, especially in women, is extremely common and results in significant lost productivity. Kidney stones are less common, but when present effectively disable the victim until the stone passes or is treated surgically.

Q **What type of pain is associated with urological emergencies?**

A The pain felt by a patient depends on the particular problem. A woman with an acute UTI will have pain over her bladder (suprapubic region). A patient with a kidney stone typically has flank pain that radiates into the anterior lower quadrant of the affected side as the stone passes through the ureter.

Assessment

Q **Is it possible to differentiate pain that is urogenital in nature from other abdominal causes of pain?**

A Sometimes—if a patient complains of typical flank pain associated with radiation into the anterior lower quadrant, nausea, and vomiting, the most likely possibility is a kidney stone. Similarly, if there is burning with urination and suprapubic pain, a UTI is likely. Otherwise, the differentiation of urogenital from abdominal pain may be difficult, even in the ED.

Q **What questions should be asked of the patient with suspected urogenital causes of pain?**

A In general, use the "OPQRST" and "SAMPLE" acronyms to determine aspects of the following:
- The nature of the pain (e.g., sharp, dull, aching).
- Time course of pain (e.g., continuous, intermittent).
- Whether dysuria (difficult or painful urination) is present.
- Urethral or vaginal discharge.
- Flank pain.
- Nausea, vomiting.
- Fever, shaking chills.

Q **What areas should be covered during the focused physical exam?**

A Specifics of the focused exam depend on the patient's complaints. Particular areas of attention in GU emergencies include:
- General appearance—in pyelonephritis, the patient looks sick; this is unusual in an uncomplicated UTI. People with a kidney stone are usually in "perpetual motion," unable to find any comfortable position.
- Abdomen—check for suprapubic tenderness.
- Flank—check for flank tenderness over the kidneys.

- Genital—follow your local protocols; as a general rule, a visual inspection of the external genitalia is only recommended when warranted by the chief complaint.
- Rectal—though helpful in the diagnosis of prostatitis, the rectal examination is not usually performed in the field.

Q **What is the management plan for the patient with a urogenital emergency?**

A As in all patients, careful attention to airway, breathing, and circulation comes first. Ice and elevation may be helpful for men with scrotal discomfort. Use pain medications, especially in people with suspected kidney stones, as per your local protocols.

Other Issues

Q **What is the significance of erectile dysfunction and what is all the "hype" about the use of prescription (e.g., Viagra®) and nonprescription medications for treatment?**

A Erectile dysfunction is relatively common. In past years, notable public figures have brought their problem to national attention. As a result, consumers are overwhelmed with media ads for various medications, both prescription and nonprescription (e.g., herbals) to ostensibly cure their problem. Whether or not the medications work is beyond the scope of this review.

Of major importance to all health care providers is a potentially deadly drug interaction between Viagra® and nitrate medications (e.g., nitroglycerin tablets, isosorbide dinitrate). Both medications cause vasodilation via a similar biochemical mechanism. With nitrates, acute cardiac conditions benefit from pre-load reduction and coronary artery dilation. Viagra® causes non-specific vasodilation, but when combined with psychological arousal, selectively affects the vessels of the genital area. The combination of both at once may lead to significant systemic vasodilation and irreversible hypotension. Most experts agree that the use of any type of nitrate is contraindicated in a patient, male or female, who has taken Viagra® within the previous 24-hour period.

CLINICAL PEARL

Most patients are not willing to freely volunteer that they are taking medications for erectile dysfunction. During the "SAMPLE" portion of the history, be certain to specifically ask about Viagra®, especially if the patient has chest pain. The administration of nitrates within 24 hours of a patient taking Viagra® may result in patient death. Morphine is far safer in treating acute pulmonary edema or suspected myocardial ischemia under these circumstances. Avoid all nitrates unless specifically instructed otherwise by medical control!

Q **What are the common sexually transmitted diseases (STDs) found in male patients and how might they present?**

A The most common STDs in both sexes are chlamydia, gonorrhea, and syphilis. Unlike women, who are commonly asymptomatic, men usually have urethral burning, especially during urination, and discharge. With syphilis, a rash or swollen area in the groin may also be present. Two other conditions, hepatitis (B and C) and HIV infection, are also thought to be sexually transmitted.

Special Thanks

Pediatric Emergency Care, 1985, Vol. 1, 123–127.

Heart and Lung, 1986, Vol. 15, 611.

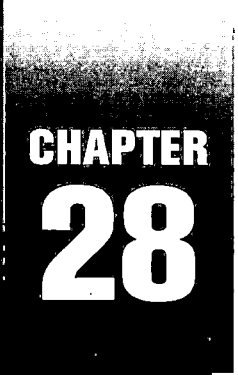

CHAPTER 28

Toxicology

This chapter discusses a wide variety of toxic exposures, both deliberate and accidental. The focus is on *why* patients present in a certain manner and *why* you need to respond in a certain way to their presenting problems.

General Statistics on Toxic Emergencies

Q What are the rates of occurrence, morbidity, and mortality of toxic emergencies?

A The latest available Poison Control Center data shows that there were 2,241,082 reported cases of toxic emergencies in the year 1998. This averages out to 8.7 exposures per thousand people in the population. The majority (88.7 percent) of exposures occurred in the patient's home. Children younger than 3 years were involved in 39.6 percent of the cases, and 52.7 percent occurred in children younger than 6 years. A male predominance is found among poison exposure victims younger than 13 years, but the gender distribution is reversed in teenagers and adults. Although the gender distribution was nearly equal for unintentional exposures, 59.4 percent of intentional exposures occurred in females, as did 64.2 percent of adverse reactions. There were 775 reported fatalities. Although responsible for the majority of poisoning reports, children younger than 6 years comprised just 2.1 percent (16) of the fatalities. Fifty-six percent of poisoning fatalities occurred in 20- to 49-year-old individuals.

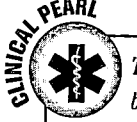

The reported fatality rate may be artificially low because only cases actually reported to the National Poison Control Center surveillance system were included.

Q What is the role of the Poison Control Center in the United States?

A Regional Poison Control Centers (PCC) are found throughout the United States. Experts agree that the PCC is the most reliable and up-to-date source of information on the assessment and treatment of toxicologic emergencies. Most have a toll-free number, easily accessible by cellular phone. Though protocols differ, many EMS systems require or encourage out-of-hospital providers to contact the PCC, either directly or via medical control.

Many EDs also contact the regional PCC routinely to obtain the most up-to-date patient treatment information. Unless a physician is a full-time toxicologist (specialist in poisoning), it is difficult to keep up with such a rapidly changing field.

What are the risk factors most predisposing to toxic emergencies?

Many factors predispose an individual to toxic emergencies. Several risk patterns are common:

- Pediatric ingestions—unattended children and a failure to "childproof" homes is the major reason that children are at high risk for toxic exposures, especially ingestion.
- Suicide attempts—poisoning has always been a common method used by people attempting suicide. Many agents are available, some of which are highly fatal.
- Occupational exposures—many workers are exposed to toxic substances and fumes on a day-to-day basis. Routine safety precautions often prevent major problems. Failure to observe these precautions results in potentially harmful exposures. Industrial accidents also account for a small but significant percentage of occupational exposures.

What organs and structures are affected by toxic emergencies?

Just about any body system may be affected by a toxic emergency. The most dangerous toxic substances affect:

- The nervous system—nerve gas and pesticides affect the transmission of nerve impulses to the muscles, essentially causing paralysis. Without prompt treatment, respiratory muscle paralysis leads to death. Narcotics and opiates depress the central nervous system. The resulting hypoventilation can also lead to respiratory arrest.
- The respiratory system—inhaled irritant gases cause pulmonary edema and severe hypoxia. If the patient survives the acute incident, subsequent scarring may lead to permanent respiratory dysfunction.
- The endocrine or metabolic system—carbon monoxide affects the ability of all cells to manufacture adenosine triphosphate (ATP), the major source of energy. When this occurs, death follows rapidly.

CLINICAL PEARL

Though any toxic exposure may affect any body system, the most significant problems occur when substances cause abnormalities in airway, breathing, circulation, or level of consciousness.

What is the difference between a poisoning and an overdose?

There is a difference between the terms poisoning and overdose:

- *Poisoning* connotes exposure to a substance that is generally only harmful and has no usual beneficial effects (e.g., cyanide).
- *Overdose* suggests excessive exposure to a substance that has normal treatment uses (e.g., aspirin). In excess, harm results.

What are the routes of entry of toxic substances into the body?

There are four routes by which poisons are introduced into the human body:

1. Ingestion—enters the body by the mouth and is absorbed by the GI tract. Ingestion is the most common poisoning route. Examples include eating poisonous mushrooms or a deliberate overdose of sleeping pills.
2. Inhalation—toxic fumes or gases may be inhaled into the lungs. The material may damage the lungs or be absorbed into the blood, leading to systemic toxicity. Carbon monoxide poisoning is an example of inhalation exposure.
3. Absorption—substances pass through the skin into the bloodstream. Many chemicals dissolve easily in the fat of the skin. These materials are the most likely to cause poisoning by absorption. Pesticides and agricultural chemicals are often absorbed this way.
4. Injection—needles or insect stingers may inject toxic material.

What is the pathophysiology of the entry of toxic substances into the body?

Once a substance enters the body, it may have only local effects (e.g., an inhaled lung irritant such as chlorine gas) or it may travel via the blood to various organs. The effects it has on the body depend on the poison. Some poisons, for example, affect the central nervous system (e.g., narcotics); others (e.g., pesticides) affect the peripheral and autonomic nervous systems.

General Assessment and Management

What important information should be obtained during the initial assessment?

When caring for a poisoning patient, try to gather information about the event:

- What substance was taken.
- How much was ingested.

- When the poisoning occurred.
- What, if anything, has been done for the patient.

Patients may state that they took a poison. If the patient is a child, the parent may be able to describe or show you the substance involved. Always bring any containers, pills, syringes, and pill bottles to the hospital with the patient. If the patient vomits, try to collect the vomitus in a plastic bag and bring it to the hospital for analysis.

Q What are some of the general signs and symptoms that should suggest a toxic exposure?

A Signs and symptoms of poisoning vary, depending on the particular substance involved. They may include:

- Burning and tearing of the eyes.
- Respiratory distress, wheezing, chest pain.
- Cyanosis.
- Nausea, vomiting, diarrhea.
- Excessive sweating or salivation.
- Weakness.
- Headache, dizziness, seizures.
- Altered level of consciousness (LOC), ranging from hyperactivity to coma.
- Pain, burning, or itching of the skin.
- Burns or stains around the mouth.

Many poisons, regardless of the route of entry into the body, result in altered levels of consciousness and alterations in vital signs.

Consider the following agents in all patients, including victims of poisoning by ingestion:

- Tachycardia—phencyclidine (PCP), anticholinergics, sympathomimetics, mushrooms, theophylline, substance withdrawal.
- Bradycardia—digoxin, beta-blockers, pesticides, clonidine, calcium channel blockers, local anesthetics, cholinergic agents.
- Hypertension—PCP, anticholinergics, sympathomimetics, substance withdrawal.
- Hyperthermia—salicylates (e.g., aspirin), sympathomimetics, PCP, anticholinergics, metal fumes.

Consider the following potential toxins (regardless of the route of exposure) when patients have alterations in the neurological examination:

- Seizures—strychnine, anticholinergics, pesticides, PCP, sympathomimetics, propoxyphene (Darvon®), carbon monoxide, phenytoin (Dilantin®), theophylline, hypoglycemia agents, local anesthetics, cyanide, lead, substance withdrawal.
- Mydriasis (large pupils)—anticholinergics, sympathomimetics, mushrooms, substance withdrawal.
- Miosis (small pupils)—pesticides, narcotics, mushrooms, nicotine, cholinergics, phenothiazines (major tranquilizers).
- Nystagmus—alcohols, barbiturates, phenytoin, PCP.

CLINICAL PEARL

The signs and symptoms of toxic exposures vary widely depending on the substance. The preceding information is generic to a wide variety of toxic exposures regardless of the route. However, assume you should always think about them.

Q How may findings on the physical exam help determine the poison involved?

A Physical findings that may help identify the poison involved include:

- Pulse—tachycardia suggests stimulant ingestion; bradycardia may be caused by various heart medications and by pesticide poisoning.
- Respiratory rate—increases in the respiratory rate, especially in children, suggest the possibility of aspirin toxicity (causes hyperventilation). Depressed respirations occur from narcotics, sedatives, and carbon monoxide poisoning.
- Temperature—elevated from aspirin and stimulants; lowered (hypothermia) with alcohol, sedatives, narcotics, and pesticides.
- BP—may be decreased if the patient took depressant or narcotic agents. The BP is often elevated if the patient has taken cocaine or amphetamines.

CLINICAL PEARL

Remember that most deliberate ingestions consist of more than one substance. Despite the utility of clinical guides, a "mixed ingestion" will result in a potentially bewildering variety of signs and symptoms. Don't assume that just because the patient's clinical findings don't fit a particular pattern that all is well.

What indications of poisoning may be present during the focused exam?

Poisonings may affect several body systems. Indications of poisoning that may be apparent during the focused exam include:

1. Respiratory system—many poisonings cause respiratory depression and partial airway obstruction. Inhaled toxins may cause respiratory distress and wheezing.

2. Cardiovascular system—some poisonings can cause irregular heart rhythm, chest pain, shock, and cardiac arrest.

3. Neurologic system—poisonings may result in changes in the pupil size. Narcotics usually cause constricted pupils, while stimulants result in pupillary dilation.

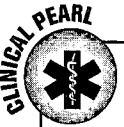

Regardless of the toxin, most poisons of significance affect the ABCs or the central nervous system (CNS).

What is a toxidrome?

Several groups of drugs present with similar clinical patterns of toxicity (e.g., cholinergics, hallucinogenics, narcotics). These syndromes are sometimes called toxidromes. They are useful for remembering the assessment and management of toxicological emergencies, but do not consider how or why the toxin has been introduced into the body. Always consider the route of entry as well as specific treatments.

What assessment findings are associated with various toxidromes?

There are five commonly described toxidromes: cholinergics, anticholinergics, hallucinogens, narcotics and opiates, and sympathomimetics. Features of each are summarized in Table 28–1.

When is there a need for rapid intervention and transport of the patient with a toxic substance emergency?

Whenever there is an actual or potential threat to the well-being of the patient or those around her. Some toxic substances have delayed reactions (e.g., tricyclic antidepressants) so that the patient appears fine initially, only to deteriorate later.

What are BLS and ALS management of toxic substances?

Cardinal principles of management for all EMS providers include:

- Ensure your own safety first.
- Maintain airway, breathing, and circulation.
- Consider decontamination (e.g., rinsing, activated charcoal) procedures as per local protocols.
- Consider specific antidotes, as per protocols and medical control (ALS).

What is the pathophysiology of poisoning by ingestion?

The substance enters the body by the mouth and is absorbed by the GI tract. From there, it travels to various organs. The toxicity exerted depends on the substance, as does the speed with which it causes harm (e.g., acute versus chronic damage).

How would the EMS provider assess the clinical significance of abnormal findings in the patient with the most common poisoning by ingestion?

The most significant findings are those that impair the integrity of airway, breathing, and circulation. Beyond the ABCs, findings that indicate impairment of CNS function (e.g., altered LOC, seizures) are also clinically significant.

TABLE 28–1

Toxidrome	Common Agents	Assessment Findings
Cholinergics	Pesticides, nerve agents	Headache, dizziness, weakness, nausea, bradycardia, wheezing, bronchoconstriction, myosis, coma, seizures; SLUDGE (salivation, lacrimation, urination, defecation, GI upset, emesis) syndrome.
Anticholinergics	Antihistamines, anti-diarrheals (contain atropine), over-the-counter cold remedies, antipsychotics, tricyclic antidepressants, mushrooms	ANTI-SLUDGE (red, hot, hyper, mad); fever, tachycardia, altered LOC
Hallucinogens	LSD, PCP, peyote, mushrooms, jimson weed, mescaline	Altered LOC, erratic behavior, active hallucinations
Narcotics and opiates	Heroin, morphine, codeine, meperidine, propoxyphene, fentanyl	Euphoria, hypotension, respiratory depression or arrest, nausea, pinpoint pupils, seizures, coma
Sympathomimetics	Amphetamines, over-the-counter diet pills, caffeine, cocaine	Tachycardia, diaphoresis, tachypnea, chest pain, stroke, myocardial

The cornerstone in the management of the poisoned patient is maintenance of airway, breathing, and circulation. Specific antidotes are available only for a few agents. Stabilizing the patient and waiting for the poison to clear from the body (including increasing excretion by activated charcoal) is adequate therapy in many circumstances.

Q What are the different treatments and pharmacological interventions in the management of the most common poisoning by ingestion?

A Care for these patients as recommended by the PCC or medical control. Some EMS systems advise giving syrup of ipecac to induce vomiting. Syrup of ipecac is not universally accepted. Consult your local protocols before giving ipecac. Do not induce vomiting if the patient is having seizures or if you suspect ingestion of acid, lye, or petroleum products. Also, do not induce vomiting if the patient has a decreased LOC or may lose consciousness. Do not delay transport to wait for ipecac to take effect.

Some protocols advise the administration of activated charcoal to absorb the poison. Do not give charcoal until ipecac has caused vomiting. Otherwise, the charcoal will absorb the ipecac and vomiting will not occur.

Q What are the factors affecting the decision to induce vomiting in a patient with ingested poison?

A Induction of vomiting by syrup of ipecac is controversial. Follow your local protocols. Do not induce vomiting if the patient:

- Is comatose or has an altered mental status.
- Is seizing or has a history of seizures.
- Is in the third trimester of pregnancy.
- Has a history of cardiac problems.

Do not induce vomiting if the patient has:

- Ingested corrosives, such as strong acids or alkali.
- Ingested petroleum products.
- Ingested iodine, silver nitrate, or strychnine.
- Ingested a drug that may cause a sudden LOC.

Q Why is activated charcoal once again recommended rather than syrup of ipecac?

A Activated charcoal has been shown to absorb many different ingested toxins from the stomach. In addition, it is able to cause the movement of toxins from the blood back into the stomach to be absorbed. This mechanism has been called "gastric dialysis"

and is effective for many common household substances and drugs such as phenobarbital, theophylline, tricyclic antidepressants, salicylates, and iron.

Q How would the EMS provider integrate the pathophysiological principles and the assessment findings to formulate a field impression and implement a treatment plan for the patient with the most common poisoning by ingestion?

A Generically speaking, look for combinations of findings (toxidromes) that suggest toxicity from ingested agents. The major considerations are:

- Protect yourself first.
- Maintain the ABCs.
- Consider gastric contamination (e.g., ipecac, activated charcoal) according to local protocols.
- Transport the patient in a timely fashion to the nearest appropriate facility.

Q What is the pathophysiology of poisoning by inhalation?

A The material may damage the lungs or be absorbed into the bloodstream, leading to systemic toxicity. This is the case with carbon monoxide poisoning where the gas competes for receptor sites on the hemoglobin molecules at a rate 200 times greater than oxygen.

Q What are the signs and symptoms related to the most common poisoning by inhalation?

A The signs and symptoms depend on the poison. Irritant substances result in bronchospasm, coughing, cyanosis, and sometimes, respiratory arrest. Systemic toxins (e.g., carbon monoxide) more often result in severe hypoxia, shock, and death.

Q How would the EMS provider assess the clinical significance of abnormal findings in the patient with the most common poisoning by inhalation?

A The most significant findings are those that impair the integrity of ABC. Beyond the ABCs, findings that indicate an impairment of CNS function (e.g., altered LOC, seizures) are clinically significant. Remember, many inhaled agents irritate the lungs, leading to bronchospasm and hypoxia. By directing your thinking toward maintaining the ABCs, these will be dealt with appropriately.

Q **What are the treatment and pharmacological priorities in the management of the most common poisoning by inhalation?**

A As in any patient, the major priorities are:

- Ensure your own safety.
- Remove the patient from ongoing exposure (using appropriate equipment and trained personnel).
- Maintain the ABCs.
- Consider specific antidotes, as provided for in local protocols (e.g., cyanide antidote kit).
- Consider bronchodilator therapy (or drugs for pulmonary edema, if present), as provided for in local protocols.
- Transport the patient in a timely fashion to the nearest appropriate facility.

Q **How would the EMS provider integrate the pathophysiological principles and the assessment findings to formulate a field impression and implement a treatment plan for the patient with the most common poisoning by inhalation?**

A Generically speaking, look for combinations of findings (toxidromes) that suggest toxicity from inhaled agents. The major considerations are:

- Protect yourself first.
- Maintain the ABCs.
- Move the patient to an area outside or with freely circulating air.
- Suspect carbon monoxide poisoning in all victims of fire.
- Help breathing as necessary and provide high-concentration oxygen by mask.
- Transport the patient in a timely fashion to the nearest appropriate facility.

Q **What is the pathophysiology of poisoning by injection?**

A Following injection, the substance is absorbed into the bloodstream and passes to various organs. Specific organ-related toxicity depends on the particular poison.

Q **What are the signs and symptoms related to the most common poisoning by injection?**

A Signs and symptoms vary widely, depending on the substance. Many poisons, regardless of the route of entry into the body, result in altered mental status (AMS) and alterations in vital signs.

Q **How would the EMS provider assess the clinical significance of abnormal findings in the patient with the most common poisoning by injection?**

A The most significant findings are those that impair the integrity of the ABCs. Besides the ABCs, findings that indicate an impairment of CNS function (e.g., altered LOC, seizures) are also clinically significant.

Q **How would the EMS provider differentiate between the various treatments and pharmacological interventions in the management of the most common poisoning by injection?**

A As in any patient, the major priorities are:

- Ensure your own safety.
- Maintain the ABCs.
- Consider specific antidotes, as provided in local protocols (e.g., naloxone, an antagonistic to narcotics).
- Transport the patient in a timely fashion to the nearest appropriate facility.

Q **How would the EMS provider integrate the pathophysiological principles and the assessment findings to formulate a field impression and implement a treatment plan for the patient with the most common poisoning by injection?**

A Generically speaking, look for combinations of findings (toxidromes) that suggest toxicity from injected agents. The most common involve narcotic or opiate injection. Respiratory depression is especially common and life threatening.

Q **What is the pathophysiology of poisoning by surface absorption?**

A Many chemicals dissolve easily in the fat of the skin. These materials are the most likely to cause poisoning by absorption.

Q **How would the EMS provider recognize the signs and symptoms related to the most common poisoning by surface absorption?**

A Signs and symptoms depend on the substance absorbed. Many poisons, regardless of the route of entry into the body, result in an AMS and alterations in vital signs.

[Q] **How would the EMS provider assess the clinical significance of abnormal findings in the patient with the most common poisoning by surface absorption?**

[A] The most significant findings are those that impair the integrity of the ABCs. Besides the ABCs, findings that indicate an impairment of CNS function (e.g., altered LOC, seizures) are also clinically significant.

CLINICAL PEARL

People suffering from a poison that has been absorbed through the skin may not be immediately aware of their exposure. Take a careful history.

[Q] **How would the EMS provider differentiate between the various treatments and pharmacological interventions in the management of the most common poisoning by surface absorption?**

[A] As in any patient, the major priorities are:
- Ensure your own safety.
- Maintain the ABCs.
- Consider specific antidotes, as provided in local protocols (e.g., atropine, L-PAM for pesticide or nerve gas poisoning; both are readily absorbed through the skin).
- Transport the patient in a timely fashion to the nearest appropriate facility.

[Q] **How would the EMS provider integrate the pathophysiological principles and the assessment findings to formulate a field impression and implement a treatment plan for the patient with the most common poisoning by surface absorption?**

[A] Generically speaking, look for combinations of findings (toxidromes) that suggest toxicity from absorbed agents. The most common poisoning by surface absorption involves pesticides or insecticides. The findings relate to three distinct aspects:
- General toxicity—nausea, vomiting, headache, AMS, bradycardia.
- Cholinergic problems—the SLUDGE syndrome.
- CNS toxicity—muscle fasciculation, paralysis.

This combination of findings, along with an appropriate clinical history (e.g., spray plane crash; working in the garden all day), strongly suggests insecticide or pesticide toxicity.

Overdose and Substance Abuse

[Q] **What are the most common poisonings by overdose?**

[A] Nonprescription pain medications (e.g., acetaminophen, nonsteroidal anti-inflammatory agents) and prescription drugs (e.g., antidepressants, antibiotics).

[Q] **What is the pathophysiology of poisoning by overdose?**

[A] The substance is absorbed into the body, resulting in greater than normal effects. It is the exaggeration of these otherwise therapeutic effects that results in harm.

[Q] **What do the following terms mean: substance or drug abuse, substance or drug dependence, tolerance, withdrawal, and addiction?**

[A] Accepted definitions are:
- Drug abuse—is the use of a drug for a nontherapeutic effect, especially one for which it was not prescribed or intended. The most common reason is to "get high." The exact meaning of this term differs from person to person. To some, "getting high" means escaping reality; to others, it may mean hallucinations. Often the term substance abuse is used, instead of drug abuse, to include alcohol and marijuana. In this same category are various substances that are taken as drugs that were not intended to be used as such (e.g., glue sniffing, gas huffing).
- Substance abuse—includes drugs, as well as alcohol and tobacco.
- Drug dependence—is a psychological craving for or a psychological reliance on a chemical agent resulting from abuse or addiction. Drug dependence is a psychological problem, not a physical one.
- Tolerance—is an acquired resistance to the therapeutic effects of usual doses of a drug. More and more drug is required to achieve the same effect.
- Withdrawal—is a set of signs and symptoms that develop in a person following abrupt cessation of taking a drug. Most times, the individual has developed a dependence or addiction to the drug. The most dangerous drug withdrawal reactions occur in people who are addicted—both physically and psychologically "hooked" on a particular drug. Classic examples include alcohol withdrawal seizures and delirium tremens. Psychological withdrawal, though severe, is often not life threatening. Withdrawal syndromes can also result from the sudden stoppage of several prescription medications that are not considered addictive by most criteria. For example, if a

person suddenly stops taking certain anti-hypertensive drugs, a rebound hypertensive emergency may develop. People who stop beta-blockers, a type of heart medicine, abruptly may develop an MI.

- Addiction—is a condition characterized by an overwhelming desire to continue taking a drug because it produces a particular effect. True addiction is both a psychological and physical event—the patient has both a physical and a psychological craving for the drug, as well as for the effect.

Q **What is the incidence of drug abuse in the United States?**

A Though the exact incidence is impossible to determine (due to the illegal nature of many illicit drugs), substance abuse, often intentional, is responsible for millions of dollars in injury and illness each year. The costs, both emotional and financial, are magnified by the loss of productive work time and property damage.

Q **What is the source of the majority of illegal drugs?**

A Many illegal drugs are imported into the United States from abroad, particularly Columbia. Some (e.g., marijuana) are more likely to be grown locally.

Q **How would the EMS provider integrate the pathophysiological principles and the assessment findings to formulate a field impression and implement a treatment plan for the patient using the most commonly abused drugs?**

A Generically speaking, look for combinations of findings (toxidromes) that suggest toxicity from common drugs of abuse. Look for altered vital signs, hallucinations, and toxidromic symptoms.

Q **How would the EMS provider develop a patient management plan based on the field impression for the patient exposed to a toxic substance?**

A Control of ABC is the first concern in poisoning management. For any type of poisoning, provide the following care:

- Assess and maintain the airway; follow the vital signs and pulse oximetry frequently.
- Place the patient on a cardiac monitor.
- Position the patient to prevent aspiration (left lateral decubitus position, head down).

- Administer high-concentration oxygen by mask. If the patient is vomiting, use a nasal cannula (3–4 lpm). If the patient is unconscious, consider ET intubation according to your local protocol.
- Use MAST/PASG for shock as necessary according to your local protocols.
- If the patient is uncooperative, violent, or suicidal, restrain according to local guidelines. Be sure to document the need for restraints on the prehospital care report (PCR). Do not be a hero, call for police assistance with violent patients.
- Notify the hospital of the suspected substances involved.

After providing life-maintaining care, consult the local PCC or your medical control center for specific advice. Depending on the patient's condition, this may be done enroute to the hospital. Bring all suspected material and containers to the hospital.

Common Drugs Involved in Out-of-Hospital Toxic Emergencies

Q **What are the clinical uses, street names, pharmacology, assessment findings and management for patients who have taken the drugs or been exposed to the substances of abuse such as cocaine, marijuana, amphetamines and amphetamine-like drugs, barbiturates, sedative-hypnotics, cyanide, narcotics or opiates, drugs abused for sexual purposes, tricyclic antidepressants, alcohols, hydrocarbons, newer antidepressants, and mushrooms?**

A The information on these substances is summarized in Table 28–2.

Q **What are the clinical uses, pharmacology, assessment findings and management for the patient who has taken the drugs (e.g., as an accidental or deliberate overdose) or been exposed to substances such as cardiac medications, caustics, common household substances, carbon monoxide, lithium, MAO inhibitors, nonsteroidal anti-inflammatory agents, salicylates, acetaminophen, theophylline, metals, and toxic plants?**

A The effects of common drug overdoses are summarized in Table 28–3.

TABLE 28-2

Assessment and Management of Commonly Abused Substances

Agent	Clinical Use	Street Names	Pharmacology	Assessment Findings	Management (ABCs assumed)
Cocaine	Local anesthetic	Blow, crack, candy, flake, nose candy, snow	Locally blocks nerve conduction (anesthetic). Prevents neuronal uptake of catecholamines and increases catecholamine release from adrenergic nerve terminals.	Restlessness, increased motor and speech activity, seizures; may provoke chest pain or cause stroke; tachycardia, tachypnea, diaphoresis.	• Diazepam • Propranolol • Active cooling
Marijuana	Pain and nausea control following chemotherapy	Weed, shit, pot, grass, dope, Mary Jane, Jane	Stimulates central cannabinoid receptors.	Euphoria; changes in mood, perception, memory, and fine motor skills.	No specific treatment usually necessary.
Amphetamines and amphetamine-like drugs	Attention deficit, narcolepsy	Crosses, white cross, whites, speed, pep pills, crank, crystal, meth, black beauties, bennies, footballs	Stimulates release of norepinephrine from adrenergic nerve terminals; directly stimulates alpha and beta receptors.	Euphoria, excess energy, extended wakefulness, anorexia, hypertension, tachycardia, sweating, palpitations, headache, mydriasis, fever, anxiety, seizures, hypertensive crisis, stroke, arrhythmias, delirium, psychosis, hallucinations.	• Supportive • Consider mixed alpha/beta blocker (labetolol)
Sedative-hypnotics (e.g., barbiturates benzodiazepines)	Seizures, anxiety disorders	Barbs, downers, goof balls, phennies, softballs, nebbies, yellows, reds, Christmas trees	Depresses sensory cortex, decreases motor activity, and produces sedation and drowsiness.	Sleep, cyanosis, areflexia, tachycardia, hypotension, anuria, hypothermia, apnea, circulatory collapse, respiratory depression, pulmonary edema.	• Activated charcoal • Avoid flumazenil (Romazicon®) • Forced alkaline diuresis (in-hospital) • Hemodialysis (in-hospital)
Cyanide	Manufacturing processes	None	Binds iron in cytochrome oxidase; this inhibits the final step of oxidative phorylation and the transfer of electrons to oxygen. All cell energy production is essentially halted.	**Inhalation:** dry mouth, air hunger, hyperpnea, apnea, coma, seizures, cardiovascular collapse. **Ingestion:** hyperpnea, vomiting, confusion, vertigo, seizures, trismus, tachycardia or bradycardia, respiratory depressions.	• Amul nitrite • Sodium nitrite • Sodium thiosulfate • Hydroxycobalamin

Agent	Clinical Use	Street Names	Pharmacology	Assessment Findings	Management (ABCs assumed)
Narcotics or opiates	Pain control, pulmonary edema, anesthesia	China white, horse, junk, M, white stuff	Binds specific receptors in the brain and spinal cord.	Drowsiness, apathy, lethargy, sedation, constipation, miosis, nausea, vomiting, respiratory depression, pulmonary edema, seizures.	• Supportive • Naloxone
Drugs abused for sexual purposes (e.g., amyl nitrate)	Angina	Aroma of men, locker room, poppers, snappers	Stimulates production of nitric oxide, leading to vasodilation.	Euphoria, hypotension, syncope.	No specific treatment usually necessary.
Tricyclic antidepressants	Bedwetting, seizures, Tourette's syndrome, depression	None	Blocks the reuptake of serotonin and norepinephrine; antiarrhythmic action in heart (prolong Q-T interval); antihistamine, anticholinergic.	Anticholinergic, sweating, headache, weakness, heat intolerance, muscle tremors, dysrhythmias, muscular rigidity, seizures.	• Activated charcoal • Sodium bicarbonate • Dilantin, lidocaine • Avoid bretylium, calcium, and beta-blockers • Beware of delayed toxicity!
Alcohol (e.g., ethanol)	Methanol toxicity	Booze, juice	Depresses inhibitory synapses in the brain, then excitatory synapses; this is why ethanol often induces euphoria initially, then acts as a depressant.	Decreased inhibitions, visual impairment, diplopia, nystagmus, muscular incoordination, slurred speech, ataxia, slowed reaction time, hypoglycemia, stupor, depression of reflexes, hypothermia, hypoventilation, hypotension.	No specific treatment necessary.
Hydrocarbons	Solvents, manufacturing	Huff, glue	Highly volatile; may function as CNS stimulants.	**Ingestion:** chemical pneumonitis, CNS depression, GI irritation. **Skin exposure:** contact burns, rash. **Inhalation ("huffing"):** CNS alteration, cardiac, renal, and liver dysfunction.	• Treatment usually supportive • Avoid activated charcoal • Avoid inducing emesis (ipecac)
Newer antidepressants (e.g., Prozac®, Welbutrin®, Effexor®)	Anxiety, depression, obsessive disorders	None	Blocks CNS neuronal uptake of serotonin; some also affect dopamine or norepinephrine.	Anxiety, dizziness, fatigue, headache, insomnia, nervousness, seizures, palpitations, diarrhea. May also result in the **serotonin syndrome:** agitation, anxiety, ataxia, coma, confusion, hyperthermia, shivering, tremor, flushing, hypotension, GI cramping, salivation.	• Cyproheptadine is a specific antidote for the signs and symptoms

(continued)

TABLE 28-2 *continued*

Assessment and Management of Commonly Abused Substances

Agent	Clinical Use	Street Names	Pharmacology	Assessment Findings	Management (ABCs assumed)
Mushrooms	No specific medical uses	Buttons, beans, cactus	CNS stimulants, causing hallucinations; affect GABA receptor in the brain. Psilocybin and Amanita mushrooms are both hallucinogenic; Amanita species potentially fatal due to acute liver toxicity.	Hallucinations, nausea, vomiting, jaundice, abdominal pain if liver toxicity occurs from Amanita.	• No specific treatment for psilocybin • Liver transplant in Amanita poisoning

TABLE 28-3

Assessment and Management of Common Drug Overdoses

Substance	Pharmacology	Assessment Findings	Management (ABCs assumed)
Cardiac medications (e.g., antidysrhythmics, beta-blockers, calcium channel blockers, digoxin)	Depends on agent	All cause dysrhythmias in excessive doses, either tachycardias or bradycardias. Syncope may also occur.	• Calcium (calcium blocker toxicity) • Epinephrine, glucagons (beta-blocker toxicity) • Digitalis antibody fragments
Caustics (e.g., acids, alkalis)	Toxicity occurs via burning	Local pain; GI distress. Alkali burns may result in chronic scarring (esophageal strictures).	• Avoid induction of emesis • Avoid neutralizing agents
Common household substances (e.g., bleach, cleaning agents)	Direct irritants; some have long-term effects (solvents)	Local pain, nausea, vomiting.	No specific antidotes
Carbon monoxide	Binds hemoglobin preventing oxygenation of tissues.	**Early:** headache, nausea, vomiting. **Late:** chest pain, coma, death.	• Removal of patient from area of exposure • High-concentration oxygen • Some recommend hyperbaric chamber
Lithium	Augments uptake of norepinephrine; interferes with hormonal responses to cyclic adenosine monophosphate (AMP, or cAMP)	AMS (agitation or lethargy), muscular fatigue, ataxia, dysarthria, tremor, nystagmus, muscle fasciculations, dystonia, athetosis, seizures, coma, and apnea; also: nausea, abdominal cramping, emesis, and diarrhea.	• Activated charcoal only of value in mixed ingestion • Whole bowel irrigation • Hemodialysis

Substance	Phamacology	Assessment Findings	Management (ABCs assumed)
Aspirin	Blocks synthesis of prostaglandins; early toxicity has respiratory stimulant effect; later, causes metabolic acidosis	Tinnitus (ringing in ears), GI distress, GI bleeding, skin bleeding, AMS, pulmonary edema, acute renal failure, fever, dehydration.	• Activated charcoal • Sodium bicarbonate • Glucose • Anti-seizure medications • Cooling
Acetaminophen	Inhibits brain prostaglandin synthesis, but not peripheral synthesis (the reason for no anti-inflammatory effect)	**Phase 1:** anorexia, nausea, vomiting, diaphoresis. **Phase 2:** liver function abnormalities, upper-right quadrant abdominal pain. **Phase 3:** jaundice, coagulation defects, hypoglycemia, altered LOC, renal failure, heart failure. **Phase 4:** abnormalities clear or patient worsens requiring liver transplant.	• Activated charcoal • N-acetylcysteine • Supportive measures
MAO (monoamine oxidase) inhibitors	Block monoamine oxidase, a major complex enzyme that breaks down catecholamines	The serotonin syndrome may occur with concomitant use of serotonin-uptake blocking drugs. Patients can develop CNS irritability, hyperreflexia, and myoclonus. The blood pressure may be normal. Fatalities have been reported. MAO inhibitors by themselves may result in motor uneasiness, agitation, violent motor activity with moaning and grimacing, profuse sweating, and hallucinations. Death may result from hyperthermia, which may peak as late as 24 hours post-presentation.	• Activated charcoal • Treatment of specific symptoms (e.g., seizures) • No specific antidote available • Avoid combination with tricyclic antidepressants or sympathomimetic amines; also certain wines and cheeses (preventative measures)
Non-steroidal anti-inflammatory agents	Inhibit production of prostaglandins	GI toxicity and bleeding; skin bleeding.	No specific antidote available
Theophylline	Inhibition of phosphodiesterase (breaks down cAMP); increased sympathomimetic action	Nausea, vomiting, AMS, cardiac dysrhythmias, seizures when levels high.	• Multiple dose activated charcoal beneficial • Charcoal hemoperfusion (All are usually done in-hospital).
Iron	Integral component of hemoglobin, cytochromes (energy production via oxidative phosphorylation)	**Phase I:** vomiting, hematemesis, abdominal pain, diarrhea, lethargy, shock, hypotension, metabolic acidosis. **Phase 2:** apparent recovery. **Phase 3:** metabolic acidosis, shock, coma. **Phase 4:** liver necrosis, widespread coagulation defects. **Phase 5:** gastric scarring, pyloric stenosis, liver cirrhosis, CNS abnormalities.	• Sodium bicarbonate • Vasopressors • Deferoxamine (All are usually done in-hospital).

(continued)

TABLE 28-3 *continued*

Assessment and Management of Common Drug Overdoses

Substance	Pharmacology	Assessment Findings	Management (ABCs assumed)
Lead	No normal body function	**GI symptoms:** crampy, diffuse, often intractable abdominal pain accompanied by nausea, vomiting, anorexia, constipation, or occasionally diarrhea. **Blood problems:** interferes with formation of hemoglobin, leading to anemia. **Nervous system problems:** irritability, incoordination, memory lapses, labile affect, sleep disturbances, restlessness, listlessness, paranoia, headache, lethargy, and dizziness. In more serious cases, manifestations include syncope-like attacks, disorientation, flaccidity, severe mental impairment, ataxia, vomiting, cranial nerve palsies, localized neurologic signs, psychosis, somnolence, seizures, blindness, and coma.	Chelation therapy: Dimercaprol is given in oil intramuscularly; calcium disodium edetate (calcium versenate) can be given either intramuscularly or IV; and D-pencillamine is administered by mouth. (All are in-hospital treatments.)
Mercury	No normal body function	Heavy aerosol exposure to mercury produces chills, fever, cough, chest pain, and hemoptysis. Oxidized elemental mercury is readily absorbed from the alveoli; subsequently it can enter the brain. With mild exposure, the manifestations are likely to be subtle: insomnia, nervousness, mild tremor, impaired judgment and coordination, decreased mental efficiency, emotional lability, headache, fatigue, loss of sexual drive, and depression. Abdominal cramps, dermatitis, and diarrhea may also occur, and the victim may complain of a metallic taste. As the poisoning becomes more severe, persistent involuntary tremors of the extremities are noted. Later signs include polyneuropathy, joint pains, swollen gums with a blue line around the teeth, and paresthesias.	Chelation therapy: Dimercaprol is given in oil intramuscularly; calcium disodium edetate (calcium versenate) can be given either intramuscularly or IV; and D-pencillamine is administered by mouth. (All are in-hospital treatments.)
Toxic plants	Depends on the plant.	Many have anticholinergic (e.g., jimsonweed) or direct irritant effects (e.g., dieffenbachia).	Usually no specific treatment is needed.

Food Poisoning

Q **What are the common causative agents, assessment findings, and management for a patient with food poisoning?**

A Food poisoning is a generic term used for any illness suspected of being caused by food eaten within the past 48 hours. Often patients have stomach pain, vomiting, and diarrhea. Common causes include:

- Bacterial infection—the best known of these is salmonella, though *E. coli* has attracted much attention in the media recently. Other bacteria, such as *staphylococci,* make a toxin that causes the symptoms. Some shellfish harbor bacteria that manufacture strong neurotoxins, though these reactions are relatively rare in the United States. Botulism is a rare, but potentially deadly, form of food poisoning with serious CNS symptoms (e.g., headache, blurred vision, respiratory paralysis).
- Viral infection—viral food poisoning is relatively common and not usually serious.
- Noninfectious—certain foods (e.g., inedible mushrooms) and substances ingested with food (e.g., pesticides) may result in symptoms.

Management guidelines are straightforward:

- Protect yourself from exposure.
- Maintain the ABCs.
- Give IV fluids to maintain adequate hydration.
- Transport the patient to the nearest appropriate facility.

CLINICAL PEARL

It is impossible to correctly determine the specific cause of a food-borne illness in the field. Treat the patient symptomatically, while collecting as much "epidemiological evidence" as possible to help local health authorities.

Bites and Stings

Q **What are the common offending organisms, assessment findings, and management for a patient with a bite or sting?**

A Many bites or stings are painful. Some are potentially dangerous. Assessment findings depend on the organism involved. Insects (e.g., bees, hornets, black widow and brown recluse spiders, ants, fleas, scorpions) can cause local or systemic reactions or have a neurotoxic effect. Allergic reactions may develop from any bite or sting. Large marine animal bites (e.g., sharks, sting rays) may cause significant bleeding, infection, and shock. Small marine animal stings (e.g., Portuguese man-of-war, lionfish, jelly fish, sea urchins) can inject painful venom into the skin. Then, of course, there are the pit viper snakes (e.g., rattlesnakes, cottonmouths, copperheads) and the coral snakes found in North America. Always ensure your own safety first before attempting to provide patient care. Use appropriately trained and equipped teams as necessary, especially to help in patient rescue. As usual, maintenance of ABC is cardinal. Generally, unless anaphylaxis is present, no certain pharmacological interventions are warranted. Treatment of allergic reactions to bites or stings is discussed in Chapter 26, Allergies and Anaphylaxis.

Special Thanks

American Association of Poison Control Centers (1999). 1998 toxic exposure surveillance system of the American Association of Poison Control Centers, *American Journal of Emergency Medicine, 17*(5), 435–487.

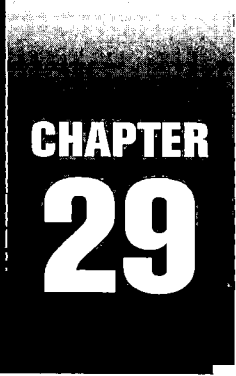

CHAPTER 29

Environmental Conditions

This chapter discusses environmental emergencies. The focus is on *why* patients present in a certain manner and *why* you need to respond in a certain way to their presenting problems.

General Principles

What is an "environmental emergency?"

An *environmental emergency* is a medical condition caused or exacerbated by weather, terrain, atmospheric pressure, or other local factors. Examples include heat stroke, hypothermia, and frostbite. By themselves, environmental emergencies may be life threatening. They may also aggravate other medical or traumatic conditions. For example, trauma patients who are hypothermic have a worse outcome (due to excess bleeding) than those who are normothermic.

> **CLINICAL PEARL**
>
> *Obvious environmental emergencies (e.g., cold water drowning) are often straightforward. Always consider the possibility of an associated environmental problem in any patient encounter (e.g., motor vehicle collision with patient trapped in a convertible, cold rain, and wind).*

What are the incidence, morbidity, and mortality associated with environmental emergencies?

Though specific figures are not available, environmental emergencies, especially those involving heat and cold illness, are common. Hypothermia, for example, may be fatal as evidenced by several well-known episodes in recent years. Loss of a limb from frostbite also takes a significant toll.

What are the risk factors that predispose patients to environmental emergencies?

As with any condition, certain preexisting factors make environmental emergencies more likely (as well as potentially dangerous). These include:

- Age—people at the extremes of age (e.g., small children, geriatric patients) are at greater risk for environmental emergencies. Small children have a large body surface area, especially the head, and a very limited ability to compensate for acute major changes in temperature. Older patients lose their ability to internally regulate their temperature and are more susceptible to temperature extremes. They get colder or warmer quicker and with less awareness than younger individuals.

- General health—anyone who has a serious underlying medical condition (e.g., heart failure, cancer), especially if he is undernourished, is more susceptible to environmental influences.

- Fatigue—when people are tired, they may not exercise appropriate judgment in potentially dangerous environmental situations (e.g., staying outside in the heat too long). In addition, fatigue may upset the body's normal regulatory mechanisms, making the person more likely to suffer harm.

- Predisposing medical conditions—though any person in poor general health is more susceptible to environmental emergencies, particularly risky conditions include diabetes (decreased sensation in the extremities), congestive heart failure (alterations of autonomic nervous system function), and thyroid disease (excess or abnormally low sensitivity to heat or cold).

- Medications—both prescription and over-the-counter (OTC) medications may predispose people to environmental injury, especially heat illness. Many common medications (e.g., antihistamines, psychotropic drugs) have anticholinergic (vagus-nerve blocking) side effects. The result is an impaired ability to sweat and dissipate heat. Heat intolerance is a common side effect of these drugs, whether they be prescription or OTC. Always obtain a careful medication history from any patient with an environmental emergency. Ask particularly about OTC and herbal or natural remedies.

CLINICAL PEARL

Many common OTC medications have anticholinergic side effects, predisposing patients to heat illness. This includes most antihistamines, cold remedies, and allergy preparations.

Q What are the environmental factors that may cause illness or exacerbate a preexisting illness?

A Though climate, season, weather, atmospheric, and terrain factors are important considerations, *anyone* can suffer an environmental emergency under the wrong conditions. For example, heat exhaustion is relatively common in fishermen off the coast of Alaska. The reason—the engine room of the boat is confined, hot, and humid. Elderly patients who fall onto a tile floor unconscious, regardless of ambient temperature, will quickly lose body heat to the tile, resulting in hypothermia. Finally, consider the effect of wind chill factor—have you ever gotten out of a swimming pool on a hot but very windy day? Magnify the chill you feel and hypothermia is inevitable. Do not exclude the possibility of an environmental emergency just because the ambient conditions don't seem to initially "fit the picture."

Q What environmental factors can complicate treatment or transport decisions?

A Any environmental "challenge" can complicate treatment or transport. These include:

- Climate and season—bad weather, especially if unexpected.
- Weather—wind, rain, snow, humidity, and temperature extremes all affect treatment and transport.
- Atmospheric pressure—high altitude or water (especially diving accidents).
- Terrain—inaccessibility (prolonged time to arrival of rescuers), difficult "carry-out" of patient.

Q What are the principal types of environmental illnesses?

A There are four principal types of environmental illnesses:

- Heat illnesses—heat cramps, heat exhaustion, heat stroke.
- Cold illnesses—hypothermia.
- Pressurization illnesses—diving illness (e.g., decompression sickness), high altitude illness.
- Localized injuries—frostbite, radiation burns (e.g., sunburn).

Q How is homeostasis influenced by environmental conditions?

A *Homeostasis* is the normal state of balance. In terms of temperature, this means that various body factors interact to maintain the body temperature at or near 37 degrees C (98.6 degrees F). These factors may fail for a variety of reasons. When this occurs, the core body temperature (CBT) rises above or falls below "safe" limits.

Q What are the normal, critically high, and critically low body temperatures?

A The normal body temperature is 37 degrees C (98.6 degrees F). Critically high temperatures, called heat stroke, are those above 40.6 degrees C (105 degrees F). Critically low body temperatures, called severe hypothermia, are those below 30 degrees C (86 degrees F).

Q What are different methods of monitoring a patient's temperature?

A CBT is measured most accurately by a rectal thermometer or by immediately measuring the temperature of freshly voided urine. Other methods of temperature measurement (e.g., oral, axillary, tympanic) are less accurate. Tactile measurement (touching the skin) is notoriously unreliable, though palpable skin temperature is important to note.

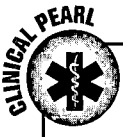

> • *Palpated skin temperature (cool, warm, hot) is important yet does not always correlate to measured CBT.*
> • *To accurately measure the temperature in a hypothermic patient, you must use a thermometer that reads low temperature values properly.*

What are the components of the body's thermo-regulatory mechanism?

The major components are:

• Hypothalamus (central regulatory center).

• Heat receptors (thermal receptors)—central, peripheral.

• Metabolic rate of the body.

• Heat balancing—loss or gain of heat by radiation, convection, conduction, evaporation, or drugs (e.g., aspirin).

• Peripheral blood vessels.

• Skin—a major portion of the body's thermal regulatory system.

What is the general process of thermal regulation?

Body heat is generated as a side effect of normal metabolic processes. This includes the breakdown of glucose, proteins, and fats to energy (e.g., glycolysis of sugar). Sensors detect if the CBT is either too high or too low.

What are the ways by which the body loses or gains heat, in general?

Thermoregulation refers to the normal body's means of heat loss (thermolysis) and gain (thermogenesis). Heat is generated by muscular activity and through metabolic reactions in the body. As the body temperature increases, changes occur in each organ system. If an individual gradually exposes himself to a hot environment, the body acclimates or becomes used to the heat.

Heat is gained or dissipated from the body by four mechanisms:

• Radiation—transmission of heat through space (e.g., warmth from a radiant heater or fireplace) as shown in Figure 29–1.

• Conduction—transmission of heat from warmer to cooler objects in direct contact (e.g., touching a cold surface, lying on a cold floor) as shown in Figure 29–2.

• Convection—transfer of heat by the circulation of heated particles (e.g., wind chill, cold water exposure, or cooling soup by blowing on it) as shown in Figure 29–3.

• Evaporation—loss of heat at the surface from vaporization of liquid (e.g., sweating, spraying water mist on the body to keep cool while sunbathing) as shown in Figure 29–4.

In humans, conduction is not a major mechanism of heat loss unless the clothing is removed and the individual lies on a cool surface. Clothing also hinders convection. At room temperature,

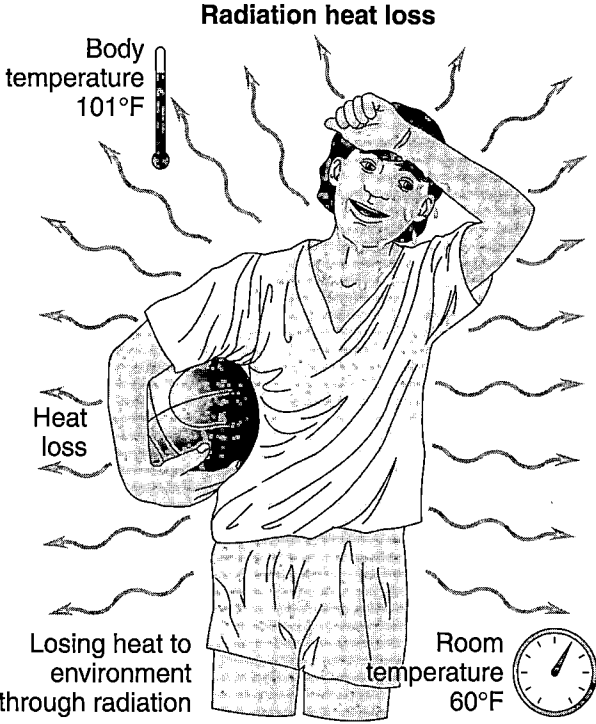

FIGURE 29–1 Radiation as a means of heat loss.

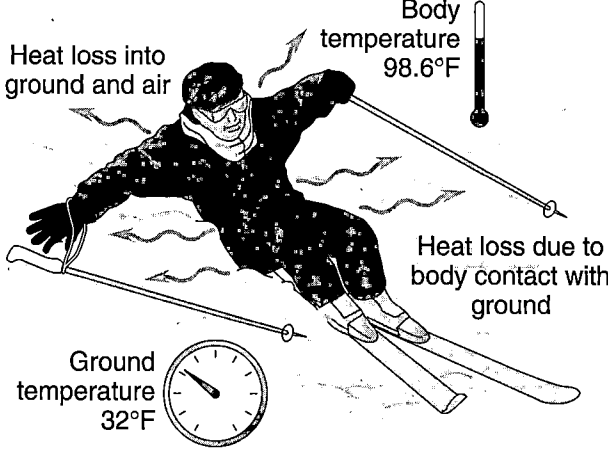

FIGURE 29–2 Conduction as a means of heat loss.

Convection heat loss

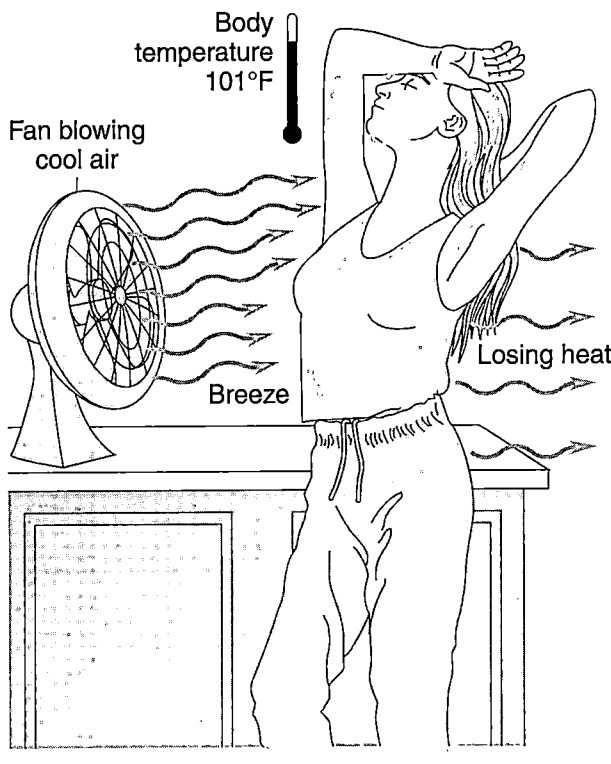

FIGURE 29-3 Convection as a means of heat loss.

Evaporation of sweat into environment

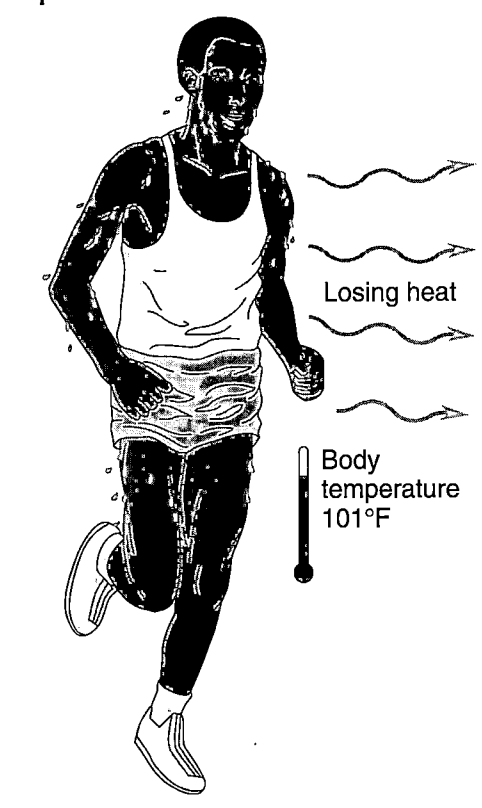

FIGURE 29-4 Evaporation as a means of heat loss.

75 percent of heat dissipation is by radiation and convection. Evaporation, the loss of moisture from the lungs and skin during respiration, accounts for about 25 percent of heat loss.

As the ambient temperature approaches body temperature, radiation is no longer effective to dissipate heat. The body may actually pick up heat by conduction and convection. At high temperatures, evaporation becomes the only effective method of heat dissipation. High humidity seriously impairs heat dissipation because evaporation occurs slowly.

Q What are the common forms of heat and cold disorders?

A Hypothermia is the most common cold disorder. Heat cramps and heat exhaustion are the most common heat problems, though heat stroke (which is uncommon) is life threatening.

Q How would the EMS provider integrate the pathophysiological principles and complicating factors common to environmental emergencies and differentiate features between emergent and urgent presentations?

A As with any situation, any feature that suggests a threat to airway, breathing, or circulation (ABC) is always emergent. In addi-

tion, alterations in mental status, when associated with heat or cold illness, indicate a need for prompt evaluation and treatment.

Heat Illness

Q What is heat illness?

A Heat illness is defined as an increased CBT due to inadequate thermolysis.

Q What is the pathophysiology of heat illness?

A In heat cramps and heat exhaustion, the underlying problem involves dehydration. The patient has lost significant fluid and electrolytes (especially sodium). The result is increased concentrations of sodium (and sometimes potassium) in the serum, with resultant symptoms.

Q What are the signs and symptoms of heat illness?

A Signs of thermolysis include diaphoresis, increased skin temperature, and flushing. Signs of thermolytic inadequacy are altered mentation or level of consciousness (LOC). Some patients have red, hot skin and fail to sweat when they develop heat stroke. This is not a universal finding, however. Findings of dehydration often accompany thermolytic inadequacy.

What are the predisposing factors for heat illness?

Extremes of age markedly increase a person's sensitivity to both heat and cold. Underlying diabetes often leads to autonomic neuropathy. This interferes with heat regulation by affecting vasodilation and perspiration. Medications, especially antihistamines, also impair the body's ability to sweat and eliminate heat.

Relevant contributing factors are the length and intensity of exposure. Ambient environmental conditions (e.g., humidity, wind) also play a significant role, whether the person is inside or outside.

What are the measures that can be employed to prevent heat illness.

It is essential that all people exposed to warm environments maintain an adequate fluid intake, regardless of thirst. Thirst is a poor indicator of dehydration, especially if the ambient temperature is not terribly warm (e.g., racing in an indoor swimming pool).

People who are acclimatized to warm temperatures are less likely to suffer heat illness. Proper acclimatization requires at least a week of gradually increasing heat exposure. This results in increased sweat production but with a lower sodium concentration than usual. The result is an increase in fluid volume in the body.

What is the pathophysiology and clinical presentation of heat cramps?

Heat cramps are cramps or pains in the muscles, especially of the abdomen and lower extremities, that occur in a hot environment. They are due to dehydration and overexertion. Heat cramps are the most common of the heat injury syndromes. They do not usually lead to heat exhaustion or heat stroke.

The cause of heat cramps is an excessive loss of salt and water in the sweat. Cramps usually occur in the young, unacclimatized individual who engages in exercise or heavy labor in hot climates and sweats profusely. Often, victims fail to drink an adequate amount of water.

Signs and symptoms of heat cramps include:

- Muscle twitching, followed by painful spasms, especially involving the lower extremities and abdomen.
- Nausea and vomiting.
- Weakness.
- Diaphoresis.

What is the pathophysiology and clinical presentation of heat exhaustion?

Heat exhaustion is a more severe loss of fluid and salt than occurs in heat cramps, usually following exertion in a hot, humid environment. Some patients simply develop dehydration without further signs or symptoms of heat exhaustion. In this case, the fluid therapy is similar.

There is a high incidence of heat exhaustion in young children, individuals on water pills (diuretics), and the debilitated who are unable to maintain an adequate oral water intake or those having prolonged bouts of diarrhea.

Signs and symptoms of heat exhaustion include:

- Lack of skin coloration (pallor).
- Profuse sweating.
- Hypotension (e.g., especially with positional changes, orthostatic changes).
- Headache, often with weakness and fatigue.
- Thirst.
- Normal or slightly elevated temperature.

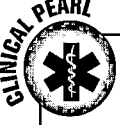

Though heat cramps do not necessarily lead to heat exhaustion, some patients have both. Assume the patient is dehydrated and treat appropriately.

What is the pathophysiology and clinical presentation of heat stroke?

Heat stroke or sunstroke, a failure of the body's temperature regulation mechanisms, is an extreme medical emergency. Heat stroke develops when the body is no longer able to get rid of heat. Unlike the heat exhaustion victim, the person with heat stroke sweats very little or not at all. Usually, the skin is hot, red, and dry. As heat accumulates, body temperature can reach a dangerously high level.

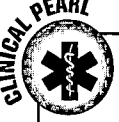

The absence of sweating is not necessary for a patient to have a life-threatening heat illness (e.g., heat stroke).

Suspect heat stroke in any individual who develops an LOC in a hot environment. Signs and symptoms of heat stroke include:

- Altered LOC.
- Increased body temperature.
- Minimal or no sweating (but not always).
- Collapse (e.g., cardiovascular or physical).
- Signs and symptoms of shock.

- Nausea and vomiting.
- Shortness of breath.

CLINICAL PEARL

Heat exhaustion rarely results in significant changes of mental status. If a patient has signs of thermolysis and an altered LOC, always consider heat stroke. Remember there are other causes of an elevated body temperature and altered mental status (e.g., meningitis or an acute hyperthyroidism).

Q How would the EMS provider assess the clinical significance of abnormal findings in the patient with heat illness?

A As with any situation, any feature that suggests a threat to ABC is always emergent. In addition, an altered mental status (AMS), when associated with heat illness, indicates a need for prompt evaluation and treatment. Pay particular attention to a patient's hydration status and LOC.

Q What is the contribution of dehydration to the development of heat disorders?

A The loss of fluid and electrolytes is a significant factor in the development of all three major heat illnesses.

Q What is the difference between classical and exertional heat stroke?

A Some heat stroke patients may have one or two days of lethargy, fatigue, weakness, nausea, vomiting, and dizziness prior to developing full-blown heat stroke ("classic heat stroke"). Other cases develop rapidly. These victims become confused or irrational, followed by an LOC within a period of minutes. This usually occurs during a period of exercise or heavy exertion and is termed "exertional heat stroke," such as during a marathon race on a hot day.

Q What is the theory on rehydration after lengthy periods of exhaustive exercise (e.g., marathons, ultras)?

A Basically, athletes who complete endurance events such as marathons (26.2 miles), Ironman® competitions (2.5-mile swim, 120-mile bike ride, then 26.2-mile footrace), triathalons (swim, bike, run distances vary), or ultra marathons (100 miles or more) can become seriously dehydrated from these events. In the past, EMS providers have staffed medical clinics at these events. The approach has been to take the athlete who was nauseated and

dizzy at the end of the race or who collapsed from dehydration and start large bore IV lines to quickly infuse two liters of normal saline.

From studying ultra marathon runners with "collapse syndrome," it has been found that this may not be the best approach. Often if the patient is allowed to lay down with their legs elevated for 10 to 15 minutes, the symptoms will subside. Clearly, they have lost a lot of sodium in their sweat. By replacing the fluid without replacing the sodium they develop hyponatremia as well as other electrolyte imbalances. The impact of the electrolyte imbalance is often worse than the impact of the relative hypovolemia from dehydration. Electrolyte disturbances can lead to cardiac tissue irritability and dysrhythmias. If, after 15 minutes, the patient does not begin to feel better, then it is appropriate to consider rehydration with IV fluids. Of course, throughout the management of the athlete, they should be monitored for dysrhythmias and have oxygen administered if they are short of breath. If you are assigned to work the medical tent at a marathon or other endurance sporting event, check with the medical director of the event, who frequently is a physician with a sports medicine background, on the latest theory on IV fluid replacement.

Prevention clearly is the answer to this problem and athletes are encouraged to drink fluids that their stomachs have become accustomed to during training, early and often during the event. Some fluids or "sports drinks" are designed to include electrolytes as well as carbohydrates and sugars.

Q What is a fever and how does it develop?

A A fever is a normal response to the release of chemicals called pyrogens. Usually, it results from an infection, though other illnesses (e.g., hyperthyroidism) may also increase the temperature.

Q What is the fundamental thermoregulatory difference between fever and heat stroke?

A The main difference is that a fever is a normal response based on an intact thermoregulatory system. Heat stroke develops when the thermoregulatory system has failed and the body is no longer able to keep the temperature from rising.

Q How can the EMS provider differentiate between fever and heat stroke?

A This is not always easy because both fever and heat stroke may cause an AMS. Sometimes a well-described history of a recent infection or illness helps favor a simple fever. On the other hand, people with an infection or illness are also more susceptible to heat stroke. When in doubt, treat for heat stroke.

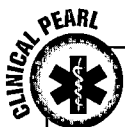

Elevated CBT and AMS is heat stroke until proven otherwise.

Q **What is the role of fluid therapy in the treatment of heat disorders?**

A Generally accepted fluid recommendations include:

- If the patient is completely conscious, give sips of cool water. Avoid liquids that are extremely cold, salty, or sweet. This may cause nausea or vomiting.
- IV lifeline; a fluid bolus of 500–1,000 cc normal saline will often decrease the pain from heat cramps. Follow your local protocols.

Q **How can the EMS provider differentiate between the various treatments and interventions in the management of heat disorders?**

A Regardless of the syndrome, always consider the following when caring for victims of a heat illness:

- Remove the patient from the predisposing environment as soon as possible.
- When necessary, use any of several available methods for active cooling. Misting and fanning appear to be the most efficient from a thermodynamic (the physics of heat) point of view—evaporation releases more energy than melting (ice bath). Many experts prefer tepid water for cooling due to the risk of reflex vasoconstriction and shivering (increases body temperature).
- Oral fluid therapy—avoid oral fluids if the patient has an altered LOC. Otherwise, cool (not cold) water or an electrolyte replacement solution may be helpful. Follow local protocols. Salt tablets are irritating to the stomach and may cause hypernatremia (excessive sodium elevation), nausea, and vomiting. Do not use them unless specifically instructed by medical control.
- IV fluid therapy—other than in extremely mild cases, people with a heat illness are dehydrated. Thus, they will benefit from administration of normal saline. Follow your local protocols.

Q **How can the EMS provider integrate the pathophysiological principles and the assessment findings to formulate a field impression and implement a treatment plan for the patient with dehydration, heat exhaustion, or heat stroke?**

A Maintain ABC. Rapid cooling is vital for the victim of heat stroke. Time is extremely important. If the victim's body temperature is not quickly lowered, permanent brain damage may result.

To care for heat stroke victims:

- Place the patient in a cool environment, such as an air-conditioned ambulance, as soon as possible.
- Remove the patient's clothing.
- Cool the patient immediately by applying ice packs to the neck, axillae (armpits), wrists, and groin. Other alternative methods for patient cooling are cold-water immersion or misting with lukewarm water and fanning the patient. Research has suggested that misting and fanning may be the most effective means of rapid cooling both in the field and the ED. Ice packs and cold-water immersion may produce reflex vasoconstriction and shivering due to their effect on peripheral thermoreceptors. Follow your local protocols.
- Give high-concentration oxygen by mask.
- IV fluids (e.g., normal saline or Ringer's lactate) at 250–500 cc/hour.
- Monitor the ECG.
- Wrap the patient with wet sheets if there is good ambient airflow present. Do not postpone transport in order to cool the patient in the field.
- Transport the patient to the hospital as soon as possible. Use the air-conditioner in your ambulance as well as any available fans to cool the patient.

Cold Illness

Q **What is hypothermia?**

A Generalized *hypothermia* is a condition in which the CBT is less than 95 degrees F due to either the decreased production of heat or the increased heat loss from the body. This may occur with or without external cold stress present. Patients lose heat by the mechanisms defined previously: radiation, convection, evaporation, and conduction.

Q **What is the pathophysiology of hypothermia?**

A The three primary causes of hypothermia are cold-water immersion, cold weather exposure, and "urban hypothermia." Cold water immersion is the principal cause of death following boating accidents. With the exception of wool, wet clothing loses 90 percent of its insulating value. Thus, soaked individuals are effectively nude. Cold weather exposure runs a close second in terms of incidence. Finally, cold stress among the aged, intoxicated, or debilitated can cause fatal hypothermia (urban hypothermia).

Conditions that may contribute to hypothermia include alcohol, the use of central nervous system (CNS) depressants (e.g., downers or alcohol), infections, endocrine system diseases (e.g., hypothyroidism, malnutrition, hypoglycemia), brain dysfunction, and burns. Hypothermia may also occur while skiing, camping, or hiking.

CLINICAL PEARL

Severe infection (sepsis) may actually result in hypothermia when the body's fever-producing centers are overwhelmed. This finding is common in people who are relatively immobile, such as in a nursing home.

What are the predisposing factors for hypothermia?

Predisposing factors to hypothermia include:

- Any elderly person living alone, especially one with chronic disease or who has suffered a stroke.
- People who are intoxicated with alcohol.
- Children less than one year old.
- Victims of submersion injury, especially in cold water.
- Patients suffering head trauma, especially if the accident occurred outdoors.
- Any patient with a history of trauma and subsequent blood loss with shock.
- Getting lost or immobilized in cold weather, especially if the individual is wet.

Many medications interfere with thermogenesis (heat production) and predispose the patient to hypothermia:

- Narcotics, phenothiazines, alcohol, and barbiturates.
- Antiseizure medications.
- Antihistamines and other allergy medications.
- Antipsychotics, sedatives, and antidepressants.
- Various pain medications including aspirin, acetaminophen, and nonsteroidal anti-inflammatory drugs (NSAIDs).

Note that some of the these medications can also lead to heat intolerance (e.g., antihistamines, antipsychotics, phenothiazines).

What are measures to prevent hypothermia?

People participating in outdoor activities should anticipate the possibility of hypothermia and prepare accordingly:

- Proper clothing.
- Proper rest.
- Adequate nutrition.
- Limit exposure time.

What are the differences between mild and severe hypothermia?

The severity of hypothermia is determined by the CBT and the presence of signs and symptoms:

- Mild hypothermia is defined as the presence of signs and symptoms with a CBT greater than 86 degrees F.
- Severe hypothermia is the presence of signs and symptoms with a CBT less than 86 degrees F.
- Compensated hypothermia is the presence of signs and symptoms with a normal CBT. In this case, the temperature is maintained by the body's intrinsic thermogenesis (metabolic processes that result in heat production) processes. As energy stores (liver and muscle glycogen) are exhausted, the CBT will drop.

How would the EMS provider describe the differences between chronic and acute hypothermia?

The onset of hypothermia parallels the cause:

- Acute onset—occurs rapidly, such as cold-water immersion; without immediate rescue, chances of survival are low.
- Subacute onset—comes on over minutes to hours, such as exposure during a winter hike. Prognosis may be better than the acute onset form unless the patient is not rescued or treated for a long period of time.
- Chronic onset—the patient has been hypothermic for hours to days, depending on the circumstances. This often is due to urban hypothermia, meaning it occurs to people who are inside but lack appropriate thermoregulation. An example is an elderly stroke victim who has fallen and is unable to move off a tile floor.

CLINICAL PEARL

Sometimes hypothermia is the primary cause of the patient's problem (e.g., cold-water immersion). Other times, hypothermia is a sign of another disease (e.g., sepsis, hypoglycemia, hypothyroidism). The differentiation may be impossible in the field.

What are the signs and symptoms of hypothermia?

There is no reliable correlation between signs or symptoms and specific CBT. Common findings include:

- Diminished coordination and psychomotor function—initially patients lose fine motor control; as hypothermia progresses, their movements become slower and less coordinated.
- Altered mentation—as hypothermia progresses, the patient's LOC decreases.

• Cardiac irritability—for years "J" waves on the ECG have been described as a sign of hypothermia. This is no longer felt to be the case and should not be relied on. On the other hand, cardiac dysrhythmias commonly accompany hypothermia. Atrial fibrillation is the most common. As the CBT continues to drop, bradydysrhythmias emerge. Ventricular fibrillation (VF) may occur, but is usually more common during the rewarming phase in a severely hypothermic patient.

CLINICAL PEARL

Severe hypothermia mimics clinical death. It may be impossible to distinguish a patient who is still alive, but profoundly hypothermic, from the victim of a cardiac arrest. Patients who have been pronounced dead from hypothermia have actually awakened in the morgue.

Q How would the EMS provider assess the clinical significance of abnormal findings in the patient with hypothermia?

A There is no reliable correlation between signs or symptoms and specific CBT. Always obtain a reliable CBT reading.

Q What is the impact of severe hypothermia on standard BCLS and ACLS protocols?

A Perform CPR as necessary. Check the pulse for 30–45 seconds before beginning chest compressions. Use normal chest compressions and ventilation. Apply the automated external defibrillator (AED) as per local protocols.

Cold may affect the potency of first-line cardiac drugs. Avoid these whenever possible until the patient is rewarmed—follow your local protocols. There is no increased risk of inducing VF from orotracheal or nasotracheal intubation as long as the patient is adequately preoxygenated. Rough handling, however, *can* induce VF.

The most common dysrhythmias in hypothermia-associated cardiac arrest are VF and asystole. The hypothermic heart is often resistant to defibrillation. The risks of VF are related both to the depth and duration of hypothermia. VF often occurs as a patient is being rewarmed when the heart temperature rises above 86 degrees F. Reasons for this are unknown.

It is generally impossible to electrically defibrillate a hypothermic heart that is colder than 86 degrees F. Avoid lidocaine and procainamide in hypothermia because they paradoxically lower the VF threshold, increasing resistance to defibrillation. Though some have recommended bretylium for hypothermic VF, the most recent American Heart Association (AHA) Guidelines 2000 have virtually eliminated this drug from many of the algorithms.

The AHA recommends that defibrillation be attempted as soon as possible. If a series of three consecutive shocks fails, continue CPR, aggressively rewarm the patient, and repeat defibrillation attempts periodically as the CBT rises.

Hypothermia and cardiac arrest in the face of near drowning are common. Rapid lowering of the CBT during cold-water immersion may protect the organs, especially the brain, during the period of anoxia. Following rescue, treat hypoxia first. Assume that all near-drowning patients are hypothermic until proven otherwise.

Q How would the EMS provider integrate the pathophysiological principles and the assessment findings to formulate a field impression and implement a treatment plan for the patient with either mild or severe hypothermia?

A The first priority, after ABC, is to stop ongoing heat loss:

• Remove the patient from the cold environment.
• If the patient is wet, dry her as much as possible.
• Provide barriers from wind, vapor, and excessive moisture in the air.
• Insulate the patient.

Specific care includes:

• Handle these patients gently. Rough handling may precipitate cardiac dysrhythmias.
• Give high-concentration oxygen by mask (10–15 lpm).
• Give warm fluids if the patient is completely conscious. Observe the patient carefully to prevent aspiration. Do not give fluids before or during an aeromedical transport.
• Start an IV lifeline—hypothermic people tend to be dehydrated. Cold stress causes peripheral vasoconstriction and increased central volume. This results in a cold diuresis and hypovolemia in many patients. Consider a fluid bolus of 500–1,000 cc normal saline as rapidly as possible if allowed by your local protocols. IV fluids are especially helpful if you are able to warm the patient to approximately 104 degrees F prior to administration.
• Care for other life-threatening injuries or conditions. Dress and protect frostbitten extremities.
• Remove wet clothing and maintain the patient in a warm, draft-free environment.
• Follow local protocols for rewarming. In some areas, rewarming is not attempted if the estimated time to arrival (ETA) to a hospital is less than one hour or there may be a chance of refreezing. Simply cover the patient with a blanket and transport him in a warm ambulance compartment to the hospital as soon as possible. Remove wet clothing prior to covering the patient.

- If local protocols include rewarming or if the ETA is greater than one hour, begin controlled rewarming with hot packs placed over the carotids, head, lateral thorax, and groin. Chemical hot packs can cause burns. Pad these with towels before placing them next to the skin.
- Warm (102–104 degrees F) moist air helps prevent heat loss, if included in your local protocols. There are several commercial devices available for this purpose. Warmed IV fluids (102–104 degrees F) serve the same purpose. The actual heat transferred to the patient is minimal, but such methods are crucial to prevent further heat loss. Warm-water immersion and other methods (e.g., heat guns, lights) have little use in the out-of-hospital setting.
- Do not try to rewarm the patient's extremities. Active external rewarming causes reflex vasodilation and may lead to rewarming shock or "afterdrop."

CLINICAL PEARL

Do NOT attempt to rewarm the extremities alone. This causes vasodilation of the arms and legs, resulting in a bolus of cold blood flowing into the central circulation. The patient's CBT may actually decrease, resulting in what is called the "afterdrop phenomenon." In addition, if the patient is somewhat dehydrated due to hypothermia (cold diuresis), then vasodilation will worsen intravascular volume status, leading to rewarming shock.

Frostbite

What is frostbite?

Frostbite is the formation of ice crystals within the tissues. These crystals damage the blood vessels and other tissues. Eventually frostbitten tissues may die. The worst tissue damage occurs when an area freezes, thaws, and then refreezes. *Trench foot* is a condition resembling frostbite that historically affected soldiers who kept their feet in wet socks and shoes for long periods. Evaluation and treatment are similar.

What is superficial frostbite (frostnip)?

Superficial frostbite occurs when there is an incomplete freezing of epidermal tissue. There is initial redness, followed by blanching. The patient typically has decreased sensation over the area for one to two hours, but recovery is the rule. Frostnip is far less severe than frostbite. A small number of people progress to full-blown frostbite, especially with continued cold exposure.

How would the EMS provider differentiate between superficial frostbite and deep frostbite?

Deep frostbitten skin has a white, waxy appearance. It feels hard (as if frozen) to palpation. Generally there is also a complete loss of sensation that does not recover within a short period (one to two hours).

What are the predisposing factors to frostbite?

Cold exposure, often involving water immersion, is the most common precipitant. People with poor circulation (e.g., elderly and diabetic patients) have a far higher incidence of frostbite, as do young children with relatively thin epidermal layers.

What are the measures to prevent frostbite?

Avoid cold weather exposure, especially water immersion, unless adequately and properly dressed. Skiers commonly get frostbite on their nose and face on bitter cold days when not wearing a mask.

CLINICAL PEARL

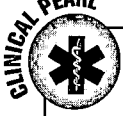

Remember that wind chill is a significant cause of both frostnip and frostbite.

How would the EMS provider assess the clinical significance of abnormal findings in the patient with frostbite?

The signs and symptoms of frostbite depend on the stage at which the patient is seen:

- Initially the frostbitten extremity appears waxy, yellowish-white, or bluish-white.
- Whether or not the skin of a frostbite victim feels soft or firm to frozen depends on the severity of injury. In severe frostbite, the area is hard to the touch, cold, and insensitive to pain.
- With rewarming, the extremity becomes flushed with a red to purple-burgundy color.
- Swelling appears within hours of thawing and may persist for days to weeks.
- Following thawing, fluid-filled blisters may form.
- After 9–15 days, a black, hard scar forms over the frostbitten area.
- If tissue death occurs, the area appears moist and weeping with pus.

Generally there is an initial cold sensation that subsides, leading to numbness. The patient may say that the affected area feels "like a stump." This feeling is due to a lack of oxygen.

Following thawing, there is severe, throbbing pain. This pain may last for several weeks. There may also be tingling and burning due to nerve damage that lasts for three to four weeks. Post-thawing pain tends to be severe, requiring strong medications for relief.

CLINICAL PEARL

Other symptoms may develop up to four years later. These consist of cold feet, excess sweating, and numbness. The symptoms are worse in the winter. Patients who have had one bout of frostbite develop an exaggerated response to cold and are, therefore, more susceptible to another episode.

Q **How would the EMS provider integrate the pathophysiological principles and the assessment findings to formulate a field impression and implement a treatment plan for the patient with superficial or deep frostbite?**

A To care for a patient with frostbite:

- Rule out the presence of other significant injuries or illnesses such as total body hypothermia, fractures, or bleeding.
- If the patient has total body hypothermia, do not care for a frostbitten extremity until the CBT is normal.
- Transport the patient to the hospital as soon as possible.
- Protect the involved site by covering it and handling it gently.
- Do not break any blisters. Cover them with dry, sterile dressings.
- Do not allow the patient to smoke. This constricts blood vessels and aggravates hypoxemia to the involved area.
- Do not rewarm frostbite in the field. An exception is if a limb is frozen to an object that cannot be moved. In this case, warm the area just enough to move the patient.
- Do not rub a frostbitten area, especially with ice or snow. This can cause severe tissue damage.
- Splint the limb.

Near Drowning

Q **What is a near drowning?**

A *Drowning* is defined as death due to asphyxiation during an immersion episode. It may occur with or without inhalation of the surrounding fluid. *Near drowning* occurs when the process of drowning is interrupted or reversed—a submersion episode with at least transient recovery.

Q **What is the pathophysiology of near drowning?**

A Causes of near drowning include swimmer exhaustion, lack of skill, and panic. An acute medical incident during swimming (e.g., myocardial infarction, seizure, trauma) can result in acute incapacitation, leading to drowning. Hyperventilation in preparation for a long underwater swim can suppress the respiratory drive sufficiently to cause anoxia while submerged. Suicide attempts are a final way that near drowning occurs. Often this is in association with jumping from a bridge or ledge and multiple serious traumatic injuries are also present. Thus, an immersion episode of unknown etiology warrants trauma management. The single *most important* factor in adult drowning is the use of alcohol and mind-altering drugs. Studies have shown that anywhere from 35–75 percent of drowning victims have elevated blood alcohol levels.

Q **What are the signs and symptoms of near drowning?**

A When examining victims of near drowning, it is important to note that they may appear initially to be normal. Usual signs and symptoms of problems include:

- Progressive dyspnea.
- Wheezing and other extraneous lung sounds.
- Tachycardia.
- Cyanosis.
- Temperature—must be taken rectally at some point in time and may be high, low, or normal. This is because of heat loss secondary to hypothermia or hyperpyrexia (increased temperature) due to hypothalamic injury (the hypothalamus is the portion of the brain that regulates temperature) from hypoxia.
- Chest pains or mental confusion may be present.
- Coma and respiratory or cardiac arrest can occur.

Q **What is the lack of significance of fresh- versus salt-water immersion as it relates to near drowning?**

A Differences between seawater and freshwater drownings have been grossly overemphasized in the past and are based on much animal work. Though the endpoints are the same, the mechanisms of lung damage from seawater and freshwater near drownings are very different. Seawater is hypertonic to blood (three to four times as concentrated in electrolytes and other osmotically active particles); its presence in the lungs causes the influx of hypotonic serum. This fills the alveoli and leads to a large shunt with profound hypoxemia (i.e., blood cannot exchange oxygen and carbon dioxide with filled alveoli, so the alveoli are bypassed).

Freshwater aspiration, on the other hand, leads to a washout of surfactant. This compound is required for the lung tissue to maintain its elasticity. Loss of surfactant results in the collapse of alveoli with subsequent hypoxemia. Aspiration of either seawater or freshwater decreases pulmonary compliance and results in pulmonary edema and hypoxia.

Cerebral hypoxia often precipitates neurogenic pulmonary edema, worsening an already bad situation. The endpoints in near drowning, no matter what type of water involved, are metabolic acidosis, pulmonary edema, and aspiration injuries.

How would the EMS provider compare and contrast the incidence of "wet" versus "dry" drownings and the differences required in their management?

There are three types of drowning. *"Dry" drowning* encompasses 10–20 percent of the victims. Here, asphyxiation is caused by anoxia as a result of a laryngeal spasm that prevents the entrance of water as well as air into the lungs. This leads to cerebral anoxia, edema, and unconsciousness. These victims have the best chance of survival. *"Wet" drowning* involves 80–90 percent of the cases. In this type of drowning, the victim makes a violent respiratory effort and fluid fills the lungs. *Secondary drowning* is defined as the recurrence of respiratory distress (usually in the form of pulmonary edema or aspiration pneumonia) after a successful recovery from the initial incident. It can occur within a few minutes up to four days later.

What are the complications and protective role of hypothermia in the context of a near drowning?

Many immersion victims are hypothermic. Cold stimulation of the vagus nerve may lead to a decreased heart rate and unconsciousness. This can lead to drowning and is potentiated by the presence of alcohol in the blood. On the positive side, cold may decrease cerebral metabolism and prolong survival.

How would the EMS provider assess the clinical significance of abnormal findings in the patient with a near drowning?

Several complications can occur following a near drowning. Persistent hypoxemia is common and usually multifactorial. Infection, especially pneumonia, may occur even several days later. Renal failure has been reported but is not overly common. The most bothersome complication is a persistent neurological deficit. The best predictor of severity is the time to the first spontaneous gasp following removal from the water. The shorter this period, the better the neurological prognosis. Patients taking more than one hour for this to occur (if it does at all) have a bleak prognosis.

How would the EMS provider integrate the pathophysiological principles and the assessment findings to formulate a field impression and implement a treatment plan for a near drowning?

Mouth-to-mouth respirations may be given in the water after clearing the airway. Remove the victim from the water as soon as possible. If there is any suggestion of neck injury (e.g., diving accident), stabilize the neck prior to removing the patient from the water. Start CPR if required. Perform the following measures:

- High-flow oxygen (10–15 lpm, mask) regardless of condition.
- ECG monitoring.
- Saltwater victims only—positional drainage of lungs (head-dependent position). This recommendation is somewhat controversial and not universally accepted. Follow your local protocols.
- IV fluids (normal saline) to keep the vein open (TKO), cardiac monitor.
- Some have recommended the immediate application of a subdiaphragmatic thrust (the "Heimlich maneuver") to all near-drowning patients. Though still controversial, the current recommendation of the AHA is that this be used only if you suspect a foreign body airway obstruction.

Overpressurization Injuries

What is SCUBA?

SCUBA is an acronym for "self-contained underwater breathing apparatus." SCUBA is also known as an aqualung—a portable breathing apparatus for divers consisting of cylinders of compressed air that automatically feed air through a mask or mouthpiece.

What are the laws of gases that relate to diving emergencies?

The most important laws are Boyle's law, Henry's law, and Dalton's law:

- *Boyle's law* states that, at a constant temperature, the volume of a gas varies inversely with the absolute pressure. In other words, as the pressure increases, the gas volume decreases. If a pair of lungs contains 2,000 cc of air at sea level, this volume decreases to 1,000 cc at 33 feet, 500 cc at 66 feet, etc.
- *Henry's law* states that, at a constant temperature, the solubility of any gas in a liquid is directly proportional to the pressure of the liquid. The deeper one dives, the greater the pressure and the greater the soluble gas (e.g., nitrogen) that becomes

dissolved in the blood and tissue fluids. The reverse occurs on ascent. It may take a much longer period of time for the gas to revaporize on ascent than it did to originally dissolve in the fluid.

- *Dalton's law* states that in a mixture of gases, the total pressure is equal to the sum of the partial pressures of each gas. Room air, for example, is a mixture of nitrogen and oxygen. The total pressure in a diving tank equals the sum of each individual partial pressure.

What is the pathophysiology of diving emergencies?

When diving, an individual is exposed to atmospheric pressures greater than those on land. This results in contraction of the gases in the lungs. As a rough estimate, pressure increases about one pound per square inch (psi) with each two feet of depth. To compensate, pressurized (compressed) air must be taken in from a SCUBA tank so that the lungs will not collapse. The events discussed here can also occur with any source of compressed air used for breathing: SCUBA gear, a hose from the surface, a bucket, or air trapped in a submerged car.

If a SCUBA tank is added to normal lungs at sea level, the volume of air in the lungs stays constant as the diver forcefully inhales supplemental air from the tank. Thus, the volume in the lungs remains constant, regardless of depth (assuming proper breathing techniques).

If the diver ascends, but forgets to exhale on the way up, the pressure decreases with ascent and the volume of gas "trapped" (due to failure of exhalation) in the lungs expands. Thus, if a diver at 33 feet with a combined lung volume of 4,000 cc ascends and fails to exhale, the total lung volume at sea level will be 8,000 cc!

What is decompression illness (DCI)?

Decompression illness is a sickness occurring during or after ascent secondary to a rapid release of nitrogen bubbles. Colloquially, it is called *the bends*. The cause is a sudden decrease in environmental pressure from a too-rapid ascent. This releases previously absorbed excess nitrogen (N_2) from the tissues into the bloodstream in the form of bubbles.

What are the different presentations of DCI?

There are a variety of symptoms that may affect many organ systems. These result both from the physical effects of N_2 bubbles in the lung tissues and the activation of numerous inflammatory mechanisms (e.g., kinin and complement systems). These responses lead to a decrease in tissue perfusion and ischemia. A vicious cycle can result with decreased perfusion leading to tissue hypoxia and interstitial edema, which further decreases perfusion.

1. A blotchy red rash on the torso may be present. The patient may complain of burning, prickly, or mottled skin (the "itches"). This is due to subcutaneous air.
2. Pain in the legs or joints is present in 90 percent of the cases. The most commonly involved joint is the shoulder, though multiple joints may be involved in serious cases. Recurrent pains are common.
3. Dizziness (the "staggers"), vertigo, visual, or hearing abnormalities may be noted in up to 5 percent of patients.
4. Paralysis occurs in 2 percent of victims; permanent sequela are possible though uncommon. The development of spinal cord manifestations may be preceded by abdominal pain.
5. Shortness of breath (the "chokes") may occur in up to 2 percent of patients. A fiery red pharynx (back of throat) is noted, and there may be pleuritic chest pain and a nonproductive cough. Spinal cord symptoms commonly accompany this, warranting careful neurologic evaluation.
6. Collapse is present in 0.5–1 percent of victims. Death, if it occurs, is usually from a cardiovascular cause. A delayed shock syndrome with pulmonary edema (adult respiratory distress syndrome) can occur one to three hours later.

A previous case of decompression sickness may increase one's susceptibility to recurrence.

What are the various conditions that may result from pulmonary overpressurization accidents?

Pulmonary overpressurization accidents may result in an air embolism or decompression sickness. Pneumothorax may occur alone or in combination with either.

What is nitrogen narcosis?

Nitrogen narcosis, often referred to as "rapture of the depths," is the development of an apathetic, slightly euphoric mental state due to the narcotic effect of dissolved N_2. This effect is analogous to excessive ethanol levels. The cause is Henry's law.

As the pressure increases (i.e., the depth of descent), so does the amount of dissolved N_2 (which is normally 79 percent of room air). The greater the depth, the greater the amount of N_2 dissolved and the greater the "high" achieved. Mild effects may be noted as low as 50 feet of water depth. This problem has been referred to as "martini's law": the mental effects of each 50 feet of descent, while breathing compressed air, are approximately equivalent to those of one dry martini. As depth increases, so does the severity of symptoms. This commonly effects divers at 100 to 125 feet.

What is an arterial gas (air) embolism?

Air embolism is defined as the presence of air bubbles in the central circulation. It is the most serious diving-related emergency. The cause is failing to exhale on ascent with a resultant expansion of air in the lungs. As the lung tissue expands, alveoli eventually rupture, resulting in the escape of air. Though it may occur, pneumothorax is not a necessary consequence of alveolar rupture. Interstitial air occurs first and can track anywhere in the body including the pleural space (pneumothorax), pericardial space (pneumomediastinum), and distant sites via the bloodstream (air embolus). Because divers most commonly ascend in a vertical position, bubbles of air in the bloodstream often travel to the brain. This can occur during an ascent from as little as four feet of water.

Air embolism may also occur in divers with lung infection, lung cysts, tumors, scar tissue, mucous plugs (asthma), and obstructive lung disease. These areas trap air that cannot be exhaled properly during ascent. Smokers, for unknown reasons, have an increased risk.

What is nitrox and a trimix?

A nitrogen–oxygen mixture in the diver's tank is called nitrox. This mixture reduces the amount of N_2 in the tank to allow the diver to attain an increased diving time. Today, standard mixtures of O_2 and N_2 are used in recreational as well as commercial diving. When commercial divers need to go to greater depths or dive for extended periods of time, they sometimes use a helium–oxygen mixture (heliox) to counteract the narcotic potency and density-induced breathing resistance at great depths.

A trimix is a mixture of O_2 and two other inert diluent gases. Technical divers who dive below 300 feet routinely use a trimix. By blending a depth-specific gas mixture, the diver can control the hyperoxia and narcotic potential of the mixture.

If your patient has been diving with a mixture in his tank, either nitrox or a trimix, be sure to inquire about the specifics of the recompression and pressure injury management from the other divers in the group or by consulting with the Diver's Alert Network (DAN®).

How would the EMS provider differentiate between the various diving emergencies?

It is extremely important to take an adequate history on any patient potentially suffering an emergency related to diving. The first question one must ask: Did the victim breathe compressed air underwater? Remember, this can occur with SCUBA gear, a surface hose, bucket, or within a submerged car. Make certain the patient was not just snorkeling and that you are really dealing with a near-drowning victim.

> **CLINICAL PEARL**
>
> *Always make certain the patient breathed compressed air underwater. If not, you may be dealing with a near-drowning victim.*

A detailed history of the entire diving day is necessary. If the patient has to be sent to a hyperbaric (decompression) chamber, this information is vital. The number of dives, depth of each, and bottom time are important. The type of equipment used as well as the diver's activities should be noted (hard work increases the risk of certain problems). Environmental factors, such as the type of water, the conditions, and the type of water entry, may be significant. It is useful to know if the diver was with a companion (who should then also be questioned) and exactly what type of gas mixture was being breathed. You also need to ask if in-water recompression was attempted. Finally, the examiner should note if the diver flew in an airplane or jogged before developing symptoms.

How would the EMS provider assess the clinical significance of abnormal findings in the patient with a diving-related illness?

As with any situation, any feature that suggests a threat to ABC is always emergent. In addition, alterations in mental status, when associated with SCUBA diving, indicate a need for prompt evaluation and treatment.

What is the function of DAN® and how may they aid in the management of diving-related illnesses?

DAN® provides a 24-hour number (919-684-8111) for assistance and referral. They will accept collect calls in an emergency situation. DAN® is considered the leading source of information regarding the treatment of diving emergencies (much as one would contact a Regional Poison Control Center for a toxic ingestion).

How would the EMS provider differentiate between the various treatments and interventions in the management of diving accidents?

Keep in mind that:

- Any complaint of joint soreness (in the absence of obvious injury) 24–48 hours after a dive should be considered for decompression therapy. At the minimum, a diving medicine (hyperbaric medicine) consultation should be obtained.

- Decompression sickness can occur at depths less than 33 feet. It is more likely if the diver has been below that depth with sufficient bottom time to permit supersaturation of the body tissues with inert N_2 gas. One should suspect air embolism in symptomatic divers who have been at depths less than 33 feet and whose symptoms occur immediately after ascent.

- If paralysis involves both sides of the body (e.g., both hands, legs) suspect decompression trauma with a spinal cord syndrome. If the loss of sensation or motion is unilateral, the odds favor an air embolus to the brain.

[Q] What are the specific functions and benefit of hyperbaric O_2 therapy in the management of diving accidents?

[A] Hyperbaric O_2 is beneficial for both air embolism and decompression sickness. Late recompression (even 10 days or greater) of decompression sickness problems can be accomplished with relief of symptoms and morbidity. Long delays are common in the lay diving population because of the lack of recognition of symptoms and "wishful thinking" that symptoms will "go away."

[Q] How would the EMS provider integrate the pathophysiological principles and the assessment findings to formulate a field impression and implement a management plan for the patient from a diving accident?

[A] It is helpful to think of a dive as being divided into five stages, each of which is associated with particular potential problems:

- The predive surface phase—may include considerable surface swimming to the site. Motion sickness, hyperventilation, physical trauma, near drowning, and marine animal encounters may occur.
- Descent phase—squeeze syndromes (excess pressure involving the ears) and gas-associated problems (e.g., carbon monoxide poisoning or hypoxia due to faulty equipment) commonly occur at this point.
- At-depth or bottom phase—physical trauma or encounters with dangerous marine life may occur. If nitrogen narcosis ensues, it is at this phase in the dive. It should also be remembered that divers are highly susceptible to the dangers of hypothermia.
- Ascent phase—barotrauma (squeeze) syndromes occur here but less commonly than with descent. Decompression sickness may begin to occur during ascent. If it does, it is usually very serious in nature.
- Postdive surface phase—there are two subphases:
  1. Immediate (within 10 minutes of surfacing)—air embolism is the cause of problems at this time until proven otherwise. Other potential problems include pneumothorax, motion sickness, or exhaustion.

  2. Delayed (after 10 minutes)—decompression is the "culprit" until proven otherwise. More than 50 percent of patients will be symptomatic within the first hour following ascent, though 1–2 percent may note their first symptoms at 24–48 hours.

Under-pressurization Illness

[Q] What is altitude illness?

[A] High-altitude illness occurs as a result of decreased atmospheric pressure, resulting in hypoxia. Many different activities may be associated with these syndromes including mountain climbing, travel to higher elevations on vacation, and flying in unpressurized aircraft. The most common altitude syndromes are acute mountain sickness (AMS), high-altitude pulmonary edema (HAPE), and high-altitude cerebral edema (HACE).

[Q] How do the gas laws apply to altitude illness?

[A] Higher altitude results in decreased atmospheric pressure and a lower inhaled amount of oxygen (FiO_2). This leads to hypoxia.

[Q] What is the etiology and epidemiology of altitude illness?

[A] The cause of all forms of altitude illness is the body's abnormal response to hypoxia at altitude. Typically, symptoms do not occur until a person is greater than 8,000 feet above sea level.

[Q] What are the predisposing factors for altitude illness?

[A] Extremes of age and underlying medical conditions are the most common predisposing factors. At particular risk are people with preexisting:

- Angina pectoris.
- Congestive heart failure (CHF).
- Chronic obstructive pulmonary disease (COPD).
- Hypertension.

[Q] What measures can be employed to prevent altitude illness?

[A] People with serious underlying medical conditions (e.g., COPD) should avoid travel to altitudes or carry supplemental oxygen. Otherwise healthy people are also susceptible to altitude illness. Problems may be avoided by:

- Gradual ascent—acclimate to the altitude over two to three days.
- Limited exertion—especially in the first 24–48 hours.
- Sleep at a lower altitude—many altitude problems seem to be precipitated during sleep.

Some experts recommend a high carbohydrate diet prior to traveling to altitude. Others recommend use of the drug acetazolamide, a prescription diuretic that speeds acclimatization and decreases the incidence of AMS. Nifedipine has also been used by people with a previous history of high altitude pulmonary edema to prevent a reoccurrence on ascent.

What is AMS?

AMS occurs after rapid ascent by an unacclimatized person to altitudes in excess of 8,000 feet. Symptoms usually develop within four to six hours of reaching altitude and may last three to four days. These include:

- Dizziness.
- Headache.
- Irritability.
- Breathlessness.
- Euphoria.

Older people and those with underlying cardiac or respiratory disorders may suffer pulmonary edema or heart failure. If AMS becomes severe, the victim may experience an altered LOC and impaired judgment. Coma often follows.

What is HAPE?

HAPE results from increased pulmonary artery pressures that develop in response to hypoxia. This leads to the release of various vasoactive substances that increase alveolar permeability. Fluid leaks into the alveoli and pulmonary edema occurs. Symptoms often begin 24 to 72 hours after exposure. At times, they are preceded by exertion. These include:

- Shortness of breath.
- Rapid respiratory rate (tachypnea).
- Cyanosis.

What is HACE?

HACE is due to increased intracranial pressure and is the most severe form of acute high-altitude illness. Patients have signs of AMS and a progressively worsening LOC. Progression from mild AMS to HACE and unconsciousness usually takes one to three days. It may occur, however, within hours of altitude exposure. Not all patients with AMS progress to HACE; it is currently impossible to predict who will. There is much overlap

between HACE and severe AMS—it is not necessary for you to distinguish the difference. HACE rapidly progresses to coma and death without treatment. Thus, the patient must be transported to an appropriate facility as soon as possible.

How would the EMS provider assess the clinical significance of abnormal findings in the patient with altitude illness?

Altered mental status suggests cerebral edema, the most severe of the altitude illnesses. Prompt treatment is essential.

What is the pharmacology appropriate to the treatment of altitude illnesses?

The most important treatments are rapid descent and oxygen. If a portable hyperbaric chamber is available, it may be life-saving. Based on applicable protocols, consider the use of the medications in Table 29–1.

How would the EMS provider differentiate between the various treatments and interventions in the management of altitude illness?

The main priorities are:

- Maintenance of ABC.
- O_2.
- Removal of the patient to a lower altitude.

How would the EMS provider integrate the pathophysiological principles and the assessment findings to formulate a field impression and implement a treatment plan for the patient with altitude illness?

Any patient who becomes ill within 48 hours of travel to an elevation over 8,000 feet has an altitude-related illness until proven otherwise. Consider cerebral edema if there are alterations of the mental status.

TABLE 29–1

Medications Used for Altitude Sickness	
Medication	Altitude Illness
Acetazolamide	AMS, HAPE, HACE
Nifedipine	HAPE
Steroids	Severe AMS, HACE
Prochlorperazine (Compazine®)	AMS, HACE
Furosemide	HAPE
Morphine	HAPE

CHAPTER

30

Infectious and Communicable Diseases

T he silent enemy can kill or permanently disable the EMS provider. This chapter discusses infectious and communicable diseases. The focus is on *why* patients present in a certain manner and *why* you need to respond in a certain way to their presenting problems.

Terminology

Q What terminology is specific to infectious and communicable diseases?

A Terminology specific to infectious and communicable diseases includes:

- CDC—Centers for Disease Control.
- Communicable disease—a disease that can be transmitted directly or indirectly from one person to another.
- Infectious disease—an illness caused by an invasion of the body by an organism such as a virus, bacteria, or fungus.
- Pathogen—an organism capable of causing disease.
- Gram stain—a testing method used to differentiate types of bacteria using a chemical stain process.
- Host—an organism (human) from which a parasite gets its nourishment.
- Parasite—an organism that lives on, within, or at the expense of another (host).

Physiology

Q What are the various types of infectious agents?

A Infectious agents are microorganisms that cause tissue damage. These agents are bacteria, fungus, helminths, protozoa, and viruses.

- Bacteria—a single-cell microscopic organism that causes an infection characteristic of its own species. Bacteria that cause disease are called *pathogens.* Nonpathogenic bacteria that live on the human skin and in the mucus membranes of the GI tract are called *normal flora.*
- Fungi—a plant-like microscopic organism.
- Helminth—a parasitic worm.
- Protozoa—a single-cell microscopic parasitic organism that causes infection.
- Virus—a parasitic organism that can only live within a cell of a living animal or plant host.

What factors influence susceptibility?

An individual's immune status and overall health are the primary factors that influence susceptibility to infection. Other factors include personal hygiene, sexual activity, heredity, gender, age, ethnic group, and nutrition.

How does the human response to infection work?

The human body has internal and external barriers to protect it against infection. External barriers include the skin and the normal flora found over the entire body and on the protective coverings of the respiratory, GI, and genitourinary (GU) systems. Internal barriers work through the inflammatory and immune responses. This is described in detail in Chapter 6, Pathophysiology, and Chapter 26, Allergies and Anaphylaxis.

What are the stages of infectious disease?

Once a host is infected, the disease progresses through several predictable stages. The duration of these stages varies by specific disease. The stages are:

- Latency period—is the period after the exposure has occurred to the host when the infection cannot be transmitted to someone else.
- Communicable period—is the time when infection can be transmitted to someone else. Signs of the disease may become apparent at this stage.
- Incubation period—is the duration between exposure to the host until signs and symptoms of the disease appear.
- Disease period—is the duration of the disease from onset of symptoms to resolution of symptoms (or death).

Health Organization

What are the public health principles relative to infectious diseases?

The study of infectious diseases takes into consideration population demographics that can effect the spread of disease. These criteria include age distributions, genetic factors, income level, ethnic group, workplace, school, geographic boundaries, and the expansion, decline, or movement of the disease.

What are the reporting requirements for infectious diseases?

The hospital or health care facility is responsible for reporting to the County Health Department communicable diseases

seen by health care providers. The Ryan White Act of 1990 further requires that all EMS providers be notified by the hospital or health care facility if they have been exposed to infectious diseases. Notification is made by an officer who acts as a liaison between the hospital and exposed EMS provider. *Notification must be made within 48 hours after exposure.*

Currently there are no requirements for hospitals to require patients to submit to tests for any infectious disease, but a request for a specific test (e.g., HIV) can be made in writing and the patient may consent.

> **CLINICAL PEARL**
>
> *Rules vary from place to place regarding which diseases must be reported to the local health department, as well as who must report them. Be aware of your local rules and regulations.*

What are the agencies and organizations involved in disease outbreaks?

Agencies involved in disease outbreak are found at many levels including federal, state, local, and private sector.

- Federal—U.S. Dept. of Health and Human Services (CDC, NIOSH), U.S. Dept. of Labor (OSHA), U.S. Dept. of Defense, and Federal Emergency Management Agency (FEMA).
- National—National Fire Protection Agency (NFPA). U.S. Fire Protection Administration (USFPA).
- State—state health departments.
- Local—county, municipal, and city health agencies.
- Private sector—local and national health maintenance organizations (HMOs), laboratories, and regional and national health care providers.

What are the recommended immunizations for EMS providers?

CDC recommends that EMS providers be immunized for diphtheria, hepatitis B (HBV), measles, mumps, rubella, tetanus, and polio. It is also strongly suggested that flu shots be considered.

What are the recommended vaccinations for children?

Polio, MMR (measles, mumps, rubella), DPT (diphtheria, pertussis, tetanus), varicella (chicken pox), and HBV. Chapter 44, Pediatrics, discusses these further.

Are any other vaccinations routinely recommended for children or adults?

Yes, hepatitis A (HAV), influenza, and pneumococcal disease vaccinations are recommended for both children and adults who are considered "at risk" for any of these diseases.

What infections can be caused by a needle stick?

Infections caused by needle stick are HBV, hepatitis C virus (HCV), and human immunodeficiency virus (HIV).

How often do needle-stick injuries occur in health care providers?

It is estimated that approximately 800,000 needle-stick injuries occur each year in the United States. It is also estimated, by NIOSH, that nearly half are not reported.

How can needle-stick injuries be prevented?

Injuries from needles and other sharps can be greatly decreased by following a few guidelines:

- Do not recap needles.
- Do not open needles unless a sharps container is immediately available.
- Use devices with safety features when possible (e.g., self-sheathing needles and needles access ports).
- Wear gloves.
- Provide training on the proper handling and disposal of sharps, and injury and infection protection.

What are BSI and Universal precautions?

Body substance isolation (BSI) is an approach that is based on the assumption that all blood and body fluids are infectious. Universal (Standard) precautions is an enhanced version of BSI recommended by CDC, OSHA, and NIOSH. The concept is to wear gloves for all patient contact.

> **PEARL**
>
> *The safest policy is to nonjudgmentally assume that every patient has something you do not want and that you have something they do not want. Act accordingly!*

How are contaminated equipment and supplies properly managed?

The exact guidelines for decontamination and disposal of contaminated equipment should be posted or easily available to reference in every EMS agency. Most single-use items can be disposed of in the trash. All needles and sharps must be discarded in puncture proof containers that are properly labeled. Biohazard wastes are disposed of in red bags that are labeled accordingly.

> **PEARL**
>
> *If all health care providers followed recommended hand washing protocols, the incidence of communicable disease probably would be decreased significantly.*

What equipment should be disinfected after caring for a patient with an infectious or communicable disease?

Nondisposable items, such as personal protective equipment (PPE), medical equipment, and the ambulance, that have become contaminated need to be cleaned and disinfected or sterilized.

Which illness does routine hand washing help to minimize the spread of?

The illnesses most commonly spread by touching droplets from sneezing and coughing are staph *(Staphyloccocal aureus)*, influenza, and colds. Hand washing is still the best preventative measure for spreading disease.

Do antibacterial products really work better than soap and water?

Some research says no. For everyday use and in some hospitals, washing with soap and water is adequate. For health care workers in contact with surgical patients, newborns, or patients with suppressed immune systems, CDC recommends the routine use of antimicrobial hand-washing products.

Infectious Diseases

What constitutes a significant exposure?

A significant exposure occurs when blood or body fluids come into contact with broken skin (e.g., cut or open sore), the eyes, or other mucous membranes or through a parenteral (needle stick) contact.

What should the assessment of a patient who has, or is suspected of having, an infectious disease include?

One of the first steps in the assessment of any patient is donning PPE. Most patients do not go around wearing a placard that says, "I have an infectious disease." You may wash your hands after using the toilet, but does your patient? This is why gloves, at a minimum, should be worn for every patient contact.

As your assessment progresses and you discover indications of an infectious or communicable disease, increase your level of PPE with masks and gowns accordingly. Signs and symptoms that indicate an infectious disease may be present include:

- Coughing and sneezing.
- Elevated temperatures (or lower temperatures in geriatric patients).
- Skin rashes, discolorations, lesions, or leaking.
- Nuchal rigidity (stiff neck).
- Swollen lymph nodes.
- Hepatomegaly (enlarged liver).
- Adventitious breath sounds.

What is the most common serious infectious disease in the United States?

Hepatitis, with 70,000 new infections annually, is the most serious infectious disease in the United States. It is estimated that 500,000 Americans are currently infected with hepatitis. This infectious disease causes inflammation of the liver, which interferes with liver functions.

How many types of hepatitis are there?

Seven types, A–G, but only the first four are common in the United States.

What is the incidence and mortality of HAV?

HAV is a highly infectious disease affecting the liver. It infects nearly 200,000 Americans each year and 30 percent of these cases occur in children. The infection is spread by direct contact with feces, usually through food or water contact by an infected person who has not washed after using the toilet. The mortality risk is low and is associated with complications such as development of chronic hepatitis, spontaneous relapse, and cirrhosis.

What are the signs and symptoms of HAV?

HAV is usually asymptomatic and is rarely serious. The course of the disease is approximately two to six weeks. The most infectious period is during the first week of symptoms. There are two vaccines available and recommended by CDC for children who live in high-risk areas. States being urged to vaccinate children are Arizona, Alaska, California, Idaho, Nevada, New Mexico, Oklahoma, Oregon, South Dakota, Utah, and Washington.

What is the incidence and mortality of HBV?

It is estimated that one million Americans carry HBV and nearly 5,000 die annually from the complications of liver disease (cirrhosis) and cancer.

What are the signs and symptoms of HBV?

Many people are asymptomatic and do not know they carry HBV. When symptoms become apparent, they include:

- Nausea and vomiting.
- Fever and night sweats.
- Loss of appetite and weight loss.
- Dark-colored urine.
- Clay-colored stool.
- Weakness and extreme fatigue.
- Yellow eyes or skin (jaundice).

What is a titer?

A titer is a test using a sample of blood to measure the amount of antibody against a particular antigen in that blood.

What are the latest recommendations from CDC about the HBV titer?

HBV titer recommendations from CDC include:

- Get a postvaccine titer one to two months after completion of the three dose series.
- If there is no response to the first series, a second series is recommended. If there is still no response after the second, no further series are recommended.
- Once a positive titer is achieved, no further titers are necessary, even after an exposure.
- After any exposure to HBV on the job, the employer must provide and pay for proper medical follow-up.

CLINICAL PEARL

The whole point of the postvaccination titer is to make sure the series of shots had its desired effect of protection against HBV.

If a person started the series of HBV vaccinations, but did not receive all three doses, does the series need to be restarted?

No, it is not recommended to start over. Just continue where the series stopped (e.g., if the first and second doses were received, only the last is needed).

Q What is the incidence and mortality of HCV?

A It is estimated that nearly four million Americans are infected with HCV, with 36,000 new infections and 8,000 to 10,000 deaths annually. The primary means of contracting HCV are through sex, needle sticks (or sharing needles), and blood transfusions.

Q What are the signs and symptoms of HCV?

A Many people are asymptomatic and do not know they carry HCV. People can carry HCV for 20 years without knowing they are infected. When symptoms become apparent, the most common symptoms are the same as HBV and less common symptoms include:

- Itching.
- Dark urine.
- Light-colored stools.
- Altered mental status (AMS).

Q Is there a preventive treatment available for HCV yet?

A No vaccine or prophylactic postexposure treatment for HCV is available currently.

Q If an exposure to HCV occurs, how is testing for a possible infection done?

A Both the EMS provider and the source patient must be fully tested to reduce the possibility of false-positive tests. The patient is tested first. If the patient is positive for HCV, then the EMS provider is tested. The first test is an enzyme immunoassay antibody test. If the test is positive, then a second test, a supplemental recombiant immunoblot assay (RIBA), is performed to confirm the results.

Q What is the incidence and mortality of hepatitis D virus (HDV)?

A HDV appears to coexist with HBV making the incidence and mortality rates high. Like HBV, it is transmitted by contact with body fluids. Fortunately, cases in health care workers are extremely rare.

Q What are the signs and symptoms of HDV?

A The signs and symptoms of HDV are similar to HBV.

Q What is the incidence and mortality of hepatitis E virus (HEV)?

A HEV is transmitted by the same route as HAV, fecal–oral. Most HEV and HAV is found in areas with poor sanitary conditions, poor hygiene, crowding, and in Third World countries. Mortality is 20 percent in pregnant women.

Q What are the signs and symptoms of HEV?

A Infections are acute and usually not life threatening.

Q What is human papilloma virus (HPV)?

A Human papilloma virus is one of the most common sexually transmitted diseases (STDs) in the United States. HPV is the cause of genital warts and cervical cancer, as well as cancer of the penis and anus. Often there are no symptoms and there is no cure for HPV. It is spread by direct contact with skin, so condoms will not prevent the spread of this disease.

Tuberculosis and Other Diseases

Q Why is tuberculosis (TB) making a comeback?

A TB was once the leading cause of death in the United States. Today, it is a major health problem throughout the world. It is not a serious threat in the United States with the exception of some serious outbreaks in some of the metropolitan areas. A reason why TB is making a comeback is that more resistant strains are developing. Estimates are that nearly eight million new cases occur each year with only one in five getting treatment.

Q How does TB progress?

A TB spreads through droplets from coughing and sneezing. The bacteria are inhaled and settle in the lungs. From the lungs, it is transported in the blood to other organs in the body. Once infected, a healthy person can remain asymptomatic for years. When the immune system is depressed, as with illness or aging, the TB becomes active.

Recently, a new case of TB infection was reported to have been transmitted from a dead body to a mortician. During embalming, the body spasmed and released respiratory secretions. This appears to be the first case of postmortem transmission.

What are the signs and symptoms of active TB?

Active TB presents with a severe cough that persists for more than two weeks, hemoptysis (coughing up blood), chest pain, fever and night sweats, chills, weakness, loss of appetite, and weight loss.

CLINICAL PEARL

> *Many patients with active TB only have a productive cough. Do not assume that TB is not a possibility because other symptoms (e.g., night sweats, fatigue, hemoptysis) are not present.*

Where in the United States is TB most prevalent?

TB is not as much of a major problem in the United States as in other countries. TB is prevalent in nursing homes, homeless shelters, hospitals, prisons, migrant farm camps, and among IV drug users and HIV-positive individuals.

How is the presence of meningitis detected and how is it treated?

A fast test (15 to 20 minutes) can be performed using a gram stain on cerebrospinal fluid (CSF) obtained from a spinal tap. The gram stain can distinguish bacterial meningitis from viral meningococcal. Bacterial meningitis requires in-hospital IV antibiotics. Viral meningitis is typically not as serious and does not usually require any specific treatment.

Is there any new test for HIV?

Currently there is an HIV test available, a single-unit diagnostic study (SUDS), that is very fast and inexpensive.

Is it true that saliva poses a risk for transmission of HBV and HCV?

No, saliva does not pose a risk of transmission. Neither does blood contact on intact skin, even for long periods.

Is it true that a bacterium causes gastric ulcers?

Yes. Until recently the cause of gastric ulcers was believed to be from stress, spicy foods, or excess stomach acid. Now we know that a bacterium, *Helicobacter pylori* or *H. pylori,* causes most ulcers. These bacteria can also cause gastritis and stomach cancer, but can be treated with antibiotics.

Is gastroenteritis a type of flu?

Gastroenteritis is often called the stomach flu. It is a general term that includes many types of infection and irritations of the digestive tract. Symptoms such as nausea and vomiting, fever, abdominal cramps, and diarrhea usually last less than 48 hours. This condition usually is not serious in healthy individuals, but children, the elderly, and patients with chronic illness can develop complications such as dehydration.

CLINICAL PEARL

> *The flu refers to influenza, a specific respiratory infection. Both laypeople and health care professionals alike incorrectly use the term flu to refer to colds as well as a variety of GI ailments.*

Why is rabies called hydrophobia (fear of water)?

Rabies is an acute viral infection of the central nervous system (CNS). Transmission to humans occurs from the saliva transferred through animal bites, most commonly by dogs, cats, bats, raccoons, and skunks. Without intervention, the disease progresses rapidly and death results. Rabies infections are characterized by irritation, paralysis, and death. It causes painful muscle spasms in the throat that interfere with swallowing, leading to dehydration and death, hence the term hydrophobia.

What is salmonella?

Salmonella are gram negative bacteria that live in the intestinal tracts of humans and other animals. To date, there are over 1,400 species of salmonella that can cause mild gastroenteritis or severe and often fatal food poisoning. Salmonella are usually transmitted to humans who eat foods contaminated with animal feces. Food may also become contaminated by an infected person who has not washed their hands after using the toilet.

How can the EMS provider recognize the presentation of Lyme disease?

Lyme disease is transmitted by ticks. Infection does not occur until an infected tick has been attached for 36 to 48 hours. Signs and symptoms begin with an expanding rash around the area of the bite. Ask about recent exposures to the outdoors, especially treed areas. Flu-like symptoms and muscle joint aches follow with or without a rash. Further progression of the infection leads to AMS, paralysis, parathesia, stiff neck, sensitivity to light, dysrhythmias, and chest pain.

What is an arbovirus?

An arbovirus is a group of virus that are transmitted to humans by mosquitoes and ticks. Diseases caused by arboviruses include the West Nile, encephalitis, yellow fever, and dengue.

What is hantavirus?

Hantavirus is any of a group of closely associated arboviruses that cause hemorrhagic fever. Rodents can carry hantavirus and exposure to humans can occur through contact with the feces, urine, or saliva of infected animals. Hantavirus pulmonary syndrome is a rare but potentially fatal pulmonary and systemic disease first recognized in 1993 in New Mexico, Arizona, Colorado, and Utah.

What are the signs and symptoms of hantavirus pulmonary syndrome?

Initial signs and symptoms are fever, fatigue, dizziness, muscle aches, abdominal pain, nausea, and vomiting. Within a week, coughing, shortness of breath (SOB), and pulmonary edema develop, followed shortly by pulmonary and cardiovascular collapse, and ultimately death.

Has anyone died from plague recently?

Yes. From 1947 through 1996, there were 390 reported cases of plague, resulting in 60 deaths.

What are the principal forms of plague?

Plague is an acute febrile, infectious, and highly fatal disease caused by gram-positive bacteria. The principal forms of plague are bubonic, septicemic (primary and secondary), and pneumonic (primary and secondary). Bubonic is the most prevalent type and is a primary disease found on rats and rodents. It is spread to humans by bites from infected fleas found on the rats and rodents. Pneumonic is less common and is spread from person to person by droplet.

Where were most of these cases of plague reported to be?

Most cases were reported in New Mexico, Arizona, Colorado, and California.

Behavioral and Psychiatric Disorders

This chapter discusses behavioral and psychiatric disorders from a practical point of view. It does not go into all of the diagnoses of psychiatric problems because EMS providers do not normally receive training in that area. The focus is on *why* patients with a behavioral problem are acting in a particular manner and *why* the EMS provider must be alert and sensitive to the patient's needs, while not dropping your guard to a situation potentially dangerous to you and your crew.

The Basics

What is an emotion?

An emotion is a strong feeling, often accompanied by physical signs (e.g., diaphoresis and tachycardia from anger).

What is an emotional disorder?

An emotional disorder (also called a "mental disorder") is any disturbance of emotional balance manifested by maladaptive behavior and impaired functioning (e.g., patients with depression).

What is the prevalence of behavioral and psychiatric disorders?

Estimates vary though some experts state that up to 20 percent of the U.S. population has some type of behavioral or psychiatric disorder. These illnesses incapacitate more people than all other health problems combined. Some researchers indicate that one in seven people will require treatment for an emotional illness at some time in their lives.

What are some common misconceptions concerning behavioral emergency patients?

Misconceptions about behavioral and psychiatric illnesses have existed for many years and most are totally unfounded. These include:

- Abnormal behavior is always bizarre—this is often the exception, rather than the rule.
- All mental patients are unstable and dangerous—many psychiatric patients are perfectly calm and never present any danger to themselves or to others.
- Mental disorders are incurable—once thought to be the case, modern medical and psychotherapeutic techniques have provided stabilizing treatment for most psychiatric disorders. Psychopharmacology (drug therapy) and advanced genetic techniques offer the potential for a complete cure in some patients.
- Having a mental disorder is cause for embarrassment and shame—though many people still feel this way, it is a result of inappropriate pressure from society, rather than any scientific evidence. Behavioral and psychiatric illnesses have an organic basis in many cases, just as a sore throat, the common cold, or a heart attack.

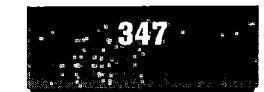

Throughout history, people with emotional illnesses have been outcast and treated as second-class citizens. We have come a long way from the "insane asylums" of earlier centuries to the current psychiatric hospitals. Unfortunately, many antiquated attitudes persist, even amongst health care providers. EMS providers can take a major lead in helping change this misconception for the better.

Q. What are each of the following types or classifications of psychiatric disorders: cognitive, schizophrenia, psychotic, mood, anxiety, substance-related, somatoform, factitious, dissociative, eating, impulse-control, and personality?

A. Each recognized type or classification of behavioral or psychiatric disorder covers a broad range of conditions of varying severity. These include:

- Cognitive disorders—affect a person's cognitive function (thinking and judgment). The most common types are delirium (acute disorientation and clouding of consciousness) and dementia (loss of appropriate thinking, judgment, social skills, and sometimes speech). Either may occur as a result of numerous medical or traumatic conditions.

- Schizophrenic and psychotic disorders—involve gross distortions of reality, often withdrawal from social interaction, and disorganized thought. Victims may hear voices (schizophrenia) or believe that someone is continually poisoning their water (paranoia). These individuals suffer from delusions and hallucinations. Often, they have nonsensical disorganized speech. Generally, they are at high risk for violent behavior.

- Mood disorders—include depression (pathological sadness, often with physical manifestations) and mania (excessive hyperactivity). Alternating periods of depression and mania is called bipolar disorder.

- Anxiety disorders—affect two to four percent of the population and usually involve increased autonomic nervous system (ANS) activity. The common theme is that apprehension, fears, and worries dominate a person's life. Common types include panic disorders (recurrent attacks of sudden, often unexplained, anxiety), phobias (exaggerated, sometimes disabling, fears), and post-traumatic stress disorder (anxiety reaction to a severe psychosocial event such as war).

- Substance-related disorders—include dependence, abuse, and intoxication. Abuse is the use of a drug for a nontherapeutic effect, especially one for which it was not prescribed or intended. The most common reason is to "get high." Addiction

is a condition characterized by an overwhelming desire to continue taking a drug to which one has become "hooked" through repeated consumption because it produces a particular effect. True addiction is both a psychological and physical event—the patient has both a physical and a psychological craving for the drug, as well as for the effect. Dependence is a psychological craving for or a psychological reliance on a chemical agent, resulting from abuse or addiction. Dependence is a psychological problem, not a physical one. Intoxication relates to the acute effects of taking a substance and may or may not be related to dependence.

- Somatoform disorders—are a group of neurotic disorders with symptoms suggesting physical disease, but with no demonstrable organic causes. The major types of somatoform disorders are somatization syndrome (recurrent and multiple physical complaints for which there is no demonstrable physical cause) and conversion disorders (a type of hysteria in which emotions are repressed and converted into physical symptoms, such as blindness, paralysis, hallucinations, or shortness of breath).

- Factitious disorders—a group of signs and symptoms that are consciously fabricated by the patient, often with a motive for secondary gain (e.g., compensation, attention).

- Dissociative disorders—type of neurosis in which emotions are so repressed that a split occurs in the personality. The result is an altered state of consciousness or confusion in the patient's identity. Also called multiple personality or schizophrenia.

- Eating disorders—involve the patient's misconception that he is too fat when, in reality, the body shape is normal or thin. The best-known eating disorders are anorexia nervosa (prolonged refusal to eat, resulting in emaciation and possibly death) and bulimia nervosa (insatiable craving for food; usually results in episodes of recurrent eating, depression, and forced vomiting).

- Impulse-control disorders—involve an abnormal inability to resist a sudden (and often irrational) urge or action. Examples include kleptomania (impulse to steal), pyromania (impulse to set fires), pathological gambling (impulse to gamble), trichotillomania (impulse to pull out one's hair), and intermittent explosive disorder (impulse to lose control and become aggressive).

- Personality disorders—large category of mental disorders characterized by inflexible and maladaptive behavior that impairs a person's ability to function in society. Often broken into three clusters: Cluster A (paranoid, schizoid, schizotypal), Cluster B (antisocial, borderline, histrionic, narcissistic), and Cluster C (avoidant, dependent, obsessive-compulsive).

What factors can alter the behavior of an ill or injured individual?

Numerous factors can alter the behavior of any ill or injured person, whether or not there is a background of emotional illness. These include:

- The patient's perceived degree of pain or severity of the illness related to the actual degree of pain or severity of the illness.
- The patient's past experiences (including friends and relatives with similar problems).
- A history of previous emotional illness.
- The presence of a current emotional illness prior to the immediate event.
- The degree of severity, treatment, and lability (unstable or adaptable) of the existing emotional illness.
- The patient's perception of care providers—the degree to which the providers empathize with the patient and how the patient feels he is being treated.

The reaction to a crisis varies from individual to individual. Once someone feels that she has "lost control" or has lost her support system (e.g., spouse, children, job), the world appears to "crash in." Some people withdraw; some become excessively active. The patient may become depressed or violent. When violent tendencies develop, these may be directed either at the patient herself, such as in a suicide attempt, or at others.

CLINICAL PEARL

Some type of psychological overlay accompanies every *illness and injury. The degree to which it affects a particular patient varies widely. Health care providers must always be aware of a person's emotional, as well as physical, needs.*

What are some of the medicolegal concerns in the management of an emotionally disturbed patient?

Generally you should act in a calm manner, but never jeopardize your own safety. Each state, and sometimes locality, has specific regulations governing the handling of mentally ill individuals, including patients who exhibit self-destructive behavior. You are responsible for following both state laws and local protocols regarding the treatment of people with a mental illness, as well as those with a temporarily impaired mental status (e.g., alcohol intoxication, drug overdose). You should be aware of local facilities and procedures for:

- Psychiatric evaluation and hospitalization.

- Alcohol and drug detoxification.
- Crisis intervention.

What is the pathophysiology of behavioral and psychiatric disorders?

The pathophysiology of behavioral and psychiatric disorders is multifactorial. Some aspects of certain illnesses are clearly genetic. A person's surroundings and circumstances affect all disorders to some extent. Many of these conditions have been shown to occur not simply due to surroundings, but due to actual chemical alterations in the brain.

Sometimes the cause of the disorder is due to an organic illness. Chemicals called neurotransmitters normally serve to convey messages between different portions of the brain. Either an excess, or more commonly, a deficit of certain of these transmitters results in some types of behavioral and psychiatric disorders, such as schizophrenia or depression.

CLINICAL PEARL

Our understanding of neurotransmitters and their significant role in emotional illness has led to many new generations of effective methods of pharmacologic treatment. Don't assume that just because a person is on a psychiatric medication that he has emotional illness. Several of these agents are useful with other conditions (e.g., antidepressants for migraine headache).

What are examples of overt behaviors typically associated with behavioral and psychiatric disorders?

During assessment, pay particular attention to the following:

- The patient's general appearance, hygiene, and dress—some people with behavioral problems (both organic and psychiatric) exhibit an abnormal lack of regard for their own personal hygiene.
- Motor activity—many behavioral emergencies are associated with abnormal motor activity. Note whether the patient appears "hyper," or abnormally lethargic. Always consider the possibility of drug intoxication, pain, blood sugar abnormality, or hypoxia when abnormal motor activity is present.
- Physical complaints—these may indicate an underlying or concomitant organic disease.
- Intellectual function—orientation, memory, concentration, judgment. This determination may require the use of some type of a "mini-mental exam" consisting of simple questions and mathematical calculations. Several variants of these have

been reported in the medical literature—consult with your physician advisor for recommendations.

- Thought content—note disordered thoughts (thoughts that seem illogical), delusions, hallucinations, unusual worries, fears, and any suicide threat or threat of injury to others.

- Language—patients with behavioral problems often speak either much faster or far slower than normal. Note the speech pattern and content. Garbled or unintelligible speech, unless the patient is actively hallucinating, is more likely to be due to an organic illness (e.g., stroke) than a psychiatric problem.

- Mood—what is the patient's level of alertness? Does he appear to be distracted (possibly hallucinating)?

Q Why are so many of the emotionally disturbed patients treated as "outpatients" rather than receiving in-patient treatment?

A There are many reasons. One of the most significant is a lack of adequate in-patient facilities for treatment. In addition, the climate of health care in the United States discourages hospitalization for many conditions, including emotional illness. Outpatient treatment is usually tried first.

Q What are phobias and how can they be unhealthy?

A Phobias are irrational, intense, and obsessive fears of specific things such as an object or a physical situation (e.g., heights, open spaces). These fears are out of proportion to reality and compel the patient to avoid the feared object or situation. This can interfere with normal daily activities, affecting both personal and societal relationships (e.g., work).

Q Does drug addition or alcoholism have an influence on psychiatric disorders?

A Yes. There is often an interrelationship between people with psychiatric disorders and substance abuse. In some cases, there is a direct cause–effect relationship. In others, the link is more anecdotal or based on stories of prior incidents. As a rule, if a person has a psychiatric disorder and then develops a drug addiction or alcoholism, the underlying psychiatric condition worsens.

Q What do the following terms mean as they relate to the EMS provider: affect, anger, anxiety, confusion, depression, suicide, fear, mental status, paranoia, hallucination, bipolar, delirium, dementia, posture?

A These terms have varying meanings, depending on their context. In the context of an EMS-related behavioral emergency, consider the following:

- Affect—the emotional tone underlying an expressed emotion or behavior. "Flat affect" means a lack of any apparent verbal or body language expression of emotion.

- Anger—an emotional reaction characterized by extreme displeasure, rage, or hostility.

- Anxiety—state of mild to severe apprehension, often without a specific cause. There are often accompanying changes in body functions such as diaphoresis and tachycardia.

- Bipolar—mental disorder characterized by alternating episodes of mania and depression.

- Confusion—state of mind in which one is uncertain of the present time, place, or self-identity. Results in bewilderment and the inability to act decisively.

- Depression—dejected state of mind with feelings of sadness, discouragement, and hopelessness. Patients often exhibit reduced activity levels, an inability to function, and sleep disturbances.

- Delirium—state of incoherent excitement, confused speech, restlessness, and sometimes hallucinations, often due to acute illness or drug intoxication.

- Dementia—progressive state of mental decline, especially of memory function and judgment. Often accompanied by disorientation and disintegration of the personality.

- Fear—feeling of dread or doom relating to an identifiable source.

- Hallucination—perception of something that is not actually present; may be auditory (hearing), visual (seeing), olfactory (smell), gustatory (taste), or tactile (touch).

- Mental status—a person's degree of intellectual, emotional, psychological, and personality function.

- Paranoia—mental disorder characterized by delusions of persecution, often centered on a specific theme (e.g., job, a specific person).

- Posture—in emotional illness, to assume a certain body language position suggestive of a particular emotion. A paranoid individual, for example, may posture by keeping the face hidden and the extremities crossed close to the body.

- Suicide—deliberate taking of one's life.

Techniques of Management

Q What are some useful verbal techniques for managing the emotionally disturbed patient?

A Establish rapport with the patient using therapeutic interviewing techniques—those that calm the patient and encourage her to cooperate with you. Therapeutic interviewing techniques include:

- Engage in active listening. This technique is discussed in detail in Chapter 13, Techniques of Physical Examination.
- Be supportive and empathetic.
- Limit interruptions.
- Avoid threatening actions, statements, and questions.
- Center your questions on the immediate problem.

Q Why is it important to take appropriate measures to ensure the safety of the patient, EMS providers, and others when dealing with a patient having a behavioral emergency?

A People having a behavioral emergency tend to have labile (unstable or adaptable) emotions. Events that would not normally lead to violence may easily trigger untoward events. In addition, these patients tend to trigger strong emotions in responding health care providers, making it even more essential that you are in total control of your emotions—remain calm and professional at all times.

Q Is it a good practice to try to remove relatives and bystanders from the scene?

A As a rule, unless the presence of another individual is necessary (e.g., when the patient will not calm down or cooperate otherwise), most experts believe that the EMS provider will be able to provide better care when relatives and bystanders are not present.

Q What techniques best allow you to obtain information from the disturbed patient?

A The management of behavioral emergencies consists, first, of maintaining scene and personal safety. If the scene is safe, your next task is to build good rapport with the patient. Speak in a calm, even voice, and exhibit a willingness to listen to the patient. Be honest because most people can easily detect a "snow job!" Describe everything you intend to do step-by-step to the patient. Avoid any sudden moves.

In the unrestrained patient, follow these guidelines to minimize the chances of a violent situation developing:

- Have physical assistance nearby. In the field, this may be your partner, additional personnel, or law enforcement (Figure 31–1). Maintain an open exit for both you and for the patient. If there is an open exit for both of you, the patient will be calmer, and you will be safer. Do NOT attempt the initial contact with a person who has a behavioral emergency in the back of a closed ambulance compartment.

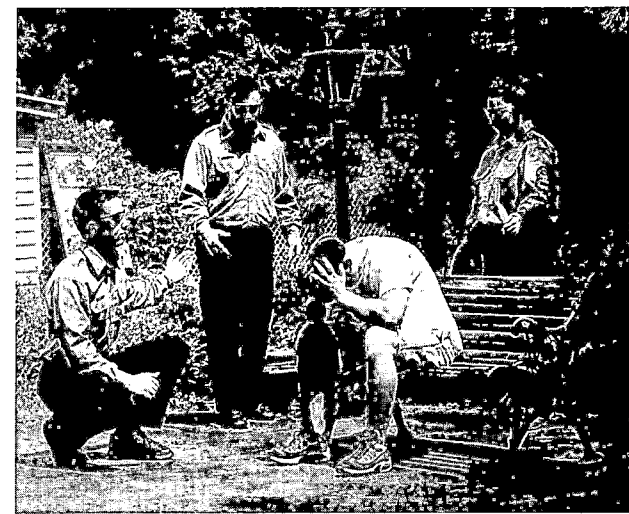

FIGURE 31–1 A show of force may be necessary to obtain the patient's cooperation. Always leave room to exit.

- Allow the patient to "vent," expressing anger and frustration verbally instead of physically.
- Form an alliance with the patient. Try to understand how the patient is feeling. You don't need to agree. For example, if a patient says, "FBI agents are following me," you might make a comment like, "That would bother me, how do you feel?"
- Avoid continuous eye contact—looking someone directly in the eye is often taken as a challenge or threat.

If the situation escalates, you have two choices: regain control or leave. If you are trapped, seek assistance and maintain safety. Try to keep talking to the patient until help can arrive. Otherwise, get away from the patient as quickly as possible, and summon assistance.

Q What are examples of situations when EMS providers may need to transport a patient against his will?

A Situations where patients must be transported against their will include any situation where the patients are a danger to themselves or to others. This determination may be made in a number of ways:

- Your local protocols together with medical control.
- In compliance with a court order.
- In compliance with a law enforcement official's mental health hold (protective custody).
- Altered mental status (AMS) patient in police custody.

Q What are examples of techniques for a physical assessment of the patient with a behavioral problem?

A Limit the physical assessment to vital signs and any other absolutely necessary evaluations:

- Approach the patient slowly and purposefully.

- Avoid threatening actions, statements, and questions.

- Respect the patient's territory—allow at least three to four feet of personal space between you and the patient whenever possible (Figure 31–2).

- Limit physical touching to necessary procedures (e.g., shaking hands, obtaining vital signs).

- Limit the number of people around the patient, isolating her if necessary.

- Always stay alert to potential danger.

- Determine the presence of life-threatening medical conditions through a rapid assessment of the ABCs, followed by rapid intervention, if necessary.

- Observe the overt behavior of the patient, as well as body language (nonverbal gestures, posture, or evidence of rage, elation, hostility, depression, fear, anger, anxiety, or confusion).

CLINICAL PEARL

Remember that organic problems can cause or worsen an emotional illness. Always be on the lookout for alternative explanations to what may, at first, appear to be an "obvious" emotional problem.

What are the methods that may be used for restraining an emotionally disturbed patient?

A number of different types are available (e.g., leather or velcro wrist and ankle restraints, full jacket restraints, handcuffs). Always follow your local protocols when using restraints. Sometimes it is helpful to create a blanket papoose to restrain a small child or elderly patient.

CLINICAL PEARL

Some EMS providers carry handcuffs to use as restraints. There are many well-documented cases of nerve injury to the wrist and hands caused by improperly applied handcuffs, even by experienced law enforcement personnel. Unless properly authorized and trained in their use, avoid handcuffs.

Is it ever appropriate to use a chemical restraint?

The decision to use a chemical restraint (e.g., sedative medication) should never be taken lightly. Used improperly, some of these agents may provoke seizures and even cause patient death. Always follow the directions of medical control, as well as your local protocols.

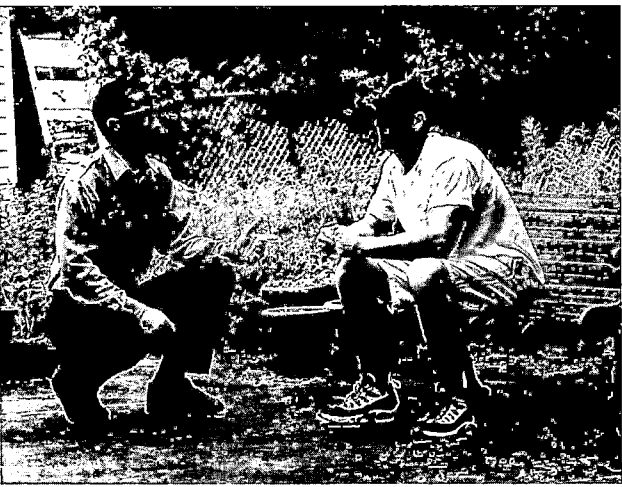

FIGURE 31–2 Never sit or kneel directly in front of a patient. Instead, crouch at least an arm's length away.

Why is it wrong to restrain a patient facedown?

Despite the fact that the technique of restraining a patient facedown in a Reeves stretcher is actually mentioned in a number of EMS texts, face-down restraint carries a high risk of patient suffocation, especially if the patient is violent.

CLINICAL PEARL

There are numerous cases reported in the medicolegal literature of serious patient injury from inappropriate restraint techniques.

What is the difference between a suicide gesture and a suicide attempt?

A *suicide gesture* is something done by a person to ask for help, rather than to die. The person performs the act in a potentially reversible way, such as taking a few aspirin or a small handful of pills. Unfortunately, small amounts of certain medications can be very poisonous—you still need to treat suicidal gesture patients as poisoning patients, as well as pay careful attention to the behavioral emergency. Sometimes people intend to kill themselves, take pills, and then change their minds.

A *suicide attempt* occurs when the patient has a true desire to die. Often the person has planned the event (e.g., purchased a gun, driven far out of town, gotten a double refill of his prescription medication).

CLINICAL PEARL

A common clinical myth is that people who engage in suicide gestures never really attempt suicide—this is a naïve and potentially deadly assumption.

What are the risk factors for suicide?

The following factors increase the risk that a person is suicidal:

- Male.
- Age is less than 19 or greater than 45.
- The presence of depression or hopelessness.
- Previous suicide attempts or psychiatric care.
- Excessive alcohol or drug use.
- Loss of rational thinking.
- Is separated, widowed, or divorced.
- An organized or well-thought-out attempt.
- Use of a firearm.
- A "life-threatening" presentation.
- Leaving a suicide note.
- No good support system (e.g., family, friends, job, or religious affiliation).
- Stated intent to try again to commit suicide.
- A major life event (e.g., recent divorce, buying a house, recent loss of job, death of spouse or other loved ones).

Do I increase a person's risk of actually committing suicide by asking if she has thought about suicide?

Whether an actual suicide attempt or a gesture, do not discount the patient's emotional state in any way. Don't be afraid to directly ask the patient, "Were you trying to kill yourself?" or "Did you want to die?" Many people are not aware of the resources available to them for help. A suicide gesture is the patient's way of seeking help.

Does divorce increase the risk of suicide more in men than women?

According to Dr. Augustine J. Kposowa of the University of California at Riverside, who recently published the National Longitudinal Mortality study on suicide, divorce or marital separation more than doubled the risk of suicide in men, whereas in women, marital status was unrelated to suicide. This is said to be due to the fact that most women have better ways of communicating and more social support networks, friends and relatives to talk to as compared to men.

Does a person's will to thrive or survive influence their recovery from disease?

Unquestionably, the "will to survive" and overlying psychological factors have been shown to affect the body's immune sys-

tem significantly. This influences a person's susceptibility to illness, as well as the ability to heal.

CLINICAL PEARL

The term "psychosomatic illness" refers specifically to physical problems brought about by underlying emotional problems. The physical ailments are very real, despite their emotional origin.

Does depression increase the risk of any other medical conditions?

Depending on the patient, severe depression may be accompanied by a lack of self-care. This, by itself, could worsen any underlying medical condition. Studies have also shown that depressed people have a higher incidence of cardiovascular disease. The exact reasons are uncertain.

How would an EMS provider differentiate between various behavioral and psychiatric disorders based on assessment and history?

Remember, it is not necessary to make a field diagnosis of the specific type of behavioral or psychiatric condition present. Rather, control the situation, maintain the ABCs, and assess rapidly for the possibility that the scene will escalate into violence. Clues that a patient may develop violent behavior include:

- Pacing back and forth; unable to keep one position for more than a couple of seconds. You may ask the patient, once, to be seated. If this fails, and you are uncomfortable, leave.
- Appearing to get more and more angry as he speaks. This behavior may simply be a reflection of the patient venting to you. If there is excessive body language, such as a red face or starting to swing the arms, you have a choice. You may try and talk with the patient, stating, "I know, you're really upset." If talking to the patient doesn't work, or if you feel uncomfortable, leave.
- Starting to act out, such as thrashing out with the arms, hitting the wall, throwing things. You may be the next target. There is no room for negotiation here. Get away from the person as soon as possible. If you notice any obvious weapons (e.g., knives, guns, baseball bats), leave immediately.
- Bragging about how tough he is; telling stories of "how many cops it took to hold me the last time." The easiest way to deal with this sort of behavior is to agree with the patient (e.g., "I'm on your side. I'm not going to mess with you.") If the patient begins implying that you'd make an easy target, making a statement like, "I could whip your butt with one hand," you have to make a choice. Either agree with the patient ("I'm sure you could") and continue the interview, or leave.

- Any domestic violence-related situation, particularly where the alleged perpetrator is still present. Police should be involved to secure the scene prior to EMS involvement. However, this is not always the case because there may not be indications of domestic violence until you have already arrived and begun to assess the patient. Try to separate the involved parties as soon as possible and call for police assistance. It is unwise to enter a scene involving domestic violence without appropriate law enforcement backup available.

- Any patient suspected of being intoxicated or on drugs. The potential for violence varies from person to person, but the mere presence of substance abuse makes violent behavior more likely to occur.

- If the patient persistently complains about your EMS system, or the service he or his family has received in the past. Statistically speaking, unhappy patients are more likely to become violent, whether or not they are in the midst of a behavioral emergency.

- Males are more likely than females to exhibit violent behavior. Do not let your guard down, however, if dealing with a female patient. Similarly, do not let the patient's age fool you because people of all ages can get violent.

[Q] What are some of the specific diagnostic points to know for common behavioral and psychiatric illnesses?

[A] The specific diagnostic points for common behavioral and psychiatric illnesses include:

- Neurosis and Psychosis—*Neurosis* is an abnormal anxiety reaction to a perceived fear. There is no basis in reality for the fear (e.g., a fear of heights so strong that it prevents a person from leaving the first floor of any building). To some degree, just about everyone has some type of neurotic fear at one time or another. This does not mean that a person is insane or crazy. Most people cope with their fears. Again, a behavioral emergency only occurs when a person is unable to cope.

Psychosis, on the other hand, is when the patient has no concept whatsoever of reality. The person truly believes his situation or condition is real. Often the psychotic person hears voices. In a drug-induced psychosis, hallucinogens or stimulant agents cause the patient to lose touch with reality. Often he develops hyperactive and dangerous behavior. The best way to deal with hallucinations is the "talk-down" technique for gently calming and reassuring the patient that everything is OK.

- *Depression*—is a common reaction to major life stresses. Several signs and symptoms may suggest that a person is depressed:

1. An unkempt appearance making it appear as though the patient doesn't care about anything.

2. Speech that is different from usual. These people may not speak or may reply in short, monotone phrases. They lack any spark or enthusiasm in their speech and actions.

3. Frequent crying bouts, often appearing to have no precipitant.

4. Abnormally increased or decreased appetite; significant weight gain or loss is common.

5. Sleep disturbances. Often depressed people fall asleep without a problem, only to wake within a couple of hours. They are then unable to fall asleep again the rest of the night.

Depression may present as another disease. Elderly people commonly appear to have an organic illness (e.g., cardiac or respiratory conditions) when, in reality, they are severely depressed.

CLINICAL PEARL

Always be on the lookout for organic causes of apparent emotional or psychiatric illnesses, especially in older patients. The most common "offenders" are medications (e.g., drug-induced sedation or psychosis) and severe infections.

Special Thanks

Kposowa, A. (2000, March). National longitudinal mortality study on suicide. *Journal of Epidemiology and Community Health.*

Hematology

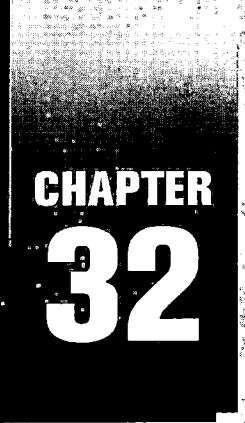

This chapter discusses diseases of the blood and blood cells. This area is basically new to the National EMT-Paramedic curriculum. The focus of this chapter is the anatomy and physiology of the hematopoietic system and the medical conditions that it may present within our patients.

Anatomy and Physiology

Q **What is the hematopoietic system?**

A The hematopoietic system produces blood cells.

Q **What are the anatomical components of the hematopoietic system?**

A The components of the hematopoietic system include the bone marrow, the liver, and the spleen. The majority of blood cells (e.g., red cells, white cells, platelets) are formed in the bone marrow. In adults, active bone marrow is confined to specific areas of bones:

- Ends of the long bones.
- Flat bones of the head and pelvis.
- Ribs.
- Vertebral bodies.

In children, active marrow is also present in the shafts of the long bones.

Q **What are the major characteristics of blood?**

A Blood is the fluid tissue that is pumped by the heart through the arteries, veins, and capillaries. Blood consists of cells and plasma. Suspended within the pale, straw-colored plasma are several types of blood cells (the "formed elements") and dissolved chemicals, minerals, and nutrients. The average pH of the blood is 7.40 (slightly lower in venous than in arterial blood). Men have approximately 70 cc's of blood per kg of body weight, whereas women have slightly less, 65 cc per kg. In an adult man, this amount equals approximately five or six liters (L) of blood.

Q **What is meant by volume and volume control in relation to the hematopoietic system?**

A Body feedback systems continuously monitor intravascular volume, as well as the numbers of circulating red and white

CLINICAL PEARL

When the red blood cell (RBC) level is lower, the kidney and liver produce erythropoietin, which stimulates the production of more RBCs by the bone marrow.

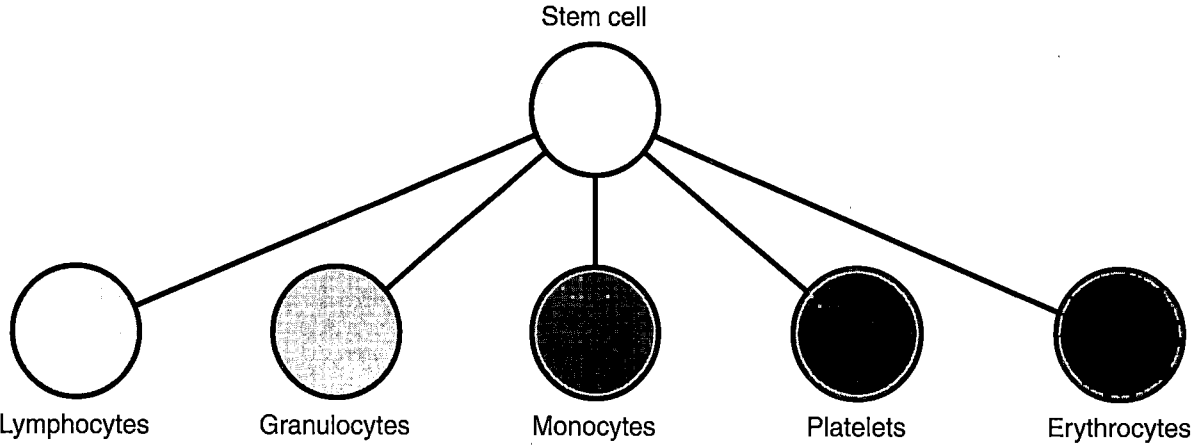

FIGURE 32–1 The stem cell is capable of reproducing into specific blood cells. (From Rothenberg, M.A. 2000, *Pathophysiology—Mechanisms of Disease.* Reproduced with permission.)

blood cells, and platelets. If more cells are needed, the kidneys and liver produce compounds that stimulate the bone marrow to manufacture additional cells.

Q What are the blood forming organs?

A Though the liver and spleen produce RBCs during fetal life, the majority of normal blood cell production after birth occurs in the bone marrow in the long and flat bones.

Q How does the bone marrow form blood cells?

A All blood cells are derived from one common stem cell as shown in Figure 32–1. This cell is capable of reproducing itself, but is also capable of differentiating (specifically developing) into any of the marrow elements (e.g., red cells, white cells, platelets). Differentiation of the common stem cell into the various types of blood cells is dependent on stimulation from a number of compounds produced outside the bone marrow, known as cytokines.

Q What is the life cycle of a normal RBC?

A Mature RBCs circulate in the blood for 120 days. After that, they are absorbed by tissues of the reticuloendothelial system (e.g., spleen, tissue macrophages). Cellular components are recycled and hemoglobin byproducts are excreted as bilirubin. Continuing production of RBCs by the bone marrow compensates for normal RBC turnover.

Q What is the significance of the hematocrit and the hemoglobin values?

A The hematocrit is a measure of the number of RBCs per unit of blood volume. If a glass tube of whole blood is spun in a cen-

trifuge, the cellular elements go to the bottom of the tube. Because there are far more RBCs than either white blood cells (WBCs) or platelets, the "cell column" height is a good indication of the number of red blood cells. The hematocrit is the percentage of the cell column height versus that of the total column of blood in the tube. This has also been called the packed cell volume as shown in Figure 32–2. Normal hematocrit (Hct) levels

CLINICAL PEARL

Mathematically, the Hct is roughly three times the Hb value. So if the patient's Hb is 12, then the Hct would be approximately 36. As a result of this predictable connection, changes in one parameter always reflect changes in the other in the same direction. If the Hct goes up, then so must the Hb, and vice versa.

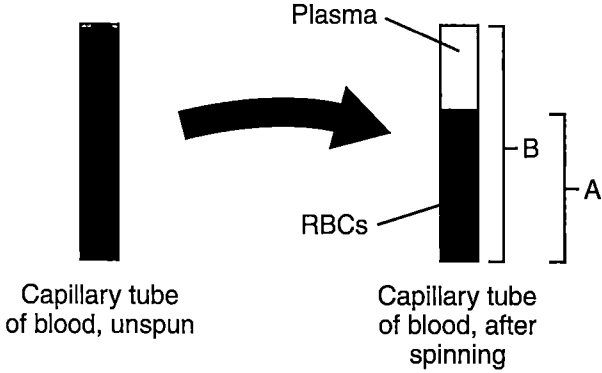

Hct = (A/B) x 100%

FIGURE 32–2 The relationship between the blood in a tube and the packed cell volume after the tube has been spun. (From Rothenberg, M.A. 2000, *Pathophysiology—Mechanisms of Disease.* Reproduced with permission.)

indicate a normal number of RBCs; a high Hct means too many (polycythemia), and a low Hct means too few RBCs (anemia). The hemoglobin (Hb) measurement is the concentration of the oxygen-carrying protein hemoglobin in the blood. If the number of RBCs is normal, so is the Hb value. If the Hb is high, there are too many RBCs; if it is low, the patient is anemic.

Q What are the normal Hb and Hct values in males and females?

A The normal values are summarized in Table 32–1. Note that the lab value RBC count is used rarely in clinical medicine—Hb and Hct have routinely replaced it.

Q What is the correlation between the RBC count, Hct, and Hb values?

A The RBC count is not used routinely in clinical medicine. However, the Hb and Hct are direct reflections of the number of RBCs. Each normal RBC contains the same amount of Hb. Thus, if we have a normal number of RBCs, the Hb concentration is *normal.* If there are too few RBCs, the Hb concentration is *low.* And, if there are too many RBCs, the Hb concentration is *high.* Because the Hct is mathematically three times the Hb, we can reach similar conclusions for Hct (e.g., three times a *normal Hb* is the *normal Hct*). Note that the Hct and Hb, when written together, are often termed the H/H or H&H (pronounced "H and H").

> **CLINICAL PEARL**
> *Either the Hct or the Hb directly reflects the number of RBCs. A normal RBC count leads to a normal H/H; a high RBC count means a high H/H; a low RBC count means a low H/H.*

Q What are leukocytes?

A There are two basic types of WBCs—granulocytes and monocytes. The generic term for both is *leukocytes. Granulocytes* contain microscopic chemical granules within the cell substance, while *monocytes* do not.

Q What are the different types of granulocytes in the blood?

A *Neutrophils* fight bacterial infections, while *eosinophils* and *basophils* are important in allergic reactions.

Q What are the different types of monocytes in the blood?

A Monocyte is a general term for cells without intracellular granules. The two types are *lymphocytes* and *mononuclear cells*

TABLE 32–1

Normal Hemoglobin and Hematocrit Levels			
Parameter	Gender	Mean	Range
Hb	Women	14.0 g/dl	12–16 g/dl
	Men	15.5 g/dl	13.5–17.5 g/dl
Hct	Women	41%	36–46%
	Men	47%	41–53%

(usually just called "monocytes"), both of which help eliminate viruses, fungal infections, and foreign bodies.

Q What is a tissue macrophage?

A When a monocyte leaves the blood vessel and migrates into the tissue, it is then referred to as a *tissue macrophage.* A macrophage is a phagocytic tissue cell that may be fixed or freely motile. Derived from the monocyte, it functions to protect the body from infection and toxins.

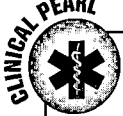

> **CLINICAL PEARL**
> *The terms* tissue macrophage *and* macrophage *are interchangeable.*

Q What is the normal WBC life cycle?

A When released from the bone marrow, granulocytes remain in the circulation for 6–12 hours. If they travel to tissues, they live for a few more days. Otherwise, they are recycled by the reticuloendothelial system, as are RBCs. Monocytes, on the other hand, are longer lived.

Q What are the functions of leukocytes?

A The main function of leukocytes is to maintain host defenses against infection, particularly bacterial infection. Monocytes and granulocytes accomplish this by ingesting and killing microorganisms, digesting tissue debris, and releasing inflammatory mediators. Lymphocytes participate in the activation and function of the immune system, aided by monocytes.

Q What are the characteristics of the inflammatory process?

A The inflammatory response is the body's reaction to injury. It consists of both a vascular component and a cellular component.

- Vascular component—blood vessels dilate and develop increased permeability. This increases blood flow, producing the signs of heat and redness. Increased permeability results in the leakage of protein-rich fluid from the vessels known as exudates. An accumulation of exudates results in tissue swelling (edema). When inflammatory edema contains neutrophils and cellular debris, it is called a purulent exudate or pus.

- Cellular component—WBCs, predominantly neutrophils, marginate to the side of blood vessel walls ("line up" along the inside wall), and then migrate through the blood vessels into the tissues.

> **CLINICAL PEARL**
>
> *The vascular and cellular components of the inflammatory response lead to the "classical" findings: rubor (red), calor (hot), tumor (swollen), dolor (pain).*

What is the difference between cellular and humoral immunity?

Humoral immunity (also known as antibody-mediated immunity) primarily involves antibodies that are produced by a specialized WBC, the B lymphocyte. *Cellular immunity* (also known as cell-mediated immunity) is the portion of our immune system that primarily involves cells (lymphocytes).

What are examples of alterations in the immunologic response?

The two main categories of alterations in the immunologic response are under-response and over-response:

- Under-response—parts of the immune system fail to respond appropriately to a foreign substance (e.g., bacteria, foreign body). As a result of this inadequate response, injury may occur to the patient. For example, people with acquired immunodeficiency syndrome (AIDS) have a failure of a portion of their cell-mediated immune component. Because these cells do not function adequately, an infection occurs from organisms that would normally be stopped. The result is often severe illness and death (e.g., atypical pneumonia).

- Over-response—the immune system responds appropriately initially, but then loses autoregulation ("control") so that mediators continue to be released. As a result, injury to the patient may occur. An example of this phenomenon is a severe allergic reaction—antibodies attempt to rid the body of the foreign antigen. As a result, histamine and other mediators are released. Positive feedback stimulates the production of even more mediators, resulting in clinical symptoms (and even death in some individuals).

What are examples of leukocyte disorders?

Generically, leukocyte disorders result from either too few WBCs, too many WBCs, or a dysfunction of the WBCs. A low number of WBCs is called leukopenia while a high number is called leukocytosis. Common causes include:

- Leukopenia—congenital problems, acquired anemia, leukemia, viral infection, drug reaction (e.g., sulfa drugs and nonsteroidal anti-inflammatory agents), immunosuppression, destruction of WBCs in the peripheral blood (e.g., immune, overresponse in severe infection), pooling of WBCs (e.g., enlargement of the liver or spleen).

- Leukocytosis—infections (usually bacterial), inflammation, tumors, drugs (e.g., steroids), tumors (e.g., leukemia, metastatic cancer).

- Abnormal WBC function—vitamin deficiency, congenital defects, drug effects (e.g., immunosuppression).

What is the life cycle of a platelet?

Platelets are formed from stem cells in the bone marrow that have differentiated into *megakaryocytes*, large multinucleated cells. In response to the cytokine thrombopoietin, megakaryocytes in the marrow divide into anuclear (without nuclei) particles known as platelets. Platelets circulate in the blood for an average of 7 to 10 days before being removed by the spleen.

What is the primary function of platelets?

Platelets form the initial "hemostatic plug" following vascular injury. Clotting proteins then "toughen" and complete the blood clot.

> **CLINICAL PEARL**
>
> *Many anti-inflammatory drugs (e.g., aspirin, ibuprofen) and some herbals (e.g., alfalfa, chinchona bark, clove oil, ginkgo, garlic, ginger, ginseng, feverfew) decrease the aggregation of platelets. Though this may have a beneficial effect (e.g., myocardial infarction or stroke prevention), these drugs may also result in a bleeding tendency. Always ask a patient about all medications, including over-the-counter and herbal preparations.*

What is the hemostatic mechanism?

The hemostatic mechanism consists of two parts. The term *primary hemostasis* refers to the initial action between circulating platelets and a damaged vascular surface. Immediately after vascular injury, the following sequence takes place:

- The vessel contracts in the vicinity of the injury.
- Vascular endothelial cells (inner lining) are exposed.
- Endothelial cells contain multiple adhesive proteins that provide binding sites for platelets.
- Platelets bind to the exposed binding sites.
- Bound platelets release granules that recruit further platelets.
- Recruitment of more platelets leads to further stimulation, aggregation, and augmentation of the platelet plug.
- The platelet surface membranes then undergo chemical changes that facilitate the binding of circulating blood clotting proteins (secondary hemostasis).

Secondary hemostasis involves the release of various factors (intrinsic and extrinsic clotting cascade) that activate chemical reactions between a set of clotting proteins, known as factors. Many of these reactions take place on the platelet surface and result in the formation of fibrin. This substance is the final "glue" that completes the blood clot, which now consists of injured vascular epithelium, a platelet plug, and intertwined strands of clot formation (Figure 32–3).

What are the extrinsic and intrinsic blood clotting systems?

Intrinsic and extrinsic clotting systems are terms based on laboratory tests that describe different, though related, sets of chemical reactions that all lead to the formation of fibrin (Figure 32–4).

- Intrinsic—in the intrinsic pathway, inactivated clotting factor XII is activated by various means (e.g., altered blood vessel surface, bacterial toxin, other mediators). This leads to the sequential activation of factors XI, IX, and VIII. Along with other necessary blood substances (called cofactors), factor X is activated. Once factor X is activated, the final process is identical for both the intrinsic and the extrinsic pathways. Activated factor X combines with factor V, catalyzing the conversion of prothrombin (factor II) to thrombin. Thrombin then catalyzes the conversion of fibrinogen (factor I) to fibrin, forming the final clot (along with the vessel endothelium and platelet plug).
- Extrinsic—in the extrinsic pathway, factor VII is activated by factor III (known as tissue thromboplastin) that is released

CLINICAL PEARL

Many clinicians now consider the differences between the extrinsic and intrinsic clotting systems to represent more of a laboratory artifact than a real life (in vivo) phenomenon. We include the pathways for enrichment value only.

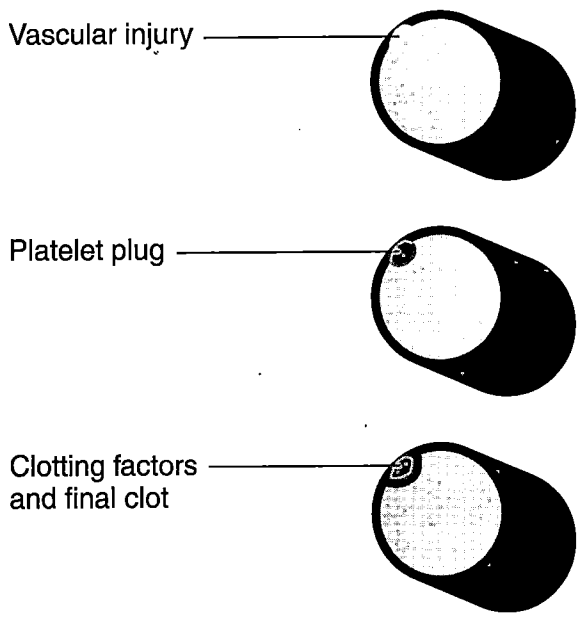

FIGURE 32–3 The formation of a clot from: 1) a vascular injury, 2) a platelet plug develops, and 3) development of the final clot with the assistance of clotting factors. (From Rothenberg, M.A. 2000, *Pathophysiology—Mechanisms of Disease.* Reproduced with permission.)

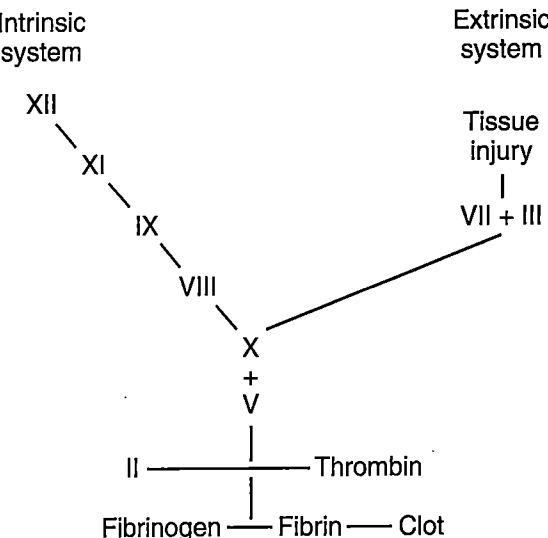

FIGURE 32–4 The chemical reactions that lead to the formation of fibrin. (From Rothenberg, M.A. 2000, *Pathophysiology—Mechanisms of Disease.* Reproduced with permission.)

from injured tissue. Activated factor VII proceeds to activate factor X. As indicated previously, activated factor X combines with factor V, catalyzing the conversion of prothrombin (factor II) to thrombin. Thrombin then catalyzes the conversion of fibrinogen (factor I) to fibrin, forming the final clot.

What are the blood groups found in the human population?

Human blood groups are determined by the presence or absence of two antigens, A and B, on the surface of RBCs. The system classifies blood into four groups:

1. Type A—contains antigen A and antibodies against antigen B.
2. Type B—contains antigen B and antibodies against antigen A.
3. Type AB—contains both antigens, no antibodies.
4. Type O—contains neither antigen; contains both antibodies.

Who can give blood to whom?

Individuals with type AB blood have no antibodies. Therefore, they may receive blood from people with any ABO blood type ("universal recipients"). People with type O blood have no antigens. Their blood may be given safely to people with any ABO blood type ("universal donors"). Transfusions between other ABO groups (e.g., Type A to Type B) are fraught with the danger of serious transfusion reactions as shown in Table 32–2.

> **CLINICAL PEARL**
> *In blood banks, numerous other antigens and antibodies are typed in addition to the "classic" ABO groups. Even if there is ABO compatibility, a reaction between other antibodies and antigens may be fatal.*

What is an acquired factor deficiency?

It occurs when a person develops a deficiency of any clotting factor or factors. The most common cause is the intake of antico-

TABLE 32–2

Who Can Give Blood to Whom		
Blood Type	Antigen	Antibody
A	Antigen A	Anti-B Antibody
B	Antigen B	Anti-A Antibody
AB (universal recipient; may receive any blood type)	Antigens A&B	No Antibodies
O (universal donor; may be given to any blood type)	No Antigen	Anti-A&B Antibodies

agulant medications (e.g., Coumadin®) that suppress the body's formation of clotting factors II, VII, IX, and X.

What is fibrinolysis?

Fibrinolysis is the body's natural and normal way of preventing excess blood clot formation. Small injuries often lead to the activation of the clotting cascade. To prevent these small clots from developing into clinically significant thrombi, plasminogen is activated to form plasmin. Plasmin lyses the clots, returning things to a "hemostatic baseline."

> **CLINICAL PEARL**
> *"Clot busters" (fibrinolytic therapy) in myocardial infarction (MI) and stroke activate the body's fibrinolytic system, resulting in clot lysis. If their effect is exaggerated, excess bleeding (a major side effect) occurs.*

How does the physical assessment relate to the hematologic system?

Specific findings during the detailed physical examination and their potential relevance to a disease of the hematologic system are summarized in Table 32–3. Further details regarding particular disease states are given in the answer to the next question.

> **CLINICAL PEARL**
> *The following are clinical "hints" to suspecting abnormalities of the blood cells:*
> - *Anemia commonly results in complaints of fatigue, lethargy, and dyspnea.*
> - *Low WBC counts (leukopenia) often leads to infections and fever.*
> - *Low platelet counts (thrombocytopenia) often causes cutaneous bleeding (including petechiae) and bleeding from mucous membranes (e.g., epistaxis, rectal bleeding).*

What is the pathophysiology and the clinical manifestations and prognoses for the following disorders: anemia, leukemia, lymphomas, polycythemia, disseminated intravascular coagulopathy, hemophilia, sickle cell disease, and multiple myeloma.

The prognoses for hematologic conditions varies widely, even within individual disease groups. As a result, it is impossible to quantify this. The information in Table 32–4 summarizes the pathophysiology and clinical manifestations for the listed disorders:

TABLE 32-3

Physical Findings and Relevance to Hematologic System Disease	
Finding	Potential Hematologic Significance
Fatigue	Anemia, leukemia
Syncope	Anemia
Prolonged bleeding	Clotting abnormalities, platelet abnormality (consider anticoagulant effect, or anti-inflammatory agent)
Bruising	Clotting abnormalities, platelet abnormality (consider anticoagulant effect, or anti-inflammatory agent)
Itching (pruritis)	Hemolysis (rupture of RBCs; itching is due to an accumulation of bilirubin in the skin and is often accompanied by jaundice)
Pallor	Anemia, leukemia
Jaundice	Hemolysis (rupture of RBCs; itching is due to an accumulation of bilirubin in the skin and is often accompanied by jaundice)
Epistaxis	Clotting abnormalities, platelet abnormality (consider anticoagulant effect, or anti-inflammatory agent)
Bleeding gums	Clotting abnormalities, platelet abnormality (consider anticoagulant effect, dilantin use, or anti-inflammatory agent), leukemia
Gum infections	Leukemia, other WBC problem (low count, inadequate function)
Oral ulcerations	Leukemia, other WBC problem (low count, inadequate function)
Melena	Clotting abnormalities, platelet abnormality (consider anticoagulant effect, or anti-inflammatory agent)
Signs of liver disease	May lead to coagulation abnormalities by decreased production of factors II, VII, IX, and X
Abdominal pain	Sickle cell crisis
Arthralgia	Joint bleeding, such as in hemophilia
Nuchal rigidity	Intracranial bleeding due to hemophilia or other coagulation abnormality
Dyspnea	Decreased oxygen-carrying capacity (anemia)
Chest pain	Decreased oxygen-carrying capacity (anemia)
Hemoptysis	Clotting abnormalities, platelet abnormality (consider anticoagulant effect, or anti-inflammatory agent)
Genitourinary infection	Leukemia, other WBC problems (low count, inadequate function)
Hematuria	Clotting abnormalities, platelet abnormality (consider anticoagulant effect, or anti-inflammatory agent)
Menorrhagia	Clotting abnormalities, platelet abnormality (consider anticoagulant effect, or anti-inflammatory agent)

TABLE 32-4

Hematologic Conditions: Pathophysiology and Clinical Manifestations		
Disease	Pathophysiology	Manifestations
Anemia	Reduction below the normal levels of the number of RBCs as manifested by a decreased H/H level. May be due to any of a number of processes; precipitating causes include blood loss, decreased erythrocyte production (e.g., chronic disease, iron deficiency), increased erythrocyte destruction (intravascular hemolysis).	Fatigue, lethargy, dyspnea, chest pain, syncope (especially with ongoing, but clinically unapparent, GI bleeding)
Leukemia	Malignant tumor of blood-forming tissues, characterized by abnormalities of the bone marrow, spleen, lymph nodes, and liver; results in the rapid and uncontrolled proliferation of abnormal numbers and forms of leukocytes.	May be acute, rapidly progressing from signs of fatigue and weight loss, repeated infections, and fever; may be chronic, progressing slowly over a period of years with few symptoms, other than decreased energy levels.
Lymphomas	Malignant tumor (neoplasm) of lymphatic tissue. Varies widely in the types of cells affected and the prognosis.	Enlarged lymph nodes, weakness, fever, weight loss, malaise, enlargement of the spleen and liver.
Polycythemia	Overproduction of RBCs, WBCs, and platelets. When all cell lines are involved, it is usually the result of a bone marrow tumor *(polycythemia vera).*	Shortness of breath; deep red-purple color to skin; pruritis (due to excessive destruction of RBCs); clotting tendencies, especially cerebral thrombosis; may be fatal.
Disseminated intravascular coagulopathy	Also known as DIC; unlikely to be seen as a primary problem in the field; common complication of severe injury, trauma, or disease. A combination of small vessel clotting (microvascular) with resultant organ dysfunction and consumption of platelets and clotting factors (due to ongoing clotting), leading to a bleeding problem in the larger blood vessels (macrovascular)	Signs and symptoms initially relate to underlying cause; patients have a failure of multiple organs (e.g., kidneys, lungs, heart) at once, accompanied by bleeding from IV sites into joints and possibly, intracranial hemorrhage.

(continued)

TABLE 32-4 *continued*

Hematologic Conditions: Pathophysiology and Clinical Manifestations

Disease	Pathophysiology	Manifestations
Hemophilia	Hereditary deficiency of clotting factors VIII (hemophilia A) or IX (hemophilia B). Gender-linked transmission (by female to the male; females are rarely affected).	Excessive bleeding after minor wounds, insignificant trauma procedures (e.g., IV start); spontaneous bleeding into joints, abdomen, or central nervous system (brain or spinal cord).
Sickle cell disease	Congenital hemolytic anemia due to the formation of abnormal Hb. More common in blacks, Puerto Ricans, and people of Spanish, French, or Mediterranean origin. The disease may mimic appendicitis or opiate withdrawal in its presentation.	People with the full-blown form (sickle cell anemia) have spontaneous sickling of RBCs in response to low-grade hypoxia, infection, or sometimes no apparent reason at all. The result is a painful and potentially deadly sickle cell crisis. Symptoms include shortness of breath and severe abdominal pain. Between crises, patients may experience minimal symptoms related to severe anemia.
Multiple myeloma	Neoplastic tumor of plasma cells (lymphocyte-like cell) that invades bone marrow.	Bone pain, pathologic fractures, skeletal deformity, anemia, weight loss, shortness of breath, kidney problems.

Special Thanks

Figures 32–1, 32–2, 32–4, and 32–5 are reproduced with
permission from *Pathophysiology: Mechanisms of Disease*
by Mikel A. Rothenberg, M.D., © 2000.

Gynecology and Obstetrics

A normal healthy out-of-hospital birth can be a very happy and exciting event, but things can go wrong very quickly. This chapter discusses the female patient with the complaint of abdominal pain or vaginal bleeding. The focus is on various obstetric and gynecological conditions that may present as emergencies.

Physiology

Q. What does a normal ovarian and menstrual cycle consist of?

A. At the time of puberty, a female has approximately 200,000 immature eggs (oocytes) that are contained in special structures called follicles where they develop. Each month, some of the eggs become active and the follicle that surrounds the egg begins to develop several layers. The oocyte grows slowly, but the follicle enlarges rapidly with fluid. After eight to ten days, only one follicle remains to be released. When the egg is released (ovulation) on day 14, the follicle cells rupture and the oocyte is carried to the fallopian tube by fluid currents directed by the fimbriae. What remains is the *corpus luteum*—an endocrine structure that develops in the ruptured ovarian follicle and secretes progesterone and estrogen. If pregnancy does not occur, the corpus luteum breaks down marking the end of a 28-day cycle.

The normal menstrual cycle is 28 days and can be divided into three phases: menses, the proliferative phase, and the secretory phase (Figure 33–1).

- Menstruation lasts from one to seven days. This is the phase of tissue sloughing and blood loss through the vagina (approximately 35 ml over this period).
- The proliferative phase follows menses and is the time when the uterine tissue is restored and the follicles begin to enlarge.
- The secretory phase begins at the time of ovulation and lasts until the corpus luteum breaks down (about 12 days after ovulation). Two days later, the cycle ends and a new one begins. Fetal development is discussed in Chapter 43, Neonatology.

Q. What is premenstrual syndrome (PMS)?

A. Premenstrual dysphoric disorder is the current term for what previously was called premenstrual tension syndrome. This condition involves both physical and emotional symptoms that occur regularly in many women during the premenstrual phase of their reproductive cycles. The cause of PMS is not clear so the current treatments are aimed at relieving the symptoms.

- Physical symptoms:
  1. Bloating with water weight gain.
  2. Headache.

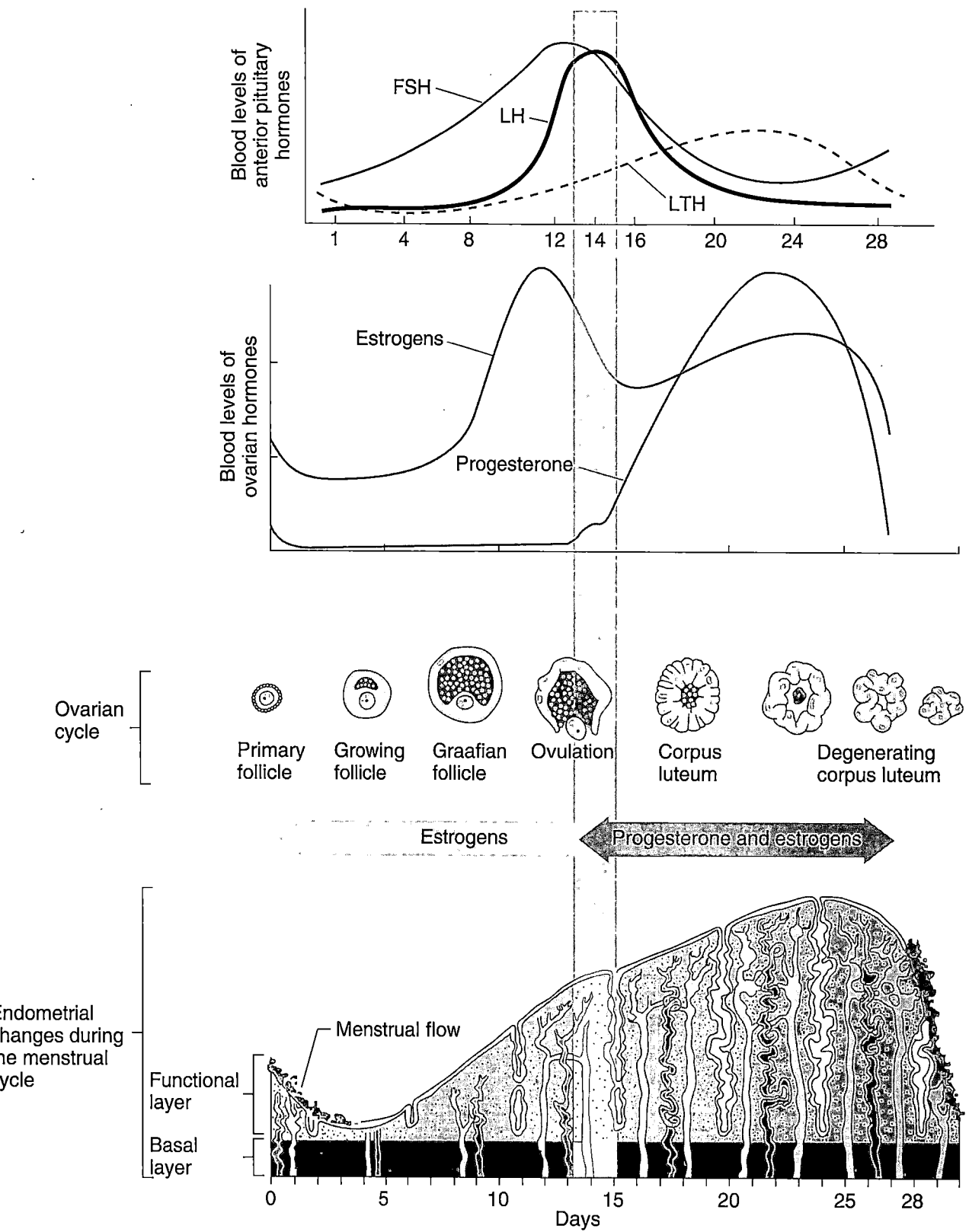

FIGURE 33-1 The menstrual cycle.

3. Breast tenderness or swelling.

4. Fatigue.

- Emotional symptoms:

1. Depression.

2. Anxiety.

3. Irritability, easily angered.

4. Interpersonal conflicts or withdrawal.

When does menstruation normally start and stop?

The average age of menarche (first menstrual period) is between 11 and 13 years of age, but can begin any time from 9 to 17 years of age. Menopause (cessation of ovarian function and menstrual activity) occurs for most women in the late 40s.

Is there anything that can stop or interrupt the normal menstrual cycle?

Yes, amenorrhea (absence of menses) occurs during pregnancy and lactation. Abnormal amenorrhea can occur with extreme exercise as seen with athletes, and in conditions of diabetes, obesity, malnutrition, starvation, stress, syphilis, TB, nephritis, hormonal imbalances, and endocrine disorders.

What are the roles of the hormones estrogen and progesterone?

Estrogens stimulate bone and muscle growth and induce the development of female sexual characteristics (e.g., maintenance of reproductive glands and organs, sex drive, distribution of hair and body fat). Progesterone is responsible for restoring and preparing the uterus for pregnancy after menses.

What is the normal process of the female reproductive system?

The average female has ovarian and menstrual cycles that continue regularly every 28 days. When fertilization occurs, these cycles are interrupted and pregnancy proceeds.

- Ovarian cycle—the production of ovum occurring on a monthly basis.

- Menstrual cycle—the 28-day cycle of changes in the endometrium in response to sexual hormone levels.

- Fertilization—union of egg and sperm to form the zygote (fertilized egg).

- Implantation—the zygote begins cell division and forms a hollow ball called a blastocyst as it moves into the uterine cavity. A few days later, the blastocyst contacts the endometrial wall,

erodes the epithelium, and buries itself in the edometrium. This initiates the development of the placenta.

- Gestation—the length of time from conception to birth (37 to 41 weeks in humans).

- Birth—the progression of a child leaving the uterus.

What is a trimester?

The human gestation period is divided into three 3-month segments called trimesters.

What are some examples of gynecological emergencies?

Typically, EMS is dispatched for a female complaining of acute abdominal pain. Possible causes of female abdominal pain include:

- Ectopic pregnancy—implantation of a fertilized egg outside of the uterus, most commonly occurring in the fallopian tubes.

- Hemorrhage—abnormal vaginal bleeding.

- Infection—either acute or chronic.

- Sexually transmitted diseases (STDs)—include more than 30 types.

- Ovarian torsion—twisting of an ovary causing ischemia.

- Renal stones—especially when obstructing the ureter.

- Ruptured ovarian cyst—fluids from the rupture cause peritoneal irritation and peritonitis.

- Sexual assault—may involve the internal or external genitalia, or rectal and peritoneal areas.

What is PID?

Pelvic inflammatory disease (PID) is an infection in the female reproductive and surrounding organs that can lead to complications including sepsis and infertility. The vagina normally contains bacteria that are part of the immune system. Typically, the cervix wards off bacteria from spreading into the internal organs. When the cervix is exposed to a STD, it becomes infected. The infection can now pass to internal organs. This condition is called PID.

What organs can PID affect?

The cervix is infected initially, and then the infection can spread to any of the following organs:

- Fallopian tubes (acute salpingitis).

- Liver.

- Ovaries (oophritis).
- Peritoneum (Peritonitis).
- Uterus or edometrium (endometritis).
- Uterine and ovarian support structures.

What signs or symptoms are associated with PID?

PID causes various signs and symptoms in different women. Some women experience none and don't even know they have it. The following is a list of possible signs and symptoms:

- Acute abdominal pains (lower quadrant) close to last menstrual period.
- Discharge (yellow or greenish, and may have an odor).
- Pain during or after intercourse.
- Guarding.
- Fever.
- Nausea and vomiting.
- Irregular periods.

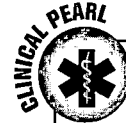

PID is the leading cause of female infertility and ectopic pregnancy.

What are some of the STDs?

Untreated STDs can cause complications, such as ectopic pregnancy, serious infections, and abscesses in female and male organs. The most common STDs are:

- Acquired Immunodeficiency Syndrome (AIDS).
- Bacterial vaginosis.
- Chancroid.
- Clamydial infections.
- Cytomegalovirus infections.
- Genital herpes.
- Genital (venereal) warts.
- Gonorrhea.
- Granuloma inguinale (donovanosis).
- Hepatitis.
- Leukemia, lymphoma, myelopathy.
- Lymphogranuloma venereum.
- Molluscum contagiosum.
- Pubic lice.
- Scabies.
- Syphilis.

- Trichomoniasis.
- Vaginal yeast infections.

What are the signs and symptoms associated with STDs?

Many STDs present without any pain or discomfort. When signs and symptoms occur they include any of the following:

- Abdominal pain, cramping.
- Lower back pain.
- Pain with urination and frequent urination.
- Abnormal discharge.
- Pain with intercourse.
- Nausea or vomiting.
- Fever.
- Emotional imbalance.

What is the most common STD?

Chlamydial infection is currently the most common of all bacterial STDs occurring in both men and women. Because many people experience no symptoms (especially men), they do not know they have it. Symptoms include abnormal genital discharge, and burning with urination. Chlamydia can be treated with antibiotics. Left untreated, it can lead to PID and is one of the most common causes of ectopic pregnancy.

Besides menstruation, what are other causes of vaginal bleeding?

Causes of vaginal bleeding include:

- Abortion or miscarriage.
- Labor.
- Lesion.
- PID.
- Abruptio placentae.
- Placenta previa.
- Sexual abuse.
- Trauma.

The most important complication of vaginal bleeding is that the underlying cause turns out to be an ectopic pregnancy. A missed ectopic pregnancy is relatively common and may be fatal.

Q **What are the complications of vaginal bleeding?**

A Uncontrolled vaginal bleeding can lead to hypovolemia, shock, or death.

Q **What is cystitis?**

A Cystitis is a bladder infection, which often occurs secondary to a urinary tract infection (UTI). This condition can be acute or chronic. The symptoms are urinary frequency and pain with urination. These infections are treated with antibiotics.

Q **What are the complications of cystitis?**

A Cystitis may lead to kidney infection (pyelonephritis) and even systemic sepsis. It may also lead to local scarring in the urinary tract that may interfere with the flow of urine.

Q **What is mittelschmerz?**

A Mittelschmerz is lower abdominal pain experienced by some women at the time of ovulation.

Q **What are the complications of mittelschmerz?**

A Mittleschmerz in itself is benign and self-limiting. The complication is making a differential diagnosis from other causes of abdominal pain.

Q **What is endometriosis?**

A Endometriosis is a condition where endometrial cells have migrated to an area in the body other than the uterus (Figure 33–2). The relocated cells respond to the same hormonal stimuli as the normal cells. The fallopian tubes are often affected, leading to tubal adhesions or occlusion and infertility. Signs and symptoms are often cyclical with the menstrual cycle and include abdominal pain, pelvic pain, lower back pain, dysuria, irregular menses, and infertility.

CLINICAL PEARL

Endometriosis may also occur within the uterus, resulting in excess growth of otherwise normal endometrial tissue. Symptoms may include excessive menstrual bleeding and severe cramps.

Endomeritis is an acute or chronic inflammation of the endometrium due to bacterial infection. The infection can originate from a STD, trauma, use of an intrauterine device (IUD), or an abortion. Signs and symptoms are lower abdominal or back

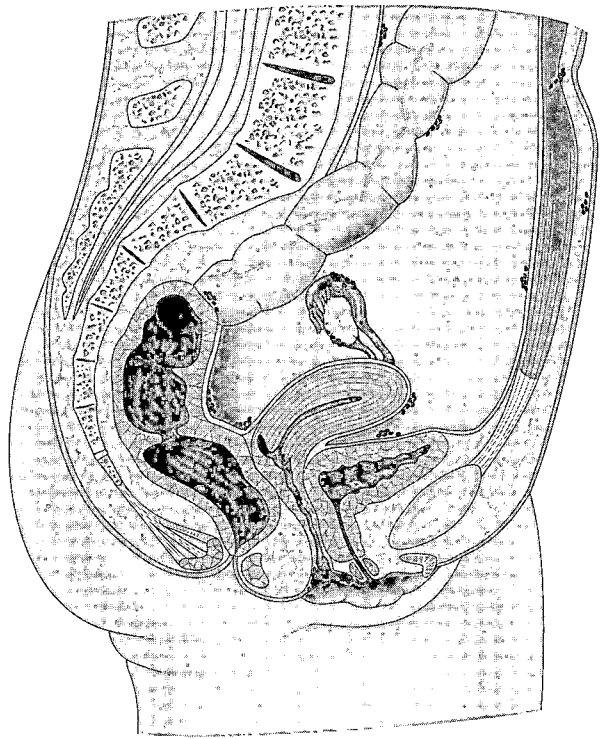

FIGURE 33–2 Endometriosis—common sites of endometrial implants.

pain, irregular menses, constipation, abnormal discharge, or infertility.

Q **What complications are associated with pregnancy?**

A There are many possible complications associated with pregnancy. This is why prenatal care is so important. When you are treating a patient who has not had prenatal care, be especially alert for signs and symptoms of the following conditions:

- Pregnancy-associated hypertension—new onset (BP is ≥140/90) is an indication of possible toxemia. Preexisting hypertension requires close monitoring. Other signs and symptoms associated with hypertension disorders during pregnancy include:
  1. Edema.
  2. Protein in the urine.
  3. Abnormal weight gain.
  4. Preeclampsia—progression of hypertension disorder in pregnancy with additional signs and symptoms of headache, epigastric pain, oligluria, pulmonary edema, and visual disturbances. Untreated preeclampsia may progress to eclampsia. The incidence of preeclampsia or eclampsia is 5–10 percent of all pregnancies.
  5. Eclampsia—the most serious condition of hypertension during pregnancy, usually between 20 weeks and one week

postpartum. Eclampsia is marked by convulsive seizures and coma and is a life-threatening condition to both the mother and fetus.

6. Other complications associated with uncontrolled hypertension in pregnancy are stroke, acute pulmonary edema, and renal failure.

- Gestational diabetes—onset of diabetes mellitus that occurs during pregnancy due to hormonal changes and usually subsides after childbirth.

- Supine hypotension syndrome—a condition that occurs when a sizeable fetus lays on the mother's vena-cava and compresses it, as when she lies on her back. This results in a decreased blood return to the heart and syncope or near syncope. The condition is easily corrected by having the mother reposition herself to a position other than supine.

- Abruptio placentae—a partial or complete premature separation of the placenta from the uterine wall after 20-weeks gestation. The premature separation causes blood loss that is not always apparent because it may be trapped behind the placenta (Figure 33–3). The mother experiences constant pain,

increased fetal movement, and possibly contractions. If the separation is complete, most often the fetus will die.

- Placenta previa—the placenta implants in the lower portion of the uterus creating either a complete or partial cover over the cervical os (opening). This condition can be detected on a sonogram before becoming a problem. The danger here is bleeding from the placenta that can be started from cervical effacing, sexual intercourse, or internal digital vaginal examination. The blood loss can be significant; however, the patient usually experiences no pain, unlike abruptio placentae (Figure 33–3).

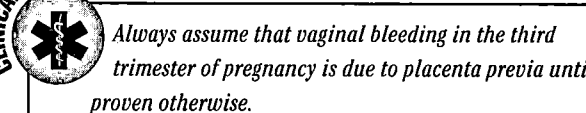

CLINICAL PEARL

Always assume that vaginal bleeding in the third trimester of pregnancy is due to placenta previa until proven otherwise.

- Spontaneous abortion or miscarriage—a pregnancy that terminates within the first 20 weeks, usually because the fetus is not developing normally. *Stillborn* is the term for the condition

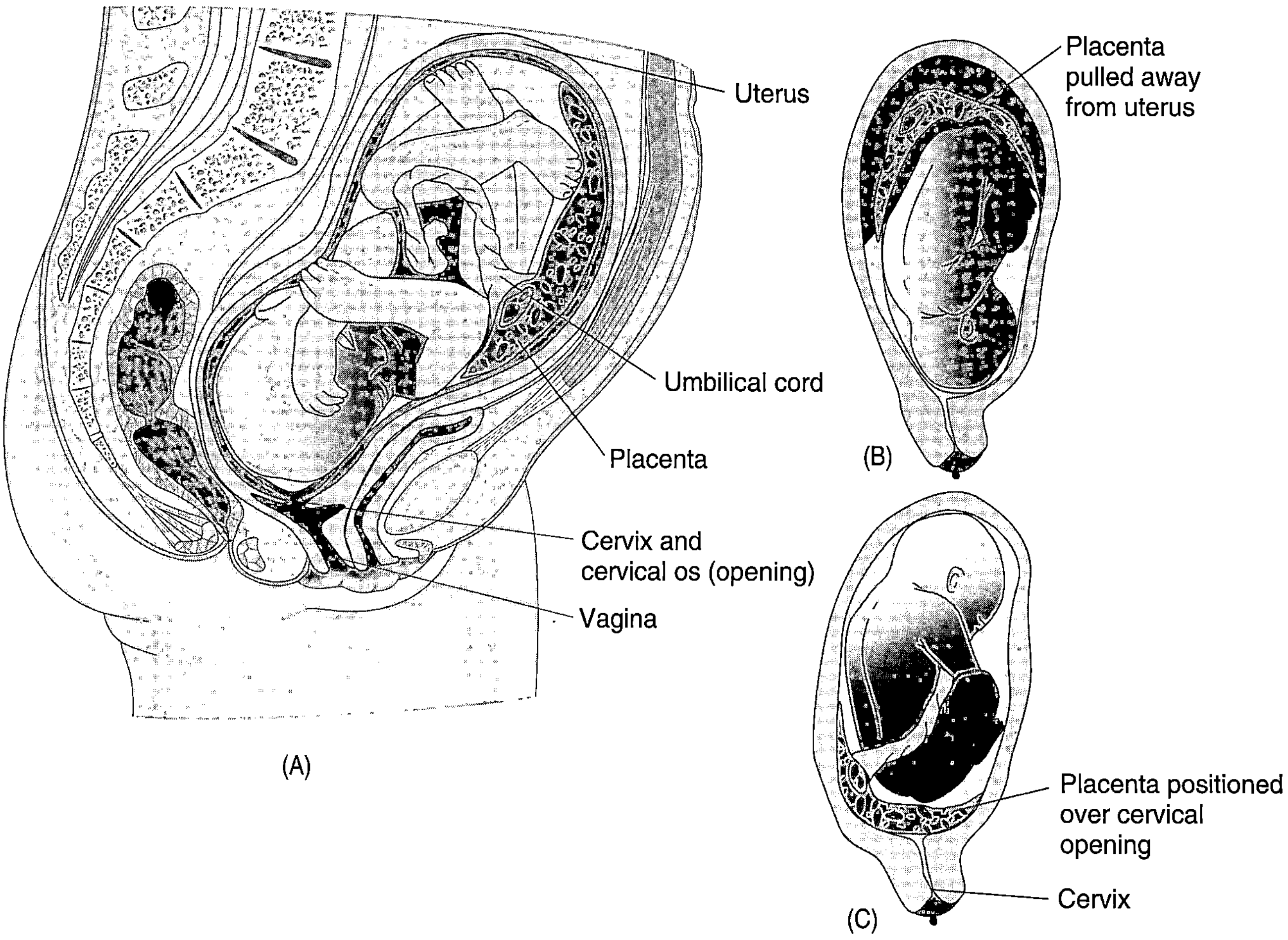

Uterus

Umbilical cord

Placenta

Cervix and cervical os (opening)

Vagina

(A)

Placenta pulled away from uterus

(B)

Placenta positioned over cervical opening

Cervix

(C)

FIGURE 33–3 (A) Normal uterine pregnancy, (B) abruptio placentae, and (C) placenta previa.

after 20-weeks gestation. Experts estimate that about half of all fertilized eggs die and are miscarried, usually even before the woman knows she is pregnant. In many cases of miscarriage, only placental tissue, not a fetus, has formed. Of pregnancies that the mother knows about, approximately 10 to 20 percent end in miscarriage, making miscarriage very common. Possible causes include uterine abnormalities or infection, problems with chromosomes or the immune system, or endocrine causes.

- Worsening of certain preexisting medical conditions (e.g., asthma, thyroid disease, diabetes).

- Cardiac—pregnancy places an extreme stress on a sick heart.

- Diabetes—a preexisting diabetic condition requires careful monitoring during pregnancy.

- Neuromuscular disorders (e.g., muscular dystrophy, multiple sclerosis, myasthenia gravis).

- Drug abuse.

What is Rh negative sensitization?

Pregnant woman with a negative Rh factor may become sensitized if her fetus has a positive Rh factor. If a fetus in any subsequent pregnancies has a positive Rh factor, Rh antibodies may cross the placenta and destroy fetal cells. Therefore, after termination of the pregnancy by either birth or abortion, the mother is given an injection of immune globuin to suppress the immune response.

What are the complications associated with childbirth?

During the birth, the fetus or umbilical cord may display an abnormal presentation. There may be meconium staining, aspiration syndrome, or hemorrhage (either maternal or fetal).

- Abnormal deliveries:
  1. Breech—feet first presentation.
  2. Limb—single arm or foot presentation.
  3. Nuchal cord—umbilical cord wrapped around the baby's neck.
  4. Prolapsed cord—umbilical cord presents before the baby.
  5. Multiple births—two or more babies (often born premature).
  6. Premature—childbirth before 38-weeks gestation increases the risk for complications in infancy.
  7. Shoulder dystocia—condition during delivery when the baby's head is out but the shoulder gets stuck against the mother's symphysis pubis.
  8. Face presentation—normally the baby's head is delivered with the face down toward the mother's perineum. Face

presentation means the baby's face is "sunny side up." Not usually a problem, just an abnormal presentation.

- Meconium—the first feces of the baby that is sometimes present in the fluids (staining) during birth. Complications, such as aspiration pneumonia, arise when the baby has aspirated (meconium aspiration syndrome) the thick green substance.

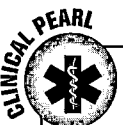

> *Consider meconium stained amniotic fluid an indication of fetal distress until proven otherwise.*

- Postpartum hemorrhage—continued heavy bleeding after childbirth due to the incomplete removal of the placenta or the failure of the uterus to contract. Can be life threatening if not corrected.

- Uterine rupture—tearing of the uterus due to trauma, extended labor, or a weakened section of the uterus from previous scarring.

- Uterine inversion—condition where the uterus turns inside out after delivery. Because ligaments and blood vessels are torn in this condition, severe blood loss and shock are the result.

- Pulmonary embolism (PE)—results from a blood clot in the pelvic circulation. This can occur during pregnancy, labor, or the postpartum phase. This condition occurs frequently and has a high mortality.

- Amniotic fluid embolism—has a high mortality rate, but is a rare condition. A clot formed of amniotic fluid crosses into maternal circulation during labor, delivery, or the postpartum phase. The clot is formed from particles (e.g., meconium, fetal hair) floating in the amniotic fluids.

Focused History and Physical Exam

What questions need to be asked in the focused history (FH)?

When the chief complaint is pain, start with OPQRST. If the patient confirms that she is pregnant, another set of questions should be asked. When a female between the ages of 12 and 60 has a complaint of abdominal pain, assume she is pregnant until proven otherwise (e.g., pregnancy test performed at the ED) even if she denies being pregnant.

In addition to OPQRST, ask about associated symptoms:

- Discharge—abnormal, color, odor, amount.
- Cramping.

- Syncope—or near syncope, light headed, or dizziness.
- Bowels—last BM, constipation, diarrhea, blood.
- Urine—frequency, urgency, dysuria, blood.
- Fever.

Do not forget the SAMPLE history; modify your history taking to include:

S—signs and symptoms of pregnancy.

A—allergies.

M—method of birth control and compliance.

P—prior pregnancy, surgeries (e.g., hysterectomy, uterine surgery, cone or excisional biopsy of the cervix), abdominal surgery (leading to scarring or adhesions).

L—last menstrual period (LMP)—menstrual history: cycles, duration.

E—events leading up to EMS being called (e.g., labor pain, water broke, trauma).

Which questions need to be asked of the pregnant patient?

Getting a good history about the present pregnancy, as well as any prior pregnancies, can help the EMS provider prepare for any possible complications during the management of the pregnant patient.

- Information about current pregnancy:
  1. Weeks of gestation (38–42 is term).
  2. Her estimated due date (EDD).
  3. Has there been prenatal care?
  4. Are there multiple fetuses?
  5. Has she used fertility drugs?
  6. Is the fetus in an abnormal position?
  7. Has there been preterm labor, either "real" or "false" (e.g., Braxton Hicks)?
- Information about prior pregnancies:
  1. Gravity—number of pregnancies.
  2. Parity—number of births.

3. Duration of gestation.
4. Number of preterm pregnancies.
5. Abortion or miscarriage—number and whether spontaneous or elective.
6. Type of delivery—vaginal (spontaneous or induced), cesarean section, forceps or vacuum extraction, episiotomy, or laceration.
7. Complications during pregnancy.
8. Length of labor(s). Precipitous delivery (labor and delivery in less than three hours).
9. Postpartum complications.
- Specific past medical history:
  1. Hypertension (preexisting or preeclampsia).
  2. Diabetes (preexisting or gestational).
  3. Medications—prenatal vitamins, recent changes in medications (if not taking prenatal vitamins, she may not have had prenatal care).
  4. Allergies.
  5. Alcohol or drug use during the pregnancy.

What are the components of the physical exam?

The EMS provider's attitude should exhibit a calm, comforting, and reassuring approach. Demonstrate compassion and be considerate by protecting the patient's modesty and privacy. The examination should include the following:
- Initial Assessment:
  1. General impression.
  2. Level of distress.
  3. Position of comfort.
  4. Skin color, temperature, and condition (CTC).
  5. Edema.
- Vital signs (if the patient is pregnant, take into consideration normal changes in pregnancy).
- Focused examination of the abdomen:
  1. Guarding.
  2. Tenderness.
  3. Masses.
  4. Distention.
  5. Absence of bowels sounds.
- Assess for discharge:
  1. Bleeding—clots, tissue.
  2. Amount.
  3. Other discharge—color, odor.

▣ What are some of the physiological changes in a woman's body during pregnancy?

🅰 There are certain normal physical changes during pregnancy that may obscure the clinical picture.

Normal changes:

- Increased heart rate (10–20 bpm).
- Decreased BP (during second trimester, returning to normal in third trimester).
- Increased cardiac output.
- Increased circulating blood volume (50 percent increase at term) without the additional hemoglobin to match (mismatch). This creates the condition known as "anemia of pregnancy." This is also a significant factor in hemorrhage as 30–35 percent of the blood volume may be lost before signs of shock become apparent. This is critical because the fetus experiences stress from hypoxia before physical signs become apparent in the mother.
- Increased abdomen size due to uterus:
  1. Slowed peristalsis (increased risk for vomiting).
  2. Decreased tidal volume due to chronic pressure under the diaphragm from the enlarged uterus.
  3. Urinary frequency.
- Varicose veins in legs or labia due to increased venous pressure.

Abnormal changes:

- Peripheral edema.
- Increased BP (preeclampsia).
- Epigastric pain.
- Dysuria (urinary tract infection).

Active labor:

- Palpate fundus during contractions.
  1. Measure duration of contractions.
  2. Measure the time of onset of contraction to onset of successive contractions to get the time between.
  3. Measure height of fundus.
- Inspect external genitalia for presenting fetus.
- Leaking amniotic fluid from ruptured membranes.

▣ How is the height of the fundus measured and why?

🅰 Measuring the height of the fundus can help determine the approximate age of the fetus. This is an important factor when considering the viability of a fetus in a critical situation such as a cardiac arrest.

To measure fundal height, place the patient in a supine position and measure from the symphysis pubis midline up over the abdomen as shown in Figure 33–4. A fundus at or above the

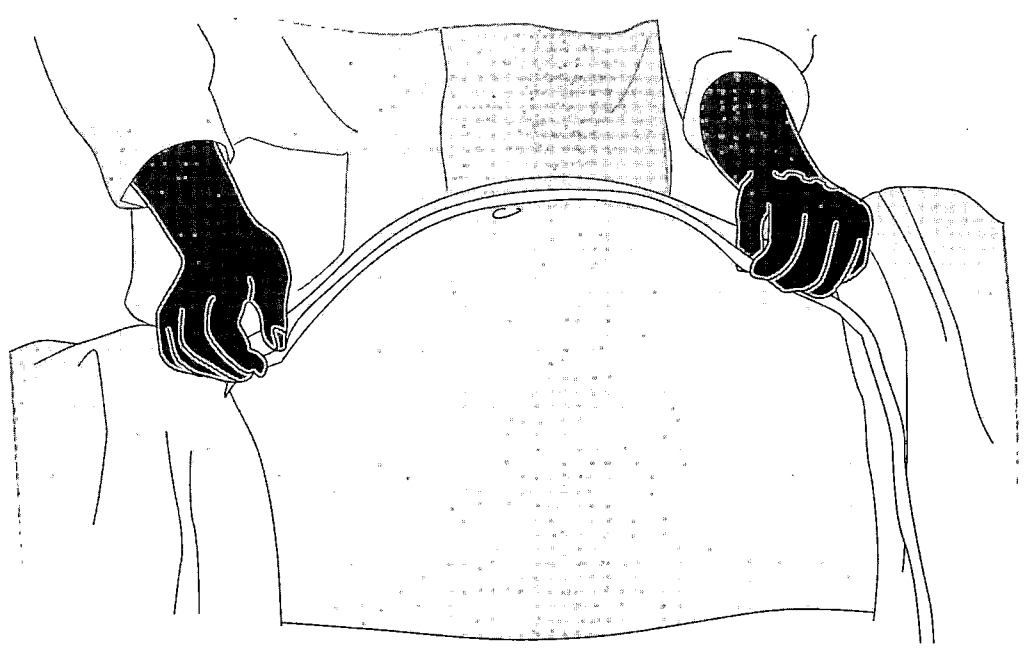

FIGURE 33–4 Measuring the fundal height.

umbilicus represents an approximate 20-week gestation. Greater than 24-weeks gestation is the age at which the fetus may survive outside the womb.

What is back labor?

Back labor is severe back pain experienced by the mother from the fetus (usually the head) pressing against the spine during labor. Some children have facial bruising (temporary) after birth from riding down the spine during the labor process.

What are the stages of labor?

There are three stages of labor. Stage 1 begins with contractions and ends with the crowning of the child's head at the vaginal opening. It is during this stage that the cervix dilates (opens) in preparation for delivery. Stage 2 begins with full dilation (8–10 cm) and crowning of the baby's head and ends with the birth of the child. Stage 3 begins after the birth of the child when contractions resume and ends with delivery of the placenta. The time of labor varies widely and subsequent deliveries for a woman typically become quicker than the one before.

- Stage 1 averages from 4 to 24 hours.
- Stage 2 ranges from minutes to an hour.
- Stage 3 averages about 15 minutes.

What happens during the labor process?

Childbirth is a passive process. The fetus relaxes and the mother's body does most of the work. Much involves involuntary muscle actions, with some active pushing near the end of the second stage until the baby is pushed out of the body. Emotional support and coaching is of great benefit to the mother.

Delivery starts as the fetus is pushed from the uterus to the birth canal (vagina). Stretch receptors in the walls of the uterus sense the increased stretch produced by the movement of the fetus. The receptors send a message to the brain that triggers the pituitary gland to secrete the hormone oxytocin into the blood stream and back to the uterus. Oxytocin stimulates the uterus to produce stronger contractions, which in turn push the baby further along. This cycle continues until the baby is pushed out of the body.

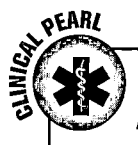

Some EMS systems use oxytocin (Pitocin®) to decrease post-delivery bleeding. Follow your local protocols.

What are the signs of imminent delivery?

Signs of imminent delivery include:

- Contractions that are strong and very close in time (1 to 2 minute intervals lasting 45–60 seconds).
- Crowning—the appearance of the infant's presenting part in the birth canal.
- The mother feels the urge to move her bowels.
- A multiparous woman tells you she is going to deliver.

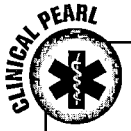

When a multiparous woman tells you that "the baby is coming," believe her!

Should an IV be started on the mother in the field?

Starting an IV routinely on women in early stages of labor is not necessary unless complications are anticipated. It is appropriate to start an IV in the field when:

- Delivery is imminent before arriving at the hospital.
- The delivery is abnormal.
- Postpartum hemorrhage is abnormal.
- The placenta has not yet been delivered. (Do not delay transport to wait for the delivery of the placenta.)
- Contractions are abnormal.
- Complications are anticipated.
- Your local protocols specify.

Some prenatal programs urge mothers to avoid unnecessary procedures, such as IVs and pain medications. If the mother is mentally competent, she has the right to refuse any proposed therapy.

How is delivery managed in the field?

When delivery is imminent, prepare the mother for delivery by having her lie down, preferably on your stretcher. Provide some privacy if possible, and have a partner coach the mother to push with the contractions and breathe deeply in between. Quickly obtain a FH and examine the opening of the vagina for crowning and leaking of amniotic fluid. Consider calling for another ambulance if multiple births or complications are anticipated. Prepare OB delivery equipment and don appropriate personal protective equipment (PPE). Follow local protocol requirements for inserting an IV at this point, if time permits.

Assist with the delivery of the baby by gently placing your hands on the baby's head to keep it from exploding out of the vaginal opening. Perineal tearing is common in childbirth, but can be minimized by preventing an explosive delivery. Once the head is out, the natural progression is for the baby's face to turn laterally from a downward position. Support the head during this process, while suctioning the mouth and nostrils. Look for the cord around the neck (nuchal cord); if present, gently lift it over the head. Next guide the shoulders through one at a time and carefully hang on to the baby because the rest of the body comes quickly and is very slippery.

Clear the airway of any remaining secretions, then dry, assess, and stimulate the baby as necessary. Keep the baby warm and if the mother is able, allow her to hold the baby on her stomach. Note the time of delivery. Clamp and cut the cord and repeat the assessment in five minutes.

Contractions will begin again for delivery of the placenta. Begin transportation and coach the mother again. After the placenta delivers, examine it for completeness. It should not have tears or patches missing. Package the placenta in a bedpan or plastic bag to be examined in the hospital. Observe for vaginal hemorrhage and save everything. Massaging the fundus with two hands or allowing the baby to suckle the mother's breast, if they are both willing, can slow bleeding.

How is the neonate assessed immediately after birth?

The Apgar score created by Virginia Apgar, an anesthesiologist, is a well-accepted assessment score chart for evaluating newborns at one minute and five minutes after birth. Table 33–1 summarizes the scoring. Each sign is rated at 0, 1, or 2. Ten is the highest score, a good to excellent score is 7 to 10, 4–6 is fair, and less than 4 at one minute is poor and indicates the need to begin aggressive assisted ventilations.

How and when is the umbilical cord cut?

There is no hurry to cut the cord; however, the baby is easier to manage and assess when the cord is cut. After assessing the

TABLE 33–1

Apgar Score			
Sign	0	1	2
Heart rate	Absent	Slow <100	>100
Respirations	Absent	Slow, irregular	Good, crying
Muscle tone	Limp	Some flexion	Active motion
Reflex	No response	Grimace	Cough or sneeze
Color	Blue or pale	Pink body and blue extremities	Completely pink

baby, clamp the cord in two places: one about four to six inches from the baby and another a few inches further away from the first clamp. Cut in between the two clamps. Assess the two ends for bleeding and adjust the clamps tighter if needed. The cord must be handled gently because it can tear. Never remove the clamps because the baby could bleed out through the cord. If the cord is not cut immediately, remember to place the infant at a lower level than the placenta prior to cutting to prevent placental transfusion.

Is it true that an IV can be started in the umbilical cord?

Yes, in fact, umbilical vein cannulation is preferred in neonatal resuscitation because the vein is so easy to identify and cannulate. The skill takes practice and a special umbilical catheter is used.

What if vascular access cannot be obtained?

Intraosseous (IO) infusion is an alternative for either fluid or medication administration. The ET route may also be used to administer medications.

Are there any other considerations in maternal resuscitation?

Yes, cardiac and respiratory arrest in the pregnant patient must be managed aggressively. When gestation appears to be second or third trimester, it is paramount that the fetus be positioned off the vena cava when the mother is placed on a backboard. This can be accomplished by manually pulling the uterus to the mother's left side or by tilting the backboard 15 degrees. When performing CPR, move the hand position for manual compression approximately one inch up from the normal position to adapt to the displaced position of the heart. Paddle placement for defibrillation should also be modified slightly by moving the lateral paddle up to accommodate the expanded uterus and elevated diaphragm. Also, some experts recommend increasing the compression–ventilation ratio from the standard 15:2. Hyperventilate with high-flow oxygen and consider aggressive resuscitation with fluids rather than drugs (follow local protocol). Transportation must begin quickly with early notification, and the destination must be one that can manage an emergency cesarean section.

Is it necessary to listen for fetal heart tones in the field?

Assessing the fetal heart rate is the standard of care in the clinical setting to determine if the fetus is in any distress.

However, in the field, don't spend too much time listening for a fetal heart beat because it is sometimes difficult to find. Loud ambient noise, and for most EMS agencies, the lack of equipment sensitive (e.g., Doppler) enough to hear fetal heart tones make it impractical in the field. If you do have the means to assess fetal heart tones, the normal range is 110 to 160 bpm.

Q Are there any other ways to assess whether a fetus is in distress?

A A moving fetus is a good sign, although it does not rule out a distressed fetus. Ask the mother when she last felt the child moving or kicking.

Q What is the significance of Braxton Hicks contractions?

A Named for a British gynecologist, John Braxton Hicks, preterm "false" labor that is irregular and most often painless is known as Braxton Hicks contractions. These contractions are practice contractions that prepare the uterus for the real thing. They can begin as early as the first trimester, but more often occur in the third trimester. Some women do not experience them at all. They are often relieved with mild exercise such as walking.

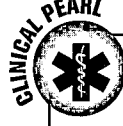

CLINICAL PEARL

Braxton Hicks contractions differ from real, but premature, labor. Unplanned early labor can be dangerous for both mother and baby. Braxton Hicks contractions, on the other hand, are relatively short lived and benign.

Q Why do pregnant women need to drink so much fluid?

A The uterus does not like to be dry. Dehydration causes contractions to begin. Mothers are told to drink 8 to 10 glasses of water a day during pregnancy.

Q What is the impact on the fetus of a state of shock in the mother?

A In a state of shock, the body's natural process to protect vital organs (e.g., brain, heart, lungs) follows a progression of systemic shunting to keep blood flowing to the vital organs. The normal process begins by shunting blood from the skin and intestines first. In pregnancy, the body perceives the fetus as a foreign object and shunts blood from the placenta before the skin. So, the fetus experiences hypoxia first and then is severely shunted as shock progresses.

Because the mother can have a significant blood loss before signs of shock appear, the fetus is in trouble long before. This is why the mechanism of injury (MOI) in pregnant women is so important.

CLINICAL PEARL

The best acute and chronic treatment for a fetus is to ensure the ideal well-being of the mother.

Q What further examinations or diagnostic testing may be performed in the ED?

A Pregnancy test, hemoglobin and hematocrit (H/H), urinalysis, electrolytes, liver function, pelvic and rectal exams, possibly a surgical consult, and ultrasound.

Sexual Abuse

Q How is the FH and physical exam completed for the sexually abused or assaulted patient?

A Sexual assault is a crime of violence with serious physical and psychological implications. It can occur in any age group and it is estimated that one in three females are raped during their lifetime with only 10–30 percent of these crimes being reported. Physical signs of abuse include bruising of the mons pubis, labia, or perineum and vaginal or rectal tears. Physical signs of the assaulted patient include swelling or new lacerations to the external genitalia. If the patient struggled, there will most likely be other associated physical injuries.

STDs present in the very young or very old may indicate sexual abuse. Emotional affect can also indicate a history of abuse. Examples are extreme anxiety, guarding, or an unwillingness to allow assessment or assume certain positions.

Most states have mandatory reporting policies for abuse. Requirements vary from state to state and are usually different for pediatrics and older patients. Be sure you understand your state's policy and know where to report suspected abuse. Preserving evidence from the crime scene:

- Bring the victim's clothing to the ED, handling the clothing as little as possible.
- Do not clean the wounds.
- Do not use plastic bags (paper bags are good) for blood-stained articles because they degrade the evidence with moisture.
- Bag each item separately.

- Ask the victim not to change clothes or bathe.
- Disturb the crime scene as little as possible.

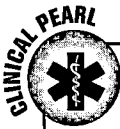 How is the victim of a sexual assault managed?

A Management after life-threatening injuries is focused on providing emotional support. Preserve evidence from the crime scene and provide a safe environment for the patient. Then respond to her physical and emotional needs.

General Management

Q How is the female with acute abdominal pain or vaginal bleeding managed?

A In the field, all abdominal complaints are managed alike, supportive treatment with care for shock. Getting a good history from these patients is paramount. In most cases, diagnosis of the cause of pain or bleeding will not be done in the field. However, the EMS provider can get a significant start on ruling out various conditions and treating for life-threatening or potentially life-threatening conditions.

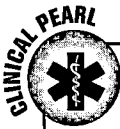

Assume a woman with abdominal pain has a leaking or ruptured ectopic pregnancy, especially if she is in shock.

All female patients of childbearing age are considered pregnant until pregnancy can be ruled out. Therefore, consider ectopic pregnancy first. Signs of shock with an unexplained source is considered and managed as intra-abdominal hemorrhage in origin until a source is found.

Treatment:

- Manage ABCs.
- Position of comfort or supine, positioning for shock.
- Provide high-flow oxygen.
- Establish IV access for fluid replacement.
- Keep the patient warm and calm.
- Consider rapid transportation.
- If the transport is long, you may want to contact medical control for their opinion on using MAST/PASG for a possible ectopic rupture.
- Transport to an appropriate facility.

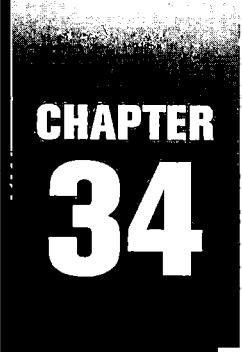

CHAPTER 34

Trauma Systems and Mechanism of Injury

This chapter discusses the makeup of trauma systems and the pathology of mechanism of injury (MOI). The focus is on *why* patients present in a certain manner and *why* some patients need an organized system of care to survive.

Epidemiology

How big a problem is trauma?

Trauma is the leading cause of death for people 1–44 years of age, with nearly 150,000 unexpected deaths occurring each year in the United States. Auto crashes account for about 44,000 and gunshot wounds (GSWs) account for 39,000 deaths each year.

What are the top five causes of trauma death?

Motor vehicle crashes, falls, poisonings, burns, and drownings are the top five causes of trauma death.

Why is so much emphasis placed on the MOI when treating a trauma patient?

Getting a complete and accurate history of the incident can help to identify as many as 95 percent of the injuries present. Many MOIs have predictable patterns for injuries. The EMS provider is trained to visualize the forces that were applied to the body and to look for specific injury patterns, even when injury is not visibly apparent.

After ensuring your personal safety and maintaining of the ABCs, the MOI is the most important information to obtain from any trauma victim.

What percent of trauma is life threatening?

Serious and life-threatening injury occurs in less than 1 percent of the trauma patients.

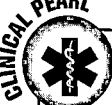

Despite the fact that few injuries are life threatening, inappropriate identification and treatment may result in high mortality rates per injury.

What are the major factors of tissue injury?

Two major factors for injuries are the amount of energy exchanged with the body and the anatomical structures that are involved. The energy that can be absorbed by the body during an impact (e.g., with an immovable object) produces damage to the patient's body. The extent of the damage caused by this energy depends on the specific organs that have been affected.

376

What are the phases of trauma care?

There are three phases of trauma care: pre-incident, the actual incident, and post-incident:

- Pre-incident—"All accidents are preventable." This phase of trauma is the "prevention" phase. EMS providers can make a big difference by setting an example and by educating the public on such things as seat belt and helmet use. Another aspect of prevention that can be influenced by EMS providers is the promotion of legislation to reduce the use of weapons.

- Incident—EMS providers can minimize further injury or death by responding and working safely on every call. This includes driving with higher safety awareness to the scene and during transport of the patient, wearing seat belts, and using appropriate personal protective equipment (PPE).

- Post-incident—The EMS provider can make a significant impact on life or death for the critical trauma patient by minimizing scene time, performing a rapid assessment and life-saving procedures, and transporting the patient to a facility that is appropriate for their needs, such as a trauma center.

Trauma Systems

What are the components of a trauma system?

The components of a trauma system are:

- Injury prevention programs.
- Out-of-hospital care—triage, treatment, and transport.
- ED care—with interfacility transport if necessary.
- Definitive care.
- Trauma critical care.
- Rehabilitation.
- Data collection—trauma registry.

What is a trauma registry?

A trauma registry is a reporting system designed to collect trauma-related data in an effort to improve the quality and cost effectiveness of care and to aid in outcome research. Two software programs produced by the American College of Surgeons (ACS) are National Tracs® and the National Trauma Data Bank™.

What are trauma centers?

A trauma center is a hospital that has the capability of caring for the acutely injured patient. Trauma centers must meet strict criteria to use this designation. The criterion delineates the

resources, personnel, equipment, and training necessary for an institution to provide quality trauma care.

What are the differences and roles of the levels of trauma centers?

Every community has different needs and resources available, so trauma centers have been classified into four levels based on the resources and programs available at each facility.

- Level I regional trauma center serves as a leader in trauma care for a specific geographical area. Most Level I trauma centers have a full range of resources, services, and programs 24 hours a day, seven days a week.

- Level II area trauma center has the capability of definitive patient care, but may not have all of the resources of a Level I trauma center. It stabilizes and transfers specialty trauma cases to the regional center.

- Level III community trauma centers are designated in communities without Level I or II trauma centers. They have the capability for stabilization, but, when necessary, will transfer patients to a Level I or II trauma center for further intervention and ongoing care.

- Level IV trauma facilities were established for rural and remote communities. A Level IV trauma facility may be a clinic rather than a hospital. The goal is to provide initial stabilization and then transfer to a Level I, II, or III trauma center.

What are specialty centers?

In addition to being trauma centers, some hospitals specialize in the following:

- Neurology.
- Burns.
- Pediatric trauma.
- Cardiac care (e.g., centers for heart transplantation).
- Microsurgery (e.g., hand and limb reimplantation).
- Hyperbaric centers.

What are the criteria for transport to a Level I trauma center?

The needs of the patient and the capabilities of that trauma center determine the criteria for transportation to any level trauma center. These criteria are based on the regional structure of the trauma care system and often can be found in local protocols. Examples of criteria for transport to a Level I trauma center are multiple system trauma, severe burns, or trauma to a pediatric, geriatric, or pregnant patient.

What is the criteria and procedure for air-medical transport?

The criteria and specific procedures for air-medical transport vary with geographic locations, however, there are typical advantages used when establishing guidelines in each county. The following is a list of indications and contraindications for the use of aeromedical evacuation.
Indications:

- Situations where the time required by ground transport pose a threat to the patient's survival or recovery.
- Access to remote areas.
- Access to specialized critical care personnel or specialty units in certain hospitals (e.g., neonatal intensive care unit, reimplantation, transplant center, burn center).
- Access to personnel with specialty skills (e.g., surgical airway, thoracotomy, and rapid sequence intubation).
- Access to specialty supplies and equipment (e.g., aortic balloon pump).

Contraindications or relative contraindications depending on the aircraft:

- Traumatic cardiac arrest.
- Inclement weather conditions.
- Extremely combative patients.
- Morbidly obese patient.
- Ground transport and appropriate level of care is available and quicker.
- Patients with barotrauma (e.g., diving injuries may necessitate lower flying altitudes).

Mechanism of Injury Energy

What physical laws of energy are associated with an MOI?

When energy is exchanged with the body, tissue damage occurs. The physical laws that apply to this are:

- Kinetic energy (KE)—This means that the more speed (motion) there is, the more energy there is. The formula for this is KE = Mass/2 × V².
- Force—Energy exchange is motion created by a force and force must stop the motion. The formulas are as follows:
  Force (Acceleration) = Mass × Acceleration; and
  Force (Deceleration) = Mass × Deceleration.
- Newton's first law of motion—"An object in motion tends to stay in motion, and an object at rest tends to stay at rest, unless the object is acted upon by an outside force." This can

easily be related to the unrestrained driver of a vehicle that suddenly crashes. As the car strikes an object, such as a pole, the car stops, but the unbelted driver continues on through the windshield and through the air until he hits the ground as gravity stops him from going further.

- Conservation of energy—This means that energy cannot be created or destroyed, only transferred or exchanged.

How is energy exchanged?

Energy exchange is the transfer of energy to another object or objects with resulting effects on motion, shape, or both. Cavitation is a good example of an energy exchange. Cavitation is the creation of a cavity in an object that can be permanent or temporary depending on the density and type of material the objects are made of. When a bullet is fired in the abdomen, the energy forces from the bullet are transferred to the tissues. This causes the tissues to move apart, creating a cavity. If the bullet was small, the cavity will most likely be temporary. This is why bullet holes are often missed during assessment. If the same bullet was fired into a plastic trash can, the energy is transferred to the thicker particles, creating a cavity and leaving an obvious hole that is permanent.

So why is speed so important to KE?

The value of the speed (the velocity) is squared in the KE formula; the value of the mass is merely divided by two. When a number is squared, it contributes greatly to the overall formula as evidenced by the comparison in Table 34–1.

An increase of 50 pounds yields an increase of 22,500 KE, while an increase of 10 mph yields an increase of 52,500 KE.

What would be the actual units for KE?

The unit is in foot/pounds, but the unit is not as important as the concept that "speed kills."

What is meant by an "index of suspicion"?

When EMS providers assess the MOI and kinematics at the scene of a trauma, they are trained to suspect that certain injury patterns have occurred. From these injury patterns, one can look

TABLE 34-1

Impact of Velocity on KE		
Velocity (Speed)	Mass (patient weight)	Total KE (foot/pounds)
30	150	67,500
40	150	120,000
30	200	90,000
40	200	160,000

for specific injuries and anticipate the potential for shock or other problems.

What are some examples of an index of suspicion?

You should suspect spinal injury when you see a cracked windshield, steering wheel or dashboard intrusion into a vehicle, or open fractured ankles after a fall.

What is the Platinum Ten Minutes?

From both Montana's and New York state's Critical Trauma Care (CTC) course, it is the goal of the maximum time spent at a scene for a critical trauma patient.

What is meant by the third collision?

Using the motor vehicle crash (MVC) analogy again, the first collision occurs when the car strikes an object, the second collision is when the body strikes the car's steering wheel or windshield, and the third collision occurs when internal organs strike against the body.

> **CLINICAL PEARL**
>
> *Any of the three "collisions" may result in severe damage. Don't forget the third one—when internal organs strike against the body. Findings are often less obvious than those from the first two "collisions," yet the injuries may be more severe.*

What is the difference between penetrating and blunt trauma?

Penetrating trauma occurs when an object penetrates the body tissues. Penetrating trauma is usually easier to recognize than blunt trauma, which creates a temporary cavity but does not penetrate body tissues. However, both types are associated with injuries and both can be lethal.

What are examples of penetrating trauma?

Typical examples of penetrating trauma injuries include knife wounds, GSWs, needle stick injuries, and missile injuries (e.g., pipe bombs or flying machine parts).

Why are GSW exit wounds larger than entrance wounds?

The exit wound is larger due to the cavitation caused by the bullet.

> **CLINICAL PEARL**
>
> *As a general rule, the entrance wound is always smaller than the exit wound. Assume that cavitation involves internal structures that are not readily visible on your clinical exam.*

Why are some bullets designed to tumble?

Tumbling creates greater tissue damage. The leading edge of the bullet does not enter the patient; rather, the bullet is tumbling through space and the entire side of the bullet enters the body. This causes a larger entry point and more tissue damage.

> **CLINICAL PEARL**
>
> *Don't assume that a projectile (e.g., bullet) followed a straight path between the entrance and exit sites. They may ricochet inside the body, especially off bones, and travel many different pathways.*

What are examples of blunt trauma?

Typical examples of blunt trauma injuries involve body tissue compression from rapid acceleration and deceleration forces as seen with MVCs, motorcycle collisions, auto–pedestrian collisions, and falls. Specific examples of blunt and penetrating MOIs and predictable injury patterns, including MVC, motorcycle, auto–pedestrian, and falls, are discussed in Chapter 15, Scene Size-Up and Initial Assessment.

What are the injury patterns associated with blast injuries?

There are three phases associated with the blast effect and each phase has a different energy pattern and potential for injury:

- Primary phase—there is a pressure wave that can cause major effects on the lungs and GI tract. This is accompanied by a heat wave that affects the eyes and skin, and can burn any exposed areas of the body.
- Secondary phase—the potential for injury comes from flying articles such as glass, wood, brick, or other people. Injuries can be blunt from compression or penetrating from lacerations.
- Tertiary phase—injuries can result from the patient becoming a flying object and striking other objects.

Why do we evaluate the MOI?

The foundation of assessment is early consideration of the MOI and kinematics of injury.

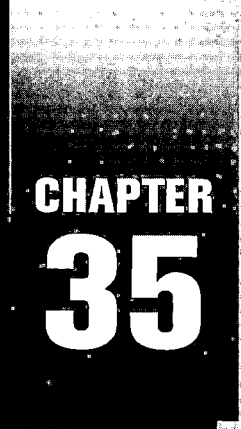

CHAPTER 35

Hemorrhage and Shock

This chapter discusses bleeding, both internal and external, and its impact on the patient. The most serious impact of bleeding, aside from immediate exsanguination, is the development of shock. The focus of this chapter is on *why* patients with serious hemorrhage and shock present in a certain manner and *why* you need to respond quickly to their presenting problems to avoid the downhill slide from blood loss.

Pathophysiology

Q What is the incidence of hemorrhage and shock?

A Hemorrhagic shock is the most common cause of death following major trauma, though the precise incidence is impossible to determine.

Q What is the mortality and morbidity of hemorrhage and shock?

A The outcome of hemorrhage and shock depends on the degree of bleeding, the patient's previous health, and the treatment. Untreated, all hemorrhage has nearly a 100 percent mortality.

Q What are the two general locations of hemorrhage?

A Hemorrhage is usually broken down into external and internal. External bleeding is usually due to trauma, whereas internal bleeding can be from either trauma or medical causes.

Q What are the most common sites of nontraumatic bleeding?

A The most common site of nontraumatic bleeding is in the GI tract (e.g., peptic ulcer, diverticulosis, esophageal varices).

> **CLINICAL PEARL**
>
> *Always think about occult GI bleeding in any person with signs of hypovolemic shock and no obvious external reason.*

Q What are the types of bleeding in anatomical terms?

A Bleeding is divided into three types: arterial, venous, and capillary. Arterial bleeding is described as spurting bright red blood. Venous bleeding is described as free flowing and a darker red or maroon color. Capillary bleeding is described as oozing and a red color.

Q What is the physiological response to hemorrhage?

A The body responds by starting to form a clot and with localized vasoconstriction. The clotting process is discussed in detail in Chapter 32, Hematology.

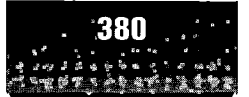

What are the stages of hemorrhage?

There are four stages, or grades, of hemorrhage:

- Stage One—involves up to 15 percent intravascular loss and is compensated by constriction of the vascular bed. The BP is maintained; there is a normal pulse pressure, respiratory rate, and renal output. The skin is usually pale and the central venous pressure (CVP) is low to normal. A person can go into Stage One by donating a pint of blood and that is why it is recommended that they rest for a half hour and do not drink alcohol or do strenuous activity.

- Stage Two—involves 15 to 25 percent intravascular loss. The cardiac output is maintained by arteriolar constriction and a reflex tachycardia. The patient also will have an increased respiratory rate, and catecholamines increase peripheral resistance. There is an increase in the diastolic pressure that is often not noticed. The pulse pressure may narrow and the patient may have diaphoresis from the sympathetic stimulation. The renal output is almost normal. This phase is also referred to as compensated shock.

- Stage Three—involves between 25 and 35 percent intravascular loss. The patient will have the classic signs of hypovolemic shock, which include marked tachycardia, marked tachypnea, a decrease in the systolic BP, and a decrease in urine output to 5 to 15 ml per hour. There may be an altered mental state (AMS), as well as cool, pale, and diaphoretic skin. This phase is also referred to as decompensated shock.

- Stage Four—involves a greater than 35 percent intravascular loss. In some instances, the patient may not have palpable peripheral pulses or may experience extreme tachycardia and pronounced tachypnea. There is a significant decrease in the systolic BP. The patient's mental status may vary from confusion to AMS. The skin is diaphoretic, cool, and extremely pale. Some texts refer to this phase as irreversible shock. Whether or not shock is irreversible is more often a function of the microcirculation in the vital organs and not the stage or grade of hemorrhage. The movement from one phase to another is a function of the volume of blood loss, interventions taking place, and when the bleeding is controlled. A specific time frame is not put on this deterioration in condition (e.g., 15 minutes, 30 minutes). The clinical signs in each phase of shock are illustrated in Table 35–1.

CLINICAL PEARL

Note that a person may suffer a significant volume loss and not have hypotension. Shock is a clinical syndrome—the diagnosis is not based on the presence or absence of hypotension; rather, it is based on a combination of all the other signs in Table 35–1.

What is a working definition of shock?

Shock is the inadequate oxygen delivery to tissues, usually as a result of inadequate perfusion.

What does perfusion depend on?

Perfusion depends on cardiac output (CO), systemic vascular resistance (SVR), and the transport of oxygen. To have perfusion, you must have blood (fluid), vessels (the pipes), and a working heart (the pump). If anything happens to impact on the blood, the vessels, or the pump, the perfusion suffers. The formula for perfusion is: Cardiac Output = Heart Rate × Stroke Volume (CO = HR × SV).

What is the stroke volume?

The stroke volume is the normal amount of blood ejected from the left ventricle with each contraction of the heart. This is

TABLE 35–1

Clinical Signs and Phases of Shock				
Test	Normal	Mild Shock	Moderate Shock	Severe Shock
Sensorium	Oriented	Slightly anxious but oriented	Anxious, confused	Lethargic, confused, incoherent
Pulse	60–100	100–120	120–150	> 140; rapid, thready
Pupils	Equal, 2–4 mm	Normal	Normal	May be dilated, slow to react
Blood pressure	120/80	110/80	70–90/50–60	< 50–60 systolic
Pulse pressure	40	30	20–30	10–20
Capillary blanch	Normal	Normal	Slow	Very slow
Respiratory rate	12–16	14–20	20–30	> 35
Urine output cc/h	40–50	30–35	15–30	Negligible
Skin	Dry	Slightly moist	Sweaty	Cool, clammy

(From Rothenberg, M.A. 2000. *Pathophysiology: Mechanisms of Disease.*)

usually approximately 70 cc of blood per beat (approximately 4,900 cc per minute).

How does stroke volume relate to the BP?

The formula is: BP = CO × SVR. Stroke volume is a component of the CO (cardiac output is equal to the stroke volume times the heart rate).

To compensate for blood loss, how does the body maintain the BP?

Based on the formula there are two options. Because it is not possible for the body to create more blood on a moment's notice, the heart rate can increase to increase the CO or the SVR can be increased through the constriction of the peripheral vessels. The body cannot increase the stroke volume on a moment's notice by a large amount. In order to increase the SV, you need to do aerobic exercise for more than 20 minutes, three or more times a week, for months. The effect of this type of exercise is the thickening of the left ventricle to increase the SV and make the muscle a more efficient pump (e.g., 100 cc instead of 70 cc).

> *An early sign of hypovolemic shock is a narrowing of the pulse pressure. The systolic pressure drops slightly (due to volume loss) and the diastolic pressure increases (representing vasoconstriction as a compensatory mechanism). This may be difficult to determine without a good baseline for the patient.*

How does the body compensate for decreased perfusion?

The body needs to compensate for decreases in perfusion. Decreased perfusion can be caused by an event that results in blood loss (either internal or external), the loss of vasomotor tone, or a tension pneumothorax that causes a kinking of the great vessels. There are a number of steps that take place, many of them simultaneously, in an effort by the body to compensate for even subtle decreases in perfusion. These steps are:

- Arterial pressure decreases—stimulates baroreceptors located in the carotid sinuses and aortic arch. They sense a decreased flow and activate the vasomotor center which, in turn, causes vasoconstriction of the peripheral vessels. In addition, the sympathetic nervous system is stimulated. If there is a decrease in systolic to less than 80 mmHg, this stimulates the vasomotor center to increase the arterial pressure.

- Sympathetic nervous system—the message from the brain makes its way down the spinal cord to the adrenal gland, which is located on top of the kidneys. The adrenal gland medulla secretes epinephrine and norepinephrine.

  1. Epinephrine has alpha and beta effects. The alpha-1 effects cause vasoconstriction, increases in peripheral vascular resistance, and an increase in afterload from arteriolar constriction. The beta-1 effects cause a positive chronotrophic, iontrophic, and dromotropic effects (affecting the conductivity). The beta-2 effects cause bronchodilation and gut smooth muscle dilation.

  2. Norepinephrine has primarily alpha-1 and alpha-2 effects that cause vasoconstriction, an increase in peripheral vascular resistance, and an increased afterload from arteriolar constriction.

- Arginine vasopressin (AVP)—also known as antidiuretic hormone. It is released from the anterior pituitary gland and increases free water absorption in the distal tubule and collecting ducts of the kidney. It also decreases urine output and splanchnic (visceral) vascular constriction.

- Renin–angiotensin system—renin is released by arterioles in the kidney. It catalyzes the conversion of angiotensinogen to angiotensin I. Angiotensin I is converted to angiotensin II via the angiotensin-converting enzyme (ACE). Angiotensin II is a potent vasoconstrictor that helps to promote sodium reabsorption and decrease urine output. It is also a positive inotrope and chronotrope.

- Aldosterone—secreted by the cells in the adrenal cortex. The aldosterone defends or protects the fluid volume and reduces urine output by promoting sodium reabsorption and water retention by the kidney.

- Insulin—secretion is diminished by circulating epinephrine. Poor perfusion impairs the effect of insulin on peripheral tissue, leading to the failure of cells to take up glucose. This contributes to the hyperglycemic states seen following injury and volume loss.

> *When the body senses hypovolemia, a number of regulatory systems are put into play to try and compensate. These include local vasoconstriction, sympathetic responses (epinephrine, norepinephrine), and endocrine responses (growth hormone, renin–angiotensin, glucagon, ACTH, anti-diuretic hormone).*

- Glucagon—stimulated by the release of epinephrine. It promotes liver glycogenolysis, gluconeogenesis, amino acid uptake for conversion into glucose, and the transfer of fatty acid into mitochondria.

- ACTH (adrenocortisopropic hormone) cortisol system—stimulates the release of cortisol from the adrenal cortex of the kidney and increases glucose production by inhibiting enzymes that break down glucose.

- Growth hormone—secreted by the anterior pituitary gland. Effects include promoting the uptake of glucose and amino acids in the muscles and stimulating protein synthesis. These hormonal changes lead to increased availability of substances that can be converted into adenosine triphosphate (ATP) to provide necessary energy.

What happens when the compensatory mechanisms fail to preserve perfusion?

When the compensatory mechanisms are overwhelmed, the preload decreases, the CO decreases, the myocardial blood supply and oxygenation diminishes, and there are capillary and cellular changes that ultimately lead to irreversible shock.

What are the capillary and cellular changes that occur in lack of perfusion states?

There are three phases the cells go through during decreased perfusion states. They are the ischemic phase, the stagnation phase, and the wash-out phase. Here is what happens in each phase:

- Ischemic phase—there is a minimal blood flow to the capillaries, so the cells switch from aerobic to anerobic metabolism. Anerobic metabolism is less efficient and produces many acids.

- Stagnation phase—the precapillary sphincter relaxes in response to lactic acid, vasomotor center failure, and increased carbon dioxide. The postcapillary sphincters remain constricted, causing the capillaries to engorge with fluid. The anaerobic metabolism continues increasing the lactic acid production that aggregates the red blood cells (RBCs) and forms microemboli. This is a vasodilator that destroys the capillary cell membrane allowing plasma to leak from the capillaries. The interstitial fluid then increases the distance from the capillary to cell that, in turn, decreases the oxygen transport. Finally, some type of "myocardial depressant factor" or "factors" are released, leading to cardiogenic shock.

- Wash-out phase—the postcapillary sphincter relaxes causing hydrogen, potassium, carbon dioxide, and thrombosed erythrocytes to wash out into the circulation. Metabolic acidosis results and the CO drops even further.

What are the "stages" of shock?

There are three stages of shock described in most textbooks: compensated, decompensated and irreversible.

What is compensated shock?

Compensated (nonprogressive shock) is characterized by the signs and symptoms of early shock (e.g., tachypnea, tachycardia, anxiety, pallor). The arterial BP is normal or high. Treatment, such as oxygenation, maintaining body heat, and fluid therapy, at this stage will typically result in recovery.

What is decompensated shock?

Decompensated (progressive shock) is characterized by the signs and symptoms of late shock (e.g., hypotension, AMS, decreased urine output). The treatment at this stage, such as aggressive fluid therapy and oxygenation, will sometimes result in a recovery.

What is irreversible shock?

Irreversible shock is characterized by the signs and symptoms of late shock (e.g., severe hypotension, shutdown of major organs, mordibund appearance), but is refractory to treatment. Even aggressive treatment at this stage does not result in a recovery.

CLINICAL PEARL

People with irreversible shock have clinical findings of late shock and are refractory to treatment. This differs from those with decompensated shock who may still respond. It is impossible to tell the difference initially in the field, so all patients should be managed aggressively.

What are the etiologic classifications of shock?

The etiologic classifications of shock include:

- Hypovolemia—hemorrhage, plasma loss, fluid and electrolyte loss, and endocrine dysfunction (e.g., insulin shock).

- Distributive—increased venous capacitance and low resistance, or vasodilation as can occur with a spinal injury. The types of shock commonly referred to as septic and anaphylactic fit under this category.

- Cardiogenic—loss of 40 percent or more of the functioning ventricular myocardium, regardless of the reason.

- Obstructive—blockage to the heart or great vessels.

Assessment

Q **What is the significance of bright red blood from a wound, mouth, rectum, or other orifice when found during an assessment of the patient?**

A Bright red blood means active arterial bleeding, usually from a laceration or the lungs. When bright red blood comes from the mouth, it is usually due to bleeding in the lungs or from the esophagus. When bright red blood is coming from the rectum (hematochezia), it is often a hemorrhoid and may not always be from the lower GI tract. Patients can bleed to death from rectal bleeding, so this condition should always be taken seriously.

Q **What is the significance of the coffee ground appearance of vomitus when found during an assessment of the patient?**

A When a patient vomits a coffee ground type substance, it can be a mix of upper GI bleeding and the digestive substances from the stomach. Upper GI bleeding causes a very pale and diaphoretic patient and should be taken very seriously. Of course, the coffee ground vomitus could be other substances that were recently eaten and aggravated the stomach, such as chocolate or too much salsa!

Q **What is the significance of dizziness or syncope on sitting or standing (orthostatic hypotension) when found during an assessment of the patient?**

A It suggests significant intravascular volume depletion. A patient can drop their BP enough to decrease the blood supply to the brain and make them temporarily dizzy or lose consciousness. If this condition occurs when they move quickly from the supine to sitting or standing position, it is known as orthostatic or postural hypotension.

CLINICAL PEARL

The presence of orthostatic changes in a person's vital signs suggests intravascular volume depletion. You should also note whether the patient has symptoms (e.g., dizziness, weakness) with postural changes. Other diseases (e.g., inner ear infections) can also cause positional symptoms.

Q **What are the assessment findings of a patient who is in the early or compensated phase of hypovolemia due to hemorrhage?**

A The patient in the early or compensated phase of hypovolemia will have many of the following findings:

- Tachycardia.
- Pale, cool skin.
- Diaphoresis.
- Mental status may be normal, anxious, or apprehensive.
- The BP is maintained.
- Narrow pulse pressure.
- Positive orthostatic tilt test.
- Dry mucosa.
- Complaints of thirst.
- Weakness.
- Possible delay of capillary refill.

CLINICAL PEARL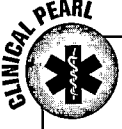

Look at the patient, not the numbers. If the patient looks "shocky," then she is in shock until proven otherwise.

Q **What are the assessment findings of a patient who is in the late or progressive phase of hypovolemic shock?**

A The patient in the late or decompensated phase of hypovolemic shock will have many of the following findings:

- Extreme tachycardia (degenerating to cardiac arrest after about a 40 percent blood loss).
- Extreme palor (white waxy looking skin), cool and clammy (diaphoretic) skin.
- Significant decrease in mental status.
- Hypotension.
- Dry mucosa.
- Nausea.

Q **How do cardiogenic shock assessment findings differ from hypovolemic shock findings?**

A Cardiogenic shock is differentiated from hypovolemic shock by one or more of the following:

- The chief complaint is usually chest pain, dyspnea, or tachycardia.
- The heart rate is usually a bradycardia or an excessive tachycardia.
- The patient may have signs of congestive heart failure (CHF) such as jugular vein distention (JVD), rales, and dysrhythmias.

Q **How do distributive shock assessment findings differ from hypovolemic shock?**

A Distributed shock is differentiated from hypovolemic shock by the presence of one or more of the following findings:

- A mechanism that suggests vasodilation, such as a spinal cord injury, drug overdose, sepsis, or anaphylaxis.
- Warm, flushed skin especially in the dependent areas.
- A lack of tachycardia may occur.

Q **How do obstructive shock assessment findings differ from hypovolemic shock?**

A Obstructive shock can be differentiated from hypovolemic shock by the presence of distended neck veins and a narrowing pulse pressure, suggesting cardiac tamponade or tension pneumothorax.

Management

Q **What is the management of hemorrhage in the field?**

A The bleeding patient should be managed in the following manner:

- Airway and ventilatory support may be necessary.
- External bleeding—control bleeding by direct pressure, elevation if possible, pressure points, and tourniquet (as a last resort to save the life). If the patient has a large gaping wound, it may be smart to pack the wound with a large sterile dressing.
- Apply a pressure bandage with a sterile dressing. Make sure the fingertips or toes can be seen to monitor the patient's distal circulation.
- Internal bleeding—if the patient has internal bleeding, military antishock trousers/pneumatic antishock garments (MAST/PASG) may be useful under certain circumstances. If the patient has bleeding from the ears or nose after a head injury, you should refrain from applying a pressure dressing. Simply apply a loose sterile dressing to protect the patient from infection.
- Consider the need for IV fluid replacement enroute to the hospital. Unless the patient is pinned or trapped, IV fluid replacement should be done while enroute to the hospital to save time. If a patient is continuing to bleed, they can easily lose more blood in the time it takes to start the IV than the IV fluids will actually replace. Indeed, only about one-third of the fluid infused stays in the intravascular space and it does not carry hemoglobin like a transfusion of whole blood does.

- Keep the patient warm.
- Position the patient in the supine or Trendelenburg position.
- Provide emotional and psychological support to the patient.
- Provide prearrival radio report so the receiving hospital will be prepared.

Q **What is the management and treatment plan for hypovolemia?**

A The management of hypovolemia includes the following support:

- Airway and ventilatory support—to include ventilation and suction as necessary. Oxygen administration and reduction of increased intrathoracic pressure in a patient with a tension pneumothorax.
- Circulatory support—hemorrhage control and IV volume expanders. An IV should be started enroute to the hospital rather than on the scene. The exception would be patients who require a lengthy extrication.
- Consider MAST/PASG—depending on your local protocols, this device may be helpful. The key is to apply it early and inflate immediately when the patient fits the protocol.
- Pharmacological interventions—besides volume expanders, positive inotropic agents and vasoconstrictors may be useful if the patient is in cardiogenic or distributive shock.

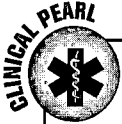 *As a rule, try a fluid challenge first prior to using pressor agents (e.g., dopamine, norepinephrine, vasopressin).*

- Psychological support—continue to communicate with the patient and make all efforts to meet their emotional and physiological needs (e.g., warmth with blankets and compassion).

Psychological support is an integral part of the treatment of any patient for any problem.

- Transport the patient as soon as possible to the appropriate facility. This may involve removal directly to a trauma center and the use of aeromedical transportation.

Q **What are the indications and contraindications, and an example of each, of certain IV volume expanders: isotonic solutions, hypertonic solutions, synthetic solutions, blood and blood products, experimental solutions, and blood substitutes?**

A There are a number of IV volume expanders used in the field or ED setting. At the time of this writing, there is still considerable controversy in some circles regarding the use of IV fluids, especially in trauma. If IV fluids are used, most agree that the best volume expander in the out-of-hospital setting is normal saline. Volume expanders include:

- Isotonic solutions—have the same tonicity (osmolarity) as plasma; normal saline or Ringer's lactate.

- Hypertonic solutions—are more concentrated than plasma; not routinely used in- or out-of-hospital; hypertonic saline.

- Synthetic solutions—are usually hypertonic, containing a high weight molecule, such as dextran and hetastarch (Hespan®); not routinely used in the field.

- Blood and blood products—plasma derivatives (Plasmanate®) or concentrated albumin solutions are used as volume expanders in out-of-hospital care in Australia and Europe. They are not used routinely in North America. Blood transfusions are beneficial for hemorrhagic shock, and are usually done in-hospital.

- Experimental solutions—several such solutions have shown promise with hypovolemic shock, but are not available for clinical use. These include stroma-free hemoglobin and combinations of hypertonic saline and high molecular weight dextran.

- Blood substitutes—"artificial blood" (Fluosol®) is available clinically and appears to be beneficial in selected patients; it is not used routinely in out-of-hospital care.

> **CLINICAL PEARL**
>
> *The fluid controversy is ongoing. In general, most EMS systems use normal saline. For trauma, the accepted approach is fluid therapy despite a few studies that have disputed this. Follow your local protocols.*

Pneumatic Antishock Garment

Q **What happened to military antishock trousers/pneumatic antishock garments (MAST/PASG)?**

A No other device used in out-of-hospital care has undergone the intense scrutiny that MAST/PASG has gone through in the past decade. In the 1960s and 70s, MAST/PASG was routinely carried on most ALS units and many BLS units as the device of choice for patients who were thought to be in shock. In the 1980s, EMS went through the "prove it to me era" where research studies were undertaken to try to prove the effectiveness of a number of devices and medications used by EMS providers. It was clear that most devices seemed to be useful, but the data did not show that they reduced the patient morbidity or mortality. Some studies, focused directly on the use of MAST/PASG in the field, have often been taken out of context and used to totally eliminate the use of the device.

So, the pendulum has swung back in the opposite direction and today MAST/PASG is rarely used. Some states have downplayed MAST/PASG from their protocols lists, while others, such as New York, have developed a protocol that dictates the device may only be used with a patient who has a systolic of 50 mmHg or less. Because a systolic of 50 mmHg is difficult to detect without a Doppler, a device rarely carried on ambulances, this narrows the utilization of the device considerably.

The authors of this text believe that there is a happy medium and the pendulum needs to swing back to the center again because there are some situations where MAST/PASG should be used. We have seen it improve the patient's BP in the presence of decompensated shock many times. With a good focus on minimizing the scene time, IV fluids enroute to the hospital, and an emphasis on adequate ventilation of the patient in shock, MAST/PASG does have its place in helping buy the patient some time until the internal bleeding can be controlled in the surgical suite.

Q **What data have "supported" the decreased use of MAST/PASG?**

A An oft-quoted study of MAST/PASG used in an urban setting with hypotensive penetrating trauma victims concluded that the suit offered ". . . no specific advantage in an urban paramedic-regional trauma center system that is closely scrutinized by full-time physician supervision that emphasizes rapid response and evacuation along with aggressive prehospital airway management and immediate in-hospital surgical intervention" (Pepe et al., 1986). It should be noted that the data in this particular study pertain to a system dealing mainly with penetrating trauma and short response times (Bickell et al., 1987; Mattox et al., 1986). These conclusions are not necessarily applicable in other localities. Medical patients were not included in the study.

> **CLINICAL PEARL**
>
> *Studies on MAST/PASG have been limited, in general, to trauma patients (usually with penetrating injuries) in specific geographic areas. It is scientifically incorrect to extrapolate these results to every EMS system in the world.*

[Q] What are the effects of MAST/PASG?

[A] Inflation of MAST/PASG leads to increased BP and increased organ perfusion to areas above the level of the suit.

[Q] What is the mechanism by which MAST/PASG works?

[A] One of the most hotly debated topics in the literature today is the physiology of MAST/PASG. Originally, it was taught that the garment increases BP due to an "autotransfusion" of up to two units of blood (500–1,000 cc). Several studies have suggested that the primary action is really increasing the SVR (constricting the blood vessels) and tamponading bleeding vessels. Other studies, though, have suggested at least a component of "auto-transfusion," though the literature must be examined carefully.

TABLE 35-2

"Classic" MAST/PASG Indications
• Hypovolemic shock.
• Cardiac tamponade.
• Pneumothorax.
• Fracture stabilization (e.g., pelvis, femur).
• Prophylactic prior to medevac.

(From Rothenberg, M. A. 2000. *Pathophysiology: Mechanisms of Disease*)
NOTE: The best accepted indication currently is stabilization of pelvic fractures.

PEARL

After reviewing this data, it is safe to conclude that many of the MAST/PASG models appear to increase the BP. It is likely that the mechanism by which hypotension is reversed differs depending on the clinical situation. It is possible that several mechanisms may be operating together. It does not appear that the "autotransfusion theory" is completely ruled out nor that the "increased SVR" is totally proven at this time.

[Q] What are the indications for use of MAST/PASG?

[A] The classic indications appear in Table 35–2.

[Q] What are the contraindications for MAST/PASG?

[A] Contraindications include pulmonary edema, CHF, pregnancy, cardiogenic shock, penetrating chest trauma, and chest injuries.

[Q] What is all the controversy with MAST/PASG?

[A] The controversy centers on whether or not MAST/PASG offers any clinical benefit. Unfortunately, current studies have been noninclusive, skewed, or otherwise biased. On balance, data supports that MAST/PASG is of benefit to people with significant hypotension (systolic BP <50 mmHg) and who do not have a penetrating chest trauma. Despite these data, many EMS systems have relegated use of MAST/PASG to the stabilization of pelvic and femur fractures.

PEARL

MAST/PASG is an alternative, albeit one used infrequently. Just because some studies are anecdotal and "nonacademic" in nature, doesn't mean that MAST/PASG might not work in certain patients. These "nonsupportive" articles continue to emerge as case reports. Remember that the American College of Emergency Physicians still recommends that the MAST/PASG suit be available for immediate use in hospital EDs (1997). Finally, military physicians (the "military" in MAST) still argue that MAST/PASG is useful in a combat setting.

Special Thanks

Table 35–1 and 35–2 are reproduced with permission from *Pathophysiology: Mechanisms of Disease* by Mikel A. Rothenberg, M.D., © 2000.

Pepe, P. E., et al. (1986, December). Clinical trials of the pneumatic shock garment in the urban setting. *Annals of Emergency Medicine, 15,* 1407.

Bickell, W. H., et al. (1987). Randomized trial on pneumatic antishock garments in the prehospital management of penetrating abdominal injuries. *Annals of Emergency Medicine, 16,* 653–658.

Mattox, K. L., et al. (1986). Prospective randomized evaluation of antishock MAST in post-traumatic hypotension. *Journal of Trauma, 26,* 779–786.

American College of Emergency Physicians. (1997, April 29). Emergency care guidelines. *Annals of Emergency Medicine, 4,* 564–571.

CHAPTER 36

Soft Tissue Trauma

This chapter discusses soft tissue injuries. It includes both open and closed injuries, as well as some minor to major wounds. The focus is on *why* patients present in a certain manner and *why* you need to respond in certain ways to their presenting problems.

Epidemiology

Q **What is the incidence of soft tissue trauma?**

A Specific figures on the incidence of soft tissue trauma are unavailable due to the many types that may occur. Any bump or bruise is technically considered "soft tissue trauma." As such, the incidence is extremely high. On the other hand, if we include only severe bruises and soft tissue hematomas, the incidence drops significantly, depending on the injury. Lacerations and contusions are, however, commonly seen in the field at motor vehicle collisions and incidents of abuse and assault.

Q **What is the mortality and morbidity from soft tissue trauma?**

A Though specific "numbers" are not available for reasons stated previously, soft tissue trauma may be fatal, even without deep injuries. Two common examples are soft tissue hematomas (e.g., bleeding into the thigh space or the scalp space) and secondary infection. Necrotizing fasciitis, which is an inflammation of the fascia causing tissue death, is essentially a gas gangrene of

the skin and fascia and may occur following an apparently minor soft tissue injury. The condition is due to a streptococcal infection of the deep tissues that results in a progressive destruction of both the fascia and fat.

Q **What are the risk factors for soft tissue trauma?**

A Any physical activity that increases the exposure of the skin to the environment and physical forces will increase the risk of a soft tissue injury. Activities such as contact sports (e.g., boxing, hockey, football) and those involving high speed (e.g., skiing, biking, rollerblading) increase the risk of soft tissue trauma. Motor vehicle collisions, falls, assaults, and violence all contribute significantly to the risk of soft tissue trauma.

Q **What prevention strategies should be considered to avoid soft tissue trauma?**

A Because it is not uncommon for trauma to occur without a corresponding soft tissue injury, all of the prevention strategies listed in Chapter 3, Illness and Injury Prevention, are appropriate. Specifically, people should be educated about the value of covering up their skin when participating in activities that could

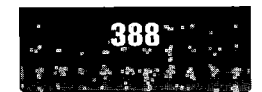

easily injure it. For example, even though it may be a hot sunny day, when riding on a motorcycle, long pants and long sleeves should always be worn to decrease the potential for a serious "road rash" abrasion in the event of a collision.

Q **What are the terms used to describe different types of skin lesions?**

A There are many names for the various lesions. They are shown and described in Figure 36–1.

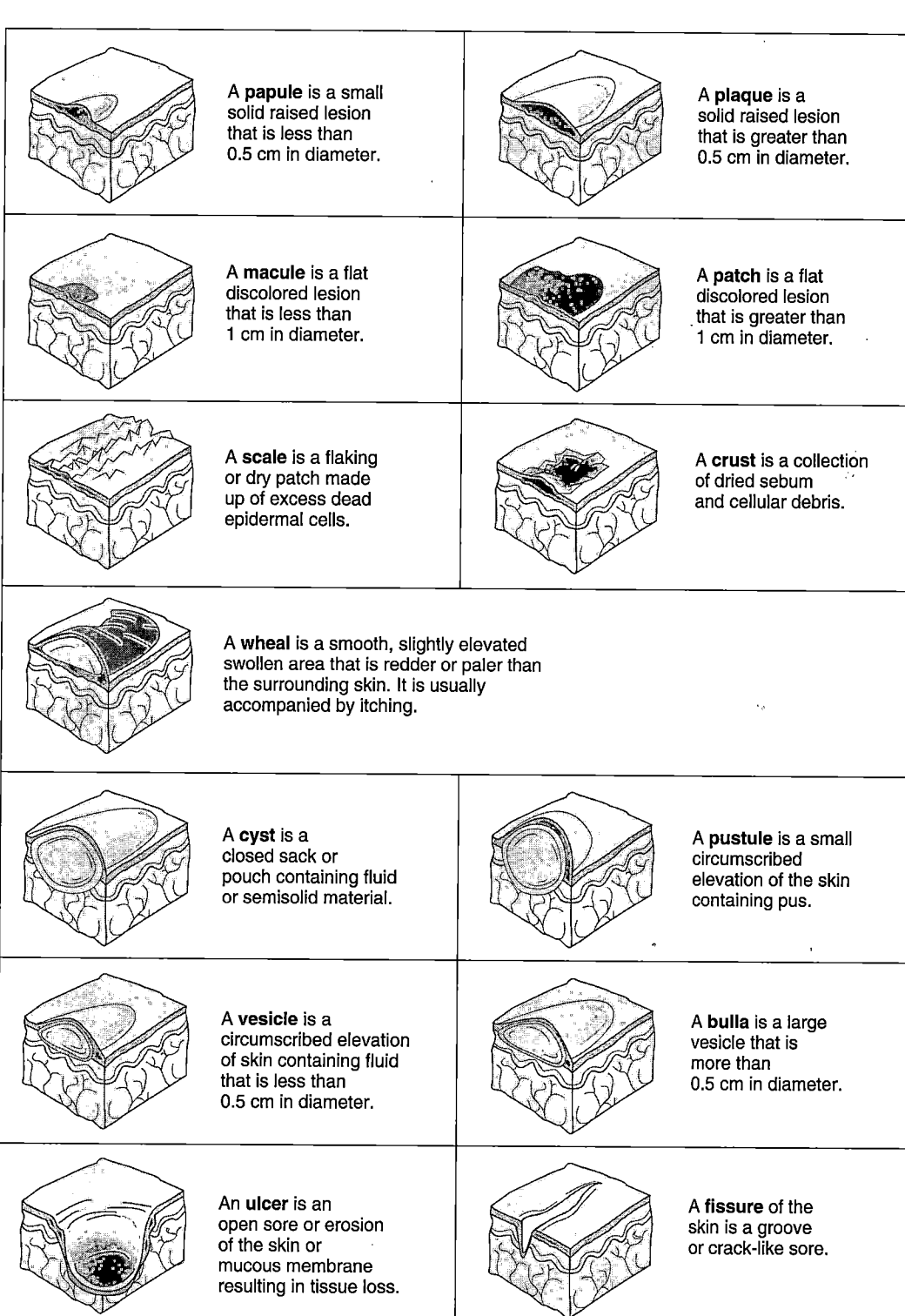

A **papule** is a small solid raised lesion that is less than 0.5 cm in diameter.

A **plaque** is a solid raised lesion that is greater than 0.5 cm in diameter.

A **macule** is a flat discolored lesion that is less than 1 cm in diameter.

A **patch** is a flat discolored lesion that is greater than 1 cm in diameter.

A **scale** is a flaking or dry patch made up of excess dead epidermal cells.

A **crust** is a collection of dried sebum and cellular debris.

A **wheal** is a smooth, slightly elevated swollen area that is redder or paler than the surrounding skin. It is usually accompanied by itching.

A **cyst** is a closed sack or pouch containing fluid or semisolid material.

A **pustule** is a small circumscribed elevation of the skin containing pus.

A **vesicle** is a circumscribed elevation of skin containing fluid that is less than 0.5 cm in diameter.

A **bulla** is a large vesicle that is more than 0.5 cm in diameter.

An **ulcer** is an open sore or erosion of the skin or mucous membrane resulting in tissue loss.

A **fissure** of the skin is a groove or crack-like sore.

FIGURE 36–1 There are many different types of skin lesions.

What is the difference between static and dynamic skin tension lines?

The skin does not just hang on the flesh; rather, it follows the contours of the underlying structures. This creates a natural stretch or tension in the skin called tension lines. There are two types of tension lines: static and dynamic. Static tension is the constant force due to taut nature of skin. Underlying muscle contraction causes dynamic tension. The effect of the tension on the skin can be seen when the skin is cut, as in a laceration, and pulls apart. Cuts that run parallel to a tension line tend to gape open very little, whereas cuts that run perpendicular to a tension line often create a wide gaping opening.

What are the phases of normal wound healing?

Wound healing involves a number of changes in the normal skin anatomy including the following:

- Hemostasis—reflex vasoconstriction for 10 minutes; then clotting begins.
- Inflammation—involves granulocytes, lymphocytes, and macrophages. These cells "invade" the blood clot and release mediators that help fight local infection, as well as initiate the healing process.
- Epithelialization—wound healing through the reestablishment of skin layers during the first 12 hours.
- Neovascularization—involves new vessel formation between 3 and 21 days.
- Collagen synthesis—involves fibroblasts; these form scar tissue that holds the wound edges tightly together.

What are examples of anatomic factors that can alter normal wound healing?

Normal wound healing may be altered by the following anatomic factors:

- Body region.
- Static skin tension—an area perpendicular to a tension line that "wants" to stay open due to the tension.
- Dynamic skin tension—an area that is prone to movement.
- Pigmented skin.
- Oily skin.

Can certain drugs taken by the patient affect normal wound healing?

Yes, normal wound healing can be slowed if the patient is taking any of the following types of drugs: corticosteroids, non-steroidal anti-inflammatory drugs, penicillin, colchicines, anti-coagulants, and antineoplastic agents.

Can certain medical conditions affect normal wound healing?

Yes, a number of medical conditions and diseases can affect normal wound healing, such as advanced age, severe alcoholism, acute uremia, diabetes, hypoxia, severe anemia, malnutrition, advanced cancer, hepatic failure, cardiovascular disease, acquired immunodeficiency syndrome, and any form of immune system suppression.

What types of wounds are considered high risk for healing problems and infection?

Wounds that have a high potential for infection from pathogens are considered high risk for healing problems. Examples include bites from humans or animals, foreign bodies, wounds contaminated with organic matter, injected wounds, wounds with significant devitalized tissue, and crush wounds.

What is keloid scar formation?

The excessive accumulation of scar tissue that extends beyond the original wound borders is called a keloid scar. These are more common in dark pigmented people and often occur on the ears, upper extremities, lower abdomen, and sternum.

What is hypertrophic scar formation?

The excessive accumulation of scar tissue confined within the original wound borders is called a hypertrophic scar formation. These are more common in areas of high tissue stress such as flexion creases across joints.

Which wounds require closure?

Large gaping wounds require closure. Plastic surgery is often requested for wounds to cosmetic regions such as the face, lip, and eyebrow. This list may involve many other body regions depending on the patient's occupation. For example, a model would be very concerned about his legs and arms. Other types of injuries that often require closure include wounds over tension areas, degloving injuries, ring injuries, and skin tears.

> **CLINICAL PEARL**
>
> *It is sometimes difficult to tell in the field whether or not a wound will require sutures. It is always best to err on the conservative side and recommend physician evaluation. The delayed closure of wounds results in an increased rate of wound infections and a less cosmetically acceptable scar.*

Pathophysiology and Assessment

Q What are the three general categories of closed soft tissue injuries?

A The three closed soft tissue injuries are contusions, hematomas, and crushing injuries.

Q What happens when a patient experiences a contusion?

A With a contusion, the epidermis remains intact. The cells are damaged and the blood vessels in the dermis are usually torn. This causes swelling and pain, which can be delayed for up to 24 to 48 hours after the injury. Blood accumulates causing ecchymosis.

Q What happens when a patient experiences a hematoma?

A There is a collection of blood beneath the skin. Generally there is a larger amount of tissue damage compared to a contusion. The vessels that are damaged are usually larger and the patient could lose one or more liters of blood in a confined space.

CLINICAL PEARL

Two soft tissue areas that are especially worrisome are the thigh and underneath the scalp. A person may bleed to death by extravasating blood within either area and the clinical findings may be minimal (except for shock).

Q What happens when a patient experiences a crushing injury?

A A crushing force is applied to the body. This pressure can cause internal organ rupture and is often associated with severe fractures. Although the overlying skin appears intact, there often is internal bleeding that can be severe and involve shock.

Q What are the types of open soft tissue injuries and what is unique to each?

A The types of open soft tissue injuries include the following:
- Abrasion—the outermost layer of the skin is damaged by shearing forces. This is a painful injury, usually superficial involving little bleeding, sometimes oozing blood, where contamination is the biggest worry.
- Laceration—breaks in the skin of varying depth that may be linear (regular) or stellate (irregular). The jagged wound is

caused by forceful impact with a sharp object and the ends usually bleed freely. A laceration may occur in isolation or together with other types of soft tissue injury and the bleeding may at times be severe.
- Incision—a break in the skin of varying depth, usually caused by very sharp objects such as a knife, sharp metal, or scalpel. These injuries are similar to lacerations except the wound ends are smooth and even. They tend to heal better than lacerations due to the constricting of the vessels.
- Major artery laceration—when a laceration occurs to a major artery, the bleeding is severe, spurting and bright red in color. The artery may spasm, decreasing the blood flow. The patient can literally spurt most of their blood volume out. The result may be shock or death when a major artery is lacerated with a gaping cut.
- Avulsion—a flap of loose torn tissue that may not be viable for reimplantation.
- Amputation—involves an extremity or other body part and the jagged skin or bone edges are typically present at the site of amputation. The patient may have massive bleeding or the bleeding may be controlled (e.g., patient run over by a subway train has a leg amputated, but there is little bleeding because the heat of the train cauterized the wound. There are three types of amputations: complete, partial, and degloving. A degloving injury is one in which the outer skin of the hand is removed in a manner similar to removing tight gloves—"inside-out."
- Blast injuries—involve an initial air blast causing compression injuries to the air-filled organs (e.g., ear drum, sinuses, lungs, stomach, and intestines). The secondary injuries are due to flying debris striking the patient. Then, tertiary injuries are caused when the patient is thrown from the blast and strikes a hard object.
- Punctures and penetrations—caused by a foreign object entering the body. The bleeding is usually minimal or absent if the injury occurs in an extremity; however, the potential for infection is great. The bleeding can be severe if the object is impaled in the thorax or abdomen. The underlying thoracic injuries can be extensive (e.g., simple open or tension pneumothorax; hemothorax; pericardial tamponade; penetrating heart wound; rupture of the esophagus, aorta, diaphragm, or mainstem bronchus). The underlying abdominal injuries can involve either hollow or solid organs with the potential for a bacterial or chemical peritonitis. The patient may also have an evisceration.
- Impaled object—this is a specific type of puncture where an instrument remains impacted in the wound and needs to be stabilized in the field. Removal is often done in the ED or surgery suite in preparation for the possibility of further damage and increased bleeding.

- Crushing injury—sustained from a compressive force sufficient to interfere with the normal metabolic function of the involved tissue. The patient may have the "crush syndrome," also called traumatic rhabdomyolysis (discussed later) and what has come to be known as "smiling death." This occurs with the patient who seems to be doing well while the concrete slab is on top of them. When the slab is removed and the pressure is lifted, they suddenly go into cardiac arrest due to the massive release of toxins (particularly potassium) from ruptured muscles into their blood stream. Field management is focused on aggressive fluid administration and the administration of sodium bicarbonate to neutralize the acids.

What is rhabdomyolysis?

Rhabdomyolysis is the destruction of muscle from a crushing type injury. There is an influx into the muscle of water, sodium chloride, and calcium from the extracellular fluid. Then, there is an efflux from the muscles into the extracellular fluid of potassium, purines from the disintegrating cell nuclei, phosphates, lactic acids, myoglobin, thromboplastin, creatine kinase, and creatinine.

The consequences of this movement of chemicals contribute to renal failure because hypovolemia, hypocalcemia, and hyperkalemia add to cardiotoxicity. The patient becomes hyperuricemic, high in phosphate, and develops metabolic acidosis and possible DIC (disseminated intravascular coagulation; a severe state consisting of concomitant activation of the clotting system and bleeding due to consumption of clotting factors). There are also increased levels of serum creatinine.

What are the causes of crush injuries?

Crush injuries can be caused by the collapse of masonry or steel structures, from earthquakes, tornadoes, or construction accidents. Other causes of a crush injury can include mudslides, avalanches, motor vehicle collisions, warfare injuries, industrial accidents, and any prolonged compression in a chronic situation (e.g., prolonged application of MAST/PASG, improperly applied cast, unconscious patient lying on an extremity).

What is the pathophysiology of a crush syndrome?

After the initial damage to the soft tissue and internal organs, continued pressure prevents adequate oxygenation of tissues. The cells in the crushed tissue are starved for oxygen and anaerobic metabolism occurs. Various compounds accumulate that are a result of local inflammation. These include oxygen free radicals, which are highly reactive chemical intermediates. They react with cell membranes, damaging them and leading to the formation of more free radicals in a process known as lipid peroxidation. Weakened cell walls allow an influx of calcium, further disrupting cellular metabolism. Enzymes, such as xanthine oxidase, are activated, leading to the formation of more toxic mediators (e.g., uric acid). Many of these compounds are released into the patient's systemic circulation when the object is suddenly lifted off the patient. The result is often acute shock and cardiac arrest.

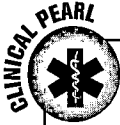

Always be prepared for "release shock" when a patient has the crush force removed.

What is the pathophysiology of compartment syndrome?

The direct soft tissue trauma causes edema and ischemia. The tissue pressure rises above the capillary hydrostatic pressure resulting in ischemia to the muscle. Edema of the muscle cells develops. A prolonged period of ischemia, greater than six to eight hours, leads to tissue hypoxia and anoxia, and ultimately cell death.

What is the clinical presentation of a compartment syndrome?

The patient may be alert to unresponsive. An affected limb may appear almost normal. The local signs and symptoms can include any of the following:

- Flaccid paralysis and sensory loss that are unrelated to peripheral nerve distribution.
- The presentation can look like a spinal cord injury.
- In the early phase, there may be rigor of the joint distal to the involved muscles, giving an appearance of a "wooden texture" to the affected skin and muscles, and the loss of voluntary contraction.
- Varying combination of pain, swelling, and sensory changes.
- The patient may have pulses and present with warm skin.

What are the *Ps* of compartment syndrome?

A patient experiencing a compartment syndrome may have the following signs and symptoms: pain, paresthesia (the sensation of "pins and needles"), paresis (weakness), pressure, passive stretch pain, and pulselessness.

What are the typical causes of blast injuries?

Blast injuries can occur from any explosion. They are often more serious when they occur inside a confined space. Examples include natural gas or gasoline explosions, firework explosions, dust in a grain elevator, and terrorist bombs.

Management

Q What are the treatment priorities for soft tissue injuries?

A The treatment priorities for soft tissue injuries include the following:

- Ensure the scene is safe for you and your crew.
- Assess and manage the mental status and ABCs before dealing with the soft tissue injury.
- Treat for hypoperfusion.
- Consider the power of the explosion in blast situations.
- Consider that both internal and external injuries are possible.
- Be aware of the possibility of multiple trauma.
- Control the hemorrhage with the most appropriate method.

CLINICAL PEARL

Some soft tissue injuries are impressive looking. Don't forget the basics—ABCs. These always come first, no matter how "fascinating" the wound may be.

Q What are the methods of hemorrhage control?

A The methods of hemorrhage control include:

- Direct pressure.
- Elevation.
- Pressure dressing.
- Pressure points.
- Tourniquet application.

Q What is the purpose of direct pressure to control a hemorrhage?

A Direct pressure is the quickest and most efficient means of bleeding control. Be sure to take body substance isolation (BSI) precautions when applying pressure directly to the wound. The purpose is to limit additional significant blood loss and promote localized clotting. Assess the effectiveness of direct pressure by determining whether the bleeding has been controlled.

Never remove a dressing once it is in place; if possible, secure it with a bandage. If direct pressure is not effective, add

more dressings layered on top of the original one. Then, consider elevation of the extremity with direct pressure. Finally, consider the application of pressure on a pressure point.

Q What is the purpose of elevation to control a hemorrhage?

A The intent is to raise the wound above the heart to allow gravity to decrease the BP in the extremity, slowing the hemorrhage and promoting clotting. Elevation is indicated in all situations where direct pressure is not enough to stop the bleeding (with a few exceptions). Do not elevate the extremity if there is a possible musculoskeletal injury to the involved extremity or a large impaled object in the extremity. If the patient has a spinal injury, it is not a good idea to elevate an extremity if it interferes with spinal immobilization.

Q What is the purpose of the pressure dressing?

A Wrapping a dressing firmly with self-adhering roller bandage or Kling® provides continuous mechanical pressure on the wound site. The pressure bandage is designed to limit additional significant blood loss with continuous pressure and to promote local clotting. It is indicated for hemorrhage control when direct pressure and elevation have not controlled the bleeding. A pressure bandage should not be used on a head wound when head injury is suspected. Do not use a circumferential bandage on the neck. After applying a pressure bandage, check for a distal pulse. The bandage should not be so tight as to create an arterial tourniquet and impede the flow of arterial blood to the distal extremity.

Q What is the purpose of using pressure point to control a hemorrhage?

A A pressure point is a location where an artery runs over a bone and is close to the skin. Generally, the pressure points are the same locations where one would palpate a pulse; however, when compressing the pressure point, the EMS provider simply presses harder to occlude the flow of blood. The most common examples are the femoral artery and the brachial artery as shown in Figure 36–2. The intent when compressing a pressure point is to decrease the flow of blood to the extremity so additional blood loss can be minimized and clotting promoted. Using the pressure point is indicated in situations where bleeding is not controlled by direct pressure, elevation, and a pressure bandage. The patient may complain of a tingling sensation in the extremity. This is normal because the blood supply is being cut off to the extremity.

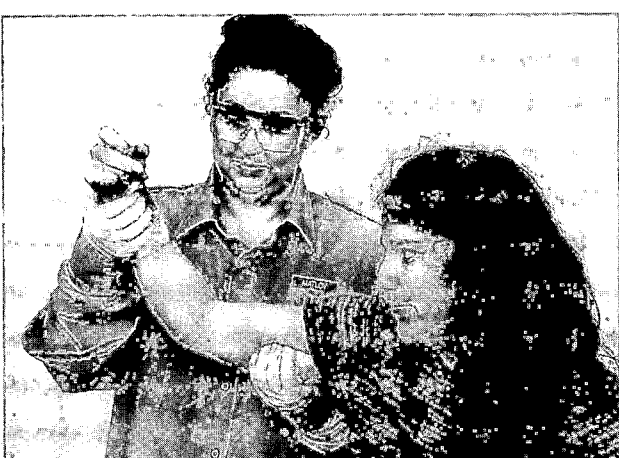

FIGURE 36-2 The EMS provider is using direct pressure, elevation, and the brachial artery pressure point to control bleeding.

What is the purpose of using an arterial tourniquet?

Arterial tourniquets are seldom used because using a pressure point is usually effective to control serious bleeding. The tourniquet is considered a last resort of bleeding control and is placed within two inches of the wound. The tourniquet should only be considered after all other means of bleeding control have been ineffective. Once applied, the result may be that you will lose the limb to save the life. Do not apply a tourniquet directly around a knee or elbow, because there is too much bone in that area and it will not adequately control the bleeding.

When applying a tourniquet, do not use wire, string, or rope because that will merely cut the skin and tissue. Use a wide band of cloth and once applied, do not loosen it. As soon as possible, make sure that the hospital knows when the tourniquet was applied.

What is the difference between a sterile and non-sterile dressing?

A sterile dressing has gone through the sterilization process to eliminate bacteria from the material and should be used when infection is a concern. A nonsterile dressing has not gone through the process of sterilization and is used when something clean is acceptable and infection is not a concern.

What is an occlusive dressing?

An occlusive dressing does not allow for the passage of air through the dressing. It is useful for wounds involving the thorax and major vessels. The application of an occlusive dressing may prevent a negative pressure that can cause air to enter the thorax or vessel. The occlusive dressing may also prevent pneumothorax and air embolism.

What is an adherent dressing?

A dressing that is designed to adhere to a wound surface by incorporating wound exudates into the dressing mesh. It can also assist in controlling acute bleeding.

What is a nonadherent dressing?

A nonadherent dressing allows the passage of wound exudates so that the dressing will not adhere to the wound surface. The dressing has been designed so it does not damage the surface of the wound when it is removed. These are often used after wound closure.

What are the complications of improperly applied dressings?

Improperly applied dressings may impede hemorrhage control, increase tissue damage, and increase the risk of a wound infection. In addition, improper technique may result in unnecessary patient discomfort.

What types of open wounds should be transported for further evaluation?

When a patient has an open wound, it should be dressed and bandaged unless the patient is so critical that your emphasis is on higher priorities. Consider transport versus patient discharge on-scene when there are open wounds. The patient may need a tetanus shot or proper cleansing and dressing of the wound. Patients should be transported for further evaluation in the ED if they present with the following:

- Wounds with nerve, vascular, muscular, tendon, or ligament compromise.
- Wounds with heavy contamination.
- Wounds with cosmetic complications.
- Wounds with a foreign body complication.

What are the immunization recommendations for tetanus?

All patients should have a tetanus shot every 10 years. The tetanus bacterium is ubiquitous. That is to say it pops up in many places at the same time. Frequent vaccination helps maintain our serum antibody levels to prevent this potentially fatal infection.

What are the causes of wound infection and how can EMS providers minimize infection?

Wounds get infected by the bacteria that enter from the device that punctured the skin, the dirt that was rubbed into them, the dirty cloth that was used to control the bleeding, and many other sources. EMS providers can minimize the infection potential by covering open wounds with a sterile dressing and clean dry bandage. Do not allow the bandage to get wet because it will act as a wick and draw bacteria into the wound. Transport the patient to the ED where the wound can be properly cleansed, debrided as needed, closed, and a topical ointment applied. If necessary, an antibiotic may be prescribed for the patient, and their immunizations can be brought current.

Q What are the special considerations for the treatment of an amputated part?

A The stump should be dressed and bandaged after the bleeding is controlled. The amputated part should be wrapped in a sterile, moist gauze pad and placed in a plastic bag. Then, place the bag on ice. Be careful to ensure that the tissue does not freeze. Never use dry ice because it can actually burn the tissue. Make sure both the patient and the amputated part are taken to the same hospital, preferably one that can do reimplantation.

Q When should a surgeon be summoned to the scene to do an emergency amputation?

A This should be done when there will be a prolonged extrication and failing to amputate would result in the patient's certain death.

> **CLINICAL PEARL**
>
> *On-scene amputations occur far more often on television than in the real world of emergency medicine. Modern extrication tools allow quicker access so that even the most entangled patient may be stabilized on-scene during extrication. If the delay would result in near certain death, a limb versus life decision must be made.*

Q What are the goals of the treatment of a crush injury?

A The goals are to prevent sudden death and renal failure, salvage limbs, institute management as early as possible in the field before the patient is actually extricated, and ensure that the ABCs are maintained.

Q How much fluid is given to the crush injury patient?

A It is not uncommon for the patient to be given 1 to 1.5 liters by bolus and up to 12 liters during the first 24 hours.

Q What is meant by alkalinization of the urine for a crush injury?

A The goal is to maintain a urine pH >6.5. Sodium bicarbonate, 50 meq, is added to the initial IV fluids. This controls hyperkalemia and acidosis to prevent myoglobinuria renal failure. Alkalinization of the urine may be started in the field on order of medical control and continued in the ED.

Q What is done to maintain urine output in the crush injury patient?

A The goal of diuresis is to have at least 300 cc per hour. With permission from medical control, the paramedic should consider mannitol (10 g or 20 percent solution to each liter of IV fluid). The use of loop diuretics, such as furosemide (Lasix®), is not recommended because they acidify the urine. The "ideal fluid" for a crush injury is D5 one-half normal saline with one ampule of sodium bicarbonate and 10 g or 20 percent solution mannitol.

Maintaining the urine output treats hypovolemia, corrects the acidosis, and treats the hyperkalemia. This prevents sudden cardiac dysrhythmias and renal failure.

Q Is there any other treatment that should be considered for the crush injured patient?

A It is helpful to treat the hyperkalemia by forced alkaline diuresis and consider insulin or glucose for severe cases (25 cc D50W followed by 10 units of regular insulin IV). This is generally not done in the field because of the inability to determine electrolyte levels in the field. The most important treatment is observing the presence of ECG changes or dysrhythmias. In that case, calcium chloride (1 to 3 cc IV in an adult) is indicated. Of course, follow your local protocols.

Q Is there any value to using hyperbaric oxygen treatment for the patient with a crush injury?

A Some experts recommend hyperbaric oxygen to prevent gangrene and improve healing in crush injuries. Contact medical control for further recommendations.

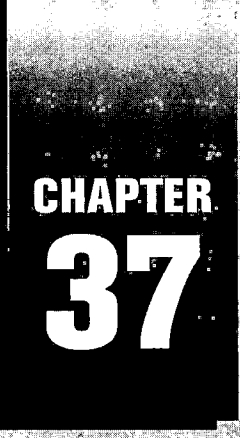

CHAPTER 37

Burns

This chapter discusses burn injuries. Burns can vary from minor to life threatening and leave patients scarred for life. The focus is on *why* patients present in a certain manner and *why* you need to respond in a certain way to their presenting problems. Actions properly done in the first few minutes can help to shorten the recovery time of the patient.

Epidemiology and Prevention

What is the incidence of burn injury?

Each year, an estimated 1.25 million people are burned severely enough to seek treatment. Those who are at the highest risk are the elderly (from impairment of mobility or sensation) and children (from child abuse).

Approximately 80 percent of the fire- and burn-related deaths are the result of a house fire. Smoke inhalation, scalds, contact, and electrical burns are especially likely to occur in children less than four years old. Burns are the leading cause of trauma in the toddler and preschool-age child. Experts advise that families should lock up matches and keep children away from outlets and stoves.

What is the impact of burn injury mortality and morbidity?

Burns account for approximately 5–10 percent of trauma deaths. Burn injuries are responsible for significant long-term morbidity in terms of work loss and scar tissue formation.

What are some of the prevention strategies promoted to decrease the number of scalding injuries in children?

According to the Burn Prevention Foundation, the number of scald injuries from hot liquids is significant; they are the number one cause of burn injury in children under the age of four. The following are examples of strategies that can be taken to prevent these injuries:

- Never leave cooking unattended.
- Cook on the back burners whenever possible and turn pot handles toward the rear of the stove so they are out of the reach of small children.
- Never drink hot liquids while holding a child.
- Keep electrical cords short on appliances such as coffee makers or deep fat fryers. The cords can be pulled off the countertop.
- Do not use a microwave to warm a baby's bottle. The hot spots could scald a tender young mouth.
- Be very careful with foods that have just been cooked in a microwave as they may be extremely hot on the inside. When the container top is removed, you can get burned by the steam that has built up inside.

- Turn down the hot water heater to approximately 100 degrees. It should never be above 120 degrees. Water at 133 degrees can cause a third degree burn in 15 seconds.
- Always test the temperature of a child's bath water with the back of your wrist or elbow prior to allowing the child to enter the water.
- Never leave a child alone in a bathtub. Besides the chance of drowning, the child can receive a scald injury by turning on the hot water.

Pathophysiology, Assessment, and Types of Burns

[Q] What are the pathophysiologic and systemic complications of burn injury?

[A] The pathophysiologic and systemic complications of burn injury are as follows:

- Fluid and electrolyte loss.
- Increased catecholamine release and dysrhythmias.
- Hypoxia, anoxia, and acidosis.
- Vasoconstriction and hypovolemia.
- Renal, liver, and heart failure.
- Formation of an eschar and the complications of a circumferential burn (burn that goes completely around a part of the body).
- Hypothermia.
- Infection.

[Q] What are the types of burn injuries?

[A] The common types of burn injuries include: thermal, inhalation, chemical, electrical, lighting, and radiation burns.

[Q] What are the depths of burn classifications?

[A] The classifications of burn injury depths include superficial burn, partial-thickness burn, and full-thickness burn.

[Q] What is the description of each classification of burn depth?

[A] A superficial burn (or first degree) involves the outer surface, epidermis layer, of the skin only. A partial-thickness (or second degree) burn involves that outermost layer of skin, the

epidermis, as well as the dermal layer. A full-thickness (or third degree) burn involves all layers of the skin and may include charring of tissue.

CLINICAL PEARL

Some burn experts also include a fourth-degree burn in the classification. This includes underlying muscle and soft tissue below the skin layer.

[Q] What are the methods for determining the body surface area burned?

[A] The rule of nines has traditionally been taught to EMS providers for many years (Figure 37–1). There is a version of the rule of nines that is designed for the pediatric patient that takes into consideration the increased body surface area (BSA) on the head. As an alternative, the EMS provider can always use the surface area of the patient's palm (minus the digits) to correspond to approximately one percent of the patient's body surface area.

[Q] What are the classifications of burns by severity?

[A] The three classifications of burn severity are:

- Minor—such as a sunburn.
- Moderate—an uncomplicated partial-thickness burn of less than 30 percent in an adult or less than 15 percent in a child.

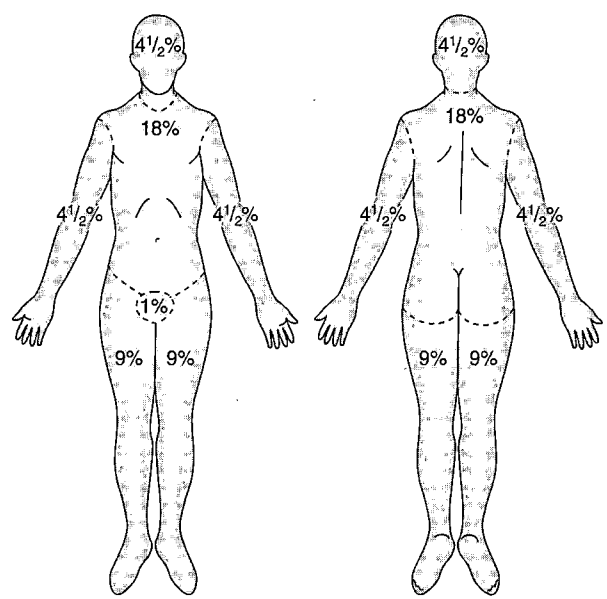

FIGURE 37–1 The rule of nines is used to determine the total body surface area burned.

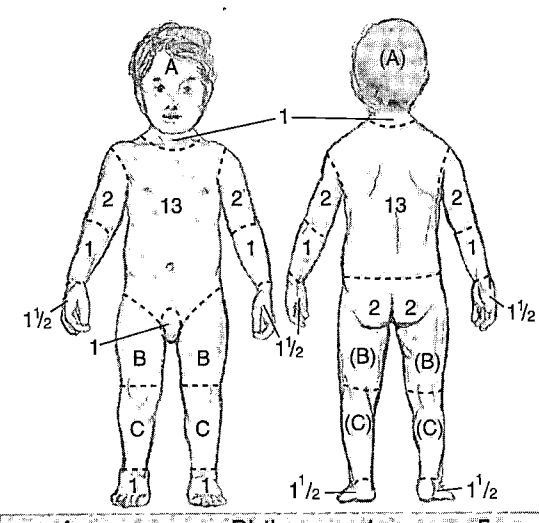

Area	Birth	1 yr	5 yr
A (head)	19	17	14
B (one thigh)	6½	7½	9
C (one leg)	6	6	6

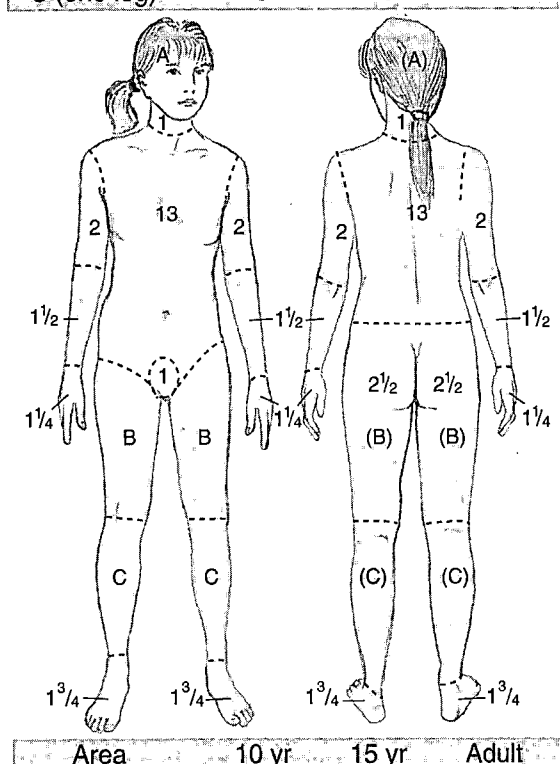

Area	10 yr	15 yr	Adult
A (head)	11	9	8
B (one thigh)	8½	9	9
C (one leg)	6	6½	7

FIGURE 37–1 *continued*

- Severe—a burn that should be transported to a burn specialty center. Examples include:

a. Burns greater than 30 percent BSA in adults, 15 percent BSA in children.

b. Burns of the head, hands, feet, or perineum.

c. Inhalation injuries.

d. Electrical burns.

e. Burns associated with multiple trauma or serious medical problems.

[Q] What considerations have an impact on the management and prognosis of the burn-injured patient?

[A] The patient's age is an important factor in how well their body can handle the burn. As a rule of thumb, a 50-year-old patient with a 25 percent full-thickness burn does as well as a 25-year-old patient with a 50 percent burn. In effect, the older the patient, the lower the percentage of total BSA burn he will tolerate. Infants and toddlers do not tolerate serious burn well either. Patients with preexisting medical problems have a more difficult time handling a critical burn. Preexisting problems with the kidneys, lungs, or heart may make it difficult for the patient to handle the tremendous movement of body fluids that occur with a burn injury.

Trauma also makes it difficult for the patient to recover from a burn. Shock from blood loss is complicated by the fluid losses from the critical burn and make the patient extremely hypotensive.

[Q] What are examples of conditions that are associated with burn injuries?

[A] Conditions associated with burn injuries include:
- Trauma (e.g., soft tissue and musculoskeletal).
- Blast injuries from explosions.
- Airway compromise from inhaling super-heated gasses.
- Respiratory compromise.
- Child abuse (e.g., dunking in a very hot bath, cigarette burns).

[Q] What are the signs and symptoms of a burn injury?

[A] There are many signs and symptoms of a burn injury. The list includes the following:
- Pain in the burn location, also may have chest pain.
- Changes in skin condition relative to the burn site.
- Adventitious lung sounds, dyspnea, or hoarseness.
- Sloughing of the affected skin.
- Dysphagia or dysphasia.
- Burnt hair or nasal hair singed.
- Nausea or vomiting.
- Unconsciousness.
- Edema or hemorrhage.
- Paraesthesia.

What is the general burn management?

In addition to management of the specific burn injury, general burn management includes attention to the airway, oxygenating the patient, and providing ventilation as is needed. Management should include IV fluids and management of pain after taking into consideration the patient's BP. The patient should be taken to the most appropriate facility to care for the burn injury.

Thermal Burns

What are the phases of "burn" shock?

Burn shock includes four general phases: the emergent phase, the fluid shift phase, the resolution phase, and the hypermetabolic phase. In these phases, the following things occur:

1. Emergent phase—this is the body's initial response to the burn injury. There is a release of catecholamines in response to the pain from the burn. The patient will have tachycardia, tachypnea, mild hypertension, and mild anxiety.

2. Fluid shift phase—there is a release of vasoactive substances from the burned tissues causing wound edema, fluid loss, and hypovolemia. During this phase, there is a massive shift of fluids from the intravascular to the extravascular space.

3. Resolution phase—usually occurs within 24 hours of the burn injury. The extravasation of fluid diminishes and an equilibrium is reached between intravascular space and interstitial space. There is also a decrease in cardiac output and an increased peripheral resistance in response to the patient's hypovolemia. This is the final phase of the burn process in which the scar tissue is laid down and healing occurs.

4. Hypermetabolic phase—if there is adequate volume replacement, the cardiac output can return to levels above normal. There is an increased metabolism to aid in the healing process.

How many of the thermal burn patients have accompanying inhalation injury?

Inhalation injury is present in 60–70 percent of all thermal burn patients who die. These patients usually have either carbon monoxide poisoning or cyanide intoxication.

What is an eschar formation?

Eschar is the scab or immediate scar that forms on the skin following a burn. It is thick and nonelastic. If large enough, it may impair circulation or respiration.

What is the problem that occurs with eschar formation?

There may be respiratory compromise secondary to a circumferential eschar around the thorax or circulatory compromise secondary to a circumferential eschar around an extremity.

What is an escharotomy?

Escharotomy is a lifesaving or limb-saving procedure used to allow expansion of the chest or restore circulation to an extremity around which the eschar has formed a tight circumferential band. The physician in the ED cuts into the eschar formed on the skin with a scalpel.

CLINICAL PEARL

Escharotomy is typically an in-hospital procedure. Under specific circumstances, it may be performed in the field with appropriate training and medical control (e.g., significant ventilatory or circulatory compromise).

What are the assessment findings in a thermal burn?

The assessment findings for a thermal burn include:

- The depth classification of the burn—is it a first (superficial), second (partial-thickness), or third degree (full-thickness) burn? Notice the depth of the injury in Figure 37–2.

- The severity of the burn—does it involve inhalation? Are the nose hairs singed or is there soot around the mouth and nose? Is the burn circumferential around the chest or an extremity? Are there other preexisting medical conditions that may be complicated by the burn? Is there multiple trauma involved? Was the 1 percent perineum involved in the burn?

- Severity of the burn—note the percentages requiring transport to a burn center (in adults 30 percent or in children 15 percent).

- Are there considerations that will impact the care and prognosis of the thermal burn injured patient—is the patient on blood thinners? Does the patient have support or homecare? Is the patient capable of keeping the injury clean and properly dressed? Is the patient very old or very young?

- What was the mechanism of injury (MOI) of the burn? Was it scalding, steam, flame, flash, retained heat, or other trauma?

What is the proper management of a thermal burn injury?

The management of a thermal burn injury includes the following:

- Remove the patient to a safe area.

- Stop the burning process. If you need to hose the patient down and remove clothing, do so right away.

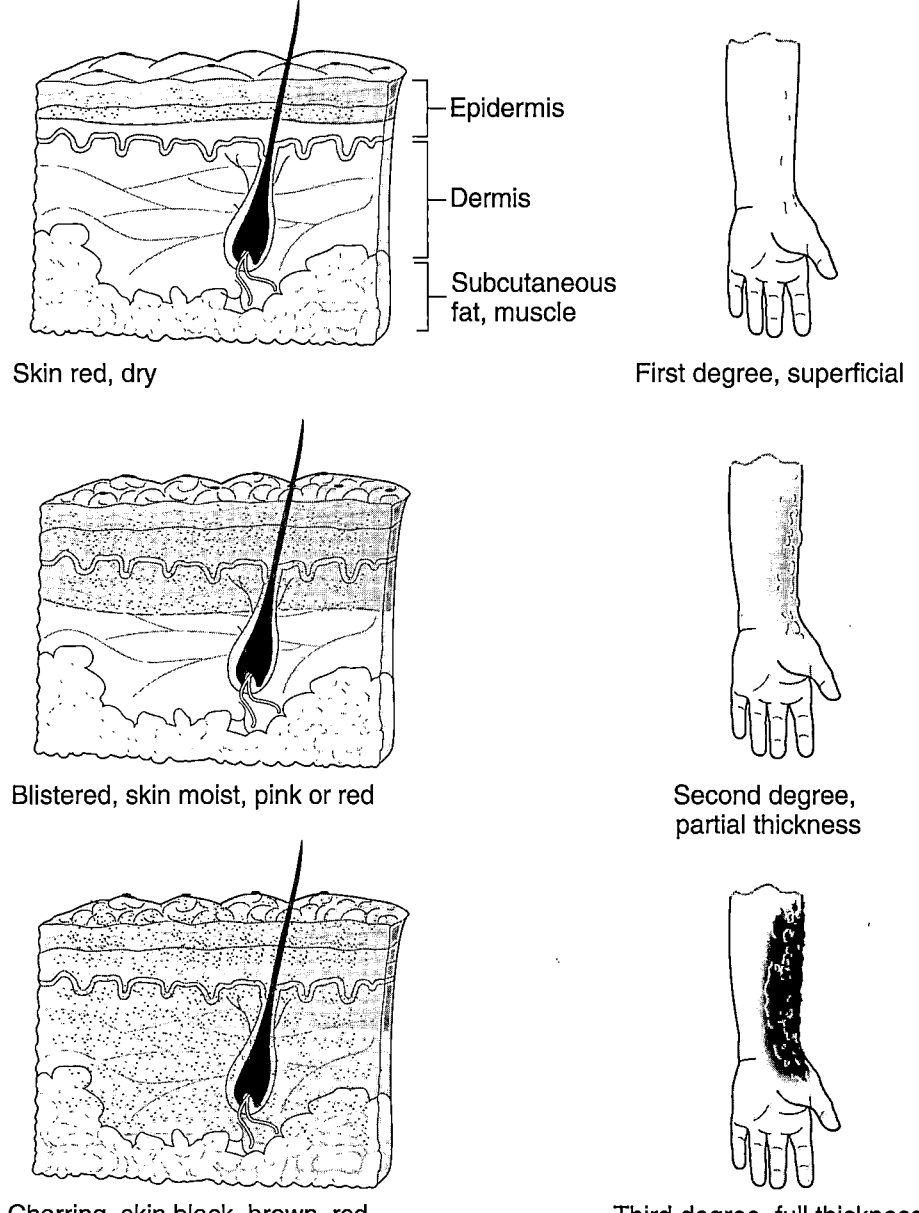

Skin red, dry

First degree, superficial

Blistered, skin moist, pink or red

Second degree,
partial thickness

Charring, skin black, brown, red

Third degree, full thickness

FIGURE 37-2 Notice the depth of the burn in each type of burn: superficial, partial thickness, and full thickness.

- Ensure the airway is clear, oxygenate the patient with high-concentration oxygen and a nonrebreather mask, and assess the need for assisted ventilation.

- Manage the circulation for shock by starting a large bore IV line (or two) and infusing fluids according to your local protocol.

- Dress the wound using a dry dressing unless it is a very small percentage or a minor injury. This may be a local protocol issue because burn centers have different opinions on the use of specific burn dressings (e.g., water jel®). You should also properly position the patient to manage shock.

- Maintain body heat so the patient does not become hypothermic.

- Transport the patient to the most appropriate facility to care for the burn injury.

- Topical applications, tetanus, and antibiotic therapy should be considered in the ED.

Q **How much fluid does the burn patient need?**

A Provided that the burn is not complicated by preexisting heart problems, fluid needs are determined using the Parkland

Formula used by most burn centers. The formula is four times the BSA times the patient's weight in kg. The first half of this amount of fluid should be administered in the first eight hours after the burn injury occurs. For example, a 100 kg patient with 40 percent BSA full-thickness burns should receive 8,000 cc's (8 liters) in the first eight hours ($4 \times 40 \times 100 = 16,000$ cc's; give half in first 8 hours = 8,000 cc's).

Inhalation Burns

What is the incidence of inhalation burn injury?

Between 20 and 35 percent of all patients admitted to burn centers have an inhalation injury. Chemical inhalation injury is more frequent than thermal inhalation injury. Factors that are associated with an increased risk of inhalation injury are standing in a room with a fire, screaming for help, and being in an enclosed area involving a fire. The coolest area of a burning room is always at the floor.

What are the MOI associated with inhalation burns?

MOIs associated with inhalation injury include toxic inhalations, smoke inhalation, carbon monoxide poisoning, thiocyanate intoxication (a form of cyanide commonly released from burning furniture), and thermal and chemical burns.

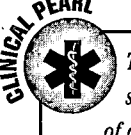

Many fires result in the generation of toxic compounds such as cyanides (thiocyanate). These are produced commonly as a result of the combustion of synthetic fabrics, such as those used in the manufacture of furniture.

What should make the EMS provider suspect that the patient may have an inhalation injury?

Always be alert for singed nasal hairs and black soot in the sputum. Any alteration to the volume and tone of the patient's voice may also be an indicator that there is swelling in the airway due to the inhalation injury. Also observe for stridor or inspiratory wheezing.

What is the current theory on the usefulness of hyperbaric chamber therapy for patients who have sustained carbon monoxide poisoning from a fire?

Regardless of the cause, hyperbaric oxygen therapy for carbon monoxide inhalation is beneficial because it helps decrease

the time it takes for the hemoglobin to become saturated with oxygen. For people with suspected carbon monoxide inhalation, consult medical control for further recommendations.

Though once reserved for only the very ill, some data suggest that treatment of patients with fairly low levels of carbon monoxide is also beneficial.

What is the appropriate management of the burn inhalation injured patient?

The management of the inhalation burn injury includes the following:

- Ensure a patent airway.
- Oxygenate the patient with high-concentration oxygen.
- Assess the need for ventilation and intubation. If it is determined that intubation is appropriate and you suspect airway swelling, have your most experienced person intubate the patient because there may not be a second chance. You may need to consider a surgical airway procedure as a backup airway in this case.
- Manage the patient for shock by maintaining warmth and appropriate positioning.
- Manage the circulation following the Parkland formula and your local protocols.
- In the event of suspected cyanide inhalation, follow your local protocols, including the administration of thiosulfate and amyl nitrate.
- Manage the thermal burn injury, if present, following your local protocols.
- Transport to the appropriate facility for management of burns in your region. If the airway is not manageable, consider transporting to the nearest facility to stabilize the airway before going directly to a regional center.
- The ED may consider the need for hyperbaric therapy.

Chemical Burns

What types of chemicals cause burn injuries?

The types of chemicals that commonly cause burns are acids, bases (alkali), dry chemicals, and phenols. Cement and dry ice are examples of chemicals that can cause a burn injury.

Where do chemical burns most frequently occur?

Most of the chemical burn injuries occur in an industrial setting. Many chemicals are used in manufacturing processes that are highly corrosive to the skin (e.g., phenols in the processing of plastics).

If a patient has been burned with a dry powder, are there any special considerations for management?

Yes! Figure out what the chemical is before just washing it off. Some chemicals react with water and produce heat or develop a substance toxic to inhale (e.g., chlorine powder). In these instances, brush the chemical off the person's body and check with the poison control center or CHEMTREC to determine the appropriate decontamination procedures. Always wear personal protective equipment (PPE) to avoid exposing yourself to the chemical.

CLINICAL PEARL

Powdered lime (a component of concrete) causes burns. Exposure to water releases significant heat and will worsen the situation. Brush off all offending material prior to rinsing the injury.

What are the considerations that impact the care and prognosis of a chemical injury to the eye?

If possible, remove contact lenses or gently wash them out if there is a chemical injury to the eye. Irrigation of most substances is recommended. Follow your local protocols. In some areas, a special lens (Morgan Lens®) may be used to facilitate irrigation. Try to keep the patient from rubbing the eye especially if dry chemical is still present on their eyes or hands. Further irritation and damage may occur.

How long do the burning effects of tear gas or pepper spray last?

The burning sensation of tear gas lasts for about an hour and pepper gas lasts about two hours. They can be minimized if

CLINICAL PEARL

Remember that both tear gas and pepper spray residue will affect you as well as the patient. Use special precautions. There is an antidote to pepper spray that is available to law enforcement agencies. Though not usually carried in the field, you may be able to acquire a supply under specific circumstances (e.g., backup duty during a suspected mass disturbance).

the patient is instructed not to rub their eyes or face. Get the patient out into the open air, and have them blow their nose and spit out any chemical residue. Consider using water to flush the eyes and to gargle. If the pepper spray is still wet on the skin, carefully sponge it off and do not spread it around.

What is the "protester facial"?

In areas that utilize pepper spray to disperse crowds, the treatment for patients exposed to pepper spray is to rub mineral oil on the skin. The mineral oil works to trap the chemical agents. Next, immediately wipe off all of the mineral oil with rubbing alcohol.

If the patient has an eye injury or burn from a chemical agent how should this be managed?

Once you are sure the agent can be diluted with water and will not react with water, flush the eye with copious amounts of water from the bridge of the nose across the affected eye to the ground or a catch basin. Do not allow the fluid to run into the unaffected eye, which would cause injury to the good eye.

What should be done if the patient has contact lenses on?

Remove the lenses with a gloved hand or assist the patient in doing so.

Can Morgan Lenses® be used for burns of the eye?

Yes, provided the eye has not been saturated with a chemical that will harm the lens and you have been appropriately trained in their use. These lenses are like a contact lens with a tube to allow for the attachment of a sterile saline solution to irrigate the eye.

Electrical Burns

Why are electrical burns often very severe?

The human body is a good conductor of electricity. The path of the electricity through the body leads to serious complications. It can cause internal injuries, as well as the entrance and exit burn. It can also cross the heart or brain and cause lethal dysrhythmias.

How many people die from electrical injuries?

In the United States, about 1,000 people die from electrical shock each year. The cause of death is usually attributed to the electrical effect on the heart, massive muscle destruction from the current passing through the body, or thermal burns from contact with the electrical source.

Does the type of current affect the severity of electrical injury?

Yes, definitely. Direct current (DC), which has zero (no variation) frequency but may be intermittent or pulsating, is less dangerous than alternating current (AC). The effects of AC on the body depend on the frequency. Low frequency currents of 50 to 60 Hz (cycles/second), which are commonly used, are more dangerous than high frequency currents and are three to five times more dangerous than DC of the same voltage and amperage.

DC tends to cause a convulsive contraction helping to force the patient away from the source. AC at 60 Hz, which is household current, produces muscle tetany and freezing of the hand to the current's source, prolonging the exposure and allowing severe burns to occur.

How does the amount of voltage and amperage relate to the extent of injury?

The higher the voltage and amperage, the greater the damage from either AC or DC sources. High voltage (>500 to 1000 V) currents tend to cause deep burns and low voltage causes freezing to the circuit. Normally you can perceive a current entering your hand at about 5 to 10 milliamperes (mA) for DC and 1 to 10 mA for AC at 60 Hz.

The maximum amperage that can cause flexors of the arm to contract but allows a person to release his hand from the current's source is termed the "let-go current." For DC the let-go current is about 75 mA for a 70 kg man and for AC it is about 15 mA (varying somewhat with muscle mass).

A low voltage (100 to 220 V) 60 Hz AC traveling through the chest for a fraction of a second may cause ventricular fibrillation at amperages as low as 60 to 100 mA (about 300 to 500 mA of DC is required). If the current has a direct pathway to the heart, such as a cardiac catheter or pacemaker electrodes, a much lower amperage (<1 mA AC or DC) can produce fibrillation.

Body resistance is also important. Body resistance is measured in ohms/cm2 and is concentrated primarily in the skin. The skin condition can alter the resistance considerably. Dry, well-keratinized intact skin averages 20,000 to 30,000 ohms/cm2 of resistance. A thickly calloused palm of the hand or sole of the foot may have a resistance of two to three million ohms/cm2. The resistance of moist thin skin is about 500 ohms/cm2. A puncture of the skin or if the current is applied to a moist mucous membrane (e.g., a child biting a cord) may have a resistance as low as 200 to 300 ohms/cm2.

What assessment findings should be considered when evaluating an electrical burn?

When evaluating an electrical burn, note if there were contact burn injuries (from directly touching the electrical source), arc injuries (a visible electrical charge generally taking the path of an arc), or flame or flash burn injury such as from a welder's flash. It is also a good idea to look for two burn locations—the electricity may have traveled through the body. The terms entry and exit are used and often are easily discernible, but it may be difficult to determine the direction of travel of the current. Some experts use the terms source and ground for the two external burn injury locations.

What are some of the symptoms exhibited by a person who has sustained an electrical shock?

The person usually has an obvious burn mark from contacting the electrical source. They may complain of some of the following symptoms:

- Fatigue.
- Trauma from falling (e.g., fractures, head injury).
- Headache.
- Hearing impairment or vision loss.
- Loss of reflex control.
- Muscle contractions or pain.
- Skin burns.

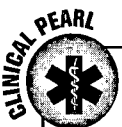

Many electrical injuries are obvious, unless the patient is unconscious and the event unwitnessed. Still, you should always consider the possibility of "occult" electrical exposure in patients with the listed findings and no obvious MOI.

Q What is my chance of being struck and killed by lightning?

A In 1990 there were 89 lightning fatalities in the United States. This means that outside of Florida, where lightning strikes are more frequent due to tropical storms, an American's odds in 1990 of being struck and killed by lightning were about 2.8 million to one. Certainly those who enjoy playing golf have a greater risk!

Q Does lightning produce exit wounds?

A Rarely. Entry and exit wounds seldom occur and rarely is there myoglobulinuria (muscle damage) because the duration of the current is too short to break the skin down.

Q How does lightning typically injure a patient?

A Lightning usually flashes over the patient as opposed to a direct hit. In these cases, it causes very little internal damage other than an electrical short-circuiting of systems.

Q What types of injuries occur due to the electrical short-circuiting?

A Lightning causes cardiac asystole, ventricular fibrillation, loss of consciousness, altered mental status (AMS), and neuropsychologic problems.

Though lightning can cause any cardiac dysrhythmia, ventricular fibrillation is most common.

Q Are there any special considerations in the management of the electrical injury?

A The number one priority with an electrical injury is not to touch the patient until you are absolutely sure that the power has been turned off and the patient is not energized. The treatment is the same as for a thermal injury. Watch the patient very closely because the internal injuries they may have sustained are hard to

determine in the field. Also make sure the patient's ECG is monitored because they may have hyperkalemia and cell death similar to that found in the crush syndrome patient.

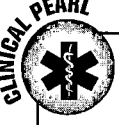

Always ensure your own safety before taking care of the patient!

Q What physiological functions can be altered by an electric burn?

A When a patient has an electrical burn, they may have involuntary muscular contractions, seizures, ventricular fibrillation, or respiratory arrest (apnea) due to central nervous system (CNS) injury or muscle paralysis. High voltage may cause significant damage to the muscle or other internal tissues between the source and the points of current.

Q What is the most common entry point for an electrical burn?

A The hands, followed by the head. The most common exit point is the foot.

Radiation Exposure

Q What are the two major classifications of radiation and what are they used for?

A Radiation is divided into ionizing and nonionizing. Nonionizing radiation includes such things as light, radio waves, microwaves, and radar. This type generally does not cause tissue damage. Ionizing radiation produces immediate chemical effects, known as ionization, on human tissue. This type includes such things as X-rays, gamma rays, and particle bombardment (e.g., neutron beam, electron beam, protons, mesons, and others). A meson is a particle of intermediate density between an electron and a proton. Because ionizing radiation is commonly used for medical testing, treatment, industrial purposes, weapons, and scientific purposes, it is not uncommon that you would respond to a location where sources of ionizing radiation are present.

Q What are the types of ionizing radiation that can cause a burn injury?

A The types of ionizing radiation that can cause a burn injury are alpha particles, beta particles, gamma rays, and neutrons.

Q **What can shield against the types of ionizing radiation sources?**

A Shielding is different for each source of ionizing radiation. The following should be a useful guide:

- Alpha particles—are slow moving and contain low energy, so things like newspaper or clothing can stop them. They are generally a minor hazard unless taken internally by ingestion or inhalation.
- Beta particles—these are small particles that are high in energy. Although they penetrate the air, aluminum or similar materials stop them. They cause less local damage than the alpha particles, yet can be dangerous if inhaled or ingested.
- Gamma rays—these are highly energized and have the ability to penetrate thick shielding. They penetrate through the body causing cellular damage and causing the cells themselves to emit alpha or beta particles. They are most commonly experienced during an X-ray. Lead shielding provides protection.
- Neutrons—are the most penetrating particles; 10 times that of gamma rays. Exposure causes direct tissue damage. In a nuclear accident, the neutron exposure is usually only near the reactor core.

Q **How is radiation detected?**

A First and foremost by the history of the event that occurred and the type of location. Be especially careful if there is a fire in a medical office that has sources of radiation (e.g., a nuclear medicine facility or research laboratory). Ionizing radiation cannot be seen, heard, or felt. The detection instrument that is used is called a Geiger counter, which measures the radiation absorbed dose (RAD).

Q **What is the difference between a RAD and REM?**

A A RAD is the radiation absorbed dose. The rate of radiation is measured in roentgens per hour (R/hr) or milliroentgens per hour (mR/hr). For example, 1,000 mR = 1R. A gauge of the likely injury to an irradiated part of an organism is called the roentgen equivalent in man or REM. For practical purposes, RAD and REM are equivalent in their clinical value to the EMS provider.

Q **What is radiation sickness?**

A Radiation sickness results when humans or animals are exposed to excessive doses of ionizing radiation. This can occur acutely from a single large exposure or chronically from exposure to dangerous levels over a period of time. Chronic exposure over a period of years usually leads to delayed medical problems such as cancer and premature aging.

Q **How much exposure causes radiation sickness?**

A As a rule, total body exposure of 100 R causes radiation sickness. The degree of illness is clearly a function of the dose, type of agent, and the rate of exposure. Here are some examples of whole body exposure and localized exposure in RADs:

- Whole Body Exposure:
  1. 100 RAD—may cause anorexia, nausea, vomiting, and fatigue in 10–20 percent of patients within two days.
  2. 400 RAD—nausea, vomiting, and diarrhea in the first several hours. Causes radiation sickness and death in half of the individuals.
  3. 800 RAD—severe nausea, vomiting, and diarrhea within a few hours. Fatal to 100 percent of patients within two weeks without prompt medical attention.
  4. 1,000 RAD or more—a burning sensation within minutes; nausea and vomiting within 10 minutes; confusion and ataxia within an hour. Fatal to 100 percent of patients within a short time without prompt medical attention.
  5. 100,000 RAD—will cause immediate unconsciousness and death within an hour.
- Local Exposure:
  1. 500 RAD—asymptomatic with a risk of altered function to exposed area.
  2. 2,500 RAD—atrophy, altered pigmentation, and vascular lesions.
  3. 5,000 RAD—chronic ulcer to area and risk of cancer.
  4. 50,000 RAD—the tissue is permanently destroyed.

Q **How is the severity of an exposure determined?**

A The best indicator, aside from taking readings of the level of radiation by properly trained personnel using a Geiger counter, is the severity of the symptoms, length of time from the exposure till symptoms begin to appear, and the changes in the body's white blood cells (WBCs).

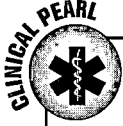 CLINICAL PEARL

WBCs are very sensitive to radiation. The higher the absorbed dose, the more depressed the WBC count.

Q **What are the symptoms of over exposure to an ionizing radiation source?**

A The patient may complain of any of the following symptoms after exposure to an ionizing radiation source: (Note that many of these are common in the patient receiving radiation therapy as a treatment for cancer.)

- Nausea and vomiting.
- Diarrhea.
- Skin burns appearing red and blistering.
- Weakness, fatigue, exhaustion, and syncope.
- Dehydration.
- Inflammation of areas (e.g., redness, tenderness, swelling, bleeding).
- Hair loss.
- Ulceration of the oral mucosa, esophagus, or GI system.
- Hematemesis.
- Bloody stool.
- Bleeding from the nose, mouth, gums, and rectum.
- Bruising or open sores on the skin.
- Sloughing of the skin.

What is the difference between a clean and a dirty accident?

There are two basic types of incidents involving exposure to ionizing radiation: a dirty accident and a clean accident. In a clean incident, the patient is exposed to an ionizing source, but is not contaminated by the radioactive substance; particles of radioactive dust; or a radioactive gas, smoke, or liquid. In this case, the

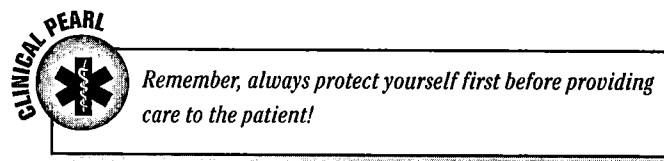

Remember, always protect yourself first before providing care to the patient!

patient is not a secondary exposure hazard to the EMS providers. However, in a dirty accident, often associated with a fire, the patient continues to be a secondary exposure hazard to the EMS provider and should be monitored with a Geiger counter and decontaminated by the appropriately trained personnel.

What is the management of a patient who has been exposed to an ionizing radiation source?

The management is the same as for any other injury or illness after first determining the type of exposure, duration, and if it was a clean or dirty accident. If it was a dirty accident, the patient can be a hazard to the EMS provider and should not be approached until the proper PPE is donned and precautions are taken by appropriately trained personnel. This discussion is beyond the scope of this text. If the patient was internally exposed, it is a good idea to save body wastes because they may contain ionizing radiation particles also. Do not do mouth-to-mouth resuscitation; use a BVM on the patient if artificial respiration is needed.

Head and Facial Trauma

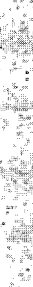

T his chapter discusses a series of injuries that can occur to the head or face as well as the sensory organs of the head. The focus is on *why* patients present in a certain manner and *why* you need to respond in a certain way to their presenting problems.

Incidence of Facial Injuries

Q What is the incidence of head and facial trauma?

A Each year, more than two million people in the United States undergo emergency evaluation for acute head and face trauma. Facial injuries are present in 5 percent to as many as 68 percent of injured people treated in EDs in various countries. The reported incidence of facial trauma among motorcycle riders involved in crashes varies between 38 percent and 57 percent, depending on the setting, the nature of the study population, and the case identification methods.

Q What is the morbidity and mortality of head and facial trauma?

A Eighty percent sustain minor trauma, 10 percent have moderate injuries, and 10 percent have severe injury. Nearly one quarter are hospitalized. Of these, nearly 200,000 die or suffer severe permanent disability. As many as 50,000 patients may die from severe head trauma before reaching the ED.

Q What are the common mechanisms of injury (MOIs) for injuries to the face and head?

A Common MOIs for blunt trauma to the face and head include motor vehicle crash (MVC), falls, body-to-body contact, and augmented force (e.g., sticks and clubs). Common MOIs for penetrating injuries to the face and head include gunshot wounds (GSW), stabbings, and human or animal bites.

Q What are the common associated injuries that accompany face or head injuries?

A Common associated injuries include airway compromise, cervical spine injury, brain injury, eye injury, and dental trauma or avulsion.

Q What is the incidence of throat injuries?

A Isolated throat injuries are unusual and often accompany more severe and often distracting injuries (e.g., cervical spine trauma). Thus, specific incidence figures are not readily available.

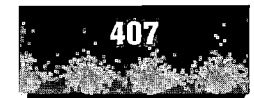

What is the morbidity and mortality of throat injuries?

Throat injuries may be fatal, usually due to associated injury to the airway or the main blood vessels (e.g., carotid, jugular). Vocal cord injury may lead to hoarseness or respiratory compromise.

What are the common MOIs for throat injuries?

Blunt trauma is commonly caused by MVC, hanging, strangulation, or a blow to the neck. Penetrating trauma is caused by GSW, stabbing, an arrow, lacerations, or punctures.

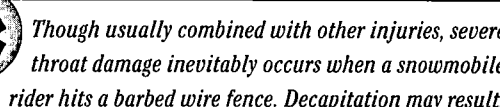

Though usually combined with other injuries, severe throat damage inevitably occurs when a snowmobile rider hits a barbed wire fence. Decapitation may result.

What are the MOIs for injury to the nose?

MVC, body-to-body contact, and falls typically cause blunt injuries to the nose. Penetrating injuries are caused by GSW, stabbing, and foreign bodies such as beans, crayons, or just about anything a child can fit in their nose!

What are the typical MOIs for ear injuries?

Blunt ear injuries occur from MVC, body-to-body contact, and augmented force. Penetrations can occur from GSW, cuttings, foreign bodies, and puncture wounds. The ears can also be injured from pressure during diving and blast injuries from explosives.

What are the common MOIs for most eye injuries?

Common cases of penetrating eye injuries are from bullets, knives, glass, arrows, and foreign bodies. Common causes of blunt eye injuries are from balls, falls, MVC, and motorcycles. Eye injuries are also caused by burns from welding, the sun, and chemicals.

What are the types of eye injuries typically caused by penetrating trauma?

Abrasions to the cornea are common from foreign bodies. These can be superficial or deep. Sometimes the eye can be lacerated by a sharp object such as glass in a collision. These cuts can also be superficial or deep.

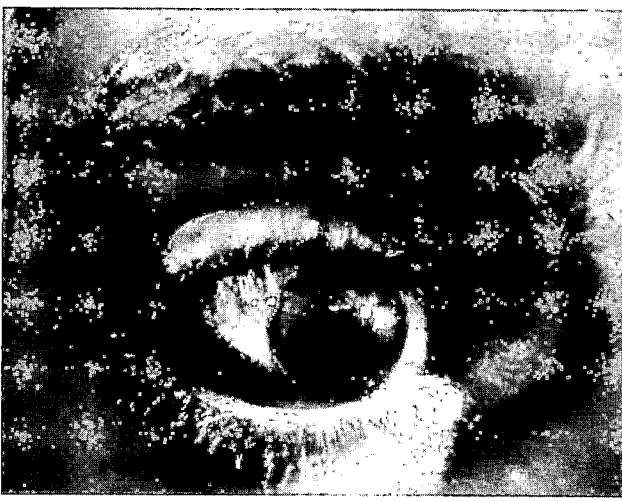

FIGURE 38-1 A hyphema is a collection of blood in the front of the eye. *(Courtesy of Dr. Kevin Reilly, Albany Medical Center, Albany, NY)*

What are the types of injuries typically caused by blunt trauma to the eye?

When the eye is struck with a blunt object, such as a ball, swelling occurs. The patient may have a conjunctival hemorrhage, which is bleeding into the conjunctiva. A hyphema (Figure 38–1) is hemorrhage to the anterior chamber of the eye.

In very serious situations, there may be a rupture of the globe allowing the aqueous humor in the anterior chamber or the vitreous humor in the posterior chamber to leak out. Sometimes the patient can have a fracture of the orbital rim. This is referred to as a "blow-out" fracture and can seriously damage the eye.

A "blowout fracture" occurs because blunt trauma is applied to the eye socket. Pressure is transmitted through the globe (eyeball) to the relatively thin bone in the medial and inferior portions of the orbit, causing it to break. By itself, the injury is not dangerous. One of the tendons of the extraocular muscles, however, may become trapped, preventing the patient from looking upward. Always check eye movement on any patient with facial trauma.

The retina can become detached, seriously interrupting the ability of the patient to see and potentially threatening the patient's sight. Limit the movement of the eye and transport the patient to a facility that has an ophthalmologist immediately available.

How can the eye be burned?

Most frequently, the eye is burned by a flash of a very bright light such as that of an arc welder. That is why eye protection is of the utmost importance. The eye can also be burned from a splashing of an acid or alkali. In the chemistry lab or whenever using chemicals, it is imperative that eye protection be used.

What other types of eye injuries can occur?

It is very common for a patient to have a lacerated eyelid, which may or may not be associated with an injury of the eye itself. Some patients may have an object impaled in their eye. In this case, the EMS provider should stabilize and pad the object. Sometimes a paper cup may be helpful to stabilize the object. The uninjured eye should be covered to limit movement from conjugate gaze. Keep in mind, the patient will be very scared of losing her sight, so you will need to provide emotional support.

What is the incidence of injuries to the mouth?

Isolated injuries to the mouth, such as from a punch, are very common, accounting for as much as 50 percent of facial trauma. More severe injuries are rare and often involve penetrating trauma.

Anatomy of Facial Injuries

What are the types of facial injuries?

The facial injuries are either an injury to a bone or soft tissue. Injuries to the bones include mandible fractures or dislocations. A maxilla fracture is further described as LeFort I, II, and III. Patients may have a fracture to the zygomatic, an orbit fracture, or nasal fracture. Injuries to the soft tissue of the face may involve the mouth, oropharynx, tongue, ear, or eye.

What are the LeFort classifications?

The LeFort classifications were named after French surgeon Leon LeFort. He classified facial fractures into three types. The higher the number, the more significant the damage and the more potential for a complicated airway in need of management.

- LeFort I—also called Guerin's fracture, involves the maxilla.
- LeFort II—also called a pyramidal fracture, involves the maxilla, nasal bones, and medial eye orbits.
- LeFort III—also referred to as craniofacial dysfunction, involves fractures of the maxilla, nasal bones, ethmoids,

zygoma, vomer, and all of the smaller bones at the base of the cranium.

> **CLINICAL PEARL**
>
> *LeFort fractures are based on X-ray or CT scan findings, not clinical impressions. Some experts now contend that the differentiation is artificial and not helpful.*

What are the associated structures that may be injured in the throat?

The associated structures of the throat that can be injured include:

- Vagus nerve.
- Thoracic duct.
- Pharynx and esophagus.
- Thyroid gland and parathyroid glands.
- Brachial plexus, which is responsible for lower arm and hand function.
- Muscles, including the platysma as the major muscle.
- Soft tissue and fascia.

What nerves are primarily responsible for central versus peripheral vision?

The rods are responsible for peripheral vision and low-light, night sight conditions. The cones are responsible for central vision and bright-light, daytime conditions. The relation between the brain and the visual pathways of the eyes is shown in Figure 38–2.

What are the typical MOIs for injuries to the mouth?

The MOIs for mouth injuries include blunt trauma, such as MVC, blows to the mouth or chin, and penetrating injuries such as GSWs, lacerations, or punctures.

What are the problems associated with lacerations to the tongue?

When a patient has a lacerated tongue, the complications include the inability to communicate and copious bleeding because the tongue is so vascular. Often the patient will have broken or avulsed teeth and blood tinged mucus. The immediate problem is often dealing with the potential airway obstruction from bleeding into the airway.

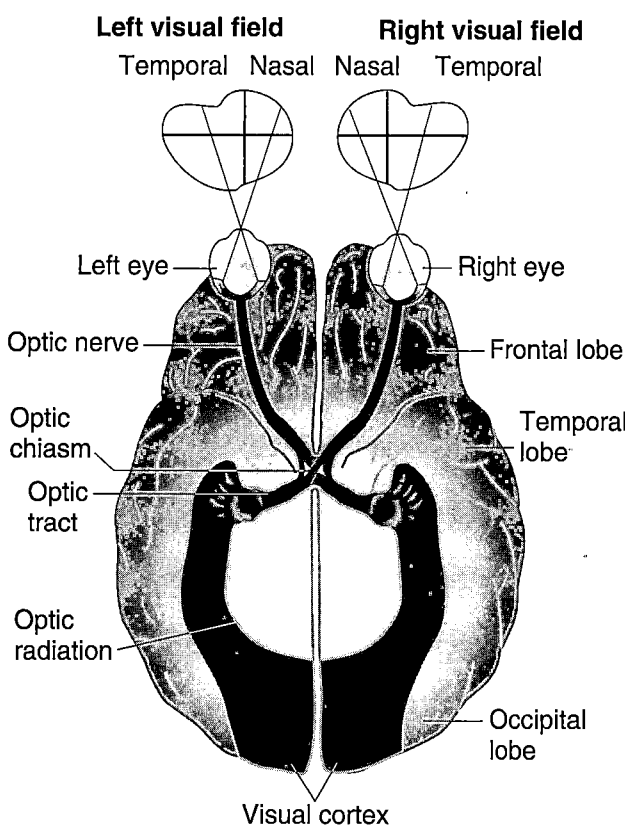

Left visual field   Right visual field

Temporal Nasal Nasal Temporal

Left eye

Right eye

Optic nerve

Frontal lobe

Optic chiasm

Temporal lobe

Optic tract

Optic radiation

Occipital lobe

Visual cortex

FIGURE 38-2 The visual pathways of the eye.

Assessment of Facial Injuries

Q **What are the assessment priorities with a facial or head injury?**

A First and foremost are airway patency and adequate ventilation. This must be done assuming that there is a cervical spine injury and maintaining spinal integrity. Next, ensure that the patient has adequate perfusion. Be aware of the possibility of an associated injury to the head involving increased intracranial pressure (ICP) and the presence of cerebrospinal fluid (CSF). Examine the patient for the presence of malocclusion (e.g., the jaws and teeth do not meet as they should), a depressed zygoma, any facial asymmetry, or diplopia (blurred vision).

Finally, examine for soft tissue injury such as open wounds, hematomas, or any broken or missing teeth. The presence of significant facial injury can be a very difficult airway to manage in the field and require all of the EMS provider's attention.

Q **What happens with a transected trachea?**

A If the trachea is completely transected, the main problem is the inability to get air into the lungs. When a trachea is cut, the larynx may be separated from the trachea or fractured. This is a serious injury that can cause vocal cord swelling or contusion. There may be a disruption of the normal airway landmarks, as well as associated soft tissue swelling. The open wound to the trachea disrupts the breathing process.

Q **What is the danger of a lacerated vessel in the throat?**

A The patient may rapidly exsanguinate. If an artery is involved, hypoxia to the brain tissue may cause an infarct. The open wound can suck air in, causing an air embolism.

Q **In addition to the routine assessment, what specifics should be noted when examining the patient with a throat injury?**

A The patient may have a pale or cyanotic face with bruising or redness of the neck. There may be a hematoma present or in cases where there is an open wound, you may see a frothy blood or sputum in the wound.

Any injury involving the throat may also have subcutaneous emphysema. The patient may complain of a tickle or a feeling of fullness in the throat or pain on palpation of the neck. Listen for voice changes such as low volume or a raspy deep voice.

Q **What is epistaxis and how is it caused or complicated?**

A Simply put, it is a nosebleed. Foreign bodies, including fingers being inserted into the nose, cause many nosebleeds. If a foreign body is still in place (e.g., pencil, peanut, or a rubber hose) do not remove it unless the airway is compromised. Epistaxis may compromise the airway if severe. The patient is more likely to bleed down the throat into the stomach causing nausea and vomiting. Anterior bleeds are from the septum and are venous bleeding. Posterior bleeds drain down the throat.

Q **Are there any special assessment points to focus on with an ear injury?**

A Try to determine if there is a gross hearing loss. If there is CSF draining from the ear, let it flow out into a loose bandage. Adequate assessment of the external ear canal, middle ear, and inner ear cannot be done in the field.

Q **What specific assessment questions should be added to the normal initial assessment for an eye injury?**

A Besides assessing the MOI and the time the symptoms began, the EMS provider should be certain to assess for the following findings:

- When did the patient first notice symptoms?
- Were both eyes affected?
- Does the patient have a past history of problems with visual acuity (e.g., glasses or contacts).
- Does the patient have a past medical history (PMH) of any diseases or conditions such as glaucoma or cataracts?
- Is the patient on any medications?

Are there any physical assessment priorities worth noting with an eye injury?

Aside from maintaining an open airway and ensuring adequate ventilation, the priorities include controlling bleeding and supporting the cardiovascular system, as well as keeping in mind the potential for a CNS injury. Observe the following for signs of injury or deformity:

- Orbital rim.
- Lids.
- Cornea.
- Conjunctiva.
- Eye movement such as disjunctive gaze (eyes going in opposite directions) or paralysis of the gaze.
- How do the pupils react?
- What is the patient's acuity?

Management of Facial Injuries

What is the key to the management of a patient with a facial injury?

Airway patency and adequate ventilation are the highest priorities. This involves a combination of suctioning, intubating, positioning, and ventilating. Next, ensure adequate circulation and cervical spine integrity.

How should an impaled object in the neck be handled?

Do not remove an impaled object unless it is obstructing the airway. You may need to prepare for an emergency cricothyrotomy.

What does the management of a throat injury involve?

The primary concerns for the management of throat injuries are airway patency and adequacy of ventilation. If an ET tube can be inserted, do so sooner rather than later, because the swelling

may make this a difficult procedure. BVM with supplemental oxygen may be needed. If you need to ventilate and the airway is crushed or grossly disfigured, look for air bubbles. That is probably the best place to insert the ET tube, lacking any other landmarks.

Maintain adequate tissue perfusion. If there is an open wound to the neck, have the patient lay on the left side in the Trendelenburg position with an occlusive dressing applied over the neck wound. Direct pressure to the wound is appropriate; however, do not use a circumferential bandage. Carefully monitor the patient for vagal stimulus because a reflex bradycardia may be developing.

Maintain cervical immobilization, but keep in mind that the use of a cervical collar may be contraindicated if it covers up the bleeding wound.

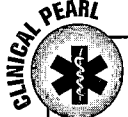

Remember the major priority in head and face injuries is the ABCs.

How should a nosebleed be managed?

The management of a nosebleed, in the anterior portions, involves direct pressure. If the patient has a nosebleed in the posterior region, it is difficult to deal with in the field and the primary concern is preventing an airway obstruction and shock. If bleeding is severe, treatment is similar to hemorrhagic shock. Provided cervical spine injury is not suspected, have the patient either sit upright leaning forward or lie in the recovery position so the blood can drain. Give the patient gauze and an emesis bag or basin and have them spit the clots out. Do not let them swallow the clots because they will upset the stomach and may result in vomiting. Ice may be helpful if applied to the bridge of the nose to promote vasoconstriction . If CSF is detected, do not apply direct pressure; simply allow the fluid to drain freely.

How should an injured ear be managed in the field?

Basically treat it like a soft tissue injury. Realign the ear into a normal position and gently bandage with sufficient padding. Cover a draining ear with a loose dressing. It is usually difficult for cartilage to heal. Infection is the prime reason for a failure to heal. Remember, if the mechanism warrants cervical spine precautions, then they should be taken.

What does the management of an eye injury involve?

If the injury is a blunt injury, position the patient with their head up to reduce the swelling, provided there is no accompanying head injury needing neck immobilization. Bandage the eyes (suggest both eyes instead of just one) to limit their movement.

Do not apply any pressure to the patient's eyes because this may damage the globe.

If the injury is penetrating, apply a moist bandage to the eye because it may not be able to close and receive tears to keep it wet. Any removal of foreign bodies (e.g., dust particles or wood chips) is a function based on your experience with carefully removing small objects from the eye. If the object is actually imbedded in the eye, stabilize and transport the patient.

CLINICAL PEARL

If a foreign body cannot be gently rinsed from the eye, do not attempt further maneuvers in the field unless you are specially trained and have the appropriate equipment (e.g., local anesthetic, magnifier, special ophthalmic burr or tweezers). Severe eye damage may occur.

If the patient has received a flash burn, cover both eyes. If they have received acid or alkali in the eye, any flushing that is done must be done from the bridge of the nose with the patient in the supine position laterally so as not to run the toxic chemicals into the uninjured eye.

Incidence and MOI of Head Injury

Q What is the incidence, morbidity, and mortality of head trauma in the United States?

A Approximately four million people sustain a head injury each year. This includes some 450,000 who require hospitalization. Most head injuries are minor with a Glasgow Coma Scale (GCS) from 13 to 15. Major head injury (GCS <8) is the most common cause of death from trauma in trauma centers. Statistics show that over 50 percent of all trauma deaths involve a head injury.

Q What is the highest risk group for head injury?

A The highest risk of a head injury is in males between 15 to 24 years of age. Infants, six months to two years, are at high risk as are young school-age children and the elderly.

Q What are the typical MOIs for head injuries?

A The most common cause of head trauma and subdural hematoma is MVC. Other MOIs for head injury include sports, falls by the elderly, falls in the presence of alcohol abuse (falls are associated with chronic subdural hematomas), and penetrat-

ing trauma (e.g., rifles, handguns, and shotguns). Sharp projectiles are not as common (e.g., knives, axes, screwdrivers).

Anatomy and Physiology of Head Injury

Q What is the importance of the scalp?

A The scalp provides a layer of protection to the skull. It is comprised of the hair and subcutaneous tissue, which contains the major scalp veins that when injured, can bleed profusely. The muscle of the scalp is attached just above the eyebrows and at the base of the occiput. The galea is a freely moveable sheet of connective tissue that helps to deflect blows. There is loose connective tissue in the scalp that contains emissary veins that drain directly into the brain and can spread infection.

CLINICAL PEARL

It is possible to bleed to death from a scalp injury. In addition, a significant hematoma may accumulate in the space between the scalp and the skull, leading to profound shock.

Q What are the key elements of the skull?

A The skull consists of the bones of the face, previously discussed, and the cranium. There are five basic regions of the skull: frontal, occipital, temporal, parietal, and mastoid. The actual bones that comprise the skull are double layered with a spongy middle layer, allowing them to be strong yet light in weight. The floor of the skull has many bony ridges that are problematic when the brain moves around inside. In essence, the skull can provide protection and can actually injure the brain too. At the base of the skull is the "big hole" or foramen magnum (Latin translation) where the spinal cord exits down the spinal column.

Q What is the significance of the middle meningeal artery?

A The temporal bone, at the sides of the head anterior to the eyes, is the thinnest part of the skull. In a groove along the side of the head just beneath the temporal bone lies the middle meningeal artery that is easily injured when the patient receives a blow to the side of the head (Figure 38–3). Because this is arterial bleeding, it develops very rapidly. The ensuing epidural hematoma can be life threatening if not recognized and cared for quickly.

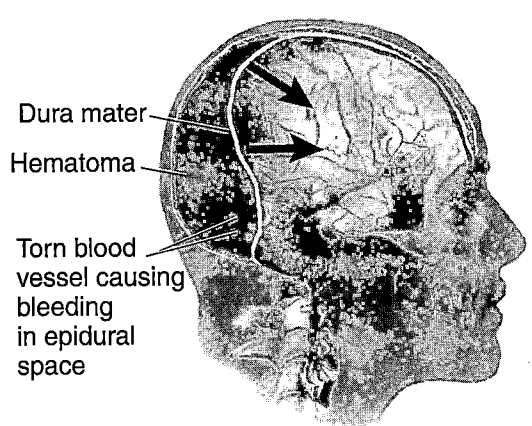

Dura mater

Hematoma

Torn blood vessel causing bleeding in epidural space

FIGURE 38-3 The pathway of the middle meningeal artery is associated with skull fracture and epidural hematoma.

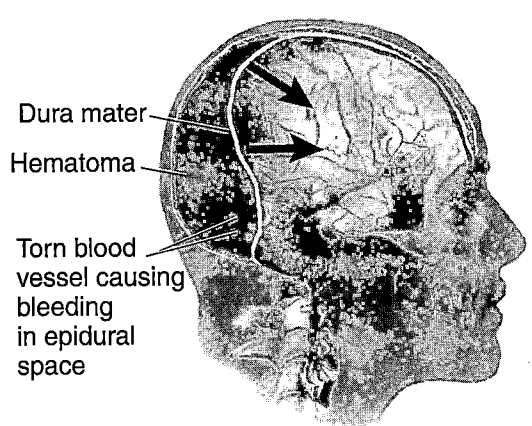

What are the functions of the sections of the cerebrum?

The lobes of the cerebrum are named by the region of the skull that they lie beneath. There are cortex controls that are responsible for voluntary skeletal movement and the level of awareness component of consciousness. Interference with the voluntary skeletal movement may result in extremity paralysis, paresthesia, weakness, or paralysis. The specific functions of the lobes are as follows:

- Frontal lobe—personality. Trauma may result in placid reactions or seizures.
- Parietal lobe—somatic sensory input, memory, and emotions.
- Temporal lobe—speech centers are located here and 85 percent of the population has their center on their left side. This also houses long-term memory, taste, and smell.
- Occipital lobe—this is the origin of the optic nerve. Trauma here may cause "stars," blurred vision, or other visual disturbances.
- Hypothalamus—holds the centers for vomiting, regulating body temperature, and water.

What is the role of the cerebellum?

The cerebellum is responsible for the coordination of voluntary movement started by the cerebral cortex.

What are the key areas of the brain stem?

The brain stem helps to connect hemispheres of the brain. The cerebellum and spinal cord are responsible for the vegetative functions and vital signs. The parts of the brain stem include the midbrain, pons, and medulla oblongata.

What are the functions of the 12 cranial nerves?

The functions of the 12 cranial nerves are described in Table 38-1.

What are the key cranial nerves for the EMS provider?

Understanding the functions of the third and tenth cranial nerves is key. The oculomotor nerve (cranial nerve III) originates in the midbrain and controls pupil size. Pressure paralyzes the nerve, rendering the pupil unreactive. The vagus nerve (cranial nerve X) originates in the medulla as a bundle of nerves primarily from the parasympathetic system. It supplies the sinoatrial (SA) and atrioventricular (AV) nodes, as well as the stomach and GI tract. Pressure on cranial nerve X stimulates bradycardia.

What area of the brain is responsible for our level of consciousness (LOC)?

The reticular activating system (RAS) is responsible for the level of arousal and must be an intact cortical function for the level of awareness to be present.

What are the meninges?

There are protective layers that surround and enfold the entire CNS called the meninges. The relation between the meninges and the hematomas that may develop around them are shown in Figure 38-4.

TABLE 38-1

The Cranial Nerves	
Cranial Nerve	Function
I. Olfactory	Smell
II. Optic	Sight
III. Oculomotor	Movement of the eyeball, pupil, and eyelid
IV. Trochlear	Movement of eyeball
V. Trigeminal	Chewing; pain, temperature, and touch of face and mouth
VI. Abducens	Movement of eyeball
VII. Facial	Movement of face and secretion of saliva; taste
VIII. Auditory	Hearing and balance
IX. Glossopharyngeal	Swallowing and secretion of saliva; taste and sensation in mouth and pharynx
X. Vagus	Sensation and movement in pharynx, larynx, thorax, and gastrointestinal system
XI. Accessory	Movement of head and shoulder
XII. Hypoglossal	Movement of tongue

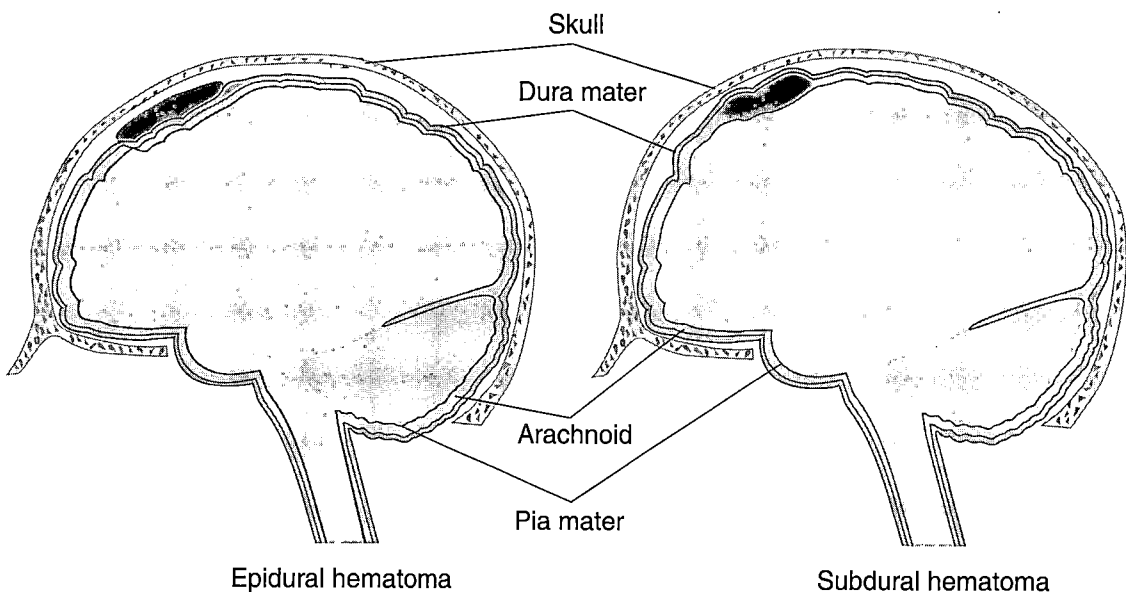

FIGURE 38-4 The relationship of the meninges and the hematomas found below or outside them, (A) epidural and (B) subdural.

What is unique about the brain's metabolism?

The brain has a very high metabolic rate. It requires many nutrients, such as glucose and thiamine, but does not have the ability to store nutrients. The brain consumes 20 percent of the body's oxygen supply.

What is unique about the perfusion of the brain?

The brain receives 15 percent of the cardiac output. A mechanism called autoregulation is responsible for regulating the body's BP to maintain the cerebral perfusion pressure (CPP). Perfusion of the brain can be affected by conditions that interfere with CPP such as edema, bleeding, or hypotension.

There must be a mean arterial pressure (MAP) of at least 60 mmHg for the brain to be perfused. Thus, the formula for CPP is CPP = MAP − intracerebral pressure (ICP). Patients with multiple system trauma involving head injury and other injuries that lead to severe shock states must have IV fluids in order for the brain to continue to be perfused adequately. With an isolated head injury, this would not be the case. Isolated head injuries do not get large volumes of fluid because the BP or intracerebral pressure should not be raised any higher than it already is.

What are the general categories of head injuries?

General categories of head injuries include:
- Coup injuries developing directly below the point of impact (Figure 38–5).

- Contra coup injuries developing in the opposite side of the point of impact. These are common when the back of the head is struck.
- Diffuse axonal injury—a shearing or tearing or stretching force to nerve fibers with axonal damage. These are more common with vehicle occupants and pedestrians struck by a vehicle.
- Focal injury—an identifiable site of injury limited to a particular area or region of the brain.

What is a head injury and what are the categories?

Head injury is a traumatic insult to the head that can result in an injury to the soft tissue, bony structures, or brain. The two major categories are blunt and penetrating. Specifically, blunt head trauma is more common and the dura remains intact. The brain tissue is not exposed to the environment, and it may result in fractures, focal brain injuries, and diffuse axonal injuries.

Penetrating head trauma is less common and usually caused by a GSW. The dura and cranial contents are penetrated often exposing brain tissue, and there are often fractures and focal brain injuries present.

What is a brain injury?

A brain injury is a traumatic insult to the brain capable of producing physical, intellectual, emotional, social, or vocational change. The categories of brain injury include a focal injury and subarachnoid hemorrhage or a diffuse axonal injury.

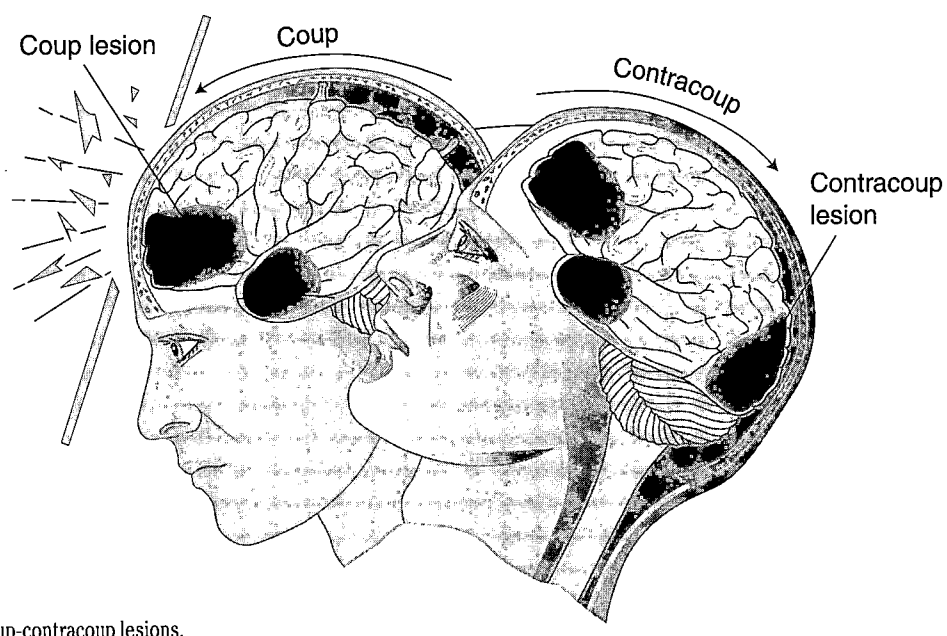

FIGURE 38–5 The coup-contracoup lesions.

What are focal injuries?

Focal injuries are specific grossly observable brain lesions (e.g., cerebral contusion, intracranial hemorrhage, epidural hematoma).

What is a diffuse axonal injury (DAI)?

DAI is the effect of acceleration or deceleration on the brain. It is often a mild or classic concussion, but it can be moderate or severe.

What is the mechanism by which ICP rises?

As the ICP approaches the MAP, the gradient for flow decreases. This reduces cerebral blood flow, which in turn decreases CPP. As the CPP decreases, cerebral vasodilatation occurs, resulting in increased cerebral blood volume leading to an increase in ICP, which again results in further cerebral vasodilatation. The hypercarbia causes cerebral vasodilatation that results in an increase in cerebral blood volume. This is a vicious cycle that is further complicated if the patient has another injury causing hypotension that also results in decreasing CPP.

What is a concussion?

A concussion is a mild DAI involving physiologic neurologic dysfunction without substantial anatomical disruption. A concussion results in a transient episode of neuronal dysfunction with a rapid return to normal neurologic activity. These injuries are most commonly the result of blunt trauma to the head. The patient is confused and disoriented and may not remember the event.

What is a contusion?

Contusions are actual structural damage to the brain from a DAI. They can be moderate or severe.

What is a skull fracture?

A skull fracture is a break in the cranium caused by a significant amount of force.

What are the types of skull fractures?

The specific type of skull fracture is determined by X-ray, but the more common types are shown in Figure 38–6 and include the following:

- Linear—80 percent of all skull fractures. These may have fluid leak out, forming a bulge. The fluid leak may not occur for 24 hours. If there are no associated injuries, there is no danger.

- Depressed—involve bone fragments that protrude into the brain. Neurologic signs and symptoms are usually evident.

- Basilar—an extension of a linear fracture to the floor of skull. A basilar fracture may not be seen on X-ray or CT. The signs and symptoms depend on the extent of damage. Most frequently, blood vessels are disrupted and CSF or blood leaks from the ear(s) or nose. The patient may have bilateral black eyes, called raccoon sign. There may also be bruising behind

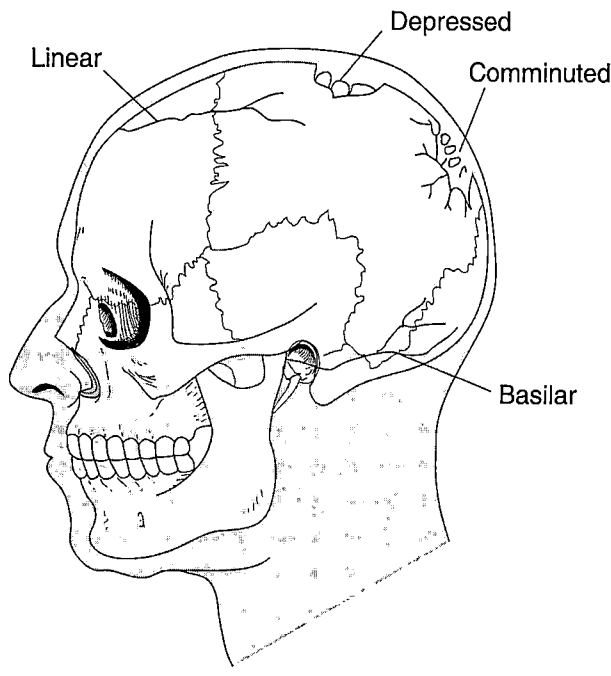

FIGURE 38-6 Common types of skull fractures.

ear(s), which is called Battle sign. These patients may have seizures due to the irritation of brain tissue by blood.

- Open skull fractures—usually due to severe force that exposes brain tissue. Neurologic signs and symptoms are usually evident.

What are the types of intracranial hemorrhage?

The types of intracranial hemorrhage are named by their location in relation to the layers of the meninges. They include epidural, subdural, intracerebral, and subarachnoid.

What is the epidemiology of an intracranial hemorrhage?

The epidemiology of intracranial hemorrhage depends on the specific location where the bleeding is occurring. For example:

- Epidural hematoma—almost always results from arterial tears, usually from the middle meningeal artery. They amount to about 0.5 to 1 percent of head injuries.
- Subdural hematoma—more common injury. Results from the rupture of bridging veins between the cortex and dura. May be acute or chronic. Chronic bleeds are more common in the elderly and alcoholics who fall down and hit their head a lot.
- Subarachnoid hematoma—results in bloody CSF and meningeal irritation.
- Intracerebral hematoma—within the brain substance. Many small, deep intracerebral hemorrhages are associated with

other brain injuries (especially DAI). Neurologic deficits depend on the associated injuries, the region involved, the size of the hemorrhage, and whether bleeding continues.

Assessment of Head Injury

What are some of the additional assessment findings with an increasing ICP that leads to the downward pressure on the brain toward the foramen magnum with potential herniation there or at the tentorium?

As the hematoma causes the brain to shift downward, the following findings may be noted:

- Cerebral cortices or the RAS is affected by movement within the skull. This causes AMS, amnesia of the event, confusion, disorientation, combativeness, or focal neurological deficits.
- The pressure on the hypothalamus causes vomiting.
- Pressure on the brain stem causes the BP to rise in an attempt to maintain MAP and CPP, vagal nerve pressure causes bradycardia. This is a late response and usually precedes death by only four to six minutes.
- Depressed respirations cause CO_2 retention, brain swelling, and hypoxemia in the brain tissue.
- Pressure on the respiratory center causes irregular respirations and tachypnea.
- Pressure on the oculomotor nerve causes unequal or unreactive pupils.
- The pressure on the brain stem also can cause posturing such as flexion or extension.

The patient may exhibit seizure activity depending on the location of the injury.

CLINICAL PEARL

The usual response to brain injury is elevated BP due to loss of cerebral autoregulation. This is the only way that the body can continue perfusion to the injured tissue. The "Cushing's reflex" of hypotension and bradycardia occurs at a late stage, and only lasts four to six minutes. Death follows shortly thereafter.

What is the impact of an increasing ICP on the cerebral cortex and upper brain stem?

When there is pressure on the cerebral cortex and upper brain stem from an enlarging hematoma, the following assessment findings may be uncovered:

- The BP rises and the pulse rate slows (Cushing's reflex).
- The pupils are still reactive.
- Cheyne-Stokes respirations may be present.
- Initially the patient tries to localize and remove the painful stimuli (pinch the arm and the patient will try to push your hand away). Eventually, as mental status further deteriorates, this sensation is lost and the patient withdraws from pain and flexion (or decorticate posturing) occurs in response to the painful stimuli.

What is the impact of an increasing ICP on the middle brain stem?

When there is pressure on the middle brain stem from an enlarging hematoma, the following assessment findings may be uncovered:

- A wide pulse pressure and bradycardia.
- The pupils are unequal, nonreactive, or sluggish.
- The patient will have the respiratory pattern known as central neurogenic hyperventilation.
- When pain is applied, the patient no longer flexes (decorticate posturing). The patient begins to extend the extremities (decerebrate posturing).
- Few patients function normally after a brain herniation gets to this level.

What is the impact when the pressure from ICP affects the lower brain stem or medulla?

At this late point in brain herniation, the patient will have a blown pupil on the side of the injury, the respirations are ataxic or erratic with no rhythm or are absent. The patient will be flaccid with no response to pain and a pulse rate that is irregular with great swings in rate. The ECG will have QRS, S-T, and T wave changes and the patient's injury is not considered survivable. Basically, the control of vegetative function and vital signs has been rendered inoperable by the tremendous pressure.

How does the severity of a head injury relate to GCS?

With GCS being an objective measure of eye opening, verbal response, and motor response with a numerical score from 3 to 15 (see Chapter 24, Neurology, for more information), a mild head injury would have a GCS of 13 to 15. A moderate head injury would be 8 to 12 and a severe injury would be less than 8 (Table 38–2).

TABLE 38–2

The Glasgow Coma Scale

	Best Response	Points
Eyes	Open spontaneously	4
	Open to verbal command	3
	Open to painful stimulus	2
	Do not open	1
Verbal	Oriented	5
	Disoriented	4
	Inappropriate words	3
	Incomprehensible sounds	2
	No response	1
Motor	Obeys command	6
	Localizes pain	5
	Withdraws from pain	4
	Shows abnormal flexion	3
	Shows abnormal extension	2
	No response	1
TOTAL		3–15

What can be expected if a patient has a moderate DAI?

A moderate DAI results from a shearing, stretching, or tearing that causes minute petechial bruising of the brain tissue. This injury occurs in 20 percent of all severe head injuries and 45 percent of all cases of DAI. It is commonly associated with a basilar skull fracture. Most of these patients survive but with neurologic impairment.

On assessment, the patient may have persistent confusion, disorientation, and amnesia of the event, extending to amnesia of moment-to-moment events. The patient may have focal deficit, an inability to concentrate, and psychological effects such as frequent periods of anxiety or uncharacteristic mood swings. They may also have sensory motor deficits (e.g., sense of smell altered).

What can be expected if a patient has a severe DAI?

This injury was formerly called a brain stem injury. It involves the severe mechanical disruption of many axons in both cerebral hemispheres and extends to the brain stem. Severe DAI represents 16 percent of all severe head injuries and 36 percent of all cases of DAI. The patient will be unconscious and may have been for a prolonged period of time. Posturing is common as are other signs of increased ICP.

What is the specific assessment of different types of skull fractures?

Basically the assessment is the same. Linear fractures may be missed unless there are symptoms of an underlying hematoma developing. Depressed and open skull fractures are usually found on palpation of the head. Be careful to use the balls of fingers to palpate and not "poke" into the fracture site, potentially driving bone fragments into the brain tissue.

The assessment should include the following:

- Airway patency and breathing adequacy must be a high priority.
- Vomiting and inadequate respirations are common in the patient with a skull fracture.
- Assess for signs and symptoms of increased ICP as previously discussed.
- Assess for an AMS and determine the GCS.
- Assess the pupils for changes in size and reaction to light from side-to-side.
- Assess the baseline vitals and monitor frequently.

What does the assessment of a cerebral contusion involve?

The assessment is the same as for all other head injuries, but pay particular attention to the following:

- Airway patency and breathing adequacy a priority.
- An AMS, such as confusion or unusual behavior, is common.
- The patient may complain of a progressive headache or photophobia (afraid of bright light).
- The patient may have difficulty remembering things, repeating the same phrases again and again.
- Be sure to assess for the signs and symptoms of increased ICP (e.g., AMS, decreased GCS, vomiting, changes in the pupils, decreased pulse rate, and increased BP).

Are there any specific assessment findings for a suspected intracranial hematoma developing?

It may be impossible to tell which type of hematoma is present. Whatever history you can obtain from the patient or bystanders is very important (e.g., What were they doing? What happened? What is wrong now? What doesn't seem right?), but is sometimes unreliable because the patient may be confused from the head injury. It is very important to recognize the presence of brain injury. Trending of mental status, vital signs, pupils, and so forth is critical to these patients.

A "classical" story of a patient with a developing epidural hematoma is the child knocked unconscious at a little league game. He was probably struck on the temporal skull. EMS was called immediately. On arrival, you find there was a lucid interval and his mental state has again begun to rapidly deteriorate. This is due to the fact that he probably injured the middle meningeal artery causing arterial bleeding into the epidural space. The blood collects very rapidly and the ensuing hematoma is life threatening if not quickly recognized by the history.

The signs and symptoms of an intracranial hematoma include the following:

- Headache that is getting increasingly severe.
- Nausea and vomiting.
- Mental state changes that range from lethargy to confusion early on to changes in consciousness from verbally responsive to unresponsive in late stages. Always pay very close attention to even subtle changes in the mental status with patients who you suspect may have a head injury.
- Changes in the size of the pupil.
- A slow pulse rate or irregular pulse rate.
- Respirations that are becoming irregular.
- Neurological posturing, paralysis of one side of the body, or seizure activity.
- The patient may have neurological deficits.
- Signs of brain irritation—change in personality, irritability, and repeating words or phrases.

Management of Head Injury

What is the appropriate management of head injury in the field?

The management of head trauma includes the following:

- Ensure a patent airway—avoid nasal intubation because it may increase the ICP.
- Ensure adequate ventilation and oxygenation. The oxygen saturation should be 95 to 100 percent. If the patient has signs and symptoms of increased ICP (confirmed with arterial blood gasses in the ED), they can be hyperventilated (no greater than 24 per minute). Make sure they are able to exhale so as not to retain CO_2, which would further contribute to the brain swelling.
- Ensure adequate circulation. Start an IV of normal saline and titrate to BP. Remember, we do not want too much fluid; however, we definitely do not want hypotension to develop. If hypotension develops, it is most likely due to bleeding from another organ or injury besides the brain.
- Conduct repeated neurological assessments (trending) and notify the ED of even subtle changes in the patient's condition (e.g., focal findings, change in GCS, or increasing ICP).
- Elevate the head end of the backboard approximately 30 degrees.

- Transport the patient to an appropriate center that can handle a neurosurgical emergency. Consider the usefulness of aeromedical transport in this case.

CLINICAL PEARL

For years, one of the recommended treatments for a person with head injury was hyperventilation, usually via ET intubation. The idea was that hyperventilation reduced the ICP. Recent studies have questioned the need for aggressive hyperventilation, suggesting that it produces a marked reduction in cerebral blood flow (CBF). Decreased CBF may lead to or exacerbate ischemia, enhancing rather than reducing injury. If hyperventilation is used, most experts recommend using arterial blood gases to follow the patient's response, along with ICP monitoring. Both techniques are not done in the field routinely.

Q Are there any pharmacological interventions worth considering?

A Studies have shown that field paralysis prior to intubation improves the outcome of combative head trauma patients. Debate remains regarding the role and timing of steroids (e.g., Solumedrol®) and diuretics (e.g., mannitol, furosemide). Follow your local protocols. Avoid glucose unless hypoglycemia is confirmed first.

Q What is the management of a suspected skull fracture or cerebral contusion?

A The management of a patient with a skull fracture or cerebral contusion is as follows:

- Take cervical spine precautions as you are ensuring a clear airway and adequate ventilation with good tidal volume.
- It is imperative that hypoxia be prevented to prevent secondary injury to brain tissue. Treat increased ICP first by ensuring adequate tidal volume. Osmotic diuretics are debatable for use by paramedics in the field.
- Ensure that the CPP is maintained by making sure the systolic BP stays over 70 mmHg. Establish an IV and manage hypotension with fluid boluses, not to exceed a systolic of 90–100 mmHg in the adult male under 40 years old (avoid shock).
- Consider elevating the head of stretcher or backboard 30 degrees.
- Keep the patient warm and comfortable.

CHAPTER 39

Spinal Trauma

This chapter discusses impacts to the spinal cord or spinal cord injury (SCI). Traumatic SCI and nontraumatic conditions, such as degenerative disc disease and low back syndrome, are reviewed. The general public rarely considers the impact of a SCI and how quickly their lives could change if they were to sustain a SCI. In recent years, this was brought to light by Christopher Reeves' tragic fall from a horse that left him a quadriplegic. Mr. Reeves has tried to make the best out of his situation by becoming an unrelenting advocate for SCI victims.

The focus of this chapter is on *why* patients present in a certain manner, the mechanisms of injury (MOIs) that often lead to SCI, and *why* you need to be attentive to the potential causes of a MOI and manage it appropriately in the field. The difference between the early recognition of a possible SCI and proper management in the field can mean the difference between a normal recovery and a lifetime in a wheelchair!

Epidemiology

Q What is the incidence of SCI?

A There are between 15,000 and 20,000 SCIs each year. The highest incidence is in men between 16 and 30 years old, primarily due to sports and inexperienced driving.

Q What are the common causes of SCI?

A There are four major categories of SCI causes. Motor vehicle crashes (MVCs) account for 48 percent, falls account for 21 percent, penetrating injuries account for 15 percent, and sports injuries account for 14 percent.

Q What is the morbidity and mortality of a SCI?

A Of the trauma patients with an initial neurological deficit, 40 percent will have a SCI. It is estimated that 25 percent of SCIs

are caused by improper handling of the patient. This includes bystanders pulling patients out of a car for fear of an explosion or fire and pulling a patient out of a swimming pool without spinal immobilization. Education in the proper handling and transportation of the SCI patient can go a long way in reducing these injuries.

Q What is the impact of a SCI on the patient?

A It is difficult to fully measure the impact of a SCI on the patient and his family. Their lifestyle is undoubtedly changed dramatically. A simple walk in the park, trip to the shopping mall, or commute to work is considerably more difficult for the SCI patient. Finally, there are the incredible medical costs of caring for the SCI patient. It is estimated that the cost of caring for a single victim with a permanent SCI is 1.25 million dollars over their life span.

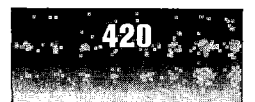

Anatomy and Physiology

Q | What are the key ligaments supporting the spine?

A | Four key ligaments support the spine: the anterior longitudinal ligament, the posterior longitudinal ligament, the cruciform ligament, and the accessory atlantoaxial ligament. The anterior longitudinal ligament runs on the anterior portion of the body and is a major source of stability. It protects against hyperextension. The posterior longitudinal ligament runs along the posterior body within the vertebral canal. It prevents hyperflexion and can be a major source of injury. The first two vertebrae are extremely important in the movement of the head. Their names are the atlas, which is vertebrae number one, and the axis, which is vertebrae number two. The cruciform ligament is a ligament shaped like a cross that supports the atlas vertebrae. The atlantoaxial ligament attaches the axis and atlas, as well as the transverse ligament that serves to hold the odontoid process close to the anterior arch.

CLINICAL PEARL

Remember that the spine consists of interconnected bones, ligaments, muscles, and tendons (as well as nerves and blood vessels). Injury to any of these components may result in neck or back pain.

CLINICAL PEARL

The lumbar spine is commonly injured. Many of these injuries involve muscle spasm and do not threaten the integrity of the spinal cord and its roots. Nonetheless, low back pain is a common problem, as well as a major cause of impairment and disability.

Q | What is the anatomical relation between the brain and spinal cord?

A | The brain, which is the largest and most complex portion of the central nervous system (CNS), is continuous with the spinal cord. The coverings, or the meninges, are also continuous between both the brain and spinal cord. The brain is responsible for all sensory and motor functions. There are 12 pairs of cranial nerves that come directly out of the brain. There are also 31 pairs of peripheral nerves, called the spinal nerves, that exit the spinal cord between each of the vertebrae and are responsible for the sensory and motor functions of the body below the head. The meninges, cranial nerves, and the brain are covered in much more detail in Chapter 24, Neurology.

Q | What is the grey and white matter in the cord?

A | The grey matter is located in the core of the cord, which resembles a butterfly with outspread wings. Most of the neurons in the grey matter are interneurons, which are small neurons that connect the larger ones. The white matter is located in the anatomical spinal tracts, which are longitudinal bundles of myelinated nerve fibers. Myelin is a soft, white, fatty substance that forms a thick sheath around certain nerves.

Q | What are the ascending nerve tracts?

A | The ascending nerve tracts carry impulses from body parts and sensory information to the brain. There are two groups of tracts involved: the fasciculus gracilis and corneatus tracts, and the spinothalmic tracts. Their specific functions are as follows:

- Fasciculus gracilis and corneatus—are part of the posterior funiculi of the cord. A funiculi is a group of nerve fibers with similar functions like a coaxial cable. They conduct sensory impulses from the skin, muscle tendons, and joints to the brain for interpretation as sensations of touch, pressure, and body movement. Due to the cross over from one side to the other at the medulla oblongata, the impulses originating from the left side ascend to the right side of the brain and vice versa.

- Spinothalmic tracts—the lateral and anterior tracts are located in the lateral and anterior funiculi. The lateral tracts conduct impulses of pain and temperature to the brain, while the anterior tracts carry impulses of touch and pressure to the brain. The impulses cross over in the spinal cord. The spinocerebellar tracts are found near the lateral funiculi. They coordinate impulses necessary for muscular movements by carrying impulses from muscles in the legs and trunk to the cerebellum.

Q | What are the descending nerve tracts?

A | The descending nerve tracts carry motor impulses from the brain to the body. There are three groups: the corticospinal, reticulospinal, and rubrospinal tracts. Their specific functions are as follows:

- Corticospinal tracts—are lateral tracts that cross over at the medulla oblongata. The anterior tract descends uncrossed. They conduct motor impulses from the brain to the spinal nerves and out to the body for voluntary movements.

- Reticulospinal tracts—these are lateral, anterior, and medial tracts that are a mix of crossed (same side works the opposite side of the body) and uncrossed fibers (same side works the same side of the body). Some of the lateral fibers cross over, while the anterior and medial tracts remain uncrossed. The motor impulses originate in the brain to control muscle tone and sweat gland activity.

• Rubrospinal tracts—these fibers cross over in the brain and then pass through the lateral funiculi. They are responsible for motor impulses from the brain controlling muscle coordination and posture.

CLINICAL PEARL

Ascending tracts are sometimes called afferent *pathways (toward the brain) and descending,* efferent *pathways (away from the brain).*

Q | What is the function of the spinal nerves?

A | The 31 pairs of spinal nerves originate from the spinal cord. These are mixed nerves that carry both sensation and motor function and provide two-way communication between the spinal cord and the rest of the body. They are named according to the level of the spine from which they originate (e.g., cervical 1–8, thoracic 1–12, lumbar 1–5, sacral 1–5, coccygeal 1 set). The spinal nerves emerge from the cord and have two short branches or roots. The dorsal root carries sensory impulses to the cord and the ventral root carries motor impulses from the cord to the body.

Q | What is the role of the motor and sensory dermatomes?

A | A dermatome is a particular area where the spinal nerve provides either motor stimulation, sensation, or both. They can be mapped out by the level of the spinal nerve (Figure 39–1). Dermatomes are a useful tool to determine the specific level of the SCI. Some examples of how the nerve roots and motor and sensory functions correlate are shown in Table 39–1.

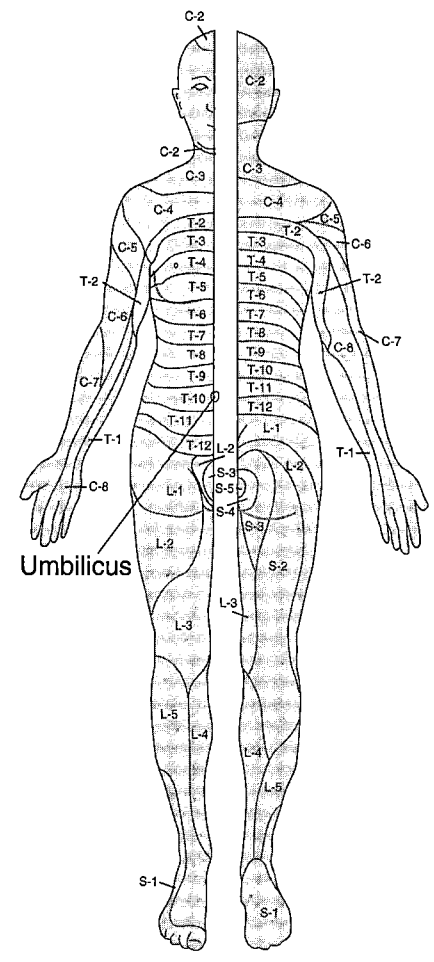

FIGURE 39–1 Dermatones.

Assessment of a Spinal Cord Injury

Q | What has traditional spinal assessment criteria included?

A | In many EMS systems, there has been a lack of clear guidelines or specific criteria to evaluate for a SCI. Assessment of the spinal-cord injured patient is evolving. Researchers are trying to establish criteria by which to "clear C-spines" in the field. Experts agree that there is a need for further research and an agreement on standardized clear criteria to assess for the presence of a SCI. Traditional spinal assessment criteria include:

• Primary MOI-based.

• Signs that suggest a SCI: pain, tenderness, painful movement, deformity, cut or bruises over the spinal area, paralysis, weakness, or paresthesias.

TABLE 39–1

Relationship between Nerve Root, Motor, and Sensory Function		
Nerve Root	Motor	Sensory
Nerve Root	Motor	Sensory
C-3, 4	Trapezius (shoulder shrug)	Top of shoulder
C-3, 4, 5	Diaphragm	Top of shoulder
C-5, 6	Biceps (elbow flexion)	Thumb
C-7	Triceps (elbow extension) Wrist/finger extension	Middle finger
C-8/T-1	Finger abduction/adduction	Little finger
T-4	Nipple	
T-10	Umbilicus	
L-1, 2	Hip flexion	Inguinal crease
L-3, 4	Quadriceps	Medial thigh/calf
L-5	Great toe/foot dorsiflexion	Lateral calf
S-1	Knee flexion	Lateral foot
S-1, 2	Foot plantar flexion	
S-2, 3, 4	Anal sphincter tone	Perianal

- Immobilization of all unconscious accident victims, immobilization of conscious accident victims until checked for a SCI prior to movement, and any patient with an injury that may have been caused by extreme motion.

It has not always been practical to immobilize every "motion" injury. Most patients with suspected spinal injuries are moved to a normal anatomical position, and placed supine on a long backboard. There has not been any exclusion criteria used for moving patients to the anatomical position with the exception of extreme pain or resistance from the bones in moving the neck. In these two rare instances, the neck should be immobilized in the position it was found.

How important is it to determine the MOI in assessing a spinal injury?

Very important. The MOI should always be evaluated because many patients do not immediately present with positive neurological deficits. The patient will either have a positive (indications found), negative (none found), or uncertain MOI when evaluated.

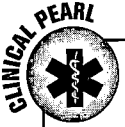

MOI is one of the most significant determinants in the assessment and treatment of any injury victim.

What are examples of a positive MOI for a spinal injury?

A positive MOI for spinal injury always requires full spinal immobilization. Examples include:

- High-speed MVCs.
- Falls greater than three times the patient's height.
- Violent injuries occurring near the spine such as stabbings or gunshot wounds (GSWs).
- Sports (high-energy impact) injuries and other high-impact situations.

Do EMS providers clear a spine in the field?

EMS providers have been choosing not to immobilize a patient with a SCI for years. Some might call that clearing the spine. Sometimes the decision was appropriate and in some instances, it may not have been. The legal implications and potential for serious harm to the patient are extremely high if a mistake is made and a patient who should have been immobilized was not. There are few objective criteria available to use in the field. In the ED, many physicians use recently published criteria to immobilize or to remove immobilization equipment all of the time. These criteria, through proven in the ED, have not yet been universally accepted in the out-of-hospital setting.

Some EMS systems have provided additional training and medical director approval for the EMS providers to determine whether immobilization is not needed on a patient who has a SCI. Several states have adopted protocols based on ED studies. Field studies are underway. Preliminary work supports the adoption of the following exclusion criteria in the field:

- The patient is reliable (to the best of your knowledge).
- There is no altered mental status (AMS) or intoxication involved.
- There are no distracting injuries.
- The patient lacks any signs or symptoms of spinal injury.

Several states and EMS systems have instituted field spinal clearance protocols with good initial results. Always follow your local protocols and medical direction.

What is meant by a negative MOI for spinal injury?

When the forces of impact do not suggest a potential spinal injury and it is determined that spinal immobilization will not be needed, the MOI is negative for spinal injury. A few examples include: dropping a rock on a foot, twisting an ankle while running, stepping into a pot hole, or an isolated soft tissue injury (e.g., laceration with a box cutter).

What is meant by the term full spinal immobilization?

This is a very misleading phrase. It leads one to believe that there is such a thing as partial spinal immobilization (e.g., applying just a collar or applying just a spine board). If the decision is made to immobilize a patient in the field, the patient should get both a collar and spine board. The only time a patient has just a collar is when they get released from the hospital with a neck muscle strain. The purpose of the collar is to remind the patient to limit movement to give the injury an opportunity to repair itself. If the patient actually had a spinal fracture, they would be placed in traction with a halo device and pins in their head.

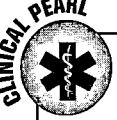

There is either full spinal immobilization or none at all. "Partial spinal immobilization" is an invitation to the courtroom for the unwary.

What are examples of an uncertain MOI for spinal injury?

A general rule of out-of-hospital medicine is that if you are unsure of the diagnosis, consider up-triaging till you have more information. Patients can have significant injuries in the absence

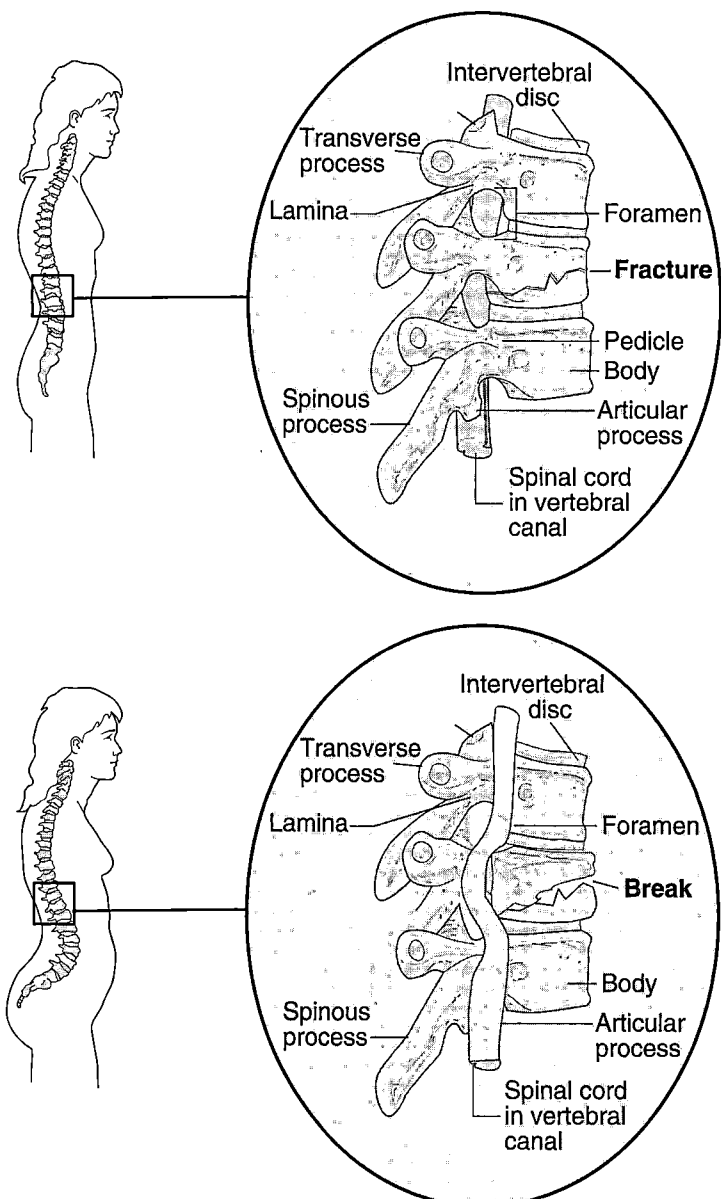

FIGURE 39-2 Even in the absence of significant neuro deficits, excessive movement of a patient with spinal injuries can cause damage to the spinal cord.

of obvious neurological deficits as shown in Figure 39–2. When you are uncertain whether the MOI could involve a spine injury, up-triage the patient to "rule out spinal injury" and go ahead and do the spinal immobilization. Examples include tripping over a garden hose and falling to the ground hitting the head, a fall from two to four feet onto a hard surface, or a low speed MVC.

Q What is a reliable or unreliable patient when considering not immobilizing in the field?

A For a patient to be considered reliable, they must be calm, cooperative, sober, alert, and oriented. An unreliable patient may have any of the following assessment findings:

- An acute stress reaction.
- Sustained a brain injury as exhibited by any temporary change in mental status.
- Uncooperative or exhibiting belligerent behavior.
- Intoxicated.
- AMS.
- Distracting injuries.
- Communication problems.

If the patient is unreliable and you suspect a questionable MOI for the spinal injury, it is essential that spinal immobilization be done.

How should a patient be assessed for spinal pain?

If there is a high impact MOI, immobilize the patient. If it is questionable, then maintain stabilization and ask the patient if he has any related spinal pain, or signs or symptoms of spinal injury. Note that the pain may be poorly localized and it may not hurt directly over the spinous process. If the patient has been moving his head and neck, ask if there was any pain with active movement. If you have any doubt, immobilize the patient. If you believe they do not need immobilization because of the minor nature of the impact or it is an "uncertain MOI," then ask the patient to slowly move his head to see if any pain occurs. If any pain is felt, have him stop moving his head and neck and immobilize the spine.

How should a patient be assessed for spinal tenderness?

If a patient is not palpated, you may never uncover tenderness. Palpate over each of the spinal processes of the vertebrae, beginning at the neck and working toward the pelvis. If tenderness is found on or next to the spine, immobilize the spine.

CLINICAL PEARL

Always palpate over the spinous processes before concluding that a patient "has no neck pain." Some providers simply ask the patient and never perform a physical exam.

How are the upper extremities assessed for neurological function?

The extremities need to be assessed for motor and sensory function, as well as pulses. Check the following:

- Assess for finger abduction and adduction. Test the interosseous muscle function, which is controlled by the T-1 nerve roots. To do this, have the patient spread the fingers of both hands and keep them apart while you squeeze the index and pinky fingers. A normal resistance should be spring-like and equal on both sides.

- Assess for finger and hand extension. Test the extensors of the hand and fingers controlled by the C-7 nerve roots by having the patient hold her wrist or fingers straight out and keep them out while you press down on the fingers. Support the arm at the wrist to avoid testing arm function and other nerve roots. Normal resistance should be felt to moderate pressure. Check both right and left sides. It is still possible to check even if the patient has an isolated finger fracture by pushing

on the hand only and not the fingers. If there is a wrist injury, support the joint and push on the fingers.

- Assess sensory function in the upper extremities. First, ask the patient about abnormal sensations such as weakness, numbness, paresthesia, or radicular pain (pain that shoots somewhere else or moves). The spinothalamic tracts control pain or pinprick sensation. It is necessary to distinguish this sensation from a light touch sensation because that sensation is carried by more than one tract. Use the end of a pen or Q-tip instead of a sharp object that may cause damage or bleeding. Have the patient close her eyes and hold out her hands. Then, have her compare between sharp and dull pain on both sides of the body.

How are the lower extremities assessed for neurological function?

The following are the ways in which to assess the motor and sensory functions of the lower extremities:

- Foot plantar flexion—the plantar flexors of the foot are controlled by the S-1, 2 nerve root. Place your hands on the sole of each foot and have the patient push against your hands. Both sides should feel equal and strong.

- Foot and great toe dorsiflexion—the L-5 nerve root controls the dorsal flexors of the foot and great toe. Hold the foot with your fingers on the toes and instruct the patient to pull the foot back or toward his nose.

- Assess pain sensation in the lower extremities—ask the patient about abnormal sensation such as weakness, numbness, paresthesia, or radicular pain. The spinothalamic tracts control pain or pinprick sensation. It is necessary to distinguish this sensation from that of a light touch, which is carried by more than one tract. Use the end of a pen or Q-tip instead of a sharp object that may cause damage or bleeding. Have the patient close his eyes and compare between sharp and dull pain on both feet of the body.

Traumatic Spinal Cord Injuries

What are the actual causes of traumatic SCIs?

The causes of traumatic SCIs include direct trauma, excessive movement, and directions of force (e.g., acceleration, deceleration, deformation, flexion, hyperflexion, extension, hyperextension, vertical compression, and distraction). It is also possible to have a SCI without a bone injury and a bone injury without a SCI.

The spinal cord may be injured with or without accompanying bone or soft tissue injury. Also, there may be bone or soft tissue injury without spinal cord damage. Some bone and soft tissue injuries are considered "unstable" (spinal cord threatening), but the determination is based on X-ray criteria. If you suspect a patient has any kind of vertebral injury, assume until proven otherwise that the spinal cord is threatened, regardless of the neurological exam.

How does an injury occur with directions of force being applied to the spine?

Injury occurs to the spinal cord depending on the specific direction of the force. Here are some examples of specifics for each of the directions of force applied to the spinal cord:

- Flexion or hyperflexion—this is the forward motion of the head. Flexion simply implies the forward bending of the head toward the body. This may be normal or may result in injury. Hyperflexion implies movement of the head toward the torso beyond the normal range of motion, whether or not an injury results. The "lip-stick sign," where a patient seems to have kissed her chest, may be observed. The cervical spine is the most common region for this type of injury. The force may cause a wedge fracture of the anterior vertebrae. It may also cause stretching or rupturing of interspinous ligaments or a compression injury to the spinal cord. It can cause a disruption of a disk with forward dislocation of the vertebrae or a fracture of the pedicle and disruption of the interspinous ligament.

- Extension or hyperextension—this is the backward movement of the head. Extension simply implies backward bending of the head toward the body. This may be normal or may result in injury. Hyperextension implies movement of the head toward the torso beyond the normal range of motion, whether or not an injury results. Extension may cause disruption of the intervertebral disks. It can cause compression of the spinal cord and compression of the interspinous ligament, as well as a fracture. The cervical spine is the most common region for this type of injury.

- Rotational—this is the normal movement of the head to the left or right from the midline. Excessive rotation is beyond the normal range of motion. It usually is caused by acceleration forces and may cause flexion-rotation dislocation, as well as a fracture or dislocation of the vertebrae. A rupture of the supporting ligaments may also occur. The cervical spine is the most common region for this type of injury.

- Vertical compression—is a force applied along the spinal axis, referred to as axial loading, usually to the top of the cranium

from a sudden deceleration such as a brick falling onto someone's head from construction on a building. It may cause a compression fracture without a SCI or a crushed vertebral body with a SCI. The most common sites are in T-12 to L-2.

- Distraction—this is from a force being applied to the spinal axis that distracts or pulls apart such as a hanging injury. It may cause a stretching of the spinal cord and supporting ligaments. The most common site of this injury is the cervical region.

What is SCIWORA?

SCIWORA is an acronym that stands for spinal cord injury without radiographic abnormalities. This situation can occur in children because the vertebrae lie flatter on top of each other, as opposed to adults where they are more curved. The child's vertebrae can easily dislocate and quickly relocate back into their normal position. This would be very difficult to accomplish with an adult's vertebrae due to the curvature of the spine and way the vertebrae sit on top of each other. The X-ray of a child who has experienced SCIWORA may show a lack of fracture and a perfectly aligned vertebral column, yet the cord itself has been compressed or transected.

SCIWORA cannot be diagnosed in the out-of-hospital setting. Even in the ED, sophisticated studies (e.g., MRI) may be required.

What are the types of spinal cord injuries?

The spinal cord can be injured in a number of ways. Here is a list of most of the ways it can be injured:

- Primary injury—occurs at the time of impact or injury. The causes are cord compression or direct cord injury produced by sharp or unstable bony structures. Another cause is an interruption in the cord's blood supply.

- Secondary injury—swelling, ischemia, or the movement of a bone fragment that occurs after a primary injury.

- Cord concussion—temporary disruption of cord-mediated functions.

- Cord contusion—bruising of the cord's tissues, swelling, and the temporary loss of cord-mediated functions.

- Cord compression—pressure on the cord causing tissue ischemia. This must be decompressed in the hospital to avoid permanent loss or damage to the cord.

- Laceration—tearing of the spinal cord tissue that may be reversed if it is a small cut with only a slight amount of damage. A laceration may result in a permanent loss if the spinal tracts are disrupted.

- Hemorrhage—bleeding into the spinal cord tissue caused by damage to blood vessels. The extent of the injury is usually related to the amount of hemorrhage. Damage or obstruction to the spinal blood supply results in local ischemia.
- Cord transection—physical disruption of the cord, either complete or incomplete; the extent of damage is a function of the portions of the spinal cord that have been disrupted.
- Chemical and metabolic changes due to a SCI.
- Spinal shock—refers to a temporary loss of all types of spinal cord function distal to the injury. The patient will be flaccid and paralyzed distal to the injury site. Spinal shock involves hypotension and vasodilatation, loss of bladder and bowel control, and priapism in the male patient. There is also a loss of thermoregulation. It is important to manage the patient carefully to avoid a secondary injury.
- Neurogenic shock—this is also called spinal vascular shock. It is a temporary loss of the autonomic function of the cord at the level of injury that controls the cardiovascular function. Although rare, shock is usually the result of hidden volume loss (e.g., chest or abdominal injuries). The patient will present with a loss of sympathetic tone, hypotension, bradycardia, and skin that is pink, warm, and dry.

What is the impact of a complete spinal cord transection?

When a patient has a complete spinal cord transection, all of the tracts are completely disrupted. All cord-mediated functions below the transection are permanently lost. This is accurately determined at least 24 hours post-injury when swelling goes down. Complete transection results in quadriplegia if it occurred at the cervical level and paraplegia if it occurred at the thoracic or lumbar level.

What is the impact of an incomplete spinal cord transection?

When a patient sustains a partial spinal cord transection, some of the tracts of the spinal cord remain intact as do some of the core-mediated functions. The patient has the potential for at least a partial recovery, depending on the extent of the injury. Function may be temporarily lost in the incomplete transection. The types of incomplete transactions include anterior cord syndrome, central cord syndrome, and Brown-Séquard's syndrome.

What is anterior cord syndrome?

Anterior cord syndrome is a partial transection caused by bony fragments or pressure on spinal arteries. It involves the loss of motor function and the sensation of pain, temperature, and heavy touch. The patient can continue to have sensation to light touch, motion, position, and vibration.

What is central cord syndrome?

In central cord syndrome, there is a partial transection that usually occurs with a hyperextension of the cervical region. The patient may have weakness or paresthesia in the upper extremities but normal strength in the lower extremities. These patients may have varying degrees of bladder dysfunction depending on which nerves have been damaged.

What is Brown-Séquard's syndrome?

This syndrome is caused by a penetrating injury that produces a partial transection of the spinal cord. It is referred to as a hemisection of the cord and involves only one side of the cord. Complete damage occurs to all spinal tracts on the involved side of the cord. The patient will have isolated loss of all types of functions (e.g., motor, pain, temperature, motion, position). Pain and temperature sensation are lost on the opposite side of the body. The motor function, motion, position, and vibration sensations, and light touch are lost on the same side of the body as the injury.

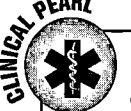

Though of interest, a definitive diagnosis of many so-called "spinal cord syndromes" is difficult in the field.

What is autonomic hyperreflexia syndrome?

Autonomic hyperreflexia syndrome is a massive uncompensated cardiovascular response to stimulation of the sympathetic nervous system. It is a life-threatening condition usually seen with injuries at T-6 or above. The characteristics of this syndrome include:

- Paroxysmal hypertension, sometimes up to 300 mmHg.
- A pounding headache.
- Blurred vision.
- Sweating above the level of the injury with flushing of the skin.
- Increased nasal congestion.
- Nausea.

- Bradycardia.
- Associated distended bladder or rectum.

These patients have stimulation of the sensory receptors below the level of the cord injury. When the autonomic nervous system is stimulated, it reflexively responds with an arteriolar spasm causing an increase in the BP. The hypertension may be treated with antihypertensives. The cerebral, carotid, and aorta baroreceptors sense hypertension and stimulate the parasympathetic nervous system to help decrease the heart rate. The peripheral and visceral vessels are unable to dilate due to the cord damage.

CLINICAL PEARL

Autonomic hyperreflexia (also called autonomic dysreflexia) usually doesn't occur immediately in the face of acute injury. It occurs in the rehabilitation or chronic phase as a result of some type of irritating stimulus (e.g., blocked catheter, appendicitis, fecal impaction). This triggers a discharge of the sympathetic nervous system without sufficient counteraction of the parasympathetic portion. The result is piloerection, severe headache, and massive elevations of both systolic and diastolic BP. Many patients with a SCI are taught to be alert for these findings and may actually alert you to the suspected diagnosis. Primary care is the alleviation of the irritant stimulus and prompt treatment of the BP, usually with IV nitroprusside or IV nitroglycerin.

Nontraumatic Spinal Conditions and Their Management

Q What are the most frequent causes of nontraumatic spinal conditions?

A The most common nontraumatic spinal conditions are: low back pain syndrome, degenerative disk disease, spondylolysis, a herniated intervertebral disk, and spinal cord tumors.

CLINICAL PEARL

A rare, but potentially deadly, cause of low back pain is an epidural abscess. The presentation is similar to other types of low back pain and diagnosis is impossible in the out-of-hospital setting. In fact, it is commonly missed in the hospital setting as well.

Q How common is low back pain?

A Low back pain affects the area between the lower rib cage and gluteal muscles and may radiate into the thighs. Approximately 1 percent of acute low back pain is due to irritation of the sciatic nerve, which runs down the back of the leg. The usual cause is a lumbar nerve root problem. The patient has pain accompanied by motor and sensory deficits such as weakness. Between 60 and 90 percent of the population experience some degree of low back pain during their lifetime. This syndrome affects men equally as often as it affects women up to the age of 60, where it increases in women.

Q What is the cause of low back pain?

A Most cases are idiopathic, where the precise diagnosis is difficult to make. The causes of low back pain include the following:

- Tension from tumor.
- Disk prolapse.
- Bursitis.
- Synovitis.
- Rising venous pressure.
- Tissue pressure due to degenerative joint disease.
- Abnormal bone pressure.
- Problems with spinal mobility.
- Inflammation caused by infection (e.g., osteomyelitis).
- Fractures.
- Ligament strains.

Q What are some of the risk factors for a low back injury?

A Occupations requiring repetitive lifting, such as EMS work, are a high risk for low back injury. Truck drivers who are exposed to vibrations from vehicles or workers exposed to vibrations from industrial machinery are at risk for low back injury. Patients who have osteoporosis are also at risk for low back pain.

Q What are the anatomical considerations for the patient with low back pain?

A The patient has pain from innervated structures that may vary from person to person. A disk has no specific innervation, however, it may compress the cord if it is herniated. The anterior and posterior longitudinal ligaments and other ligaments are richly supplied with pain receptors. The muscles of the spine are also vulnerable to sprains and strains.

"Classical teaching" has been that intervertebral disks have no sensory nerve fibers. This has been disproven in the chiropractic, neurologic, and orthopedic literature since 1985, but is still not widely known by other health care professionals. Sensory nerves have been shown to extend into the disc at least one-third the radius of the outer rim, the annulus fibrosis. In the clinical setting, either in- or out-of-hospital, it is impossible to tell if low back pain is coming solely from the irritation of these nerves. Remember, it is always a possibility, even if standard tests (e.g., MRI, CT) show no damage. Injury to these nerves occurs at a microscopic level that is undetectable on "standard tests."

Q What in-hospital procedures assist in the diagnosis of low back pain?

A Although precise diagnosis is difficult for low back pain, the diagnosis is based on history and the following in-hospital tests: CT scan, electromyelography, and MRI.

Though electromyelography (EMG) is still suggested in some venues in the workup of back pain, most experts rely on a combination of clinical findings and the results of either a CT scan or an MRI scan.

Q What is degenerative disk disease?

A Degenerative disk disease is common in patients over 50 years of age. It is a narrowing of the disk that results in variable segment instability. It is caused by biomechanical alterations (e.g., degeneration) of the disk. Because the disk provides cushioning between the vertebrae, the degeneration of a disk may cause the vertebrae to come in closer contact with each other.

Q What is spondylolysis?

A Spondylolysis is a structural defect of the spine involving the lamina or vertebral arch. It usually occurs between the superior and inferior articulating facets. Heredity is considered

It is impossible to tell without an X-ray that a person has spondylolysis. Even if the defect is present, it may not be responsible for a person's back pain.

to be a significant factor. In most individuals, it is congenital. Rarely, it may be acquired, but rotational fractures may more commonly occur at the affected site.

Q What is a herniated intervertebral disk?

A Also referred to as a herniated nucleus pulposus, the herniated intervertebral disk is a tear in the posterior rim of the capsule (annulus pulposus) enclosing the gelatinous center of the disk. Trauma, degenerative disk disease, and improper lifting may cause it. Men, ages 30 to 50, are more prone to this problem than women. It commonly affects L-5, S-1, L-4, and L-5 disks, but it may also occur in C-5, C-6, and C-7.

Q What are some of the symptoms of a herniated disk?

A The patient usually has pain with straining, coughing, or sneezing. He may have a limited range of motion in the lumbar spine and tenderness on palpation. There may be alterations in sensation, pain, and temperature due to nerve root pressure. Cervical herniations may include upper-extremity pain or paresthesia increasing with neck motion. A slight motor weakness may also occur in the biceps and triceps.

There is no way to clinically (in- or out-of-hospital) tell with certainty whether a patient has a herniated disk versus any other cause of back or neck pain.

Q What is the management of a patient with low back pain?

A Management is primarily palliative to decrease any pain or discomfort from movement. The EMS provider may elect to immobilize the patient to aid in comfort on either a long backboard or a vacuum-type stretcher. Full spinal immobilization is not required unless the condition is a result of trauma.

Some patients with acute low back spasm are literally "paralyzed" with pain. The best way to move them is to use a "scoop-type" metal stretcher that fits under the patient. Administration of IV diazepam (Valium®), as per protocols or medical control, may be extremely helpful.

Q What are the causes of spinal cord tumors?

A The most common cause of spinal tumors is metastases, usually from breast cancer in a woman or the prostate in a man.

Management of the Suspected SCI Patient

Q **What are the general principles of spinal immobilization?**

A The techniques of spinal management may differ but the principles remain the same. The following are the general principles of SCI management:

- The primary goal is to prevent further injury.
- The spine should be treated as if it were a long bone with a joint at either end (the head and the pelvis).
- 15 percent of secondary spinal injuries are preventable with proper immobilization.
- Always use complete spinal immobilization of the head and neck and the remainder of the column.
- The spinal stabilization should begin with the initial assessment and continue until the patient is completely immobilized on a long backboard.
- The head and neck should be placed in neutral, in-line position unless contraindicated.

Q **Why should the patient be placed in a neutral, in-line anatomical position?**

A Neutral positioning allows for the most space for the cord. The diameter of the cord is approximately 10 mm and the diameter of the spinal column is approximately 15 mm, so the room for "play" is very small. Neutral positioning will help reduce cord hypoxia and reduce excess pressure. This is the most stable position for the spinal column, reducing instability.

Q **What are the devices commonly used to immobilize the spine in the field?**

A In the field, the commonly used devices for spinal immobilization are the rigid cervical collar, the long backboard or full-body vacuum splint, and an interim immobilization device such as the vest-type device (e.g., KED, Kansas Board, XPl).

Q **How is the cervical spine immobilized in the field?**

A To immobilize, the first thing used is a set of hands holding manual in-line stabilization. Once the neck has been assessed and priorities have been dealt with, the EMS provider should apply a rigid collar. These are also referred to as extrication collars. They help to minimize the movement of the neck if

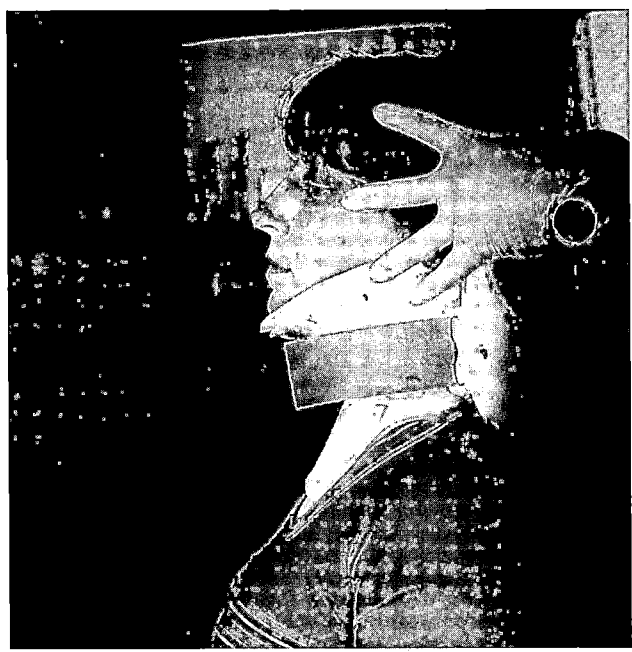

FIGURE 39-3 Continuous manual stabilization should be maintained, even after the collar has been applied, until the torso and then the head and neck are attached to the immobilization device.

properly sized. No collar totally eliminates neck movement. That is why it is important not to let go of the manual stabilization until the patient is completely immobilized (Figure 39–3). The next step is to immobilize the torso and then the head and neck to the KED (vest-type device) or long backboard being utilized in the field.

CLINICAL PEARL

Don't expect cervical collars to eliminate neck movement. The best use for the collar is to remind both the patient and the EMS provider that there is a potential vertebral or spinal problem and to take special caution.

Q **Why do we no longer use soft collars like the hospital uses?**

A Some folks refer to the soft collars as "neck-warmers" because that is about all they do. They do not immobilize the neck; they merely remind the patient not to move his neck. They serve a purpose, but they should only be used on patients who do not have a fracture or ligament tear that could allow a dislocation of the vertebrae. In the field, we have no way of knowing if these injuries actually exist, so we must use a collar that limits movement such as a Stiff Neck® or Philadelphia collar®.

Should padding be used when immobilizing the spine in the field?

Yes—to fill voids, which will ultimately make the patient more comfortable. Some patients, when placed on a wooden or plastic long backboard in the supine anatomical position, will have some voids that can be filled with towels or small pillows. Lying on a hard surface is uncomfortable for even the healthiest back! Patients who have preexisting back problems will be very uncomfortable by the time they reach the ED. Of course, this does not mean we should skip the long backboard because the consequences are much more severe for a spinal injured patient who was not appropriately immobilized. This just means we should be sensitive to the treatment, which may actually be causing some pain, and pad if needed as long as it does not take too much time for the critical patient.

Some services have switched to a full-body vacuum splint that, when the air is rapidly evacuated or pumped out of the splint, conforms to the actual anatomy of the patient. These devices are used extensively in European countries and its use is spreading in the United States.

> **CLINICAL PEARL**
>
> *An interesting study recently showed that uninjured patients who are immobilized on a backboard all develop a significant headache and back pain within 20 minutes. This does not mean to avoid immobilization. It simply implies that the technique may be uncomfortable, even without underlying injury. Do everything in your power to minimize the injured person's discomfort.*

What is the best way to strap a patient to a long backboard?

There is no best way, just many acceptable techniques that work. The principle here is that the head, upper-rib cage, pelvis, and legs must be attached to the board in such a way that if the board were turned on its side (e.g., to clear the airway of a vomiting patient), there would be little movement. Some EMS providers have developed techniques that crisscross straps across the upper chest and the pelvis that work well. You may also use three Velcro straps, so the length can easily be adjusted, across the upper chest and arms, directly on the pelvis, and across the thighs together with a rigid collar, two compressible head blocks, and 2-inch tape across the forehead and the collar. No amount of crisscrossing or strap tightening, however, is going to hold down straps placed in the wrong spot. You must affix bones to the board, not soft tissue or fat. If the patient has a big abdomen, don't bother trying to strap it down, search for the pelvic bones and tie them down! If the patient is pregnant,

immobilize bones to the board, then turn the board on its side to take the weight of the uterus off the vena cava.

If it is necessary to stand patients upright to move them, make sure the straps under the arms are extra tight and that the feet are tied in so they will not slide down on the backboard. This may be especially uncomfortable for the patient, but you can loosen up the extra straps once the patient is in the supine position on your stretcher.

What is the proper order in which to immobilize and then remove the immobilization equipment, on authorization of the ED physician, from the spinal injured patient?

Always provide manual in-line stabilization right away. After assessment of the patient, she must be carefully lifted with plenty of help or with a scoop-type device to a long backboard or a full-body vacuum splint, or log-rolled to a long backboard. When it is time to actually strap the patient to the immobilization device, the torso should be strapped first, then the head and neck. Keep in mind that patients with a CNS injury are prone to vomit. The order of immobilization, torso then head, relates to the possibility that the patient who is not yet immobilized may move, especially if he feels the urge to vomit. The patient is a lot easier to control if you need to quickly roll him to his side should he begin to vomit, if the torso is strapped and the head is manually stabilized. If the head were tied down and the torso was not yet secured, and the patient needs to be quickly rolled to his side, it would be very difficult to control the patient without twisting their injured neck!

Removing the straps in the ED after physician approval should be done in just the reverse order. Remove the head first, then the torso.

What can be used to immobilize the head and cervical spine?

Just about anything, if it works and doesn't add time. The principle here is that the device should limit movement of the head and neck and not actually require movement of the head and neck to apply. It is also helpful for the device to be either disposable or disinfectable because it is not uncommon for these patients to have facial lacerations and bleed all over. Another useful feature is for the device to be useable in the cold and rain.

Commercial devices such as the Ferno® head immobilizer and the CID® are useful because they apply quickly, tie down with Velcro straps, and clean up easily. A blanket roll can be used or small compressible pillows and tape. The downside of these supplies is that they will need to be properly laundered after each use (following your agency's infection control plan). Many services now use a combination of a commercial plastic-covered disposable block or pillow and tape. The one thing that should not be used in the field for spinal immobilization is sand bags. They have some use in the ED with patients who are not moving around, but are useless in the field. Imagine someone placing a sandbag on the sides of your head and then turning the backboard on its side when you start to vomit! If you are still carrying these devices on your EMS unit, replace them. Their only use might be to throw under the tires when the vehicle gets stuck in the snow!

What types of helmets are found on patients in the field?

In most cases, when a patient who was wearing a helmet for motorcycling or sports has been injured, the patient has already removed the helmet. In some cases, the helmet may still be in place because the patient was unable to remove it or bystanders or an athletic trainer advised against removing the helmet. There are many types of helmets used to decrease the chance of head injury. Examples include:

- Full face, half, or three-quarter motorcycle or auto racing helmets.
- Skiing and snowboarding helmets.
- Kayaking, water sports helmets.
- Helicopter flight crew helmets.
- Cycling helmets.
- Horseback riding, polo helmets.
- Football helmets.
- Baseball batter's helmets.
- Hockey, lacrosse helmets.
- Rock climbing helmets.
- Boxing.
- Skateboarding, ATV, in-line skating helmets.
- Some toddlers wear soft helmets to bed because of sleep disorders.

If the patient has a helmet on and a SCI is suspected, should it be removed in the field before immobilization?

Much controversy exists as to whether or not to remove helmets in the field. What the issue boils down to is the urgency of airway management, the fit of the helmet, and where the best trained hands are to take it off. Consider the following:

- The airway rules! If for any reason you are not able to adequately manage the airway with the helmet on, then take it off using the proper technique.

- The helmet must fit to provide any form of immobilization. If the helmet is not the proper size, the head will move around. If the head moves around inside the helmet, it should be removed using the proper technique. This commonly occurs with motorcyclists who carry a rider helmet. Because it is not practical to carry a full set of sizes, a large is often carried. When a rider jumps on and dons the helmet, they are often wearing the wrong size.

- Use the best-trained hands. If the helmet is going to be taken off, it is a good idea to do it where the best-trained hands are available. In the field, it is not uncommon to have the assistance of an athletic trainer who is very knowledgeable about the technique for removal and the specific brand of sports helmet they use for their team. In addition, EMS providers are all trained and practice the proper technique for helmet removal and the health care providers in the ED are not. Keep in mind that if a patient has on football gear, the shoulder pads take up a lot of space behind the shoulders. If the helmet is removed and the shoulder pads are left in place, it will be necessary to pad behind the head to avoid hyperextension of the neck because the shoulders are not flat on the backboard.

What are the indications for leaving the helmet in place?

Reasons for leaving a helmet in place and immobilizing the patient include:

- A good fitting helmet with no head movement within the helmet.
- No impending airway or breathing problems.
- Removal may cause further injury.
- Proper spinal immobilization can be performed with the helmet in place.
- There is no interference with the ability to assess and reassess the airway.

What are the indications for immediately removing the helmet?

The helmet should be immediately removed, using the proper technique, if any of the following findings exist:

- Inability to assess or reassess the airway and breathing.
- Restriction on adequate management of the airway or breathing.
- Improperly fitted helmet with head movement within the helmet.
- Proper spinal immobilization cannot be performed with the helmet in place.
- Cardiac or respiratory arrest.

What about the use of steroids for traumatic sports injuries?

The use of steroids in suspected spinal injury is not as popular as it once was. They were used to reduce the swelling and often take hours to begin to have an effect. Follow your specific local protocols.

What are the indications for the rapid takedown technique?

The patient who is walking around at a collision scene or who has sustained a significant MOI to the spine needs to be immobilized. They should not be asked to sit down on a long backboard. The proper technique requires three EMS providers who have been appropriately trained in the rapid takedown (standing takedown) technique.

Why not just apply the long backboard while the patient is standing up?

Most of the patients who just sustained a potential spine injury who are standing up at a collision scene still need to be immobilized. It is strongly suggested that the rapid takedown technique be employed. The reason why they are not just backboarded in the standing position is because many of these patients will not stand still for the amount of time it takes to complete the immobilization. Many of these patients are dizzy, weak, or intoxicated and will not just stand there patiently while the board is applied. In addition, patients who have sustained head trauma may have a head injury. Also, if the backboard is applied and then the patient is placed in the supine position, it is not uncommon for the straps and padding to loosen up as the patient lies down.

What are the indications for rapid extrication?

Rapid extrication should only be used with the critical patient (e.g., the unconscious patient; cardiac or respiratory arrest; decompensated shock; serious head trauma; or a penetrating injury to the chest, head, neck, or abdomen).

When should a child be removed from a car seat to immobilize the spine?

In most instances, a toddler can be immobilized in a child seat. If it becomes necessary for the child and seat to be placed in a supine position, it is necessary for the child to be rapidly extricated out of the car seat. This is because when the child lies supine with the legs raised in a sitting position, it causes extra pressure on the abdomen and reduces the lung expansion.

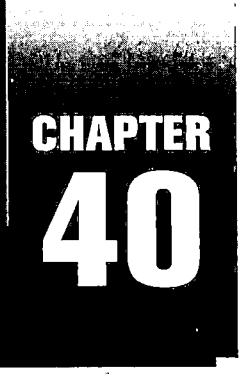

CHAPTER 40

Thoracic Trauma

C hest trauma can result in life-threatening injuries in a short time. The focus is on *why* patients present in a certain manner and *why* you need to respond in a certain way to their presenting problems. It is imperative that you always suspect and be alert for thoracic trauma in the field.

Epidemiology

Q **What is the incidence of thoracic trauma?**

A The true incidence depends on the definition of "thoracic (chest) trauma." If we consider only life-threatening injuries (e.g., massive damage to the chest wall, and injuries to the intrathoracic viscera and vessels), the incidence is 3.5 percent of all trauma cases.

Q **What is the morbidity of thoracic injuries?**

A Chest injuries are the second leading cause of trauma deaths each year.

Q **What are some of the risk factors associated with thoracic trauma?**

A The risk factors involved in thoracic trauma involve the potential for serious life-threatening injury to the mechanical

process of breathing. Injuries as minor as one rib fracture to a major crushed chest cavity can impact the patient's ability to breathe. In addition, the heart and great vessels are common targets of injury.

CLINICAL PEARL

Injuries to the chest—whether severe or seemingly slight—often give rise to elusive findings that are overshadowed easily by associated injuries.

Q **What are some of the prevention strategies associated with thoracic trauma?**

A Prevention strategies include:
- Educating the public to safely use and store guns.
- Outlawing Kevlar-piercing bullets.
- Requiring the police to wear bulletproof vests.
- Ensuring that the proper safety equipment is used for sporting events (e.g., safety vest for horse racing).
- Requiring passenger restraints in motor vehicles.

Injury Patterns

[Q] What are the classifications of thoracic trauma mechanisms of injury (MOI) and examples?

[A] The MOIs of a thoracic injury involve blunt trauma caused by deceleration or compression and penetrating trauma. Various injury patterns can cause chest trauma. The following are examples of injuries that may occur to the thorax:

- Thoracic cage—an injury to the rib cage from crushing up against an object or being struck with a blunt object such as the steering column or a baseball bat.
- Cardiovascular—an injury to the heart or great vessels from compression or blunt trauma.
- Pleural and pulmonary—compression of the chest can cause massive lung contusion. Compression against a closed glottic opening can cause a pneumothorax from a "paper bag" injury. Moments before the car collides, almost instinctively, the patient takes a deep breath and closes the glottic opening while the chest is compressed. This is just like blowing up a paper bag, closing the opening, and then popping the bag. It is also possible to cause air to enter the potential space between the visceral (lining the lung) pleura and the parietal (lining the inside of the chest wall) pleura when the chest wall is punctured.
- Mediastinal—the major problem with the injury to the mediastinal area is the tearing of a great vessel.
- Diaphragmatic—these injuries cause the contents of either the thorax or abdomen to rupture the diaphragm. Abdominal organs may herniate into the chest through the rupture site. This will seriously impact on the mechanics of breathing.
- Esophageal injury—tears may occur to the esophagus when the throat or upper chest is perforated.
- Penetrating cardiac trauma—injury directly to the heart muscle can cause massive bleeding into the pericardial sac and pericardial tamponade. This condition may be fatal rapidly.

[Q] What is the impact of the MOI from a blast injury to the chest?

[A] The shock wave or pressure wave from the blast injury can cause serious compression of the chest. When an explosion occurs within a confined space, the pressure injures the lung tissue causing massive lung contusions to develop. There is also a potential for respiratory burn injuries from the inhalation of heated gases. Contusion or bruising reduces the area available to exchange oxygen and carbon dioxide (CO_2). There also can be

blunt or penetrating injuries from the bomb parts or debris in the vicinity.

Anatomy and Physiology

[Q] What takes place during ventilation?

[A] The mechanical process of ventilation involves the following steps:
- During inspiration, the diaphragm and intercostal muscles contract.
- Diaphragmatic contraction creates a vacuum (negative intrathoracic pressure) in the chest cavity.
- Negative intrathoracic pressure (the vacuum) "sucks" air into the lungs, expanding them.
- Expiration is a passive process—the lungs "snap closed" due to their natural elasticity.

Any injury that affects the diaphragm, intercostal muscles, or accessory muscles of breathing can affect the mechanics of ventilation severely.

[Q] What is the neurochemical control of respiration?

[A] Chemoreceptors, which are located in the aortic arch and carotid sinus, are constantly measuring the CO_2 levels in the blood. Respiratory centers in the brain adjust the rate and depth of breathing to maintain normal CO_2 concentrations. The normal impetus to breathe is a function of the percentage of CO_2. If the CO_2 gets too high, the respiratory rate increases in order to "blow off" the excess.

[Q] What are the key components in gas exchange during respiration?

[A] The ability to exchange gas during respiration is a function of the following elements: the alveolar–capillary interface, capillary–red blood cell (RBC) interface, pulmonary circulation, cardiac circulation, and the acid–base balance.

[Q] What types of thoracic trauma may impair cardiac output (CO)?

[A] Thoracic trauma may impair CO due to any of the following mechanisms: overall blood loss, increased intrapleural pressures, blood collecting in the pericardial sac making it difficult for the heart to fully fill with each contraction, myocardial valve damage, or vascular disruption.

How may thoracic trauma impair ventilations?

Thoracic trauma may impair ventilation in any of several ways:

- Interruption in the chest "bellows action"—can be the result of pain, such as a rib fracture restricting chest excursion, air entering the pleural space from an open or closed pneumothorax, or the chest wall failing to move in unison. This is commonly referred to as paradoxical respirations from a flail chest.

- Bleeding into the pleural space (an intercostal artery can bleed 50 cc's a minute into the chest cavity causing a massive hemothorax).

- Ineffective diaphragmatic contraction from an injury to the major muscles of breathing or damage to the nervous system's control of the diaphragm itself (e.g., spinal injury).

What are impairments in gas exchange that can occur from thoracic trauma?

Examples of impairments in gas exchange from thoracic trauma can include:

- Atelectasis from inadequately inflating all of the alveoli.
- Contusion to the lung tissue from compression of the chest.
- Disruption of the respiratory tract from a cut to the trachea or major respiratory anatomy.

Assessment of the Chest Trauma Patient

What history is most significant when assessing a patient who has experienced chest trauma?

Ascertain the following significant elements of the history:

- The presence of dyspnea and chest pain (OPQRST).
- Associated symptoms including other areas of pain or discomfort or symptoms that occurred prior to the incident.
- Past medical history of cardiorespiratory disease.
- MOI (e.g., bent steering wheel) and the use of restraint in a motor vehicle crash (MVC).

What are examples of significant assessment findings when evaluating a patient who has experienced thoracic trauma?

Assessment findings of the patient who has experienced thoracic trauma may include:

- Pulse—there may be tachycardia from shock, bradycardia from a cardiac conduction problem, or a deficit from damage to a great vessel.

- BP—there may be a narrow pulse pressure, which is the mathematic difference between the systolic and diastolic, due to pericardial tamponade. The patient may have hypertension from the anxiety of the chest trauma or pulmonary hypertension. Hypotension from shock or an obstruction to cardiac flow may be present. The patient may have pulsus paradoxus, which is a pulse that weakens abnormally during inspiration and is symptomatic of various abnormalities. This produces a variation of the pulse with the respirations.

- Respirations—there may be tachypnea or bradypnea, labored respirations, retractions, or other evidence of respiratory distress such as hemoptysis.

- Temperature—the patient may be hypothermic.

- Skin—the patient may be diaphoretic and the skin color can be pale or cyanotic. There may be open wounds to the chest, which need to be sealed, or ecchymosis and other evidence of trauma. The neck may exhibit subcutaneous emphysema from air under the skin.

What are physical examination findings that may become evident when examining the patient with chest injury?

The patient with a chest injury may have any of the following physical findings:

- Contusions, tenderness, or asymmetry.

- Lung sounds that are absent or decreased bilaterally or unilaterally, the presence of bowel sounds in the thorax possibly indicating herniation of the diaphragm.

- Abnormal findings on percussion (e.g., hyperresonance or hyporesonance from excessive or minimal air in the chest).

- Heart sounds may be muffled, distant, or have a regurgitant murmur; this suggests hemothorax, pericardial effusion, or cardiac injury. There may also be a shift in the apical pulse location.

- Observe for open wounds involving a hole, penetration, perforation, or impaled object. Feel and listen for crepitation.

- Observe for paradoxical movement of the chest wall.

- Observe for a scaphoid abdomen (a normal finding indicating inward curvature of the abdomen).

- Note any decreased mental status.

- Observe the ECG for ST–T wave elevations or depressions, conduction, or rhythm disturbances.

- Observe for subcutaneous emphysema.

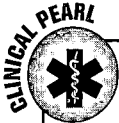

Some patients with serious chest injuries have minimal findings. Always consider the MOI. Untoward anxiety and unexplained tachycardia may be the only signs of a potentially life-threatening injury.

What modalities does the management of thoracic trauma involve?

The management of chest trauma depends on the specific injury the patient has sustained. In general, the treatment plan may involve many of the following modalities:

- Airway and ventilation management can involve: sealing the chest wall with an occlusive dressing, oxygen therapy or positive pressure ventilation (a ventilator with positive end expiratory pressure is inappropriate for this patient), stabilizing impaled objects or flail segments, evaluating need for ET intubation, and evaluating the need for a surgical airway or needle cricothyrotomy.

- Managing lethal cardiac dysrhythmias and obtaining intravenous access.

- Considering the need for analgesics or antidysrhythmic medications.

- Determining the need for a needle thoracostomy (chest decompression) or in-hospital management by a tube thoracostomy or pericardiocentesis.

Always consider maintenance of ABCs your first priority.

Specific Chest Injuries

What are the typical chest wall injuries found in the field?

Typical chest wall injuries include rib fractures, flail segments, and sternal fractures.

What is the epidemiology of rib fractures?

Rib fractures require significant force to occur unless there is preexisting bone disease present. They are rather infrequent until adult life and increase in elderly patients. A rib fracture can lead to serious consequences especially associated with underlying pulmonary or cardiovascular injury. Complications from rib

Remember, it is nearly impossible to make a definitive diagnosis of a rib fracture in the field. Even when X-rays are available, small fractures are often missed. If you suspect that rib fractures may be present, evaluate carefully for associated injuries (e.g., lung or heart contusion, great vessel injury). The fractures alone are painful, but not particularly dangerous to the patient.

fractures increase with age, the number of fractures, and the location of the fractures.

What is the pathophysiology of rib fractures?

The most frequent cause of a rib fracture is blunt trauma that creates a "bowing effect" causing a midshaft fracture. Ribs four to nine are most often fractured because they are thin and poorly protected. When there is respiratory restriction due to pain, splinting the patient can cause atelectasis and a ventilation–perfusion mismatch. Rib fractures can be associated with an underlying lung or cardiac contusion and intercostal vessel injury. Sternal fractures are second in frequency.

What are the associated complications of rib fractures?

Associated complications of rib fractures can include the following:

- Fractures of the first and second ribs indicate injury by severe trauma and may also involve a rupture of the aorta, a tracheobronchial tree injury, or a vascular injury. Fortunately these injuries are rare due to the protection provided by the clavicles.

- Fractures of the lower-left ribs are often associated with a splenic rupture and lower-right ribs with a hepatic injury.

- Multiple rib fractures can cause atelectasis, hypoventilation, inadequate cough or inability to clear out the lower airways, and pneumonia.

- Open rib fractures are rare and when they occur, they are usually associated with a visceral injury.

- Posterior ribs (fifth to ninth) are most frequently injured. The lower rib fractures are associated with spleen and kidney injuries.

What are the assessment findings in a patient with a rib fracture?

These patients have localized pain or point tenderness (they can point to with one finger). The pain worsens with movement such as deep inspiration and coughing. There may be a feeling of crepitus or an audible crunching noise, the so-called "snap, crackle, pop" of Rice Krispies® on examination. The patient can often be observed "guarding or self-splinting" the injured area by limiting their respiratory excursions. This causes hypoventilation. If anteroposterior pressure is applied, it elicits pain.

What is the appropriate field management of a patient with rib fractures?

Once the airway has been secured, oxygen therapy begins and the patient must be assessed for the need for positive pressure ventilation. Some experts advocate encouraging the patient to cough and breathe deeply to expand all of the air sacs and prevent pneumonia from developing. This is very painful and can probably wait until admission to the hospital. An analgesic may be appropriate to help the patient relax, provided it does not alter their mental status. Avoid circumferential splinting of rib fractures because it limits respiratory excursion and may alter the gas exchange.

What is the epidemiology of a flail segment?

The most common cause of a flail segment is a MVC. Other causes include falls from heights, industrial accidents, assaults, and birth trauma. A flail segment is a very serious chest injury and has a mortality rate of 20–40 percent due to the associated injuries and impact on ventilations. Mortality is increased with advancing age, seven or more ribs fractured, three or more associated injuries, shock, or a head injury.

What is the pathophysiology of a flail segment?

The flail segment involves three or more ribs fractured in two or more places that produce a free-floating segment of chest wall (Figure 40–1). The patient experiences respiratory failure from the underlying lung contusion, inadequate bellows action of the chest, and associated intrathoracic injury. If the flail segment is small, the paradoxical movement is minimal due to muscle spasm. Larger segments can have a very serious effect by compromising ventilation.

Pain is a contributing factor to the severity of this injury because it greatly reduces thoracic expansion and decreases venti-

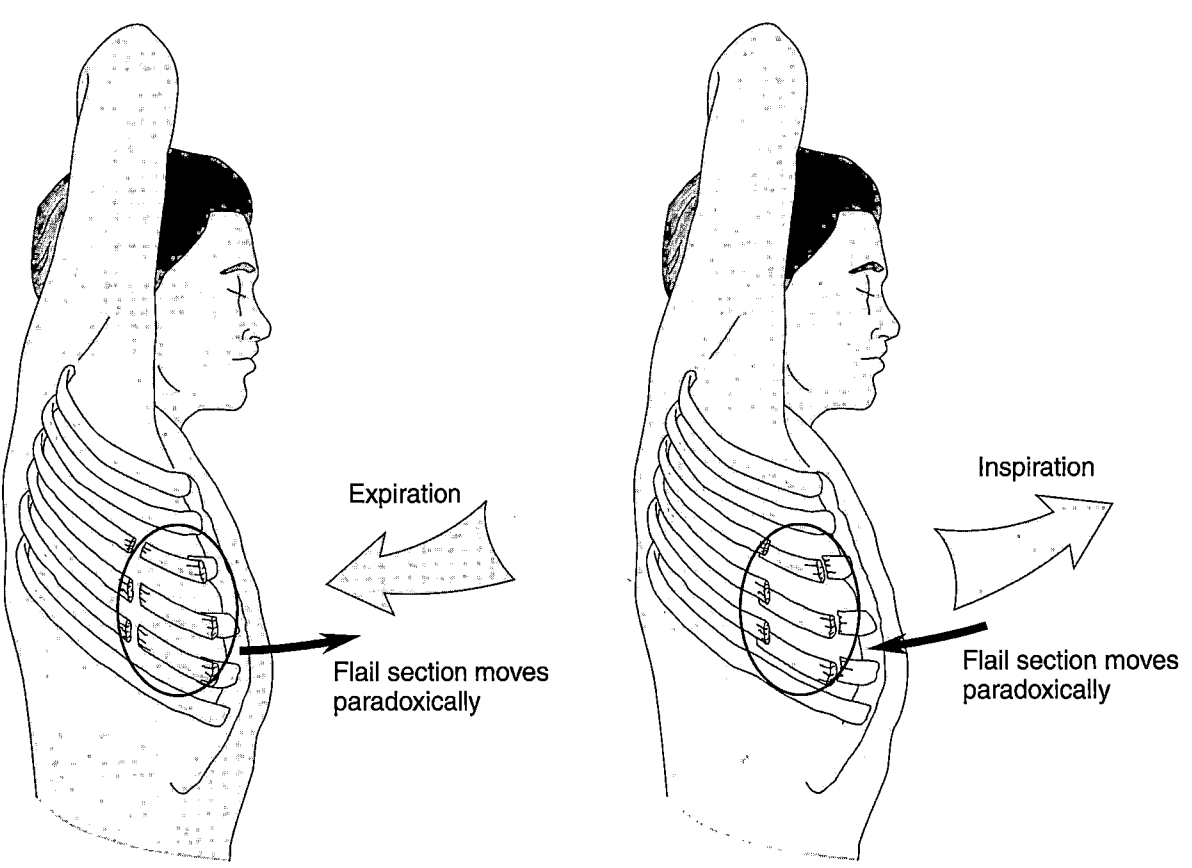

FIGURE 40–1 The flail segment impairs breathing because of its paradoxical motion.

lation. The venous return is impaired, resulting in a ventilation–perfusion mismatch from the hypercapnia and hypoxia that develops.

What are the associated complications of a flail segment?

It is common to develop a pulmonary contusion along with a flail segment. The contusion causes a decrease in the lung compliance and hemorrhage in the intra-alveolar capillaries and alveolus, making it even more difficult to ventilate and exchange gases at the cellular level.

What are the assessment findings in a patient with a flail segment?

On assessment of the patient who has a flail chest, the EMS provider may note the following findings:

- Chest wall contusion.
- Respiratory distress.
- Paradoxical chest wall movement.
- Pleuritic chest pain.
- Crepitus.
- Pain and guarding or splinting on the affected side.
- Tachypnea.
- Tachycardia.
- Possible bundle branch block or ectopy on the ECG.

What is the appropriate field management of a patient with a flail segment?

The management of the patient with a flail segment involves, first and foremost, airway and ventilation control. Positive pressure ventilation may be needed for an internal splinting effect. Administer high-concentration oxygen and evaluate the need for ET intubation. Consider this a trauma intubation involving in-line manual stabilization of the spine throughout the procedure. This is due to the amount of trauma required to fracture multiple ribs. Stabilize the flail segment with wide tape extending from stable portions of the chest wall, over the flail segment, and to other stable portions. If stabilization is controversial in your community, contact medical control enroute to the hospital for advice.

Restrict fluids to avoid pulmonary complications from excessive volume. Analgesics may be helpful provided the patient is not hypotensive or does not have an altered mental status (AMS). Transport the patient to an appropriate facility.

What is the epidemiology of a sternal fracture?

About five to eight percent of blunt chest trauma patients have a sternal fracture. The most common cause is a deceleration compression injury caused by the steering wheel or dashboard in a MVC. Other causes include blunt blows to the chest and severe hyperflexion of the thoracic cage. The most common site of the injury is at or below the manubriosternal junction. This is a very serious injury that involves a 25 to 45 percent mortality rate.

What is the pathophysiology of a sternal fracture?

Rarely is the fracture displaced posteriorly to directly impinge on the heart or vessels. The break in the sternum is usually not the cause of the morbidity and mortality. The associated injuries that contribute to the severity of this problem include pulmonary and myocardial contusion, flail chest, vascular disruption of the thoracic vessels, intra-abdominal injuries, and head injuries.

CLINICAL PEARL

The main reason why a sternal fracture has such a high mortality rate is associated injuries. The sternum is a thick bone. If the thorax receives enough force to fracture the sternum, then we must assume that the same force was transmitted to the heart, great vessels, lungs, and diaphragm.

What are the assessment findings in a patient with a sternal fracture?

Patients will complain of localized pain and tenderness over the sternum. They may also have crepitus and tachypnea. Any patient with a history of blunt trauma to the chest should have their ECG monitored because myocardial contusion is often associated with sternal fracture.

What is the appropriate field management of a patient with a sternal fracture?

The management of the patient with a sternal fracture involves, first and foremost, airway and ventilation control. Administer high-concentration oxygen and evaluate the need for ET intubation. Positive pressure ventilation may be useful. Because there has been sufficient energy to break the sternum, this may be a trauma intubation involving in-line manual stabilization of the spine throughout the procedure.

Fluids should be restricted and analgesics may be helpful provided the patient is not hypotensive or does not have an AMS. This patient should be transported to an appropriate facility that can handle major trauma.

What is the epidemiology of a "simple" pneumothorax?

Between 10 and 30 percent of the patients with blunt chest trauma have a simple pneumothorax and close to 100 percent of the patients with a penetrating chest trauma have a pneumothorax (Figure 40–2). The term "simple" is used here to differentiate between a "sucking chest wound," a hemopneumothorax, and a tension pneumothorax. The morbidity and mortality is a function of the extent of the atelectasis and associated injuries that develop. Patients with a simple pneumothorax that is small in size do well if managed appropriately.

CLINICAL PEARL

Pneumothorax is an abnormal accumulation of air, in any amount, in the pleural space. Pleural effusion is a similar accumulation of fluid.

What is the pathophysiology of a simple pneumothorax?

The lung is actually between one and three cm from the chest wall. If a patient has developed a pneumothorax, there may be a stable amount of air accumulation in the pleural cavity. A simple pneumothorax may develop due to the bursting of small blebs on the lung surface. This is often found in very thin frail people and athletes. The development of an internal wound, such as a rib fracture, may allow air to enter the pleural space. The small tears often self-seal, while the larger ones may cause a tension pneumothorax. The other cause of a pneumothorax is the "paper bag" effect of rapidly inhaling, closing the glottic opening, and then crushing the chest cavity, as is often the case in a collision with the steering wheel.

If the standing air accumulates, it often collects in the apexes. The EMS provider should check there first for diminished or absent breath sounds. If the patient is supine, it accumulates in the anterior chest. Tracheal shift may be present in a tension pneumothorax, but its absence does not preclude the diagnosis. When a large pneumothorax develops, the patient will have a subsequent ventilation–perfusion mismatch. In a small pneumothorax, the ventilation–perfusion deficit is negligible.

CLINICAL PEARL

As long as a tension pneumothorax is not present, the degree of respiratory impairment caused by a simple pneumothorax varies considerably. Large collections of pleural air may cause significant ventilation–perfusion abnormalities, as well as impair diaphragmatic movement.

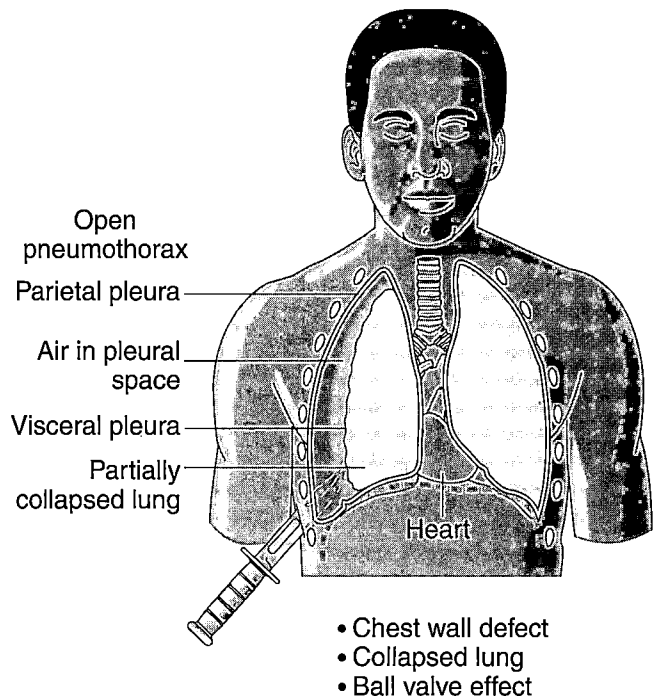

Open pneumothorax
Parietal pleura
Air in pleural space
Visceral pleura
Partially collapsed lung

Heart

- Chest wall defect
- Collapsed lung
- Ball valve effect

FIGURE 40–2 A pneumothorax is created when air enters the chest.

What are the assessment findings in a patient with a simple pneumothorax?

When evaluating the patient with a simple pneumothorax, the EMS provider should look for the following: tachypnea, tachycardia, respiratory distress, dyspnea, and absent or diminished breath sounds on the affected side. The patient may have decreased chest wall movement and slight pleuritic chest pain, which may be referred to the shoulder or arm on the affected side.

What is the appropriate field management of a patient with a simple pneumothorax?

The management of the patient with a simple pneumothorax involves, first and foremost, airway and ventilation control. Positive pressure ventilation may be useful, but should be carefully used because it could increase the volume of air in the chest, worsening the condition. Administer high-concentration oxygen and evaluate the need for ET intubation. Monitor the patient for the development of a tension pneumothorax. If the pneumothorax involves most or all of the lung, based on a lack of breath sounds in all lung fields, or is beginning to proceed to a tension pneumothorax, the paramedic must consider a needle decompression early because the procedure may be required. Of course, this procedure can only be done by trained, appropriately certified paramedics who are authorized by medical control.

Fluids should be restricted if lung contusion is also suspected. Analgesics may be helpful provided the patient is not hypotensive or does not have an AMS. Transport the patient to a facility that can handle major trauma.

What is the epidemiology of an open pneumothorax?

In cases of penetrating trauma to the chest, open pneumothorax occurs. This is most common due to a penetrating trauma from either a knife or gunshot wound (GSW). Profound hypoventilation can result, leading to death if the management is delayed.

What is the pathophysiology of an open pneumothorax?

The open pneumothorax is an open defect in the chest wall. This defect causes the following actions to occur: communication between the pleural space and the atmosphere, interference with the development of negative intrapleural pressure, collapse of the ipsilateral lung, inability to ventilate the effected lung, and a ventilation–perfusion mismatch due to shunting, hypoventilation, hypoxia, and a large functional dead space developing.

As the patient inspires, air enters the pleural space. Air may exit during the expiratory phase. If the resistance to air flow through the respiratory tract is greater than through the open wound, the respiratory effort is ineffective. If the size of the hole is greater than the glottic opening, little to no air comes in through the glottis. A one-way flap valve may develop, letting air in but not letting it out, resulting in a buildup of pressure in the pleural space.

As the volume of air in the chest increases, the mediastinum begins to move in the direction of the healthy lung, causing the great vessels to sway and kink. This decrease in the preload from shutting down the inferior vena cava can quickly cause a cardiovascular collapse.

What are the assessment findings in a patient with an open pneumothorax?

The examination of a patient who has an open pneumothorax includes finding a see-sawing or to and fro motion of air out of the affected lung. A penetrating injury that may not seal itself may be obvious or may be difficult to find. The patient may have a sucking sound on inhalation. He may also have tachypnea, tachycardia, and respiratory distress. Be sure to palpate for subcutaneous emphysema and listen for decreased breath sounds on the affected side.

What is the appropriate field management of a patient with an open pneumothorax?

The management of the patient with an open pneumothorax involves, first and foremost, airway and ventilation control. Occlude the open wound using an occlusive dressing. If a dressing is not quickly available, the EMS provider can use an exam glove. Positive pressure ventilation may be needed. Administer high-concentration oxygen and evaluate the need for ET intubation.

Closely monitor the patient for the development of a tension pneumothorax. If a tension develops, you may want to consider "burping" the dressing by opening up one of the four taped sides. Field management by appropriately trained and authorized EMS providers may involve a needle chest decompression. The patient needs in-hospital management with a tube thoracostomy for definitive therapy.

Fluids should be restricted and analgesics may be helpful; however, this patient is probably going to be hypotensive or may already have an AMS. This patient should be transported to a facility that can handle major trauma.

CLINICAL PEARL

Remember that by sealing an open chest wound completely, a tension pneumothorax may develop. Always leave a small side open to act as a "ball valve" and allow air to escape.

What is the epidemiology of a tension pneumothorax?

A tension pneumothorax develops in situations of penetrating trauma and blunt trauma. Morbidity is common; this injury should be considered an immediate life-threatening condition. Mortality is related to delayed management.

What is the pathophysiology of a tension pneumothorax?

There is a defect in the airway allowing communication with the pleural space. In cases of blunt trauma, there is a penetra-

CLINICAL PEARL

Though respiratory compromise is usually significant following a tension pneumothorax, the increased pressure compresses the great vessels. This results in decreased venous return and shock. Many experts feel that decreased preload and shock are the major potentially fatal results of tension pneumothorax.

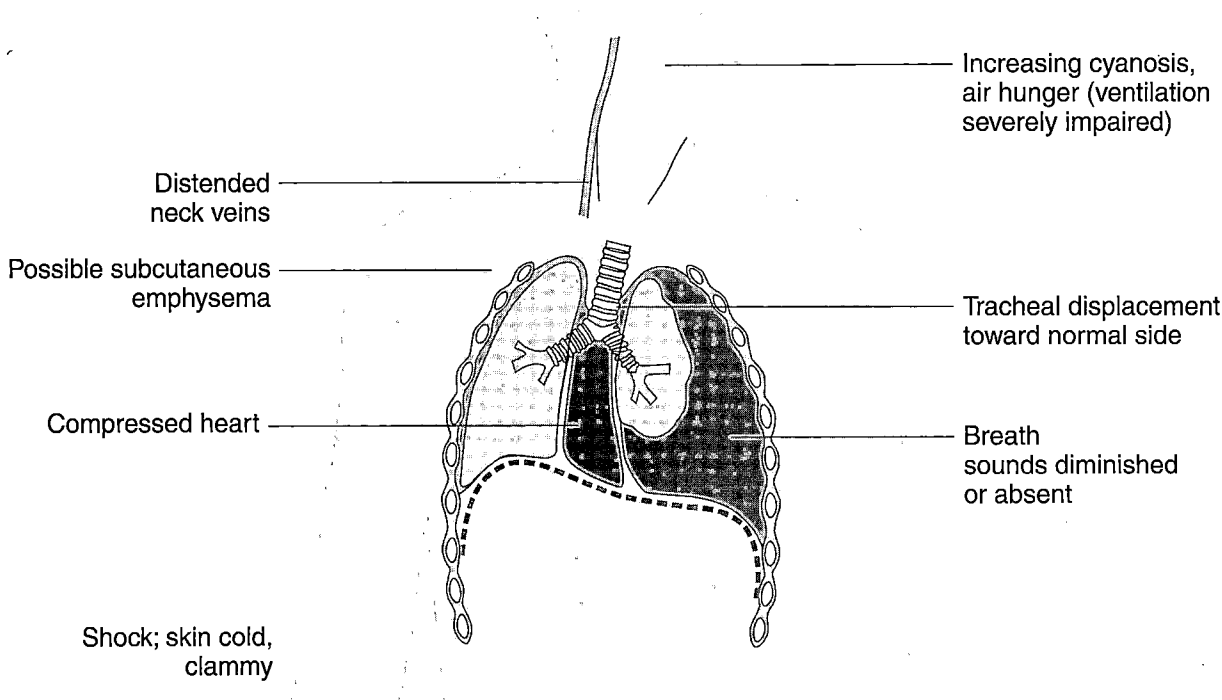

Increasing cyanosis, air hunger (ventilation severely impaired)

Distended neck veins

Possible subcutaneous emphysema

Tracheal displacement toward normal side

Compressed heart

Breath sounds diminished or absent

Shock; skin cold, clammy

FIGURE 40–3 A tension pneumothorax is initially a respiratory problem that proceeds to a cardiac problem as the mediastinum shifts, kinking the great vessels.

tion by a rib fracture, a sudden increase in the intrapulmonary pressure, or the bronchial disruption from shear force. Air becomes trapped in the pleural space with a buildup of pressure. The lung collapses on the affected side with mediastinal shift to the contralateral side (Figure 40–3). The lung collapse then leads to right-to-left intrapulmonary shunting and hypoxia. Finally, there is a serious reduction in CO due to the increased intrathoracic pressure and deformation of the vena cava, reducing preload.

What are the assessment findings in a patient with a tension pneumothorax?

When evaluating the patient who you suspect has a tension pneumothorax, findings may include the following:

- Unilateral decreased or absent breath sounds, dyspnea, respiratory distress, and hyperresonance.
- Tachypnea, cyanosis, and extreme anxiety.
- Tachycardia, hypotension, and a narrow pulse pressure.
- Jugular vein distention (JVD), tracheal deviation, and subcutaneous emphysema.

CLINICAL PEARL

In the appropriate clinical setting, shock (a late sign), decreased breath sounds, and hyperresonance to percussion on the same side of the chest means a tension pneumothorax until proven otherwise!

What is the appropriate field management of a patient with a tension pneumothorax?

The management of the patient with a tension pneumothorax involves, first and foremost, airway and ventilation control. Relieve the tension pneumothorax to improve CO. Positive pressure ventilation may be needed. Administer high-concentration oxygen and evaluate the need for ET intubation.

Field management by appropriately trained and authorized EMS providers may involve a needle chest decompression. Reassess the need for additional needles to be inserted. The patient requires in-hospital management with a tube thoracostomy for definitive therapy. Restrict fluids and consider analgesics based on the mental status. Transport the patient to the closest appropriate facility.

[Q] What is the epidemiology of a hemothorax?

[A] A hemothorax is associated with either blunt or penetrating trauma. A pneumothorax may or may not be present. Rib fractures are a frequent cause. A life-threatening hemothorax is an injury that frequently requires urgent chest tube and surgical intervention. A hemothorax is associated with great vessel or cardiac injury. Statistics show that 50 percent of these patients die immediately, 25 percent live 5 to 10 minutes, and the other 25 percent may live 30 minutes or longer.

[Q] What is the pathophysiology of a hemothorax?

[A] Basically, there is a large volume of blood that has accumulated in the pleural space. The bleeding may be from a penetrating or blunt injury to the lung, the chest wall vessels, the intercostal vessels, or the myocardium itself. It is not uncommon for an intercostal artery to bleed as much as 50 cc's per minute into the chest. Bleeding from a pulmonary contusion generally causes 1,000 to 1,500 cc's of blood loss although the chest cavity can hold some 2,000 to 3,000 cc's of blood.

Intrapulmonary hemorrhage occurs in either the bronchus or the parenchyma. The pulmonary parenchyma is a low-pressure vascular system. When there is a massive hemothorax, it usually is an indication of a great vessel or cardiac injury causing the collapse of the ipsilateral lung. The degree of respiratory insufficiency and hypoxia is dependent on the amount of blood in the chest.

[Q] What are the assessment findings in a patient with a hemothorax?

[A] When evaluating the patient with a hemothorax, expect to find the signs and symptoms of shock, decreased breath sounds, respiratory distress, and a chest that is dull on percussion.

> **CLINICAL PEARL**
> *The major problem following a massive hemothorax is the development of hypovolemic shock and respiratory compromise.*

[Q] What is the appropriate field management of a patient with a hemothorax?

[A] The management of the patient with a hemothorax involves, first and foremost, airway and ventilation control. Positive pressure ventilation may be helpful to reexpand the injured lung, which in turn may help reduce the bleeding. Administer high-concentration oxygen and evaluate the need for ET intubation.

The patient requires in-hospital management with a tube thoracostomy to evacuate the blood from the chest. Surgery is often required, as well. Restrict fluids and consider analgesics, based on the mental status. Transport the patient to the closest appropriate facility.

[Q] What is a hemopneumothorax?

[A] A combination of blood and air in the pleural space.

[Q] How is a hemopneumothorax managed?

[A] The same as a hemothorax.

[Q] What is the epidemiology of a pulmonary contusion?

[A] One of the most common serious injuries from blunt thoracic trauma is a pulmonary contusion. It is estimated that 30 to 75 percent of the blunt trauma patients develop a pulmonary contusion. It is an injury that is commonly associated with rib fractures, high energy shock waves from explosions, rapid deceleration, high-velocity missile wounds, and low-velocity injuries such as an ice pick stabbing. Pulmonary contusions can be missed due to the high incidence of other associated injuries. The mortality is between 14 and 20 percent.

> **CLINICAL PEARL**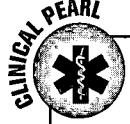
> *Remember that significant thoracic trauma may injure any organ in the pathway of the missile or the force.*

[Q] What is the pathophysiology of a pulmonary contusion?

[A] There are three physical mechanisms involved in the pulmonary contusion:

- An overexpansion effect—from an excess of air trapped in the lungs secondary to positive-pressure concussive waves outside the chest. This can cause a rapid excessive stretching and tearing of the alveoli.
- An inertial effect—causes the stripping of the alveoli from heavier bronchial structures when accelerated at varying rates by a concussion wave from an explosion or blunt trauma to the chest.
- The Spalding effect—the liquid–gas interface is disrupted by a shock wave, caused by external blunt trauma to the chest, releasing energy. The differential transmission of energy causes a disruption of the tissue in the lung.

There is alveolar and capillary damage with interstitial and intra-alveolar extravasation of the blood. The patient develops interstitial edema and increased capillary membrane permeability. There are also gas exchange disturbances. The patient develops hypoxemia and has CO_2 retention. The ensuing hypoxia causes a reflex thickening of mucous secretions and both bronchiolar obstruction and atelectasis.

Finally, the blood is shunted away from the unventilated alveoli, leading to further hypoxemia.

What are the assessment findings in a patient with a pulmonary contusion?

On examination of the patient who has a lung contusion, the EMS provider finds the following:

- Tachypnea, respiratory distress, dyspnea, and cyanosis.

- Tachycardia, apprehension, and evidence of chest trauma.

- A cough and hemoptysis. (The lack of hemoptysis does not exclude lung contusion.)

- Decreased breath sounds.

- Decreased oxygen saturation of arterial blood (SpO_2).

What is the appropriate field management of a patient with a pulmonary contusion?

The management of the patient with a lung contusion involves, first and foremost, airway and ventilation control. Positive pressure ventilation may be needed. Administer high-concentration oxygen and evaluate the need for ET intubation.

Fluids should be restricted because they can contribute to the developing pulmonary edema. However, if patients are hypovolemic, they require the volume replacement. Restrict fluids and consider analgesics, based on mental status. Transport the patient to the closest appropriate facility.

CLINICAL PEARL

Patients with pulmonary contusions also tend to have other severe thoracic and abdominal injuries. Always assume multiple potential injuries are present.

What is the epidemiology of a pericardial tamponade?

The incidence of a pericardial tamponade is rare with a blunt trauma, but common with a penetrating trauma. Less than two percent of chest trauma patients sustain a pericardial tamponade. The mortality is higher with GSWs compared to stab wounds and lower if the tamponade is the only injury present.

What is the function and structure of the pericardium?

The pericardium is a tough fibrous sac that encloses the heart. It attaches to the great vessels at the base of the heart and

has two layers: the visceral layer forms the epicardium and the parital layer is regarded as the sac itself.

The purpose of the pericardium is to anchor the heart and restrict excess movement. It also prevents the kinking of the great vessels. The parietal layer is acutely nondistensible, but can slowly distend by as much as 1,000 to 1,500 cc's with gradual accumulations of fluid over days to weeks. The space between the parietal and visceral layers is a potential space, just like in the pleura, and is normally filled with 30–50 cc's of straw-colored fluid secreted by the visceral layer. The fluid is designed for lubrication, lymphatic drainage, and to provide immunologic protection for the heart.

What is the pathophysiology of a pericardial tamponade?

Fluid, usually blood due to cardiac bleeding, is rapidly accumulated over a period of minutes to hours in the potential space between the two membranes. This leads to increases in the intra-pericardial pressure. The increased pressure impairs diastolic filling of the heart, with a subsequent decrease in CO. Venous return is also impaired. The removal of as little as 20 cc's of blood can drastically improve the patient's CO.

CLINICAL PEARL

The major reason for pericardial tamponade is an impairment of ventricular diastolic filling. This significantly decreases the amount of blood the heart is able to pump out (CO). As a result, severe shock occurs.

What are the assessment findings in a patient with a pericardial tamponade?

On examination of a patient who has a cardiac tamponade (Figure 40–4), the EMS provider may locate many of the following:

- Tachycardia, a narrow pulse pressure, pulsus paradoxus, and ECG changes.

- Respiratory distress and cyanosis of the head, neck, and upper extremities.

- Kussmual's sign (increased venous distension during inspiration).

- The Beck triad, found in 30 percent of the patients, involving hypotension, JVD, and muffled heart tones.

- Muffled and distant heart sounds.

Basically, cardiac tamponade is an injury that may require a patient history to recognize. For example, if a patient was stabbed with an ice pick, you may not find the tiny wound unless you very thoroughly assessed the trunk or received a tip from a bystander as to what happened. A number of these patients go

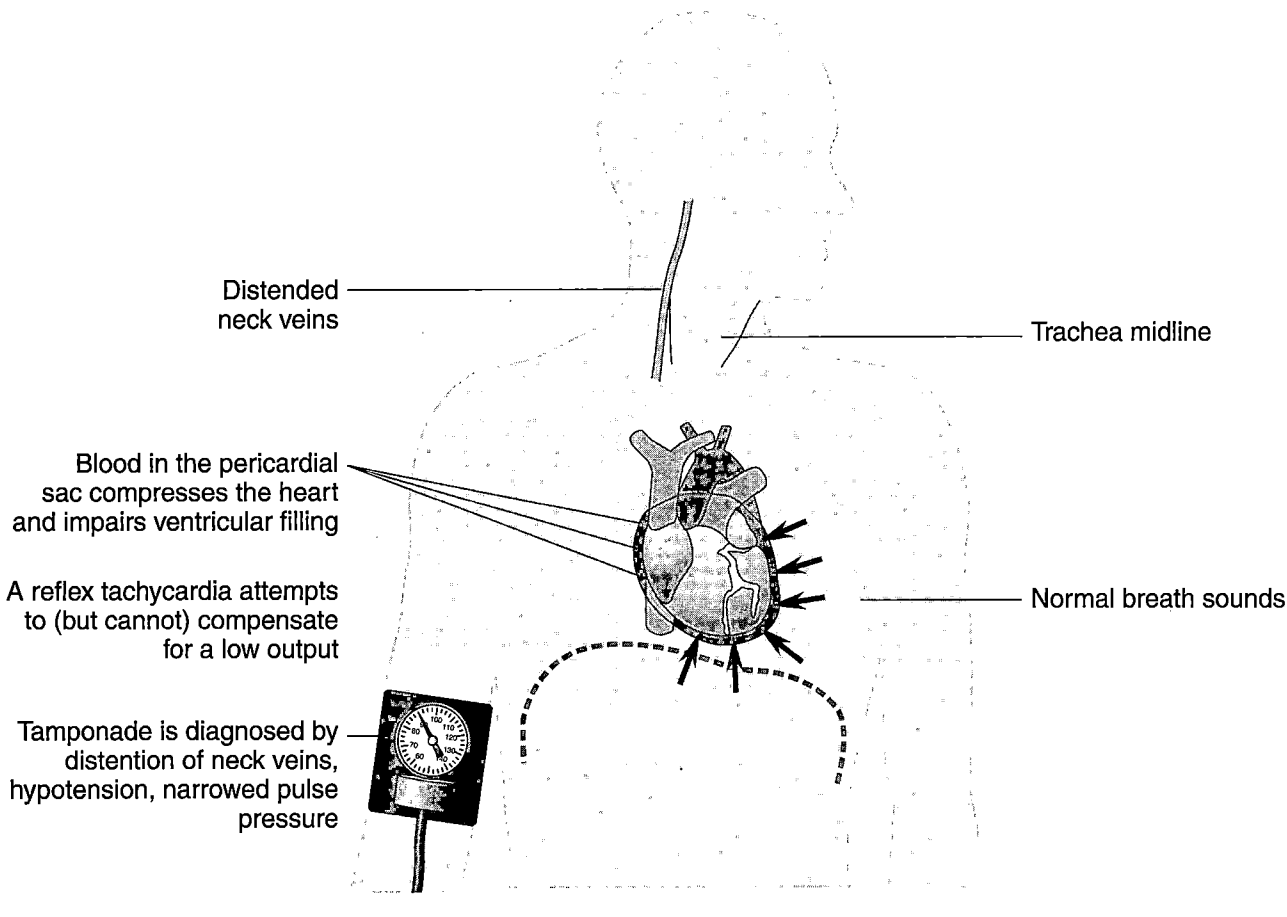

Distended neck veins

Trachea midline

Blood in the pericardial sac compresses the heart and impairs ventricular filling

A reflex tachycardia attempts to (but cannot) compensate for a low output

Normal breath sounds

Tamponade is diagnosed by distention of neck veins, hypotension, narrowed pulse pressure

FIGURE 40-4 A narrowed pulse pressure and neck vein distension are signs of pericardial tamponade.

into cardiac arrest, so you must get the history right away or you may never get it until the autopsy.

PEARL

Despite the many signs described for pericardial tamponade, few are present together in any one patient. Hypotension and distended neck veins in the presence of normal lung sounds (ruling against pneumothorax), combined with an appropriate history, suggests tamponade until proven otherwise.

What is the appropriate field management of a patient with a pericardial tamponade?

The management of the patient with a pericardial tamponade involves, first and foremost, airway and ventilation control. Positive pressure ventilation may be needed. Administer high-concentration oxygen and evaluate the need for ET intubation.

Field management involves a fluid challenge and the rapid removal of the patient to the ED. Be sure to call ahead so that on your arrival, a physician can be waiting at the doorway to do a

pericardiocentesis. This procedure of removing fluid from within the sac can be lifesaving. Most patients, however, still require definitive surgery to repair the myocardial bleeding. Transport the patient to the closest appropriate facility.

What is the epidemiology of a myocardial contusion?

Between 16 and 76 percent of the patients with blunt trauma experience a myocardial contusion. This is a significant cause of morbidity and mortality in the blunt chest trauma patient.

What is the pathophysiology of a myocardial contusion?

The contusion causes a hemorrhage with edema and fragmented myocardial fibers. There is cellular injury and vascular damage may occur. If the epicardium or endocardium are lacerated, a hemopericardium can develop. The fibrinous reaction at the contusion site may lead to a delayed rupture or ventricular aneurysm. The areas of contusion are usually clearly demarcated and may cause conduction defects on the ECG.

Q What are the assessment findings in a patient with a myocardial contusion?

A When evaluating the patient with a suspected cardiac contusion, the EMS provider should locate many of the following:

- There are associated injuries usually involving a sternal fracture or one to three rib fractures.

- The patient may complain of a retrosternal chest pain.

- There may be a cardiac murmur and a pericardial friction rub in the later stages of the contusion's development.

- ECG changes may include persistent tachycardia, S-T elevation, T wave inversion, right bundle branch block, atrial flutter or fibrillation, and premature ventricular contractions (PVCs) or premature atrial contractions (PACs).

CLINICAL PEARL

Many patients with a myocardial contusion are relatively asymptomatic, at least initially. Accompanying injuries may present more dramatically. Helpful signs are ECG changes, if present, and persistent sinus tachycardia without obvious hypovolemia.

Q What is the appropriate field management of a patient with a myocardial contusion?

A The management of the patient with a myocardial contusion involves, first and foremost, airway and ventilation control. Administer high-concentration oxygen and evaluate the need for ET intubation.

Administer fluids. Consider anti-dysrhythmics and vasopressor agents, according to local protocols. Transport the patient to the nearest appropriate facility.

Q What is the epidemiology of a myocardial rupture?

A A myocardial rupture is either associated with immediate trauma or delayed for some two to three weeks. The injury is associated with a compression between the sternum and the vertebrae or a penetrating trauma involving a rib, missile, bullet fragment, or the sternal bone. Other causes include patients who have a history of trauma with a presentation of congestive heart failure (CHF) and cardiac tamponade.

Q What is the appropriate field management of a patient with a myocardial rupture?

A The field management is supportive and involves managing the ABCs. Pay close attention to a patient with an onset of CHF or pulmonary edema following trauma. This may be due to a rupture of cardiac valves or an intraventricular septal rupture.

Q What is the epidemiology of an aortic dissection or rupture?

A The causes are primarily MVCs and falls. Aortic dissections are present in 15 percent of all blunt trauma deaths. This is a very critical injury where 85 to 95 percent of the patients die instantaneously. Ten to 15 percent of the patients survive to arrive at the hospital.

Q What is the pathophysiology of an aortic dissection or rupture?

A An aortic dissection or rupture is a shearing injury involving a separation of the aortic intima and media. The blood enters the media through a small intima tear. The tears occur as a result of high-speed deceleration on portions of the aorta at points of relative fixation. The thinned out layers may rupture due to increased intraluminal pressure from the impact. The descending aorta at the isthmus just distal to the left subclavian artery is the most common site of rupture. This is called the ligamentom arteriosum. Ruptures of the ascending aorta are much less common.

Q What are the assessment findings in a patient with an aortic dissection or rupture?

A Patients with an aortic rupture die very quickly. Those who survive have formed a pseudohematoma that may rupture at any time. When examining a patient who the EMS provider suspects may have an aortic dissection or rupture, the following findings may be present:

- Retrosternal or interscapular pain.

- Dyspnea and dysphagia.

- Ischemic pain of the extremities.

- Upper-extremity hypertension with absent or decreased amplitude of femoral pulses.

- A harsh systolic murmur over the interscapular region.

- A different BP on each arm.

Q What is the appropriate field management of a patient with an aortic dissection or rupture?

A The management of the very critical patient involves airway management and ventilation. The patient will probably need ET intubation and oxygen administration. Provide IV fluids, but do not overhydrate and monitor the ECG. Do not pass an NG tube on this patient because it may perforate the hematoma that has developed, leading to immediate exsanguinations. Transport the patient to a hospital that can handle this type of injury.

What is the impact of a developing hematoma in the chest?

Hematomas may cause the compression of any structure such as the vena cava, trachea, esophagus, great vessels, and the heart.

What is the pathophysiology of a diaphragmatic injury?

There is a high-pressure compression to the abdomen with a resultant intra-abdominal pressure increase. There is a diaphragmatic rupture with extravasation of abdominal contents into the chest. This can produce very subtle signs and symptoms such as bowel obstruction and strangulation. The lung expansion is restricted by a diaphragmatic injury, resulting in hypoventilation and hypoxia. The injury can cause a mediastinal shift with the resultant cardiac and respiratory compromise.

What are the assessment findings in a patient with a diaphragmatic injury?

When evaluating a patient with a suspected diaphragmatic injury, the EMS provider should look for the following:

- Tachypnea, decreased breath sounds, and respiratory distress.
- Tachycardia and bowel sounds in affected hemothorax.
- Dullness to percussion and a scaffold abdomen.
- Pain or discomfort.
- Nausea or vomiting.

What is the appropriate field management of a patient with a diaphragmatic injury?

The field management of a patient with a diaphragmatic injury involves airway management and ventilation with high-concentration oxygen. Positive pressure ventilation may be necessary and if so, use it with caution because it may worsen the injury. Do not place the patient in the Trendelenburg position because this may make the respiratory distress much worse. Also be alert for vomiting.

What is the epidemiology of an esophageal injury?

The most frequent cause of an esophageal injury is a penetrating trauma by a missile, bullet, or knife. It is rare from a blunt trauma. If an esophageal injury is missed, it can be life threatening.

What are the assessment findings in a patient with an esophageal injury?

On examination of the patient with an esophageal injury, the EMS provider may find the following:

- Pain and fever.
- Hoarseness and dysphagia.
- Respiratory distress and shock.
- A cervical perforation may have local tenderness, subcutaneous emphysema, and neck resistance on passive motion.
- Intrathoracic perforation may have mediastinal emphysema, mediastinitis, subcutaneous emphysema, and a splinting of the chest wall.
- May present as a cardiac event.

What is the appropriate field management of a patient with an esophageal injury?

The management involves airway management and ventilation with high-concentration oxygen. If the patient is hypotensive, fluids should be administered. The patient should be taken to the most appropriate facility.

What is the epidemiology of a tracheobronchial injury?

Tracheobronchial injury is rare, occurring in less than three percent of the chest injuries and both penetrating and blunt trauma. It has a high mortality rate of greater than 30 percent.

What is the pathophysiology of a tracheobronchial injury?

The majority of the injuries occur within three cm of the carina, although the tear can occur anywhere along the tracheal–bronchial tree. There is a rapid movement of air into the pleural space, often making the tension pneumothorax refractory to a needle decompression. There is a continuous flow of air from the needle in a decompressed chest. This patient has severe hypoxia.

What are the assessment findings in a patient with a tracheobronchial injury?

On examination the EMS provider may note these findings in the patient with a tracheobronchial injury:

- Tachypnea, dyspnea, and respiratory distress.
- Tachycardia and hemoptysis.
- Signs of tension pneumothorax that does not respond to a needle decompression.
- Massive subcutaneous emphysema.
- The patient is difficult to intubate.

🔘 What is the appropriate field management of a patient with a tracheobronchial injury?

🅰 The management of the patient with a tracheobronchial injury involves airway management and ventilation with high-concentration oxygen. If the patient is hypotensive, administer fluids. Transport the patient to the closest appropriate facility.

🔘 What is the epidemiology of traumatic asphyxia?

🅰 This injury results when chest movement is impaired to the point that the patient is unable to breathe effectively. The most common cause is a crush injury. The incidence of these injuries is low, though a specific figure is impossible to determine because of varied definitions in the medical literature.

🔘 What is the pathophysiology of traumatic asphyxia?

🅰 The sudden compressional force squeezing the chest backs the blood up into the head and neck. The jugular veins engorge and the capillaries rupture. In addition, the chest is unable to expand to create the negative intrathoracic pressure necessary for the inflow of air.

🔘 What are the assessment findings in a patient with traumatic asphyxia?

🅰 When examining the patient with a traumatic asphxia, the EMS provider may locate any of these findings:

- Cyanosis to the face and upper neck.
- JVD.
- Swelling or hemorrhage of the conjunctiva.
- The skin below the area remains pink.
- There is hypotension when the pressure is released.
- Petechia, bleeding beneath the skin, in the upper chest, neck, and face.

🔘 What is the appropriate field management of a patient with traumatic asphyxia?

🅰 The management of a patient with traumatic asphxia involves airway management and ventilation with high-concentration oxygen. When the compression is released, there is hypotension that should be managed with IV fluids. The patient should be taken to the most appropriate facility.

Abdominal Trauma

T he abdomen contains the major vessels of the circulatory, digestive, endocrine, and urogenital systems. When trauma to the abdominal cavity occurs, the extent of the injury can be difficult to appreciate in the out-of-hospital setting. Major hemorrhage can occur rapidly and be unrecognized. This is why abdominal trauma is a major cause of trauma death and the second leading cause of *preventable* trauma death.

This chapter discusses the structures and areas of the abdominal cavity, the pathophysiology of abdominal trauma, and the assessment and treatment priorities for the patient with abdominal trauma.

Pathophysiology of Abdominal Trauma

Q **What are the most common causes of abdominal trauma?**

A Injuries to the abdominal cavity result from blunt trauma, penetrating trauma, or both. Most commonly, the injuries are a result of motor vehicle crashes (MVCs), falls from heights, gunshot (GSW) and stab wounds, abdominal compression, and blows to the abdomen. Because the bladder is in the pelvic cavity, technically it is called the abdominopelvic cavity. For the purposes of this chapter, the term abdominal cavity also includes the pelvic cavity.

Q **What types of injuries occur with abdominal trauma?**

A There are numerous types of injuries that result from abdominal trauma, as well as associated injuries to the chest and spine, due to the close proximity. Therefore, these patients are often managed as multisystem trauma victims. Abdominal injuries may involve any or all of the following structures:

- Bladder.
- Diaphragm.
- Reproductive structures and fetus (in pregnancy).
- Bowel.
- Liver.
- Pancreas.
- Kidneys.
- Spleen.
- Pelvis.
- Spine.
- Blood vessels.

What is the morbidity and mortality rate of abdominal trauma?

Abdominal trauma is the second leading cause of trauma death. There are a few reasons for this. When the mechanism of injury (MOI) is penetrating trauma, the obvious wound is the clue to underlying injury. However, when the MOI is blunt, the potential for injury is often underappreciated or not recognized at all. Even when penetrating trauma is obvious, such as a bullet entrance wound, the extent of injury may be underappreciated because an exit wound was missed on examination.

Another reason for the high mortality is the potential for injury to any of the major organs, as well as multi-trauma. Consequently, severe bleeding can progress rapidly. The adult abdominal cavity can hide a significant blood loss (1.5 liters) easily before showing any signs of distention.

CLINICAL PEARL

Always remember the concept of "associated injuries." Based on the MOI, certain "syndromes" are common. For example, people with abdominal injuries (especially upper abdomen) often have a chest injury as well.

What are the primary concerns for abdominal trauma?

Immediate concerns, after the ABCs, are hemorrhage, major organ damage, and associated chest injuries. Later concerns are loss of blood, peritonitis, sepsis, and loss of organ function.

Why is it important to recognize abdominal trauma early?

Late recognition of abdominal trauma can be a fatal mistake. Abdominal trauma often goes unrecognized because the MOI is often not fully appreciated or goes unrecognized. The solid organs are very vascular and when injured, create a large blood loss that is not easily recognized due to the size of the abdominal cavity. Therefore, when a patient has shock with an unexplained source or the extent of shock is greater than explained by the injuries present, assume there is an abdominal injury.

CLINICAL PEARL

Isolated head injury rarely causes hypotension. If a trauma patient is hypotensive and has a head injury, look for a pelvic fracture or intra-abdominal bleeding.

What type of injuries can be predicted with blunt or penetrating trauma?

When you understand the anatomy of the abdominal cavity, it is reasonable to predict certain types of injuries with specific MOIs. For example, MVCs often involve rapid deceleration forces that compress internal organs and cause a shearing of organs that are suspended by ligaments. Injuries from stab wounds can be narrowed down if the length of the object and the direction of thrust are known.

Why is rapid intervention and transport of a patient with abdominal injuries so important?

Surgical intervention is the definitive treatment for many abdominal injuries. In the out-of-hospital setting, it is not important to determine the specific organ(s) injured because the treatment is the same for all abdominal injuries. Consider what the patient needs and what you can do. Assess the MOI, maintain a high index of suspicion of the injury, treat shock, and transport the patient rapidly to an appropriate facility.

The out-of-hospital care provider can make the difference between life and death from abdominal injuries. Recognizing the potential for life-threatening injury and providing rapid transport to definitive care will make all the difference for a successful patient outcome.

What are the common terms associated with the abdomen?

The terms associated with the abdomen include:

- Closed injury—an internal injury without breaking through the skin.
- DPL—diagnostic peritoneal lavage.
- Guarding—reflex muscle tensing over an injury or inflammation of the peritoneum. There are two types of guarding: voluntary guarding, which is conscious and intentional, and involuntary guarding, which is reflexive and automatic.
- Hematuria—blood in the urine.
- Ileus—decreased motility.
- Open injury—an internal injury with a break through the skin.
- Peritonitis—signs and symptoms include abdominal tenderness, rebound tenderness, and involuntary guarding. Treatment may be surgical or supportive depending on the cause. If there is a perforation, it presents with acute symptoms. If there is an infection, it produces a slower onset (several hours) of symptoms.
- Rebound tenderness—cough, severe pain from bouncing on stretcher.

- Retroperitoneal cavity—the posterior of the abdominal cavity.
- Viscus—an internal organ enclosed within a body cavity, such as intestines within the abdomen.

Assessment

What are the key aspects in the initial assessment?

The essential aspects of the initial assessment are knowing the anatomy of the abdomen and fully appreciating the MOI. These two essential aspects should lead the out-of-hospital provider to have a high index of suspicion of injury to abdominal organs and associated structures. Consider that a patient presenting with shock not consistent with obvious injuries or from an unexplained source has intra-abdominal bleeding until proven otherwise.

Information obtained from the initial assessment is critical for deciding on a rapid transport to an appropriate facility. After recognizing the need for a rapid transport, treat the shock and begin transport.

What are the key aspects of the focused history (FH) and rapid trauma exam?

The FH and rapid trauma exam should be performed simultaneously. During the FH, obtain more specific information about the MOI if possible (e.g., approximate speed of a crash, direction of a blow or stabbing, how many gunshots were fired, and the time the incident occurred).

Use the information obtained about the MOI at the scene and during the FH while performing the rapid trauma exam. Be observant for predictable injury patterns associated with the MOI. For example, when a GSW is present, look for entrance and exit wounds. Obtain serial vital signs during the rapid transport and notify the ED early (on scene if possible) so they can prepare accordingly.

What does an abnormal abdomen feel like?

The normal abdomen should feel warm and soft without any lumps, distention, or hardness. There should be no pain (not tender) for the patient during palpation or after palpation. Rebound tenderness is when the sudden release of pressure hurts more than the pressure itself.

Abnormal findings of the abdomen include masses (whether pulsating, suggesting aneurysm, or not), distention (e.g., gas, fluid), rigidity or hardness (e.g., ascites, muscle spasm), and pain, either direct or rebound.

When should the abdomen not be palpated?

If the patient is experiencing severe abdominal pain, use only a very light touch to determine skin temperature, abdominal rigidity, and areas of significant tenderness. (Rebound tenderness is discussed in Chapter 27, Gastroenterology and Urology). Locate the exact area of pain or discomfort by asking the patient to show you where it hurts. If they indicate one particular quadrant, you can avoid that quadrant and palpate the three remaining quadrants during the exam.

What is the difference between somatic and visceral pain?

Somatic pain is due to a direct irritation of the parietal peritoneum. As such, it is more localized. Visceral pain is due to an irritation of the visceral peritoneum, which receives input from both sides of the spinal cord. Thus, visceral pain is more diffuse.

What about listening for bowel sounds?

Listening for bowel sounds in the field is not helpful. To properly auscultate bowel sounds, it is necessary to listen for several minutes; in the field, there is often no time for this and the ambient noise is too great.

In the clinical setting, listening for bowel sounds is helpful. An abnormal or absent bowel sound may indicate obstruction or peritonitis. The bowel sounds are usually hyperactive in an intestinal obstruction (ileus).

What are Cullen's and Grey-Turner's signs?

Cullen's sign is a black and blue discoloration (ecchymosis) in the umbilical area caused by peritoneal bleeding from any cause (e.g., ruptured spleen, ruptured ectopic pregnancy). Grey-Turner's sign has ecchymosis in the lower abdominal and flank regions. These are both caused by intra-abdominal bleeding found 12 to 24 hours after the initial injury. If found, they may be seen in the victim of trauma who either delayed calling EMS or was not found immediately after the incident.

CLINICAL PEARL

Cullen's and Grey-Turner's signs are in all the books, but rarely in any patients. Their presence is helpful, and their absence does not rule out life-threatening abdominal hemorrhage.

What is Kehr's sign?

It is pain in the abdomen that radiates to the left shoulder and may be an indication of intraperitoneal bleeding.

> **CLINICAL PEARL**
>
> *Pain from irritation of the diaphragm is often referred to the shoulder. Gallbladder disease is the most common cause on the right side. On the left, intraperitoneal bleeding, especially a ruptured spleen, may lead to Kehr's sign.*

> **CLINICAL PEARL**
>
> *Anecdotal cases of the successful use of MAST/PASG with ruptured aortic aneurysms and ectopic pregnancy abound, especially in areas with prolonged transport times. Always follow your local protocols.*

[Q] Aside from managing the ABCs, shock management, and rapid transport to an appropriate trauma center, is there any other treatment that can be done in the out-of-hospital phase?

[A] Yes, treat all life threats as they become identified during the rapid trauma assessment and ongoing reassessment. Then, treat noncritical injuries as manpower and time permit.

- Cover open wounds and control bleeding where necessary.
- Stabilize impaled objects in place unless they interfere with the patient's airway or CPR.
- Immobilize patients with suspected spinal injuries.
- Cover eviscerations with moist sterile dressings and keep the area warm. Never attempt to replace eviscerated organs.
- Stabilize suspected pelvic fractures with a backboard and military antishock trousers/pneumatic antishock garment (MAST/PASG) where appropriate. Check your local protocols for MAST/PASG use.
- Always suspect and check for associated chest injuries. The specific management depends on the injury (see Chapter 40, Thoracic Trauma).
- Remember that an abdominal aortic aneurysm (AAA) requires rapid, but gentle, handling and transport, IV fluids enroute, and early ED notification.

Enroute to the trauma center, continue reassessing the ABCs and providing high-concentration oxygen. Be alert for vomiting. Provide assisted and advanced airway management if indicated. Initiate an IV of normal saline (NS). If hypovolemia is suspected, administer a 250–500 cc fluid bolus and titrate the IV drip rate to the patient's hemodynamic status. (Follow your local protocols). Contact medical control for additional fluid bolus authorization or other orders.

[Q] What is the current role of MAST/PASG in the field?

[A] MAST/PASG are helpful in stabilizing and decreasing bleeding in pelvic and long bone fractures of the lower extremities. MAST/PASG is harmful to trauma patients with moderate hypotension (systolic BP 50–90 mmHg) and short transport times, especially when accompanied with penetrating chest trauma. The MAST/PASG is discussed in detail in Chapter 35, Hemorrhage and Shock.

[Q] What types of abdominal surgery might be necessary with abdominal trauma?

[A] Exploratory surgery may reveal a number of specific or multi-trauma injuries that require repair. Common abdominal surgical interventions include:

- Appendectomy—removal of the appendix.
- Colostomy—an opening made in the large intestine.
- Cesarean section—delivery of a fetus through an incision through the abdomen into the uterus.
- Gastrectomy—removal of all or part of the stomach.
- Hernioplasty—surgical repair of a hernia.
- Laparotomy—surgical opening of the abdomen, used as an exploratory procedure.
- Dilation and curettage (D&C)—surgical procedure that enlarges the cervical canal so the lining of the uterus can be scraped.

> **CLINICAL PEARL**
>
> *In the past, the complete removal of the spleen (splenectomy) was routine for any splenic injury. The surgical approach has changed radically in recent years. The spleen provides an important immune function; without it, people are susceptible to life-threatening infections from organisms that would otherwise not be a problem. Surgeons have devised numerous methods of "splenic salvage," ranging from the simple suturing of lacerations to grinding up residual splenic tissue and reimplanting it into the omentum ("splenosis"). Both splenic preservation techniques eliminate the risk of sepsis (overwhelming infection). Patients who have had the spleen completely removed (splenectomy) are at risk to develop severe infections from common organisms. A physician must evaluate any post-splenectomy patient with an infection (e.g., sore throat, cold, flu).*

[Q] What special considerations are there for the pregnant patient?

[A] Direct trauma to the abdomen of the pregnant patient may result in premature labor, abortion, abruptio placenta (premature separation of the placenta from the uterine wall), uterine rupture, and fetal death.

Seat belt injuries are especially common with pregnancy. They should not be a reason to rationalize going without a seat belt!

Rapid transport and early notification of the facility that is capable of handling this type of injury is paramount. The administration of high-concentration oxygen early is a high priority because the patient can lose up to 35 percent of blood volume before signs of shock are evident. Position the patient on her left side to keep the fetus from compressing the vena cava and creating supine hypotension. If the patient is immobilized on a backboard, tilt the board 15 degrees to the left to achieve the same effect. Be alert for vomiting due to decreased peristalsis and the frequent full stomach.

Sexual Trauma

What is vaginal insufflation syndrome?

This is a type of cunnilungus that incorporates blowing air into the vagina. With orogenital insufflation, air overflows from the vagina into the fallopian tubes and then to the peritoneal cavity, creating pneumoperitoneum.

Vaginal insufflation syndrome may result in fatal peritonitis. Patients are usually embarrassed to divulge the exact circumstances of their situation. Even if you do not discuss this possibility directly with the patient, alert ED personnel of your suspicion.

What is pneumoperitoneum?

Pneumoperitoneum is free air in the abdomen that may present as acute abdominal pain. This can occur for a number of reasons such as:

- Douching.
- Gynecological procedures.
- Orogenital insufflation.
- Perforated viscus.
- Peritonitis with gas-forming organisms.
- Pneumomediastinum.
- Recent surgical procedures.

What is pneumoscrotum?

Pneumoscrotum is subcutaneous air in the male scrotum that occurs as a result of severe subcutaneous emphysema. The most common cause is the dissection of air subcutaneously from a massive pneumothorax.

In rare cases of severe localized infection (necrotizing fasciitis), gas-forming organisms cause similar scrotal swelling. Pneumoscrotum by itself is very unusual. If there is no evidence of subcutaneous emphysema anywhere but the scrotum, localized infection or direct trauma is more likely.

What types of injuries are seen with sexual trauma?

The physical and emotional injuries associated with rape often come to mind first when sexual trauma is mentioned. However, many traumatic injuries occur during consensual sex:

- Pierced body jewelry is very popular and may be ripped free during sexual excitement, creating lacerations and tears.
- Restraint injuries—bondage injuries, such as lacerations and bruising, may result from a variety of restraints including whips, chains, handcuffs, leg irons, and ropes.
- Autoerotic injuries—a syndrome of young males (10 to 30 years old) resulting from transient asphyxia induced to heighten erotic sensation or sexual fantasies. A common method is by hanging. Complications arise when the patient is unable to self-rescue due to a mechanism failure, drugs, or alcohol.
- Perforations—common in both male and female, they are caused by natural and foreign objects inserted into the vagina or rectum. Signs and symptoms include acute abdominal pain, tachycardia, tachypnea, fever, and a rigid abdomen.
- Fractured penis—is a real injury that occurs when an erect penis is severely struck or bent. Although there is no bone in the penis, the patient often hears and feels a loud "snap or

A strange, though prevalent, practice consists of placing the closed fist and wrist into a body orifice (either vagina or rectum) for sexual stimulation. This is referred to as "fisting." Whether the patient is male or female, organ rupture (vagina, rectum) is likely. Life-threatening peritonitis may result. As with other sexually related injuries, patients are often reluctant to divulge correct historical information.

pop," and then loses the erection. The injury is obvious with a deviation away from the tear in the tunica albuginea of one of the corpora cavenosa, although it is possible to tear both. Swelling, discoloration, and bleeding from the urethra may also be present. Splinting is not recommended, but pain management should be considered.

What is the management of external foreign objects on the genitalia?

Sometimes people place a tight ring around the penis, scrotum, or both to enhance erection. Severe problems arise when the patient cannot remove the object. The complications that can result are unrelieved swelling, edema, and if prolonged, ischemia, tissue loss, or amputation.

Out-of-hospital management is limited to a position of comfort and pain management. Depending on the ring's material, removal of the object may be performed using a standard ring cutter, depending on local protocols and transport time. Generally, this treatment is done in the ED setting.

What if something has gotten stuck in a woman's vagina?

Out-of-hospital management includes placing or keeping the patient in a position of comfort, monitoring the patient for signs and symptoms of shock, and treating for shock if present. Do not attempt to remove vaginal foreign objects in the field. Most objects will be removed in the ED; few require surgical removal.

How do you deal with an anal foreign body in the field?

Out-of-hospital management for this is the same as for vaginal foreign bodies. The complications associated with these types of emergencies are perforations and hemorrhage. The signs and symptoms of perforation into the intraperitoneal area include acute abdominal pain, rigid abdomen, tachycardia, tachypnea, and elevated body temperature. All are due to contamination by fecal matter.

What is the treatment for bleeding from the male or female genitalia?

Direct pressure and positioning are the primary treatment for controlling bleeding of male or female genitalia. Monitor the airway and breathing and observe for signs of shock. As with all shock patients, provide high-flow oxygen and watch for nausea and vomiting. Begin IV fluid replacement; if shock is present, run IV fluids according to your local protocols.

What is the management for an amputation of the penis?

If the proximal penile stump is bleeding, use direct pressure to control it. If you recover the amputated distal penis, place it in a clean plastic bag. Seal the bag and immerse it in cold saline, if available. The repair of a severed penis is possible up to six hours after amputation. Beyond this period, local reshaping plastic surgery is usually recommended.

What is testicular torsion and how is it managed?

Testicular torsion occurs when a testicle twists on its pedicle (a combination of nerves, blood vessels, and spermatic vessels), leading to acute ischemia. This usually occurs spontaneously in males under 40 years of age. Many individuals have an underlying anatomic abnormality that predisposes them to torsion, but it cannot be detected in advance without surgery. The patient presents with acute, usually excruciating pain, nausea, diaphoresis, and, sometimes, vomiting (much as if hit in the groin, but worse. The patient's pain may be out of proportion to the degree of tenderness on palpation.

Out-of-hospital treatment consists of the ABCs, IV fluids, and pain medications as per local protocol, and rapid, yet gentle, transport to the nearest appropriate medical facility. Though some emergency physicians advocate attempting a manual detorsion, do not attempt this in the field. The treatment is prompt surgery in almost all cases. A delay of more than a few hours can lead to the loss of both testicles and permanent infertility.

Special Thanks

McSwain, N., Jr., et al. (1999). *Prehospital trauma life support* (3rd ed.). St. Louis: Mosby.

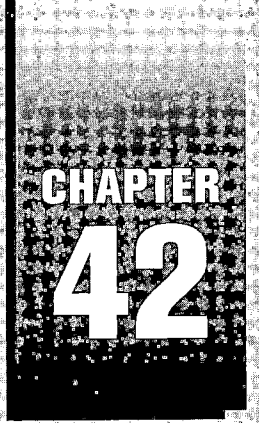

Musculoskeletal Trauma

This chapter discusses the injuries that can happen to the muscles and bones. It discusses the pathophysiology of the musculoskeletal (MS) system. The focus is on *why* patients present in a certain manner and *why* you need to respond in a certain way to their presenting problems.

Epidemiology

Q What is the incidence of MS trauma?

A Between 70 and 80 percent of the multiple-trauma patients suffer MS injuries.

Q What is the mortality and morbidity of MS trauma?

A Upper-extremity injuries contribute to long-term impairment, but rarely are life threatening. Lower-extremity injuries are associated with higher magnitudes of injury. They have more significant blood loss and are more difficult to manage in the multiple-trauma patient. Femur and pelvic injuries may constitute life threats.

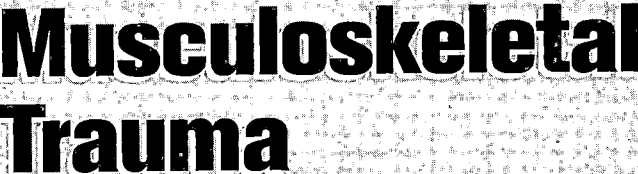

CLINICAL PEARL

The biggest risk in patients with MS trauma is that we miss other injuries not related to the MS system (e.g., overlooking abdominal trauma).

Q What are some of the prevention strategies to minimize the number of MS injuries?

A There are many prevention strategies that can be implemented to reduce the number of MS injuries. The following are examples:

- Proper sports training.
- Wearing seat belts.
- Child safety seats.
- Airbags.
- Gun safety and education.
- Motorcycle driver education.
- Fall prevention.
- High-rise window guards.

Physiology

Q What are the age-associated changes to bones?

A As we age, our bones change in a number of ways. There are morphological changes and changes that affect the bones

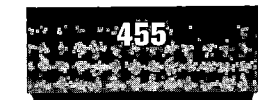

causing increased chances of fracture. Specifically, the changes are as follows:

- Morphological changes—the water content of the intervertebral disks decreases and there is an increased risk of disk herniation. A loss of between one-half to three-quarters of an inch in overall stature can occur due to aging. Bone tissue disorders also tend to shorten the trunk, and the vertebral column gradually assumes an arc shape. The costal cartilage ossifies, making the thorax more rigid and causing more shallow breathing due to the rigid thoracic cage. In addition, the contours of the face change.

- Fractures—the bones are more prone to fracture because they are more porous and become brittle. It is not uncommon for patients to fracture the vertebrae or the femoral neck. The development of osteoporosis (thinning of the bone) is related to an increased incidence of fractures.

What is the purpose of cardiac muscle?

Cardiac muscle is unique because it can generate an impulse and contract rhythmically on its own. This attribute, being able to generate an impulse, is referred to as automaticity. Cardiac muscle is also excitable and conducts electrical impulses.

What is the purpose of a smooth muscle?

Smooth muscle is found in the lower airways, blood vessels, and intestines. It is under the control of the autonomic nervous system (ANS). Smooth muscle can relax or contract to alter the inner lumen diameter of vessels.

What is the purpose of skeletal muscle?

Skeletal muscle is under conscious control. It includes the major muscle mass of the body and allows for mobility.

What provides the muscular support of the skeleton?

The muscular support of the skeleton is provided by the tendons, cartilage, and ligaments. Their functions are as follows:

- Tendon—is a band of connective tissue binding muscle to bone (M-T-B). The tendon allows for power of movement across the joints.

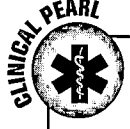

Remember, bones articulate at joints where they are padded by cartilage. Ligaments hold the joints together.

- Cartilage—is connective tissue covering the epiphysis that acts as a surface for articulation. Cartilage allows for the smooth movement at the joints.

- Ligament—is connective tissue that support the joints. It is designed to attach to the bone ends and allow for range of motion (B-T-B).

What is the purpose of the bones?

The bones serve many functions. They protect the vital organs and provide a structure for muscles to allow movement. They are responsible for producing red blood cells (RBCs) and storing salts (e.g., calcium) and metabolic materials. Bones also act as a point of attachment for tendons, cartilage, and ligaments.

What are the structural classifications of the joints?

Structurally, the joints are classified into fibrous, cartilaginous, and synovial joints.

What is the purpose of fibrous joints?

Fibrous joints are those connected by fibrous tissue such as the sutures that are immovable and located in the skull. Syndesmoses are articulations in which the bones are united by ligaments. Gomphoses are immovable joints; one bone is fitted into the socket of another bone that is not intended for movement. An example is a tooth.

What is the purpose of cartilaginous joints?

A cartilaginous joint is one in which there is cartilage connecting the bones. Synchondrosis is an immovable joint having surfaces between the bones connected by cartilage. This could be temporary, because the joint ultimately becomes ossified, or it could be permanent. A symphysis is a line of fusion between two bones that were separate in early development.

What is the purpose of synovial joints?

A synovial joint is a joint filled with fluid that lubricates the articulated surfaces. Examples of synovial joints include plane, hinge, pivot, condyloid, saddle, and ball and socket (Figure 42–1).

What are some of the movements allowed by synovial joints?

Synovial joints allow gliding, rotation, and angular movements such as flexion, extension, abduction, adduction, and circumduction.

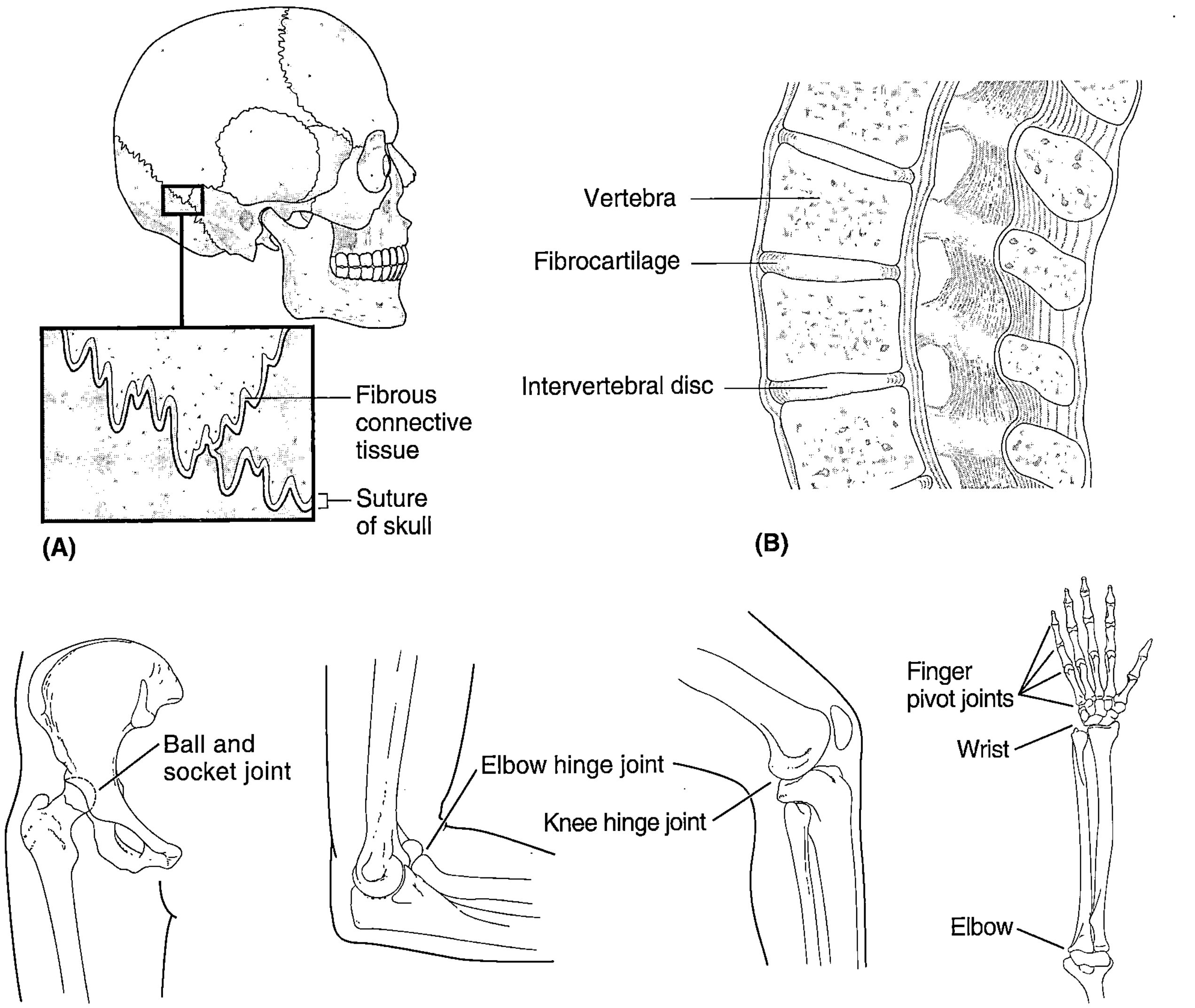

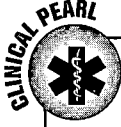

(A)

(B)

FIGURE 42-1 The types of joints: (A) an immovable fibrous joint, (B) a slightly movable cartilaginous joint, (C–F) freely movable hinge or ball-and-socket joints.

Pathophysiology

What are some of the problems associated with MS injuries?

When a patient has an MS injury, the associated injuries may include hemorrhage, instability, loss of tissue, simple lacerations and contamination, interruption of blood supply, and long-term disability.

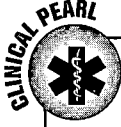

Often, though not always, associated injuries are more life threatening than the MS trauma itself.

What is the difference between an open and closed fracture?

An open fracture has a break in the skin that presumably was caused by the bone ends. These are also called compound fractures. Simple fractures or closed fractures do not involve a break in the skin.

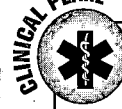

Sometimes the bone breaks the skin and then retracts back due to muscle spasm. Any break in the skin overlying a fracture is an open fracture until proven otherwise.

What are the X ray descriptions of fractures?

These descriptions used to be taught in the EMT course and appeared in earlier textbooks. The descriptions usually are not taught any longer because an EMS provider would not know what type of fracture a patient had in the absence of an X ray. You may not know there is an actual fracture unless there is a bone protruding. Once the fracture is X-rayed, the ED physician can verify that the patient has one or more fracture types (Figure 42–2).

- Greenstick—a fracture that tears away the outer covering of the bone, often most of the length of the bone; similar to how a live green tree splits.
- Oblique—the bone is broken in a slanted or diagonal direction from one side to the other.
- Transverse—the break is at a right angle to the axis of the long bone.
- Comminuted—the bone is broken or splintered into many pieces. Consider the combined blood loss and potential for other injuries with this type of fracture.
- Spiral—the break follows a helical line around the bone, usually caused by a twisting motion.
- Epiphysial fracture—occurs in young children involving the separation of the majority of the long bone from the growth plate at the ends of the bone.
- Incomplete—the break has not gone completely from one side of the bone to the other.
- Complete—the break extends from one side of the bone to the other.

Can a patient go into shock from a broken bone?

Yes. Uncomplicated fractures bleed about 500 cc from a tibia or fibula, 1,000 cc from a femur, or 2,000 cc from a pelvis over the first two hours after the fracture. If the patient has multiple fractures of long bones, you can quickly add up a considerable blood loss. If the fracture is complicated, such as one that severs the femoral artery, the patient can easily bleed to death.

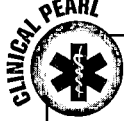

Consider pelvis and femur fractures as potentially life-threatening injuries.

What is a sprain?

A sprain is an injury to the ligaments around a joint and is marked by pain, swelling, and the dislocation of the skin over the joint. Sometimes it is difficult to distinguish between a fractured

leg and a sprained ankle. This is not really a problem because the out-of-hospital management is the same.

CLINICAL PEARL

A strain is an injury of the muscles and tendons. Remember the spelling: "S" "T"—"T" stands for tendon. A sprain, on the other hand, is an injury of the ligaments. A sprained ankle involves partial or complete tears of the many ankle ligaments.

What causes a sprain?

Excessive movement of the joint that tears the ligament.

What is a stress fracture?

A stress fracture is a break in the bone, typically one or more of the foot bones, caused by repeated long-term or abnormal stress.

What is a pathological fracture?

A fracture through an already abnormal area of bone is referred to as a pathological fracture. The underlying disease can be metastasis from cancer, cancer of the bone, or osteoporosis.

What is a dislocation, a subluxation, and a luxation?

When the bone is moved from its normal position within a joint, it becomes dislocated. A dislocation is a disruption of the integrity of a joint; a partial dislocation is generally called a subluxation. Complete disruption is termed a dislocation. A subluxation is a partial dislocation of a joint that usually has a great amount of damage and instability. A luxation is a complete dislocation of the joint.

What are examples of dislocations found in the field?

Common dislocations that can be found in the field include acromioclavicular, shoulder, elbow, wrist, metacarpal–phalangeal joint, hip, knee, ankle, foot, and hand.

What are the most serious dislocations?

Although they may look grotesque, dislocations are usually not life or limb threatening. There are two exceptions that should be taken very seriously in the field. The knee dislocation (Figure 42–3) can completely disrupt the blood supply to the

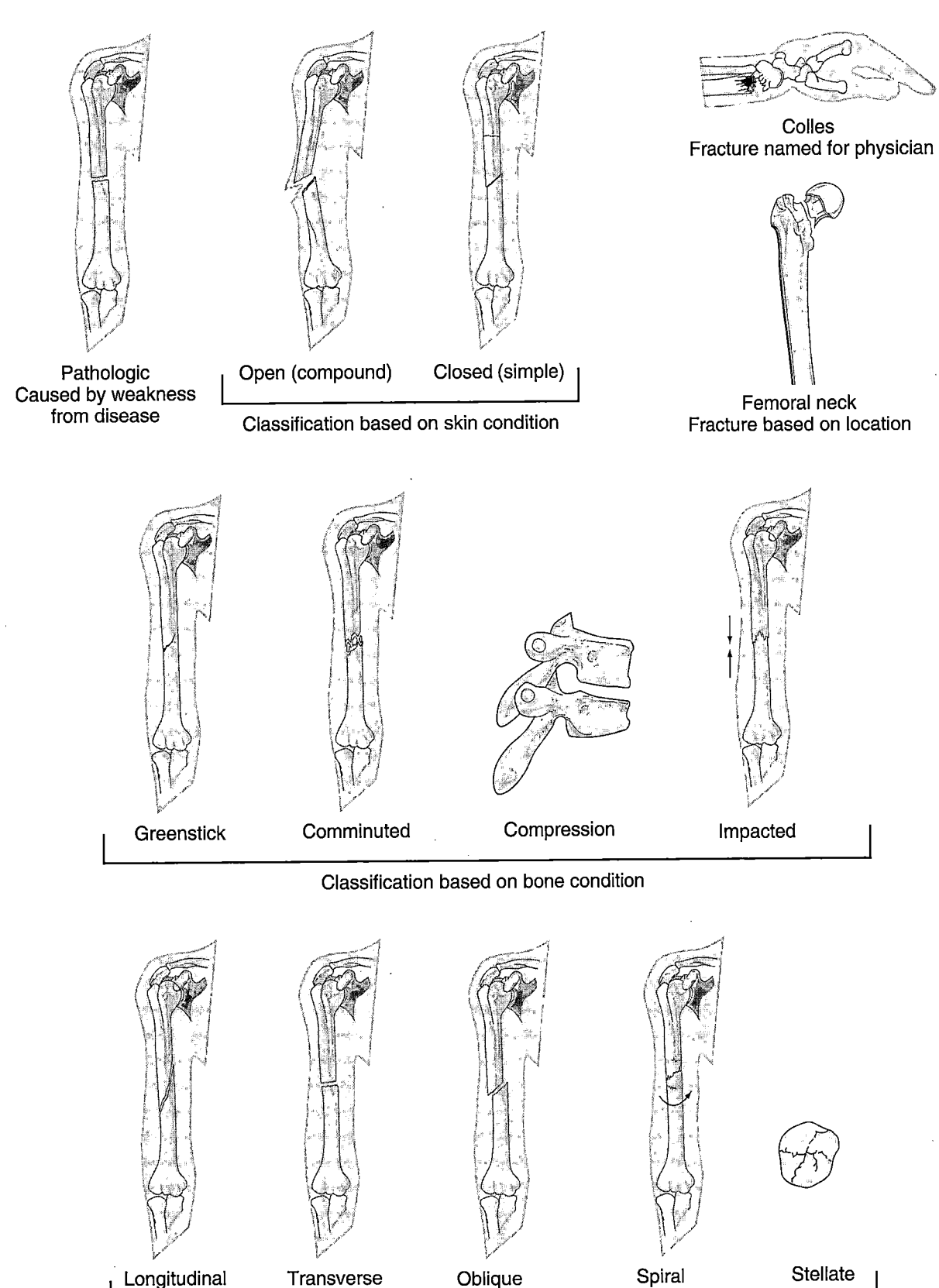

Pathologic
Caused by weakness
from disease

Open (compound)   Closed (simple)

Classification based on skin condition

Colles
Fracture named for physician

Femoral neck
Fracture based on location

Greenstick   Comminuted   Compression   Impacted

Classification based on bone condition

Longitudinal   Transverse   Oblique   Spiral   Stellate

Classification based on position of fracture line

FIGURE 42–2 The types of fractures.

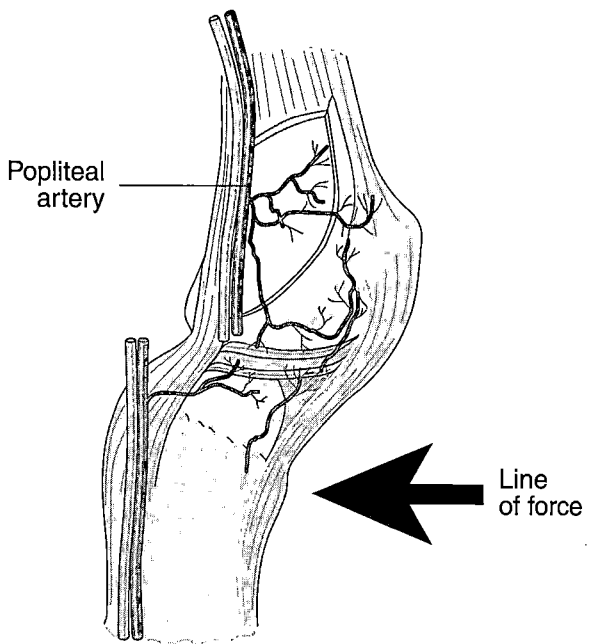

Popliteal
artery

Line
of force

FIGURE 42–3 The knee dislocation can be limb-threatening due to the lack of bloodflow to the extremity.

lower leg when the tibia is displaced to the posterior, compressing the posterior tibial artery. The elbow, when dislocated, can threaten the brachial artery and blood supply to the arm.

What are the three grades of sprains?

A sprain is a ligament injury, usually involving a tear. Sprains are classified in Table 42–1.

CLINICAL PEARL

This grading system is used for both sprains and strains. Of course, the "tear" involves different structures. Many times there is less pain but more swelling from a Grade III injury because the nerves are also torn. In Grade II injuries, the nerves are usually intact.

TABLE 42–1
Classifications of Sprains

Injury	Definition	Clinical
Grade I	No visible tear but microscopic injury has occurred	Pain, swelling; often able to bear weight
Grade II	Partial ligament tear	Severe pain and swelling; may not be able to bear weight
Grade III	Complete ligament tear	Significant swelling; often less pain than Grade II (nerves also torn); usually unable to bear weight

What constitutes a complicated fracture?

A fracture is considered complicated if it involves one or more of the following conditions:

- An accompanying laceration to an artery that could cause exsanguination.
- Major blood loss occurring at the break point.
- Decreased distal pulse.
- Diminished distal sensory or motor function.
- A crushing injury.

What are examples of inflammatory and degenerative conditions?

Patients can have a number of conditions that cause inflammation and degeneration of the joints: bursitis, tendinitis, osteoarthritis, rheumatoid arthritis, or gouty arthritis.

What is the concern with an elbow injury?

Injuries to the elbow have a high probability for blood vessel and nerve damage. This is especially true in children with supracondylar fractures. A Volkman's contracture, which is due to ischemia and usually affects the hand, may also result from this injury.

Musculoskeletal Assessment

What are the four classes of patients who have MS trauma?

There are four classes of patients with MS injuries. They are patients with:

- Life–limb-threatening injuries or conditions, including life–limb-threatening MS trauma (e.g., fractured pelvis, crushed chest, and shock).
- Other life–limb-threatening MS injuries and only simple MS trauma (e.g., fractured spine).
- Life–limb-threatening MS trauma and no other life–limb-threatening injuries (e.g., compound femur fracture).
- Only isolated nonlife–limb-threatening injuries (e.g., simple ulnar fracture).

What is the first part of the assessment of a patient with obvious fractures?

Conduct the initial assessment first to determine if there are any life threats that must be dealt with in the usual manner. Just as you should not overlook life–limb-threatening MS trauma, you also should not be distracted by a severely deformed extremity and overlook the ABCs.

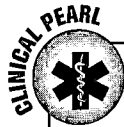

CLINICAL PEARL

Regardless how "impressive" an obvious MS injury may be, the initial priorities are unchanged: ABCs.

What are the five "Ps" of MS assessment?

The five "Ps" of MS assessment include:
- Pain or tenderness.
- Pallor—pale skin or poor capillary refill.
- Paresthesia—pins and needles sensation.
- Pulses—diminished or absent.
- Paralysis—the inability to move.

What are the general assessments when an MS injury is suspected?

When evaluating for an MS injury, be sure to inspect and palpate for DCAP-BTLS (deformity, contusions, abrasions, penetrations or punctures, burns, tenderness, lacerations, and swelling).

What specific findings should be noted on inspection and palpation of an MS injury?

In addition to assessing DCAP-BTLS, also look for the position the extremity was found in; the presence of a hematoma, dislocation, or cyanosis; the presence of motion or reduced range of motion; bleeding; guarding or self-splinting; and crepitus.

What are the assessment findings determined on palpation of the extremity?

When palpating the extremity for the presence of an MS injury, look for all of the following: tenderness or pain, deformity, crepitation, swelling and skin tension, pulses, capillary refilling, and sensation and movement.

Musculoskeletal Injury Management

When managing a closed fracture what is the key objective?

The key objective is to carefully splint the long bone fracture in a straight "splintable" position without allowing the bone

to protrude through the skin. Hospital care of an open fracture requires surgery; setting a closed fracture may be a matter of a few hours in the ED. Sometimes splinting is very difficult because certain bones are very close to the surface of the skin. Reach down and feel your tibia. That bone is very close to the surface and can easily break through the skin.

What are the general principles of MS injury management?

The general principles of management include:
- Splint the bone ends and the two adjacent joints.
- Immobilize open and closed fractures in the same manner.
- Cover open fractures to minimize contamination.
- Check distal pulses, motor function, and sensation (PMS) before and after applying the splint.
- Stabilize the fracture with gentle in-line traction to a position of normal alignment.
- Immobilize the patient where he is found. If the patient is found at the bottom of the stairs, the immobilization should occur at the base of the stairs. This does not mean that the fractures are immobilized in the position they are found. Long bones have to be moved with gentle traction to a "splintable" position. It makes the most sense to move a long bone injury into a "splintable" straight position.
- Immobilize dislocations in a position of comfort and good vascular supply.
- Immobilize joints in the position found unless there are no distal pulses. If there is no distal pulse, the joint should be moved once slightly to try to return the pulse. Always follow your local protocols because they may differ somewhat from these guidelines.
- Apply cold to reduce swelling and pain.
- Once splinted, consider elevation of the extremity.

What are the types of splints used in the field?

There are many types of splints used in the field. The most common are cardboard, wood, air, traction, vacuum, pillows and blankets, short spinal immobilization devices, and the ultimate body splint: the long spinal immobilization device.

What are the types of traction splints?

Traction splints are either unipolar (one pole) (e.g., the Sager® splint or KTD®) or bipolar (two poles) (e.g., the Hare® traction splint). The principle underlying these splints is that in-line traction can help to control the spasm of the strong muscles surrounding the femur and help to minimize overriding by the broken bone ends.

How are dislocations realigned?

The realignment of dislocations should be considered if distal circulation is impaired or if transportation is long or delayed. Typically, dislocated joints are immobilized in the position of injury and transported for reduction. Delayed or prolonged transport may require a different approach. Check circulation and nerve function before and after any manipulation of any injured bone or joint. Discontinue an attempt at repositioning if the pain is increased significantly by manipulation or resistance to movement is encountered.

What is the procedure for the realignment of a finger dislocation?

If you are going to attempt to realign a dislocated finger in the field, first assess PMS distal to the injury site before manipulating the injury. The procedure should include:

- Only one attempt if there is severe neurovascular compromise.
- The realignment should be attempted as soon as possible after the injury occurs.
- Do not attempt if the dislocation is associated with other severe injuries.
- Consider analgesics prior to manipulation.
- Pull traction above and below the dislocated joint along the shaft of the finger.
- The pull should be steady and slow to relax the muscle spasm.
- If successful, the ball pops into the joint and there is a sudden relief of pain that allows the finger to return to a normal position in a relatively painless fashion.
- Immobilize the fully extended finger in an appropriate splint and reevaluate PMS.
- Apply cold.

How is a hip dislocation realigned?

If you are going to attempt to realign a dislocated hip in the field, first assess PMS distal to the injury site before manipulating the injury. The procedure should include:

- Only one attempt if there is severe neurovascular compromise.
- The realignment should be attempted as soon as possible after the injury occurs.
- Do not attempt if the dislocation is associated with other severe injuries.
- Consider analgesics prior to manipulation.
- Pull traction at the hip and knee (90 degrees) along the shaft of the femur.
- The pull should be steady and slow to relax the muscle spasm.

- If successful, the ball pops into the joint and there is a sudden relief of pain that allows the leg to be painlessly returned to full extension.
- Immobilize the fully extended leg on a long backboard and reevaluate PMS.
- Apply cold.

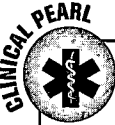 CLINICAL PEARL

Remember—only attempt the field reduction of a dislocation if there is an obvious threat to neurovascular integrity.

What is the difference between a knee dislocation and a patella dislocation?

The patella is the kneecap. Some people can literally pick their kneecap up and move it around. A knee dislocation involves the tibia literally popping out of the knee joint.

How is a knee dislocation realigned?

First, do not confuse a patella dislocation with a knee dislocation, which is a misalignment of the tibia. The distal PMS should be assessed before manipulating the injury. The procedure includes:

- Only one attempt should be made as soon as possible after the injury occurs.
- Only attempt to reposition the knee into its anatomical position if the transport time is long or delayed more than two hours, even if the distal circulation is normal.
- Do not attempt if the dislocation is associated with other severe injuries.
- Consider analgesia for the patient.
- Apply gentle and steady traction, and then move the injured joint into normal position.
- Carefully place the knee into full extension with a steady pull to relax the muscle spasm.
- Success occurs when the knee pops into the joint, relieving the pain and deformity, and making the knee now more mobile.
- Immobilize the knee in the full extension position using a long-board splint and no traction.
- Reassess PMS.
- Apply cold.

How is an ankle realigned?

Before realigning an ankle, the distal PMS must be assessed. The procedure includes:

- Only one attempt should be made as soon as possible after the injury occurs.
- Do not attempt if the dislocation is associated with other severe injuries.
- Consider analgesia for the patient.
- Apply gentle and steady traction on the talus while stabilizing the tibia. Slow and steady traction is designed to relax the spasm.
- Success occurs when there is a sudden rotation to the normal position.
- Immobilize the ankle as if it were fractured.
- Reassess PMS.
- Apply cold.

Q | How is a shoulder dislocation realigned?

A | Before realigning the shoulder, the distal PMS should be assessed. The procedure should include:

- One attempt should be made as soon as possible after the injury occurs.
- Do not attempt if associated with other severe injuries.
- Consider analgesia for the patient.
- Apply gentle and steady traction in the normal anatomical position only.
- Reassess PMS.
- Apply cold.

Q | What is the recommended procedure for immobilizing a pelvic fracture?

A | A combination of a long backboard and MAST/PASG are used for a pelvic fracture. These patients can easily go into decompensated shock from the normal blood loss accompanying a fracture of the pelvis (approximately 2,000 cc).

Q | What are the recommended methods of splinting various long bone fractures?

A | The following fractures are immobilized as indicated:
- Femur—unipolar or bipolar traction splint.
- Proximal femur or anterior hip—long backboard.
- Tibia or fibula—either a pneumatic splint, a long-board splint, or a cardboard splint.
- Ankle—air splint or a pillow splint and leg immobilization.
- Foot—pneumatic splint, cardboard splint, or a ladder splint.
- Shoulder dislocation—be creative and try using a rolled blanket with a cravat through the center to create something for the patient to rest the dislocated shoulder on. This can be done with a combination of sling and swathe to prevent movement.

- Knee—any fracture within three inches of the joint should be treated similar to a dislocation. Use triangulation with two long-board splints and cravats. Do not apply a traction splint to this injury. If the leg is found straight, use two long-board splints and cravats or a cardboard splint.
- Humerus—this is difficult to immobilize and is best stabilized with a sling and swathe and a padded arm board. If the patient has a neck injury, do not put the sling around the neck.
- Elbow—use a padded wire splint and a sling and swathe.
- Forearm—this injury may involve the radius or ulna, or both. A Colle's fracture from falling on an outstretched arm may be found in the "silver fork" deformity position. This is a "splintable" position and it is not necessary to straighten it further. The injury should be splinted with two boards and padding or a cardboard splint and padding.
- Hand and wrist—these are common with direct trauma and have a noticeable deformity. There is a high incidence of nerve and vessel damage. Splint the injury on a padded board splint with the hand in the position of function (as if you were holding a tennis ball).
- Epiphysial fracture—the growth plates or ends of the long bone are the weakest part of the child's joint, presenting as a sprain in an adult. The fractures may result in a permanent angulation or a deformed extremity, and may also cause premature arthritis.

Q | When should heat or cold be used on an MS injury?

A | Cold is used during the first 48 hours after the injury to reduce swelling. Heat can be useful to improve circulation to the area, but only after the initial swelling has gone down—no earlier than 48 hours after the injury and perhaps longer.

Q | Should all possible MS injuries be seen in the hospital?

A | All MS injuries should be evaluated to determine the need for immobilization and an X ray. Some of these patients may wish to refuse medical aid. Due to the potential of injury to the circulatory and nervous systems and permanent disability, patients should be strongly encouraged to seek medical attention.

CLINICAL PEARL

As a general rule, people with any significant MS injury (i.e., enough to be seen by EMS) should be evaluated further. Whether this is in an ED or an office setting is not "set in concrete." Many offices lack X ray facilities, requiring the patient to make a separate trip. Hospital EDs are better equipped to handle a suspected fracture or neurovascular compromise.

CHAPTER 43

Neonatology

The arrival of a new baby is an exciting and rewarding experience for the family and EMS provider. However, when a neonate is born with a health problem, suddenly the experience becomes very challenging. The focus of this chapter is on *why* we need to identify the potential for neonatal injury and illness and *why* you need to respond in a certain way to manage the presenting problems.

Anatomy and Physiology

Q What is the difference between a newborn and a neonate?

A A baby is considered a newborn for the first few hours of life and a neonate is a newborn up to six weeks of age.

Q What is neonatology?

A Neonatology is the medical specialty concerned with the diagnosis and treatment of disorders of the newborn.

Q What do the terms antepartum, intrapartum, and extrauterine mean?

A These terms are used in reference to the mother. Antepartum is before the onset of labor, intrapartum is during labor, and extrauterine is outside the uterus.

Q What are the stages of fetal development?

A The pre-embryonic period (weeks one and two) is when fertilization and the implantation of the embryo into the endometrium occurs. The embryonic period (weeks three to eight) is when all of the body's organ systems form. The fetal period (weeks 9–40) is the term of rapid growth and development of all organ systems.

Q What is fetal circulation?

A Maternal and fetal circulation are separate and do not mix throughout pregnancy. During fetal development, auxiliary vessels are needed to allow the exchange of oxygen and nutrients from the mother to the fetus and exchange (remove) waste from the fetus to the mother.

These vessels include:

- Placenta—where the exchange of oxygen and other substances between maternal and fetal circulation occurs.
- Umbilical cord:
    1. Two umbilical arteries—two extensions of the iliac arteries of the fetus that carry fetal blood to the placenta.

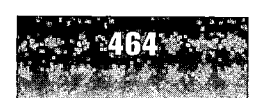
464

2. One umbilical vein—returns oxygenated blood from the placenta to the fetus. The vein extends and branches out and under the liver of the fetus and continues as the ductus venosus and empties into the inferior vena cava.

- Ductus arteriousus—a small vessel that connects the pulmonary artery with the descending thoracic aorta and diverts blood away from the lungs and into systemic circulation.
- Ductus venosus—the continuation of the umbilical vein that empties into the inferior vena cava.
- Foramen oval—the opening in the septal wall between the right and left atria in the fetus. A valve at the opening of the inferior vena cava diverts blood away from the lungs and through this opening.

How can I tell if twins are identical or fraternal at birth?

You can usually tell by the placenta. Identical twins develop from the same zygote. They usually share the same placenta, but each has their own umbilical cord. Fraternal twins develop from two separate zygotes and each has a placenta.

What changes occur in fetal circulation after birth?

After the umbilical cord is cut, the auxiliary vessels described previously are no longer needed and stop functioning. The placenta is expelled from the mother. The foramen oval closes and shunts blood to the lungs after the baby takes its first breath, and then closes permanently after nine months of age. The ductus arteriousus and ductus venosus turn into fibrous cords that serve as ligaments.

Pathophysiology

What is persistent fetal circulation?

Newborns are very sensitive to hypoxia and if they experience hypoxia or severe acidosis, a condition called persistent fetal circulation may occur. The hypoxia or acidosis can trigger the pulmonary vascular bed to constrict and reopen the ductus arteriousus, creating fetal circulation as in utero. The danger here is that the majority of the circulation is then shunted from the right heart to the left heart, bypassing the lungs. This has a severe impact on the initial development of the lungs. This condition can be corrected or avoided altogether by stimulating the newborn to breathe, keeping it warm, and assisting with oxygenation and ventilation when required.

What is the difference between primary and secondary apnea?

When hypoxia and persistent fetal circulation continue, the newborn becomes apneic, the heart rate drops, and the child becomes limp. This condition is referred to as primary apnea. If the condition is allowed to continue without intervention, the child progresses to secondary apnea, recognized by a few last gasps of breath, continued bradycardia, unresponsiveness, and finally death. Unless prompt intervention is begun, brain damage or death results.

What are the incidence, morbidity and mortality, and risk factors for neonatal apnea?

Neonatal apnea is rare and may be due to many primary diseases that affect neonates. Such disorders produce a direct depression on the central nervous system's (CNS) control of respiration (e.g., hypoglycemia, meningitis, drugs, hemorrhage, seizures), disturbances of oxygen delivery by perfusion (e.g., shock, sepsis, anemia), or ventilation defects (e.g., pneumonia, persistent pulmonary hypertension, muscle weakness). It appears to be more common in premature infants. Unless severe and prolonged, apnea does not usually alter an infant's prognosis.

What is apnea of infancy?

Apnea of infancy (AOI)—occurs in infants that were born full term and are less than one year old. When the cause of apnea can't be found, it is given the catch-all diagnosis of AOI. This condition usually resolves itself, but does need to be monitored until such time.

What is an ALTE or AOP?

An event that is a combination of apnea, choking, gagging, and change in color and muscle tone, and is not a sleep disorder, is called an apparent life-threatening event or ALTE. ALTEs are associated with medical conditions that cause apnea such as infections and neurological disorders.

Apnea of prematurity (AOP) is a condition that may occur in babies who are born before 34-weeks gestation. Because of the immature brain or respiratory system, the baby is unable to normally regulate its own breathing. AOP can be central, obstructive, or mixed. The out-of-hospital management includes managing the ABCs. In-hospital management may entail the use of a ventilator and the administration of surfactant to help the baby expand its lungs until its own supply of surfactant kicks in.

What are the types and causes of apnea?

There are three types of apnea: central, obstructive, and mixed.

- Central—results when the part of the brain that controls breathing doesn't start or maintain the breathing process properly.
- Obstructive—caused by an obstruction of the airway, commonly caused by enlarged tonsils and adenoids or genetic syndromes such as Pierre Robin syndrome or Down syndrome.
- Mixed—a combination of central and obstructive apnea that may occur when the baby is awake or asleep.

What is the Pierre Robin syndrome?

The Pierre Robin syndrome is a birth defect that is characterized by a cleft palate and unusually small jaw. The tongue is displaced downward and the infant has no gag reflex. The problems for the infant are that sucking and swallowing are difficult due to the cleft palate, and excessive fluids are present in the larynx due to the loss of the gag reflex.

What is a cleft palate or cleft lip?

A cleft palate and cleft lip are birth defects. A cleft palate (Figure 43–1) is a split in the palate that creates an opening between the mouth and nose. The opening may be unilateral, bilateral, complete, or incomplete. This type of birth defect interferes with sucking, feeding, and speech. A cleft lip is mostly a cosmetic problem that appears as a separation in the lip as illustrated in Figure 43–2. Both types of defects can be corrected with plastic surgery.

What is Down syndrome?

Down syndrome is a chromosomal abnormality that occurs in one of every 800–1,000 live births. In 1997, more than 1,600 babies were born with Down syndrome. The most common cause of Down syndrome occurs when a baby is born with three, rather than two, copies of the twenty-first chromosome. This extra genetic material disrupts their physical and cognitive development. Down syndrome can occur in any pregnancy, but the risk increases with the mother's age, especially over age 35. There is no way to prevent Down syndrome, but it can be detected during the pregnancy by amniocentesis and other tests.

How can an EMS provider recognize Down syndrome at the time of birth?

There are certain traits of Down syndrome infants that vary, but can be recognized at birth (Figure 43–3). Distinguishing facial features include:

- Tongue is proportionately larger in relation to the size of the mouth.
- Flat facial profile with a small nose and a depressed nasal bridge.
- Upward slant of the eyes and small folds on the inner corners of the eyes (epicanthic folds).
- Small ears with an abnormal shape (dysplastic ears).

Other distinguishing features:

- There is a single deep crease across the palm of the hand (simian crease).
- There is an excessive space between the large and second toe (sandal gap).

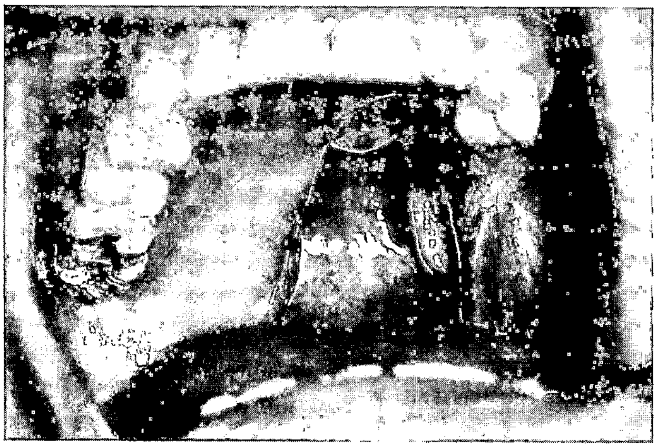

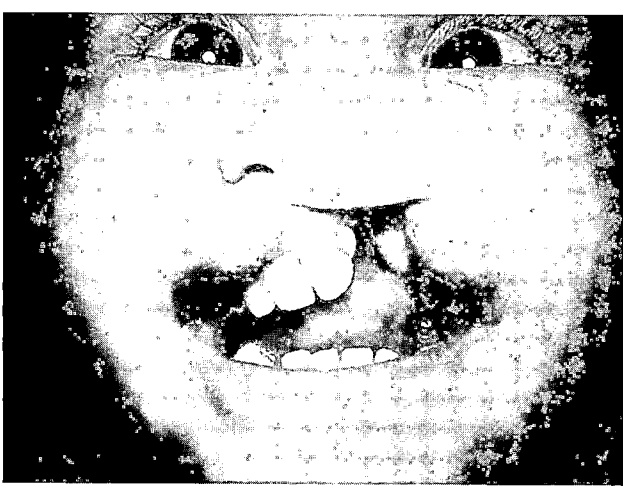

FIGURE 43-1 The cleft palate. *(Courtesy of Dr. Joseph Konzelman, School of Dentistry, Medical College of Georgia)*

FIGURE 43-2 The cleft lip. *(Courtesy of Dr. Joseph Konzelman, School of Dentistry, Medical College of Georgia)*

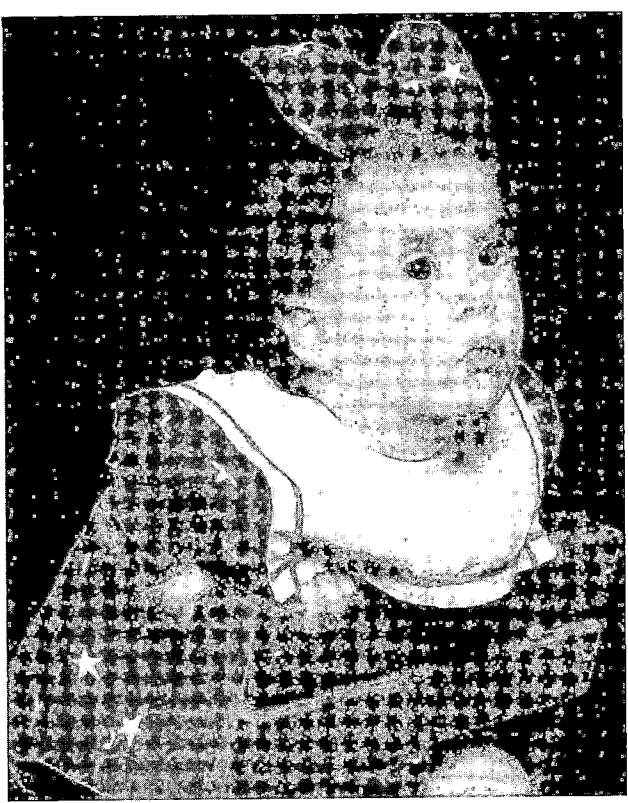

FIGURE 43–3 A child with Down syndrome.

- Overall body muscle tone is weak (muscle hypotonia).
- The infant has an excessive ability to extend the joints (joint hypermobility).

What is spina bifida and how can the EMS provider recognize this condition at birth?

Spina bifida is a birth defect. The infant is born with exposed spinal structures. In 1997, more than 900 babies were born with spina bifida. There are three common types: occulta, meningocele, and myelomeningocele (Figure 43–4):

- Occulta—a defect in the vertebra that does not affect the meninges or spinal cord. There may be a dimple or hair growth on the skin over the malformed vertebra and the infant is usually asymptomatic.
- Meningocele—can be recognized by an external sac on the spine. The sac is filled with protruding meninges and cerebrospinal fluid (CSF) and is covered with skin.
- Myelomeningocele—the most serious form, it affects the spinal cord, meninges, and spine. At birth, there may be a round and raised sac on the spine. The sac can be bluish in color and may be leaking. Associated findings may include kyphosis (deformed spine), deformed joints, loss of motor and sensory function below the level of the lesion, and incontinence with a constant dribbling of urine.

What is the difference between tonsils and adenoids?

Tonsils are lymph glands located on both sides of the throat. Tonsils trap bacteria and viruses that enter through the throat and produce antibodies to help fight infections. Tonsilitis is common in children and can be recognized by the symptoms of fever, sore throat, pain when swallowing, raspy voice, and swollen glands.

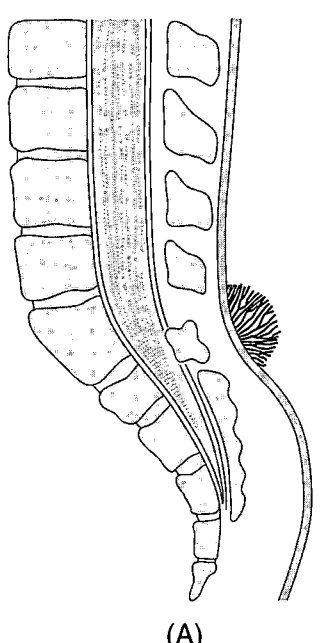
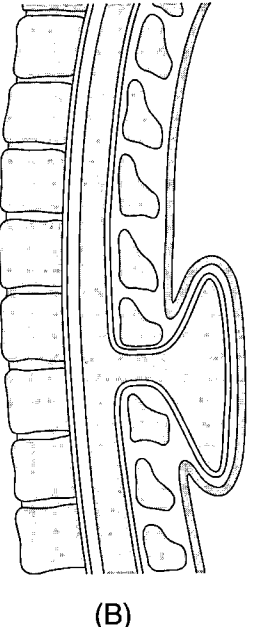
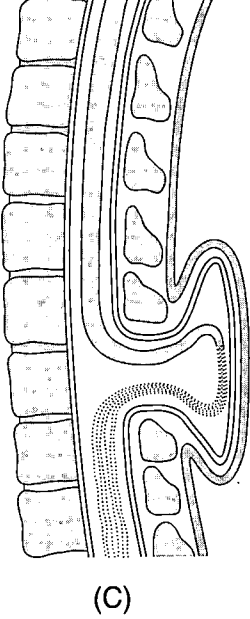

(A)   (B)   (C)

FIGURE 43–4 The types of spina bifida: (A) occulta, (B) meningocele, and (C) myelomeningocele.

Adenoids are also called pharyngeal tonsils, but are not the tonsils located in the throat. The adenoids are located in the passage that connects the nose and throat, and they look like tiny clusters of grapes. Also lymph glands, the adenoids trap bacteria and viruses that enter through the nose and produce antibodies to help fight infections. The adenoids can become enlarged or infected creating various problems for a child, including sleep apnea, difficulty breathing, recurrent infections, and nasal speech. Additional symptoms associated with enlarged or infected adenoids include noisy breathing, breathing through the mouth, and snoring.

Q | What significant antepartum factors can affect childbirth?

A | There are many. Some are avoidable, such as substance or alcohol use, and others are not; for example, the onset of gestational diabetes. A list of factors affecting childbirth includes:

- Maternal use of drugs, alcohol, and cigarettes.
- Multiple fetuses.
- Placenta previa or abruptia.
- Post-term gestation.
- Inadequate or no prenatal care.
- Hypertension syndromes.
- Diabetes.
- Mother's age is under 16 or over 35.

Q | What are significant antepartum factors that classify the newborn as "high risk"?

A | The list of high-risk factors for the newborn includes:

- Third trimester hemorrhage (treated as placenta previa until proven otherwise).
- Premature labor.
- Prolonged labor.
- Prolapsed cord.
- Abnormal limb or fetal presentation.
- Meconium staining or aspiration syndrome.
- Mother's use of narcotics just before delivery.

Q | What factors are associated with premature birth and low birth weight?

A | In 1998, 11.6 percent of births in the United States were preterm births and 298,208 babies were born with a low birth weight (500–2,500 grams). Examples of factors associated with premature birth and low birth weight are:

- Maternal use of drugs, alcohol, and cigarettes.
- Multiple fetuses.
- Inadequate or no prenatal care. .
- Hypertension syndromes.
- Gestational diabetes.
- Mother is under 16 or over 35.
- Third trimester hemorrhage.
- Premature labor.
- Various preexisting medical and neurological conditions.
- Maternal hormonal imbalance.
- Structural abnormality of the uterus.

Q | What is the incidence and mortality of birth defects?

A | Approximately three to five percent of the four million infants born annually in the United States are born with birth defects. Birth defects account for 20 percent of all infant deaths, which is more than from any other single cause.

Q | What was the impact of thalidomide on births in the 1960s?

A | Thalidomide is a sedative that was banned in the 1960s because it caused severe birth defects. Used in Europe, 125 cases of birth deformity were reported. Although it was never approved in the United States, some people received it as a sample. It was prescribed to pregnant women to combat the nausea of morning sickness in the first trimester.

Major deformities included growth and mental deficiencies; defects in the eyes, ears, and nose; and characteristic deficient limb development affecting the arms and the legs. Some infants had no legs at all, just toes sprouting from their hips, along with foreshortened, flipper-like arms. Today, thalidomide appears to treat a particularly lethal type of bone marrow cancer called myeloma.

CLINICAL PEARL

Thalidomide seems to be reemerging for completely different reasons than its original use. Under these circumstances, the likelihood of arm and leg deformities is negligible.

Q | What has been the impact of crack and cocaine use in pregnancy?

A | The use of crack and cocaine during pregnancy has many effects on the fetus and mother. The risk of miscarriage is increased during early pregnancy. In late pregnancy, premature labor, fetal stroke, or death may occur. The drugs increase the risk for abruptio placenta. For the infant, the risks increase for low birth weight, birth defects, feeding problems, sleep disorders, SIDS, and the slowed development of motor skills.

What other drugs are dangerous during pregnancy?

Drugs and agents that can cause fetal malformations are called teratogens. The following is a list of teratogens that mothers may be taking, abusing, or exposed to during pregnancy that could cause harm to the fetus:

- Alcohol.
- Androgens and testosterone derivatives.
- Angiotensin-converting enzyme (ACE) inhibitors (e.g., enalapril, captopril).

> **CLINICAL PEARL**
>
> *Though ACE inhibitors have many great uses in medicine (e.g., hypertension, congestive heart failure, acute myocardial infarction), their use is* absolutely *contraindicated in pregnancy.*

- Coumarin derivatives (e.g., warfarin).
- Carbamazepine.
- Folic acid antagonists (e.g., methorexate and aminopterin).
- Diethystilbestol (DES).
- Lead.
- Lithium.
- Organic mercury.
- Phenytoin.
- Streptomycin and kanamycin.
- Tetracycline.
- Trimethodione and paramethodione.
- Valproic acid.
- Vitamin A and its derivatives.

Assessment and Management

What are newborns assessed for at birth?

Newborn assessment performed immediately after birth evaluates respiratory effort, heart rate, and skin color for perfusion. The APGAR (appearance, pulse, grimace, activity, reflex) score is a well-accepted assessment tool for evaluating newborns at one minute and five minutes after birth. Weight, length,

and other physical dimensions such as head circumference (32–38 cm) and chest circumference (34–40 cm) are measured as well. The APGAR score is described in chapter 44, Pediatrics.

What are newborns screened for at birth?

Newborns are screened for genetic and metabolic disorders, but specific tests vary from state to state. The more common screening tests are:

- Phenykletonuria (PKU)—caused by a baby's inability to use the amino acid phenylalanine; leads to brain and nerve damage and mental retardation.
- Congenital hypothyroidism—caused when a baby is born without enough thyroid hormone; can lead to poor growth and mental retardation.
- Biotinidase deficiency—can lead to seizures; skin infections; loss of hearing, vision, and hair; mental retardation; and possibly coma and death.
- Galactosemia—caused when a baby cannot digest the sugar found in milk; can lead to cataracts, liver damage, mental retardation, and death.
- Homocystinuria—caused when a baby is unable to use the amino acid methoinine found in the proteins of foods; leads to mental retardation, seizures, and death.
- Sickle cell disease—caused by an inherited abnormality of hemoglobin, leading to abnormal red blood cells (RBCs), especially during stress (e.g., hypoxia). Causes anemia and may lead to infections, pain, poor growth, stroke, and death.

    Premature infants must be examined for many more disorders until they catch up with normal weights and sizes.

What is fetal alcohol syndrome (FAS) and how can it be recognized?

FAS results from maternal alcohol consumption. Even the consumption of very small amounts of alcohol during pregnancy can have serious effects on a developing fetus.

FAS is distinguished by congenital abnormalities—microcephalia (small head), low birth weight, developmental disabilities, cardiovascular defects, or death. The physical characteristics of FAS, in addition to microcephalia, include small eye openings, receded upper jaw, and thinned upper lip. After birth, the child's breathing may be depressed and require immediate resuscitation.

How can you recognize a newborn with narcotic depression?

Maternal narcotic use within four hours of delivery can depress the fetus and is associated with respiratory depression at birth. Low birth weight is also associated with maternal narcotics use. After birth, the child can experience withdrawal symptoms such as decreased mental status and tremors, and is startled easily. Treatment is similar to adult narcotic overdose. Provide high-flow oxygen assisted with ventilations and administer naloxone.

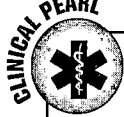

Medications given to the mother during labor may also affect the fetus, especially pain medicines (e.g., morphine).

What are examples of common birth injuries?

Childbirth is very traumatic for the baby. A wide range of injuries can occur as a result of the birthing process. The management of injuries from childbirth is focused on the airway and providing adequate oxygenation, ventilation, and chest compressions, if needed. Listed are possible complications resulting from childbirth:

- Hypoxia.
- Shock.
- Spinal cord injury.
- Cerebrovascular accident (CVA).
- Fractured clavicle from shoulder dystocia.
- Bruising and swelling of soft tissues.
- Conehead from prolonged labor.
- Forceps trauma to the head.
- Brachial plexus injury (from overstretching the arm).

What is meconium?

Meconium is the baby's first bowel movement. If it occurs while the fetus is still in utero, it is considered a sign of fetal distress. Meconium staining of the amniotic fluid is a danger sign. In addition, the baby may aspirate the meconium, leading to respiratory distress syndrome. Dark-greenish to black meconium stool is normal immediately following birth.

What are the causes of fetal distress?

Possible causes of fetal distress are postterm gestation over 42 weeks, maternal supine hypotensive syndrome, eclampsia, umbilical cord obstruction or prolapse, placental insufficiency, hypoxia, drug effects, or bacterial sepsis.

What are the incidence, morbidity, and mortality, and the risk factors for meconium aspiration?

Meconium staining and aspiration occurs in 9–16 percent of all births (primarily postterm) and 20 percent of these cases develop further complications such as pneumonia or pneumothorax. Meconium aspiration accounts for a significant number of neonatal deaths. The risk factors for the aspiration of meconium are not recognizing the presence of meconium and not managing the newborn's airway accordingly.

What is the pathophysiology of meconium staining?

The presence of meconium staining in the amniotic fluid indicates that the fetus has experienced stress during the pregnancy. If particulate meconium is present at birth, the distress has probably just occurred and now the baby is at risk for respiratory problems because the newborn may have meconium in the airway. During delivery, if the baby takes its first breath through the mouth, the meconium can be aspirated into the lungs. The particulate meconium results in a small airway obstruction and aspiration pneumonia.

What are BLS and ALS management of the presence of meconium during childbirth?

Remember, the presence of meconium at birth indicates fetal respiratory distress. All of the meconium must be removed from the mouth, nose, and trachea before stimulating respirations. Begin the removal of meconium when the head of the newborn appears and before delivery of the body. Using a portable suction unit, quickly suction the mouth, nose, and pharynx while watching for signs of distress. Repeat suctioning until the meconium clears.

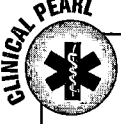

Suction, suction, suction—meconium aspiration is avoidable and often fatal.

ALS management involves ET tube placement and a meconium aspirator (a special adapter for suctioning) attached to the ET tube (size 2.5 for premature neonates and 3.0 for full term) for suctioning. The ET tube is placed for deep suction rather than ventilating purposes. Repeat suctioning using a new ET tube until no meconium appears in or on the ET tube. This means that it is necessary to carry lots of small ET tubes. A bulb syringe or French catheter is not very effective for suctioning because the meconium is very thick and sticky.

How can the EMS provider recognize signs of neonatal respiratory distress?

Signs of respiratory distress can occur within minutes or hours of birth. Tachypnea, sternal retractions, grunting, and cyanosis are all signs of respiratory distress in the neonate.

When is it necessary to begin ventilations on a newborn?

Any time that an infant has signs of respiratory distress and is not responding to supplemental oxygen, it is paramount to assist with ventilations.

When is it appropriate to begin chest compressions?

The neonate's adequacy of respirations is determined by the heart rate. If the heart rate falls below or remains below 60 bpm despite adequate assisted ventilations for 30 seconds, then provide chest compressions.

What is the pathophysiology of neonatal cardiac arrest?

Respiratory arrest is the leading cause of cardiac arrest in all ages of pediatric patients.

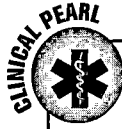

Most neonates, infants, and children suffer cardiac arrest as a result of respiratory events and hypoxia.

What are BLS and ALS resuscitation steps for the distressed neonate?

Neonatal resuscitative efforts are directed at airway management and ventilation. The inverted pyramid for newborns is the accepted standard for resuscitation steps. Proceed from simple BLS interventions to ALS management. ALS interventions are begun only after airway, ventilation, and oxygenation are done. Begin the initial assessment during initial stabilization.

- Using a bulb syringe, suction the mouth first and then the nose. (Suctioning the nose first may stimulate the newborn to take its breath, which will be through the mouth.)
- If meconium is present, manage accordingly. Do not use the bulb syringe to try to suction meconium out, use a meconium aspirator as previously described.
- Warm and dry the baby with a warmed towel if possible. This stimulates the baby to breathe. Continue to keep the baby warm and provide additional stimulation if needed by slapping the bottom of the feet or rubbing the back.

- Position the baby on its back and place a towel under the shoulders to align the neck in a neutral position.
- Reassess respiratory rate and effort. If the baby is responding slowly, provide blow-by oxygen (oxygen blowing by the face, as opposed to a mask on the face).
- If the baby does not respond to tactile stimulation within three to five seconds, provide positive pressure ventilation (PPV). Be careful! Assisted ventilations and PPV can easily cause barotrauma and pneumothorax.
    1. Ventilate using a BVM (without a pop-off valve) at a rate of 40–60 bpm.
    2. Assess the adequacy of the ventilations by watching the chest rise and fall.
    3. If the baby improves with PPV, slowly decrease the rate and pressure of the ventilations. Watch for signs of adequate perfusion and respiratory effort before stopping altogether.
- If the baby does not improve, proceed to ET intubation, if available. Suction as needed. Intubation is preferred when PPV by BVM is inadequate or prolonged ventilation is required and is a route for medication administration.
- Assess the pulse rate. The adequacy of respirations is judged by the heart rate and the newborn's response to stimulation. If the heart rate falls below or remains below 60 bpm despite adequate assisted ventilations for 30 seconds, then provide chest compressions.

What is postarrest stabilization for the neonate?

In the field, the essential aspects of postarrest stabilization are keeping the baby warm and ensuring oxygen delivery. Follow local protocols and medical direction for additional interventions.

What is in the NALS course and for whom is it designed?

Neonatal advanced life support is an American Heart Association course for critical care providers who work in neonatal intensive care units.

Other Medical Emergencies

How can the EMS provider recognize a premature newborn?

Premature neonates are born before 38-weeks gestation and weigh less than 5.5 pounds (2.2 kg).

What are the major risks associated with premature birth?

The premature newborn is at increased risk for complications from hypoxia, hypothermia, hypoglycemia, hypovolemia, and respiratory and cardiac arrest. In the field, problems with poorly developed lungs and respiratory muscles and drive increase the need to provide assisted ventilations.

What is the role of surfactant?

Premature infants often have immature lungs because the lungs are one of the last organs to develop in utero. Some preemies lack enough surfactant, a chemical that prevents the alveoli (air sacs) from collapsing when a baby exhales. Surfactant is not present in adequate quantities until after 34-weeks gestation. Preemies less than 34-weeks gestation often have to be placed on ventilators after birth.

Why is the newborn at risk for hypothermia?

Neonates can lose body heat rapidly because they have a larger body surface area (BSA) in relation to their weight. They also have much smaller amounts of subcutaneous fat to keep them warm. Their temperature regulating mechanisms are immature (i.e., they cannot yet shiver to produce body heat).

In the field, it is paramount to prevent heat loss by quickly drying the newborn. Remove wet linens, wrap using warm blankets, and turn up the heat in the ambulance!

What is the pathophysiology of neonatal seizures?

Hypoxia, fever, infection, and hypoglycemia are the most common causes of seizures in neonates. An infection can be obtained from the mother before, during, or after birth. Additional causes of seizures include alcohol or drug withdrawal, and less commonly, genetic or metabolic disorders.

What is the pathophysiology of fever in the neonate?

An infection from a virus or bacteria is the most common cause of fever in neonates. Due to the immature thermoregulatory system, any fever is serious and requires evaluation. High ambient temperatures are a factor as well.

CLINICAL PEARL

Assume that a fever in the neonate represents neonatal sepsis (severe overwhelming infection) until proven otherwise.

What is the pathophysiology of neonatal hypoglycemia?

Newborns have higher glucose requirements per kilogram of body weight than children and adults. Therefore, they show a progressive decrease in blood glucose. Following birth and within a short period of fasting, liver glucose stores (in the form of glycogen) become insufficient. Newborns must rely primarily on gluconeogenesis to meet glucose requirements. Signs of hypoglycemia in the neonate may include irregular respirations or apnea, twitching or seizures, acidosis, poor muscular contractility or limpness, eye rolling, high-pitched cry, and sometimes cyanosis. A similar presentation may be seen with several other disorders, including septicemia, brain injury, severe respiratory distress, and congenital heart disease.

What is the pathophysiology of neonatal jaundice?

Jaundice occurs when a baby's immature liver can't dispose of excess bilirubin (a yellow pigment produced by the normal breakdown of red blood cells) in the blood. Approximately 60 percent of full-term infants and 80 percent of premature infants develop jaundice in the first two to three days of life. This condition usually disappears within five to seven days. The most common treatment is exposing the infant to ultraviolet lights to help break down the extra bilirubin so the baby's liver can process it.

What is the pathophysiology of vomiting in the neonate?

Vomiting in the neonate is caused by infections, increased intracranial pressure (ICP), and drug withdrawal. It is less commonly caused by genetic or metabolic disorders. Complications can result from the aspiration of vomitus, an electrolyte imbalance, or dehydration due to the loss of fluids. A congenital abnormality of the pyloric valve (pyloric stenosis) leads to vomiting within a few days after birth.

What is the pathophysiology of diarrhea in the neonate?

Diarrhea in neonates is difficult to assess because all stools are loose. A general guideline is to consider more than six stools to be excessive. Common causes of diarrhea in neonates include infections, lactose (milk) intolerance, gastroenteritis, cystic fibrosis, and, less commonly, genetic or metabolic disorders. Complications can result from an electrolyte imbalance and dehydration due to loss of fluids.

CLINICAL PEARL

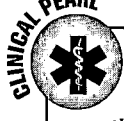

Besides airway problems, fluid imbalance problems are the most common potentially life-threatening disorder that affects neonates.

What is the pathophysiology of abdominal distention in the neonate?

Air, air, air—neonates are prone to gastric and fluid distention due to immature digestive systems. Air fills the stomach and impacts on the baby's lung expansion. Other causes of distention are associated with intestinal obstruction, hernias, and other congenital abnormalities. Full stomachs and vomiting go hand in hand with babies. Babies are belly breathers, so the impact of the distended abdomen is decreased lung capacity. Therefore, the management for a distended abdomen is to watch the airway and ensure adequate oxygenation.

Do babies get hernias?

Yes, some babies, especially preemies, are born with small openings in the body that are supposed to close, but do not. Nearby tissues can squeeze into that opening and present as a bulge or lump; this is a hernia. Sometimes the hernias are only apparent when the child cries or coughs. The most common type of hernia in neonates is the umbilical hernia (an opening or weakened muscles around the belly button permit a bulge when the infant cries, coughs, or strains). An umbilical hernia is most frequently seen in female, African American, and low birth weight babies.

What are the incidence, morbidity and mortality, and the risk factors for a diaphragmatic hernia?

The diaphragmatic hernia is a rare condition that is caused by a defect in the pleuperitoneal canal. As a result, a protrusion of abdominal viscera into the thoracic cavity occurs in varying degrees. Infants usually present following delivery with respiratory distress, cyanosis, decreased breath sounds on the side of the hernia, and a shift of the mediastinum to the side opposite the hernia. The infants are often difficult to resuscitate and require early intubation. The rapidity and severity of respiratory distress presentation is dependent on the degree of associated lung compression. Both lungs are compressed and often underdeveloped in utero because of the hernia. If the neonate has no respiratory distress during the first 24 hours of life, the survival rate is excellent. The survival rate for the infant requiring PPV during the first 18 to 24 hours is approximately 50 percent.

What are the complications of ET intubation?

A misplaced ET tube is the most common complication of intubation. Uncuffed tubes are recommended for neonate and children under eight years old. The uncuffed tube does allow for air to blow back up and into the esophagus, creating a distended abdomen. Therefore, anytime a neonate is intubated, a gastric tube should be placed as well. Barotrauma and pneumothorax are always a potential complication of PPV.

What are the routes for medication administration?

In the neonate, medications may be administered via the ET tube, peripheral IV, intraosseous (IO), and scalp vein. In the newborn, the umbilical vein is another route.

If peripheral IV access is not available quickly (within 90 seconds), gain access via the IO route. It is a safe, reliable, and accepted route for medications and fluids. The administration of medications via the ET tube can lead to low plasma levels and should be the last choice for a medication route.

CHAPTER 44
Pediatrics

Not only do children differ from adults generally, but children in one age group differ from children in other age groups. This chapter discusses the anatomical, cognitive, and emotional differences between children and adults. The focus is on trauma and medical emergencies in pediatric patients, *why* assessment and management of these patients is performed in a certain manner, and *why* you need to respond in a certain way to their presenting problems.

Anatomy and Physiology

Q What are the differences in airway anatomy?

A Young and older infants alike have distinct physiological and anatomical differences from older children or adults. They are obligate nose breathers until six months of age, and they might not open their mouths to breathe even when their nose becomes obstructed from a cold, creating periods of apnea. Their tongue is very large in relation to the size of their mouth. It can fall back and obstruct their airway much easier than in an adult. The small trachea is more anterior than an adult's airway, increasing the likelihood of obstruction, either by foreign bodies or when the infant's head is hyperextended. The smallest diameter of the airway is the cricoid ring.

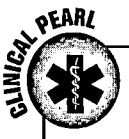

CLINICAL PEARL

The cardinal pediatric problem is airway, airway, and airway.

Q What are the soft spots?

A The fontanels are the membrane-covered spaces between the incomplete ossified cranial bones of an infant. These bones have not yet fused at the joints. Infants have an anterior and posterior fontanel (Figure 44–1). Parents commonly call them the "soft spots." In a healthy child, the fontanels are normally soft and flat. The fontanel can be used as a diagnostic aid when assessing for shock, dehydration, or a head injury by observing whether it is sunken or swollen. The posterior fontanel normally closes at four to six months of age and the anterior fontanel closes at 12 to 18 months of age.

Q What are the characteristics of the infant's chest?

A An infant's respiratory muscles are not well developed. The immature muscles cannot sustain a rapid respiratory rate for long periods of time. The infant becomes fatigued easily. It is normal for infants to be abdominal or "belly breathers." In cases of severe respiratory distress, as the child attempts to compensate, sternal retractions occur.

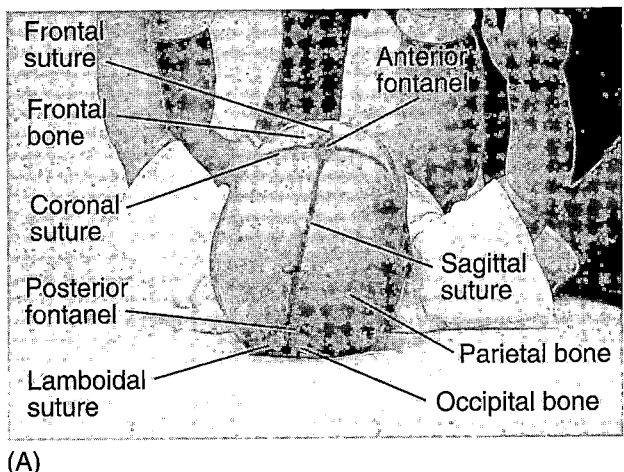

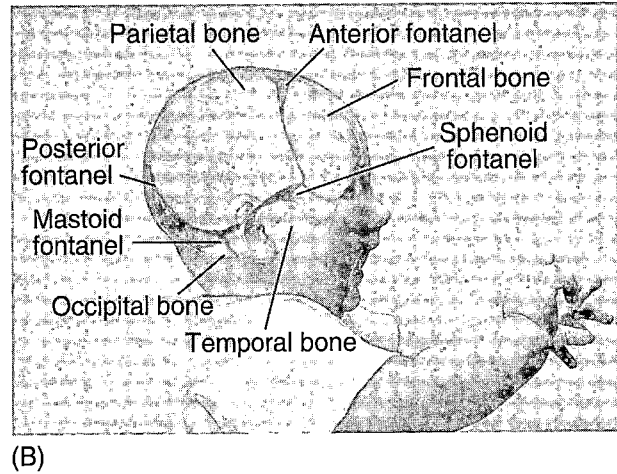

(A)

(B)

FIGURE 44-1 The (A) superior and (B) lateral view showing the fontanels on an infant's head.

[Q] How is temperature regulation different in infants?

[A] It is important for us to be aware that infants have immature and underdeveloped thermoregulatory systems, making it difficult for them to maintain their body temperature. They do not have the ability to shiver to create body heat. In the field, it becomes our job to keep the infant warm when they are in our care. Skin color is a good indicator of hyper- or hypothermia; red and flushed or pale, bluish or mottled, respectively. When a thermometer is not available, estimate a child's temperature by feeling the infant's forehead and extremities with the back of your hand.

Pediatric Trauma

[Q] What is the leading cause of death in children?

[A] Trauma is the number one cause of death in children over one year old. The leading causes of trauma death in pediatrics are motor vehicle crashes (MVCs), abuse, auto–pedestrian accidents, bicycle injuries, falls, burns, drowning, and firearms.

[Q] How are trauma emergencies in pediatrics different from adults?

[A] As children develop, they have unique and dynamic anatomical, physiological, and psychological characteristics that not only differ from adults, but also differ between various age groups. This creates certain predictable types of injuries in each age group. Several differences are:

- Due to the relatively larger size of the child's head, face, and neck, these areas are injured more frequently than in adults

(Figure 44–2). Injuries to the chest and abdomen are the second cause of child mortality. Their bones are not fully developed and do not have the strength of mature bones. This puts internal organs at a high risk for injury. Trauma to the chest and abdomen often results in injuries to the spleen, liver, and thorax. Pneumothorax and hemothorax can and do occur, as in an adult.

- Management of the pediatric trauma emergency requires meticulous support of the airway because it is more easily occluded than an adult's.

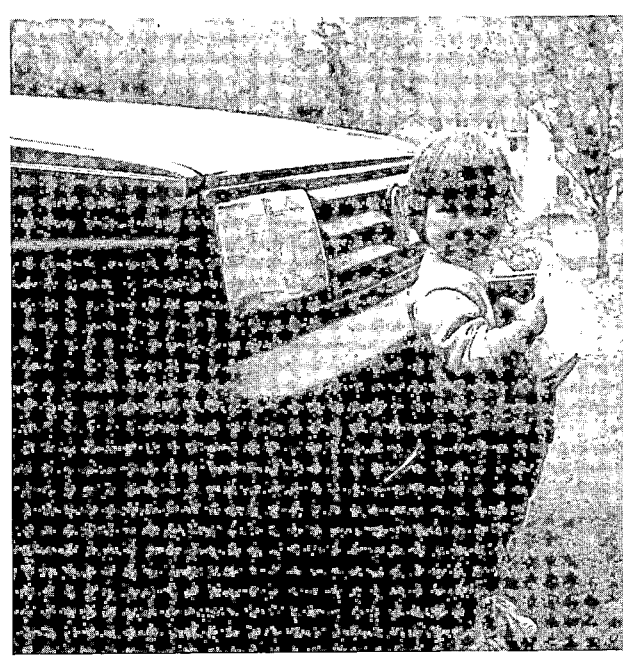

FIGURE 44-2 Notice the relatively larger size head of this toddler and her height in comparison to the automobile bumper. *(Courtesy of Bob Elling)*

Poisonings, Toxins, and Substance Abuse

Q What are the types of poisons that children ingest?

A Although children can often figure out childproof containers, it is not always the prescription medications that children ingest. The most common ages of curiosity are two and three years old (Figure 44–3). Children at this age tend to explore packages they are familiar with, like food containers.

Products stored under the kitchen counter, such as household cleaners, alcohol, and petroleum-based products, are common problems. So are over-the-counter (OTC) products such as aspirin, diaper care products, lotions, soaps, and cosmetics.

Q What household plants are poisonous?

A Contrary to popular belief, a poinsettia is not poisonous to humans, but it may cause a skin rash. Poisonous plants found around the home include:

- Angel's Trumpet (Datura meteloides).
- Azalea (Rhododendron).
- Jerusalem cherry (Solanum pseudocapsicum).
- Jimsonweed.

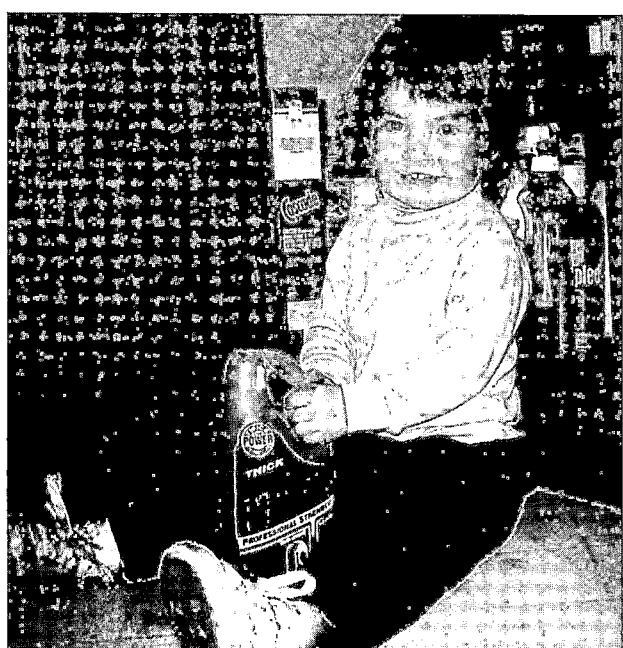

FIGURE 44–3 Toddlers and preschoolers are inquisitive and can easily get into unlocked cabinets that contain poisons. *(Courtesy of Bob Elling)*

Q What are the drugs most often used by school-age and adolescent children?

A Drug overdose can be accidental or an intentional suicide attempt. Listed are the common drugs used by these two age groups:

- Alcohol.
- Nicotine (smoking).
- Marijuana, LSD, PCP, hashish.
- Central nervous system (CNS) stimulants (e.g., cocaine, crack, and amphetamines).
- CNS depressants (e.g., barbiturates).
- Hydrocarbons and fluorocarbons (e.g., kerosene, naphtha, glue, chloroform, aerosol propellants).

Q What is the immediate concern in poisoning and drug overdoses?

A Many poisons and drug overdoses, but not all, can cause respiratory depression. Respiratory depression is the initial concern in the out-of-hospital setting. Many of these products cause life-threatening symptoms in the respiratory, CNS, and circulatory systems.

Pediatric Suicide and Psychiatric (Behavioral) Problems

Q What is the incidence of pediatric suicide?

A The statistics show that suicide has increased dramatically over the past decade! In 1997, according to the National Institute of Mental Health, suicide:

- Was the third leading cause of death in 15 to 24 year olds with a rate of 11.5 per 100,000 and the gender ratio was 5 males to every female.
- In the 10 to 14 year olds, the death rate was 1.6 per 100,000.
- In the 20 to 24 year olds, the death rate was 13.6 per 100,000 and the gender ratio was 7 males to every female.

Q What are the major risk factors for suicide?

A The risk factors are shown in Table 44–1.

Q What are the warning signs of suicidal intentions?

A The warning signs of suicidal intentions that should be discussed in the focused history (FH) are listed in Table 44–2.

TABLE 44-1

Risk Factors for Pediatric Suicide

- Access to lethal weapons.
- Access to drugs and alcohol.
- Greater access to motor vehicles.
- Inadequate support system.
- Family history of depression or alcoholism.
- Exposure to domestic violence.
- Abuse or neglect.
- Divorce in the family.
- Loss of loved one (death in family).
- Break up of a romantic relationship.

TABLE 44-2

Warning Signs of Suicidal Intentions

- Talk of suicide.
- Expressing signs of depression, hopelessness, or excessive guilt.
- Withdrawal from family and friends.
- Lack of interest in favorite activities.
- Dramatic changes in personal appearance.
- Self-destructive behavior.

- Attentional, conduct, or learning disorder.
- Loss of a loved one.

Q What is the out-of-hospital management for the attempted suicide patient?

A A patient's self-inflicted injury is managed the same as any other injury. The special considerations for this type of call are:

- Preserve evidence.
- Ensure good documentation and reporting of the entire call.
- Provide psychological support:
  1. Provide a safe and private environment (usually the ambulance).
  2. Offer compassion, support, and understanding.
  3. Question the child about the attempt. Don't be afraid to ask direct questions (e.g., "Did you intend to harm yourself?") Listen carefully to what they say.
  4. Take the attempt seriously.
  5. Follow your local protocols and state laws concerning any requirements to notify law enforcement. Remember, if they were planning on killing themselves, especially by violent means, they may not have any concern about committing a homicide as well.

CLINICAL PEARL

It is a myth that asking a person about suicide will "put the idea into their head" and make them actually "do it!" Always ask under appropriate circumstances.

Q What is the incidence of depression in adolescents?

A Studies are showing that 8.3 percent of the adolescents in the United States suffer from depression. Risk factors include:

- Girls 2:1 over boys in adolescence.
- Stress.
- Smoking.
- Abuse or neglect.
- Chronic illness.

Q What are the signs associated with depression in children and adolescents?

A Signs that may be associated with depression in children and adolescents are:

Physical complaints:

- Headache.
- Muscle ache.
- Stomach ache.
- Lack of energy.

Other signs may include:

- Unexplained irritability.
- Lack of interest in friends or family, boredom.
- Alcohol or substance abuse.
- Reckless behavior.
- Increased anger or hostility.
- Running away from home.
- Fear of death.
- Extreme sensitivity to rejection or failure.

Child Abuse and Neglect

Q What is child abuse?

A Child abuse and neglect occurs when a child is injured or allowed to be injured by someone who was entrusted with their care. The injury can be physical, sexual, or emotional in nature.

Q What is the incidence of child abuse?

A The incidence of reported child abuse in this country is over three million reports a year. Experts suggest that the numbers of actual child abuse cases are grossly underreported.

What are some of the risk situations surrounding abuse?

Risk situations found to be a common denominator in many abuse situations are:

- Lack of financial support.
- A colicky child.
- Lack of emotional support.
- Misunderstandings of the normal child developmental stages leading to unrealistic expectations of the child's behavior.

Who are the high-risk children?

An ill infant or a developmentally delayed or a chronically ill child may cause enough stress in the family to induce an abusive situation. The biggest risk is being the sibling of an abused child or having a parent who was abused as a child.

What are some clues suggesting child abuse?

Although the presence or absence of the clues listed in Table 44–3 do not positively prove or disprove an abusive situation, they can prompt you to suspect abuse and encourage you to perform a detailed physical assessment and obtain an objective detailed history that will aid you in treating your patient.

What are examples of child neglect?

Children who may be shut in and denied proper nourishment or medical care for a variety of reasons are examples of child neglect.

TABLE 44–3
Clues Suggestive of Child Abuse

- Multiple bruises of various ages—estimate the age of a bruise by its color. Document the location and the color of each bruise, not the age estimation, on your PCR.
- Unusual burn injuries such as skin burns (e.g., stocking or glove distribution) from dunking in hot water, burns on genitalia.
- CNS injuries—the main cause of pediatric abuse deaths. Protect the patient's spine if you suspect a shake injury or other related trauma.
- The shaken baby syndrome—is an often fatal internal brain injury that occurs when an infant is shaken vigorously. An infant's large head and weak neck muscles contribute to shearing the bridging veins and the meninges in the skull.
- Mouth injuries—caused by direct trauma from being struck. You may also find mouth and gum lacerations resulting from a bottle being shoved too hard, repeatedly, into an infant's mouth.
- Injuries to the eye, ears, or nose affecting the sensory functions.
- Inappropriate interaction with the caregivers.
- A child who is not comforted by a parent.

What is shaken baby syndrome?

Shaken baby syndrome (SBS) is a group of signs and symptoms associated with severe head trauma and is usually caused by child abuse. The injury occurs when the child is physically shaken. Because infants have weak neck muscles and heads that are disproportionately larger than their bodies, small rips and tears occur in the brain. The result is subdural hematomas from the bleeding, swelling of the brain (edema), and retinal hemorrhages in the eyes. Signs and symptoms of SBS are listed in Table 44–4.

Is any particular child at risk more than others?

Yes, the statistics show that most children with SBS are:

- Under one year old.
- Male (60 percent).
- From families below the poverty level.
- From young parents.
- Baseline with a preexisting medical or physical disability.

What are some of the signs of sexual abuse?

Physical indications include bleeding, cuts, bruising, swelling, pain, or itching on external genitalia, perineum, buttocks, or thighs. Difficulty walking or sitting is another clue. A common form of abuse is tying a string around the penis of a male bed wetter. Emotional signs include avoidance of eye contact, anxiousness, and being uncooperative with certain aspects of the assessment. In suspected cases of sexual abuse or rape, remember, do not allow the patient to wash or shower.

How is child abuse reported?

Child abuse is a crime. It is highly recommended that you document all of your assessment findings on the prehospital

TABLE 44–4
Signs of Shaken Baby Syndrome

- Irritability, altered mental state (AMS) or seizures.
- Vomiting or decreased appetite.
- Poor sucking or feeding.
- Irregular breathing or apnea.
- Rigidity.
- Unequal or dilated pupils.
- Pale or cyanotic skin.
- Unexplained bruising.
- Injury or bleeding from the mouth.
- Inability to lift head.
- Limp extremities.
- Death.

care report (PCR) and provide the ED with your findings. The ED physician, other health care providers, and teachers are obligated by law in most states to report the incident. The failure to report is a Class A misdemeanor in some states.

Be aware of your state's reporting laws. In some states, EMS providers are required to report suspected child abuse independently of the hospital or physician.

What observations should be recorded?

You are in a unique position to observe the child in his own environment during an EMS call. Record your observations in an objective manner and provide the hospital staff with the condition of the child's home environment. Examples of environmental conditions suggesting child abuse include the following:

- Evidence of alcohol or drug use.
- Report of mechanism of injury (MOI) does not fit the scene (e.g., a child with a head injury from falling off the couch onto a carpeted floor).
- Family members giving different accounts of the accident.

What is the field management of potential child abuse?

You should perform an initial assessment and focused physical exam (PE) as you would for any other ill or injured child. Remember to document your findings on the PCR. Avoid judging the family or parent and do not take sides. Avoid confrontation, be nonjudgmental and do not make any accusations. Be aware of the family that is constantly switching hospitals to avoid detection for repeated calls.

Injuries and Injury Prevention

Does injury prevention make a difference?

Yes, injury prevention is working! The National SAFE KIDS Campaign, the only national organization dedicated to the prevention of unintentional childhood injury, reports a decline in unintentional injury–related death rates from 1987–1997 in children under the age of 14 in the following categories:

- MVC (9 percent).
- Bicycle injury (48 percent).
- Pedestrian injury (42 percent).
- Drowning (37 percent).

- Residential fire injury (50 percent).
- Foreign body airway obstruction (FBAO; 15 percent).
- Firearm injury (49 percent).
- Fall injury (33 percent).
- Poisoning (27 percent).

What is SCIWORA?

Spinal cord injury without radiograph abnormality (SCIWORA) is associated with traumatic spinal cord injury in children. This condition is discussed in detail in Chapter 39, Spinal Trauma.

Medical Emergencies

What is the leading medical complaint with children?

Respiratory distress is the leading complaint in the medical category. Assessing and managing a patient's airway is paramount in the out-of-hospital setting. That is why we spend quite a bit of time on this topic.

The pediatric airway is proportionately smaller than the adult's at all levels. The smaller openings are prone to obstruction from secretions, head positioning, and foreign bodies. Control of the infant's proportionately larger tongue is important to prevent frequent obstructions.

Pneumonia, infections, and other causes of airway swelling can drastically reduce the inner diameter of the pediatric airway. Even minor degrees of swelling may cause severe narrowing of the smaller airway to the point of complete obstruction in some cases.

Airway obstruction may result from:

1. Tongue—most common cause, falls back and occludes the pharynx.
2. Larynx—its high position in the child facilitates aspiration.
3. Epiglottis—edema and swelling from an infection or irritation may cause an obstruction.
4. Foreign bodies—are easily trapped in the narrow airway passages.

What are the most common respiratory emergencies?

Respiratory emergencies are one of the most common and stressful types of calls for the EMS provider. In the case of a sudden onset of respiratory distress or stridor, an aspirated foreign body should be suspected first (especially in children one to three years of age). If air exchange is adequate, be alert for signs of deterioration and be prepared to manage the airway. Handle the child gently and transport the child for removal of the object. If air exchange is inadequate, make vigorous attempts to clear the airway following obstructed airway procedures. The causes of respiratory emergencies for each age group are described in Table 44–5.

[Q] What are asthma, bronchiolitis, croup, epiglottitis, and pneumonia and how is each managed?

[A] Never look in the throat. Do not attempt to visualize or manipulate the airway in any manner. Handle the child gently, avoiding agitation or crying. Aggressive maneuvers may startle the child and that could result in a complete obstruction.

- Asthma—is a lower-airway disorder characterized by recurrent episodes of reversible narrowing of the smaller airways of the lungs. An asthma "attack" can be caused by a wide variety of conditions. Asthma can occur at any age, but is prominent in the 3- to 12-year age group. Onset can vary from sudden to slow. Asthma is a recurring lung disorder that usually includes a history of the illness. Allergies differentiate this disorder from croup, epiglottitis, and foreign body airway obstruction.

  Early Asthma Symptoms—A patient in the early stages of an asthma "attack" experiences air trapping in the lungs. This is when the child is able to inhale, but has great difficulty exhaling, resulting in the trapping of the residual air in the lungs. The child compensates by increasing their rate and effort of breathing.

  Late Asthma Symptoms—When the patient becomes physically exhausted and can no longer compensate, the child experiences ventilatory failure. A child with a low heart rate and a sharp decrease in mental status in the face of an acute asthmatic attack is in imminent danger of arrest.

CLINICAL PEARL

A major warning sign is a quiet-sounding chest in a patient who is obviously tachypneic and short of breath. The patient is "too tight to wheeze"—respiratory failure may be imminent.

Field management is to keep the child calm, provide high-flow oxygen, and administer aerosolized bronchodilators. When the attack is severe, subcutaneous epinephrine and IV corticosteriods may be given. Follow your local protocols.

- Bronchiolitis—is an infection of the bronchioles that results in a swelling of the lower airways that causes tachypnea, retractions, and cyanosis. Bronchiolitis is produced by a viral

TABLE 44–5

Causes of Respiratory Emergencies	
Infant	Asthma, croup, bronchiolitis, foreign body.
Toddler	Asthma, croup, pneumonia, foreign body, epiglottitis.
School-age	Asthma, pneumonia, foreign body, epiglottitis.
Adolescent	Asthma.

infection. Symptoms are often indistinguishable from asthma. The flexible chest walls in young infants make it extremely difficult to compensate for the increased work of breathing. Bronchiolitis occurs in children less than two years of age during the winter and spring seasons. Onset of dyspnea occurs after a few days of sneezing, coughing, and a runny nose. Bronchiolitis differs from asthma in that it does not recur and it is not precipitated by an allergic reaction.

In addition to all of the symptoms listed for asthma, look for signs of a respiratory infection. These may include nasal congestion and a low-grade fever. Brief periods of apnea are common in young infants.

Field management of pediatric patients experiencing an asthma or bronchiolitis attack includes all of the recommendations listed earlier for respiratory distress. Oxygen is the single most important out-of-hospital treatment that we can provide for this patient. Solicit a detailed history to determine the presence of an infection and always be prepared to assist the child's respirations as indicated.

- Croup—is caused by viral or other infections, including ear infections, that may cause the tissue of the upper airway to swell. The swelling of the vocal cords, trachea, and the tissue directly under the epiglottis can result in a partial airway obstruction. Croup usually occurs in children in the three-month to three-year age group. Its duration of onset is generally from two to three days following a recent upper-respiratory infection (URI) that has progressed into difficult breathing. The patient may have a mild or severe seal-like barking cough. There will be no noticeable drooling. When home remedies fail, the family then calls EMS.

- Epiglottitis—is a relatively rare, potentially life-threatening infection that causes a severely inflamed and swollen epiglottis. The swollen epiglottis has the potential to completely obstruct the airway. Infection can occur at any age, but three to six years of age is the most common. The child has a history of mild flu-like symptoms and within one to two hours develops severe respiratory distress. Signs and symptoms include pain and difficulty swallowing, profound drooling, a sore throat, little or absent cough, and difficulty breathing. The child experiencing respiratory distress can pose an out-of-hospital dilemma: it is difficult to tell the difference between croup and epiglottitis in the field. Therefore, always treat each situation as if epiglottitis is present.

Croup causes the tissue under *the glottal opening to swell, whereas epiglottitis causes the tissue* above *the glottic opening to swell, resulting in a higher risk of complete airway obstruction.*

Field management of croup and epiglottitis: Keep the child calm and always maintain an adequate airway. Provide 100 percent humidified oxygen without agitating the child and be prepared to ventilate the child if necessary. Allowing a parent to assist may aid in your management. Transport the child in a safe but comfortable position. Avoid alarming the child by slamming the ambulance doors, excessive speed, or siren use.

- Pneumonia—may be caused by viral or bacterial infections and is associated with recent URIs. Signs and symptoms include fever, tachypnea, rales, consolidation in one or more lobes, and cough. Field management is to keep the child calm, provide high-flow oxygen, and transport for further evaluation.

Why does the prevalence of asthma decrease as children get older?

As their airways get bigger, some children actually grow out of the disease.

What are the signs of respiratory distress?

Although it may be difficult to obtain an accurate respiratory rate for a pediatric patient, the respiratory rate by itself is not the best indicator of the severity of respiratory distress unless it is very slow and gasping.

Early signs of respiratory distress, regardless of cause, usually induce a noticeable change in the child's general appearance. This includes increased agitation, nasal flaring, changes in skin color, and increased respiratory rate and effort. As the distress progresses, the child begins to use her accessory muscles in an attempt to compensate for the increased work of breathing. In addition to using neck and abdominal muscles, you often see retractions of the sternum in a pediatric patient. Indications of respiratory distress are:

- Always suspect a child with altered mental status (AMS) to be experiencing respiratory difficulties until proven otherwise.
- Skin color—cyanotic or mottled is a result of poor oxygenation and decreased perfusion.
- Respiratory effort—nasal flaring, the use of accessory muscles, sternal retractions, and an overall physically tired-looking child are signs of poor respiratory effort.
- Respiratory sounds—stridor with grunting on expiration is abnormal and indicates distress.

What is pediatric respiratory failure?

As respiratory distress progresses, the child deteriorates to respiratory failure, which is when the child is unable to maintain satisfactory blood oxygen and carbon dioxide levels to meet the body's needs. The child is more than just tired; the child is becoming exhausted! Intense intervention is required. When the child can no longer compensate and becomes physically exhausted, ventilatory failure and respiratory arrest quickly follow.

The most prominent indicator of respiratory failure is the child's decreased level of consciousness!

What are the other common medical emergencies seen in pediatrics?

The most common causes of medical emergencies are:

- Seizures—may be caused by infections, fever (febrile seizure), epilepsy, poison ingestion, increased intracranial pressure (ICP), electrolyte disturbances (e.g., loss of sodium, calcium, or glucose), toxic encephalopathy, or tumors. Often the cause is unknown.
- Dehydration—a common childhood condition caused by one or a combination of the following: fever, nausea, vomiting, diarrhea, burns, loss of appetite, and poor feeding. A child's reserves are low to begin with and they do not tolerate fluid loss well. Other signs to look for include sunken fontanels or eyes, recent weight loss, poor skin turgor, decreased urine output (using fewer diapers), decreased oral intake, no tears with crying, and tachycardia.
- Nausea and vomiting—these are symptoms of an illness or injury. Persistence of these symptoms can lead to dehydration.
- Diarrhea—may be caused by viral or bacterial infections and is very common in infants and children. Persistence of diarrhea can lead to dehydration.
- Rotavirus—this virus is one that almost all children get by age two. Symptoms, such as vomiting and watery diarrhea, last from 24 hours to days. The primary concern is dehydration, especially in infants. Signs include extreme lethargy, decreased urine output, sunken eyes, poor skin turgor, and dry mouth.
- Hypothermia—may be caused by exposure to cool or cold temperatures, ingestion of drugs or alcohol, metabolic disorders (e.g., hypoglycemia), prolonged infection (e.g., sepsis), or brain disorders affecting thermoregulatory center.
- Hyperthermia—may be caused by exposure during hot weather, toxic dose of certain medications (e.g., aspirin, antihistamines), but more often is caused by viral or bacterial infection with a resulting fever.
- Hypoglycemia—may be caused by too much insulin without adequate food intake, increased physical stress (e.g.,

exercise, fever) without adequate food intake or reduced insulin intake.

- Hyperglycemia—may be caused by too little or missed insulin dosing, undiagnosed new onset of diabetes mellitus.

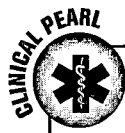

> *Remember that diabetic ketoacidosis (DKA) can present with abdominal pain in older children.*

- Shock—may be caused by dehydration, sepsis, burns, poison ingestion, anaphylaxis, DKA, adrenal insufficiency (adrenogenital syndrome), or meningococcemia.

- Ataxia—may be caused by poison ingestion, infection, or tumor.

- Delirium or coma—may be caused by infection (e.g., encephalitis, meningitis), Reye's syndrome, DKA, hypoglycemia, hepatic failure, substance abuse, or head trauma.

- Congenital heart defects—causes of congenital heart defects are unknown. There may be one or multiple defects present.

- Apnea—may be caused by seizure disorder, cardiac arrhythmia, SIDS, acute life-threatening event (ALTE). These are discussed more in Chapter 43, Neonatology.

- Special needs—children at home may be on life support equipment such as oxygen, ventilators, and apnea monitors. They may have tracheostomies, vascular access devices, feeding tubes, and use suction, feeding pumps, and medication pumps. The family will be very familiar with the equipment and very knowledgeable about the patient. They are often calling for transport or additional assistance. For more information on this area, review Chapter 47, Acute Interventions With the Home-care Patient.

What is the pathology of congenital heart defects?

Congenital heart defects are deformities of the structures of the heart, or the heart itself, that occur while the fetus is developing and are present at birth. There are more than 35 types of heart defects. The structures of the heart that may be defective are the valves, aorta, pulmonary vein, and septal wall. These defects disrupt normal blood flow and can cause irregular mixing of oxygenated and deoxygenated blood. This mismatch leads to hypoxemia and metabolic acidosis. These defects can range from simple, self-correcting problems to devastating, cardiomyopathy and CHF, to life-threatening deformities. Many conditions can be corrected surgically due to significant advances in surgery.

The child may not show signs for days after birth or even until adulthood, depending on the defect. The child may present as *cyanotic* with associated signs, such as cold hands and feet, or *acyanotic* with other symptoms such as CHF, murmur, high BP, cardiomegaly, tachycardia, poor feeding, failure to thrive, weak pulses, low energy, shortness of breath (SOB), and fainting.

Major congenital heart defects include:

- Patent ductus arteriosus (PDA)—the ductus arteriosus is a channel that allows circulation between the pulmonary artery and the aorta in the fetus. This normal structure involved in fetal blood circulation sometimes does not close properly after birth. If left open, a significant amount of the blood bypasses the lungs and is not oxygenated.

- Coarctation of the aorta—a lesion that narrows the aorta and can interfere with the normal closing of the ductus arteriosis. Also commonly associated with aortic stenosis, ventricular septal wall defects, and transposition of the great arteries.

- Aortic or pulmonic valve stenosis—valves may be absent, too small, or do not close completely.

- Aorta and pulmonary artery—may be deformed or in the wrong position. Transposition of the great arteries is a common heart defect that has the aorta rising from the right ventricle and the pulmonary artery from the left ventricle. This condition appears in the first week of life with signs of cyanosis and murmur and symptoms of CHF. Truncus arteriosus is a rare defect where the aorta and pulmonary artery share a common semilunar valve that is usually abnormal. This condition appears within the first two months of life with symptoms of CHF and mild cyanosis.

- Ventricular septal defect (VSD)—an abnormal opening in the ventricular septal wall. VSD is not usually cyanotic and may or may not be associated with tetralogy.

- Atrial septal defect—most often diagnosed in older children.

Which cardiac dysrhythmias occur in children?

In the setting of acute emergencies, the most common dysrhythmias seen in children are rhythms that are too fast (tachycardias), too slow (bradycardias), or the absence of a rhythm (asystole). This is because children usually have not yet developed atherosclerotic heart disease. Therefore, irregular rhythms, murmurs, and bundle branch blocks are generally not as common in children as adults.

- Tachycardias—children tolerate tachycardias well for the most part, but not indefinitely. First, determine if the complex is wide (rare) or narrow. When a narrow complex is present, determine the rate. Distinguishing between an ST and an SVT can be difficult, so rate is used to make the distinction.

Sinus tachycardia (ST):

> Infants <220 bpm
>
> Children <180 bpm

Supraventricular tachycardia (SVT):

> Infants >220 bpm
>
> Children >180 bpm

Once the rate has been determined, treatment is guided by the status of the child's perfusion. Treatment for ST is aimed at correcting the underlying problem (e.g., fever or pain). ACLS recommended for the treatment of SVTs is similar to adults and includes the use of adenosine and cardioversion.

- Bradycardias—children do not tolerate bradycardias well. The number one cause of bradycardia is hypoxia. Hypoxia leads to acidosis and suppression of the SA node, causing the brady-cardia. AV blocks are rare. Correction of the hypoxia with oxy-gen usually corrects the bradycardia. If oxygenation fails, then the use of epinephrine, atropine, and pacing are the ACLS standard of treatment for correction of bradycardia in children.

> **CLINICAL PEARL**
>
> *Always consider hypoxia to be the underlying cause until proven otherwise in a child with cardiac dysrhythmias.*

- Asystole—bradycardias left untreated deteriorate to asystole. Follow BLS and ALS with pediatric advanced life support (PALS) guidelines for resuscitation in asystole.

[Q] Do children have strokes?

[A] Yes, they do. We don't often think of stroke as a condition that a child might have, but the signs and symptoms are the same as an adult. Risk factors for stroke in children include prematu-rity, sickle cell anemia, congenital heart disease, coagulation dis-orders, trauma (including birth), and arteriovenous disorders.

[Q] What are the common childhood diseases that the out-of-hospital care provider should be familiar with?

[A] Table 44–6 lists childhood infectious diseases, type of exposure, and recommended field personal protective equip-ment (PPE).

[Q] What are febrile seizures and how are they managed?

[A] Febrile seizures are associated with a rapid rise in body temperature, usually above 39 degrees C (102 degrees F). They are most common in children between the ages of three months

TABLE 44–6

Infectious Diseases With Exposure Risk and Field PPE Recommendation

Disease	Type	Exposure	PPE
Meningococcemia Meningitis	Life threatening	Highly contagious	Isolation technique
Meningitis viral (aseptic)	Nonlife threatening	Moderately contagious, contact with respiratory secretions	Use gloves and mask
Infectious mononucleosis	Nonlife threatening	Modestly contagious virus with fever, fatigue, and pharyngitis	Use gloves and avoid contact with saliva or blood
Conjunctivitis (pink eye)	Nonlife threatening	Highly contagious bacterial and viral types with discharge from eyes	Use gloves and avoid contact with discharge or eyes
Impetigo	Nonlife threatening	Highly contagious bacterial skin infection	Use gloves and avoid contact with blisters
Coxsackie virus (hand, foot, and mouth syndrome)	Nonlife threatening	Highly contagious virus with fever and skin rash on hands, feet, mouth, and buttocks	Use gloves and avoid contact with rash and feces
Pertussis (whooping cough)	Preventable disease	Highly contagious respiratory infection with fever and cough	Use gloves and mask
Measles	Preventable disease	Highly contagious virus with fever and rash	Use gloves and avoid contact with rash
Tetanus	Preventable disease	Highly contagious bacteria, direct contact in cut or wound	Use gloves
Diphtheria	Preventable disease	Highly contagious bacteria, direct contact with respiratory secretions	Use gloves and mask
Rubeola	Preventable disease	Highly contagious virus with fever and rash	Use gloves and avoid contact with rash
Rubella (German measles)	Preventable disease	Highly contagious virus with fever and rash	Use gloves and avoid contact with rash
Mumps	Preventable disease	Contagious viral disease with fever and swollen salivary glands	Use gloves
Polio (Poliomyelitis)	Preventable disease	Moderately contagious virus with or without flu-like symptoms	Use gloves
Varicella (Chickenpox)	Preventable disease	Highly contagious virus with itchy rash and blisters	Use gloves and avoid contact with rash and blisters

and five years. Most febrile seizures are generalized and last only a few minutes. The seizure is very frightening for the parent or caregiver because the child's eyes roll back in the head and he appears to have stopped breathing. The postictal period is usually brief, but the child will be tired. There are no lasting neurological deficits for the child and the child may never have another one.

Management is supportive with attention to the airway. Remove any excess clothing to cool the child and consider administering acetaminophen for the temperature. If the seizure is prolonged or the patient has status epilepticus, diazepam is usually given. The parent or caregiver often needs supportive attention after witnessing the child seize. Follow local protocols and medical control recommendations.

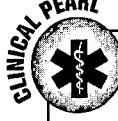

CLINICAL PEARL

Rectal diazepam gel, if available and covered under your local protocols, is very helpful in children with status epilepticus.

What causes asthma in children?

To date, it is still unknown what causes asthma. Various triggers of asthma are well known and differ from person to person. Common triggers include:

- Exercise—symptoms develop after rigorous exercise such as running, biking, or swimming.
- Allergies—75–80 percent of patients with asthma have allergies.
- Respiratory infections—common triggers.
- Viral infections—colds or flu are the most common triggers.
- Exposure to smoke, irritants, or strong odors.
- Stress or emotions—real triggers that are often believed to be psychosomatic by others.

What happens when asthma is triggered?

Three important changes in the airway occur. First, the airway becomes inflamed, then excess mucus production results, causing the airway to become congested and clogged (plugged). Lastly, bronchoconstriction of the smooth muscle lining the airway develops causing the classic wheezing that is heard with asthma. The absence of wheezing does not mean that the problem is gone. Severe asthmatics move very little air and become too tight to wheeze. If the patient looks sick, it means that the patient is no longer moving any air.

What is SIDS?

Sudden infant death syndrome (SIDS), also called "crib death," is the unexpected death of an infant from an unexplained etiology. Though victims range in age from two weeks to one year, SIDS rarely occurs in infants older than six months. In many cases, the infant has died during sleep and is not discovered immediately. Approximately 3,000 infants in the United States are stricken each year. There are no symptoms and the cause of SIDS is unknown. Epidemiological studies have revealed the following information about SIDS deaths:

- The greatest incidence of SIDS occurs during the winter months.
- Premature and low birth weight infants are at a greater risk.
- Males are at greater risk.
- Infants with respiratory infection are at risk.
- Lack of prenatal care is a high risk.
- Maternal smoking is a high risk.
- Placing the infant on the stomach is a high risk.
- Certain ethnic backgrounds have an increased risk, especially Native American Indians, African Americans, and Native Alaskans.
- Family history of SIDS is a high risk.

Current research is looking at possible causes that include brain abnormalities, specifically the "arcuate nucleus," a portion of the brain that is likely to be involved in controlling breathing and waking during sleep; conditions that decrease oxygenation such as maternal smoking, respiratory infections; and metabolic disorders.

How should this type of call be managed?

The psychological aspect is paramount in this type of call. However, like most EMS calls, each case will vary. Most parents will want to see you do everything possible, even if it is apparent that the child has been dead for a while. Others may not. Supportive care must include the emotional aspect for the family and caregivers.

Another consideration is the effect on the responders. The death of a child is traumatic and very few of us are immune to the feelings of such loss. This must not be ignored or overlooked. Talking about the call is the first step in working through such an event.

What is Reye's syndrome?

Reye's syndrome is an acute and potentially fatal disease of childhood. This disease process affects multiple body systems and is characterized by severe edema of the brain, increased ICP, hypoglycemia, and liver dysfunction.

The cause of Reye's syndrome is unknown, but it is usually associated with a previous viral infection. There is also an association between the administration of aspirin for fever, particularly with flu and chickenpox, and the subsequent development of Reye's syndrome. This is why children should not be given aspirin for fevers or infections. Acetaminophen is used as an alternative to decrease fevers.

Signs and symptoms include URI, nausea and vomiting, and AMS ranging from confusion to coma. Out-of-hospital treatment is supportive of the ABCs, with IV fluids and seizure precautions.

Assessment

What are the essential aspects of pediatric assessment?

Gearing your approach to the age of the patient is key to obtaining an accurate patient assessment and providing the best appropriate medical care. Use common sense in cases where the child's chronological age does not match the appropriate emotional age.

The initial assessment—the performance of the initial assessment of a child is essential to rapidly determine the severity of the illness or injury and begin intervention, stabilization, and safe transportation of the patient.

Children are very dependent on the quality of their home environment. This includes their interactions with other family members. Therefore, the EMS provider should routinely assess the child's environment as part of the general assessment of the child. This should be done with a professional attitude, keeping the provider's emotions in check.

What is the approach to take with infant patient assessment?

If a spinal injury is not suspected and the older infant's general appearance does not indicate a life-threatening injury, it is best to perform your exam of the child in the parent's lap. The child in this age group may be anxious if separated from her parents by a stranger. Start the exam at the patient's toes and work your way up to her head to avoid causing the older infant to constantly cry during your assessment.

Keeping the patient and parents calm is vital to both an accurate assessment and preventing the child from agitating the condition. Approach the child in this age group slowly and kneel on his level. Encourage the parents to perform as many tasks as possible for you in the care of the child. You should see a slight decrease in the heart rate, respiratory rate, and BP in the older infant as compared to the younger infant.

Is it necessary for the parent to hold the patient during the assessment?

The exam need not take place in the parent's arms. Be calm and reassure the parents that you are doing everything possible to help their child. A parent should accompany the child in the ambulance.

Is the approach for assessment of the toddler different?

Your primary concerns and approach to this age group are the same as that of the infant. You must establish trust with the child and the family in order to be successful. If all attempts to examine the child fail, this is probably a good indication that the child is really not very ill. Consider taking along one the child's toys for comfort and distraction.

How should the preschooler be approached?

Your approach to this age group is similar to that of a toddler. Remember, it is important to emphasize that the child did nothing wrong. Simple and truthful explanations reassure the child and parents. Clean up a visible injury, especially blood, as soon as possible. Do not say, "Big kids don't cry" to the tearful child. It is better to tell the child that you would probably cry too if you hurt as much, and it's okay to cry!

What is the approach technique for the grade-school age group?

Involve the child in the history-taking process even if it is not necessary. Allow the child to make minor choices in order to increase her sense of control. It is very important that a child in this age group not feel different from other children. Prepare the child for the ED by explaining what she will see and hear at the hospital.

How should the teenager be approached?

Approach the patient in this age group as you would an adult. Try to remain neutral and avoid taking sides in any disputes between the parents and the child. If possible, interview and assess the teenager without the parent nearby because teens often withhold information they do not want their parents to know.

What are the special considerations when taking pediatric vital signs?

Normal values must be age appropriate. Don't rely on memory, use a pocket reference or Broslow tape and keep it handy or with the pediatric equipment.

- With all pediatric equipment, proper size is a factor; this is especially true with the BP cuff. Too big or too small gives false readings.
- Taking BP is not necessary to determine that the patient is in shock. Because children have such good circulation, their skin CTC will tell you they are in shock.
- Capillary refill is a reliable indicator in children. A capillary refill greater than two seconds is significant. Assess the capillary refill on the bottom of the foot with infants.

How is a child's weight estimated?

Whenever you can, ask the parent about the child's weight; most of the time he or she knows. However, when you have to guess the weight, there are a couple of ways you can do it. If you have a pediatric pocket guide or chart, such as the Broslow tape, use that first. Or you can use this simple formula to estimate the body weight for pediatric patients: (Child's age × 2) + 8 = weight/kg. To estimate the expected normal systolic BP for your patient, multiply the child's age by 2, then add 80 to the answer.

What do we look for in the general appearance assessment?

One of the single most important parameters used when assessing a pediatric patient's severity of illness or injury is her general appearance. Your evaluation of the child's appearance should take only a few seconds as you first approach the patient. A child's general appearance is usually a very reliable indicator of actually how ill the child may or may not be. This is your opportunity to see the child prior to the fear, thrashing, and crying that usually results when you begin a hands-on assessment.

Consider the following questions:

- How responsive is the child?
- Can a person or object get the child's attention?
- Is the cry strong, weak, or absent?
- Does the child appear flaccid or lethargic?
- Look for cyanosis or mottling of the skin.
- Assess for nasal flaring and other signs of increased respiratory effort.
- Does the child appear to gaze aimlessly or does he maintain eye contact with objects or people?

A child who is smiling, moving spontaneously, and has a nice pink color is not in acute distress. This child certainly does not need a "lights and siren" ride to the hospital. The child who does not react or vocalize at your approach, is lethargic, and whose color is poor is at least moderately ill and in need of EMS intervention.

CLINICAL PEARL

One of the most dangerous things to record regarding mental status is "A&O times 3" (meaning alert and oriented to person, place, and day) for a small baby (less than 1 year old) who can't even talk.

What approach can be taken to handle complex pediatric calls?

You must have a plan and the first component of your plan is for you to be prepared to handle critically injured children at very emotional emergency scenes. A calm approach helps keep the child and the family calm as well. We need a clear set of priorities and discipline in order to follow our assessment plan. Tips on handling this type of situation include assigning a team member to inform and deal with the parents. It is important that one person assess the patient and delegate the management to other team members. Avoid overwhelming the child with a swarm of EMS providers. Clearly, one person has to be in charge. Having the necessary and correctly sized equipment readily available at the patient's side is extremely important.

What are the essential aspects of the initial assessment?

The key to performing an effective assessment is being organized and systematic in your approach. Refer back to the plan (MS-ABC) if you get side tracked. Patient assessment is a dynamic process. Pediatric patients can deteriorate quickly, so it is necessary to constantly reassess your patient and reprioritize treatment status decisions.

Treat as you go! While performing the initial assessment, the EMS provider must always be aware of the patient's needs. Therefore, they must assess as needed and provide necessary medical treatment at each step of the assessment plan before continuing on to the next step.

Immediately open the patient's airway if it is not open and ensure that the airway stays open throughout the remainder of the call. Be prepared to treat all possible airway obstructions caused by blood, vomitus, foreign bodies, or the patient's tongue.

Always assume a cervical spine injury in a pediatric patient who sustains a traumatic injury. Apply and maintain manual stabilization of the patient's head and neck throughout the remainder of the call.

The equipment must be at the patient's side so that it is immediately available when an airway emergency occurs. Caution must be used so as not to injure an infant's soft palate and oral pharynx when using rigid suction catheters. When using an oropharyngeal airway (OPA), insert it straight in and don't flip it over.

Is the patient's breathing adequate and does anything endanger it? Often, it is difficult for us to count an accurate respiratory rate in infants. A method that works well is to expose the patient's chest and watch the chest and abdomen rise and fall. Note any indications of breathing difficulty. If you are having a difficult time watching the chest move, ventilate first and rationalize later!

Listen and feel. A child who is unable to speak or cry may be in imminent danger of respiratory arrest. Listen with a pediatric stethoscope at the midclavicular line, no lower than the nipples, on each side of the chest to assess for adequate breath sounds.

If a child is moving air adequately, provide 100 percent oxygen by non-rebreather mask. If air movement is not adequate or the respiratory rate is below the acceptable rate for the child's age, assist ventilations with 100 percent oxygen by BVM. Treat all chest trauma as needed.

Regardless of the type of shock present, the signs and symptoms are the same. Even small volumes of blood loss are significant in pediatric patients. Capillary refill is an excellent indicator for measuring the perfusion of blood to vital organs and extremities. A capillary refill greater than two seconds indicates that the patient is in shock. In addition, the child will have cool, clammy, and pale skin. Pulse differences between the central and peripheral pulses may indicate hypoperfusion (Figure 44–4). Cyanosis of the extremities is also considered an early indicator of shock

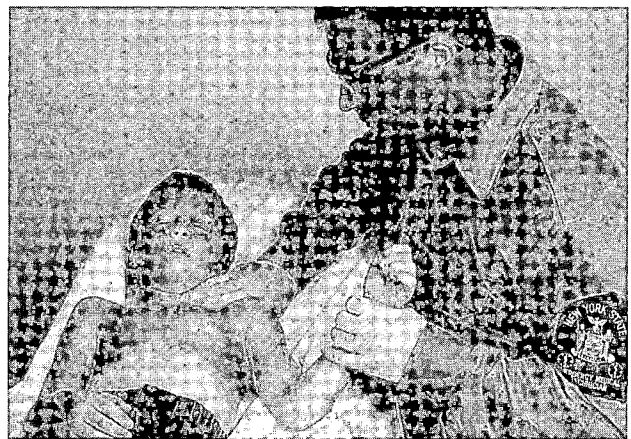

FIGURE 44–4 Pulse differences between central and peripheral pulses may indicate hypotension.

in children. The BP is one of the last indicators of shock in children. Thus, it is not a good indicator of the child's circulatory status.

Your treatment of poor perfusion and shock includes administering 100% oxygen, the use of MAST/PASG per your regional protocol, and positioning the child's head lower than his body when there is no accompanying head trauma or airway difficulties. It is also very important to make an early patient status decision to facilitate transportation as soon as possible.

Mental status is a good indicator of the severity of the illness or injury. Based on the behavior of the infant or toddler: alert means moves spontaneously, verbal, or crying; verbal means responds to verbal stimuli appropriately or inappropriately; pain means responds to painful stimuli only (tickle the young child and avoid applying pain); unresponsive means the patient does not respond to any stimuli. Based on the physical findings: check the patient's pupils for reactions and symmetry. A bulging fontanel is indicative of ICP secondary to a head injury. Quickly assess the patient's ability to feel and move all four extremities.

If not done already, apply a rigid extrication collar provided it does not interfere with the management of the patient's airway. Document all pertinent patient information on the PCR regarding the patient's neurovascular response before and after spinal immobilization.

Minimize exposure by removing only as much clothing as needed for your assessment and treatment of the patient. Avoiding body heat loss is of primary concern for the pediatric patient. Quickly replace all clothing when possible to assist the infant to maintain body heat.

What is the pediatric CUPS status tool?

The CUPS (critical, unstable, potentially unstable, and stable) acronym is used to classify the patient according to the severity of the illness or injury. "C" and "U" patients require immediate resuscitation and transportation. "P" patients are potentially unstable; therefore, they require an early transportation decision and secondary assessment and management enroute to the hospital. "S" patients have not sustained a potential life-threatening injury and they should receive a secondary assessment prior to transporting to the hospital.

What are some examples of critical patients?

The "C" patient category is any patient needing ventilatory assistance. This includes respiratory or cardiac arrest. Cases of pediatric respiratory or cardiac arrest usually stem from a few common problems. The most common causes are injuries or illnesses associated with maintaining adequate oxygenation and ventilation.

What are some examples of unstable patients?

An unstable patient is any patient who presents with life-threatening injuries. These injuries usually affect the ABCs. Many of the injuries or illnesses that affect adults and are classified as being potentially unstable are classified differently for children. You will find that many of these same injuries or illnesses place the pediatric patient into the unstable category.

Why is temperature an important vital sign in pediatrics?

A fever in the first three months of life is a serious symptom and any temperature over 38 degrees C (101 degrees F) most likely warrants a hospital visit and a complete work-up. Infants and children are especially susceptible to rapid changes in temperature (febrile seizure) and many pediatric illnesses are accompanied by a fever.

The temperature of a sick child should be considered the fourth vital sign and should be taken routinely in the field.

Management Tips

How can the EMS provider manage the large head of a child when they are in a supine position?

A towel placed under the shoulders of infants, toddlers, and small children when managing an airway or performing spinal immobilization will help keep the larger head of the child in proper alignment. Because an infant's head is proportionally large in relation to its body, the infant's head will flex forward and cause the chin to rest on the chest when the infant is lying on its back. The flexion will partially obstruct the airway. To avoid this problem, place the patient's head in a neutral or sniffing position. To aid you, a small blanket or towel can be placed under the infant's shoulders, allowing the head to naturally fall back to the neutral position.

When should children be suctioned?

Infants naturally produce large amounts of secretions. Children who have difficulty maintaining their airway or who have an AMS need to be suctioned often. Do not perform blind suctioning! Look at what you are suctioning.

Are OPAs used on all age children?

Yes, use an OPA on all unconscious patients and on all children who do not have a gag reflex. Always use the proper size air-

way. Using the wrong size can push the patient's tongue back and create an obstruction. To size the airway, measure the distance between the corner of the patient's mouth and the bottom of the ear, or measure from the center of the patient's mouth to the angle of the jaw. In infants, insert the OPA in the same anatomical position as the child's oral pharynx. Do not attempt to insert the airway backward and rotate it as you would in adults.

Why isn't the OPA rotated during insertion as in adults?

Because it may tear the tonsil and soft palate in infants causing bleeding and tissue damage.

Why is the proper size BVM important?

Use the proper BVM for the size of the patient. Too large or too small a bag can cause harm or insufficient ventilation of the patient. The key to ventilating a child is to slowly and gently squeeze the bag to cause the patient's chest to rise. As soon as you see the chest rise, stop! Use caution so as not to overinflate the patient's lungs.

The correct BVM is one used with an oxygen reservoir and clear air-cushioned mask that makes a snug fit over the patient's nose and mouth. The most important aspect of ventilating a pediatric patient with a BVM is to ensure that the patient's chest is rising with each ventilation.

Why don't we use BVMs with pop off valves?

The use of pop-off valves has never been recommended by the American Heart Association (AHA) for use on pediatric or adult patients. You risk underinflating the lungs and not delivering proper ventilation.

Can powered positive pressure ventilation be used on small children?

Never use a high-pressure ventilatory device, such as a demand valve resuscitator, on a child. The high pressures from these devices can actually do more harm than good in children. Pneumothorax and tension pneumothorax are injuries that can result from the high pressures.

Is it true that giving a child too much oxygen can make them go blind?

Not in the field. This misconception is from treatment precautions in the hospital where continued high-flow oxygen use (over 24 hours) in the neonate patient has resulted in blindness. Out-of-hospital BLS and ALS protocols call for the use of high-concentration, high-flow oxygen to treat pediatric patients who are experiencing respiratory distress or suffering from trauma.

The downward spiral of respiratory distress is caused by hypoxia or a lack of oxygen. Therefore, the use of high-concentration oxygen will benefit the pediatric patient who is already experiencing respiratory distress, as well as help prevent the patient from beginning this downward slide.

How is ALS different for children?

The basic difference in the care of the pediatric patient is that specific treatment is based on weight or size. Because there are so many ages, weights, and sizes associated with pediatrics, there are many charts, formulas, and pocket references available so that it is not necessary to memorize it all.

- Drug doses are administered by weight per kilogram (e.g., epinephrine is 0.01 mg/kg).
- Joules for defibrillation and cardioversion are weight based (2 j/kg for defibrillation and 0.5 to 1 j/kg for cardioversion).
- IV access is expanded to include intraosseous (IO) and scalp veins.
- Volume replacement is weight based (10 cc/kg for neonates and 20 cc/kg for infants).
- Equipment, such as ET tubes, is available in several sizes.

What special considerations are there for intubating the pediatric patient?

Special considerations for intubating the pediatric child include selecting the appropriate equipment, positioning the head, verifying tube placement, and reassessing.

Selecting equipment:

- When choosing the ET tube size, use the formula 4 + (age in years) / 4.
- It is appropriate to have one size smaller and one size larger ready should this formula not fit the child.
- Cuffed versus uncuffed tube. For children less than eight years of age, the recommendation is to use uncuffed tubes. The reason for this is that the smallest part of the airway is the cricoid ring. A cuffed tube does not easily pass through the ring and may cause trauma; therefore, uncuffed tubes are used. However, this does leave a small space that air can escape past and overflow to the stomach. This creates the need to use a nasogastric (NG) or orogastric (OG) tube to decompress the stomach.
- Blade size and type. Due to the anterior anatomy of the pediatric airway, the straight blade is recommended. Pediatric size blades are 0, 1, and 2.

- Handle size—there are two standard sizes, large and small. Although the small size handle is often called the pediatric handle, either size is appropriate. It is entirely a matter of personal comfort and preference.
- NG or OG tube. Water-soluble jelly and an appropriately sized tube.
  >8 years of age = Salem Sump (R)/ 14 Fr./ 10 cc syringe/ 10 cc air.
  1–8 years of age = Argyle (R) Feeding/ 8 Fr./ 3 cc syringe/ 2 cc air.
  <1 year of age = Argyle (R) Feeding/ 5 Fr./ 3 cc syringe/ 1 cc air.

Verification of tube placement:

- Because of the small chest size, auscultation of lung sounds is diffuse.
- Rely on visual chest rise and fall.
- An extended abdomen is a problem. The air trapped in the stomach distends the diaphragm up, pressing it against the lungs and heart and limiting ventilation.
- Placing an NG or OG tube to decompress the stomach allows for improved ventilation.

How can the pediatric patient be transported safely?

The safe way to transport the pediatric patient under 40 pounds is in a car seat. Use the child's car seat whenever possible. A child experiencing respiratory distress should be transported in a safe, upright, sitting position. The use of a child restraint seat allows you to accomplish this.

How do we manage the family of an ill or injured child?

When a child expresses discomfort or pain, the parents suffer almost equally in their anxiety and feeling of apprehension. When treating an injured or ill child, you are also treating the family. Often, the key to performing a good assessment depends on your ability to deal with the reactions and emotions of the entire family.

Grief is the primary reason for any reaction or behavior exhibited by the parent. Reinforce that the treatment of the injured child is your first priority. Honestly explain procedures and keep the family informed. Allow the family to assist you in the treatment of their child and always maintain a professional composure by not passing judgment.

Why do some pediatricians say with kids the priority is AAA not ABC?

Airway, Airway, and Airway!!! Basically, most life-threatening problems in children are usually related to the airway and not a breathing or cardiac event.

Q What resources are available for continuing education about pediatrics?

A There are several good continuing education programs available for providers and instructors:

- Pediatric Advanced Life Support (PALS) by AHA.
- Neonatal Advanced Life Support (NALS) by AHA.
- Pediatric Basic Trauma Life Support (PBTLS).
- Teaching Resources for Instructors of Prehospital Pediatrics (TRIPP).

- Pediatric Education for Prehospital Professionals (PEPP) by the American Academy of Pediatrics.
- Pediatric Prehospital Care Program (PPC) by the National Association of EMTs.
- Prehospital Pediatric Care Course (PPCC) by NYS EMS Bureau.
- State and national EMS education conferences.
- Regional and local seminars and conferences.

Geriatrics: Abuse and Assault

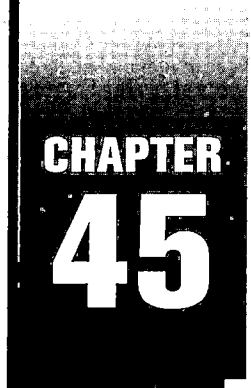

CHAPTER 45

T his chapter discusses the normal and abnormal physiological changes in the older patient. The focus is on *why* the ill or injured geriatric patient presents in a certain manner and *why* you need to understand these changes and respond in a certain way to the presenting problems.

Anatomy and Physiology

Q What is gerontology?

A Gerontology is the study of the problems of all aspects of aging.

Q What are gerontological variations?

A The skin and hair provide the most visible signs of aging. Many more are not so apparent unless you know where and how to look for them.

- Skin—loss of the elastic fiber causes sagging and wrinkles. The loss of sebaceous glands and vascularity in the skin affects thermoregulation (increased risk of hypothermia).
- Musculoskeletal (MS)—decreased muscle and bone mass.
- Eyes—loss of vision, cataract opacification (forming of opacities), loss of accommodation.
- Ears—loss of hearing and sense of balance.
- Inflammatory response—loss of T-cell function, healing takes longer.

- Pain response—diminished perception of pain increases the risk of injury especially from cold and heat.
- Respiratory—ventilation and gas exchange is affected as lung compliance diminishes with the loss of elasticity. Chest wall becomes stiff and rigid and the ribs are susceptible to fractures. A decrease in cilia and diminished cough and gag reflexes increase the risk of infectious pulmonary diseases.
- Cardiovascular—cardiac output (CO) decreases with age; a decreased catecholamine response affects the ability to increase the heart rate in response to stress and exercise. Coronary artery disease predominates in the elderly.
- Central Nervous System (CNS)—brain shrinks (atrophy), memory impairment, slower reflexes.
- Renal—decreased blood flow and elimination of waste.
- Endocrine—decrease in thyroid and reproductive functions.
- GI—decrease in the ability to chew, salivate, digest, and excrete.
- Genitourinary (GU)—incontinence and increased urinary tract infections (UTIs).
- Psychological—loss of support system, increased isolation and depression.

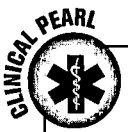

As a general rule, body systems become less effective with advancing age. The aging rate varies widely between people.

Q What is menopause?

A Menopause is the period of time in a woman for the gradual transition from childbearing years to postmenopausal years. In the years before menopause (perimenopause), the ovaries begin to produce less of the three sex hormones: estrogen, androgen, and progesterone. During perimenopause, 90 percent of women experience irregular menses and begin to experience symptoms due to the drop in hormone levels.

Q What are the symptoms of menopausal syndrome?

A In addition to the classic symptoms of hot flashes and irregular menstrual periods, 80 percent of menopausal women experience other symptoms; collectively they are called menopausal syndrome:

- Night sweats.
- Vaginal atrophy (thinning of vaginal walls).
- Vaginal dryness.
- Decreased sexual drive.
- Stress incontinence (leaking of urine during coughing and sneezing).
- Insomnia.
- Fatigue.
- Depression.
- Headaches.
- Irritability and nervousness.

Demographics

Q What is the number of the elderly population in the United States?

A In 2000, the estimated number of people age 65 or older was 35 million, nearly 13 percent of the total population. In 2011, the "baby boom" generation (born between 1946–1964) will begin to turn 65, and by 2030, it is projected that one in five people will be age 65 or older.

Q Are people living longer?

A The statistics clearly show that the number of people age 85 and older is steadily increasing. Projections by the U.S. Census

Bureau suggest that the number of people age 85 and older could grow from about 4 million in 2000 to 19 million by 2050. In 2000, there were approximately 65,000 people age 100 or older.

Q Who is living longer?

A Women are still living longer than men, but the gap is closing slowly. Married people, cohabiting people, and people with higher levels of education also are living longer. Living arrangements and the availability of caregivers are significant factors in the health status of older Americans. Higher education is usually associated with higher incomes, higher standards of living, and above average health status among older Americans.

Q Does social activity influence health and longevity?

A Yes, people who continue to interact with others tend to be healthier, both physically and mentally, than those who become socially isolated.

Q How do these numbers impact society's views of aging?

A The increase in the population age 65 and older has affected every aspect of our society. With the projection of the "baby boomers" reaching the greatest number of older Americans just around the corner, we are faced with new challenges, as well as opportunities for health care providers, policy makers, families, and businesses.

Q How is it estimated that the geriatric population's mental health care will be affected by this shift to an older America?

A As the baby boomers grow older, it is estimated that treating psychiatric illnesses, including everything from depression to alcohol abuse to schizophrenia, is going to become a "crisis" in the United States. The number of mentally ill seniors is expected to quadruple by 2030.

Common Diseases of the Elderly

Q What are the leading causes of disease in people age 65 or older?

A The leading causes of death in the geriatric population are:

- Heart disease—the actual number of people dying from heart disease has risen by 37 percent since 1950, and it remains the number one cause of death in the United States. In 1997, 60 million Americans had some form of heart disease. Forty-one percent of all deaths are due to heart disease. Risk factors for heart disease include obesity, hypertension, diabetes, smoking, elevated cholesterol, poor diet, and lack of exercise.

- Cancer—more than 60 percent of cancer patients are over age 65.

- Stroke—nearly 500,000 Americans suffer a stroke each year, making it the third leading cause of death. High risk factors include hypertension, smoking, and diabetes.

- Chronic obstructive pulmonary disease (COPD)—nearly all cases of COPD (e.g., chronic bronchitis, emphysema, asbestosis, black lung, or a combination) are caused by smoking or exposure to smoke. Those with COPD are at risk for developing other respiratory infections and pneumonia.

- Pneumonia and influenza—people age 65 and older are at high risk. It is the fifth leading cause of death by disease in the United States. Nearly 20–30 percent of people over age 65 who have pneumococcal pneumonia develop bacteremia and 20 percent of the patients die from it.

- Diabetes—complications of diabetes leads to many other diseases. Diabetes-related deaths are associated with stroke and heart disease two to four times more than those without diabetes. Hypertension is estimated at 60–65 percent in those with diabetes. Diabetes is the leading cause of new onset of blindness and end-stage renal disease. Sixty to seventy percent of diabetic patients have neuropathy. Other complications are associated with dental disease, amputations, impaired healing of infections, and pregnancy.

Q **What are the most prevalent chronic diseases for older Americans?**

A Chronic diseases are long-term illnesses that are rarely cured. Five of the six leading causes of death among older Americans are chronic diseases: arthritis, hypertension, heart disease, cancer, diabetes, and stroke.

Q **What is the difference in the pathology of pulmonary diseases in the older patient from that of younger adults?**

A Though the pathophysiology varies for each disease, pulmonary emergencies typically arise due to a lack of oxygen exchange and the resulting dyspnea and hypoxia. The pulmonary function gradually deteriorates with age, making relatively insignificant alterations in pulmonary function that cause more dysfunction in the elderly.

Q **What general assessment findings are associated with pneumonia, COPD, and pulmonary embolism (PE)?**

A Pulmonary emergencies usually present with complaints of dyspnea (respiratory distress). Getting a good history helps to differentiate, but usually does not change the treatment in the field. Remember that the patient can have concurrent problems with confusing findings. Additional signs and symptoms for each problem include:

- Pneumonia—coughing, fever, adventitious or diminished lung sounds, recent respiratory infection.

- COPD—may or may not have fever or coughing, adventitious or diminished lung sounds.

  1. Emphysema—may have a recent weight loss, barrel chest, cough (mostly in the morning), clubbing of the fingers or toes, signs of right heart failure, wheezing, and rhonchi.

  2. Chronic bronchitis—history of smoking, constant coughing, respiratory infections, often overweight.

- PE—patients present with difficulty breathing that progressively increases, pleuritic chest pain, anxiety, leg pain, usually no fever or cough. Often overweight with a history of heart failure, recent surgery, immobilization, or estrogen use.

Q **How can the EMS provider integrate the pathophysiological and assessment findings to formulate a field impression and implement a treatment plan for the patient with respiratory distress due to pneumonia, COPD, and PE?**

A After ensuring your own safety, especially personal protective equipment (PPE) for respiratory infections, get a good history while performing a physical exam, keep the patient in a position of comfort and provide high-flow oxygen. ALS treatment usually includes the use of aerosolized bronchodilators (e.g., albuterol and Atrovent®) and corticosteriods (e.g., Solu-medrol®). For further information on this topic, review Chapter 22, Pulmonary and Respiratory.

Q **What is the difference in pathology of cardiovascular emergencies from that of younger adults?**

A Cardiovascular emergencies such as heart failure, myocardial infarction (MI), dysrhythmias, aneurysm, and hypertension arise when the carbon dioxide level is insufficient to meet metabolic demands. The older patient does not have the reserves that younger adults do. The significant difference between young and older adults is heart failure (HF) is more common in those under 65 years. The underlying cause of HF may be from an MI, dysrhythmia, aneurysm, anemia, fever, or hypertension. The younger adults tend to die of acute MI rather than HF. For further information on this topic, review Chapter 23, Cardiology.

Q What are the assessment findings associated with cardiac emergencies in the older patient?

A Cardiac emergencies may result in a variety of signs and symptoms. Often the signs and symptoms are vague and atypical, without the classic Levine's sign of the fist clenching at the chest due to chest pain. Obvious and subtle assessment findings include:

Obvious Assessment Findings:

- Severe shortness of breath (SOB).
- Diaphoresis.
- Syncope.
- Dizziness.
- Nausea and vomiting.
- Heartburn and indigestion.
- Back-neck-jaw pain.
- Tingling or numbness.

Subtle Assessment Findings:

- Mild SOB, especially with exertion.
- Fatigue or weakness.
- AMS, confusion, or syncope.
- Weakness or fatigue.
- Epigastric, back, or neck pain.
- Irregular heart beat.
- Fever.

Q How can the EMS provider integrate the pathophysiological and assessment findings to formulate a field impression and implement a treatment plan for the patient experiencing a cardiac emergency?

A Any problem that affects the ABCs needs immediate intervention. For the patient with a cardiac emergency, circulation or carbon dioxide is the problem. Alterations in vital signs (e.g., dyspnea, bradycardia, tachycardia) or level of consciousness (LOC) need immediate intervention.

Q What is the prevalence of hypertension in the elderly?

A Arterial hypertension is currently the single greatest health problem in the United States. It is estimated that nearly 55 percent of all Americans will have hypertension by age 60. Women and African American men have an even higher prevalence.

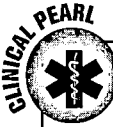

One of the main problems associated with hypertension (high BP) is that it is often asymptomatic until severe complications (e.g., stroke) occur.

Q What is the mortality rate of Parkinson's disease?

A Parkinson's disease is the fourth most common nerve cell damaging disease of the elderly, affecting one percent of those over 65. The average age of onset is about 57 years.

Q How can the EMS provider integrate the pathophysiological and assessment findings to formulate a field impression and implement a treatment plan for the patient with Parkinson's?

A Emergencies in Parkinson's patients usually result from falls, dementia, and dysphagia. Symptom-based assessment and treatment, as well as careful attention to the ABCs, are essential. Always consider hypoglycemia as a potential cause of AMS.

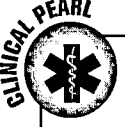

Medication toxicity may result in an exacerbation of symptoms.

Q What is the mortality rate of Alzheimer's?

A Alzheimer's, a chronic and progressive neurological condition that robs memory and intellect, is the fourth leading cause of death in American adults. It can run its course in just a few years or last as long as 20 years; the average is 9 years. It strikes over 21,000 in the United States each year. It is the sixth leading cause of death among white women, age 85 or older.

Q How can the EMS provider integrate the pathophysiological and assessment findings to formulate a field impression and implement a treatment plan for the patient with Alzheimer's?

A Emergencies with Alzheimer's patients fall in the three categories: behavioral, psychiatric, and metabolic.

- Behavioral—anxiety, paranoia, hostility, wandering, and uncooperativeness.
- Psychiatric—depression.
- Metabolic—dehydration, infection, and drug toxicity.

Symptom-based assessment and treatment, as well as careful attention to the ABCs, are essential. For further information on Alzheimer's and Parkinson's diseases review Chapter 24, Neurology.

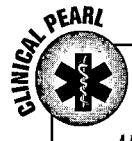

Always consider medications as a cause of new or worsened symptoms in any patient, including those with Alzheimer's disease.

What are some nonacute causes of confusion in the elderly?

When confusion is not acute, get a good history from the family or caretakers and do a thorough physical exam to begin to rule out the following conditions (discussed in detail in Chapter 24, Neurology):

- Dementia—a gradual onset (months to years) of impaired memory and at least one other area of cognition: judgment, abstract thinking, aphasia (inability to comprehend words), apraxia (difficulty moving), agnosia (unable to recognize familiar objects), or constructural ability.
- Delirium—a mildly acute onset (hours to days) of disorganized thinking and decreased attention span. Most causes are reversible.
- Depression—complaints are more somatic than psychologic. Loss of self-esteem, apathy, and withdrawal are common, as are an inability to concentrate, impaired memory, and decreased cognitive functions.
- Transient ischemic attack (TIA)—warning signs of stroke often, but not always, precede a stroke days or months before the actual stroke.

How can the EMS provider integrate the pathophysiological and assessment findings to formulate a field impression and implement a treatment plan for the patient with diseases of the nervous system?

Obtain a good history and consider the duration of onset; perform a focused mental status exam and always consider hypoglycemia as a potential cause of AMS. Symptom-based assessment and treatment and careful attention to the ABCs are essential.

How does depression affect the health of older Americans?

Depressive symptoms are an important indicator of the general well-being and mental health of older Americans. Higher levels of depressive symptoms are associated with higher rates of physical illness, functional disability, and higher health care resource usage.

What are the common causes of depression in older Americans?

There are physiological and psychological factors that can cause depression, including:

Physiological Factors:
- Dehydration.
- Electrolyte imbalance.
- Fever and infection.
- Hyponatremia.
- Hypoxia.
- Metabolic disorder.
- Medications.
- Organic brain diseases.
- Thyroid diseases.

Psychological Factors:
- Loss of their support system (e.g., spouse, family, and friends).
- Decreased quality of life.
- Disfigurement.
- Reduction or loss of mobility.
- Lowered or lost self-esteem.
- Decreased independence.
- Fear of dying.
- Significant illness or injury.
- Financial insecurity.

What are the signs and symptoms of depression in the older patient?

The signs and symptoms of depression are similar to those in other age groups, but do vary by the individual and include any of the following:

Physical complaints are vague:
- Headache.
- Muscle ache.
- Stomachache.
- Lack of energy.

Other signs:
- Unexplained irritability.
- Loss of weight.
- Alcohol or substance abuse.
- Loss of appetite.
- Recurrent thoughts of death.
- Fear of death.

- Extreme isolation.
- Sleeplessness.
- Feelings of worthlessness or guilt.

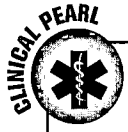

Depression is common in the elderly. Always remember to ask about suicidal thoughts.

How does thyroid disease affect the elderly?

As the body ages and organ systems begin to decline and fail, the thyroid undergoes atrophy (shrinking) and can become affected by abnormalities. Thyroid hormones tell the body how fast to work and use energy. When the thyroid produces too many hormones (hyperthyroidism), the body uses energy faster than it should. Too little hormone production (hypothyroidism) makes the body use energy slower than it should, predisposing the patient to risks such as hypothermia. The thyroid can become inflamed (thyroiditis) or enlarged (goiter) or develop thyroid cancer. The incidence of hypothyroidism is nearly five percent in patients over 65 years old. Hypothyroidism is 10 times more common in women than in men, and one out of five women over the age of 74 has Hashimoto's thyroiditis, the most common cause of hypothyroidism.

How can the EMS provider recognize and manage the older patient experiencing a thyroid problem?

Recognizing a thyroid problem is not easy in the elderly. It masquerades as many different conditions. For most, symptoms are vague and nonspecific and can include confusion, incontinence, changes in appetite, weight loss or gain, decreased mobility, muscle aches and pains, weakness, and falling. Assessment and management are symptom based and supportive, as well as careful attention to the ABCs.

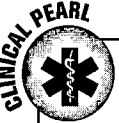

A new onset of atrial fibrillation may be the only presentation of hyperthyroidism (overactive thyroid).

What are the special considerations for diabetes in the elderly?

Diabetes is highly prevalent in the elderly, nearly 20 percent. Because of the changes associated with aging, the elderly are at high risk for complications from diabetes. Cognitive and physical impairments may hinder an older person from preparing meals. Declining senses of thirst, taste, and appetite are also contribut-

ing factors that can make getting nutritious meals at the appropriate time a problem.

Neuropathy is more prevalent in the elderly. They have an increased susceptibility to certain infections and slowed healing. Slower metabolism affects carbohydrate absorption, often without signs or symptoms.

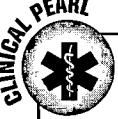

Elderly patients are more prone to develop hyperosmolar coma (see Chapter 25, Endocrinology) than are younger individuals.

What are the most common GI bleeds in the elderly?

The most common causes of major GI bleeds are peptic ulcer, diverticular disease, and angiodysplasia. The most common causes of minor GI bleeds are hemorrhoids and colorectal cancer.

Angiodysplasia and diverticular disease are the most common causes of significant lower GI bleeding.

What other GI problems are prevalent in the elderly?

Bowel obstruction is worth mentioning. In the elderly, cancer, adhesions, or hernias most often cause the obstruction. Other conditions that may present as a bowel obstruction include acute appendicitis, cholecystitis, diverticulitis, pancreatitis, and pneumonia. Signs and symptoms of a bowel obstruction are acute onset of pain, cramps, vomiting, distention, and constipation.

Alcohol and Substance Abuse

What age group is more susceptible to substance abuse?

Some experts feel that the "baby boomer generation" has shown a higher susceptibility to substance abuse compared to previous elderly population groups.

Are the elderly at risk for alcoholism?

Yes, alcoholism is particularly insidious among the elderly. Often, symptoms are not easily recognized until the affected person becomes truly alcohol dependent.

What are the symptoms of alcoholism?

Symptoms associated with alcohol abuse include:

- Headaches.
- Insomnia.
- Flushed skin and ruptured capillaries in the face.
- Social anger.
- Temporary blackouts or memory loss.
- Anxiety.
- Shaking hands (tremors).
- Chronic diarrhea.

What physical ailments can result from alcoholism?

Alcoholism can lead to a number of illnesses, including hypoglycemia, heart and brain damage, chronic gastritis, pancreatitis, impotence in men, cirrhosis, and enlarged blood vessels in the skin.

Bone Diseases

What is osteoarthritis and who gets it?

Osteoarthritis is a degenerative joint disease and the most common type of arthritis. Basically, it is a breakdown of the cartilage in joints. Osteoarthritis affects nearly 16 million men and women in the United States, most of whom are over the age of 65. EMS providers are often called to assist the patient with a move from the floor to their couch or bed because a flare up of this condition has caused them to fall or not ambulate well that day.

What are the risk factors for osteoarthritis?

Factors that increase the risk for developing osteoarthritis include:

- Heredity.
- Obesity.
- Injury to a joint.
- Overuse of a joint.
- Spine abnormalities (e.g., scoliosis, kyphosis).

What is osteoporosis and who gets it?

Osteoporosis, often called the "the silent thief," is a disease distinguished by low bone mass and the deterioration of bone tissue. This condition leads to the bones becoming fragile and at risk for fractures, especially the hips, spine, and wrists. One in four women and one in eight men over the age of 50 has osteoporosis.

Osteoporosis affects 24 million Americans and young people get it too. Estimates are that another 18 million are believed to have below-average bone mass. The cost of treating osteoporosis and the fractures it causes is astronomical. About 1.3 million fractures are attributed to this condition each year. The condition reduces the quality of life significantly through the effects it produces (e.g., disfigurement, reduction or loss of mobility, lowered self-esteem, and decreased independence). Complications from surgery and the lengthy period of immobilization often lead to blood clots or pneumonia.

CLINICAL PEARL

Hip and vertebral fractures are the most common complications of osteoporosis. Hip fractures in older people increase mortality significantly over the next year, even if the victim is in good health prior to suffering the fracture.

What is Paget's disease and who gets it?

Paget's disease is a chronic inflammatory disease of the bones that results in the thickening, softening, and eventual bowing of the bone and is second only to osteoporosis in frequency, affecting 2.5 million in the United States. Paget's disease of the bone affects men more than it affects women, especially those over age 40.

There may or may not be symptoms with this condition, and the most commonly affected bones are the femur, tibia, skull, clavicles, lumbosacral spine, and ribs. Neurological complications develop when the spinal cord is affected. Other complications include loss of hearing from nerve damage, kidney stones from an increase in bone turnover, and cancer of the bone.

Medication Problems

What are the problems that occur with the elderly and medications?

The older generation frequently takes multiple medications for their multiple medical problems. These medications can interact with other medications, potentiating side effects or neutralizing each other. Other complications include:

- Geriatric patients have a higher risk of an adverse reaction. The elderly patient can have a poor response to drug therapy due to a decline in liver and kidney functions, which often occur with a coexisting disease process. Many medications are a predisposing factor for hypothermia, especially when the patient's thermoregulatory system is already depressed.

- If a physician prescribes medication without knowing that another doctor has prescribed another medication, the chance of drug interaction is enhanced.

- Taking over-the-counter (OTC) medications, borrowed medications, or leftover medications can lead to drug interactions.

- Noncompliance with medications—forgetting to take medications because of AMS or memory loss, skipping doses to save money, or no resources to obtain more medications.

- Poor vision and no one to assist with doses.

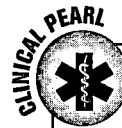

> Sometimes patients have medications that were dispensed as generic and as trade names. Thus, patients have the same medications, though the labels on the bottles are different and the pills look different from each other.

How are the common signs and symptoms of adverse drug reactions in the elderly?

Common signs and symptoms include:

- Confusion.
- Constipation.
- Depression.
- Falls.
- Incontinence.
- Loss of memory.
- Restlessness.

What are examples of medications that cause problems for the elderly?

The following is a list of problem drugs for the elderly:

- Analgesics—pentazoxine, propoxyphene.
- Antidepressants—amitripyline.
- Antiemetic agents—trimethobenzamide.
- Antihypertensives—methyldopa, propranolol, reserpine.
- Dementia agents—cyclandelate, isoxsuprine.
- Muscle relaxers—carisoprodol, cyclobenzaprine, methocarbamol, orphenadrine.
- Nonsteroidal anti-inflammatory drugs (NAIDs)—indomethacin, phenylbutazone.

> If a patient is on a medication, assume that it could be contributing to just about any health problem.

- Oral diabetes agents—chlorpropamide.
- Sedatives—chlordiazepoxide, diazepam, flurazepam, meprobamate, pentobarbital, secobarbital.

How does the elderly patient develop toxicologic or poisoning problems?

Disease can slow the absorption of a medication. Geriatric patients often have concurrent illnesses that decrease their cardiac function, circulation, and renal and liver functions. This has an effect on decreasing the rate of metabolism of drugs. When this goes unrecognized or unchecked, it leads to an increase of drugs in their system. The increased amount of drugs in the system can reach lethal levels commonly referred to as drug toxicity. Some of the most common drugs that produce drug toxicity are digitalis, lidocaine, and various beta-blockers.

Resources

What are some examples of services available for the elderly living at home?

There are a number of community services available that can provide care at home. Over 5,000 home health agencies in the United States provide services either directly or indirectly under a physician's supervision. These agencies may be private (profit and nonprofit), hospital based, or affiliated with public health agencies, neighborhood health centers, local and county health departments, or community and church groups. Reimbursement for home health services may be available through Medicare, Medicaid, and private insurance plans.

- Home care—adult day care, day hospitals, mental health day care, social day care, nutrition services (Meals on Wheels), educational and recreational activities.

- Home health services—skilled services such as nursing, physical therapy, speech and hearing therapy, dental care, and nutritional counseling and case management. Support services such as housekeeping, meal preparation, shopping service, transportation, and personal care (e.g., dressing, bathing, and grooming).

- Pharmacies and medical supply houses—medications can be delivered to the home. Oxygen equipment and hospital beds can be rented for the home.

- Hospice programs—palliative and supportive services for the terminally ill patient. Hospice care emphasizes comfort measures and counseling to meet physical, spiritual, social, and economic needs. This care is under medical supervision.

What are the different types of nursing homes?

There are more than 19,000 nursing homes in the United States. Federal regulations apply broad standards for the physical environment, medical and nursing requirements, and staffing design for three different types of nursing homes. State clarification of these standards varies widely. The three types are:

- Intermediate care facilities—independent living with limited nursing care, social and recreation activities, and rehabilitation programs.

- Residential care facilities—semi-independent living with meals and some medical monitoring provided.

- Skilled nursing facilities—24-hour nursing care by RNs, LPNs, and nurses' aides.

Trauma

Why is falling a serious health problem among elderly people?

In the elderly, falling is widely recognized as a major life- and health-threatening problem. Approximately 30 percent of people over the age of 65 experience falls each year. Injuries resulting from falls are the sixth leading cause of death among the same group. Common injuries include hip and upper-limb fractures, and result in an estimated $7 billion of medical care costs each year.

What are examples of preventive measures for falls in the elderly?

The EMS provider can make suggestions and recommendations to the customers they serve in their community either while responding to a call in the home or through public awareness programs. Consider the following factors the next time you respond to a call at the residence of an elderly person.

Seeing:

- Is there adequate lighting in all areas (especially stairs and doorways)?

- Is there adequate night lighting for halls, bathrooms, and bedrooms?

- Remove clutter and clear pathways.

Slipping:

- Remove throw rugs and mats.

- Tack down carpet edges.

- Use nonslip mats around sinks, bathtubs, and showers.

- Use nonslip footwear.

- Make sure ice and snow are removed from walkways and stairs.

- Install grab bars in the bathrooms.

- Move frequently used items to areas at or below waist level.

- Install a lifeline or a phone in each room.

Stairs:

- Is there adequate lighting?

- Ensure handrails are in place and firmly attached.

- Remove any items on steps.

- Apply nonskid treads to surfaces that are slippery.

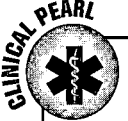

Special hip pads are available to reduce the incidence of hip fracture in at-risk people.

How do affective disorders increase the risk of injury?

Affective disorders (AD), such as forgetfulness, distractibility, or difficulty following directions, interfere with the tasks of daily living. Injuries commonly occur with driving, falls, wandering, and cooking (burns or fires).

Is suicide a high risk for the older population?

Yes, the rate of completed suicide for the older American is higher than the general population. The loss of a support system (family and friends), a decreased quality of life, disfigurement, reduction or loss of mobility, lowered self-esteem, and decreased independence are all contributing factors.

What are pressure sores and how are they managed?

Pressure sores are ischemic, and sometimes necrotic, damage to the skin, subcutaneous tissue, and often muscle. The sores develop as a result of intense pressure on a body part over a short period of time or low pressure exerted over a long period. People most often get pressure sores from long periods of immobilization as when hospitalized or confined to a bed. The greatest incidence occurs in those over 65 years of age. Prevention is the best medicine, and EMS is not often called to respond for pressure sores. However, when caring for a patient with these sores, it is important to keep the affected areas clean, dry, and padded. Avoid putting any pressure on or against the injury area.

Why do severe burns result in increased mortality with advancing age?

Because of changes in the skin, a decreased immune response, and preexisting illness, the elderly are at an increased risk of morbidity and mortality from burns. After managing the ABCs and treating the burn, the approach is to begin fluid therapy to prevent renal failure.

> *Burns result in significant dehydration. Due to an increased risk of underlying cardiovascular disease, fluid replacement in the elderly is tricky. Follow your local protocols.*

Why do head injuries result in poor outcomes in the elderly patient?

The brain is another organ that atrophies with age. As the brain shrinks, the subdural space enlarges and veins become stretched. When the patient experiences rapid acceleration or deceleration forces, the brain and the vessels tear on the sharp bony edges inside the skull. Bleeding leads to a subdural hematoma. When a loss of consciousness occurs with the injury, the outcome is usually worse.

Abuse of the Elderly

What group of elderly are at risk for abuse?

Any older person could become a victim of abuse.

Who are the abusers?

Abusers can be anyone that an older person comes in contact with. Most commonly, the abusers are family members, but caregivers, landlords, neighbors, and friends are not excluded.

What are the various types of abuse of the elderly?

The following are all considered abuse:
- Physical abuse—hitting, punching, pushing, physical restraint, grabbing, hair pulling, or forced sexual activity.

- Mental abuse—threats, ridicule, humiliation, or destruction of personal property.
- Financial abuse—theft, misappropriation of money, or the sale of property without consent.
- Physical or emotional neglect—withholding food, medicine, medical care, or support.
- Care giver or institutional abuse—this type of abuse can occur at home or in a nursing home and can include any of the types of abuse listed earlier.

Why do victims resist reporting abuse?

Because the abuser is most often someone they know and rely on to meet their needs. There are many other reasons that include:
- A fear that things will get worse if they tell.
- Hope that the abuse will stop, especially if promised it will never happen again.
- A fear of being placed in a nursing home.
- Being embarrassed or ashamed of their family members.
- Denial of what is happening.
- Memory or language problems.

Assessment

What are the essential aspects of the initial assessment?

The essential aspects of assessing the elderly patient in the field are to care for emergent problems first, but also to assess the medical, psychosocial, and functional problems and capabilities. These additional components are important for the overall health of the complex and frail aging patient. The EMS provider sees the patient in their home environment and can relay or report to the ED essential information (e.g., a progressively failing patient living alone without assistance). Determine whenever possible:
- What the baseline is for the geriatric patient, especially mental status (MS) and physical limitations.
- Have there been any changes in the activities of daily living, either acute or progressive? Be alert for subtle changes!

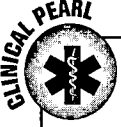

> *Knowing the patient's baseline MS is essential to perform an accurate assessment.*

The key to performing an effective assessment is being organized and systematic in your approach. Patient assessment is a dynamic process and the EMS provider does not always have the time or manpower to assess all of the aspects discussed here.

- Medical assessment—MS-ABCs, focused history, and physical exam based on the chief complaint and initial assessment findings. Treat as you go!
- Psychological assessment—MS and affect.
- Social assessment—adequate support system: spouse, family, friends, caretakers, or support services.
- Functional or physical limitation assessment—ability to perform activities of daily living: bathing, dressing, feeding, and toileting.

Why are some geriatric patients difficult to assess?

The older patient very often has concurrent illnesses that can present with confusing signs and symptoms. Many of the normal physiological changes of the human body, such as loss of sensation, can obscure findings during the assessment. Serious problems for the patient are often underestimated.

Obtaining a good history is often difficult due to the patient being a poor historian or the lack of a family member or caretaker being available with the needed information.

What other factors make assessment difficult?

Older patients are often cold and wear many layers of clothing or wear supportive clothing (e.g., the full body girdle). Just gaining access to their body for an evaluation is often a challenge.

It is important to respect the patient's modesty and to explain what you are doing. The older patient must be handled gently so as not to cause any additional injury. These things can take extra time, especially when the patient has a vision or hearing impairment or is confused.

What are examples of new symptoms or physical changes that should be evaluated by a physician?

Any change in a person's usual physical or mental condition, especially if it is a sudden change, is something never experienced before, or affects their ability to go about their daily routine. Examples of changes requiring evaluation include:

- SOB or chest pain (especially on exertion).
- Headache or dizziness.
- Depression.
- Confusion or AMS.
- Weakness or shaking of extremities.
- Vague aches and pains.
- Swelling in joints and legs.
- Ability to ambulate.
- Oral intake.
- Urine and bowels.
- Fever.

Why is temperature an important sign in the elderly?

Because of a decrease in the function of the thermoregulatory system and the body's impaired ability to maintain homeostasis, even a modest elevation or subnormal temperatures are indications for concern, especially when it is associated with confusion, loss of appetite, or other behavioral changes. Slight elevations in temperature are consistent with pneumonia, UTIs, and sepsis.

CLINICAL PEARL

Unless there is an obvious environmental explanation, assume that hypothermia in the elderly is due to severe infection until proven otherwise.

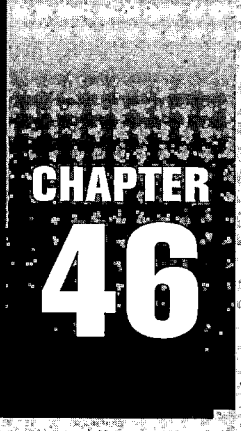

CHAPTER 46

The Challenged Patient

This chapter discusses the general approach to people with "special challenges." This group encompasses a broad spectrum of patients with problems ranging from hearing impairment to financial impairment. Each group has particular needs that must be addressed in addition to routine medical care. The focus is on *why* patients present in a certain manner and *why* you need to respond in a certain way to their presenting problems.

Q **What are the different types of hearing impairments?**

A There are two types of hearing impairments and it may be impossible to differentiate between them in the field setting:

- Conductive deafness—sound waves traveling through to the inner ear are blocked by an obstruction, usually in the external ear canal. Common causes include infection, injury, ear wax, and foreign bodies. Often the defect is curable once the obstruction is removed.

CLINICAL PEARL

> Do not attempt to remove foreign bodies from the ear unless you are properly trained and covered by protocols and medical control.

- Sensorineural deafness—the nervous system is unable to perceive or transmit sound impulses due to damage to nerve or brain tissue. This type of deafness is often not curable, and depending on the cause, may be progressive. Causes include congenital hearing abnormalities, birth injury, disease (e.g., meningitis), medications (especially some antibiotics), viral

infection (e.g., meningitis, measles, mumps), tumor, prolonged exposure to loud noises, and aging.

Q **How does the EMS provider recognize a patient with a hearing impairment?**

A Sometimes the presence of a hearing aid makes the diagnosis clear. In recent years, however, hearing aids have become smaller and more difficult to see. People with long-standing hearing deficits may have poor diction and hard-to-understand speech. Another clue to a hearing impairment is a patient's inability to respond to verbal communication unless you are making direct eye contact.

CLINICAL PEARL

> Many people with borderline hearing impairment are unaware that they have a problem. These defects are more obvious in the presence of distracting noises, such as a noisy accident scene. If a patient frequently asks you to repeat what you said, suspect hearing impairment.

Q **What are examples of the accommodations needed in order to properly manage the patient with a hearing impairment?**

A Hearing impairment is common; the EMS provider must be prepared to deal with this situation frequently. Accommodations that may be helpful or necessary include:

- Asking patients if they have a hearing aid—make sure you bring it to the hospital.
- Written communication—writing notes to the patient, and then allowing her to answer verbally is effective.
- Lip reading—many deaf people are able to read lips. Ask the patient, "Can you read lips?" If so, make eye contact prior to speaking. Speak slowly, but do not exaggerate your lip movements—lip readers are trained to read normal lip movements, *not* exaggerated ones.
- Sign language—only use American Sign Language (ASL) if you are trained and appropriately certified. Attempts to communicate with only a few signs may result in improper information being given to the patient, and received by you. Notify the receiving facility as early as possible if you need an ASL interpreter.

CLINICAL PEARL

Sometimes a patient's friend or relative is able to interpret. Remember that unless you are using the services of a certified interpreter, any conclusions you reach based on this information may not be completely valid.

- Avoid shouting—80 percent of hearing loss is related to the loss of high-pitched sounds, which are exaggerated by shouting and speaking loudly. Use low-pitched sounds directly into the ear canal.

CLINICAL PEARL

Some people with a hearing impairment have overly sensitive ears to loud noises, especially when close to their ears. Use a normal tone of voice.

- Use of an "amplified" listening device—there are several commercially available ear amplifiers available for the hearing impaired.

CLINICAL PEARL

An easy makeshift hearing amplifier is your stethoscope. Place the ear pieces in the patient's ears and speak in a normal tone into the bell of the stethoscope. Be certain the patient understands what you intend to do prior to using this technique.

- Use of a picture book that illustrates basic needs or procedures. There are several of these available—they also work to communicate with people who are not fluent in English.

Q **What are the different causes of visual impairments?**

A The two most common etiologies of visual impairment are:

- Injury—the most common injuries involve blunt or penetrating trauma to the eyeball (globe). Some patients wear a patch or other protective covering over the affected eye. Sometimes acute head injury may cause transient blindness.
- Disease—numerous diseases may cause visual impairment, both temporary and permanent. Acutely, strokes and central nervous system (CNS) infections are the most likely ones the EMS provider will see. Any of a number of degenerative diseases (e.g., optic neuritis, multiple sclerosis, glaucoma) cause progressive chronic vision loss. Congenital abnormalities (e.g., congenital cataracts), infections (e.g., cytomegalovirus) or complications of metabolic conditions (e.g., diabetics with a hypoglycemic reaction) may cause significant vision impairment.

Q **How does the EMS provider recognize the patient with a visual impairment?**

A The recognition of visual impairment may be difficult. People who are completely blind often fail to make eye contact when speaking. Some patients have obvious abnormalities of the eyes. In other situations, it may be necessary to ask the patient if he is able to see you properly.

CLINICAL PEARL

Not wearing prescribed corrective lenses (e.g., glasses or contact lenses) is the most common cause of impaired vision in the field. If possible, allow the patient to use these and bring them to the hospital with her. The situation is compounded even further in an elderly patient who is scared and confused.

Q **What are examples of the accommodations needed in order to properly manage the patient with a visual impairment?**

A Always describe everything you are going to do before actually doing it. If the patient wears glasses or contacts, get them and allow the patient to use them, if possible. If the patient is ambulatory, have her take your arm while you lead—avoid pushing. People who are chronically visually impaired expect to be led—don't be afraid to ask patients about the best way you can help them "navigate." If a patient has a leader dog ("seeing eye dog"), allow the animal to remain at the patient's side during the entire encounter, including transportation to the hospital.

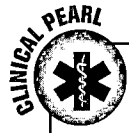

> *Remember that leader dogs are "working dogs." Don't allow bystanders to play with the animal or distract it in any way unless the patient initiates the interaction.*

What are the different types of speech impairments?

There are four types of speech impairments:

- Language disorders—the patient has difficulty understanding language, forming language, or expressing language. Collectively, these disorders are referred to as *aphasia.* Common causes are stroke, head injury, brain tumor, delayed development, hearing loss, lack of stimulation, or emotional disturbance. Sometimes a slowness to understand or express speech makes aphasia fairly obvious. Other patients have difficulty with vocabulary and sentence structure. It may be difficult to distinguish expressive aphasia (patient is unable to say what he means) from an articulation disorder.

- Articulation disorder—the patient is able to understand language and form speech patterns, but is unable to express them properly due to a physical impairment of the speech pathways *(dysarthria).* Damage to the nerve and muscle pathways anywhere from the brain to the muscles in the larynx, mouth, or lips may cause dysarthria. Patients often have slurred, indistinct, slow, or nasal-sounding speech.

- Voice production disorders—though the neuromuscular pathways are intact, voice production disorders result from factors that impair the proper functioning of the vocal cords. Patients are able to understand language and formulate speech patterns. Infections (e.g., laryngitis), trauma (e.g., laryngeal injury), tumors, and polyps are common causes. In addition, hormonal or psychiatric disturbances may affect a person's ability to produce a normal vocal tone. People with a severe loss, particularly long-standing, often speak in an abnormal tone of voice because they are unable to hear themselves (lack of normal "vocal feedback"). Patients with voice production disorders may exhibit hoarseness, have a harsh quality to the voice, an inappropriate pitch, or an abnormal nasal resonance.

- Fluency disorders—fluency disorders, manifested primarily by stuttering, are poorly understood. Recent evidence indicates an organic basis that may be related to seizure disorders or a deficiency of neurotransmitters (e.g., dopamine, serotonin). Stuttering may also be associated with psychiatric or developmental disorders.

What are examples of the accommodations needed in order to properly manage the patient with a speech impairment?

The most important factor is to assume that the patient is aware of the problem. He is likely as frustrated by the inability to communicate as you may be. Allow the patient time to respond to questions and provide any aids (e.g., writing tablet, pictures) necessary, if available.

What are the etiologies of obesity?

Obesity (defined as being 20 to 30 percent over normal body weight) results when a person's caloric intake exceeds the calories burned. There are numerous underlying and often related causes. Some people have a low inherent metabolic rate (basal metabolic rate). There is also a genetic predisposition to body type and the distribution of fat cells. Current thinking has shown that many obese people have an underlying metabolic defect involving excess insulin secretion—many of these individuals gain weight even on normal or moderately reduced-calorie diets. Several drugs (e.g., steroids) favor weight gain, as does cessation of cigarette smoking (nicotine stimulates a compound that breaks down fat). In addition, many obese people have psychological problems relating to their body image.

What are examples of the accommodations needed in order to properly manage the patient with obesity?

In many cases, moderately obese individuals present no special challenge to EMS personnel. Some obese people have a complicated medical history consisting of numerous related health problems (e.g., asthma, hypertension, heart disease). Other than maintaining professionalism, practical accommodations may include:

- Using appropriate sized diagnostic equipment—a regular-sized BP cuff will falsely elevate the pressure reading if the person's arm is large. This is true whether the patient is obese or simply muscular. Always have a variety of different-sized cuffs available to choose from.

- Moving and transporting a very large person may present special challenges. Some EMS systems have contingency plans prepared in advance for known obese patients who are frequently sick. In lieu of a preset "action plan," consider assis-

> *When transporting a large person, make certain you alert the facility in advance of the need for special accommodations (e.g., two gurneys tied together).*

tance from other public safety providers, including EMS, law enforcement, and fire service personnel. In rare circumstances, flatbed trucks and other non-EMS vehicles have been used to transport extremely obese individuals to the hospital.

What are the causes of paraplegia or quadriplegia?

Paraplegia is the weakness or paralysis of both legs, while *quadriplegia* is paralysis of all four extremities and the trunk. The most common cause of either is spinal cord injury (SCI).

What are examples of the accommodations needed in order to properly manage the patient with paraplegia or quadriplegia?

These accommodations refer to people with preexisting conditions—those with acute para- or quadriplegia require full spinal immobilization as discussed in Chapter 39, Spinal Trauma. Consider special arrangements to accommodate the following:

- Airway management, including portable ventilators.
- Traction devices, such as halo traction.
- Special care may be necessary when packaging the patient's extremities to avoid injury or pressure sores because the patient will not be able to feel them.
- Ostomy care—tracheostomy, cystotomy, colonostomy.

Remember that some males with a chronic SCI may exhibit priapism (persistent, nonsexually-oriented erection of the penis). This is often embarrassing—respond in a professional manner.

> **CLINICAL PEARL**
>
> *Always involve the alert and oriented patient in any decisions made regarding movement and transport. He may know more about his own particular needs than you do.*

What is mental illness?

"Mental illness" is a catchall term for a large variety of psychiatric disorders ranging from incapacitating behavioral conditions to acute stress reactions.

What are the causes of mental illness?

In general, the causes of mental illness are differentiated into the psychoses and the neuroses:

- Psychoses—Psychosis is when the patient has no concept of reality. Often, there is complex underlying biochemical brain disease (e.g., deficiency of neurotransmitters). The person

truly believes her situation or condition is real—often the psychotic person hears voices. In a drug-induced psychosis, hallucinogens or stimulant agents cause the patient to lose touch with reality. Often, he develops hyperactive and sometimes dangerous behavior. The best way to deal with hallucinations is the "talk-down" technique—gently calming and reassuring the patient that everything is alright.

- Neuroses—Neurosis is an abnormal anxiety reaction to a perceived fear. There is no basis, in reality, for that fear (e.g., a fear of heights so strong that it prevents a person from leaving the first floor of any building). Neuroses are related to personality disorders more than to underlying biochemical defects. To some degree, just about everyone has some type of neurotic fear at one time or another—this does not mean that a person is insane or crazy. Most people cope with their fears. Again, a behavioral emergency only occurs when a person is unable to cope.

What are the presenting signs of the various mental illnesses?

It is impossible to specifically diagnose most mental illness in the field. Various factors should suggest the potential presence of such a condition. During assessment, pay particular attention to the following:

- The patient's general appearance, hygiene, and dress—some people with behavioral problems (both organic and psychiatric) exhibit an abnormal lack of regard for their personal hygiene.
- Motor activity—many behavioral emergencies are associated with abnormal motor activity. Note whether the patient appears "hyper" or abnormally lethargic. Always consider the possibility of drug intoxication, pain, blood sugar abnormality, or hypoxia when abnormal motor activity is present.
- Physical complaints—these may indicate an underlying or concomitant organic disease.
- Intellectual function—orientation, memory, concentration, judgment. This may require use of some type of a "mini-mental exam" consisting of simple questions and mathematical calculations. Several variants of these have been studied in the medical literature—consult with your medical control for recommendations.
- Thought content—note disordered thoughts (thoughts that seem illogical) delusions, hallucinations, unusual worries, fears, any suicide threat, or threat of injury to others.
- Language—patients with behavioral problems often speak either much faster or slower than normal. Note the speech pattern and content. Garbled or unintelligible speech, unless the patient is actively hallucinating, is more likely to be due to an organic illness (e.g., stroke) than a psychiatric problem.

- Mood—what is the patient's level of alertness? Does she appear to be distracted (possibly hallucinating)?

Q **What are examples of the accommodations needed in order to properly manage the patient with a mental illness?**

A Dealing with these situations presents a challenge to health care providers. A major reason is the prevalence of several common misconceptions about behavioral emergencies:

- Abnormal behavior is always bizarre.
- All mental patients are unstable and dangerous.
- Mental disorders are incurable.
- Having a mental disorder is cause for embarrassment and shame.

None of these are uniformly correct in any given patient, though some may be partially applicable under specific circumstances. Specific accommodations and "hints" include:

- Don't be afraid to ask about a history of mental illness, prescribed medications, whether the patient is taking the medications as prescribed, and concomitant ingestion of alcohol or other drugs. If you do so in a professional and caring manner, the information obtained may be enlightening.
- Be certain to ask the patient's permission before approaching too closely or touching him.
- Treat the person with a possible mental illness as you would any other patient, especially if the call is not related to the emotional problem. Remember that patients with a mental illness also have physical problems (e.g., myocardial infarction, hypoglycemia, dislocated shoulders).

Q **What is a developmental disability?**

A Developmental disability refers to an impaired or insufficient development of the brain, resulting in an inability to learn at the usual rate.

Q **What are examples of the accommodations needed in order to properly manage the patient who is developmentally disabled?**

A Always act in a gentle and calm manner. Explain everything before you do it. Attempt to get the history from the patient first, but also use information from bystanders, relatives, and other caregivers. Generally, no other special accommodations are necessary. Remember that many individuals with developmental disabilities may not be legally capable of making informed decisions. Follow your local protocols.

Q **What are examples of the accommodations needed in order to properly manage the patient who has Down syndrome?**

A In addition to comments made earlier for a developmentally disabled patient, remember that people with Down syndrome have an IQ that may vary from 30–80. Many (25 percent) have a congenital heart defect, so always include this topic in the history. They also have unique airway anatomy, which sometimes makes it a difficult airway to manage.

Q **How does intelligence quotient (IQ) relate to mental retardation?**

A A standardized intelligence test is a common method to identify mental retardation. When the IQ exam is administered, a tested IQ 70 is usually considered the upper line for those needing special care and training. Retardation is classified according to severity and the categories take into account an individual's physical and social development, which in turn corresponds roughly to their IQ scores. The categories are as follows:

- Scores from 53 to 70—the upper range of retardation. The majority of retarded people fall in this category. At this level, they are able to learn academic and prevocational skills with some special training.
- Scores from 36 to 52—the moderate range of retardation. They are able to talk and care for their own basic needs. These patients are able to learn functional academic skills, and undertake semi-skilled work under sheltered conditions.
- Scores from 21 to 35—the severe range. They show slow motor development, limited communication skills, possible physical handicaps, the ability to talk and care for their basic needs, and contribute to their own maintenance with supervision in work and living situations.
- Scores below 21—the profound range. They comprise the smallest number of retarded patients. These patients demonstrate minimal responsiveness, secondary to physical handicaps, poor motor development and communication skills, and the ability to perform only highly structured work activities. Institutionalization in this case is almost inevitable.
- Educators have coordinated IQ scores with school capabilities: educable, 50–75; trainable, 25–50; and custodial, 0–25.

Q **What is meant by emotional or mental impairment?**

A Emotional or mental impairment refers to actions and thought patterns that deviate from society's norms and expectations. Typically, these interfere with a person's well-being and ability to function, though an individual may not be aware of it. Sometimes, though not always, the resultant behavior is harmful to the patient or other people. A more practical term for emotional or mental impairment is maladaptive behavior, indicating that a person is unable to properly adapt to various challenging circumstances for a variety of different reasons.

How does the EMS provider recognize a patient who has an emotional or mental impairment?

Recognition may be difficult. Some patients may exhibit anxiety or perform tasks repetitively (e.g., twisting their hair). Others appear hysterical. Whether this indicates maladaptive behavior or an appropriate response to a bad situation requires professional judgment.

What are examples of the accommodations needed in order to properly manage the patient who has an emotional or mental impairment?

As long as you always keep control of the situation and remain alert for violent behavior, a calm and professional manner is the best accommodation for any challenging situation.

Describe the following diseases, the common presenting signs, and examples of the accommodations needed in order to properly manage the patient: arthritis, cancer, cerebral palsy, cystic fibrosis, multiple sclerosis, muscular dystrophy, myasthenia gravis, poliomyelitis, spina bifida, and previously head-injured patients.

Table 46-1 summarizes the relevant information for each disease.

TABLE 46-1
Management of Chronic Conditions

Disease	Description	Signs	Accommodations
Arthritis	Inflammation of a joint	Pain, stiffness, swelling, redness of one or more joints	• Decreased range of motion may limit physical exam • Take complete medication history prior to giving meds • Limited ability for motility • Make your equipment fit the patient, not vice versa • Pad all voids
Cancer	Growth of malignant cells; details depend on primary site	Vary with tumor and the degree of involvement of various organs	• Assess specifics on history • Look for transdermal pain medications • Look for external vascular sites (e.g., Mediport®)
Cerebral palsy	Nonprogressive disorders of movement and posture usually due to hypoxia in the perinatal period	Spastic paralysis (abnormal stiffness and contraction of groups of muscles), athetosis (involuntary writhing movements), ataxia (loss of coordination and balance); some people may have mental retardation, though many with athetosis and spastic paralysis are highly intelligent	• Assume patient understands everything you say and do, regardless of the physical appearance • May require additional resources for transport • May need suctioning due to increased oral secretions • Pad contractures, don't force extremities to move
Cystic fibrosis	Inherited metabolic disease of the lungs and digestive system resulting in abnormal clogging of mucus glands	Patients have history of disease; may be oxygen dependent; productive cough usually present	• May require respiratory support, frequent suctioning, oxygen
Multiple sclerosis	Progressive autoimmune disease of the CNS resulting in the destruction of scattered patches of myelin in the brain and spinal cord (demyelination)	"Multiple lesions in space and time;" may exhibit fatigue, vertigo, clumsiness, muscle weakness, slurred speech, ataxia, blurred or double vision, numbness, weakness, or facial pain. With spinal cord involvement, there may be tingling, numbness, or a feeling of constriction in any part of the body. The extremities may feel heavy and weak; spasticity may be present	• Recognize characteristic presentation (patient history helpful) • Assess for muscle spasm, urinary tract infection, constipation, skin ulcerations, mood disorders • Consider need for respiratory support • Though often capable, don't expect patient to ambulate

(continued)

TABLE 46–1 *continued*

Management of Chronic Conditions

Disease	Description	Signs	Accommodations
Muscular dystrophy	Inherited muscle disorder of unknown cause with slow but progressive degeneration of muscle fibers	Progressive muscle weakness; usually begins in either shoulder girdle (arm weakness) or pelvic girdle (wobbly gait, difficult walking)	• Consider need for respiratory support in later stages • Don't expect patient to ambulate
Myasthenia gravis	Disease characterized by chronic fatigability and weakness of muscles, especially in the face and neck region	Gradual onset of weakness; drooping eyelids and facial muscle weakness. Patients may have double vision, difficulty speaking, chewing, or swallowing. Extremity muscles may also be involved. Characterized by exacerbations and remissions, some of which may lead to respiratory arrest.	• History very important; many common medications may worsen an exacerbation—always contact medical control prior to administering any drugs other than oxygen • Other accommodations vary depending on the presentation
Poliomyelitis (polio)	Infectious disease of the CNS; also known as polio. Now largely prevented by vaccination	Many patients are asymptomatic; some have fever, malaise, headache, and GI distress; may lead to development of paralysis, usually of the lower limbs, though respiratory failure is possible	• If lower extremities are paralyzed, patient may have (require) bladder catheter • Respiratory paralysis requires airway control and mechanical ventilation (originally, the "iron lung" was used on these patients)
Spina bifida	Congenital defect in which part of one or more vertebrae fails to develop, leaving a portion of the spinal cord exposed	Presentation depends on degree of spinal cord exposure; some people are totally asymptomatic. Others have bladder and bowel dysfunction and altered motility of the lower extremities	• Management of catheters, if present • Don't expect patient to ambulate, even though some are able
Previously head-injured patients	Residual effects from prior head injury	Varies widely, depending on the degree of brain damage. Some patients have behavioral abnormalities only; others have cognitive defects and motor problems. There is no "typical" clinical appearance. Short-term memory loss is common	• History (old injury) • Note if there has been a recent change in patient's condition • Calm, professional, and understanding manner essential

What is meant by cultural diversity?

Though there are many definitions of "cultural diversity," the most important for EMS providers is the concept that ethnicity, religion, gender, homelessness, and other differences between human beings may dictate various acceptable medical practices. A patient's culturally based preferences may conflict with the learned medical practice of the EMS provider. Language barriers often compound cultural differences.

How does an EMS provider recognize a patient who is culturally different?

Certain differences may be obvious. Others, such as religious belief systems, may only emerge during treatment.

CLINICAL PEARL

Don't assume that just because a person is "culturally different" from you, his needs, wants, aspirations, or desires are any different. Be aware of cultural differences, but not to the point of limiting your thinking about the other person.

What are examples of the accommodations needed in order to properly manage the patient who is culturally different?

Always obtain permission to treat when possible. A calm and professional manner goes far to overcome many cultural differences. If the patient is non-English speaking, obtain a reliable interpreter as soon as possible. Sometimes phrase books (e.g., *Medical* Spanish) may be helpful. Don't expect to become an "instant interpreter" with these—use them as guides only. Also notify the receiving facility of the need for an interpreter as soon as possible, especially if the patient's native language is not spoken commonly in your area. Consider using the AT&T Language Line® if no "live" interpreter is present and the need is urgent.

CLINICAL PEARL

Though "phrase books" and hand-held translating devices are helpful, neither incorporates idiomatic language. Sometimes a literal translation from one language to another results in hurt feelings and the miscommunication of information. Remember that a pleasant demeanor and caring presence does not require a translator!

Q **What is meant by a patient being called terminally ill?**

A The phrase "terminally ill" is subject to widespread interpretation. In a sense, we are all "terminally ill" because death is inevitable. For the EMS provider, a working definition of "terminally ill" usually means that the patient has a condition that, regardless of any currently available treatment, will result in her death within the next 6 to 12 months.

Q **How would an EMS provider recognize a patient who is terminally ill?**

A Patient appearance is a poor guide to the presence of a terminal condition. The best way is if a patient or relative tells you (e.g., "My doctor gave me six months to live.").

CLINICAL PEARL

Unless you need to make treatment decisions (e.g., do not resuscitate) based on the presence of a terminal illness, such information should not alter your care of a patient.

Q **What are examples of the accommodations needed in order to properly manage a patient who is terminally ill?**

A The most important consideration is a clear understanding of the patient's "end of life" decisions—follow your local protocols for "No Code," "living will," and other related determinations. Always offer the patient compassion, remembering that your medical priorities may differ radically from his "end of life" priorities. Whenever possible, follow the patient's wishes—of course, follow your local protocols and consult medical control when necessary.

CLINICAL PEARL

Pain control is a major issue for people with terminal illness, especially cancer. Though you should always follow your local protocols, remember that when we are no longer able to "defeat" the disease, we can still attempt to make the patient as comfortable as possible. "Death with dignity" should be a goal of all health care providers for their patients.

Q **What are examples of patients with communicable diseases?**

A The majority of communicable diseases involve either bacterial or viral infection.

CLINICAL PEARL

The most "dangerous" people with communicable diseases, in terms of transmitting them to unwary health care providers, are those with "minor" symptoms. The typical example is a minor cough in an otherwise healthy older person. I have seen this type of patient unknowingly transmit tuberculosis to 12 of my colleagues within 10 minutes!

Q **How does an EMS provider recognize a patient who has a communicable disease?**

A Assume that any person with signs or symptoms of any type of infection (e.g., cough, fever) has a communicable disease until proven otherwise. Also, consider the possibility in people with an altered mental state (e.g., bacterial meningitis).

Q **What are examples of the accommodations needed in order to properly manage a patient who has a communicable disease?**

A Use of body substance isolation (BSI) precautions (standard precautions) is mandatory for all patients.

CLINICAL PEARL

Always assume the patient has something we do not want, and that we have something they don't want either!

Q **What is meant by the term financial impairment?**

A For EMS purposes, financial impairment means that a patient lacks the financial resources (including health care insurance), at least in her opinion, to pay for appropriate medical care. As a result, some people are apprehensive about seeking necessary care.

What are the special considerations to accommodate the financially impaired patient?

An understanding manner may be the most helpful. If the patient really needs care, you should try to convince him that this should be the first priority. Remember that competent patients have the right to refuse. Be aware of local resources (e.g., shelters, social workers) that might be able to help out.

CLINICAL PEARL

Before making assurances about "free care" or "they'll lower your bill," be certain you are correct. False assurances in an attempt to get patient cooperation usually backfire. Remember that a patient's priorities are not your priorities. Some patients may be more concerned about leaving an animal at home uncared for if they go to the hospital than dying. Remember that the competent patient has a right to refuse care.

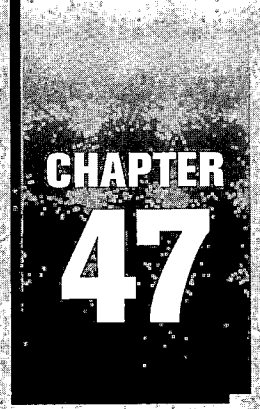

Acute Interventions with the Home-Care Patient

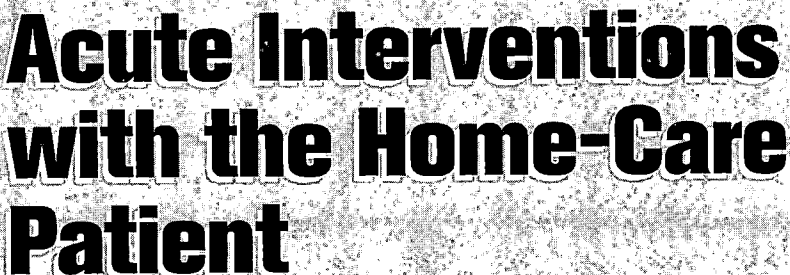

This chapter discusses aspects of acute intervention with the home-care patient by the EMS provider. The focus is on *why* you need to be aware of the special considerations of home health care, the professionals and family members you interact with, and the special equipment you may encounter, and *why* you need to respond in a certain way to their presenting problems.

Q How do the primary objectives of the EMS provider compare to those of the home care professional?

A Both professions cater to the field of supportive health care for the patient living at home.

Q How do the primary objectives of the EMS provider differ from those of the home care provider?

A The home care provider's expertise is in supportive care, assessment, and routine monitoring. They address nonemergent care for the patient living at home. The EMS provider's expertise is in the rapid assessment and intervention of acute or deteriorating problems.

Q What types of patients require home care?

A There is a great spectrum of patients who require home care. The most common patient conditions are listed in Table 47–1.

Q What are examples of diseases or conditions typical to the home-care patient?

A Examples of diseases or conditions typical to the home-care patient are:

TABLE 47–1

Patients Requiring Home Care

- Chronic obstructive pulmonary disease (COPD) and cystic fibrosis patients.
- Patients using hospice care—palliative care, comfort care, or grief care.
- Maternal or infant care—postpartum hemorrhage, sepsis, or pulmonary embolus. Infants with failure to thrive.
- Progressive dementia patients.
- Chronic pain management patients.
- Chemotherapy patients.
- Transplant candidate patients.
- Cerebrovascular accident (CVA) or other neurologically and muscularly disabled patients.
- Patients with psychological disorders.

- Airway conditions—obstructed airway and birth defects, sleep apnea, bronchopulmonary dysplasia, increased airway secretions, and patients who are lung transplant candidates.
- Circulatory pathologies—cardiomyopathy, post-myocardial infarction (MI) insufficiency, obstructed shunts or vascular devices, embolus, and anticoagulation disorders.
- Infections—complications, sepsis.
- Wound care—open wounds requiring dressing changes, wound packing, or drainage.

What are examples of home health care providers?

There are a number of community services available that can provide care at home. These agencies may be private (profit and nonprofit); hospital based; or affiliated with public health agencies, neighborhood health centers, local and county health departments, or community and church groups. Examples are:

- Home health services:
  1. Skilled services—nursing, physical therapy, speech and hearing therapy, dental care, maternal and infant care, and nutritional counseling and case management.
  2. Support services—housekeeping, meal preparation, shopping service, transportation, personal care (dressing, bathing, and grooming), educational and recreational activities, and companions.
- Pharmacies and medical supply houses—medications can be delivered to the home. Oxygen equipment, hospital beds, respirators, and wheelchairs can be rented for home use.
- Hospice programs—palliative and supportive services for the terminally ill patient. Hospice care emphasizes comfort measures and counseling to meet physical, spiritual, social, and economic needs. This care is under medical supervision.

Why is home health care important?

With the help of the aging baby boomers, home health care is one of the fastest growing segments of the health care system. These services can help to reduce or prevent expensive hospitalizations or nursing home placements, as well as shorten inpatient stays. For most patients and their families, the preference is to receive services in their own homes and communities, rather than in institutional settings.

How do the primary objectives of acute care, home care, and hospice care differ?

The primary objectives for each group vary to certain degrees, but often overlap in the supportive care for patients at home.

- Acute care—usually provided by EMS. Provides rapid intervention for conditions related to acute respiratory and cardiac events, acute sepsis, or GI and genitourinary (GU) crises.
- Home care—provides supportive care, comfort care, and referral for patient conditions such as chemotherapy, pain management, or daily activities.
- Hospice care—provides psychological, physical, spiritual, and pain management support for terminally ill patients and their families. Other services include help with Do Not Attempt Resuscitation (DNAR) orders and other patient directives and bereavement care.

What is hospice?

The word "hospice" means a place of shelter for travelers on a difficult journey. Hospice programs and services provide the ultimate in support for the dying person and for the family members as the death experience comes to a culmination. Most hospice patients are at home; they usually do not die in the hospital. Hospice also provides a place for the patient so the family can get a break for a day or two.

What are examples of home care that have the potential to become a detriment to the quality of care for a given patient?

Any patient who requires high maintenance has the potential of receiving care or a lack of care that can become detrimental to the patient. Neglect and abuse are high risks for this group of patients.

What are examples of complications seen in the home-care patient that result in their hospitalization?

Examples of complications include infections and sepsis, respiratory and cardiac failure, emergencies with defective or inoperative equipment and access devices (e.g., plugged catheters, dislocated or accidentally removed tubes).

How do the costs, mortality, and quality of care for a given patient compare between in-hospital versus the home-care setting?

As a general rule, the cost of home health care is less than hospital care. Though difficult to study on a direct comparative basis, mortality in the home-care setting may actually be lower due to a decreased chance of hospital-acquired infections. Quality of care in any setting depends on the professionals involved. The average cost per day of a nursing home stay is $153 according to research by the Metlife Mature Market Institute.

What is palliative care and how does it relate to the home-care setting?

Palliative care is the work toward the relief of pain and suffering and the provision of care for chronically ill patients and their family and friends. This includes ease of pain, distress, and many other physical, emotional, and spiritual problems that are

CLINICAL PEARL

Palliative care is intended to maximize the quality of a patient's life. Generally, no further attempts are actually made to "treat" the actual disease process.

present with a terminal illness. Home care is a huge aspect of palliative care and often accompanied with hospice care.

What is "comfort care"?

Comfort is another term for palliative care. The goals of comfort care are to alleviate pain and other distressing symptoms for patients with potentially life-threatening illnesses and their families and friends.

What are examples of airway devices typically found in the home-care environment?

Airway devices found in the patient's home include nasal cannulas, face masks, tracheostomies, and suction devices to clear airways. Problems arise with airway devices when they are improperly placed, become obstructed, when oxygen tubing becomes blocked, or the oxygen runs out.

What are examples of devices that provide enhanced alveolar ventilation found in the home-care setting?

Devices that enhance ventilation and are found in homes are pulmonary function meters (exercisers) and ventilators. Problems that arise with ventilators are due to power failures and pressures that are either too high or too low.

What are BiPAP, CPAP, and PEEP?

BiPAP (biphasic continuous positive airway pressure), CPAP (continuous positive airway pressure), and PEEP (positive end-expiratory pressure) are modifications of traditional positive pressure ventilation. Each is often effective in increasing the patient's oxygenation.

CLINICAL PEARL

> *Both CPAP and BiPAP may be administered by nasal or face mask without ET intubation. These techniques are often referred to as "noninvasive ventilation."*

What is an apnea monitor and when are they usually sent home with a patient?

Apnea monitors are devices that detect changes in thoracic or abdominal movement and heart rate. Parents use these monitors at home with babies that have infantile apnea. They are also used with adults who have sleep apnea.

How does the EMS provider identify the failure of a ventilatory device found in the home-care setting?

Assessment findings may include dyspnea, decreased breath sounds, decreased tidal volume, decreased peek flow or SpO_2 or respiratory failure or arrest.

What are examples of vascular access devices found in the home-care setting?

Vascular access devices (VADs) and medication ports are common in home-care settings. They are used to administer medication, maintain long-term vascular access (e.g., chemotherapy or dialysis), and provide nutritional support. VADs include central venous catheters (Port-A-Cath®, Hickman®, Groshon®) (Figure 47–1) that are surgically implanted under the skin, dialysis shunts, peripheral vascular catheters (PICC®, Intracath®). Sometimes patients are sent home with atrial catheters. These catheters are found on the chest and can be recognized as a thin white cord with a Leur plug protruding from a small incision. The patient keeps this covered with a dressing. Problems that arise with VADs are due to infection, clotting, dislodgment, extravasation, hemorrhage, embolism, or an infusion given too rapidly.

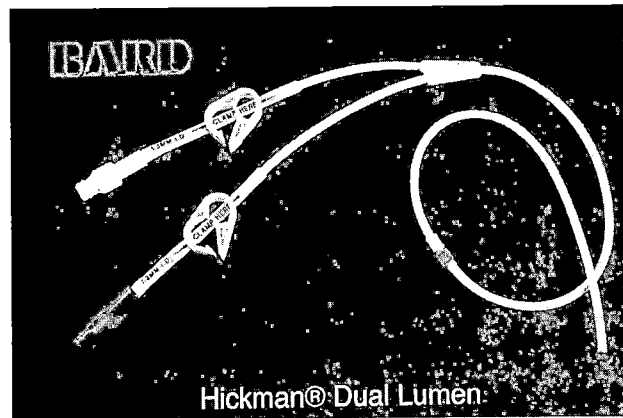

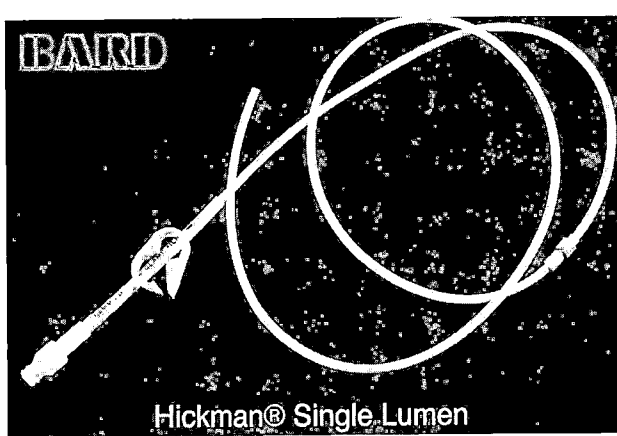

FIGURE 47-1 The Hickman® central intravenous catheter is commonly used. *(Photo provided by Bard Access Systems)*

❓ How does the EMS provider identify the failure of a VAD found in the home-care setting?

🅐 Assessment findings may include signs of infection at the site (e.g., redness, swelling), hemorrhage, hemodynamic compromise, angina, or signs of embolus.

❓ Can VADs be used in a cardiac arrest situation?

🅐 Yes, when a patient is unstable and no other vascular access is available, these access devices may be used. Special care should be taken to avoid contamination. First, use a needle attached to a syringe to aspirate blood from the port. Then remove the syringe, connect the IV tubing, and begin the infusion.

❓ What are examples of devices used in the home-care setting to empty, irrigate, or deliver nutrition or medication to the GI or GU tracts?

🅐 External urinary catheters (Condom catheter® or Texas catheter®), indwelling urinary catheters (Foley catheters® or Coudé catheters®, Figure 47–2) or surgical urinary catheters (e.g., suprapubic catheters or urostomy) are devices for the GU tract. NG tubes, feeding tubes, PEG tubes, J-tubes, G-tubes, and a colostomy (Figure 47–3) are all used to access the GI tract for feeding or emptying in the home-care setting (Figure 47–4).

❓ What are the problems that occur with GI and GU devices?

🅐 A GI or GU crisis can result from improper patient positioning, gastric feeding, or emptying problems; urinary tract infection (UTI); urinary retention; and urosepsis. However, these same

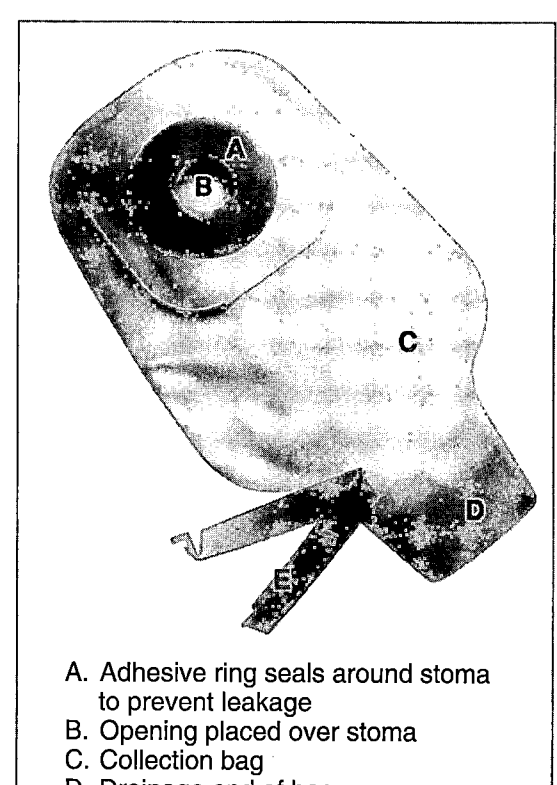

A. Adhesive ring seals around stoma to prevent leakage
B. Opening placed over stoma
C. Collection bag
D. Drainage end of bag
E. Secures drainage end of bag to prevent leakage

FIGURE 47–3 The colostomy appliance has an adhesive ring to prevent leaks.

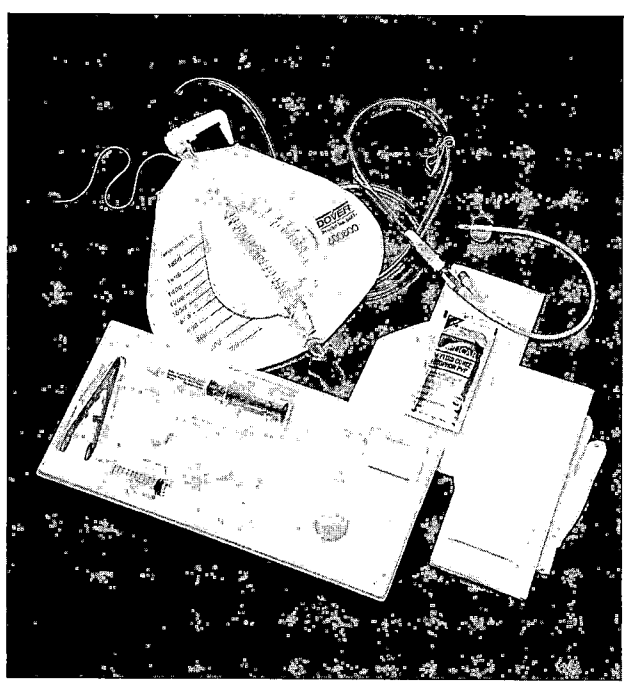

FIGURE 47–2 The indwelling catheter kit. *(Courtesy of Sherwood-Davis & Geck)*

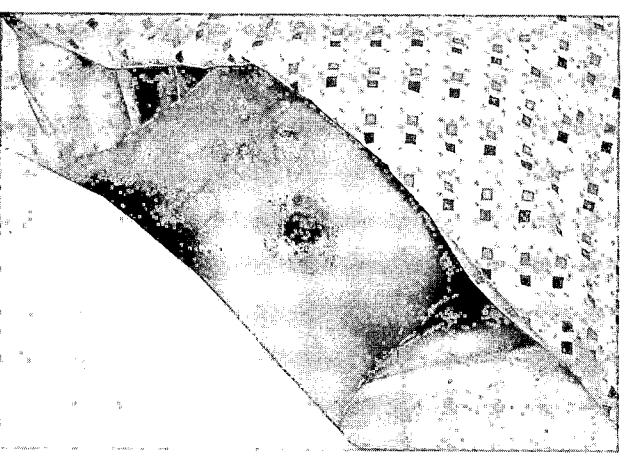

FIGURE 47–4 The colostomy stoma.

conditions can be the reason for using these devices. UTI and urinary retention are the primary reasons for placing a urinary catheter.

How does the EMS provider identify a failure of a GI or GU device in the home-care setting?

Assessment findings may present as signs of aspiration, abdominal pain, distention, decreased or absent bowel sounds, distended bladder, dysuria, or changes in urine output or color.

What is the importance of interacting with the family members who take care of the home-care patient?

Home care is a great responsibility for the family, in addition to being emotionally and physically stressful. They must deal with administering medical care, special diets, as well as fulfilling all of the emotional needs of the patient. Family members often know more about the patient and their special needs than anyone else. They can provide you with the focused history and all of the information about the patient's care. Listen carefully to them and what they have to say about the patient's wishes when the patient cannot speak for herself.

What are the rights of the terminally ill patient?

These rights are as follows:
- He has the right to know the truth.
- He has the right to confidentiality and privacy.
- He has the right to consent to treatment.
- He has the right to choose the place to die and time of death.
- He has the right to determine the disposition of his body.

How do the stages of the grief process relate to an individual in hospice care?

There are five stages a dying person goes through, much like the grieving process after death. When a person first learns they are dying, they experience "shock and disbelief." Then, acceptance comes after moments or months and they enter the second stage, "anger." Bargaining is the third stage, which is followed by depression. Finally, acceptance is achieved in the final stage of detachment.

How do different individuals accept and cope with their own impending death?

The individual's ability to move through the stages about how they feel about dying vary as much as the individual's ability to grieve. People move through these stages at different paces and some do not successfully move on at all. Acceptance often comes when the patient realizes that something is wrong. They may be suffering pain, be hospitalized, or be receiving uncomfortable treatments. Coping with one's own impending death comes as the stage of depression and sense of loss are worked through.

CHAPTER 48

Ambulance Operations and Multiple Casualty Incidents

This chapter discusses EMS operational issues such as standards for ambulances, response standards, staffing and deployment, safe driving strategies, aeromedical evacuation, and handling multiple casualty incidents. The focus is on safety and the proper management of resources.

Ambulance Standards and Design

Who is responsible for setting the standards for ambulances?

There are various standards, administrative rules and regulations, that have an influence on the design of ambulances, the medical equipment carried on an ambulance, and the staffing levels and deployment of EMS agencies. Oversight for EMS usually lies in the domain of state government. Many of the requirements for ambulance services are written in state statutes or regulations. National standards and trends do have an influence on the development of these laws (e.g., the federal KKK1822 Ambulance Specifications have been adopted by many states).

Are the ambulance standards written directly into the laws?

Typically, state laws are broad and the corresponding regulations are much more specific. For example, the public health law may authorize the state's Department of Health, through its EMS Bureau, to issue regulations, often referred to as the State EMS Code, that list specific equipment to be carried on ambulances.

Why are most state ambulance equipment standards very simple and basic?

In most cases, equipment lists promulgated by states are very basic because the government standards tend to be generic enough to be "palatable," affordable, and politically feasible to all EMS agencies in the state.

What is the difference between minimum standards and gold standards?

State standards are minimum standards and are not considered "gold standards." Minimum standards specify the worst they could let things get and still be allowed to operate. When the local or regional EMS system gets into the position of requiring equipment for ambulances, their lists tend to be much more detailed and often approach a gold standard. Gold standards are the goal of giving ample resources to meet the standard.

Which agency issues the ambulance design specifications?

The U.S. General Services Administration's Automotive Commodity Center issues the federal regulations specifying ambulance design and manufacturing requirements. These specifications are an attempt to influence safety standards, as well as standardize the look of ambulances. The specifications are not only used for the purchase of ambulances by the federal government; a few states refer to the specifications in their own state regulations.

What is the effect of a state referring to the federal specifications in their state regulations?

When this is done, the latest version of the federal specifications becomes the state standard for ambulance services to follow when specifying ambulances they plan to purchase. In effect this makes the federal specifications apply to the state.

What is the reference to the latest federal specifications?

The most recent version was issued in November, 1994 and is called the DOT-KKK-1822D specifications.

What are the types of ambulances designated in the federal specifications?

The specifications describe the following basic ambulance designs:

- Type I—conventional truck cab–chassis with a modular ambulance body.
- Type II—standard van, forward control integral cab–body ambulance.
- Type III—specialty van, forward control integral cab–body ambulance.
- There also is a medium duty ambulance rescue vehicle that is designed to handle heavier loads and has a gross vehicle weight of approximately 24,000 pounds.

Are there any other organizations that influence ambulance standards?

There are many other federal agencies and national organizations that influence standards. Some of them are:

- Air ambulance standards are usually designed with input from representatives of the National Flight Nurses Association (NFNA) and National Flight Paramedics Association (NFPA).

- The Federal Communications Commission (FCC) has rules that specify the radio bands and types of equipment that may be used in ambulances.
- The Occupational Safety and Health Administration (OSHA) is the federal agency that is charged with setting and enforcing standards for worker safety.
- The National Institute for Occupational Safety and Health (NIOSH) is also involved in setting safety standards and has an influence on the lists of equipment carried on ambulances.
- There are also voluntary standards set by peer groups, such as the National Fire Protection Association (NFPA), that have in many cases been referred to in local ordinances and thus become the standard for the municipality.

Medical Equipment Standards

Who determines what equipment must be carried on an ambulance?

Some city, county, or district ordinances actually specify standards for equipment that should be carried on the ambulance. Locally, medical control boards that provide off-line or indirect medical control specify the medications carried and the specific ALS equipment and supplies on an ambulance. For example, in areas where paramedics are trained to obtain a 12-lead ECG, the medical control board may have specified the actual brand of equipment they want used in their region to standardize the system.

Is there a national "gold standard" for ambulance equipment?

At the national level, the Commission on Accreditation of Ambulance Services (CAAS) is a voluntary "gold standard" within the EMS community. CAAS is often specified in the requests for proposal issued by municipalities. CAAS requires that onboard medical equipment and supplies be consistent with the state and local guidelines.

In the absence of state or local guidelines, what should a service use to determine the equipment to carry on the vehicle?

The service should develop guidelines that meet or exceed those established by the American College of Surgeons (ACS). The ACS Committee on Trauma issued its first list of "essential equipment" to be carried on an ambulance back in 1970 and revised the list in 1994. Even the first version of the list included

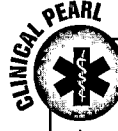

CLINICAL PEARL

Lists of "essential equipment" have been admitted into court as evidence when EMS services were missing certain devices and patient harm resulted.

ALS equipment and the emergency drugs and fluids to be used on ALS calls.

Checking the Ambulance

Q | Why should the ambulance equipment and supply checklist be completed each shift?

A | During each shift, an essential part of the EMS provider's responsibilities includes completing the ambulance equipment and supply checklist. It serves a number of functions:

- Aside from reminding the EMS providers exactly where all equipment and supplies are stored on the vehicle, the shift checklist helps to ensure that all equipment and supplies are available and in working order when needed for patient care.
- This helps make the work environment safer for the EMS provider by ensuring personal protective equipment (PPE) is available.
- The ambulance is in proper driving condition.
- The warning devices are all operating.

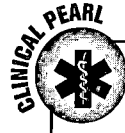

CLINICAL PEARL

Documented checks each shift are mandatory both for good practice and as a risk management tool.

Q | What are the components of a typical vehicle and equipment checklist?

A | These checklists usually include the following:

- Patient infection control, comfort, and protection supplies.
- Initial and focused assessment equipment.
- Equipment for the transfer of the patient.
- Equipment for airway maintenance, ventilation, and resuscitation.
- Oxygen therapy and suction equipment.
- Equipment for assisting with cardiac resuscitation.
- Supplies and equipment for immobilization of suspected bone injuries.
- Supplies for wound care and treatment of shock.
- Supplies for childbirth.

- Supplies, equipment, and medications for the treatment of acute poisoning, snakebite, chemical burns, and diabetic emergencies.
- ALS equipment, medications, and supplies.
- Safety and miscellaneous equipment.
- Information on the operation and inspection of the ambulance itself.

Q | What is an example of a preventative maintenance program that reduces the risk of injury to EMS providers?

A | Ambulance service risk management can be minimized with detailed routine shift checks of the ambulance. Because a faulty stretcher can easily cause a patient to be dropped and cause EMS personnel back injuries, many services have "stretcher day" once a week where preventative maintenance is done and documented on all stretchers.

Q | What are examples of special considerations for EMS providers who carry medications on their vehicles?

A | Medications carried on the ambulance expire, so their expiration dates should be checked each shift and the older unexpired drugs marked appropriately so they are used first. This is another reason to check out the equipment and supplies daily. In services that use scheduled medications, such as narcotics, the EMS providers routinely sign for these medications at the beginning and at the end of each shift.

Q | What should the EMS provider do if equipment is not working properly when checked?

A | The ambulance should be checked routinely so it is always in working order. If the ambulance or any equipment is found inoperable or in need of repair, it is the responsibility of the EMS provider to report the equipment failure to his supervisor in the manner prescribed by the service SOPs.

Q | Are there any special requirements for cleaning the vehicle or its contents?

A | OSHA requires that the ambulance be properly disinfected after the transport of any patient with a potential communicable disease. Most services routinely clean the ambulance after each call and some agencies actually document this being done. Each service is required by OSHA, or the state equivalent of OSHA, to have an exposure control plan that specifies cleaning requirements and how the personnel clean up a blood spill in the ambulance.

What are examples of equipment that should always be checked on a regular basis?

Specific equipment that should always be checked and may require routine calibrating on a schedule includes:

- The automated external defibrillator (AED).
- The glucometer.
- The cardiac monitor.
- Any battery-operated equipment, oxygen systems, the automatic transport ventilators (ATVs), the pulse oximeter, suction units, laryngoscope blades, lighted stylets, and penlights.

Ambulance Deployment and Staffing Standards

What is ambulance deployment?

The strategy used by an EMS agency to maneuver its ambulances and crews in an effort to reduce response times is referred to as deployment.

What is an ambulance deployment strategy based on?

Deployment is often based on the location of existing facilities to station the ambulances in, location of hospitals, geographic considerations, and the anticipated call volume in each area of the community. Most services are not in the position to just move their station to a better location in town. This requires years of budgeting, acquiring land, zoning, community relations, designing, and a capital construction project. The ideal decision on the placement of ambulances must take into consideration the data showing the history of responses in the community, as well as projected population changes.

How is the call volume described?

The call volume, "peak load," should be described by data analysis in terms of the day of the week and the time of the day (e.g., the busiest day and time of the week is Friday from 16:00 hrs to 20:00 hrs and the slowest day and time is Sunday from 07:00 hrs to 09:00 hrs).

What is a primary area of responsibility for ambulance unit coverage?

In communities that do not have multiple strategically located stations, ambulances are often deployed to wait for calls at a specific location, referred to as the primary area of responsibility (PAR). These same ambulances may then be relocated throughout the day as the population moves and other ambulances in the community are assigned on calls. The size of the PAR may vary from a few city blocks to the "northeast sector of town" depending on the number of ambulances available and the call volume expected.

How can computers be used to assist with ambulance deployment strategies?

Some sophisticated EMS systems use computers to assist the dispatch center in relocating the ambulances, as well as vehicle tracking systems that tell the computer exactly where each vehicle is located at any given time. The deployment of ambulances also needs to take into consideration the daily movement of the population. For example, in many suburban areas, a large percentage of the population travels to work in the city and then returns home in the evening. This moves the call volume onto the highway during the morning and evening commute times.

What is the impact of temporary traffic conditions on the deployment of ambulances?

Traffic congestion should be taken into consideration, as well as special situations like a ground level railroad traveling through the center of town. In some communities, it is actually necessary to move one ambulance to the other side of the tracks before the freight train splits the town in two for the 15 minutes it takes to pass through.

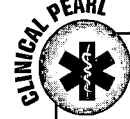

The failure to consider, in advance, the effects of a long train "splitting a town" may be fatal.

What other considerations should be looked at on a daily basis for the ambulance deployment strategy?

Other considerations for ambulance deployment involve a daily analysis of the activities within the community. Additional crews are often necessary for sporting event coverage, VIP coverage, mass gatherings, community days, and other special events.

How should the staffing take into consideration the peak load?

The number of ambulances and EMS providers should be taken into consideration during the peak load of the system. Some services actually vary the shift change times for some of their units based on the peak load to ensure ample coverage during the busiest times of the day and days of the week.

What is reserve capacity?

Reserve capacity is the ability to muster additional crews should all of the regularly staffed ambulances be on calls or a multiple casualty incident (MCI) overtax the system's resources. Some services ask off-duty personnel to carry pagers or sign up for backup coverage. Whatever the plan, each service must consider how they will deal with reserve capacity.

What is system status management?

One system of deployment that has become popular in the past decade is known as system status management (SSM). SSM is a computerized personnel and ambulance deployment system designed to meet service demands with fewer resources and to ensure appropriate response time and vehicle location.

What is an appropriate response time?

An appropriate response time has to be determined by each community based on their resources. National standards dictate that the cardiac arrest victim receive defibrillation and CPR within the first four minutes and ALS within eight minutes. The standards of reliability of a response agency take into consideration the percentage of the time that high priority calls are responded to within an agreed on system response time. The medical director must have direct input into this system standard because it may be the difference between life or death for the citizens of the community. An example of a response time standard for a community is a service that is able to respond within four minutes to 90 percent of the priority-one calls (e.g., a cardiac arrest, motor vehicle collisions [MVCs], and respiratory complaints).

How can a "tiered response" help improve the communities' response time to emergencies?

Some communities employ a tiered response to achieve a four-minute arrival by using public safety agencies trained as first responders who carry an AED to the patient's side. The first tier of response is then backed up with a second tier of response that is an ALS unit positioned to arrive within eight minutes. Other communities add in a third tier of response by separating their paramedics from their ambulances.

Is there a single best deployment strategy?

This, of course, is always a controversial topic. However, there is no single best deployment strategy for all communities. The best deployment strategy for your specific community must take into consideration the resources, personnel, facilities, available training, medical direction, and many other factors.

Is there a single best staffing protocol for ambulances in communities providing ALS care to their citizens?

For as long as EMS providers have been trained to the advanced level, the controversy has existed over how many paramedics should be on a unit. This too is a complex decision that must take into consideration the other crews being dispatched to each priority-one call. Clearly, a crew that has two paramedics on it, which is the only responder to a cardiac arrest (no additional backup), is limited in the amount of care they can provide to the patient.

Some communities combine an EMT-Intermediate with a paramedic to make an ALS unit. Other communities argue that a unit must have two paramedics on it so they can back each other up when making decisions on the scene. The controversy will continue to rage because no one can show that what works in one community is guaranteed to work in every other community because the available resources and personnel vary so much.

CLINICAL PEARL

Despite a number of highly opinionated arguments favoring a particular "set-up" of EMS personnel, different areas have different requirements. Needs must be established on a local or regional level. A "national standard" is impossible to define because there are many differences between areas and systems.

Preventing Ambulance Collisions

Are there standards for the operators (drivers) of an ambulance?

Ambulance operator (driver) and driving standards are usually spelled out at the local service level. There are some states that have specific requirements as to the type of license that an operator of an emergency vehicle must have.

What is the number one rule of medicine and how does that relate to driving an emergency vehicle?

The number one rule of medicine, no matter what level of health care professional you are, is the same: "Do no harm!" This clearly relates to driving an emergency vehicle because patients, family members, other motorists, and fellow EMS providers are often injured, sometimes fatally, in ambulance collisions.

What are some of the other costs of ambulance collisions?

In addition to personal injuries, there are many other costs of ambulance collisions such as:

- Vehicle repair or replacement.
- Lawsuits.
- Down time.
- Increased insurance premiums.
- The effect on your agency's fine reputation in your community.

Is there an "acceptable" rate of ambulance collisions?

No, especially if you consider the number one rule of medicine! Because there is no national database with 100 percent of the states contributing similar data on ambulance collisions, it is difficult to establish any form of "acceptable" ambulance collision rates per calls or miles driven.

Is there research that shows how to reduce ambulance collisions?

There are very few scientific studies published attempting to prove what strategies, if any, work at reducing ambulance collision rates. Some localities show that using low priority, non-lights and siren responses can decrease the number of emergency vehicle collisions four-fold.

Is your service leadership accountable for strategies to prevent ambulance collisions?

When your agency experiences the sometimes devastating effects of a serious ambulance collision, the question of how proactive your agency was to prevent ambulance collisions and train the EMS providers to be safe operators of the vehicle will undoubtedly be raised!

The leadership needs to ask themselves a few very serious questions. Do you have an aggressive proactive training program or have you taken the reactive approach, saying, "We will just deal with it as it comes up"? When the message, "Ambulance collides with car, killing three small children and seriously injuring mother and sister: Ambulance operator arrested on three manslaughter counts," goes out over Associated Press, there definitely will be some serious questions raised about your training program.

So, how big is the problem of ambulance collisions?

The first part to any prevention education is defining and owning up to the extent of the problem. In the absence of a national database, this is easier said than done. The statistics referred to here come from an analysis of 22 years of reportable MVCs in New York state. The data used here is not intended to be scientific evidence that can be generalized to the other 49 states; rather, it serves a descriptive purpose based on large numbers of collisions. During the years 1974 through 1996, there were 7,756 ambulance collisions involving 64 fatalities and 10,636 injuries.

So, what can be gleaned from all of these collisions?

An analysis of the data actually helps to develop a profile of the typical ambulance collision. It also helps to review the weather conditions, amount of daylight and visibility, direction of travel, location of the collision, types of collisions, and road conditions.

What was the analysis of weather conditions and daylight visibility?

Inclement weather accounts for only a small number of collisions (e.g., 16 percent cloudy days; 18 percent rainy days; 6 percent snow, sleet, hail, and freezing rain days). The majority (55 percent) of the collisions occurred on clear days and 67 percent of the collisions occurred during daylight hours.

What types of collisions were most common?

Although head-on collisions can be very serious, fortunately, they only account for some one percent of the collisions. The majority of the collisions (41 percent) occurred when the vehicle was struck or did strike another vehicle laterally or at a right angle intersection. Approximately 21 percent of the collisions occurred from side-swiping or overtaking another vehicle. Collisions involving the ambulance making a right or left turn occurred 12 percent of the time.

What types of road conditions were reported for these collisions?

One might expect road conditions to be a large contributing factor. Actually, only eight percent of the collisions occurred on snowy or icy roads. About 24 percent occurred on wet roads, but the majority (60 percent) occurred on dry roads.

What is the most important observation from the data?

Probably the most important observation from the data is that 72 percent of the collisions occurred in an intersection. Most safety conscious ambulance operators agree that the days of "blowing through intersections" at high speed with the lights blaring and sirens blasting have come and gone.

How often were these intersections controlled with a stop sign or traffic light?

Although half of all collisions occurred at locations with a traffic control device, nearly a third were at locations with no traffic device or sign at all. Locations with stop signs only accounted for seven percent of the collisions.

In the data presented, what was a "reportable collision?"

Reportable collisions involve over $1,000 of vehicle damage or a personal injury. This means that many of the crashes from backing the ambulance are not reported in this data because they cost less to repair, there was no injury involved, or the service decided not to report the collision to their insurance company for fear their rates would increase.

How can slow-speed backing collisions be eliminated?

Requiring a spotter who is always visible to the driver in the left side mirror can eliminate most of the slow-speed backing collisions.

So, what would the profile of a typical ambulance collision look like?

The profile of an ambulance collision would most likely involve a clear day, daylight hours, and a dry road with a lateral collision in an intersection that has a traffic light.

CLINICAL PEARL

> REMEMBER—the profile of an ambulance collision would most likely involve a clear day, daylight hours, and a dry road with a lateral collision in an intersection that has a traffic light.

How can the "profile of the typical collision" be a useful tool to focus the development of a service-level ambulance operator training program?

The first step in implementing prevention strategies is to identify the extent of the problem and determine when it is most apt to occur. That is why the "profile" is helpful to focus your precious training time away from skidding around in a snowy parking lot and onto handling the vehicle during normal driving conditions.

When developing strategies to help reduce ambulance collisions in your community, what should your service leadership consider?

Consider the following areas:
- Establishing driver qualification checklists and running license checks with the local police or Department of Motor Vehicles.
- A clear understanding of the preventative maintenance program for the ambulances, the need for shift vehicle operator checklist completion, and the procedure for reporting any problems found during the check or when driving the vehicle.
- Plenty of driver hands-on training using experienced and qualified field training officers. A 10,000 to 24,000 pound ambulance has a much longer stopping distance than your EMS provider's 2,500 pound compact car! In some instances, inexperienced operators have been surprised that the ambulance slid right through the intersection and was stopped by a light pole.
- A slow-speed skills course to ensure that the operator is proficient in use of the mirrors, backing, turning radius, braking distance, parking, and handling a vehicle the size of an ambulance.
- Ensuring that operators have the knowledge of the proper reaction to emergency situations such as the loss of brakes or power steering, a stuck accelerator, a blowout, and the procedure for dealing with a vehicle breakdown.
- Demonstrated knowledge in the primary and backup routes to all hospitals from your service response area.
- An understanding of the state Department of Motor Vehicles' rules, regulations, and laws pertaining to the operation of an ambulance.

Are there any specific standard operating procedures (SOPs) that ambulance services should have in place that deal with driving the vehicle?

Yes, well-thoughtout SOPs are good. Just remember that all the operators need to be trained in the SOPs and comply with them! Here are some examples to consider:
- The procedure for qualifying as an ambulance operator.
- The procedure to follow in case an ambulance collision occurs.
- The review, investigation, and quality assurance process that will be followed after each ambulance collision.
- The use of a spotter for backing the vehicle. Make sure the driver of the vehicle can always easily see the spotter.
- The use of seat belts in the ambulance and how to transport a child passenger weighing less than 40 pounds.
- What constitutes an emergency response and what exemptions may be taken under your state's laws and under what specific circumstances?

- The use of prudent speed, properly traveling in the oncoming lane, and how to negotiate an intersection properly.
- Your service's SOP on escorts.
- A zero-tolerance policy on driving the vehicle under the influence of any drugs or alcohol.

Q What is the "due regard" concept?

A Most state motor vehicle laws were developed from a model law; therefore, there is a lot of similarity. One concept that appears in most statutes that deal with emergency vehicle operation is the concept of due regard. Due regard is a responsibility that the operator of an emergency vehicle takes on when operating an emergency vehicle.

Where the laws are often rather liberal in what exemptions they allow, there usually is very specific language that clearly puts the responsibility on the shoulders of the ambulance operator. The laws often say, "The foregoing provisions and exemptions do not relieve the operator of an emergency vehicle from acting with due regard for the safety of all persons." This language sets up a higher standard for the operator of an emergency vehicle than for any other driver on the road. Nowhere in the motor vehicle laws does it say any other driver is responsible for the safety of all other motorists!

Q What do the typical state laws allow the operator of an ambulance to do?

A Typical laws allow the operator of an ambulance, while in emergency operation, to be exempted from the posted speed limit, the posted direction of travel, the posted parking regulations, and the requirement to stop and wait at a red light. Rarely do the exemptions include passing over a railroad crossing with the gates down or passing a school bus with the blinking red lights on. In the latter case, you should wait till the school bus operator secures the safety of the children and then turns off the red flashing lights to allow you to proceed past the bus.

We strongly suggest that you obtain a copy of your state's motor vehicle regulations and read them very closely. If you have any questions, ask your service's attorney for an interpretation.

Q How is the investigation of an ambulance collision (e.g., involving the death of a pedestrian who darted out in front of the ambulance) different than that of a normal collision between an automobile and a pedestrian?

A When the police arrive, they take statements from all involved, ensure that the operator of the ambulance was sober, check the vehicle's inspection, and measure skid marks. In some states such as New York, they will then turn over the investiga-

tion to the County Grand Jury to investigate further. The operator of the ambulance will most likely be questioned by the grand jury, which is likely to involve scrutiny of his/her personal and professional driving record, habits, service SOPs, rules of the road, etc.

Always be cognizant that you will be held to a higher standard as the operator of an emergency vehicle and always be prepared and attentive to the responsibilities you have chosen to shoulder.

Q How well can the other motorists see or hear the oncoming ambulance?

A Studies have shown that most other motorists do not see or hear your ambulance until it is within 50 to 100 feet of their vehicle. Do not rely solely on the lights and siren to alert the other motorists. Be sure to leave plenty of room around your vehicle and get a face-to-face commitment from other drivers that they understand where your vehicle is going.

Q What effect does a siren have on the driving public, our patients, and the EMS provider?

A A siren has the following effects on other motorists:

- Motorists are less inclined to yield to an ambulance when the siren is continually sounded.
- Many motorists feel that the right-of-way privileges granted to ambulances are being abused when the siren is sounded.
- The continuous siren sound can worsen a sick or injured patient's condition by increasing their anxiety.
- Ambulance operators have experienced anxiety themselves from long runs with the siren operating and have developed long-term hearing impairments.
- Tests have shown that inexperienced ambulance operators tend to increase their driving speed by 10 to 15 miles per hour when the siren is sounded.

Q What are some guidelines for the proper use of a siren?

A Some states have specific laws, or services have SOPs, that address the actual use of the siren. Here are some guidelines to consider:

- Use the siren sparingly and only when you must.
- Never assume all motorists hear your siren.
- Assume that some motorists hear your siren, but choose to ignore it.
- Be prepared for panic and erratic maneuvers by drivers when they finally do hear your siren.
- Do not pull up close to a vehicle and then sound your siren.
- Never use the siren to scare someone.

Q Many of the vehicles on the road today always have their headlights on. Should we do the same in the ambulance?

A Yes! Whenever the ambulance is on the road, day or night, turn on the headlights to increase its visibility. Alternating headlamps should only be used on nighttime calls if they are installed in a secondary lamp.

Q What is the most effective light so a citizen can see the ambulance approaching behind him?

A Probably the most useful light is the one in the center of the cowling on the front hood that can easily be seen in the rearview mirror of the car in front of you.

Q What other lighting should be specified for an ambulance?

A Each corner of the ambulance should have flashers that are large and blink in tandem or unison to help oncoming vehicles identify the location and size of the ambulance. Although the controversy over the use of strobes continues to remain unresolved, consider the latest research when designing the lighting on your ambulance. It is suggested that the lighting system consist of a combination of single-beam bulbs and strobes rather than using only one lighting system or the other. The vehicle must be clearly visible from 360 degrees to all other motorists and pedestrians.

Q Should ambulances use a police escort?

A Most EMS agencies no longer recommend the use of a police escort for ambulances except in those circumstances where the ambulance is providing service to an unfamiliar district and needs to be taken to the patient or hospital. The acceleration speed and braking distance of the ambulance is very different than that of a police car. Often the ambulance follows too closely behind the police car and can easily rearend the car when they both attempt to come to a quick stop. In other instances, the ambulance operator may have difficulty keeping up with the car and leave too big a cushion between the vehicles, allowing other vehicles to pull in between them.

Also, the ambulance operator should never assume that the other motorists realize the ambulance is following the police car.

Many vehicles actually pull out right in front of the ambulance after having watched the police car speed by and thinking the coast is now clear.

Q What is the danger associated with a multiple emergency vehicle response?

A In multiple vehicle responses, the dangers are the same as with an escort. Another danger occurs when two emergency vehicles are approaching the same intersection at the same time. Besides totally confusing the driving motorists and pedestrians, the potential for an intersection collision is increased dramatically. Often motorists fail to yield the right-of-way to the first emergency vehicle, the second emergency vehicle, or in some instances, both. It is a good habit to pay attention to the other calls in your district, but do not assume you know all of the responses taking place. The police often respond to incidents without announcing their response so as to not warn the perpetrators of their arrival.

Q So, what is a good policy when approaching an intersection to prevent a collision with another emergency vehicle?

A Always approach every intersection cautiously and with the thought that you could be meeting another emergency vehicle at that intersection.

Q Where should the ambulance be positioned at the scene of a highway incident if you are the first to arrive?

A When arriving at the scene of a highway incident, if you are the first to arrive, take steps to size up the scene for potential hazards to you, your crew, and the patients. Consider establishing a danger zone, parking at least 100 feet from the wreckage, upwind and uphill (if possible) to avoid fire or any escaping hazardous liquids or fumes, and deal with the traffic till the police arrive to relieve you of that task. If there is no fire or escaping liquids or fumes, park at least 50 feet from the wreckage. Park in front of the wreckage if your ambulance is the first emergency vehicle on the scene so your warning lights can warn approaching motorists before flares can be set up (Figure 48–1).

Q Where should the ambulance be positioned at the scene of a highway incident if you are not the first to arrive?

A If the scene has already been secured, park beyond the wreckage to prevent your ambulance from being exposed to the

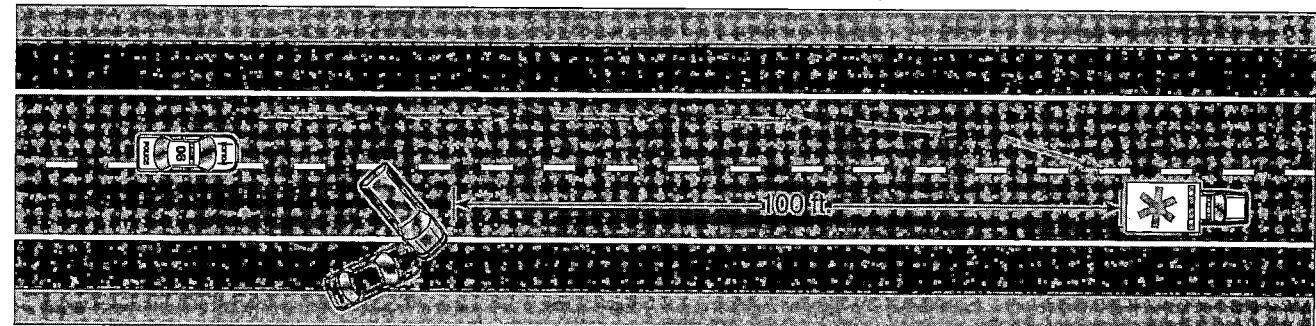

FIGURE 48-1 If, upon your arrival, the scene is already shielded, the ambulance should be positioned just beyond the collision scene to allow for an easy exit and to limit the exposure of the crew and patient when loading the ambulance.

traffic. You may also receive arrival instructions if a first arriving EMS unit at the scene has already declared medical command. The arrival instructions may have specific instructions as to where the medical commander would like you to park your ambulance and to whom you should report.

How can the proper positioning of the ambulance at the scene of the highway incident actually prevent injuries to your crew?

EMS providers have been seriously injured, and some even killed, while working at the scene of an incident when they were struck by passing motorists. Do not expose your crew or the patient to the traffic. Be aware that the rear doors of the ambulance often obstruct the view of the warning lights when the doors are open to load the patient. Studies show that red revolving beacons attract intoxicated or tired drivers. Consider pulling off the road, turning off your headlights, and using just the amber rear-sealed beam blinkers that flash in tandem to help the oncoming motorist identify the size of your ambulance.

CLINICAL PEARL

Always assume that oncoming traffic does not see you and that even if they do, they often won't move over or slow down.

With 72 percent of the ambulance collisions occurring in an intersection, this clearly is a very unsafe, if not deadly, place to be. What are some examples of tips for safely negotiating an intersection?

The following tips might be useful:

- Stop at all red lights and stop signs and then proceed with caution.

- Always proceed through an intersection slowly, one lane at a time, and make eye contact with the motorists to ensure that they understand your intentions.

- If you are using any of the exemptions offered to you as an emergency vehicle during an emergency operation, such as passing through a stop sign or red light, make sure you are using your lights and siren appropriately to warn the motorists.

- The lights and siren "ask" the public to yield the right-of-way to your ambulance. If the public does not yield, it may be because they misunderstand your intentions, cannot hear your siren due to the noise in their own vehicle, or cannot see your lights. Never assume that just because you are using your lights and siren on an emergency call the other motorists know how to properly react to you!

- Always go around cars stopped at the intersection on the driver's side. This may involve, in some instances, passing into the oncoming lane, which should be done slowly and very cautiously. To just sneak past a group of cars stopped at an intersection using a clear right lane invites trouble. Remember, if the motorists are doing what they are supposed to be doing, they might actually pull to the right into the lane you are attempting to pass through.

- Know how long it takes for your ambulance to cross an intersection. This will help you judge whether you have enough time to accelerate from a stop through the intersection.

- Watch the pedestrians at the intersection carefully. If they all seem to be staring in another direction and not at your ambulance, it is probably at the fire truck you are about to meet in the intersection.

- Remember that there is no such thing as a rolling stop in an ambulance weighing in at over 10,000 pounds and in some instances with medium duty vehicles, 24,000 pounds. The vehicle simply will not stop on a dime at a speed as little as 30 mph. Consider "covering the brake" to shorten the stopping distance when negotiating all intersections.

Aero-medical Transport

Q What does the term aero-medical transport include?

A Aero-medical transport includes both fixed-wing aircraft and rotorcraft, which are more commonly referred to as helicopters. These missions are also referred to as medevac or airmedical evacuations.

Q When are fixed-wing aircraft used?

A Fixed-wing aircraft are used as the primary means of emergency transport in remote regions such as parts of Alaska. In addition, these aircraft are often used to bring critical patients, who sustain a serious medical emergency or injury while traveling, from far away places back to a hospital closer to their home. Fixed-wing aircraft are generally used for over 100-mile distances from the tertiary hospital facility.

Q What are the advantages of aeromedical evacuation?

A The advantages include:
- Rapid transport in situations where the time required by ground transport poses a threat to the patient's survival or recovery.
- Access to remote areas.
- Access to specialized critical care personnel or specialty units in certain hospitals (e.g., neonatal intensive care unit, reimplantation or transplant center, burn center).
- Access to personnel with specialty skills (e.g., surgical airway, thoracotomy, rapid sequence intubation).
- Access to specialty supplies and equipment (e.g., aortic balloon pump).

Q What are the disadvantages of aeromedical evacuation?

A The disadvantages to aeromedical evacuation include:
- Weather and environmental restrictions on flying, altitude limitations, and airspeed limitations.
- Depending on the specific aircraft used, the cabin size can place limitations on the number of crew members, equipment carried, and configuration of the stretcher in the aircraft. In the smaller aircraft, such as the commonly used Bell LongRanger®, besides restricting the number of flight crew members to one pilot and a flight-medic or flight nurse, the procedures that can be done on the patient in flight are limited.

- Flight climate control systems may not meet normal expectations. The thin walls of the fuselage do not allow much space for thermal insulation. The ship is hot in the summer and cool in the winter.
- It is also important that no glare from inside lights enters the pilot's compartment because this could severely affect her eyesight. Even though there is a curtain between the patient compartment and the pilot, often the lights still must be kept low, making ongoing patient assessment a challenge for the flight crew.
- Helicopter transport is very expensive. Some communities simply cannot afford to have a program.
- Due to the extensive preventative maintenance that must be done on the aircraft, there is also a considerable amount of down time.

Q How should the helicopter be accessed?

A Just as the public should access EMS by a single point (e.g., 911), there should be a single access point for the helicopter(s) in the region. In order for a helicopter program to be effective, the front line first responders, EMT-Basics, and EMS providers must be willing to consider the need for the helicopter as early as possible in each call when it may be warranted. The final decision on whether a mission is taken always takes into consideration the pilot's input on the safety of flying the aircraft during specific weather conditions, as well as the potential landing sites and terrain.

Q What are the indications for patient transport by helicopter?

A In most programs, the indications include:
- Medical life-threatening emergencies.
- Trauma life-threatening emergencies.
- Search and rescue missions.
- Anatomic or physiologic compromising factors that may warrant the need for air medical transport, including:
  1. Unconsciousness or decreased mental status.
  2. A Glasgow Coma Scale (GCS) of less than 10.
  3. A systolic BP less than 90 mmHg with signs of shock.
  4. A respiratory rate of less than 10 or greater than 30.
  5. Compromised airway.
  6. Penetrating injury to the chest, abdomen, head, or neck.
  7. Multiple long bone fractures.
  8. Flail chest.
  9. Paralysis or suspected spinal cord injury (SCI).

10. Severe burns with or without trauma.

11. Chest pain or shortness of breath.

12. Active seizures.

13. Amputated extremities.

- Injury factors that may warrant the need include:

  1. Lengthy extrications.

  2. Falls of 15 feet or more.

  3. MVC with a severe mechanism of injury (MOI).

  4. Rearward displacement of the front of the car by 20 inches or greater.

  5. Rearward displacement of the front axle.

  6. Passenger compartment intrusion of 15 inches or more.

  7. Ejection of the patient from a moving vehicle.

  8. Rollover with an unrestrained occupant.

  9. Gross deformity of a patient's contact point with the vehicle such as a bent steering wheel.

  10. Death of any occupant in the same vehicle.

  11. A pedestrian hit at 15 mph or more.

  12. A child less than 12 years old who is struck by a vehicle.

Why don't all helicopter programs do rescue missions?

Technically, the FAA does not license commercial operators to do rescue missions involving a special means of access such as rappelling out of the helicopter to access the patient. These missions are usually undertaken by highly trained teams who respond with police agencies under a public safety provision of the regulations.

How can EMS personnel learn the needs of the flight crews?

Once the decision has been made that a patient will be transported by helicopter, EMS personnel should keep in mind any special considerations or limitations that will be necessary prior to loading the patient. It is strongly suggested that EMS agencies set up in-service training so all of their personnel can become familiar with the flight personnel and their procedures before any mission occurs and review this information on a regular basis.

Are there any special packaging considerations if a patient is going to be transported in the helicopter?

Yes, there may be, depending on the regional program's procedures and the size of the ship. The patient may need to be immobilized on a specific type of backboard that fits into the

ship. Smaller helicopters only accept a specific size board. Larger helicopters may actually be able to take an entire stretcher. Some helicopter services have limitations on the length of the patient when supine, which could alter your method of immobilizing a fractured femur because a standard bipolar splint may extend the leg too long to fit in the ship.

Are there any special infection control procedures for a patient in the helicopter?

Yes, there may be. Some programs have infection control procedures designed to limit the spread of blood-borne pathogens in the helicopter such as wrapping the packaged patient in a disposable blanket or packaging the patient in a body bag.

Are there any special treatment considerations if a patient is going to be transported by helicopter?

It will be necessary to convert IV bags over to pressure infuser bags. Some flight crews need to intubate the patient prior to flight due to the limited area around the airway once the patient is loaded in the aircraft. Depending on the altitude that the helicopter flies, it may be useful to replace air with fluid in the air cuffs of tubes, such as ET tubes or Foley catheters, because the fluid will not expand or contract as a gas will under certain flight conditions. The MAST/PASG may also be affected by pressure changes. The problem arises during descent when the volume of gas in the chambers decreases, so it is important to maintain the pressure in the device on descent. The reverse is the case when ascending and is the reason why even a small pneumothorax is often managed with a prophylactic placement of a Heimlich valve or chest tube. When the helicopter rises, the injury could easily enlarge due to the changes in the pressure of the atmosphere at higher elevations.

Does the extreme noise have an impact on the patient care that can be administered in some helicopters?

Yes. Noise adds to the difficulty in assessing the patient's lung sounds in a helicopter. For this reason, it is imperative that tube placement be ensured by visualization, the use of an esophageal intubation device (EID), observing symmetrical chest expansion and condensation in the ET tube, and positive color changes or a reading with an end-tidal CO_2 detector. The use of the pulse oximeter is common to assist in ongoing patient assessment and monitoring the patient.

How safe is helicopter transport?

The medical helicopter industry has had a number of very serious crashes, especially in the mid-1980s. Great strides have been made in improving the safety of helicopter transport over the past decade. The focus on the safety of the flight personnel has been a key factor in bringing about these changes. The Commission on Accreditation of Air Medical Services (CAAMS) was developed as a voluntary process for aeromedical services to strengthen the safety of the aviation transport environment and to promote the highest quality of patient care.

PEARL

Several services have installed wire-strike equipment and adhered to a firm policy that the fly–no fly decision is based first on safety (e.g., fog), not on patient needs.

What is a landing zone or "LZ" and how is it established?

The flight crews should train all EMS personnel in the region on their procedures and expectations to maintain a safe scene and define a safe landing zone for the helicopter. A helicopter requires an LZ of approximately 100 by 100 feet (approximately 30 large steps on each side) (Figure 48–2) on a ground with less than an 8-degree slope. All EMS providers should be capable of selecting an LZ and describing the terrain, major landmarks, estimated distance to the nearest town, and other pertinent information to the pilot of the helicopter on a designated frequency.

How is the LZ properly marked?

The LZ and approach and departure path should be clear of wires, towers, vehicles, people, and loose objects. Most flight

crews suggest marking the LZ with a single flare in an upwind position. During night operations, never shine a light into the pilot's eyes as this could temporarily blind him or interfere with depth perception.

How should EMS providers approach the helicopter that has landed?

First, wait for the approval of the flight crew. Use extreme caution and follow the instructions that were discussed in your orientation with the flight crew and ship prior to any actual call involving patients. There are some general rules to follow:

- Make sure all loose objects are secured, such as pillows and linens on your stretcher.
- Allow the flight crew to direct the loading of the patient.
- Stay clear of the tail rotor at all times (Figure 48–3).
- Approach crouched down as a sudden gust of wind can cause the main rotor of a helicopter to dip to a point as close as four feet from the ground.
- If the helicopter is parked on a slight incline, approach it from the downhill side (Figure 48–4).
- Keep all traffic and vehicles 100 feet or more away from the helicopter.
- Do not allow anyone to smoke within 200 feet of the aircraft.

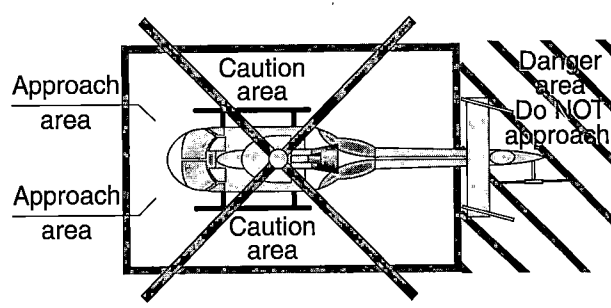

FIGURE 48-3 All EMS providers should be familiar with the danger zones around a helicopter.

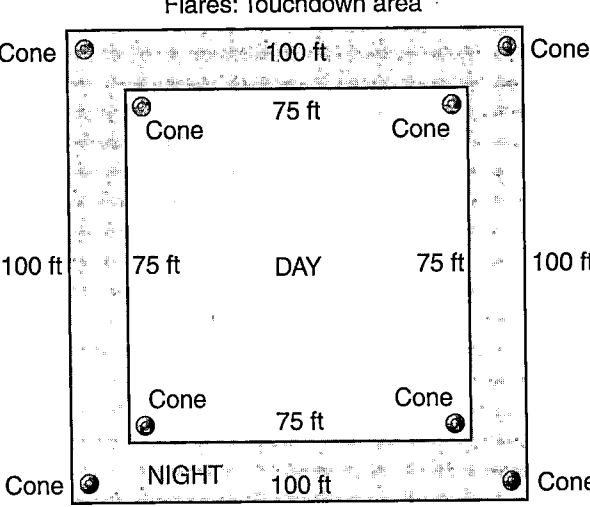

FIGURE 48-2 The marking of an LZ should be clear to the pilot from the air.

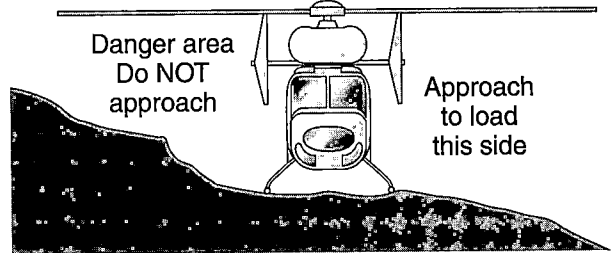

FIGURE 48-4 When approaching a helicopter that has landed on a slope, always approach from the downhill side to avoid injury.

Medical Incident Command Structure

Q Why is an incident management system (IMS) needed for handling major emergency medical services incidents?

A Any incident that involves multiple units responding to an incident requires management of the resources and personnel for a timely and efficient operation. When multiple agencies, especially from different jurisdictions, are involved, it is even more urgent that a system be in place to manage the incident and coordinate the response. EMS providers are trained to manage a single patient with multiple priorities. This is practiced on a daily basis. When the situation arises that they must manage multiple patients and deal with multiple units responding, which is not a daily practice, they need to fall back on an IMS that is simple and well understood by all providers. Each community needs to have an IMS that has been practiced and is understood by all of the providers in each of the agencies that may be asked to respond to any major incidents.

Q What is an MCI?

A An MCI is a multiple casualty incident that results in casualties that severely burden or exceed the normal EMS resources of an agency in whose area the event occurs. Some people use the term "mass" casualty incident for MCI. This is misleading because it gives providers the impression that the MCI plan should be saved for the "big one," such as a plane crash or bombing. It is strongly recommended that the MCI plan be practiced with all incidents involving a response of greater than two ambulances or more than two critical patients.

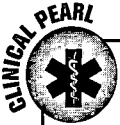

MCI plans work effectively in smaller, as well as in larger, incidents.

Q What should be sized up on arriving at the scene of an MCI?

A The scene size-up is the same as you have learned in prior chapters of this book. In addition, on the arrival at an MCI, the first unit should make immediate contact with fire and police representatives to gather facts and start coordination and effective communication. Gather information and report to your dispatcher a "first in size-up report" of the incident.

Q What should the first in size-up report include?

A The first radio report to your dispatcher is very important. Be sure to include the following:

- Incident location—be specific and give cross streets or distances from known locations.
- Extent of the incident—What do you see? What does the fire officer or police officer, who arrived prior to you, report has occurred? Gather an accurate description of the incident.
- Is the incident contained or continuing, open or closed?
- Location of the command post.
- Approximate number of patients.
- Access routes and the best location for a staging sector.
- Additional number of BLS or ALS units needed.

Q What is an open incident?

A An open incident is one where the patients are accessible and the EMS providers will have safe access to the patients. An example is a residential fire where all of the patients are out on the front lawn of the home.

Q What is a closed incident?

A A closed incident is one where the patients need to be rescued or extricated to gain access to them. An example is an overturned bus where there is limited access to the passengers inside.

Q What is a continuing incident?

A A continuing incident is one where the danger continues, such as a leaking tanker car with anhydrous ammonia or a terrorist bombing with the threat of secondary devices.

Q What is a contained incident?

A A contained incident is one where the cause has ceased and everyone who was going to be injured has already sustained her injury. An example is a ferryboat crashing under foggy visibility conditions into the dock, throwing many passengers down the metal stairwells.

Q What is the role of the EMS providers and agencies in planning for MCIs?

A The role of EMS providers and their agencies in planning is that of active participants. EMS agencies must participate in the local and regional planning for MCIs. They must educate all of their providers about the response plan and the IMS that is put in place during an MCI. The failure to be involved in this planning, educating, and drilling process will spell definite disaster for all involved. It is best summarized in the saying, "Failure to plan is planning to fail!"

What is the history of the ICS?

As a result of a series of devastating wildfires that roared across Southern California, burning over 600,000 acres and 772 structures in the fall of 1970, a task force was formed to develop a management system that allowed multiple agencies in multiple jurisdictions to work together with a common goal of life, safety, and property conservation. The task force that developed the original ICS consisted of representatives from the California Department of Forestry and Fire Preventions through the U.S. Forest Service and the Federal Emergency Management Agency (FEMA), along with the California State Fire Marshal's Office, the Office of Emergency Services, and FIRESCOPE (Firefighting Resources of California Organized for Potential Emergencies).

Though originally developed for fire services, ICS has been adapted to serve all emergency response disciplines. The system consists of procedures for controlling personnel, facilities, equipment, and communication. It is designed to begin developing from the time an incident occurs until the requirement for management and operations no longer exists.

In the early 1980s, Chief Alan Brunacini of the Phoenix Fire Department (PFD) was very active throughout the country presenting a series of workshops on the function of the fire service incident commander. In 1982, Captain Gary Morris, also from PFD, published an article in *JEMS* magazine broaching the issue of MIC. Ironically, this milestone in EMS occurred after a series of MCIs across the United States, including the MGM Grand and Hilton fires in Las Vagas, the Kansas City Hyatt Regency skywalk collapse, and the Washington, D.C., combined aircrash and subway accident.

According to Morris, the most effective commander must be a manager who is experienced in managing under emergency conditions on a daily or frequent basis. He must be familiar with the disaster plan, the EMS system, and the SOPs of each agency responding. The command, as well as all sector officers, should be clearly designated by a colorful vest and should simply use the radio designation "command." The early establishment of command and transferring command were addressed in the article, as well as a medical operation and fire operation branches for the ICS during a combined fire and EMS incident.

Brunacini went on to document his views in the excellent book, *Fire Command,* published by the NFPA in 1985. Many of the principles in this book are a detailed elaboration of the essential components of an ICS. In 1986, OSHA was directed by the Superfund Amendments and Reauthorization Act (SARA) to establish rules for operations at hazardous materials incidents. OSHA

requires, in 29 CFR 1910.120, that all organizations that handle hazardous material incidents use an ICS.

In 1987, NFPA developed standard 1500 that establishes a fire department occupational safety and health program. This standard states the following:

- That all departments should establish written procedures for an ICS.
- That all members be trained in ICS and that the responsibility for safety be specified for all supervisory personnel.
- That a system of accountability of all personnel at an incident be developed.
- That the department outline the safety requirements.
- That sufficient supervisory personnel be provided to control the position and function of all employees operating at the scene of an incident.

In 1990, NFPA issued standard 1561 that defines fire department emergency management systems. This standard provides guidelines for what should be included in an emergency management system. It emphasizes the importance that agencies and jurisdictions that work together in emergency operations have a common emergency management system.

Why is there an essential need for common terminology in an ICS?

Because there may be units from many different jurisdictions, it is easier to use simple sector titles based on the function they serve (e.g., staging, command, operations, triage, treatment, transportation, extrication). During an MCI is not the time to begin figuring out another agency's "code system." Plain English works best in these situations. It is much easier for responding units to report to the Incident Commander instead of trying to remember that the medic on unit 620 is the person commanding the EMS units at the scene.

What is meant by ICS organizational structure developing in a modular fashion?

Each incident may be different and not need all of the components of IMS or ICS. The organizational structure develops in a modular fashion at each incident. The development of the organization is top down, meaning that an Incident Commander (IC) is always designated for all incidents. As the incident needs dictate, additional responsibilities may be assigned by the IC. If they are not assigned, the IC serves in all of the roles.

What is an integrated communications plan?

The management of communication at an incident requires integrated communication. An integrated communication plan includes standardized procedures, the use of clear instructions with common terminology, two-way confirmation that the messages are received, and status reports on the assignments given to keep the IC updated. Radio frequencies should be set up ahead of time so that all arriving units have common frequencies. There are also tactical and command frequencies that can be used at the incident.

What are the purposes of the functional components of an IMS?

For larger or lengthy incidents any one or more of the functional components of an IMS may be implemented. There are five functional components (Figure 48–5); one is command, which is implemented at all incidents. The others are as follows:

- Operations—is responsible for all tactical operations at an incident. At a large-scale incident, this may include up to five branches, 25 divisions or groups, and 125 single resources, task forces, or strike teams.
- Planning—is responsible for the collection, evaluation, dissemination, and use of information about the development of the incident and the status of the resources. This includes situation status, resource status, documentation, and demobilization units, as well as technical specialists.

- Logistics—is responsible for providing facilities, services, and materials for the incident. This includes the communication unit, medical unit, food unit, service branch, supply unit, facilities unit, and ground support units within the support branch.
- Finance—is responsible for all costs and financial considerations at the incident. This includes the time unit, the procurement unit, compensations and claims unit, and the cost unit.

What is the difference between singular and unified command?

A singular command usually only works well when there is one emergency service agency responsible for the entire operation and no need for other disciplines to be involved. A unified command structure is more common and a key component of an ICS. This means that all involved agencies contribute to the command process by determining the overall goals and objectives, joint planning for tactical activities, and maximizing the use of all assigned resources at the incident.

How should the type of command relate to an on-scene command post?

At many larger incidents, a command post is set up so it is easy to find the commanding officer and so the necessary tools

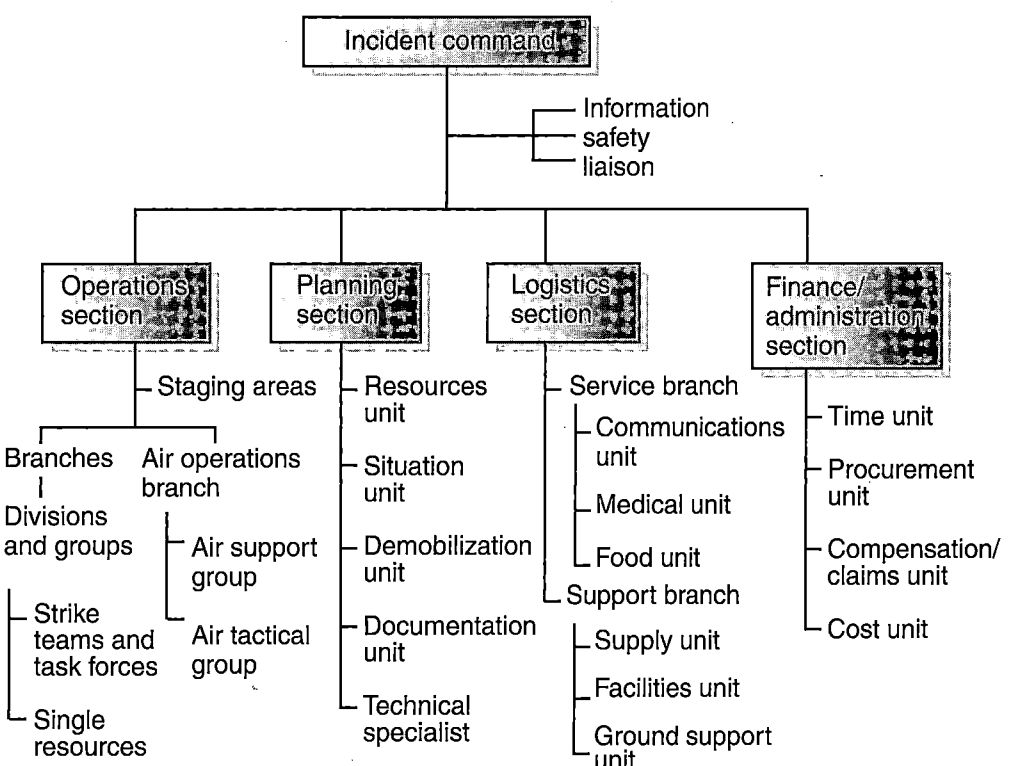

FIGURE 48–5 This chart demonstrates the IMS modular organizational components.

(e.g., maps, status boards, phones, radios, computer connections) for managing resources can be handled from one location. When setting up a command post, a unified command structure is best achieved by setting up one command post instead of a separate one for police, fire, and EMS services.

What is a consolidated action plan?

Every incident needs a consolidated action plan. This should be developed at the unified command post. It makes no sense for every sector to order up their own idea of how many additional units they think are needed at the scene. This approach can quickly deplete the resources of the entire region and add to a duplication of efforts. Complex incidents may require written action plans that cover all strategic goals, tactical objectives, and support activities for the entire operational period of the incident.

What is span of control?

Another key component of an ICS is the span of control. A manageable span of control is the number of subordinates that one supervisor can manage effectively. The desired range is from three to seven, with five being optimal. It can be very easy to lose track of your workers at an incident if they are not assigned to small units.

What is the role of the IC?

The IC is the individual with the overall responsibility for managing the incident. This responsibility includes:

- Assessing incident priorities.
- Determining the strategic goals and tactical objectives.
- Developing an incident action plan and the appropriate organizational structure.
- Managing incident resources.
- Ensuring personnel safety.
- Coordinating the activities of outside agencies.
- Authorizing the release of information.

What is the role of the EMS command or medical command?

In an incident that is primarily an EMS incident, the EMS Command or Medical Command is the first crew leader on the first arriving unit. His responsibilities include:

- Confirming the incident to dispatch.
- Managing the EMS response.

- Establishing a command post and remaining there.
- Designating the EMS division or sector officers.
- Working cooperatively with other agency commanders.

What is the importance of a transfer of command?

At an incident, as supervisory personnel arrive, sometimes it is logical to transfer command to a different person. Brief the person who will be assuming the command face-to-face on what has gone on and what is needed. The transfer of command should be seamless and all sector officers, dispatch, and arriving units need not know there is a new person commanding the incident. The radio designation remains the same, Command, EMS Command, or Medical Command.

What are some of the differences between the command structures at small, medium, or large incidents?

Smaller incidents may have EMS or Medical Command, triage, and transport sectors. A medium-sized incident may require a treatment and field hospital sector, a safety officer, and an extrication sector.

The larger incidents or incidents that need an IMS for long periods of time may have a public information officer and the additional sections such as operations, logistics, finance, or planning.

Operating at an MCI

What is involved in establishing command at an MCI?

Establishing command at an MCI involves a number of very important tasks. The following is a list to be considered:

- Perform a scene size-up.
- Locate police and fire officers and establish a unified command post.
- Don the EMS command vest.
- Notify the EMS dispatcher of the first in size-up report.
- Designate a triage officer.
- Designate a staging officer and notify the dispatcher to have additional ambulances respond to the staging sector.
- Request that the dispatcher call hospitals for bed availability.
- Designate a treatment officer and location for this sector (as needed).
- Designate a transportation officer and location for this sector (as needed).

- Consider the need for aeromedical evacuation and find an appropriate landing zone near the scene.
- Consider the usefulness of a school bus to transport low-priority patients. Make sure everyone on the bus is medically examined and that medical personnel also ride on the bus.
- Consider need for an extrication sector (if not already established).
- Consider the need for a safety officer.
- Consider the need for follow-up critical incident stress management (CISM) and rehab of personnel.
- Keep the dispatcher and other service chiefs in close contact throughout the incident.
- Along with police and fire officers, consider need for a public information officer to work with arriving media.

What is the purpose of bibs or vests?

The bibs or vests make it easy to identify the command officers at the scene of an MCI. They can be easily donned over the uniform and outer coat. As the saying goes, the IC wears all of the vests until she begins to delegate the responsibility for the command positions.

What other sector officers are helpful at an MCI?

The following sector officers may be necessary, depending on the size of the incident: safety, logistics, rehabilitation, staging, treatment, triage, transport, extrication and rescue, morgue, communication, and the public information officer (PIO).

What is the value of a scribe at an MCI ?

Some ICs like to have a scribe or a support person, similar to a chief's driver in large city fire departments, to help assist with their communication and to take notes. This is especially helpful when the command post is being operated out of the back of a car or there are many units to keep track of.

How important is staging?

At some incidents, it is absolutely essential! An analysis of an incident where staging was not done often reveals very cluttered scenes without ample time to establish a flow of vehicles. If a staging sector is set up, as an ambulance is needed at the scene, they pull up, pick up their patient as assigned, and then transport to the facility assigned to them. There have been MCIs where the ambulances could not leave the scene because the streets were so congested with emergency vehicles—they literally had to tow parked units off the scene to make a pathway.

Staging is also helpful because personnel can report to staging and not the scene. Typically if the personnel show up at the scene and the command structure at the scene is not yet prepared for them, freelancing and chaos often occurs. Long-range basic needs can be attended to in the staging sector also (e.g., restrooms, food, a place to rest).

CLINICAL PEARL

> *A lack of restroom facilities is inconvenient and potentially dangerous for all responders. Include this as one of your major planning needs.*

Where should the command post be set up?

It should be set up in a safe location that is visible from the scene, but not directly in the middle of all the action. For example, the tower at the airport where all of the key players can be located with all of the resources needed.

The Function of Triage

What is triage?

Triage is a French word that means "to sort." All EDs have a triage desk where a nurse or other qualified health care professional asks a few key questions of every patient coming in the door to determine what priority they should be for treatment. At an MCI, triage is done on all patients to ensure that the most serious patients are treated and transported first. In situations where there are many serious patients and limited ambulances, the very critical patients who have a small chance of survival are given the lowest priority (e.g., cardiac arrest, mortal head wound).

What is the best place to put physicians and nurses who show up at the scene of an MCI?

It is not uncommon for physicians and nurses to stop at the scene of an MCI and offer assistance. Use them where their expertise can help best. Put them in the treatment sector managing patients or in the triage sector evaluating priorities. It is not a good idea to take a physician or nurse who is not familiar with the workings of your EMS system and put them in a sector officer position.

What is the value of triage tags?

Triage tags can be very useful tools. The hardest part is getting the crews to pull them out and start using them! Some EMS agencies have tag days where all patients are tagged to give the crews practice using the tags. Typically there are a few different types of triage tags commercially available for services to purchase. Some states have actually designed their own tags and issued supplies to all EMS agencies. Most tags have four priorities: P-1 (immediate or red), P-2 (delayed or yellow), P-3 (hold or green; often referred to as the "walking wounded,"), and P-0 (deceased, no priority, or black). One very useful aspect to triage tags is that it helps to eliminate the need to reassess each patient over and over again. Once the patient is tagged, it is clear that an EMS provider has seen them at least once.

What are some helpful tips that can smooth out the operations at an MCI?

There are lots of tips that can help smooth out the operations at an MCI. Here are a few:

- Cones are always helpful to control the flow of patient movement.
- Colored tarps are a great idea for designating triaged patients placed in a field hospital or treatment sector. If each vehicle carries red, yellow, green, and black tarps, there will be plenty to use.
- Rather than tie up the radios with each ambulance calling into the hospital, the transport sector officer should designate a communication staff person to call into the hospitals with an abbreviated report of how many patients and what priority they have assigned to the hospital.
- The driver, keys, and stretcher should never leave the ambulance.
- Limit radio communication. When on the scene, walk over and talk face-to-face.
- Have dispatch call mutual aid for availability.
- Use the media for their lighting equipment and to make appropriate traffic notifications.

What is START?

START is an acronym for simple triage and rapid treatment. This is a method of triaging that was developed in Newport Beach, California, in the early 1980s. Under START, the first concept is to clear an area and tell all of the walking wounded to get up and walk over to that location. After clearing the scene of many of the walking wounded, the next step is to triage each patient in less than 60 seconds, assessing their respiratory status, hemodynamic status, and their mental status (Figure 48–6). Basically, patients who have an adequate respiratory status, hemodynamic status, and are alert are classified as "delayed." If they do not have an adequate respiratory status or hemodynamic status or are not alert, they are usually classified as "immediate."

The START process permits a few rescuers to triage large numbers of patients very rapidly. If this is the system used in your region, check with your medical director for more specifics on how to use the system.

Which patients fit into the following triage categories: immediate, delayed, hold, and deceased?

Here are some examples:

- P-1, Red—airway or respiratory compromise, severe burns, cardiac, severe bleeding, open chest or abdominal wounds, severe head injuries, severe medical problems (e.g., heart attack, strokes).
- P-2, Yellow—burns, multiple fractures, spinal injury, uncomplicated head injury.
- P-3, Green—minor fractures and wounds, burns <10 percent of the body surface area (BSA), psychological emergencies.
- P-0, Black—expired or cannot be saved.

What are some tips for dealing with lots of low-priority patients?

Some systems like to put them on a school bus and take them to a hospital that is not being used for the high-priority patients. This is an acceptable idea provided that all patients are examined and cleared to ride on the bus and that medical personnel ride on the bus with a supply of equipment in case a patient's condition changes enroute to the hospital.

What should be done to manage stress at an MCI?

MCIs are one of the indications for CISM. Keep this in mind and call for the team in your area to consider the need for debriefings or defusings. For more on this topic see Chapter 1, The Well-Being of the EMS Provider.

What modifications to radio traffic should be done at an MCI?

As much as possible, limit radio traffic so the command officers can do their job. Face-to-face communication is helpful whenever possible.

Practice, Practice, Practice

What is the value of drills?

Practice makes perfect. It is not wise to practice only once every few years when your region has the big airport drill. Prac-

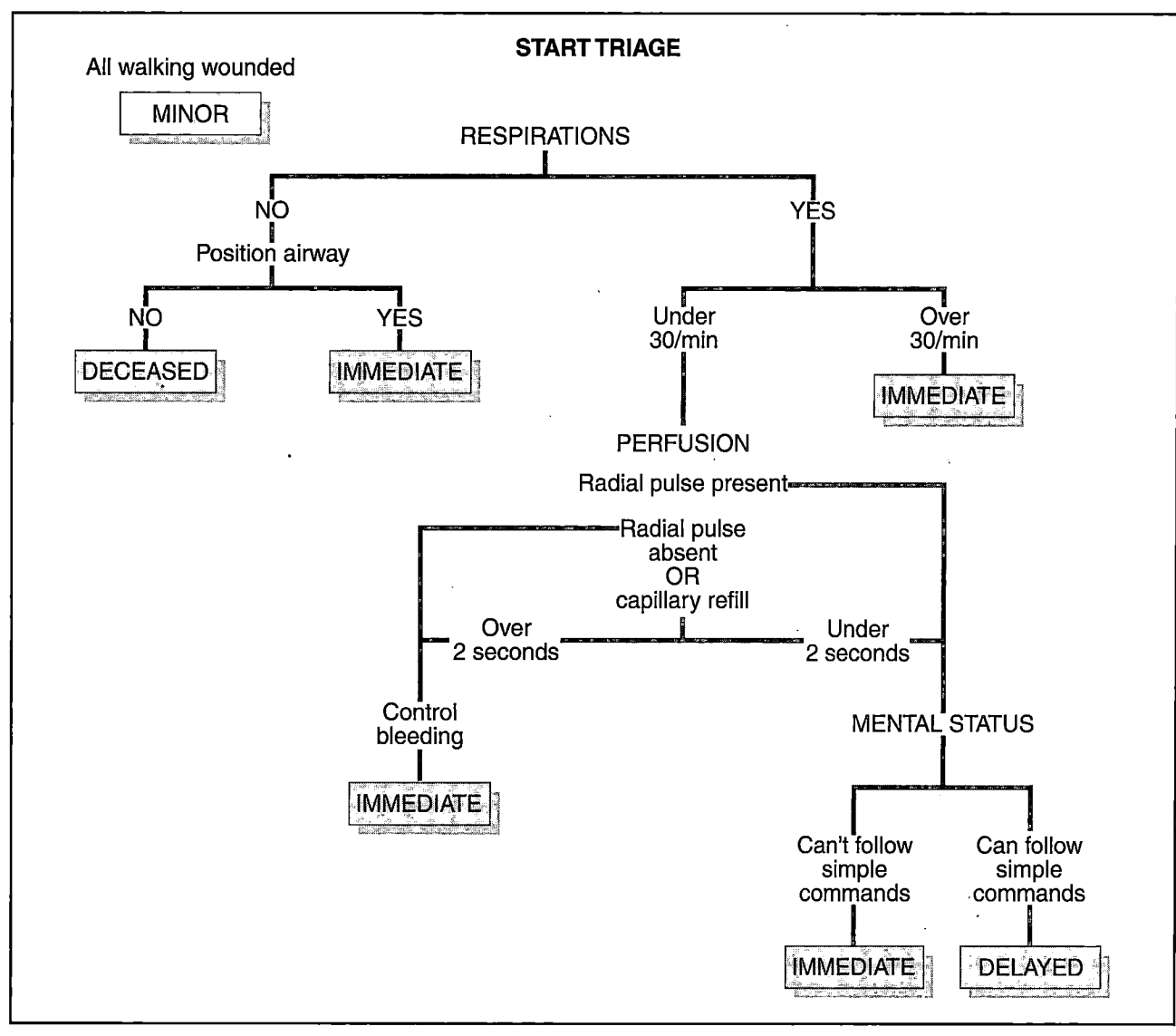

FIGURE 48-6 START stands for *simple triage and rapid treatment.* Here is an algorithm used for START triage.

---

tice should be done frequently with small drills that involve two or three agencies with small numbers of patients, such as the van crash drill with six critical patients.

What is the value of tabletop simulations?

Some areas have developed rather elaborate tabletop simulations involving HO scale cities and vehicles. This is good practice especially if radio communication is used and the different emergency services work together through realistic problems that could happen in your community. It is also helpful to use as a tool to get the commanders and supervisory personnel used to working together.

What lessons have been learned from the analysis of previous MCIs?

Each incident is different and has its unique challenges. There are a few common themes that seem to pop up in many of the critiques, such as:

- Separate radio frequencies are helpful.
- There is too much radio traffic.
- The local media tie up all of the cellular phone channels.
- Staging should be set up earlier.
- A separate PIO to brief the media helps relieve the IC of that responsibility.
- Recent planning and drills pay off!

- Limit the uninvited EMS units or personnel by sending them to the staging sector.
- The proper staging of vehicles allows for a good flow of ambulances to the scene.
- Staging and dropping off extra equipment at a central point is helpful.

Q **What is the value of a post-incident critique?**

A There is something to be learned from each incident so we can do a better job the next time. In a non-threatening manner, the commanders of each emergency service should schedule a critique to discuss the incident. This is not a media event and is not to be confused with a CISD, which serves a totally different function.

Rescue Awareness and Operations

This chapter discusses "rescue" and operating at scenes that involve specialty rescue teams. The focus is on *why* specialty teams can be helpful and how not to get hurt by taking on a rescue that is over your head in terms of training or equipment capabilities. All EMS providers should be trained to the awareness level in rescue specialties so they clearly know when to call for the right backup to mitigate a complex rescue situation.

Rescue and the Role of the EMS Provider

What exactly is "rescue?"

The definition of *rescue* according to Webster is "the act of delivery from danger or imprisonment." Humans who are traumatized or stranded are in need of rescue.

What should drive the priorities of every rescue?

Because there is no rescue if there is no patient, all rescues should be driven by patient need. It is just as frustrating to have a specialized rescue team that has no idea about patient care as it is frustrating to have a team of EMS providers who have no concept of rescue! Although it is not practical to train every EMS provider in the detailed operational-level skills and knowledge for each rescue specialty, it is important that each EMS provider be trained to an "awareness level."

What is awareness level training?

Awareness level training implies enough knowledge to comprehend the hazards and realize that additional expertise is needed to effect the rescue.

What is the problem with not training EMS providers to the rescue awareness level?

Failing to train EMS providers in rescue awareness eventually ends in injury or death to the EMS personnel or patient.

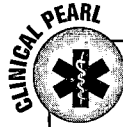

Just as in patient care, the first concern in rescue is rescuer safety.

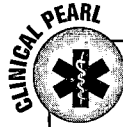

One of the major benefits of rescue awareness training is to avoid a provider attempting a rescue for which he is not trained.

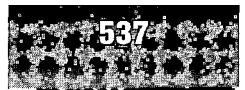

Q Why is medical and mechanical training needed to effect a successful rescue?

A Rescue involves a combination of medical and mechanical skills, with the correct amount of each applied at the appropriate time. The patients must be accessed and assessed for their treatment needs. Treatment must begin at the site of the incident while the patient is being released from their entrapment or imprisonment. The medical care must continue throughout the incident. The medical and mechanical skills must be carefully balanced to ensure that patients obtain effective treatment and timely extraction. Rescue efforts must be driven by the patient's medical and physical "needs."

Q What is the role of the EMS provider at a rescue operation?

A The role of the EMS provider in a rescue operation may differ by locality and the specific additional training beyond the awareness level that your agency has provided. In general, however, all EMS providers should have the proper training and personal protective equipment (PPE) to allow them to access the patient and provide assessment and management at the site of the incident, as well as throughout the incident.

Q What hazards should the EMS provider be aware of at a rescue scene?

A As the "first responder" to many types of incidents, the EMS provider should understand the hazards associated with various environments (e.g., hot, cold, below grade, toxic atmosphere, in the water, and structurally unstable situations). It is essential that the EMS provider know when it is safe and when it is not safe to gain access to the patient or attempt a rescue.

Q How much training should the EMS provider have in rescue?

A The amount of training beyond the awareness level is clearly a function of the role that the EMS provider will be taking in your community. This is something that needs to be well thought out by the leadership of the EMS and rescue agencies before an actual incident occurs because it may involve policy development, equipment purchases, and extensive training.

When it is deemed a safe environment, the EMS provider should be trained in the appropriate skills to effect a rescue or at least participate in the rescue under the guidance of individuals with additional expertise. The EMS provider should understand the rescue process and when various techniques are indicated or may be contraindicated.

Rescuer and Patient Protective Equipment

Q How important is PPE for the EMS provider when responding to rescue scenes?

A PPE is very important to the EMS provider! Personal safety must be the paramount issue in any rescue situation. The EMS provider will jeopardize her own safety and the safety of the patient without the appropriate protective gear. In a rescue situation, the PPE is more extensive than the typical gloves, eye-shield, and mask worn for body substance isolation (BSI).

Q Is there one set of PPE that fits all situations?

A Unfortunately, there is not! The PPE needs to be appropriate for the situation encountered as shown in Table 49–1. For example, full firefighting gear is inappropriate in a water rescue situation. Your PPE may not prevent exposure to infectious disease, but it does minimize the risk. Most PPE has not been specifically designed for EMS workers. The typical EMS provider's PPE has historically been adapted from other fields such as firefighting, mountaineering, and occupational safety.

Q What types of helmets should be available for the EMS provider?

A The best helmets have a four-point, nonelastic suspension system, in contrast to the two-point system found in construction hard hats. Most of the four-point suspension helmets are designed to withstand more severe impacts than hard hats. Avoid helmets with nonremovable "duck bills" in the back because a helmet should be compact enough to wear in tight spaces. A compact firefighting helmet meeting NFPA standards is adequate for most vehicle and structural applications. Climbing helmets are often used for confined spaces and technical rescue situa-

TABLE 49–1

Personal Protective Equipment for Rescue
All rescues—helmet, eye protection, hearing protection, respiratory protection, gloves, boots, turnout gear, appropriate lighting, PPE for BSI.
Water rescues—kayaking helmet, specialized personal flotation device (PFD), knife, whistle.
Ice rescue—exposure suit, ropes, PFD.
Confined space—self-contained or supplied air breathing apparatus (SCBA or SABA) (for those appropriately trained in their use), full body harness.
Off road or high angle—climbing helmet, harness, backcountry survival gear (if needed).
Hazardous materials—specialized exposure suits depending on training and the substance involved.

tions. A padded rafting or kayaking vented helmet is more appropriate for a water rescue.

What types of eye protection should be available for the EMS provider?

The eye protection should include both goggles, vented to prevent fogging, and industrial safety glasses held by an elastic band. These should be ANSI (American National Standards Institute) approved. The faceshield on most fire helmets is inadequate protection for your eyes.

What types of hearing protection should be available for the EMS provider?

From a purely technical standpoint, high-quality earmuff-style hearing protectors, similar to those worn by aircraft landing ground crews, provide the best protection. Practicality, convenience, and availability also play a role in the choice of hearing protectors. The multi-baffled rubber earplugs used by the military and sponge-like disposable earplugs are good choices. They should be used by crews or patients whenever working in high noise areas, especially if superior hearing protectors are either unavailable or impractical.

What types of respiratory protection should be available for EMS providers?

Surgical masks or commercial dust masks are adequate for most occasions. These should be routinely supplied to all EMS units.

What types of gloves should be available for EMS providers?

In addition to disposable rubber or latex gloves for BSI purposes, leather work gloves, such as those used for gardening, are usually best for protection against cuts and punctures. They allow the free movement of the fingers, as well as provide good protection. Heavy, gauntlet-style firefighting gloves are too awkward for most rescue work.

What types of boots should be worn by EMS providers?

High-top, steel-toed or shank boots with a coarse lug sole to provide traction and prevent slipping are preferred for EMS providers. For rescue operations, lace-up boots provide greater stability and better ankle support by limiting the range of motion. They also don't pull off as easily as pull-on boots in deep mud. Insulated boots may be helpful in some colder environments.

What type of "turnout gear" should be used by EMS providers?

Turnout gear, coveralls, or jumpsuits add some arm and leg protection and can be put on quickly. They also protect the uniform pants and shirt if they are not the actual uniform. Strong consideration should be given to using Nomex®, PBI®, or flame-retardant cotton to provide limited flash protection. They can be designed with bright colors (e.g., orange or lime) with reflective trim and symbols for high visibility. Some services have a standard operating procedure (SOP) that highly visible gear or orange or lime safety vests must always be worn during highway operations both day and night. Insulated gear or jumpsuits are helpful in cold weather; however, they can also increase heat stress during heavy working conditions or high ambient temperatures. Typical firefighting turnout gear provides the best protection against the sharp, jagged metal or glass that is found when extricating a patient from vehicle wreckage or structural collapse.

Why are PFDs recommended as necessary PPE for the EMS provider?

PFDs that meet the U.S. Coast Guard standards for flotation should be available on the EMS unit that responds to bodies of water. There may not be a major lake or river in your district, but there certainly are residential swimming pools. PFDs should always be worn when operating on or around water (Figure 49–1). The Type III PFD is preferred for rescue work. A knife that can be easily accessed, a strobe light, and a whistle should be attached to the PFD.

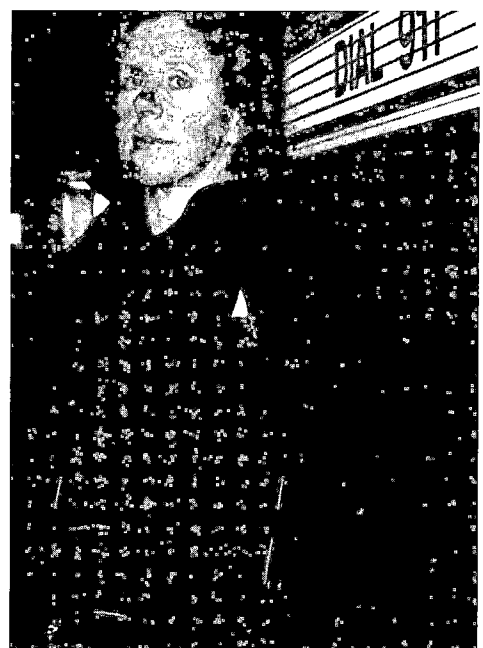

FIGURE 49–1 A PFD should be worn by all EMS providers whenever operating around a body of water.

![Q] Why is lighting recommended as PPE for the EMS worker?

![A] Depending on the type of rescue involved and the location, EMS providers should have access to portable lighting. Carry a flashlight or consider carrying a headlamp that can be attached to a helmet for hands-free operation.

![Q] Should hazardous material suits or SCBA be provided to the EMS provider for rescues?

![A] Hazardous material suits or SCBA should only be made available to personnel who are thoroughly trained in their use. These items are often supplied on specialty support vehicles, such as hazardous material (hazmat) response units.

![Q] When should a survival pack be considered PPE for the EMS provider?

![A] If your unit has the occasion to provide EMS coverage to a remote or wilderness area, have a backcountry survival pack available. This compact backpack should be prepacked with PPE for inclement weather conditions (e.g., cold, rain, snow, wind) and have provisions such as a water purifier, or actual personal drinking water, snacks for a few hours, potential shelter, and a light source.

![Q] What equipment should be available at the rescue scene for patient personal protection?

![A] Many of the considerations for EMS provider safety also apply to patients. Patient safety equipment should include the following items:

- Helmet—There is usually no need for patient helmets to be as heavy duty as those of the EMS providers. The less expensive, construction-type hard hats are adequate. If you anticipate severe hazards, outfit patients with the same high-grade helmets that the EMS providers use for the situation.
- Eye protection—A set of vented goggles, held in place by an elastic band, are ideal for the patient. They are not as easily dislodged as safety glasses. Workshop faceshields also may be useful for the patient.
- Hearing protection—The hearing and respiratory protection used by the EMS providers is adequate for the patient.
- Protective blankets—A variety of protective blankets should be available to shield patients from debris, fire, or weather. Inexpensive vinyl tarps do a good job of protecting patients from water, weather, and most debris. Aluminized rescue blankets should be available for protection from fire, heat, or glass dust. Commercially available wool blankets provide excellent

insulation from the cold. Plastic sheeting (e.g., the kind used by landscapers) is inexpensive, durable (usually 3–4.5 millimeters thick), and comes in large rolls. Trash bags of many sizes and thickness are also useful. One 55-gallon drum liner is large enough to cover a single patient. It also can be used as a disposable blanket, poncho, or vapor barrier.

- Protective shielding—The circumstances may call for protective equipment more substantial than blankets or plastic sheets. All EMS providers should be trained to use backboards and other commonly found equipment as shields to protect patients from fire, weather, falling rock or debris, glass, or other sharp-edged objects. The shield that is specifically designed for a Stokes® basket should be available. Keep in mind that a device that shields a patient from debris or the elements may also limit the EMS provider's access to the patient.

Safety Procedures

![Q] Why should rescue teams have written SOPs?

![A] All teams should have written safety procedures or SOPs that are familiar to every team member. The contents should include sections on all types of anticipated rescue. Procedures should specify the required safety equipment, particular actions required or prohibited, and any rescue-specific modifications in assignments. SOPs should include a statement requiring a safety officer and describing his relationship to command.

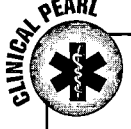

CLINICAL PEARL

The need for SOPs in rescue is identical to the need for policies, procedures, and protocols in any EMS system.

![Q] What is the role of a safety officer at a rescue operation?

![A] The safety officer is part of the command structure for the incident. The safety officer should be someone with the knowledge and authority to intervene in unsafe situations. This person makes the "go–no go" decision for the operation.

![Q] What else can be done to minimize the safety hazards to the EMS providers at the scene?

![A] In addition to written procedures and the selection of a safety officer, an EMS unit must anticipate crew assignments and special needs in advance. These tasks can be done through personnel screening and careful preplanning.

What is the value of personnel screening for an assignment to specialty rescue units?

Search and rescue planners often use personnel screening to determine the participants in the rescue process. Programs are available that identify the physical capabilities of crew members. The findings of these programs could have significant impact on personnel assignments. In addition, psychological testing is recommended. It may even be desirable to screen for specific traits, such as phobias. For example, a rescuer's inordinate fear of heights or small spaces should be considered in assigning rescue duties.

What is the purpose of a rescue plan?

A rescue plan contributes greatly to personnel safety and operational success. Preplanning starts with the identification of potential rescue locations, structures, or activities. Effective preplanning then evaluates the specific training and equipment needed to manage each of these incidents. The preplan also generates ideas on the efficient use of existing personnel and equipment and anticipates the need for additional equipment, rescuers, or expertise.

What other considerations for the health and well-being of the EMS provider and rescue personnel should be made at a rescue that will take a long time to complete?

Provisions must be made for the maintenance and rotation of EMS providers and rescue personnel at lengthy operations. Plans should be made for "stand-by" or staging sites that offer protection from the weather. Sites should be away from the immediate operation area and secure from bystanders and the media. Personnel should be rotated at controlled intervals. The crew should follow predetermined policies regarding food and hydration. To maintain maximum personnel performance, rescuers should eat frequently, but in small amounts. The diet should be high in complex carbohydrates and low in complex sugars and fats that "hype" the rescuer up and are difficult to digest. This is not the time for coffee and doughnuts! Fluid replacement should consist of plain water or relatively dilute electrolyte solutions (e.g., Gatorade®, XLorate®, PowerAde®).

Phases of a Rescue Operation

What are the phases of a rescue operation?

The seven phases of a rescue operation are shown in Table 49–2.

TABLE 49–2

Phases of a Rescue Operation
• Arrival and size-up.
• Hazard control.
• Gaining access to the patient.
• Medical treatment.
• Disentanglement.
• Patient packaging.
• Transportation.

What responsibilities does the EMS provider have during the arrival and size-up phase of a rescue operation?

Size-up begins with the dispatcher's call and subsequent arrival at the scene. Although the dispatch message may indicate a rescue situation, the responding crew must understand the environment and potential risks. They must rapidly establish medical command and conduct a scene size-up to determine the number of patients and appoint a triage officer and other personnel as necessary. Notify dispatch if the magnitude of the incident exceeds the capability of either the EMS unit or routine backup. Initiation of multiple casualty incident (MCI) response procedures, implementation of mutual-aid agreements, and the contact of off-duty personnel can be an unfamiliar, and hence slow, process. Also, as the principal on-scene medical personnel, you have to estimate the severity of the injuries, the need for ALS, and patient transport needs.

What is the importance of the EMS provider in identifying the type of rescue?

The EMS provider should quickly identify the type of emergency or rescue operation. For example, you arrive at a structural collapse, vehicle rescue, water rescue, or climbing accident. Each situation can necessitate specialized crews, additional medical supplies, or the need for sophisticated equipment.

What is meant by determining the need for a rescue versus a body recovery?

The decision whether the incident is a search, a rescue, or a body recovery must be made. Often this involves a quick "risk versus benefit" analysis based on the conditions found on arrival. Be careful not to overestimate your capability to handle a rescue situation. Individual acts of courage may be called for, but rescue operations involve safety first, not heroics. If in doubt, always err on the side of precaution and safety.

Q What are the responsibilities of the EMS provider during the hazard control phase of a rescue?

A On-scene hazards need to be identified with equal speed and clarity. Often the EMS provider must deal with these hazards prior to attempting to reach the patient. To do otherwise places everyone at the scene at risk. Control as many of the hazards as possible. Some situations involve hazardous materials, chemical spills, radiation, or gas leaks. These types of incidents require a specialized hazmat team, so the EMS provider's approach should be limited to creating a safe perimeter, attempting to identify the substance involved from a safe position, and keeping bystanders and EMS personnel away from the hot zone. Other situations pose the potential for fire or explosion. Only a spark is needed to set off a gas leak or oil spill. Electric wires hold a "double threat" for fire and electric shock.

Q Can the actual environment be the hazard?

A Yes, the very environment in which the EMS provider is standing can be risk filled. Look around to determine the possibility for lightning, avalanche, rock slides, cave-ins, and so on. Manage and minimize the risks from uncontrollable hazards as soon as possible to avoid other injuries.

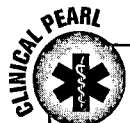

CLINICAL PEARL

The failure to heed environmental hazards is dangerous for both you and for the patient.

Q What safety precautions should be taken at all rescue scenes?

A Ensure that all EMS providers are in the PPE appropriate for the situation. Make sure all EMS personnel are clearly visible and always alert to traffic at the scene. Intoxicated drivers attracted to the bright lights have killed EMS providers at highway incidents.

Q What are some other examples of hazards that may exist at the scene of a rescue?

A Other potential hazards include the following conditions:
- Poisonous or caustic substances.
- Biological agents or germ-infested materials.
- Water hazards such as swift-moving currents, floating debris, or toxic contamination.
- Confined spaces such as vessels, trenches, mines, or caves.
- Extreme heights, particularly in mountainous situations.

- Possible psychological instability such as those experienced in hostage crises, urban violence, mass hysteria, or individual emotional trauma on the part of either the patient or the crew.

Q What responsibilities does the EMS provider have to gain access to the patient at a rescue incident?

A Once the hazards have been controlled, the EMS provider should gain access to the patient(s). Determine the best method to gain access to the patient. Command needs to deploy personnel to the patient. It may be first necessary to stabilize the physical location of the patient (e.g., structural collapse, cave-ins, vehicle rollover).

CLINICAL PEARL

Though you may need to gain access to the patient, do so only with appropriate assistance from trained rescue personnel. Do not risk your own safety simply to access the patient.

Q What should be considered if the patients are hidden from view?

A On rare occasions, you will come across rescue situations that "hide" patients. Such conditions involve entrapment in vessels, cave-ins, avalanches, and structural mishaps. If possible, ask dispatch to send an on-scene specialist (e.g., search and rescue [SAR] team member) to meet the crew. Search dogs, electronic detection devices, or an experienced search manager may be required to find the patients.

Q What is meant by developing the rescue plan?

A During the access phase, key medical, technical, command personnel, and the safety officer must agree on the strategy that will be used to accomplish the rescue. To ensure that everyone understands and supports the rescue plan, a quick formal briefing should be held for rescue personnel before the operation begins. Even with well-trained personnel and adequate equipment, rescue efforts are often poorly executed because team members do not understand the "big picture" or do not know what they, or their fellow rescuers, are supposed to do.

Q What is the responsibility of the EMS provider during the medical treatment phase of the rescue?

A After gaining access, medical personnel can begin to make patient contact. No EMS provider should enter an area to provide patient care unless they are protected from hazards with PPE and have the technical skills to reach, manage, and remove patients safely. In a rescue, an EMS provider has the following three major responsibilities:

- Initiation of patient assessment and care as soon as possible.
- Maintenance of patient care procedures during disentanglement.
- Accompaniment of the patient during removal and transport.

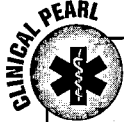

> *No EMS provider should enter an area to provide patient care unless they are protected from hazards with PPE and have the technical skills to reach, manage, and remove patients safely.*

In a rescue situation, what is the focus of the patient assessment conducted by the EMS provider?

To the extent possible, quickly conduct an initial assessment (MS-ABC and c-spine status) on each patient (discussed in detail in Chapter 15, Scene Size-Up and Initial Assessment). The next critical steps include rapid trauma assessment for the trauma patient with a significant mechanism of injury (MOI), detailed physical exam, and medically oriented recommendations to evacuation teams. Because a long time may pass before patients are ready for transport, their condition can change significantly during disentanglement and removal. As a result, the EMS provider should perform the patient assessment with two goals in mind. First, identify and care for existing patient problems. Second, anticipate changing patient conditions and determine the assistance and equipment needed to cope with those changes.

What is disentanglement?

Disentanglement is a rescue term that means to remove, sometimes piece by piece, the debris or parts of the vehicle from around the patient(s) so they may be freed for removal from the vehicle or structure.

> *Disentanglement literally means removing the wreckage from the victim, not the other way around!*

What are examples of situations where the priority of patient care is BLS and not ALS?

In many situations, the best overall patient care requires the rapid basic stabilization and immediate removal of the

patient rather than ALS interventions done at the site of the incident. Medical management should be provided appropriate to the situation. Final positive patient outcome may depend on the initial sacrifice of definitive patient care so the patient and rescuers can be removed from imminent danger. Example of such situations include:

- Injured, stranded high-rise window cleaners; workers on water, radio, or TV towers; high-rise construction workers.
- Patients involved in a trench cave-in.
- People stranded in swift running, rising water.
- Patients entrapped in vehicles with an associated fire.
- Patients overcome by life-threatening atmospheres.

In all of these cases, rapid transport of a nonstabilized patient to a safer location is justified by the risk of injury to the rescuers and the possibility of worsening patient injuries by applying "definitive" patient care at the scene. This rapid movement might be required even though the transport itself will aggravate the patient's injuries.

Is the treatment of a patient being rescued the same as all other patients?

Specifics of patient management during a rescue are often the same as protocols and procedures used "on the street." However, some specifics may be, or should be, significantly different. Differences are based mainly on the effects of lengthy time periods required to access, disentangle, or evacuate the patient. EMS providers are trained in rapid stabilization and transport, particularly with trauma patients. However, during a rescue mission, the desire to achieve speedy transport, as well as to obey the cherished "Golden Hour and Platinum Ten" rules, may be irrelevant. The EMS provider must be able to "shift gears" mentally to an extended care situation.

How should the EMS provider be prepared to provide more in-depth psychological support for the patient?

The EMS provider should be prepared to provide psychological support for the patient during a rescue. This is especially true in situations where the patient is entrapped for a considerable amount of time. Establish a solid rapport with the patient, striking up a constant reassuring conversation. In quieting the fears of rescue patients, try to use the following tips:

- Learn and use the patient's name.
- Be sure the patient knows your name and knows that you will not abandon her.
- Be sure that other team members know and use the patient's correct name. The term "it" should never be substituted for the patient's name in any out-of-hospital setting.

- Avoid negative comments regarding the operation or the patient's condition within earshot of the patient.
- Explain all delays to the patient and reassure her if problems arise.
- Ask special rescue teams to explain technical aspects of the operation that could directly impact the patient's condition. Translate these operations into clear, simple terms for the patient.

What is the responsibility of the EMS provider during the disentanglement phase of the rescue?

The disentanglement phase may be the most technical and time-consuming part of the rescue. During this phase, the EMS provider has the following three responsibilities:

- Personal and professional confidence in the technical expertise and confidence that the gear needed will function effectively in the active rescue zone (also referred to as the hot zone or inner circle).
- Readiness to provide prolonged patient care.
- Ability to call for and use specialty rescue resources.

If an EMS provider or another member of the rescue team cannot fulfill these requirements, reassess available rescue personnel and call for backup. This is not a place for the claustrophobic or squeamish because sometimes the only means of disentanglement may be a field amputation. The methods used to disentangle the patient must each be analyzed for their risk versus benefit to the patient's medical needs and the estimated time they take to perform.

What is the responsibility of the EMS provider during the patient packaging phase of the rescue?

The patient packaging needs to take into consideration the means of egress (e.g., a litter carry through the woods versus walking a patient out), as well as the time the patient has to live based on the medical conditions (e.g., rapid extrication technique versus Kendrick extrication device application). Some patient packaging can be more complex than others considering the specialized rescue techniques required to get them out of the situation they were found in (e.g., being lifted out of a hole in a Stokes® by a ladder truck, being vertically hauled up through a manhole in a SKED®). In situations where the patient may be vertical or suspended in a Stokes® basket, it is essential that the EMS provider know how to properly package the patient to prevent any additional injury.

What are the responsibilities of the EMS provider during the transportation phase of the rescue?

The removal of the patient may be one of the most difficult tasks to accomplish or may be as easy as placing him on the stretcher and wheeling him 50 feet to the ambulance. Activities involved in the removal of a patient require the coordinated effort of all personnel. Transportation to a medical facility should be thought out well in advance, especially if you anticipate delays. Decisions regarding patient transport, whether by ground vehicle, by aircraft, or by being manually carried out, should be coordinated with advice from medical control. Enroute to the hospital, do the ongoing assessment, repeating vitals every five minutes for an unstable patient and 15 minutes for a stable patient. Update the patient's condition and administer additional therapy as ordered by medical control.

What disciplines are considered by EMS providers to be "special rescue operations" or "special ops?"

The rescue operations that include technically difficult procedures, very specialized equipment, or both are considered special ops. *Only personnel with special training and experience in these areas should attempt these rescues!* Special rescue operations include:

- Surface water rescue—including moving water or flat water.
- Hazardous atmospheres—including confined space, hazardous material incidents, trenches, and cave-ins.
- Highway operations—also called vehicle rescue.
- Hazardous terrain—including high-angle rescue and off-the-road rescue.

Water Rescues

What are the typical incidents involving water rescues?

The usual water rescue involves a body of water where a patient has gotten into trouble. This may include pools, rivers, streams, lakes, canals, or even the ocean. Some communities have drainage systems, which are usually dry, but flash floods can create raging rivers in these systems.

What can EMS providers do to prepare for water rescue incidents?

Incidents in or around water are preventable and each EMS provider should do his part to become familiar with aquatic practices by learning to swim, carrying PFDs (and wearing them whenever around the water or ice), and taking a basic water rescue course.

What is the significance of cold-water rescues?

Compared to the normal human body temperature of 98.6 degrees F, almost any body of water is colder and causes heat loss. The temperature in smaller bodies of water varies widely with the seasons and snow runoff. Even on warm days, the temperature can be quite cold in most places. Water temperature and heat loss are contributing factors to the demise of both the patient and the improperly equipped EMS provider.

Immersion in cold water can rapidly lead to hypothermia. Humans cannot maintain body heat in water that is less than 92 degrees F. The colder the water, the faster the loss of heat. Compared to the air, water causes a heat loss at a rate 25 times faster. Immersion for more than 15 to 20 minutes in 35 degree F water is likely to be fatal. Contributing factors to the hypothermic patient's demise are an inability to attempt self-rescue due to becoming incapacitated, an inability to follow simple directions, an inability to grasp a line or flotation device, and the sudden immersion may trigger a laryngospasm and increase the likelihood of drowning.

CLINICAL PEARL

Remember that hypothermic patients tend to be dehydrated due to the "cold diuresis." Remove them from the water in a horizontal position to avoid orthostatic stresses. Also, removing a person from water, regardless of the temperature, is like suddenly removing MAST/PASG—the circumferential hydrostatic pressure of the water is suddenly lost.

What is the value of a PFD on the EMS provider at a water incident?

The use of a PFD lessens heat loss and conserves the energy required for flotation. It may save a life even if someone is a good swimmer.

What is the HELP position?

If you become suddenly submerged, you should assume the heat-escape lessening position (HELP). This position involves floating with the head out of the water and the body in a fetal tuck (Figure 49–2). Researchers estimate that someone who has practiced with HELP can reduce her heat loss by almost 60 per-

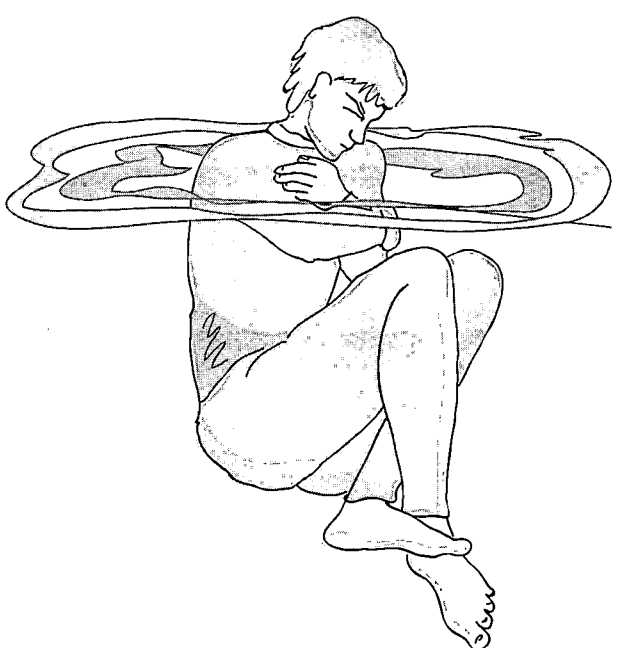

FIGURE 49–2 The heat-escape lessening position (HELP).

cent as compared to treading water. When in the water with a group, it is suggested that victims huddle to decrease the heat loss and provide a better target for rescuers.

What is a survivability estimate at a water rescue?

A survivability estimate should be done as quickly as possible after arriving at the scene of the incident to help weigh the risk of the rescue against the benefit of the rescue. Determine if this is a rescue or a body recovery. The estimate should include the best available information on the following factors:

- The number of patients.
- The number of trained and equipped rescuers.
- The environmental conditions present and expected.
- Age of the patients.
- The length of submersion of patients.
- Any known trauma to patients.
- The temperature and speed of water.

What are the subtypes of water rescues?

Rescues involving water are usually broken into moving water and flat water (nonmoving). If your EMS unit is a responder to frozen bodies of water, consider additional ice rescue training and obtaining the proper cold-water entry dry suits.

What is the water rescue model and responsibility of the EMS provider?

The water rescue model is Reach-Throw-Row-Go. All EMS providers should be trained in reach and throw techniques. A PFD must be worn, even for shore-based rescues. If at first you are unable to talk the patient into a self-rescue, then reach with a pole or long rescue device. If this is not effective or the patient is too far out, try throwing a flotation device. All EMS providers should become proficient with a water throw bag for a shore-based water rescue. Water throw bags are designed to carry a polypropylene line that can easily be thrown to the patient in the water with good accuracy. Both boat-based rescues and swimming techniques require specialized water rescue training.

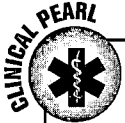

Do not attempt a swimming rescue unless you are specially trained and there is no other alternative.

What are the special capabilities of swift-water rescue teams?

The competency to cope with swift-water rescue situations comes only through extensive experience. Trained swift-water rescuers should have a background in the technical operations required by high-angle rope rescue. In addition, they must also be able to adapt these techniques to the specific demands of swift water. To prepare for technical rope rescues, swift-water rescuers must be competent and well practiced in the skills of crossing, defensive swimming, negotiating strainers, using throw bags and boogie boards, shore-based swimming, boat-based rescue techniques, the ability to manage water-specific emergencies, and the ability to package the patient with water-related injuries and illnesses for transport.

What are the hazards of moving water?

People are drawn to moving water for recreation. This is especially dangerous when combined with alcohol, which contributes to a considerable number of drownings each year. Many people, as well as EMS providers, underestimate the power of the water. The force of moving water is very deceptive and it cannot be overstated that EMS providers should not enter moving water without specialty training. The hydraulics of moving water change with variables such as depth, velocity, and obstructions to flow.

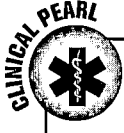

Alcohol or drug abuse underlies many of the drownings that occur each year.

What is the "drowning machine effect" of moving water?

Water moving over a uniform obstruction to flow, such as a large rock or low head dam, can literally create a "drowning machine." On appearance, a low head dam seems very tame and often fishermen are seen on the downstream side casting into the recirculating water (Figure 49–3) This is a good place to catch fish because they can often be seen just below the dam. If you stop for a moment and think about this, if the fish with their natural ability to swim get stuck in the recirculating currents, why is it so hard to believe that the same thing will happen to humans who get too close to the dam? Once caught in the recirculating current, it is very difficult to escape and the rescue can be a very hazardous one even for specially trained rescuers.

What is a strainer and what hazards does it present?

Water moving through obstructions to flow, such as downed trees, grating, or wire mesh, is referred to as a "strainer." The current can force a patient up against a strainer, making it difficult to be removed due to the power of the water. The current may be flowing into a drainage pipe under the surface that is protected by a metal grate. A patient can get sucked into the grate with the force of the water pinning her up against the object.

What should the rescuer do if he accidentally falls into swift-moving water?

If you fall into water floating swiftly downstream and see yourself potentially getting pinned by a tree or obstruction, it is suggested that as you approach the object you attempt to swim over it. It is extremely unsafe to walk in fast moving water over knee depth because an extremity can get trapped. When this occurs, the weight and force of the water knocks the victim down, often pinning them face down in the water. In order to be

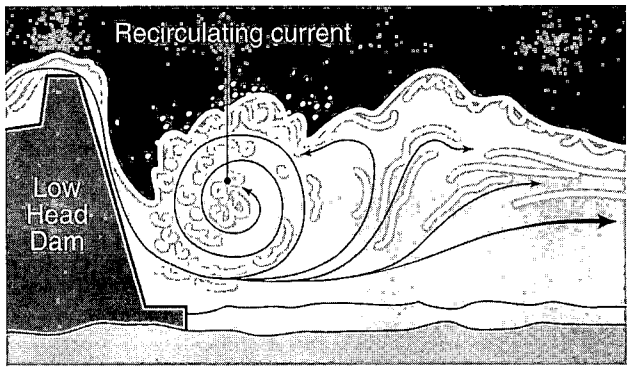

FIGURE 49–3 The low head dam produces a "drowning machine" as the water recirculates, making it nearly impossible to swim clear of the dam.

removed from an extremity pinning, the limb must come out the way it went in and the force of the water often makes this extremely difficult.

What techniques of self-rescue should the EMS provider be aware of when working around water?

The EMS provider should be aware of self-rescue techniques should he inadvertently fall into the water. First, cover your mouth and nose during entry, then protect your head and keep your face out of the water. In moving water, do not attempt to stand up. Float on your back and point your feet downstream. Steer with your feet and point your head toward the nearest shore at a 45-degree angle or continue to float downstream until you come to an area where the water slows enough for you to swim to the river's edge.

When water turns a bend in the river, the outside of the curve moves faster than the inside of the curve. If you are being carried rapidly downstream, steer to the inside of the next curve in the river. Also there are often large objects, such as rocks, that block the flow of the water and cause the water to circulate back upstream around the downstream side of the obstruction. This back current is called an eddy, and the currents are slower and sometimes will actually sweep you toward the river's edge to safety.

What is the greatest problem with flat water for the EMS provider?

The greatest problem with flat water is that it seems so tame. Two out of every three drowning victims are non-swimmers who never planned on entering the water. Alcohol is a very large contributory factor to as many as 50 percent of the boating fatalities. Many states have enacted tough laws to restrict the operation of a boat while intoxicated.

How can drowning incidents be prevented?

Wearing PFDs whenever around water can reduce drownings considerably. Merely having PFDs available is not enough; they must be worn. One study showed that of the boating accident fatalities in 1987, 89 percent were not wearing a PFD. The same goes for EMS providers; all agencies responding to bodies of water should have PFDs available and a very strict policy that they be worn.

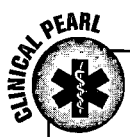

PEARL

PFDs that are not worn are not helpful.

What is the protective response when submerged in cold water?

The water temperature contributes considerably to death in patient submersions because hypothermia can quickly incapacitate the patient and lead to drowning. The human body has a protective response to cold water referred to as the mammalian diving reflex, which can increase the chances of a cold-water drowning patient's survival. Due to this reflex, saves have been documented from cold immersion of up to 66 minutes. The colder the water, the more it seems to increase the chances of survival. Another factor can be how long the head was above the water during the cooling process.

The actual protective physiologic response involves the following: face immersion causing parasympathetic nervous system stimulation, a heart rate decrease to a bradycardic rhythm, peripheral vasoconstriction and shunting of the blood to the core of the body, and a drop in the BP.

What aspects can affect the patient's survivability profile?

Age, posture, fat (adipose tissue), lung volume, and the water temperature affect the patient's survivability "profile." Due to the number of survivors from cold-water submersion, the saying is, "You are never cold and dead, you are only warm and dead." Hypothermic patients should be presumed salvageable with resuscitation efforts continued until they are rewarmed so an accurate assessment can be made.

On arrival at a water rescue, what should you ask the bystanders right away?

Try to establish a location of the submerged patient based on quick interviews with witnesses. Try to separate the witnesses and ask them to return to the locations where they were during the incident and to describe exactly where they noticed the victim go under the water. Ask each witness to try to locate an object across the water to form a line. Then, use the point of convergence of the lines to locate the most accurate "last seen point," which is then used as the "datum" point to begin searching for the patient. Search patterns should form larger circles away from this point at least the distance equal to the depth of the water.

How should the patient who is found in a swimming pool or body of water be immobilized and removed from the water?

First, assume there is a spinal injury. The patient should be immobilized in the water. Because this technique is not routinely described in EMS textbooks, we have included it here. The procedure is similar to the long-board application with a few modifications:

- Phase One—In-water spinal immobilization (can be done with one EMS provider)

    1. Approach the patient from the side to use the head-splint technique. There are other techniques, but they do not work as well when the EMS provider is wearing a PFD.

    2. Move the patient's arms over her head.

    3. Hold the patient's head in place by using the patient's arms as a "splint."

    4. If patient was found face down, after steps 1–3, rotate the patient toward the EMS provider into a face-up position.

    5. Ensure an open airway.

    6. Maintain this position until a cervical collar is applied.

- Phase Two—Rigid cervical collar application (requires two EMS providers)

    1. The second EMS provider should determine the proper collar size.

    2. The second EMS provider then holds the collar open under the patient's neck.

    3. The primary EMS provider maintains immobilization and a patent airway.

    4. The second EMS provider brings the collar up to back of patient's neck as the primary EMS provider allows the second EMS provider to bring collar around the patient's neck and throat, while the primary EMS provider maintains the airway.

    5. The second EMS provider secures the fastener on the collar, while the primary EMS provider maintains the airway.

- Phase Three—Back boarding and extrication from the water (requires at least three EMS providers in the water and additional EMS providers at the water's edge)

    1. Submerge the board under the patient at his waist. It is strongly suggested that you use a floating backboard for water rescue.

    2. Never lift the patient to the board, allow the board to float up to the patient.

    3. Secure the patient with straps, cravats, or other devices.

    4. Move the patient to an extrication point on shore or a boat.

    5. Always extricate the patient head first so that body weight will not compress the possible spinal trauma.

    6. If possible, avoid the extrication of the patient through surf because the board could capsize and dump the patient back into the water. Consider using bystanders who can swim as a breakwall behind the patient.

    7. Maintain airway management during the extrication.

Hazardous Atmospheres

What is the difficulty with confined-space rescues?

The major problem with confined spaces is that they often are oxygen deficient. Most confined spaces appear, at first glance, to be relatively safe. As a result, rescue procedures may appear far less difficult, time consuming, or dangerous than they actually are. Consequently, as a rescue category, confined-space rescues have the highest fatality rate among potential rescuers. In fact, NIOSH estimates that 60 percent of the fatalities associated with confined spaces are people attempting a rescue of a patient.

What is the definition of confined space?

The definition of a confined space in the OSHA regulation (CFR 1910.146) is "a space with limited access or egress that is not designed for human occupancy or habitation." Examples of confined spaces include:

- Storage or transport tanks.
- Grain bins.
- Silos.
- Wells and cisterns.
- Vessels.
- Manholes.
- Pumping stations.
- Drainage culverts.
- Pits.
- Hoppers.
- Underground vaults.

CLINICAL PEARL

> *Confined spaces (e.g., manholes) are deceiving. They look habitable, but may contain little oxygen or deadly invisible toxins.*

What are some of the ways that confined spaces can pose a threat to their occupants?

Confined spaces present threats to occupants for the following reasons:

- They are often oxygen deficient—rescuers often do not see the threat and presume the atmosphere is safe. Prior to entering a confined space, specially trained entry teams always must monitor the atmosphere to determine the following: oxygen concentration, hydrogen sulfide level, explosive limits, flammable atmosphere, and toxic air contaminants.

- They may contain toxic or explosive chemicals—some chemicals are very toxic to inhale, while other chemicals displace oxygen in the red blood cells (RBCs). Some chemicals are highly explosive. The types of gases found in confined spaces include hydrogen sulfide, carbon dioxide, carbon monoxide, exceptionally low or high concentrations of oxygen, methane, ammonia, and nitrogen dioxide.
- They may create an engulfment hazard—the patient can get buried in fine solid materials that can flow like sand such as grain, coal, or dust. Dust also creates an explosive hazard.
- They can get entrapped in machinery—confined spaces often have machinery, such as augers or screws, that can entrap the patient.
- They can electrocute the patient—confined spaces often have motors and materials to manage equipment that has electrical power. Sometimes this machinery can have stored energy. It may be necessary to dissipate all stored energy prior to the rescue team entering the space and "Lockout–Tagout" procedures (an OSHA safety requirement) must always be followed to prevent further hazards when rescuers are in the confined space.

- They may present limited access due to structural concerns—often these spaces have structural supports, such as "I" beams, that can cause injury due to limited light and height. Not all spaces are cylindrical. Spaces that are "L," "T," or "X" shaped can present difficult extrication problems. In addition, an air supply is needed for the rescuers. Due to limited access, sometimes through small manholes and tight tubes, SCBA use is difficult. SCBA has a limited air supply and many entries are not possible with standard SCBA on. Confined-space rescue teams often use SABA lines and need to be lowered into the hole with a full body harness on for ease of retrieval should something go wrong (Figure 49–4).

Does industry have any responsibility in preventing hazards with confined spaces?

Yes—most employers are required to develop a confined-space rescue program that includes providing training for their employees who work in and around confined spaces. These employees may be called on to perform on-site rescues. The typical emergencies in confined spaces involve: falls, medical

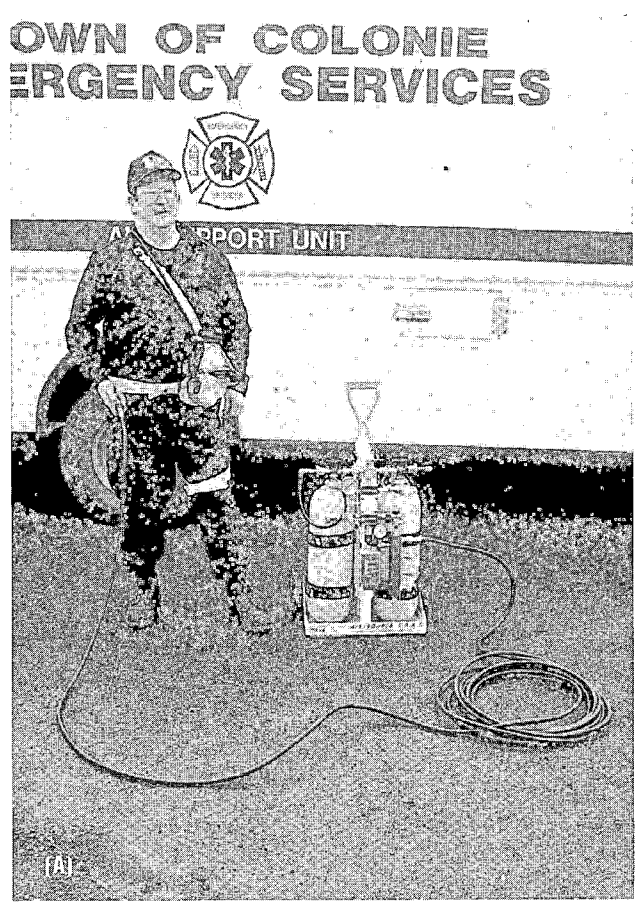
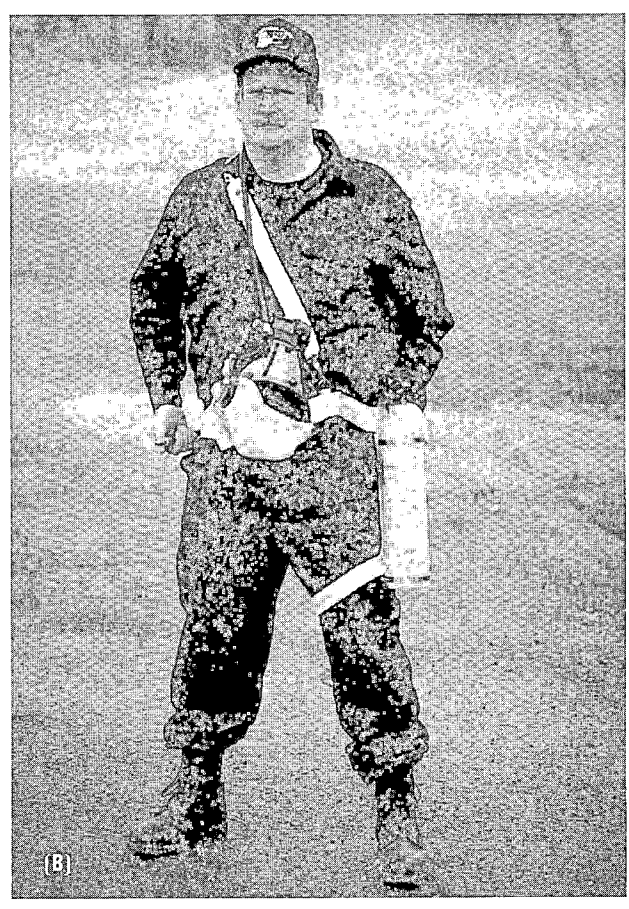

FIGURE 49–4 Confined-space rescue requires the use of supplied air. (A) A supplied air respirator with face piece, hose, and air supply. (B) Note the emergency escape cylinder on his hip.

emergencies, oxygen deficiency or asphyxia, explosions, or entrapment. OSHA requires a permit process before workers may enter a confined space. Most industries have strict requirements such as continuous atmospheric monitoring, posted warnings, and work-site permits with detailed data on hazard management. The area must be made safe or workers must don PPE. Retrieval devices must be in place when workers enter the spaces. The non-permitted sites are likely locations for emergencies because no atmospheric monitoring is done and the entrants are likely to encounter oxygen-deficient atmospheres. EMS providers should never be allowed to enter a confined space to perform a rescue unless they have training, equipment, and experience specific to this environment.

How common are trench rescues?

Although it certainly is very dramatic to watch rescues from cave-ins or structural collapses every time the earth quakes in California, rescues from trenches or cave-ins occur in all communities. Most trench collapses occur in trenches less than 12 feet deep and 6 feet wide. Patients are suddenly covered with heavy soil, resulting in asphyxia. A typical cubic foot of soil weighs 100 pounds and two inches of soil on the chest or back can weigh between 700 and 1,000 pounds.

What are the usual reasons for a trench cave-in?

The reasons for a cave-in or collapse typically include:

- Contractors disregarding safety regulations to save money. Federal law requires either shoring or a trench box for excavations deeper than five feet.
- The lip of one or both sides of the trench caves in.
- The wall falls in or shears away.
- The soil pile (dirt removed from the hole) was piled too close to the edge of the trench, causing the sides of the trench to collapse.
- Water seepage.
- Ground vibrations.
- Intersecting trenches.
- Previously disturbed soil.

What should be the EMS provider's initial response to a trench rescue or cave-in?

The initial response to a trench rescue or cave-in should involve sizing up the scene, establishing command, and securing a perimeter. If the collapse caused burial, a secondary collapse is likely to occur. Call for the team specializing in trench rescue and

do not allow entry into the trench or cave-in area. Specially trained personnel should make safe access only after shoring is in place.

Highway Operations and Vehicle Rescue

What is the greatest hazard when working a highway operation?

The greatest concern is the traffic itself. Emergency vehicles have been struck and motorists driving right into the scene of a collision have killed EMS providers. Studies have shown that drivers who are drugged, intoxicated, or tired actually drive right into the emergency lights. EMS providers must work closely with the law enforcement on the scene to ensure that the scene is as safe as possible and that the traffic is being routed properly away from the area where they are working. The police should quickly take control over the flow of traffic to avoid unnecessary congestion, especially when the collision is on a limited access highway where congestion can easily impede access by other emergency vehicles assigned to the scene.

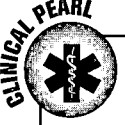

Always assume that oncoming traffic is unable to see you and act accordingly.

What are examples of strategies that can help to reduce traffic hazards?

The reduction of traffic hazards involves the combination of the following strategies:

- Staging—always consider staging emergency vehicles away from the scene and have command bring them in when there is an appropriate place for them and assignment for the crew. The staging area should be within a minute or two of the scene in a large parking lot or much less congested location. This is especially helpful on limited access highways.
- Positioning emergency vehicles—place the vehicles in a position to assist with protecting the scene and disrupt the least amount of traffic flow. The ambulance loading area should not be directly exposed to traffic and should not solely rely on the ambulance lights to warn traffic because they are often obstructed when the doors are open for loading.
- Emergency lighting—only a minimum of warning lights should be used to make it clear to the oncoming traffic that there is a hazard and to define the actual size of your vehicle. When too many lights are used, it is very confusing and blinding to the

oncoming traffic. It is strongly advised that your headlights be turned off when parked at the scene. Many services have switched over to large amber lights placed on the top corners of their emergency vehicles to signal a hazard.

- Redirect traffic—as soon as the first unit arrives on the scene, flares or cones should be placed to direct traffic away from the collision. If the police have not yet arrived, this may be your responsibility. Remember, this is hazard control, which is always an early phase of rescue. The flares should create a safety zone and move traffic away from the emergency workers. Take caution not to place flares too close to the scene due to the danger of igniting fuel on the street or brush on the side of the road. Once flares have been lit, let them burn themselves out. Attempting to pick up flares once lit can cause very severe chemical burns.

- Stay visible at all times—all EMS providers should be dressed in highly visible clothing. Because many EMS, police, and fire agencies wear a dark-colored uniform, it is strongly advised that either a turnout coat, which is very visible, or an orange vest with retro-reflective tape be donned at the scene of the collision.

What additional hazards should EMS personnel be aware of at the scene of a highway operation?

In some communities the EMS providers are trained to manage hazards at the scene of a highway operation. In other communities, they are trained to be aware of these hazards and call for rescue personnel to manage the hazards. No matter what the procedure may be in your response area, it is essential that all EMS providers be able to recognize the potential hazards at a highway operation to avoid becoming injured.

Examples of non-traffic hazards found at highway operations include:

- Fire and fuel—fuel spilled at the scene increases the chance of a fire. Be very cautious when you smell fuel or see liquid on the ground at a collision. Keep in mind that bystanders who are smoking can cause a bigger problem than the original crash if there is spilled fuel. Do not drive your emergency vehicle over a fuel spill or park on one! Remember that under each vehicle is a catalytic converter (which has a temperature around 1,200 degrees F) that is a good source of ignition for a fire. Be especially careful sizing up a collision where the vehicle has gone off the road onto tall dry grass that could be ignited easily by the catalytic converter.

- Alternate fuel systems—be aware of alternate fuel systems in vehicles involved in a collision. There may be a natural gas or high-pressure tank at risk of fire or explosion. Electrically powered vehicles have storage cells that may be very dangerous. Even a loose oxygen cylinder in the trunk of an EMS

provider's personal vehicle can be extremely dangerous when involved in a collision if it is not properly secured.

- Sharp objects—at the scene of a collision, there often are lots of sharp metal or glass objects that can injure rescuers. Wear leather gloves, protective gear, and eyewear and be very careful of glass.

- Electrical hazards—a downed power line is often obvious, yet rescuers still get too close to this lethal hazard. If it is in contact with the vehicle, consider the vehicle to be "charged" and call the power company immediately. In most new communities, the electric lines are no longer overhead; they are underground. This can present a hazard if a vehicle runs up onto a generator or electrical feed box. This may not be very obvious, so always look under the car and around all four sides during your size-up before coming in contact with the vehicle.

- Energy absorbing bumpers—the bumpers on many vehicles have pistons in them and are designed to withstand a slow speed collision to limit the damage to the front or rear of the vehicle. Sometimes these bumpers become "loaded" in the crushed position and do not immediately bounce back out. When exposed to a fire or simply tapped just the right amount by rescuers working around the vehicle, the spring can rapidly become unloaded. There have been cases where a bumper was thrown 100 feet from the vehicle. If this happens, you do not want anyone to be nearby or they may get seriously injured. EMS providers must properly deal with loaded bumpers before the area around a loaded bumper can be considered safe. If you see a loaded bumper, stay away from it unless you are properly trained to deal with it.

- Supplemental restraint systems (SRS)—air bags, which have not deployed during a collision, have been known to deploy in the middle of extrication. Rescuers have been seriously injured by the accidental deployment of the SRS. If the patient removal involves a mechanical disentanglement and extrication, consider deploying the SRS so it does not inadvertently go off. The auto manufacturers can provide information about the power removal or power dissipation of their brand of SRS. Many newer vehicles are now also installing side impact bags.

- Hazardous cargo—most hazardous substances travel by highways across our nation. Always be suspicious when collisions involve commercial vehicles, vans, and trucks. There are many outlaws who transport hazardous cargo without properly placarding the vehicle. If you see a placard, read it from far away with binoculars, before actually approaching the scene.

- Unstable vehicles—on arrival at a highway operation, size up the vehicles involved to determine if they are in a safe position. Don't overlook the subtle situations that can occur. For example, many people involved in a collision forget to place their vehicle in park. You arrive at the scene and see a vehicle on all four wheels and consider it in a stable position.

Someone from your crew jumps into the rear seat to manually stabilize the patient's neck and suddenly the vehicle starts rolling down the street because the transmission is not in park. Some vehicles need to be stabilized on their side or roof or on an incline, embankment, or unstable terrain. Don't forget to turn off the ignition and be aware that some cars have remote ignition starters on their key rings. EMS providers should learn the proper techniques of temporary stabilization with ropes, chocks, or a come-a-long until the vehicle rescue team has arrived at the scene (Figure 49–5).

🅠 What auto "anatomy" should the EMS provider become familiar with?

🅐 There is a limited amount of auto anatomy that every EMS provider should know. Obviously, the specifics of each automobile are different and members of vehicle rescue teams need to be in-serviced on a regular basis on the changing vehicle designs and functions. The EMS provider should be knowledgeable about the following parts of a vehicle:

* Roof support posts—are named from the front of the vehicle toward the back of the vehicle with the first post, supporting the roof at the windshield, called the "A" post. The next post is "B" and the third post, found in a sedan or station wagon, is "C." Station wagons also have a "D" post. After removing the plastic moulding on the posts, the remaining steel can easily be cut with a hacksaw and some power steering fluid to reduce the heat of the cutting. Vehicles with unibody construction require that all posts, floor, firewall, trunk support, and windshield be intact to maintain the integrity of the vehicle. If you cut a post to remove the roof, remember this could affect the entire vehicle depending on where else the frame has been stressed, causing it to bend or fold. Most vehicles are unibody construction these days. The older vehicles and light trucks are frame construction.

* Firewall—separates the engine and occupant compartment. The firewall can collapse on a patient's legs when involved in a high-speed head-on collision. Sometimes the patient's feet may go through the firewall. Movement of other parts of the vehicle, such as cutting a post or rocker panel, can cause additional pressure on the patient's feet.

* The battery—the engine compartment usually contains the battery. This can cause a fire hazard, so many rescue teams cut the cables to eliminate this hazard. It is a good idea to move electric seats back and lower power windows prior to disconnecting the power.

* Safety glass—the glass that is used in the windshield and is designed to crack when struck with an object such as a flying stone. It is a combination of two layers of glass with a plastic laminate layer in the middle. When shattered or broken, safety glass stays intact. It does produce glass dust and shards of

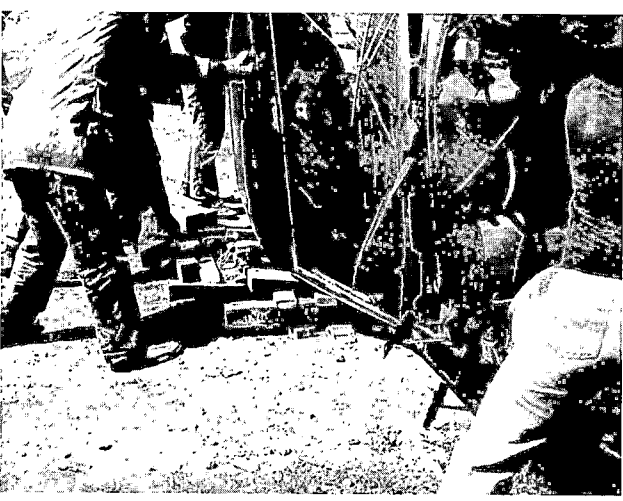

FIGURE 49–5 Training to stabilize a vehicle on its side with cribbing prior to gaining access. *(Courtesy of Bob Elling)*

glass that can easily cause cuts or get into the eyes, nose, mouth, or wounds, so it is essential to cover the patient whenever removing this type of glass.

* Tempered glass—is the glass designed to withstand blows with a blunt object without breaking. This glass is used in the side and rear windows of a vehicle. When tempered glass is struck with a sharp object, it shatters into many small beads.

* Door reinforcement bars—the doors of most newer automobiles contain a reinforcing bar designed to provide protection to the occupant in a side impact collision.

* Nader pin—to help keep the doors from blowing open during a collision, there is a case-hardened pin, named after the consumer advocate who lobbied to mandate them on cars, called a Nader pin. The Nader pin must be disengaged to make it possible to pry the door open unless hydraulic jaws are used.

🅠 What steps are involved in accessing a patient through the doors at a vehicle collision?

🅐 To assist in accessing the patient through a door, the EMS provider should be trained, by a rescue instructor, to take the following steps:

* Try all four doors first.
* Gain access through a window furthest away from the patient.
* Be aware of how to open a door using simple hand tools: peel back the outer sheet metal on the door, expose the lock mechanism, unlock the lock, pry the cams from around the Nader pin, and then pry the door open. This can be helpful in situations where there is a delay in the arrival of the vehicle rescue team and the patient needs to be removed from the vehicle through the door.

What is an example of a well-thought-out "rescue strategy" for highway operations?

A rescue strategy for highway operations should include the following steps:

- Initial scene size-up—establish command, call for appropriate backup, locate and triage the patients (this may need to be delayed until hazards are controlled).

- Control the hazards—remember, traffic can be your worst enemy at a collision.

- Assess the degree of entrapment and fastest means of access, disentanglement, and removal. It may be necessary to break the glass to access the patient. Always try all of the doors before deciding to break a window or remove a door. Although the EMS providers may not have the operational responsibility for actually using heavy hydraulic equipment to access or disentangle the patient, it is important that they observe these procedures and learn the capabilities that are available to them should the patient need them. Be aware of the techniques of door removal, roof removal, making a third door, and a dashboard or firewall roll up.

- Establish an inner circle and an outer circle—the inner circle is where the rescue takes place. Limit the number of workers in this area to those actually assigned to either patient care or operating a rescue tool. The outer circle is where equipment staging and additional personnel should wait until they are assigned a duty. Aside from one or two EMS providers inside the vehicle actively stabilizing the patient, this is where the rest of the crew should be preparing equipment for the moment when the patient is disentangled from the vehicle.

- Provide patient care, package and remove—provide just the right amount of patient care so as not to impede the progress of the mechanical side of the rescue so the patient can be rapidly removed from the wreckage. EMS providers should be well practiced in the application of spine boards for removal of the patient through the door or vertically when a roof has been removed.

Hazardous Terrain Rescue and Packaging

What are the types of hazardous terrain?

The types of hazardous terrain are divided into low angle, high angle, or flat with obstructions. A steep slope or "low-angle" terrain is capable of being walked up without using your hands. This terrain can become more dangerous due to difficult footing especially when carrying a patient in a basket on snow or ice, or on rocks or in mud. Vertical or "high-angle" terrain usually

involves a cliff, building side, or terrain that is so steep that hands must be used for balance when scaling the terrain. There is total dependence on a rope or aerial apparatus for litter movement in a high-angle situation.

What additional training is involved in the operations specialty of high-angle rescue?

High-angle or vertical rescuers must constantly contend with the nondiscriminatory effects of gravity. Any organization that can be assigned a vertical technical rescue must have extensive initial training, additional advanced training, frequently supervised practice, and top-of-the-line equipment. Members of a vertical rescue team should have individual competency in such techniques as rappelling, ascending, belaying, knot tying, hauling systems, rigging, patient packaging, and self-rescue (Figure 49–6).

What should all EMS providers know about high- and low-angle rescue?

All EMS providers should be trained in the procedures for accessing the high-angle rescue team in their region and how to

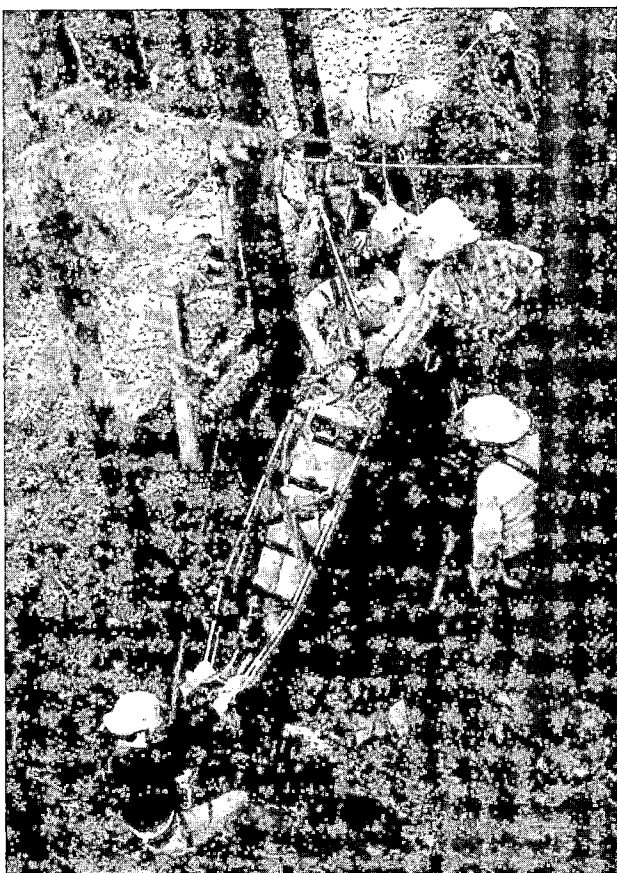

FIGURE 49-6 High-angle rescues can be quite complex, involving rappelling, belaying, rigging, packaging, and hauling skills. *(Courtesy of Bob Elling)*

determine when the team is needed. Many EMS agencies have trained their employees in the skills of low-angle rescue or "off-the-road" rescue, which include assessing the situation, a hasty rappel to access the patient and assess his condition, providing a hasty harness tied from two-inch tubular webbing for each of the basket team, belaying the basket to the patient, packaging the patient, and providing a simple hauling system to assist the litter team up the embankment. Sometimes ropes are used to simply provide a hand line to assist with rescuer balance in a low-angle situation. These skills should be learned and practiced and the appropriate equipment obtained to make this procedure as safe as possible. Low-angle situations are not the same as high-angle situations. In high-angle rescues, much more training is required and the consequence of an error may be fatal.

When should a Stokes® basket be used?

The basket "Stokes®" stretcher is the standard for rough terrain evacuation. It provides a rigid frame for patient protection and is easy to carry with an adequate number of personnel.

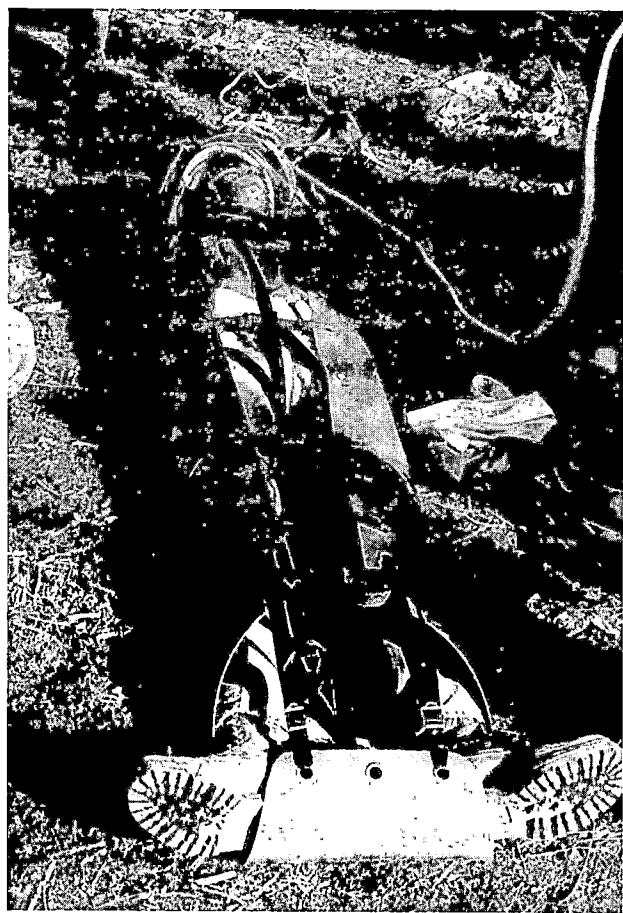

FIGURE 49-7 The SKED® can be a useful substitute for a Stokes® in tight places. If the patient has a possible spine injury, place him on the long backboard first, then put him into the SKED®. *(Courtesy of Bob Elling)*

There should be a minimum of six personnel on the Stokes® and extra teams of six should be rotated in situations where there is a long way to carry the Stokes®. The standard EMS patient handling devices, such as a wheeled ambulance stretcher or scoop stretcher, do not work over rough terrain. Alternative spinal immobilizers can be used in a Stokes® basket such as the KED® or the LSP Halfback®. The Stokes® can be used as a spinal immobilizer by itself as a last resort. A SKED® can also be used in tight places, such as a confined space or pipe shaft, to remove a patient (Figure 49–7).

What is the difference between the types of Stokes®?

Stokes® baskets come in wire and tubular, as well as plastic. The wire mesh Stokes® baskets are the stronger of the types and provide better air and water flow through the basket. They tend to be less expensive and when the flotation (material designed to help the device float) is applied, they are better for water rescue. The older "military-style" wire mesh Stokes® will not accept a backboard due to the leg separator. The plastic basket stretchers are generally weaker than steel baskets, often rated for 300 to 600 pounds, yet they provide better patient protection. The baskets have a plastic bottom and a steel frame. They are very versatile—they can also slide in the snow. Most Stokes® baskets are not equipped with adequate restraints and require additional strapping or lacing for rough terrain evacuation or extraction (Figure 49–8). A plastic litter shield can be purchased to provide patient protection from dust and objects dropping in the patient's face.

What additional precautions should be taken to package the patient into a Stokes® basket?

When a patient is placed in a Stokes® for removal over flat rough terrain, the patient should be laced in to limit their movement. For high- or low-angle evacuation in a Stokes® basket, the following additional preparations should be taken:

- A harness should be applied to the patient.
- Leg stirrups should be applied to the patient.
- Lifters should be applied to prevent the patient from moving around in the basket.
- The tail of one litter line gets tied to the patient's harness.
- A helmet or litter shield should be used to protect the patient.
- Fluids (IV or PO) should be administered to the patient to keep them from dehydrating if the walk out will take a long time.
- Maintain accessibility to the patient's arm for BP, the airway for suction, and the ability to do distal perfusion assessment.
- Padding is a crucial consideration.
- A patient heating and cooling system should be considered.

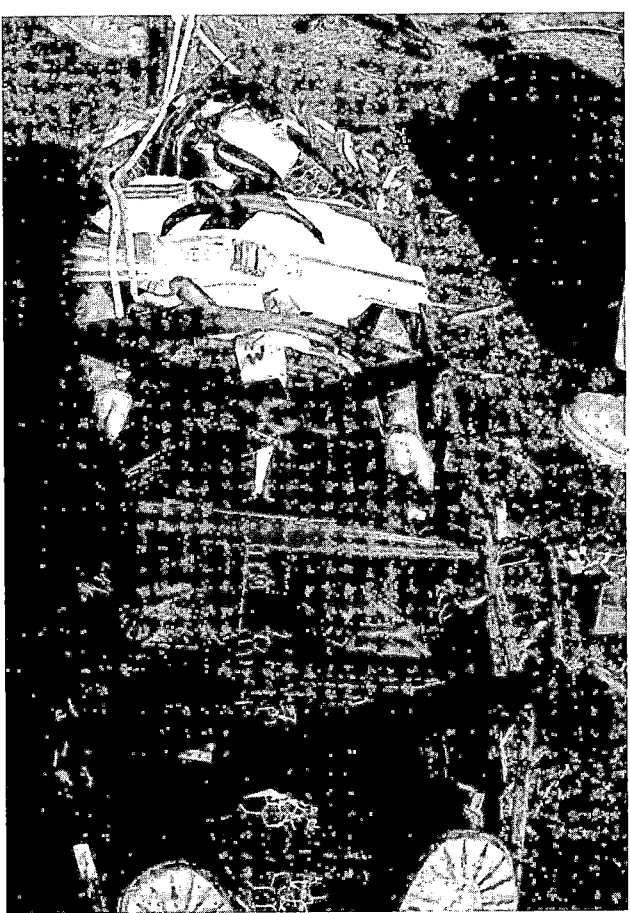

FIGURE 49-8 Strapping a patient into a Stokes® basket. *(Courtesy of Bob Elling)*

How many rescuers should be available for a long carry out of the woods with a Stokes® basket?

Lots! For long litter carries it is helpful to have numerous teams to "leapfrog" ahead of each other to save time and rotate rescuers. An adequate number of litter bearers in this case would be two or better yet three teams of six. It is also helpful to use load lifting straps tied to the Stokes® and stretched across your shoulder to be held by your outside hand. This helps to minimize the strain on the back from bending over sideways to carry the Stokes® for long periods of time.

At a high- or low-angle rescue, are there things for the nontechnical rescue trained EMS providers to assist the specialty team with?

Absolutely, there is a lot to do! When using either low-angle or high-angle evacuation techniques, it is necessary to use combinations of rope anchors and lowering and hauling systems that require specialized knowledge and skill. Any rescue requiring hauling needs plenty of "helpers" to assist with the hauling.

Can a ladder truck be used to remove the Stokes® basket from a building roof?

Yes, in certain situations. Some fire department ladder companies are practiced in the use of an aerial apparatus, tower ladder, or bucket to assist in the removal of a patient in a Stokes® basket. This is usually done in a structural environment, but can be adapted to hazardous terrain if there is access for the truck. It is necessary to provide a litter belay (method of protecting the basket with a rope) during the movement to the bucket and it's important to know the proper procedure for attaching the litter to the bucket. When aerial ladders are used, there is a restriction because the upper sections are usually not wide enough to slide the litter down the steps of the ladder. If being slid down a ladder, the litter must always be belayed to prevent it from falling off. Finally, ladder or aerial apparatus should not be used as a crane to move a litter because they are not rated to do this and it can seriously stress the ladder, causing it to fail.

Is there a role for a helicopter in rough terrain rescue?

Yes—helicopters can be useful in a hazardous terrain rescue. It is important that EMS providers understand the capabilities of their local helicopter system and know who does rescue in their region. There is a difference in mission, crew, training, and capabilities between helicopters that only do air medical care versus rescue helicopters. EMS providers should learn from their local rescue helicopter crew if there are any restrictions for boarding, deboarding, and non-crew members riding along. Inquire if they use a cable winch for rescues, whether they have weight restrictions or restrictions on hovering rescues, and whether they practice one-skid rescues. Many rescue helicopters use short hauls or sling loads of equipment or personnel as opposed to rappel-based rescues, which can be very dangerous.

Extended Care Assessment and Environmental Issues

What should EMS providers know about the management of patients who require an extensive evacuation time?

If your situation warrants (e.g., you cover a backcountry area), at least some EMS providers from your agency should have formal training in managing patients whose injuries have been aggravated by a prolonged lack of treatment. If your agency responds to patients requiring extended care, your medical director should consider protocols that at least address the following areas:

- Long-term hydration management.
- Repositioning of dislocations.
- Cleansing and care of wounds.
- Removal of impaled objects.
- Pain management.
- Assessment and care of head and spinal injuries.
- Hypothermia management.
- Termination of CPR.
- Crush injuries and compartment syndromes.

What are examples of environmental issues that can affect assessment and management?

Environmental issues that can affect your assessment and management include:

- Weather and temperature extremes—may present difficulty in completely exposing patients for full assessment and treatment, and may compromise physical examination and leave the patient susceptible to hypo- or hyperthermia. The rescuer mobility can also be restricted due to clothing and PPE in extreme temperature environments.
- Access to the patient may be limited—you may not be able to access all parts of the patient when they are pinned or stuck under a rock. Cramped space or low-lighting conditions may make assessment difficult. Bring a light or head lamp with you to help with assessment in the dark.
- Street equipment is not easily transported to the patient—tackle boxes and heavy equipment may be inappropriate to take into a confined space, into the backwoods, or down a

hasty rappel. Downsize your equipment and use backpacks for hands-free carrying.

- EMS provider PPE is just as essential but cumbersome—the PPE must be used and, in some instances, it might need to be removed to perform skills. Remember to reapply your PPE as soon as possible.
- Exposure of patients—cover the patient and ensure thermal protection as soon as possible. During the extrication, place hard protection, such as a spine board, to protect the patient and prevent glass shards from contacting patient with an aluminized blanket.
- ALS skills should be limited to only those really necessary—the more wires and tubes, the more complicated the extraction process. Definitive airway control and volume replacement may be essential; as practical, consider continuous oxygenation of the patient. You can't really carry lots of oxygen tanks into the backwoods, so the tank you use should be limited to essential use at a slower flow rate so it will last for a longer period of time.
- Patient monitoring—in high-noise areas, take the BP by palpation. Compact pulse oximeters are now available and may be very helpful. An ECG monitor is cumbersome during extrication. Throughout the rescue, continue talking to the patient, establish a rapport, explain what is being done, and answer the patient's questions.
- Improvisation is common—to minimize the amount of equipment carried into the backwoods, you may want to consider improvising, such as tying upper extremity fractures to the torso, or tying lower extremity fractures to the uninjured leg. SAM® splints can be very useful and are lightweight.

Hazardous Materials: Issue Awareness

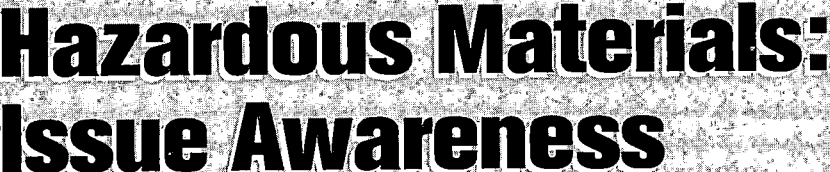

This chapter discusses hazardous materials and issue awareness for the EMS provider. The focus is on situations you may encounter in the field from a scene safety perspective. Because EMS providers are rarely in the position to be responsible for mitigating the incident, the focus is on an awareness of the hazmat hazards.

Hazmat Terminology

What is a hazmat?

The National Fire Protection Association (NFPA) standard number 704 defines a hazardous material (substance or waste) as: "Any substance that causes or may cause adverse effects on the health or safety of employees, the general public, or the environment; any biological agent and other disease-causing agent, or a waste or combination of wastes."

What are some of the basic terms used in hazmat?

The following is a list of terms commonly used in the field of hazmat. These terms have important relevance to the risk assessment process:

- Alpha radiation—large radioactive particles that have minimal infiltrating potential.
- Beta radiation—small radioactive particles that can be inhaled or can infiltrate the skin and subcutaneous layers.
- Boiling point—the temperature at which liquid changes its phase to a vapor or gas. This is the temperature at which the pressure of the liquid equals atmospheric pressure.

- Ceiling level (TLV-C)—the maximum concentration to which a healthy adult can be exposed without risk of injury.
- Flammable or explosive ranges—a specific concentration of flammable vapors in the air for a particular material at which combustion will occur. There is a lower flammable limit and an upper flammable limit at which the vapors are either too lean to burn or too rich.
- Flash point—the minimum temperature at which a material produces enough vapors, in air, to form an ignitable mixture near the surface of the material.
- Gamma radiation—the most dangerous form of radiation particles that can infiltrate the body and cause internal and external injury.
- Ignition (autoignition) temperature—the minimum temperature required to ignite gas or vapor without a spark or flame being present.
- Immediately dangerous to life and health (IDLH)—the concentration of a chemical in the atmosphere that poses an immediate threat to life or health. If a person were to escape immediately, he could survive without harm. IDLH is expressed in parts per million (ppm) or mg/cu meter.
- Parts per million/billion (ppm/ppb)—the number of units of a particular material present in a total volume of one million

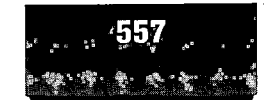

or one billion units. One part per million is the equivalent of 1/10,000 of 1 percent; one part per billion is 1/10,000,000 of 1 percent.

- Permissible exposure limit (PEL)—a time weighted average concentration that must not be exceeded during any 8-hour work shift or a 40-hour work week.

- Short-term exposure limit (TLV-STEL)—measured over a 15-minute period.

- Specific gravity—the ratio of the mass of a unit volume of a substance to the mass of the same volume of a standard substance at a standard temperature.

- Threshold limit value (TLV)—the maximum average concentration (averaged over eight continuous hours) to which a healthy adult may be exposed.

- Vapor density—the weight of a specific volume of gas or vapor compared to an equal volume of air at the same temperature and pressure. Air has a vapor density of one. Gases with vapor densities less than one are lighter than air, and vapor densities greater than one are heavier than air.

- Vapor pressure—a measure of the tendency of a liquid to vaporize into a gas.

- Water solubility—the quantity of a chemical that will mix or dissolve in water.

Hazmat Regulations and Guidelines

[Q] What are the standards that guide hazmat operations?

[A] The National Fire Protection Association (NFPA) has published voluntary standards for the fire service that are often adopted by local municipalities. These standards are referred to by their NFPA number in this book. These standards address competencies for first responders to hazardous materials incidents and the role of EMS providers at hazmat incidents. The relevant NFPA standards are as follows:

- NFPA 472: Professional Competence of Responders to Hazardous Materials Incidents—this preceded and set the stage for the OSHA 1910.120 regulations.

- NFPA 473: Competencies for EMS Personnel Responding to Hazardous Materials Incidents—established two levels of EMS hazmat responders above the awareness level and was the first standard to specifically address EMS workers.

- NFPA 1500—established health and safety standards for the fire service, as well as incident command training and the role of the safety officer.

- NFPA 704—established a system of placarding and labeling fixed facilities for hazardous materials.

[Q] What are the regulations that agencies must follow for hazmat operations?

[A] The Occupational Safety and Health Administration (OSHA) regulations are published in the Code of Federal Regulations (CFR). The EMS provider agencies must follow CFR 1910.1200 (the "Right to Know Law") and CFR 1910.120 (Emergency Response to Hazardous Substance Releases). The latter regulation contains the following rules:

- Sets out training requirements for five levels of responders to hazmat incidents.

- Specifies who can teach the training programs.

- Sets out refresher training requirements.

- Specifies medical surveillance and consultation requirements.

- Specifies chemical protective clothing and postemergency response operations.

[Q] What are the different levels of training required by OSHA regulations?

[A] There are five levels of hazmat training; the first four listed are defined under NFPA 472:

- First responder awareness—training to recognize a hazmat incident, back off, and call for help.

- First responder operations—the level to which many EMS providers and fire personnel are trained. At this level, the responder can perform risk assessment procedures; select and don appropriate personal protective equipment (PPE); carry out basic control, containment, and confinement operations; and carry out basic decontamination procedures.

- Hazardous material technician—has additional training in the use of specialized instruments, PPE, and containment and confinement operations.

- Hazardous material specialist—has advanced training in all aspects of hazmat operations, including working as a liaison with local, state, and federal government.

- On scene incident commander—trained to assume control of a hazmat incident. This training includes an understanding of the incident command system. For more information on this topic, review Chapter 48, Ambulance Operations and Multiple Casualty Incidents.

[Q] What is the role of the EMS provider in the incident scene size-up, the assessment of toxicologic risk, the determination of appropriate decontamination methods for the patient and the responders, and the transportation considerations of these patients?

[A] The role of the EMS provider is to first keep herself and the crew from being exposed or injured. Then, a scene size-up is performed to assess for risks of primary or secondary contamination of the patient and the responders, to determine the need for additional resources, and to decide what safety parameters must be immediately established. Depending on the role your agency plays in local hazmat response plan and the level of training provided, the EMS provider may also assess the level of decontamination, treatment, and transportation considerations.

Q How does the EMS provider size up a hazmat incident to determine the potential hazards, the risk of primary contamination to patients, and the risk of secondary contamination to rescuers?

A On arrival at any scene, the EMS provider performs a scene size-up that entails recognizing that the incident involves hazmat. From an upwind position, using binoculars if necessary, observe

labels or placards. If possible, stay clear of all spills, vapors, fumes, and smoke. The identity of the substance should be made using any resources immediately available such as the *North American Emergency Response Guidebook* (NAERG). After identification and referencing has been made, the EMS provider can now determine the need for immediate evacuation (as shown in the NAERG Figure 50–1), the need to establish safety zones, and how to manage ambulatory patients. The need for decontamination decision is made using hazmat references (e.g., consulting with CHEMTREC). Method, treatment, and transport decisions are made in a similar fashion.

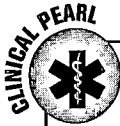

Recognizing that you are dealing with a potential hazmat incident is the first and most important step.

TABLE OF INITIAL ISOLATION AND PROTECTIVE ACTION DISTANCES

ID No.	NAME OF MATERIAL	SMALL SPILLS (From a small package or small leak from a large package) First ISOLATE in all Directions Meters	(Feet)	Then PROTECT persons Downwind during- DAY Kilometers (Miles)		NIGHT Kilometers (Miles)		LARGE SPILLS (From a large package or from many small packages) First ISOLATE in all Directions Meters	(Feet)	Then PROTECT persons Downwind during- DAY Kilometers (Miles)		NIGHT Kilometers (Miles)	
2420	Hexafluoroacetone	60 m	(200 ft)	0.3 km	(0.2 mi)	1.0 km	(0.6 mi)	215 m	(700 ft)	0.8 km	(0.5 mi)	3.5 km	(2.2 mi)
2421	Nitrogen trioxide	60 m	(200 ft)	0.2 km	(0.1 mi)	0.5 km	(0.3 mi)	155 m	(500 ft)	0.5 km	(0.3 mi)	1.6 km	(1.0 mi)
2438	Trimethylacetyl chloride	60 m	(200 ft)	0.2 km	(0.1 mi)	0.5 km	(0.3 mi)	155 m	(500 ft)	0.5 km	(0.3 mi)	1.9 km	(1.2 mi)
2442	Trichloroacetyl chloride	60 m	(200 ft)	0.3 km	(0.2 mi)	1.0 km	(0.6 mi)	215 m	(700 ft)	0.8 km	(0.5 mi)	3.4 km	(2.1 mi)
2474	Thiophosgene	95 m	(300 ft)	0.3 km	(0.2 mi)	1.1 km	(0.7 mi)	215 m	(700 ft)	1.0 km	(0.6 mi)	4.2 km	(2.6 mi)
2477	Methyl isothiocyanate	60 m	(200 ft)	0.2 km	(0.1 mi)	0.6 km	(0.4 mi)	185 m	(600 ft)	0.6 km	(0.4 mi)	2.4 km	(1.5 mi)
2480	Methyl isocyanate	125 m	(400 ft)	0.5 km	(0.3 mi)	2.3 km	(1.4 mi)	305 m	(1000 ft)	1.9 km	(1.2 mi)	8.2 km	(5.1 mi)
2481	Ethyl isocyanate	185 m	(600 ft)	1.3 km	(0.8 mi)	6.1 km	(3.8 mi)	520 m	(1700 ft)	5.0 km	(3.1 mi)	11.0+ km	(7.0+ mi)
2482	n-Propyl isocyanate	155 m	(500 ft)	1.3 km	(0.8 mi)	5.8 km	(3.6 mi)	490 m	(1600 ft)	4.7 km	(2.9 mi)	11.0+ km	(7.0+ mi)
2483	Isopropyl isocyanate	155 m	(500 ft)	1.3 km	(0.8 mi)	5.8 km	(3.6 mi)	490 m	(1600 ft)	4.7 km	(2.9 mi)	11.0+ km	(7.0+ mi)
2484	tert-Butyl isocyanate	155 m	(500 ft)	1.1 km	(0.7 mi)	5.3 km	(3.3 mi)	460 m	(1500 ft)	4.3 km	(2.7 mi)	11.0+ km	(7.0+ mi)
2485	n-Butyl isocyanate	155 m	(500 ft)	1.1 km	(0.7 mi)	5.3 km	(3.3 mi)	460 m	(1500 ft)	4.3 km	(2.7 mi)	11.0+ km	(7.0+ mi)
2486	Isobutyl isocyanate	155 m	(500 ft)	1.1 km	(0.7 mi)	5.3 km	(3.3 mi)	460 m	(1500 ft)	4.3 km	(2.7 mi)	11.0+ km	(7.0+ mi)
2487	Phenyl isocyanate	155 m	(500 ft)	1.1 km	(0.7 mi)	4.8 km	(3.0 mi)	460 m	(1500 ft)	4.0 km	(2.5 mi)	11.0+ km	(7.0+ mi)
2488	Cyclohexyl isocyanate	155 m	(500 ft)	1.0 km	(0.6 mi)	4.7 km	(2.9 mi)	460 m	(1500 ft)	3.9 km	(2.4 mi)	11.0+ km	(7.0+ mi)
2495	Iodine pentafluoride	DANGEROUS: When spilled in water, see list at the end of this table.											
2521	Diketene, inhibited	60 m	(200 ft)	0.2 km	(0.1 mi)	0.6 km	(0.4 mi)	155 m	(500 ft)	0.5 km	(0.3 mi)	2.3 km	(1.4 mi)
2534	Methylchlorosilane	60 m	(200 ft)	0.2 km	(0.1 mi)	0.8 km	(0.5 mi)	185 m	(600 ft)	0.6 km	(0.4 mi)	2.9 km	(1.8 mi)

FIGURE 50–1 One of the most important sections of the NAERG is the one covering initial isolation and protective action distances. Any chemicals highlighted in the yellow or blue sections are listed here.

[Q] What resources can the EMS provider use to identify hazardous materials during the scene size-up?

[A] There are several methods for identifying hazardous materials. Many EMS agencies are required to carry some form of reference to identify hazardous materials.

- *North American Emergency Response Guidebook*—provides the names of substances, UN (United Nations) numbers, placard facsimiles, an emergency action guide, and evacuation and isolation information.
- NFPA 704 placard system—this is a fixed placard system used in many fixed facilities. The placards are colored and indicate specific hazards. Red = fire hazard, blue = health hazard, and yellow = reactivity hazard (Figure 50–2).
- UN numbers and DOT placards (Figure 50–3)—placarding vehicles is required by law, although many people do not

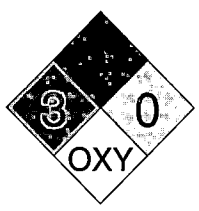

FIGURE 50–2 An NFPA 704 placard.

comply. These placards classify substances in the following categories:

1. Corrosives.
2. Explosives.
   a. Explosives A.
   b. Explosives B.

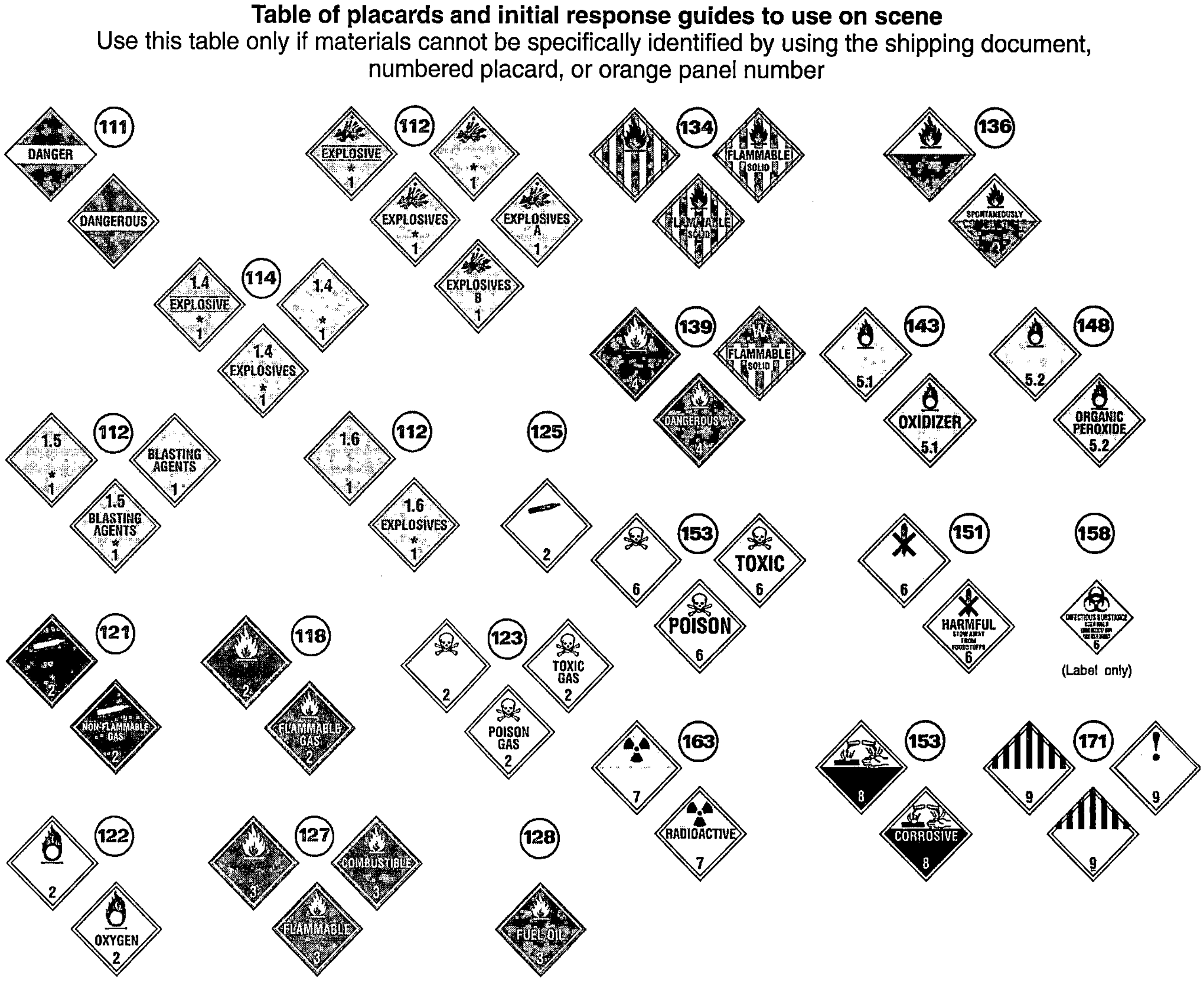

Table of placards and initial response guides to use on scene
Use this table only if materials cannot be specifically identified by using the shipping document, numbered placard, or orange panel number

FIGURE 50–3 Here are examples of the placards and labels that indicate transit of hazardous materials.

c. Explosives C.

d. Blasting agent.

3. Flammable liquids.

a. Flammable liquid.

b. Combustible liquid.

4. Flammable solids.

a. Flammable solid.

b. Flammable solid (dangerous when wet label only).

5. Gases.

a. Poison A.

b. Flammable gas.

c. Nonflammable gas.

d. Corrosive gas.

6. Other regulated materials (ORM).

a. ORM—A.

b. ORM—B.

c. ORM—C.

d. ORM—D.

e. ORM—E.

7. Oxidizers.

a. Oxidizer.

b. Organic peroxide.

8. Poisonous.

a. Poison B.

b. Irritant.

c. Etiologic.

9. Radioactive materials.

a. Class I.

b. Class II.

c. Class III.

- MSDS—a list of detailed information about a substance to be used when exposure occurs with that product. MSDSs are used throughout industry as a means of identifying chemicals and complying with the employee's right to know. These must be readily available for employees to review.

- Packaging labels.

- Shipping papers (e.g., bill of lading or waybill)—are carried by the shipper when transporting substances and contain the name of the product.

- Textbooks, handbooks.

- Dispatcher—when resources are not immediately available to the EMS provider, the dispatcher may be able to obtain information for you.

- Assistance from CHEMTREC (an information resource available through an 800 phone number with detailed information on the chemicals involved and the manufacturer of the chemical).

Where would the shipping papers be found?

These documents should be with the operator of the vehicle of transportation. For surface transportation via tractor-trailer, the driver should have these papers. In a train, they should be in the engine car, and on a ship or sailing vessel, they should be near the Captain's mailbox.

What information does the EMS provider need to reference immediately?

After identifying the substance, the EMS provider has to determine what type of chemical is involved and the actions of the chemical. If the chemical is a hazard that requires immediate evacuation, distance parameters must be immediately established. Then, assess the potential for secondary contamination and what treatment can be given in the field. Determine if there is a need for special approach suits or self-contained breathing apparatus (SCBA).

What is the difference between primary and secondary contamination?

Primary contamination is exposure to the substance that is harmful to the individual with little chance of exposure to others. Secondary contamination comes from exposure or contact with others who were primarily exposed to the substance. It is easily transferred to another, as when a patient is touched. The rescuer or hospital personnel may get secondary contamination if they are not careful.

What are the properties of hazmats?

Flammability, health hazards, and reactivity are the properties of potential hazards, and are listed for chemical substances on placards and in references. Health hazards include descriptions such as "may be fatal if inhaled, contact may cause burns to skin and eyes, and fire may produce irritating or poisonous gases." Reactivity is the ability of a substance to interact with other substances and body tissues. Flammability is the capacity of a substance to ignite and burn rapidly. Flammability hazard warnings include fire or explosion; may be ignited by heat, sparks, or flames; may ignite other combustible materials; reaction with fuels may be violent.

Q What are safety zones?

A Prior to working at an incident where hazmat is present, zones are established to prevent injury and unnecessary exposure to the substance. From the location of the substance, there are three circular zones established in an outward pattern similar to a bull's-eye target (Figure 50–4). The inside zone closest to the substance is the *hot* zone; this is the dangerous area. Working outward is the *warm* zone; this is the entry point and decontamination area (corridor). Farthest out is the *cold* zone; this is the safe area for personnel trained to the awareness level or higher. The public belongs even farther back.

Q What are examples of scenes for which the EMS provider should have a high degree of awareness for a hazmat?

A Motor vehicle crashes (MVCs) are one of the most common scenes for possible hazmat exposure, especially crashes that involve commercial vehicles, tankers, tractor-trailers, pest control trucks, or cars with alternative fuels such as natural gas. Other scenes to be aware of are railroads, pipelines, farms, industrial work sites, chemical plants, fires, fertilizer facilities, warehouses, and hardware and agricultural stores.

Q What other clues can the EMS provider use to detect hazmats?

A Placards and labels, markings and colors, occupancy or location, shipping papers, and other documents.

Q How does the EMS provider research information about a specific hazmat, suggest the appropriate medical response, and determine the risk of secondary contamination?

A The EMS responder can use a reference such as the NAERG. On the first page is information about how to quickly use the book. It gives you three methods to reference the substance, then leads you to a guide. The guide lists potential hazards, public safety precautions, emergency response procedures, and first-aid treatment. Whenever possible, use multiple resources, such as contacting CHEMTREC. From the information collected from the resources, the responder is able to suggest the appropriate medical response and determine the risk of secondary contamination.

Q What is CHEMTREC?

A CHEMTREC is a service operated by the Chemical Manufacturers Association to provide information about emergency responses that involve chemicals and transportation. The telephone number is 1-800-424-9300.

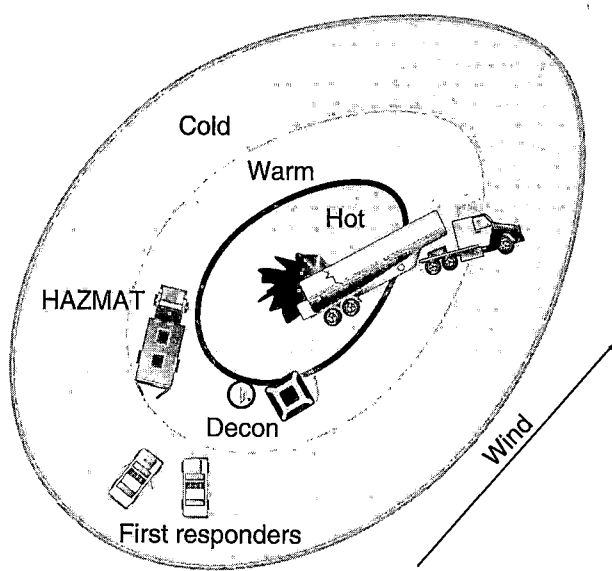

FIGURE 50–4 The establishment of zones is usually based on the types of hazards that may be present. For general chemical spills, the zones established are referred to as the hot, warm, and cold zones.

Q What are examples of emergency actions an EMS provider can take at a hazmat incident?

A Examples of emergency actions are:

- Keep unnecessary people away; isolate hazard area and deny entry.
- For small fires, use a dry chemical, CO_2, water spray, or regular foam.
- For a spill or leak, shut off ignition sources—no flares, smoking, or flames in the hazard area.
- Do not touch or walk through spilled material.
- First aid—move victim to fresh air.
- Remove and isolate contaminated clothing and shoes at the site.
- Keep victim quiet and maintain normal body temperature.

Physiology

Q How are poisons metabolized?

A The stages of the metabolism of a poison are the same as with any drug. *Absorption* is the time the substance takes to get into the bloodstream. *Distribution* is the movement of the substance in the blood to target organs, creating effects. *Biotransformation* usually occurs in the liver and *elimination* or excretion is made through the kidneys, lungs, or GI tract. This process is explained in further detail in Chapter 7, Pharmacology.

What are poison actions?

Poison actions are how and what a poison does to the body.

- Dose response—this is how much substance it takes to cause a physiologic response. Understanding this determines the level of decontamination.
- Route of exposure (local or systemic)—exposure can cause effects at the site of contact such as rashes, burns, or wheezing, and the effects can reach body systems such as the cardiovascular, neurologic, renal, and hepatic.
- Synergistic effects—combined effects can result from more than one substance or from treatment with drugs.
- Toxicity (acute and delayed)—toxicity can be immediate (acute) with signs and symptoms rapidly apparent or delayed with effects appearing later.

Are there any other factors that can influence how an individual is affected?

Yes, factors such as age, gender, general health status, pre-existing medical conditions, and medication use can influence the exposure response.

How does the specific substance and route of contamination alter triage and decontamination methods for the EMS provider?

The type of substance and route of absorption determines how fast the effects of the product are on a patient or responder. This information prioritizes (triages) how quickly a patient requires treatment. Decontamination is not a quick process, but there are different levels of decontamination taking more or less time.

PPE and DECON

What is decon?

Decontamination or decon is the physical or chemical process of removing hazardous material from an exposed person and equipment at a hazardous materials incident.

What are the limitations of field decontamination?

Training requirements are a significant factor that limits field decontamination. Most EMS providers are trained to the awareness level and do not have the training to operate or participate as a hazmat technician or specialist. There is no single type of PPE that is compatible with all chemicals. Patient condition can also limit the decontamination process. The more stable a patient is, the more thorough the decon that can be completed.

What are the various types of PPE used by EMS providers and what are their limitations?

The use of many of the PPE required for hazmat operations requires training, recertification, and appropriate fit testing to conform to OSHA regulations. Because no one piece of PPE can protect against all substances, manufacturer's guidelines and recommendations must be followed.

PPE used by EMS providers includes protective respiratory devices—respirators, filtration devices, SCBA, and supplied air breathing apparatus (SABA). Protective clothing includes turnout gear, coveralls, boots, gloves, hard hats, safety glasses or goggles, and shields made from materials such as Tyvek®, nitrile rubber, Teflon®, and Viton®.

What are the levels of protective suits?

OSHA and the Environmental Protection Agency (EPA) have classified levels of protection as level A, level B, level C, and level D.

- Level A is the highest level of protective equipment and is designed to be vapor tight to protect against gases or vapors (Figure 50–5).

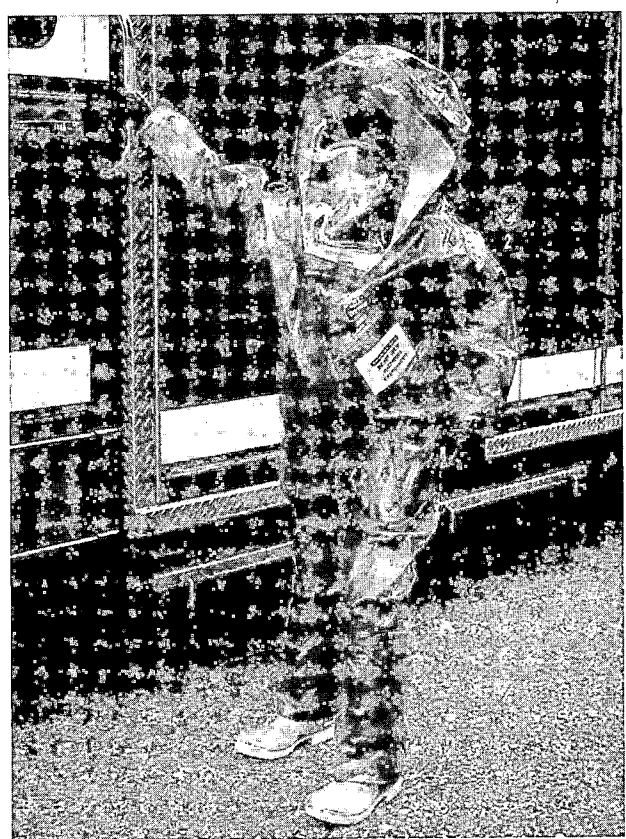

FIGURE 50–5 The Level A suit offers good protection from chemicals.

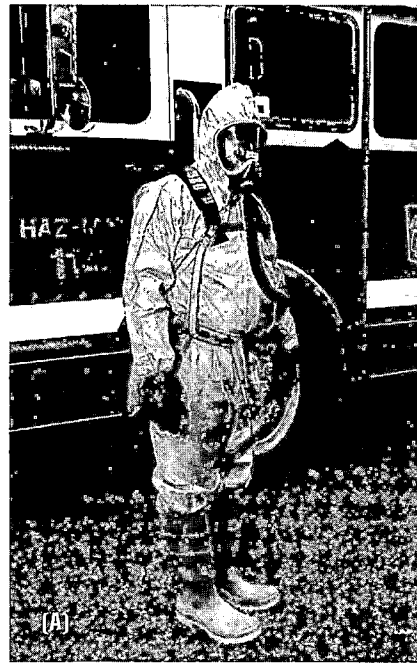 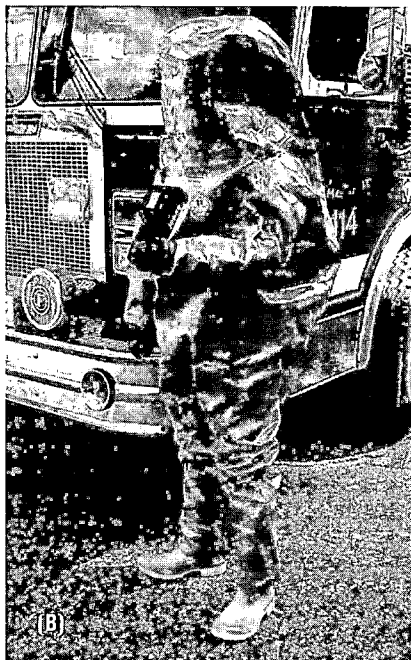 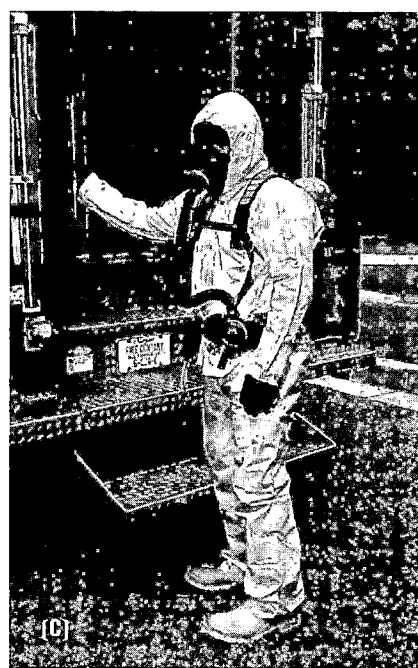

FIGURE 50–6 The suits here all represent Level B suits: (A) coverall style, (B) an encapsulated suit, and (C) two-piece style. Level B is intended to offer splash protection and is not gastight like a Level A suit.

- Level B is the second highest level of protective equipment and is designed to be liquid tight to protect against splash hazards (Figure 50–6).
- Level C is the third level of protective equipment and is designed to be used when hazards are known and controlled and not for emergency response.
- Level D is the lowest level, providing no protection, and typically consists of street clothing or standard EMS uniforms.

What are the stages of a decon corridor?

The stages of a decon corridor (Figure 50–7) are:

- Stage 1: Single entry point and hot zone.
- Stage 2: Gross decon.
- Stage 3: Protective clothing removal.
- Stage 4: SCBA removal.
- Stage 5: Personal clothing removal.
- Stage 6: Body washing.
- Stage 7: Dry off.
- Stage 8: Medical assessment.

What are the procedures for decon of critical and noncritical patients?

The critical patient gets a rapid decon, which is a two-step process. The first step is to remove the patient from danger and the second is to perform a gross decon. The noncritical patient can be approached in a more guarded fashion. The latter method consists of all of the eight stages listed earlier.

What are the most common decon solutions used by EMS providers?

The most common decon solutions are water, water and tincture of green soap, isopropyl alcohol, and vegetable oil. Water is a universal decon solution that dilutes and reduces topical absorption.

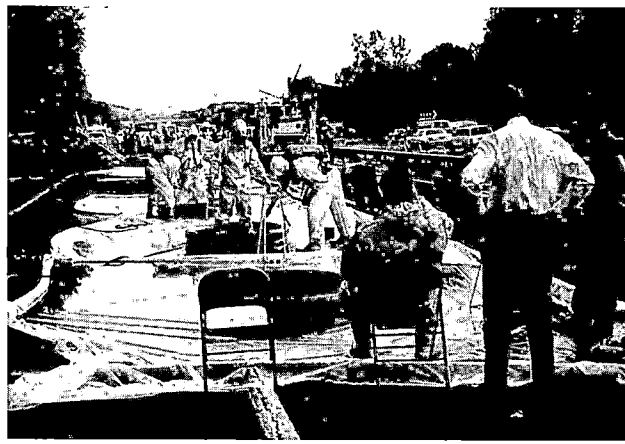

FIGURE 50–7 The decontamination corridor is located in the warm zone. *(Courtesy of Baltimore County Fire Department)*

[Q] With what substances is water not to be used to decontaminate?

[A] Water-reactive metals, also called alkaline metals, include calcium, lithium, magnesium, and sodium. These substances react with water, creating severe burns. If these metals ignite due to contact with skin, smother the flame using sand or a class D fire extinguisher and cover with vegetable oil.

[Q] What are the difficult body parts to decontaminate?

[A] Difficult body parts to clean thoroughly include:

- Axilla.
- Behind the knees, between the toes, and toenails.
- Buttocks.
- Ears.
- Groin.
- Hair and scalp.
- Navel.
- Nostrils.

Management

[Q] How can the EMS provider determine where and when to treat a patient exposed to a hazmat?

[A] The decision of where and when to treat a patient is determined by assessing the substance toxicity, patient condition, and availability of decontamination.

[Q] What are the common signs and symptoms, as well as treatment considerations, for the following hazardous materials: corrosives, pulmonary irritants, pesticides, chemical asphyxiants, and hydrocarbon solvents?

[A] Signs and symptoms for specific exposures vary. Be alert for any of the following signs and symptoms:

- Anxiety.
- Dizziness or lightheadedness.
- Confusion or any altered mental status (AMS).
- Vision disturbance.
- Coughing, drooling, or rhinorrhea.
- Respiratory distress.
- Chest pain.
- Loss of coordination.
- Nausea or vomiting.
- Changes in skin color, temperature, or condition (CTC).
- Abdominal cramping, diarrhea, or incontinence.

Hazmat substances can produce external and internal injuries. Injury examples are:

External:

- Corrosives—acids and alkalis.
- Thermal—cold and heat.

Internal:

- Carcinogens—burning wood products and other products that produce dioxins.
- Chemical asphyxiants—cyanide and carbon monoxide.
- Hepatotoxins—hydrocarbon solvents such as xylene and methlyene chloride.
- Nerve agents—nerve gas, nitrous oxide, and pesticides such as carbonates and organophosphates.
- Neurotoxins—arsenic, lead, and mercury.
- Pulmonary irritants—ammonia and chlorine.

[Q] How does the EMS provider manage a patient who has indications of exposure?

[A] The EMS provider should don the appropriate level PPE for the specific type of substance exposure. Then, an initial assessment can be performed. A gross decontamination may be appropriate before initiating treatment other than putting on an oxygen mask. Further assessment and treatment can follow the decontamination process. Contamination of the ambulance and equipment can be minimized by a thorough decontamination process and taking a few steps to prepare the ambulance.

Prepare the ambulance by removing any equipment that is outside closed compartments and covering it with plastic. Use disposable items whenever possible and get any equipment you may use out of closed compartments before loading the patient. Then keep the cabinets closed.

Early notification of the hospital should be made, and a clear discussion about decontamination protocols should be reviewed and confirmed.

[Q] What are the risks associated with invasive procedures performed on contaminated patients?

[A] The risk of exposure increases significantly whenever invasive procedures are performed. Procedures such as starting an IV can pose an additional risk for needle sticks. When reviewing the resources and establishing a treatment plan, consider the risk versus the benefit when it comes to invasive procedures on contaminated patients.

What is medical monitoring?

Medical monitoring is a basic medical evaluation of emergency response personnel. EMS providers determine and record basic vital signs, neurological status, and general health. It may also include body weight and ECG. Medical monitoring is typically conducted prior to and after entry into an incident (hazmat, confined space, fire entry) to determine if any significant changes have occurred.

What information about hazmat medical monitoring and rehabilitation operation must be documented?

The type of substance involved, its toxicity, and the danger of secondary contamination must be documented. Additional information to record includes appropriate PPE and suit breakthrough time, appropriate antidote, medical treatment, and transportation method.

What factors influence the heat stress of hazmat personnel?

The factors that directly influence how heat stress affects rescue personnel include:

- Hydration.
- Physical fitness.
- Ambient temperature.
- Activity.
- Level of PPE.
- Duration of activity.

Can hazmat patients be transported to any hospital?

Not every hospital has the resources to sufficiently decon patients. The hazmat preplans of your area should take into consideration hospitals that have the capacity to decontaminate patients.

Crime Scene Awareness

This chapter discusses an awareness of the human hazard of crime and violence. The focus is on *why* perpetrators may focus their anger at the EMS providers and how to minimize your chance of being injured or killed. The emphasis is on how the EMS provider should operate at the scene and *why* you need to act in a certain way at crime scenes and other emergencies.

Hazard Awareness Control and Avoidance

Q **What are the potential exposures for EMS providers in the area of scene violence?**

A Violence continues to be a threat to the EMS provider during calls. Types of exposures include street violence including assaults and robberies, groups threatening citizens and government (e.g., terrorists), domestic violence, drug trafficking and drug users, street calls with exposure to crowds and unruly mobs.

In most communities, a violent crime draws the response of both police and an EMS unit. Sometimes the EMS unit arrives on the scene prior to the police personnel. This can be a very dangerous situation for the EMS providers.

CLINICAL PEARL

As a general rule, if the scene is at all suspicious (i.e., potentially unsafe) stage out of sight and wait for law enforcement personnel before entering.

Q **How can your approach to the scene be an important part of the scene size-up?**

A As a part of hazard awareness, the EMS provider should make every effort to identify and respond to dangers before they become threatening. Safety concerns should begin with the information that was obtained from the dispatcher. Try to use all available resources, such as the police, prior to arrival at the scene.

Q **What should the EMS provider do if the scene cannot be made safe?**

A While on the scene, if the EMS provider becomes aware of a potential threat, weapons, or any violent or abusive actions toward the EMS personnel or the patient, retreat right away. Return to the ambulance and drive away until such time as the police have arrived and notified the EMS providers that the scene is secured. Do not intercede in a violent scene and attempt to break up a fight. That is the responsibility of law enforcement personnel who have other tools, such as pepper spray and firearms, at their disposal. There is no such thing as a dead hero!

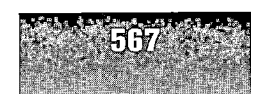

Q: While responding to the scene, what pieces of information can be helpful clues that there may be violence?

A: Some dispatchers maintain records in the computer that there was previously a problem with violence at a specific address. Information from other crews who have previously responded to the address may be helpful in giving you the "heads up" that there may be a dispute at the location.

Q: When should the EMS provider begin to size up the potential crime scene?

A: As soon as you are in the neighborhood, begin to make observations of the scene you are approaching. Some examples of what you should be looking for are:

- Is there a crowd in front of the residence?
- Is there someone running from the residence?
- Is there a vehicle speeding away from the residence?
- As you pull up outside, can you hear screaming inside?
- As you begin to approach the home, is there broken glass around the front door?

Q: What is the effect of the use of the lights and siren on arrival at the scene?

A: It is a good practice to turn off the siren a few blocks from the scene and to turn off the red lights as you approach the scene. This helps to minimize announcing your presence in the community. It may also help keep the crowd small. If the call is on a busy highway and traffic has not been controlled, keep the warning lights on.

Q: What other hazards should the EMS provider be alert for on arrival at the scene?

A: There are many nonviolent dangers such as hazardous materials, power lines, and dangerous pets, which are discussed in detail in Chapter 15, Scene Size-Up and Initial Assessment.

Q: Once on the scene, if there does not appear to be a threat to the EMS providers, can you move on to other things?

A: Yes, turn your attention to assessing the patient. However, there should always be someone on the crew who keeps an eye

CLINICAL PEARL

Never let your guard down at any scene. "Thinking things were OK" has resulted in injury and death to public safety providers.

open for potential hazards and a situation with the bystanders that may change very quickly.

Q: Do you have an escape plan?

A: As you enter any building or residence, it is important to size up the passageway that you walk through and look for other potential exits should you need to retreat. It is also important to observe your access points closely since they will help you determine the most appropriate transport device to use to remove the patient from the scene.

Q: What are examples of things that can change at an incident, making it hazardous to you and your crew?

A: Violence that was occurring prior to your arrival can resume. A crowd can gather or someone on the scene may become angry at the care you are administering to their friend or family. Even though the police are on the scene with you, violence can still occur. Don't let their presence be a false sense of security for you. If someone shows up on the scene and pulls out a handgun, it's the police who have a bulletproof vest on, not you!

CLINICAL PEARL

Some EMS personnel routinely wear body armor depending on the location in which they work. Follow your local protocols.

Q: Is it common for EMS providers to be mistaken for police officers?

A: Some EMS agencies wear uniforms that look a lot like the police uniform in their community. The EMS providers arrive in a vehicle that has lights and a siren and are often the first to arrive on the scene. They also wear a badge and holsters with medical equipment in them. To the criminal, especially in a low-light situation, if they are afraid of the police or looking to strike out at the police, it may be easy to confuse the uniform. This could cause aggression toward the EMS providers as authority figures. In a number of communities, the medical personnel wear white shirts and bright colored jackets with retro-reflective stripes and large clear lettering that says "EMS."

Q: If you are dispatched to a known violent scene, where should you stage?

A: The EMS unit should be staged out of sight of the scene. If it is within sight, people may come out to you and start entering your vehicle. By entering an unsafe scene, you add additional potential victims, yourself and your crew. Do not put yourself or your crew in harm's way because you may be seriously injured or killed. It is also possible that you could be grabbed as a hostage by the perpetrator at the scene.

Q **Do only certain types of calls require a scene size-up for violence hazards?**

A No, all scenes, including the everyday response, require a level of awareness that the scene may be dangerous or pose a threat to you or your crew.

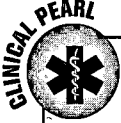

Always perform a proper scene size-up, regardless of the apparent nature of the call.

Q **What are some of the warning signs of danger in residential calls?**

A The following are a number of warning signs to be alert for and avoid to prevent injury to yourself and your crew:

- Past history of problems or violence at the address.
- A known drug or street gang area of town.
- Hearing loud noises or items breaking.
- Seeing or hearing fighting.
- Observing signs of intoxication with drugs or alcohol.
- Observing evidence of potentially dangerous pets such as droppings, barking, signs, or chains.
- Noticing an unusually quiet or darkened residence with the front door ajar.
- Your approach should use tactics that match the threat or situation (e.g., it may be necessary to avoid walking in front of windows or the driver's door for safety).

Q **What are some safety strategies to employ to minimize your exposure to violence-related hazards at the scene?**

A The following is a list of safety strategies to use on calls:

- Always carry a portable radio with you and do not leave your crew inside without a means of communication.
- If actual danger is present, retreat and call the police.
- Do not broadcast your approach with lights and siren.
- Consider using a foot approach on an unconventional path instead of the sidewalk up to the front door.
- Do not backlight yourself by getting between the EMS unit and the residence.

- Stand to the side of the door on the doorknob side.
- Listen for signs of danger before announcing your presence or knocking on the front door.

Responses Involving Motor Vehicles

Q **What are some of the potential dangers when responding to a patient in a vehicle on the side of the road?**

A The notorious "man slumped over the wheel" calls sound perfectly harmless, yet they can prove to be very dangerous. The occupants of these vehicles or of a crashed vehicle on the side of the road may be intoxicated or drugged, wanted by the law, armed, or violent or abusive from an altered mental status (AMS). Look out for some of the following clues that there may be a dangerous condition:

- Are there suspicious movements within the vehicle?
- Does it look like someone inside the vehicle is trying to hide or grab an item, such as a weapon?
- Is there arguing going on between the occupants of the vehicle?
- Is there a lack of activity where activity is likely?
- Are there any signs of alcohol or drug use?
- Is there an open or unlatched hood or trunk?
- Does it look like they are trying to hide a person inside the vehicle?

Q **What is the safest way to approach a vehicle on the highway?**

A Pull behind the vehicle and use the ambulance lights to illuminate the car if it is nighttime. One partner remains in the ambulance, which is elevated and provides greater visibility. The EMS provider who is going to approach the car should have a portable radio in hand. Before getting out of the ambulance, it is a good idea to notify the dispatcher of the situation, the exact location, and the vehicle license plate number and state. Approach from the passenger side of the vehicle. This is done because the driver normally expects the police to approach on the driver's side and it does not expose the EMS provider to traffic.

It is smart not to walk between the ambulance and the car, as the backlighting shows exactly where you are all the time and the vehicle could back up and injure you. If the EMS provider who is the driver of the unit is going to approach the car, walk around the rear of the EMS unit, then approach the car from the passenger side. The posts in the vehicle provide a limited amount of ballistic protection. As you approach the car, observe the rear seat. Do not move any farther than the C post unless there are no threats in the back seat. Next, move forward and observe the front seat from behind the B post. Only move forward after you are sure it is safe. If there is any sign of violence, retreat right away.

Violent Scenes in General

Q **What is the danger of an injury at the scene of a murder, assault, or robbery?**

A These types of incidents often involve dangerous weapons. Sometimes the perpetrators are on the scene and you do not even know it. Other times, the perpetrators can return to the scene to finish off your patient. In these situations, even the patient may be violent toward EMS providers.

Large Crowds

Q **What dangers do large crowds pose to the EMS provider?**

A A crowd may quickly become large and volatile. It may start out as a party of celebration, but can turn violent. In 1999, when the Denver Broncos won the Super Bowl, the jubilant crowd went on a rampage turning over vehicles and starting fires throughout the city. Violence can be directed against everything and everyone in its path. During the LA riots after the Rodney King trial decision, there were firefighters shot at and injured by the unruly mobs roaming the streets. EMS providers are not immune from the effects of this type of violence.

Q **What are some of the warning signs of danger at street scenes?**

A It is often an indicator when the voices begin to get louder and pushing and shoving starts. Any development of hostility toward any other person (e.g., police, perpetrator, victim) at the scene can begin to escalate the mood of the crowd. When the police are having difficulty controlling the crowd and begin to call for reinforcements, you know there is going to be some serious trouble and probably should retreat.

Q **What is the best approach to take with a crowd?**

A Constantly monitor the crowd. Do not antagonize anyone in the crowd; treat people with respect. Retreat if necessary and, if

possible, take the patient with you to a safe spot. If you are able to get the patient removed quickly from the scene, you will not have to go back later.

Street Gangs

Q **What are some of the street gangs that are controlling many of the inner-city streets?**

A Usually, the presence of certain types of graffiti marks the territory and identifies the presence of street gangs. Some of the names of the gangs that appear in many U.S. cities are the Crips, the Bloods, the Latin Kings, Hell's Angels, the Outlaws, the Pagans, and the Banditos. Most of the gangs are heavily involved in drug trafficking and use underage children to do most of the violence. A child can actually move closer to the inner circle or core of the gang by committing a homicide.

Q **What is the significance of the clothing and "colors" of the gangs?**

A Each of the gangs has unique clothing that identifies the group. Often the "colors" represent the gang member's status within the group. These "colors" are very important to the gang members and an EMS provider must be careful to show respect to the colors or face deadly repercussions. If a gang member is shot and you are treating him and it becomes necessary to cut off his clothes, such as the leather jacket of a Hells Angel, make sure that the other gang members understand this is a life-threatening situation and cut along the seams so the garment can be repaired if necessary. Better yet, do it after the gang member is out of sight of the rest of the group in your "office" (the ambulance), where it is quieter and more private.

CLINICAL PEARL

Gang experts recommend that you always explain why and ask permission before "cutting the colors" in front of other members of the gang. Even if you do it in your "office" (the ambulance), bad repercussions may ensue if other gang members find out later. Regardless of your personal beliefs, gangs have a strong system of their own values, based on "respect." As long as the gang members perceive that you respect them, everything is usually OK. If you "dis" (disrespect) them at any time, trouble is likely.

What is the significance of gang graffiti?

Gangs use graffiti to mark their presence in a community. If you learn how to read it, you can understand who was marked for a hit and when it happened. They also mark their numbers in the graffiti. Generally, the younger members of the gangs are responsible for the graffiti as directed by the gang leadership.

Should communities inhabited by gangs be considered dangerous?

Absolutely! Gang presence increases the potential for street violence. Some younger members have been known to slash the face of citizens for no reason other than a show of power. The slashing is to the face so the injured will never forget the mark left by the gang every time he looks in the mirror. Other hazards include clandestine drug labs that may have booby traps (e.g., light socket booby trap that has a shotgun shell in it) set to go off when anyone approaches the location. EMS providers who look like law enforcement officers are a definite threat to the gang members. You should be very cautious when working in the gang's territory.

Clandestine Drug Labs

What are clandestine drug labs?

A drug lab is a location where illegal drugs are manufactured. "Clandestine" means secret. Some are referred to as "meth" labs. Usually, the process involves highly flammable chemicals that can explode easily. EMS providers may respond to an explosion at one of these labs or, when on a routine call, stumble across one of these labs.

How might the EMS provider determine that there is a clandestine lab?

There may be chemical odors or chemistry equipment such as glassware, chemical containers, heating mantles, or burners. There may be suspicious people, activities, or deliveries occurring at the lab location. Usually, the location of a clandestine lab

is in an area that affords a considerable amount of privacy and has access to utilities and ventilation.

What are the types of labs?

Some labs are designed to do chemical synthesis and create drugs, such as LSD or metamphetamine, from chemical precursors. Other labs are designed to do chemical conversion, changing drugs from one form to another, such as cocaine HCl to the base form. There are also labs that do chemical extraction and prepare tablets.

What are the hazards of clandestine labs?

These labs can be very dangerous locations. The hazards include toxic inhalation and the potential for fire or explosion due to the chemicals being "cooked" at the lab. It is not uncommon for booby traps to be set to warn the criminals of the approach of intruders. Remember, the occupants of the labs are often armed and otherwise violent people.

What actions should be taken if you believe you have arrived at the scene of a clandestine drug lab?

The safest response is to leave the area immediately, then notify law enforcement. It is suggested that the incident command system be initiated and hazmat asked to respond, as well as the fire department. The police may notify the Drug Enforcement Administration (DEA), which has responsibility for and expertise in this particular area. Chemical specialists may be used to advise on the status of any reactions that may be occurring. Never touch anything, stop any reaction, or alter any reaction that is occurring because there can be an explosion.

Domestic Violence

What is domestic violence?

Violence between people in a domestic relationship such as spouses, boy–girlfriend, or same sex relations. The victims of domestic violence may be male or female and the violence may be physical, emotional, sexual, verbal, or economic.

What are the indications of domestic violence?

The indications of domestic violence include the following:
- Apparent fear of a household member.
- One party preventing the other from speaking.

CLINICAL PEARL

Suspect illicit activity if a residence has an unusually large number of security systems or devices, including guard dogs (e.g., steel doors, barbed wire fences). Avoid entering the scene without backup from law enforcement on the scene.

- Differing accounts by parties at the scene.
- A patient who is reluctant to speak.
- Injuries that do not match the mechanism of injury (MOI).
- Unusual or unsanitary living conditions or hygiene.

What actions should the EMS provider take if domestic violence is suspected?

First and foremost, treat the patient. Do not be judgmental about the situation. Provide the phone number for a domestic violence hot line or a shelter when the injured person is not in sight of the perpetrator.

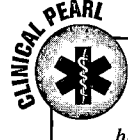
> *One of the most potentially dangerous situations to be in is the "middle" of a domestic disturbance. Always have police backup at your side.*

When is it appropriate to consider notifying the authorities about suspected domestic violence?

If it is the policy or regulation that governs your service, you may be required to report incidents of suspected domestic violence to law enforcement personnel. EMS providers should be aware of the phone number for the domestic violence hot line or shelter in your district. Mandatory reporting may be required in your state. Check with your state EMS code or medical director if you are unsure about being a mandatory reporter. In a non-judgmental fashion, notify ED personnel if you suspect domestic violence.

Tactics for Safety and Patient Care

What is one of the most important rules of tactical safety?

Avoidance is always preferable to confrontation. Become a keen observer and maintain a knowledge of the warning signs of violence. Be aware of the proper tactical response to avoid danger and know how to deal appropriately with danger in situations where it cannot be avoided. Always consider staging your unit until law enforcement has responded and the scene is considered secure.

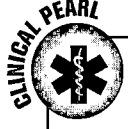
> *Better to have not entered the scene in the first place, than to have entered and wished you didn't.*

When and how should retreat be considered the safest option for the EMS provider?

Leaving the scene is an appropriate thing to do when violence or indicators of violence are observed. An immediate decision has to be made and the retreat should be done in a calm, safe manner. Be aware of the danger that is now behind you. Your retreat may be on your feet or in the ambulance or EMS unit. Remember, there is nothing in the vehicle that is worth your life! Choose a mode and route of retreat that provides the least exposure to danger.

How far should the EMS provider retreat?

The location that you retreat to must protect you and your crew from any potential danger. If possible, you should be out of sight. The location must be protected from gunfire, provide cover, and be out of the "kill zone." The kill zone is the area where a shotgun could reach if it was fired by the perpetrator. Be sure you are far enough from the scene that you have time to react if danger approaches. Be sure to notify all other responding units that you have repositioned to a specific location and make sure the dispatcher does not send any further EMS units directly into the scene.

Are there any special documentation requirements for an incident involving violence and your retreat?

It is strongly suggested that the EMS provider document objectively on the prehospital care report (PCR) any observations of danger, who was notified of the danger, your actions, and the time you left and returned to the scene. This is helpful in reducing liability should your agency be sued. Retreat for appropriate reasons is not abandonment.

> *Remember that a refusal to enter a scene or leaving a scene out of concern for your own personal safety is not patient abandonment, especially if you have not yet begun patient care.*

What is concealment?

Concealment is positioning yourself or crew behind an object that hides you from the view of others. Concealment offers no ballistic protection should the perpetrator begin firing a weapon at you. Examples of concealment include bushes, wallboard, the vehicle door, or drapes.

What is cover?

Cover hides your body and also provides ballistic protection. Examples include large trees, telephone poles, a brick wall, or the vehicle engine block.

When should cover and concealment be used?

As you retreat, it is smart to use cover and concealment. Also use them when you are "pinned down" while attempting to retreat. Cover and concealment should be used properly. Place as much of your body as possible behind cover. Constantly look to improve your protection and location. Be aware that the reflective clothing you may be wearing makes you stand out to the perpetrator.

If an aggressor seems to be chasing the retreating EMS provider, what should you do?

Try to wedge the stretcher in the doorway to block the aggressor. Throw the equipment to slow or trip the aggressor. Use an unconventional path while retreating and anticipate the moves of the aggressor.

When in a suspected dangerous situation, what can the EMS providers do to minimize the risk?

Some experts advocate preassigning the roles of cover and contact. The contact provider is responsible for initiating and providing direct patient care, assessment, and handling most of the interpersonal scene contact.

The cover provider, in a tactical context, has the main function of covering or observing the scene for danger while the contact provider takes care of the patient. The cover provider generally avoids patient care duties that prevent observation of the scene. The cover provider is also responsible for keeping the exit accessible. In small crews, the cover provider is likely to have other functions like obtaining and carrying equipment.

It is also a good idea for the EMS providers to have some signals for when there is danger and when they think it is appropriate to retreat. These signals should not alert the aggressor and should also involve the dispatcher as soon as possible.

Finally, use common sense! Do not wear items, such as a stethoscope or a tie or a radio strap, that can be used to pull you closer to the aggressor or to strangle you. Keep your hands free and out of your pockets. Keep a safe stance with your feet apart, ready to react.

CLINICAL PEARL

If you are required to wear ties, use snap-on ties with quick release fittings that will tear away easily if you are grabbed.

What is the purpose of body armor and is it appropriate for EMS providers?

Body armor, also known as a bulletproof vest, has been worn for many years by law enforcement personnel. The vest offers protection from most handgun bullets and most knives. It also reduces the blunt trauma from being struck with an object such as a bat or the steering wheel in a collision. Body armor does not offer protection against high velocity rifle bullets or thin or dual-edged weapons such as an ice pick. For it to work, it must be worn, not kept in your locker. The material that body armor is made from, Kevlar®, has reduced protection when wet.

When wearing body armor, remember it is not a superhero cape! Do not get a false sense of security from the vest that might lead you into situations you normally would not enter. They can always shoot you in the head or neck and kill you just as fast! Wearing body armor does not go without injuries. The cavitation and blunt trauma from a bullet striking, but not penetrating, the outside of the armor can be serious.

CLINICAL PEARL

Even with body armor in place, bullets transmit significant energy to the areas of the body underneath the vest. Significant injuries can still occur, though they are usually far less severe than if the vest was not worn in the first place.

Tactical EMS

What is "tactical EMS?"

Tactical EMS is provided in a violent or tactically "hot" zone. All armies take medics to the front line to care for and evacuate the wounded soldiers. In the urban crime fight in some cities, a limited number of EMS providers are trained in special tactics to accompany the police on high-risk operations. This requires a working relationship with the law enforcement team, as well as special training. Tactical medics wear body armor and special uniforms. Their equipment is often more compact and functional in small cases compared to the typical portable equipment carried by most EMS providers. They are trained to use mace and a metal clipboard as defensive tools. This assignment may require risks that are not normally taken in the routine EMS situation.

Are there differences in patient care when practicing tactical EMS?

When someone is shooting at you and your objective is to drag the patient out of sight under cover, patient care is different! Extrication of the patient from the area safely is a major concern of tactical medics. They frequently care for trauma patients and rarely deal with medical emergencies. Care must be modified to meet tactical considerations and the means of evacuation. All medical and transport interventions must be coordinated with the incident commander. Once the patient is moved to a cold zone where there is no hazard, complete patient care can proceed, as well as transportation.

Q Where can an EMS provider learn more about tactical medic responsibilities?

A Many cities have joint law enforcement agency (LEA) teams that include EMS providers. Some of the designations and courses that have been available in the past include LEA/SWAT team, CONTOMS, SWAT-Medic, EMT-T. Start by talking with your local police department to see what they already have in place for extremely violent situations.

The CONTOMS Program

Q What is the CONTOMS program?

A CONTOMS stands for Counter Narcotic and Terrorism Operational Medical Support program. Funded by the Department of Defense, the CONTOMS program started in 1989. The program was designed to provide the specialized medical training to support law enforcement operations. The concept has application in a broad range of law enforcement special operations including counternarcotics, counterterrorism, protective operations, hostage rescue, explosive ordnance disposal, maritime operations, civil disorder, and major events. The program includes a family of courses including EMT-Tactical, The Advanced School, Commanders Course, Medical Director's Course, and the Instructor Development School.

During the 11 years the programs were offered, over 4,000 responders from more than 750 agencies and support law enforcement agencies from all 50 states, the District of Columbia, Guam, and Puerto Rico were trained. More than 40 local, state, and federal law enforcement agencies mandate this certification as a condition of employment for their SWAT medics.

Q What is the CONTOMS program designed to offer?

A The CONTOMS program is designed to:
- Provide access to urgently needed training for state and local law enforcement agencies.
- Ensure a national standardized curriculum, certification process, and quality improvement procedure to meet the

needs of EMS providers who operate as part of tactical law enforcement teams.
- Transfer military medical science and technology to users in the civilian community.
- Serve as the primary academic and scientific resource in the development of Tactical Emergency Medical Support (TEMS) as a discipline.
- Reduce death and injury to officers, innocent bystanders, and suspects.
- Reduce lost work time and duty-related disability.

EMS at Crime Scenes

Q What is a crime scene?

A A crime scene is a location where any part of a criminal act has occurred or where evidence relating to a crime may be found.

Q What are examples of evidence that can be found at a crime scene?

A We have all watched TV. Whether you still watch the reruns of *Dragnet* or are an *NYPD Blue* fan, you have seen examples of how law enforcement officers attempt to limit access to the crime scene so it is not tainted or disrupted. EMS providers are often called to manage an injured or dying patient at a crime scene. By understanding what evidence is important to law enforcement personnel, EMS personnel can both manage the patient and not disrupt the crime scene.

Examples of evidence include the following:
- Fingerprints—everyone has a unique fingerprint, so the characteristics left behind on a surface with oils and moisture from the skin can help to identify the perpetrator. They also can identify the EMS provider as touching various things at the scene if you were not wearing disposable gloves. It is highly recommended that EMS providers wear disposable gloves while at a crime scene. Remember that the gloves may prevent you from leaving your own prints, but they do not prevent you from destroying or "smudging" the perpetrator's prints. So, touch as little as possible!
- Footprints—many times specific shoes leave a mark on the floor or in the mud that can help to distinguish the type of shoe or sneaker and the size of the foot. Sometimes the imprint of the gas or brake pedal can be found on the bottom of the shoe.
- Blood and body fluids—the location and type of blood splatter can help the investigators understand how the injury occurred. DNA tests and ABO blood typing are done to confirm that this

was in fact the victim of the crime. Sometimes the blood may be from the perpetrator who was also injured. Finding the perpetrator's blood or DNA at the scene is extremely important evidence. Other particulate evidence is important too, such as hairs, carpet, and clothing fibers. Be very careful not to step in a pool of blood at a crime scene and leave tracks all over the location.

- Other forms of evidence include clothing stained with blood or body fluids, such as semen. When removing the clothing of an injured person, be careful to place it in a paper bag. Better yet, have the law enforcement officer assist you so it is handled in the manner that they prefer. Never cut through a knife or bullet hole in clothing because this area of the clothing is useful as evidence. Do not move weapons, bullets, or touch the telephone at a crime scene. If you suspect that a sexual assault occurred, be very careful if any clothing is removed because it may have semen stains that can be used to identify the perpetrator.

- Unattended deaths—leave the body in the position found. If you have to move it, note the position and report that to the responding police officer.

What if a person is found hanging, should I cut them down?

If you suspect the hanging is recent and you are going to attempt resuscitation, then cut the rope. Use gloves and avoid cutting right through the knot, cut at least six inches above the knot if possible. If the police are present, let them deal with the rope.

Are the EMS provider's observations important to solving the crime?

They may be very important. Try to get a good picture of the scene as you enter. Don't have tunnel vision on the patient. Observing the entire scene also helps keep you from getting hurt should there still be any danger at the scene. Pay close attention to the position the patient was found in, the lights that were on, the position of the curtains or windows, and any signs of a forced entry into the residence. Keep in mind that patient care takes priority.

Listen carefully to statements you may hear from others at the scene as you arrive and treat the patient. Document on the PCR, in quotes, any dying statements of the patient. Documentation is very important and your PCR will undoubtedly be used as evidence in the case if it goes to trial. Be especially careful to note observations objectively not subjectively. As Officer Friday said many times, "Just the facts." Avoid opinions that are not relevant to medical care. In some states, there may be a requirement mandating the EMS provider to report certain types of crimes (e.g., domestic violence, child abuse, geriatric or elder abuse, rape, violent acts). Check with your medical director to determine the proper reporting requirements, as well as how to maintain patient confidentiality.

In some communities, EMS providers are called to the scene of a crime where a patient is obviously dead and the police need a medical person to tell them that the patient is dead. In that case, be very careful when entering the room, disrupt as little as possible, and do your job. If there is any chance that the patient is viable or does not meet your local protocol definitions of obvious death, then it is necessary to resuscitate the patient. Work together with the police to carefully remove the body from the crime scene, disrupting as little as possible.

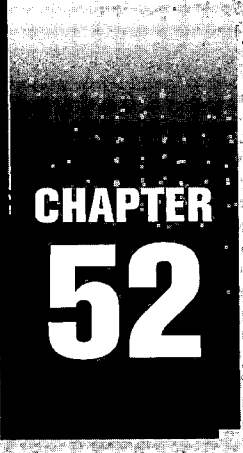

CHAPTER 52 Advanced Cardiac Life Support

This chapter discusses the International Resuscitation Guidelines for advanced life support (ALS). The focus is on the latest changes and updates in ALS, as well as *why* the changes have been made.

Q What are the differences between basic life support (BLS) and ALS?

A ALS is the generic term for care that goes beyond the scope of a basic EMT level. BLS is EMT-Basic level care. As applied to cardiac emergencies, BLS includes CPR, early defibrillation, and early recognition of myocardial infarction (MI) and stroke. ALS encompasses BLS, as well as various drug treatments, airway adjuncts, and other skills not included in the EMT-Basic training. It is also a part of the emergency cardiac care (BLS and ALS) provided to patients experiencing symptoms of a heart attack. ALS when used in the context of cardiac care is the same as ACLS (advanced cardiac life support).

Q What are the Class I guidelines for ALS interventions?

A Examples of Class I ALS interventions include:

- Tracheal suctioning in the delivery of an infant with meconium-stained amniotic fluid if the infant has any of the following: absent or depressed respirations, heart rate below 100, poor muscle tone.
- Angioplasty is an alternative to fibrinolytic therapy in centers with high volume and experienced operators.

- Patients under 75 years old in cardiogenic shock should be transported to a facility that can provide primary angioplasty and intra-aortic balloon placement (door to balloon time 90 minutes or less).
- Acute MI patients, including non-Q wave MI, should receive aspirin and beta blockers in the absence of contraindications.
- IV recombinant tissue plasminogen activator (RTPA) improves the neurologic outcome of stroke patients meeting fibrinolytic criteria within three hours of symptom onset.
- Administration of nitrates for cocaine overdose.

Q What are the Class IIa guidelines for ALS interventions?

A Examples of Class IIa ALS interventions include:

- To prevent tracheal tube dislodgement in the adult patient, a commercially manufactured tracheal tube holder should be used (Figure 52–1).
- Secondary confirmation with end-tidal CO_2 detectors should be used for tracheal intubation of adult patients with spontaneous circulation.
- The laryngeal mask airway (LMA) and esophageal tracheal combitube (ETC) are listed as acceptable alternate advanced airway devices.

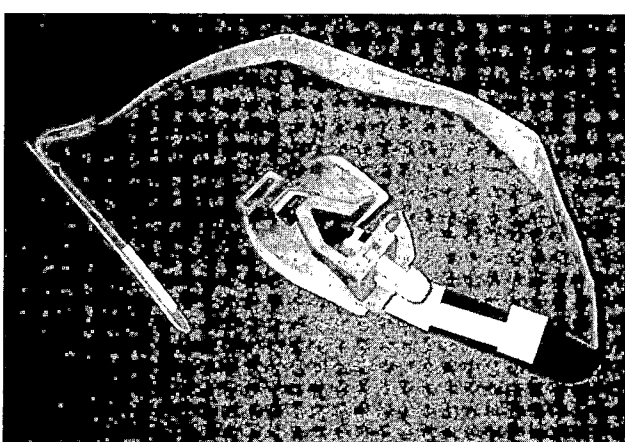

FIGURE 52-1 The Guidelines 2000 strongly suggest that a commercial tube restraint be used whenever an endotracheal tube is placed. Here is one example of a device. *(Courtesy of Bob Elling)*

- The pediatric advanced life support (PALS) course uses the suggested 90-second limit for the establishment of vascular access in a cardiac arrest situation. After 90 seconds, the EMS provider should use the intraosseous (IO) technique.

- Pediatric ET tube confirmation using primary confirmation (i.e., visualization of the tube entering the vocal cords, and observing the chest rise with ventilation), plus one or more of the following secondary confirmation techniques: qualitative end-tidal CO_2 detectors and quantitative and continuous CO_2 measurement, as well as devices that specifically detect tube placement in the esophagus (e.g., chest X ray).

- Post-resuscitation monitoring of normal ventilation and treating hyperthermia in pediatrics.

- Twelve-lead ECG should be standard equipment on all ALS units.

- Patients who are not eligible for fibrinolytic therapy should be considered for transport to a special cardiac facility.

- Patients with large anterior infarctions, systolic BP <100 mmHg, and pulse >100 or rales greater than one-third of the lung fields should be considered for transfer to a special cardiac facility.

- Antiplatelet therapy with glycoprotien IIb and IIIa inhibitors for patients with non-Q wave MI and high risk unstable angina.

- Febrile patients postarrest should be treated with antipyretics.

- Post-resuscitation patients who require mechanical ventilation should have ventilatory parameters in the normal range.

- Benzodiazipines for cocaine overdose.

- Induction of systemic alkalosis (pH 7.50 to 7.55) in tricyclic antidepressant overdoses.

- Rapid reversal of opiate overdose with mechanical ventilation and naloxone.

Q   What are the Class IIb guidelines for ALS interventions?

A   Examples of Class IIb ALS interventions include:

- Secondary confirmation of tracheal intubation using esophageal detector devices on adult patients in cardiac arrest.

- Detection of tracheal tube dislodgement is done using an end-tidal CO_2 monitor (either capnometer or capnography).

- Post-resuscitation, allow a mild hypothermia to exist in pediatric patients.

- Vagal maneuvers (e.g., ice water or ice to the face) for pediatric supraventricular tachycardia (SVT) as long as it does not delay cardioversion or adenosine administration.

- High dose epinephrine for adult and pediatric cardiac arrest.

- Vasopressin in refractory ventricular fibrillation (VF) or pulseless ventricular tachycardia (VT) in adults.

- Amiodarone for shock refractory VF or pulseless VT.

- Magnesium for VF or pulseless VT, torsade de pointes, and dysrhythmias with known hypomagnesemia.

- Diabetic patients who are undergoing reperfusion therapy should also have metabolic manipulation of the infarction with glucose-potassium-insulin.

- EMS systems should implement out-of-hospital stroke protocols to evaluate and rapidly identify patients who may benefit from fibrinolytic therapy.

- Stroke patients who are candidates for fibrinolytic therapy should be transported to hospitals identified as capable of providing acute stroke care including 24-hour CT scan and interpretation.

- Patients who are mildly hypothermic postarrest should not be actively rewarmed.

- Alpha adrenergic blocking agents for cocaine overdose patients who do not respond to nitrates and benzodiazipines.

- Plunger CPR.

- Interposed abdominal compression CPR in-hospital.

- Vest CPR in-hospital.

- Mechanical piston CPR.

- Direct cardiac massage CPR in-hospital after external chest compressions have failed and arrest is still in 30-minute window.

- Impedance threshold valve with the active compression–decompression Cardiopump®.

Q   What are the Class Indeterminate guidelines for ALS interventions?

A   Examples of Class Indeterminate ALS interventions include:

- Under alternate advanced airway devices the pharyngotracheal lumen airway (PTL) and the cuffed oropharyngeal airway (OPA) are listed.

- The LMA is used for cardiac arrest in pediatric patients. It has received this class due to the current lack of studies to support a higher class at this time.
- The use of amiodarone is introduced into the pediatric care plans for pulseless arrest on the basis of extrapolated evidence from adult, not pediatric, studies.
- The LMA can be used in newborns where BVM ventilation is ineffective or there is a failed ET intubation.
- The fluid of choice for volume expansion is an isotonic crystalloid solution (e.g., normal saline or Ringer's lactate).
- Epinephrine for refractory VF or pulseless VT. It has been given this class because its effectiveness has not yet been shown in prospective randomized human clinical trials.
- Lidocaine for shock refractory VF or pulseless VT.
- Antithrombin therapy with low molecular weight heparins is an alternative for unfractionated heparin in high-risk unstable angina or non-Q wave MI.
- Use of RTPA and prourokinase (separately) are being investigated in stroke patients in the three to six hour window.
- Active hypothermia postarrest is under clinical investigation.
- Lidocaine or procainamide for ventricular dysrhythmias from tricyclic antidepressant overdose.

What are the Class III guidelines for ALS interventions?

Examples of Class III ALS interventions include:
- Post-resuscitation hyperventilation for adult and pediatric patients.
- Hyperthermia in newborns.
- Beta blockers for cocaine overdose patients with acute coronary syndromes.

What is the goal of the new American Heart Association's (AHA) Advanced Cardiac Life Support for Experienced Providers (ACLS-EP) Course?

Since 1994, the ACLS course has concentrated on 10 core situations. In a typical course, there simply is not enough time to cover the special situations that arise and the resuscitation problems that occur. In addition, the new course covers patients on their way to cardiac arrest instead of just patients in cardiac arrest (the concentration area of the traditional ACLS course). Examples of the topics discussed in the ACLS-EP include:
- Asthma.
- Anaphylaxis.
- Electrolyte disturbances.
- Toxicology-induced disturbances in rhythm and BP.

- Submersion.
- Lightning strikes.
- Electrical injury.
- Arrest associated with pregnancy.
- Arrest associated with trauma.

What is the new "primary and secondary ABCD survey"?

In ACLS, the new unifying approach to assessment and management involves the combination of a primary ABCD and a secondary ABCD survey. The basic and advanced EMT curricula stopped using these terms in the 1990s and replaced them with the terms initial assessment and detailed physical exam.

- The primary survey includes airway (is it open?), breathing, circulation (chest compression), and defibrillation (use the automated external defibrillator [AED]).
- The secondary survey includes airway (advanced use of tracheal tube), breathing (placement confirmed and effectiveness checked), circulation (gain access to the circulation and give indicated medications), and differential diagnosis.

The Guidelines 2000 require the use of the BVM by all health care providers, as well as recommend the use of the LMA and Combitube® as alternative advanced airway devices for health care providers. Previous standards were very much in favor of the ET tube as the gold standard. What is the latest research on EMS providers placing ET tubes in the field that has led to this change in emphasis?

Studies have shown that when used by properly skilled BLS providers, a BVM attached to supplemental oxygen and continuous cricoid pressure can be as effective as an ET tube in terms of oxygenation, ventilation, and protection from aspiration for short transportation times.

CLINICAL PEARL

> *The reduced tidal requirements in the new guidelines make one-rescuer BVM ventilation reasonable to perform. Previously, it was nearly impossible to achieve the recommended tidal volumes.*

The DOT EMT-Basic curriculum allows ET intubation to be an optional skill. Many service medical directors have held back from training their EMT-Basics on this optional skill. New evidence reveals that unrecognized, uncorrected esophageal intubations or tube dislodgements occur with unacceptable frequency. One study of EMS providers providing pediatric field intubations revealed that eight percent of patients arriving at the ED had a tube in their esophagus. Another study in a large adult group of cardiac arrests revealed that 25 percent of the tubes were in the esophagus or pharynx.

❓ What do the Guidelines 2000 recommend to deal with this problem of misplaced tubes?

🅰 The Guidelines 2000 make recommendations on tube placement confirmation, and continuous monitoring of the position of the tube to avoid its becoming dislodged. To ensure that the tube is inserted in the correct location, the Guidelines 2000 recommend both primary and secondary tube confirmation techniques. The primary techniques include:

- Direct visualization of the tube going through the vocal cords.
- Physical examination of the tube placement.
- Bilateral chest expansion.
- Five-point auscultation (two in each lung and epigastrium).
- Tube condensation.

The secondary techniques include:

- Use of the esophageal detector device (EDD).
- End-tidal CO_2 monitors may be helpful after the first five or more ventilations.

❓ To detect whether an ET tube has become dislodged, especially during the transfer of the patient, what do the Guidelines 2000 recommend?

🅰 The Guidelines 2000 recommend the use of continuous end-tidal CO_2 monitoring to provide early detection of any tube dislodgement. These devices come in two types: capnometers, which have a numerical value, and capnographs, which provide a continuous visual display of the level of expired CO_2. The latter is more accurate, but is also more expensive.

❓ Were any devices recommended as acceptable alternative advanced airway devices?

🅰 Yes. The LMA and the Combitube® are both recommended for all health care providers.

❓ How do the LMA and Combitube® compare to the gold standard of ET intubation?

🅰 In some settings, it is felt that these devices are superior to the BVM technique for ventilation and oxygenation. Surprisingly, the research shows that both devices are equivalent to the ET

tube in the adult patient. Other ways in which these two devices are similar include:

- Both are advanced airway techniques.
- Both are placed orally and inserted past the hypopharyngeal space.
- Both are inserted blindly.
- The Combitube® offers protection from aspiration of the stomach contents into the lungs.
- Both are easy to use and do not require extensive training in the difficult skill of laryngoscopy.
- Training selected EMS providers on the use of either of these devices may expand the number of patients who are afforded an advanced airway when one is needed.

❓ Can the LMA be used in pediatrics?

🅰 LMAs are widely used in the operating room and provide an effective means of ventilation and oxygenation (Figure 52–2). With proper training, they can be used in the pediatric patient. They come in infant and child sizes and are thought to be simpler than ET intubation.

❓ Besides the LMA and the Combitube®, were any other alternative advanced airway devices evaluated?

🅰 Yes. The PTL and the cuffed OPA were evaluated. The Guidelines 2000 list these as class indeterminate and do not recommend the devices.

❓ What is an ETC?

🅰 The ETC is an abbreviation for the esophageal tracheal combitube or Combitube®. This device is discussed in detail in the respiration section of this book.

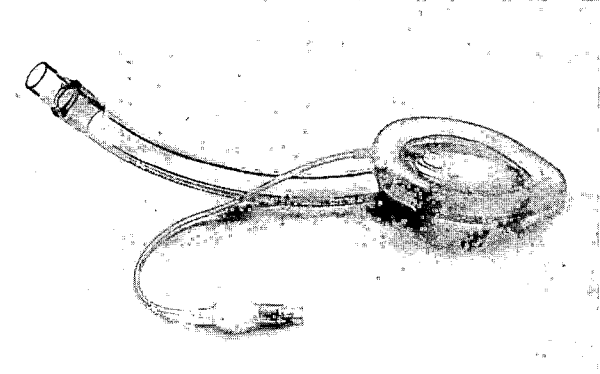

FIGURE 52–2 The LMA was introduced to the field in the Guidelines 2000. *(Courtesy of LMA North America, Inc.)*

Pediatric Advanced Life Support

Q What is the primary emphasis of the Guidelines 2000 in the area of ALS for pediatrics?

A Early identification of critical illnesses such as respiratory failure and shock, and the prevention of cardiac arrest continue to be the emphasis of the Guidelines 2000.

Q What is the default sequence of PALS intervention based on?

A The default is based on the most common cause of arrest for specific age groups. The program now also emphasizes cardiovascular emergencies related to special resuscitation circumstances such as drug overdoses, toxins, electrolyte abnormalities, asthma, and anaphylaxis.

Q Why is there more emphasis on the cardiovascular effects of drug toxicity and poisonings in the Guidelines 2000?

A There is more knowledge about specific dysrhythmias and the cardiovascular effects of drugs, such as cocaine. Because more PALS providers have mastered the previous course content, it is a logical time to enrich the program with this new knowledge in the area of managing common poisonings, toxicological problems, and electrolyte abnormalities.

Q Is the de-emphasis on ET tubes similar in the pediatric training as it is in the adults?

A The Guidelines 2000 take a stronger stance in favor of the health care provider using the BVM with supplemental oxygen as opposed to an ET tube in a pediatric patient for short transports. This is because studies have shown that most EMS providers are not sufficiently practiced in pediatric ET tube placement. Studies confirm that, in some EMS systems, the success rate for pediatric intubation had an unacceptable level of complications. One study showed that 1 out of 11 tubes were placed in the esophagus.

Q What are the recommendations for proper tube placement confirmation for pediatric patients?

A Any time a pediatric tube is placed, the health care provider must ensure that the tube has been properly placed by using primary confirmation (i.e., visualization of tube entering the vocal cords and observing the chest rise), plus one or more of the following secondary confirmation techniques: qualitative end-tidal CO_2 detectors or quantitative and continuous CO_2 measurement,

as well as devices that specifically detect tube placement in the esophagus (e.g., chest X ray).

Q Are specific approaches to prevent tube dislodgement addressed in the pediatric ALS portions of the Guidelines 2000?

A Yes, they are. Commercially manufactured tube holders should be used instead of tape or string tie-downs. In the out-of-hospital setting, movement greatly increases the chance for tube dislodgement. A dislodged tube can be a fatal error if not recognized rapidly. That is why breath sounds should be reassessed after each patient move and continuous end-tidal CO_2 monitoring is necessary. The Guidelines state that the sensitivity and specificity of these devices are lower than when a perfusing rhythm is present. Be aware of this issue as a low end-tidal CO_2 reading can mislead the EMS provider into mistakenly suspecting esophageal intubation in a child in cardiac arrest even though the tube is actually in the trachea. That is why continuous monitoring is recommended. It actually takes five ventilations to begin to get a reliable reading.

Q Are there any pediatric post-resuscitation interventions that may improve the neurological outcome?

A In the past, patients were hyperventilated. This is no longer recommended because studies show hyperventilation reduces cerebral blood flow and may create cerebral ischemia. Both hypo- and hyperglycemia are detrimental and should be avoided in the post-resuscitation patient. The Guidelines 2000 recommend the following for post-resuscitation:

- Maintain normal ventilation rates and volume.
- Monitor body temperature, treating hyperthermia and allowing a mild hypothermia to exist.
- Manage postarrest myocardial ischemia dysfunction.
- Maintain normal blood sugar levels.

Q Are there any other reasons not to hyperventilate the patient?

A Yes, hyperventilating increases the risk of gastric inflation in both pediatrics and adults.

Q What is the age limit for the use of IO venous access in children?

A The Guidelines 2000 have removed the previous age limit of six years old. They state that venous access should be established in the cardiac arrest situation within a reasonable amount of time. The PALS course used 90 seconds as the limit for establishing a peripheral line. If one cannot be established within this time period, then IO should be attempted. The success rate for older children is less than that of infants, but this is still a viable and acceptable means of venous access that should be considered. There is more flexibility as far as time is concerned if the patient is stable.

Q Is it true that the Guidelines 2000 recommend applying ice water to the face of an infant or young child?

A Yes, in very specific circumstances. This is one of a number of acceptable vagal maneuvers that can be tried in the child with poor symptomatic perfusion from an SVT. The vagal maneuvers are done while preparing to cardiovert or use adenosine and should not delay these "electrical" treatments.

CLINICAL PEARL

This maneuver is not as strange as it may sound at first. The cold leads to vagal stimulation in a relatively benign fashion. This may break an SVT.

Q Are there any new medications added to pediatric treatments of potentially lethal dysrhythmias?

A Amiodarone has been added to the management of both supraventricular and ventricular dysrhythmias. Although successful experience with this drug is currently accumulating because there were no prospective, randomized trials in pediatric cardiac arrest, all recommendations are extrapolations of adult studies. This is the reason why the Guidelines 2000 gave amiodarone an indeterminate class.

Q The previous guidelines recommended higher doses of epinephrine for the second and subsequent doses in the pediatric cardiac arrest patient. Is this still the case?

A In the Guidelines 2000, the use of high-dose epinephrine for pediatric cardiac arrest has been de-emphasized. Basically, the initial dose of 0.01 mg/kg by IV or IO or 0.1 mg/kg by the ET route should be repeated every three to five minutes of the arrest. Higher doses are mentioned (IV or IO) as a consideration but not a recommendation. This is because a number of large multi-institutional adult studies, well-controlled animal studies, and uncontrolled retrospective pediatric data failed to show a benefit from high-dose epinephrine. Actually, the high-dose epinephrine can have adverse effects, such as increased myocardial oxygen demand, hyperadrenergic state, tachycardia, hypertension, and myocardial necrosis.

Neonatal Care

Q Are there any recommendations for the care of the neonate in the Guidelines 2000?

A Yes, a few are:

- Ventilation—the importance of establishing adequate ventilation was reaffirmed in the newly born infant who presents with a heart rate less than 100 bpm.
- Meconium-stained amniotic fluid—the Guidelines 2000 no longer recommend tracheal suctioning of infants who are active and vigorous and present with meconium staining. It has been shown that some infants aspirate in utero and tracheal suctioning does not improve the outcome and may cause complications if the infant is active and vigorous. The procedure, when meconium is observed in the amniotic fluid, is to deliver the head and suction the meconium from the hypopharynx. If there is meconium staining and the infant has absent or depressed respirations, heart rate below 100, or poor muscle tone, then direct tracheal suctioning should be done.
- The chest compressions of CPR should be started if the heart rate is absent or if the heart rate is less than 60 after 30 seconds of ventilations.
- The compression to ventilation ratio and rate should be 3:1 at a rate of 120 events per minute (90 compressions and 30 ventilations).
- The two-thumb and encircling fingers method is the preferred method for two-rescuer infant CPR. This has been shown to generate higher peak systolic and coronary perfusion pressures.
- The LMA can be used, by properly trained providers, in newborns where BVM ventilation is ineffective or there is a failed ET intubation. However, an ET tube is still needed if meconium needs to be suctioned from the newborn.
- Secondary confirmation of tracheal tube placement by the monitoring of exhaled CO_2 can be useful in the newborn with equivocal clinical assessment. There must also be consideration for the fact that there are false negative results leading to the removal of a good tube and false positive results leading to thinking an esophageal intubation is in the correct location.
- The fluid of choice for volume expansion is an isotonic crystalloid solution (e.g., normal saline or Ringer's lactate). Albumin-containing solutions are rarely used due to limited availability, a potential for infectious disease transmission, and an association with increased mortality.
- Hyperthermia should be avoided because it has been associated with perinatal respiratory depression.
- The use of 100 percent oxygen for assisted ventilations was reaffirmed.

- Personnel capable of starting CPR should attend every delivery.

Are there any special circumstances where the initiation of CPR on the newborn may not be appropriate?

The Guidelines 2000 list a few special circumstances where the initiation of a resuscitation may not be appropriate or the discontinuation of a resuscitation may be the most appropriate course of action. These are ethical decisions that should be made in conjunction with discussions with the parents and family members. Specific examples include infants with confirmed gestation <23 weeks, birthweight <400 grams, anencephaly (absence of all or a major part of the brain), confirmed trisomy 13 (CNS defects and mental retardation called Patau's syndrome), or trisomy 18 (mental retardation and skull abnormalities, also known as Edward's syndrome).

Advanced Cardiac Life Support for Adults

What is the difference between the International Liaison Committee on Resuscitation (ILCOR) algorithm and the AHA algorithms for ACLS?

The international resuscitation community prefers a simple format with the items listed representing just a hint of the unseen details. In the ILCOR algorithm all cardiac arrest conditions are found in one universal algorithm. The algorithms used by the AHA tend to be more detailed with teaching aids and four separate cardiac arrest conditions: VF, pulseless VT, asystole, and pulseless electrical activity (PEA).

What are the key changes in the management of VF and pulseless ventricular tachycardia?

In the primary ABCD survey, the emphasis is on phone first to activate the EMS system to get the defibrillator to the VF patient as fast as possible. The new changes in the secondary ABCD survey include:

- Recognition that the LMA or Combitube® are acceptable advanced airway alternatives.
- Emphasis on both primary and secondary confirmation of tube placement (discussed previously).
- De-emphasis on high-dose epinephrine. Repeat initial dose of 1 mg every three to five minutes. High dose is still considered acceptable but only after 1 mg of epinephrine has failed.

- Vasopressin is a vasopressor agent that appears to be as effective as epinephrine in cardiac arrest. It lasts between 10 and 20 minutes, so only one dose is recommended. If no response, resume epinephrine in 5 to 10 minutes.

- Amiodarone is the antiarrhythmic for shock refractory VF or pulseless VT. It is not produced in a preloaded syringe because the medication is too caustic for the plastic. Realize that it will take a moment or two to draw it up from the ampule. The alternate antiarrhythmic is lidocaine. Due to supply problems and a high incidence of side effects, bretylium is no longer included in the algorithm.

- Magnesium has been shown to be effective for VF or pulseless VT, torsade de pointes and dysrhythmias with known hypomagnesemia.

What are the key changes in the management of PEA?

The PEA algorithm contains the following key changes:

- Recognition that the LMA or Combitube® are acceptable advanced airway alternatives.
- Emphasis on both primary and secondary confirmation of tube placement (discussed previously).
- De-emphasis of high-dose epinephrine. Repeat initial dose of 1 mg every three to five minutes. High dose is still considered acceptable, but only after 1 mg doses have failed.
- The changes are teaching tips to help the EMS provider remember the potential causes of PEA (e.g., hypovolemia, hypoxia, hydrogen ion, hyper- or hypokalemia, hypothermia, tablets, tamponade, tension pneumothorax, thrombosis).

What are the key changes in the management of asystole?

The management and medications used for asystole remain the same. However, the key changes are in the area of determining the presence of a Do Not Attempt Resuscitation order because asystole often occurs in terminally ill patients expecting to die. It is emphasized that each community needs to have protocols for stopping CPR after consultation with medical control and provisions for leaving the body at the scene. Other arrangements should be made to transport the body directly to a funeral home and the focus of care should be toward supporting and comforting the family.

What is the treatment for symptomatic bradycardias?

Clinical research has not identified the need for any changes in the way bradydysrhythmias are managed using atropine, transcutaneous pacing, dopamine, and epinephrine.

Has the management for tachycardia changed?

There has been considerable change. The changes adhere to five principles:

- Anti-dysrhythmics are now known to also have pro-arrhythmic effects.
- The use of more than one anti-dysrhythmic is no longer recommended due to the increased risk of complications.
- If the patient has impaired myocardial function, most anti-dysrhythmics will make the cardiac function worse. The selection of the optimal medication requires a knowledge of the patient's underlying ventricular function.
- Electrical cardioversion should be the intervention of choice or second anti-dysrhythmic. The rule of thumb is: "When an anti-dysrhythmic is administered to a patient with persistent tachycardia, and the tachydysrhythmia remains, that patient should then be considered unstable."
- Arriving at a diagnosis is a high priority, if time permits, in the acute setting.

Are there any changes in the management of atrial fibrillation?

There are a number of new medications that have been introduced in the Guidelines 2000 for use in the patient with atrial fibrillation who is symptomatic (e.g., amiodarone, flecainide, propafenone, sotalol, and ibutiulide). The algorithm suggests considering the following questions:

- Is the patient clinically unstable?
- Is cardiac function impaired?
- Is Wolff-Parkinson-White syndrome present?
- Has the duration of the rhythm been greater than 48 hours?

The treatment depends on the following rule of thumb: "If unstable, cardiovert, otherwise first control the rate then convert the rhythm."

Are there any changes in the management of a narrow complex SVT?

Although adenosine still starts the management for these dysrhythmias, the algorithm then sorts the rhythms into junctional tachycardia, paroxysmal SVT, and multifocal atrial tachycardia.

Are there any changes in the management of stable VT?

The management depends on whether the VT is stable or unstable, polymorphic or monomorphic. Polymorphic VT management is further divided into normal and prolonged Q-T inter-

vals. Amiodarone is the first-line drug for stable VT with procainamide as the second-line choice. If the patient has a wide complex VT, amiodarone is first line.

Are there any post-resuscitative care recommendations in the Guidelines 2000?

Yes, there are, and they are summarized as follows:

- If the patient is mildly hypothermic after the arrest, they should not be actively rewarmed. Active hypothermia is currently being investigated, but is not a recommendation.
- If the patient is febrile, they should be treated with antipyretics.
- If the patient requires mechanical ventilation, they should be maintained within a normal rate and volume.
- Hyperventilation should only be considered for patients who have signs of cerebral herniation after resuscitation.

Do the Guidelines 2000 make any recommendation for new devices to use as adjuncts to mechanical CPR?

Yes, there are a number of devices or techniques that are given a Class IIb so that they can be further studied for effectiveness. The following is a list of alternatives to traditional CPR that should only be used when an adequate number of rescuers properly trained in the techniques are available:

- Plunger CPR—the active compression–decompression.
- Interposed abdominal compression CPR for in-hospital resuscitation.
- Vest CPR—an alternative for hemodynamic support and short-term (six hour) survival.
- Mechanical (piston) CPR that is used in many areas already incorporating a Thumper®.
- Direct cardiac massage is an alternative to be considered in-hospital after external chest compressions have failed and the time of the arrest is still within 30 minutes.
- The impedance threshold valve has been shown to enhance negative thoracic pressure during the decompression phase of chest compression with the active compression–decompression Cardiopump®.

Acute Coronary Syndromes

What does the term acute coronary syndrome include?

AMI and unstable angina are now recognized as a part of a spectrum of disease known as acute coronary syndromes or ACS.

Q Do the Guidelines 2000 take a strong stand on the use of 12-lead ECGs?

A Yes, they do. In fact, they state that the out-of-hospital 12-lead ECG should become standard equipment on all ALS units handling ACS patients.

Q Are there any medications recommended for the out-of-hospital management of the ACS?

A All patients with AMI, including non-Q wave MI, should receive aspirin and beta blockers in the absence of contra-indications.

Q What is the focus of the Guidelines 2000 on the use of thrombolytics for ACS patients?

A Clotbusters or fibrinolytic therapy is beneficial in the out-of-hospital phase of care if the transport time is prolonged (60 minutes or longer).

Q Are there any other reperfusion therapies recommended for the ACS patient?

A In the hospital phase of care, antiplatelet therapy with glycoprotein IIb and IIIa inhibitors should be administered to patients with non-Q wave AMI and high-risk unstable angina. Another is antithrombin therapy with low molecular weight heparins as an alternate agent for unfractioned heparin for high-risk unstable angina or non-Q wave MI.

The weight adjusted dose of unfractioned heparin indicated as an adjunct therapy with fibrin specific lytics (e.g., alteplase, reteplase) has been reduced to 60 U/kg (with a maximum of 4,000 U and 12 IU/kg/h infusion) to minimize the incidence of intracerebral hemorrhage with these agents.

CLINICAL PEARL

Platelets have surface receptors (IIb and IIIa) that facilitate aggregation during clot formation. The receptor inhibitors block, to at least some degree, this adhesion. These agents have demonstrated significant efficacy, with or without concomitant thrombolytic therapy, in people with ACS.

In patients, especially those with diabetes, the metabolic manipulation of the infarct with glucose-insulin-potassium is currently being investigated. Patients with a large anterior infarction, left ventricular dysfunction, and ejection fraction under 40

CLINICAL PEARL

Glucose-insulin-potassium (GIK) infusions have been used on and off for many years. Though they had fallen into disfavor, recent data again supports their use.

percent should receive early ACE inhibition in the absence of hypotension.

Q Do the Guidelines 2000 make any statement about where ACS patients should be taken for their condition to be acutely managed?

A Patients less than 75 years old who are in cardiogenic shock should be transported to a hospital that can do primary angioplasty and intra-aortic balloon placement. The door to balloon time should be less than 90 minutes.

Patients who are not eligible for fibrinolytic therapy due to exclusionary criteria should be considered for transport or transfer to a hospital with these specialty facilities. Patients with large anterior infarctions, systolic BP <100 mmHg, heart rates over 100, or rales greater than one-third of the lung fields should also be considered for transfer to these specialty facilities.

Stroke

Q Do the Guidelines 2000 take a more aggressive approach to the management of strokes?

A Yes, they do. In fact, IV fibrinolytics have been shown to improve the neurological outcome of stroke patients who meet the criteria if they are administered within three hours of the onset of the symptoms. These patients should be triaged with the same urgency as acute S-T-elevation MIs.

The use of RTPA, as well as an agent called prourokinase, in patients in the three- to six-hour window from onset of symptoms is under investigation but not currently recommended.

Q Do the Guidelines 2000 make any recommendation for the out-of-hospital management of the stroke patient?

A Yes, they recommend that EMS systems implement a stroke protocol to evaluate and rapidly identify patients who may benefit from fibrinolytic therapy similar to ACS patients. These patients, if they qualify, should be transported to hospitals capable of providing acute stroke care, including 24-hour CT scan and interpretation.

Toxicology

What do the Guidelines 2000 say about cocaine overdose?

Cocaine has been shown to be associated with serious ventricular dysrhythmias and ACS. The standards make the following recommendations:

- Nitrates should be first-line therapy as well as benzodiazipines. Alpha adrenergic-blocking agents should be second-line therapy only if the patient does not respond to the first-line drugs. Be cautious because these agents may cause tachycardia and hypotension.

CLINICAL PEARL

Cocaine has both alpha and beta stimulatory effects. Just blocking beta receptors may lead to unopposed alpha stimulation, vasoconstriction, and hypertension. A better choice for cocaine toxicity is labaetolol, a mixed alpha–beta blocker.

- Beta-blocking agents should not be administered in the cocaine overdose with an ACS history.

What do the Guidelines 2000 say about tricyclic antidepressant overdoses?

An overdose of tricyclic antidepressants has been shown to cause hypotension or ventricular dysrhythmias. The treatment of choice is the induction of a systemic alkalosis with a pH of 7.50 to 7.55. The use of antiarrhythmic agents, like lidocaine or procainamide, has not been studied in this setting, so no recommendation is made.

What do the Guidelines 2000 say about opiate overdose?

Opiate or narcotic overdoses can cause acute respiratory failure. It is recommended that the patient receive an expeditious reversal of these abnormalities by the combination of mechanical ventilation and naloxone administration. This will reduce the incidence of acute pulmonary edema and lethal dysrhythmias.

Resources

Abrams, W., & Berkow, R. (1995). *The Merck manual of geriatrics* (2nd ed.). Rahway, NJ: Merck Sharp & Dohme Research Laboratories.

American College of Emergency Physicians. (1997). Emergency care guidelines. *Annals of Emergency Medicine, 29* (4), 564–571.

Anderson, D. (1994). *Dorland's illustrated medical dictionary* (28th ed.). Philadelphia: W. B. Saunders.

Auerbach, P., & Geehr, E. (Eds.). (1989). Management of wilderness and environmental emergencies (2nd ed.). St. Louis, MO: Mosby.

Bates, B., Bickley, L., & Hoekelman, R. (1995). *A guide to physical examination and history taking* (6th ed.). Phildelphia: Lippincott.

Bickell, W., Pepe, P., Bailey, M., Wyatt, C., & Mattox, K. (1987). Randomized trial on pneumatic antishock garments in the prehospital management of penetrating abdominal injuries. *Annals of Emergency Medicine, 16*, 653–658.

Bledsoe, B., Porter, R., & Cherry, R. (2000). *Paramedic care: Principles & practice, volume 1: Introduction to advanced prehospital care.* Upper Saddle River, NJ: Prentice Hall.

Bledsoe, B., Porter, R., & Cherry, R. (2000). *Paramedic case: Principles & practice, volume 2: Patient assessment.* Upper Saddle River, NJ: Prentice Hall.

Bledsoe, B., Porter, R., & Cherry, R. (2001). *Paramedic case: Principles & practice, volume 3: Medical emergencies.* Upper Saddle River, NJ: Prentice Hall.

Bledsoe, B., Porter, R., & Cherry, R. (2001). *Paramedic case: Principles & practice, volume 4: Trauma emergencies.* Upper Saddle River, NJ: Prentice Hall.

Bledsoe, B., Porter, R., & Cherry, R. (2001). *Paramedic case: Principles & practice, volume 5: Special considerations and operations.* Upper Saddle River, NJ: Prentice Hall.

Brody, T. (1999). *Nutritional biochemistry* (2nd ed.). San Diego, CA: Academic Press.

Brown, E. (1998). *Basic concepts in pathology: A student's survival guide.* New York: McGraw-Hill.

Campbell, J. (1998). *Basic trauma life support for paramedics and other advanced providers* (3rd ed.). Upper Saddle River, NJ: Prentice Hall.

Castro, W., Skarin, R., & Roscelli, J. (1985). Orthostatic heart rate and arterial blood pressure changes in normovolemic children. *Pediatric Emergency Care, 1,* 123–127.

Cotran, R., Kumar, V., & Collins, T. (1999). *Robbins pathologic basis of disease* (6th ed.). Philadelphia: W. B. Saunders.

Cummins, R., & Hazinski, M. F. (Eds.). (2000, August 22). Guidelines 2000 for cardiopulmonary resuscitation and emergency cardiovascular care. *Circulation, 10* (American Heart Association Suppl.).

Dernocoeur, K. (1998). *Streetsense: Communication, safety and control* (3rd ed.). Redmond, WA: Laing Research Services.

Eichelberger, M., Pratsch, G., Ball, J., & Clark, J. (1998). *Pediatric emergencies: A manual for prehospital care providers* (2nd ed.). Upper Saddle River, NJ: Prentice Hall.

Elling, B. (2001). *Pocket reference for the EMT-B and first responder* (2nd ed.). Upper Saddle River, NJ: Prentice Hall.

Elling, B., & Guerin, R. (1990, October). Getting there. *Emergency,* 52–92.

Elling, B. (1989, July). Dispelling the myths about ambulance accidents. *Journal of EMS,* 60–64.

Elling, B., & Politis, J. (1987, September). Backboarding the standing patient. *Journal of EMS,* 64–66.

Elling, B., & Politis, J. (1983). An evaluation of EMT's ability to use manual ventilation devices. *Annals of Emergency Medicine, 12*(12), 765–768.

Estes, M. E. (1998). *Health assessment and physical examination.* Albany, NY: Delmar Thomson Learning.

Foltin, G., Tunik, M., Cooper, A., Markenson, D., Treiber, M., Phillips, R., & Karpeles, T. (1998). *Teaching resource for instructors of prehospital pediatrics.* The Center for Pediatric Emergency Medicine.

Ghajar, G. (1999). Guidelines for prehospital management of traumatic brain injury. Brain Trauma Foundation.

Ginsburgh, W. (1998). Prepare to be shocked: The evolving standard of care in treating sudden cardiac arrest. *American Journal of Emergency Medicine, 16*(3), 315–319.

Goldfrank, L. (1986). *Goldfrank's toxicologic emergencies* (3rd ed.). Norwalk, CT: Appleton-Century-Croft.

Gray, H. (1977). *Gray's anatomy* (16th ed.). London: Bounty Books.

Guyton, A. (1986). *Textbook of medical physiology* (7th ed.). Philadelphia: W. B. Saunders.

Henry, M., & Stapleton, E. (1992). *EMT prehospital care.* Philadelphia: W. B. Saunders.

Huszar, R. (1995). *Basic dysrhythmias interpretation and management* (2nd ed.). St. Louis, MO: Mosby.

Keuhl, S. (1994). *Prehospital systems and medical oversight* (2nd ed.). National Association of EMS Physicians.

Kposowa, A. (2000). Marital status and suicide in the national longitudinal mortality study. *Journal of Epidemiology and Community Health, 54*(4), 254–261.

Kübler-Ross, E. (1969). *On death and dying.* New York: MacMillan.

Limmer, D., Elling, B., & O'Keefe, M. (2001). *Essentials of emergency care: A refresher for the practicing EMT-B* (3rd ed.). Upper Saddle River, NJ: Prentice Hall.

Limmer, D., O'Keefe, M., Grant, H., Murray, R., & Bergeron, J. (2000). *Emergency care* (9th ed.). Upper Saddle River, NJ: Prentice Hall.

Litovitz, T., Klein-Schwartz, W., Caravati, E., Youniss, J., Crouch, B., & Lee, S. (1999). 1998 annual report of the American Association of Poison Control Centers toxic exposure surveillance system. *American Journal of Emergency Medicine, 17*(5), 435–487.

Martini, F., & Bartholomew, E. (1997). *Essentials of anatomy and physiology.* Upper Saddle River, NJ: Prentice Hall.

Mattox, K., Bickell, W., Pepe, P., & Mangelsdorff, A. (1986). Prospective randomized evaluation of antishock MAST in post-traumatic hypotension. *Journal of Trauma, 26*(9), 779–786.

Merriam-Webster's medical desk dictionary. (1996). Albany, NY: Delmar Thomson Learning.

Mitchell, J., & Bray, G. (1990). *Emergency services stress: Guidelines on Preserving the Health and Careers of Emergency Services Personnel.* Upper Saddle River, NJ: Prentice Hall.

Moore, K., & Newton, K. (1986). Orthostatic heart rates and blood pressures in healthy young women and men. *Heart and Lung, 15*(6), 611–617.

National Association of Emergency Medical Technicians (1998). *Prehospital Trauma Life Support* (4th ed.). St. Louis, MO: Mosby.

Nelson, D., & Cox, M. (2000). *Lehninger principles of biochemistry* (3rd ed.). New York: Worth Publishers.

Pepe, P., Bass, R., & Mattox, K. (1986). Clinical trials of the pneumatic shock garment in the urban prehospital setting. *Annals of Emergency Medicine, 15*(12), 1407–1410.

Rothenberg, M. (2001). *Pathophysiology: A plain English approach.* Eau Claire, WI: PESI HealthCare.

Thibodeau, G., & Patton, K. (1998). *Anthony's textbook of anatomy & physiology* (16th ed.). St. Louis, MO: Mosby.

Tintinalli, J., Ruiz, E., & Krome, R. (Eds.). (1992). *Emergency medicine: A comprehensive study guide* (3rd ed.). New York: McGraw-Hill.

Towler, J. (1997). *A love affair with life.* Navarre, FL: American College of Prehospital Medicine.

U.S. Department of Transportation. (1997). *Paramedic: National Standard Curriculum.* Washington, DC: Author.

U.S. Department of Transportation. (1997). *Intermediate: National Standard Curriculum.* Washington, DC: Author.

Venes, D., & Thomas, C. (Eds.). (2001). *Tabor's cyclopedic medical dictionary* (19th ed.). Phildelphia: F. A. Davis.

Wills, M., Gould, G., & Watson, L. (2000). *MedEMT: A learning system for prehospital care.* Upper Saddle River, NJ: Prentice Hall.

Index

AAA (abdominal aortic aneurysm), 249
Abandonment, 43
ABCD survey, 578
Abdominal pain, 297, 300–301, 366, 367
Abdominal trauma, 449–54
  assessment, 451–53
  pathophysiology, 449–51
  sexual trauma, 453–54
  terminology, 450–51
Abnormal gaits, 272
Accommodations, in patient management, 507–8
ACE inhibitors, 87, 229
ACLS (advanced cardiac life support), 104, 576–85
Acquired factor deficiency, 360
ACS (acute coronary syndromes), 583–84
Activated charcoal, 314
ADA (Americans With Disabilities Act), 51
AD (affective disorders), 499
Adams-Stokes syndrome, 246
Addiction, 4–5, 317
Adenoids, 467–68
Adherent dressing, 394
Adolescents
  development of, 120–22, 126–28
  milestones, 128
  vital signs, 120, 126
Adrenal gland disease, 287–89
Adrenal insufficiency, 288–89
Adrenergic receptor, 84–85
Adults
  development of, 122–25, 126–28
  milestones, 122, 128
  vital signs, 122, 123, 126
Advance directive, 46, 56

AED (automated external defibrillator), 19, 107–8
AEIOU-TIPS, 172, 267
Aeromedical transport, 182, 378, 526–28
AHA (American Heart Association), 54, 106, 578
Air embolism, 337
Airway management and ventilation, 129–44
  airway control, 131–34
  airway devices, 513
  physiology, 129–31
  respiratory distress, 134–44
Albuterol, 221
Allergies, 72, 81, 290–95
ALS (advanced life support), 50, 181, 489, 576–78
ALTE (apparent life-threatening event), 465
Altitude illness, 338–39
Alzheimer's disease, 75, 494
Ambulance operations, 51–54, 516–25
  checking ambulances, 518–19
  deployment and staffing standards, 519–20
  medical equipment standards, 517–18
  preventing collisions, 520–25
  standards and design, 516–17
AMI (acute myocardial infarction), 228, 238–39, 241
Aminophylline, 221
Amnesia, 260–61
Amputation, 395
AMS (acute mountain sickness), 339
Analog transmission, 199
Anaphylaxis, 290–95
Angioneurotic edema, 291

ANS (autonomic nervous system), 84
Antepartum factors, 468
Anterior cord syndrome, 427
Antibody, 290
Antigen, 290
Antisocial behavior, 121
Anxiety, 5
Anxiety-hyperventilation syndrome, 217, 233
AOI (apnea of infancy), 465
AOP (apnea of prematurity), 465–66
Aortic dissection, 446
APCO (Association of Public Safety Communications Officials), 197
APE (acute pulmonary edema), 250–51, 252
Apgar score, 373
Apical pulse, 154
Apnea, 143
Apnea monitor, 513
Apothecary system, 100–101
Appropriate response time, 520
Arbovirus, 346
Arterial gas (air) embolism, 337
Arterial tourniquet, 394
Ascending nerve tracts, 421
Ascites, 66
Aspiration, 131
Aspirin, 248
Assault and battery, 50
Assessment-based curricula, 171
Assessment-based management, 185–88
Asthma, 218–20, 480, 481, 484
Asystole, 245, 582
Atelectasis, 140
Atherosclerosis, 241, 242
Atrial fibrillation, 583
Atrophy, 60
Attachment theory, 117

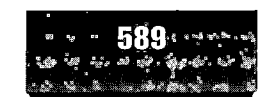

ATV (automatic transport ventilator), 139
Auscultation, 151–52, 153
Autoimmunity, 81
Automaticity, 236
Autonomic hyperreflexia syndrome, 427–28
AVPU, 268
Awareness level training, 537

BAAM® (Beck Airway Airflow Monitor) adapter, 143
Back labor, 372
Bacteria, 62–63
Barrel chest, 215–16
Barton, Clara, 17
BCLS (basic cardiac life support), 104–12
Beck's triad, 252
Behavioral and psychiatric disorders, 347–54
Biological clock, 122
Birth injuries, 470
Bites and stings, 323
Black stool, 303
Blast injuries, 392
Blood, 355, 360
Blood-brain barrier, 86
Blood forming organs, 356
Blood gas report, 212–13
Blood glucose, 157
Blood pressure, 154–55
Blood samples, 93–95
BLS (basic life support), 104, 181, 576
Body recovery, 541
Bone marrow, 356
Bones, 456
Bowel sounds, 304, 451
Boyd, David, 182
Brain, 253–57, 259–61, 414
Brain abscess, 266
Brain herniation, 274–75, 416
Brain stem, 413
Braxton Hicks contractions, 374
Breathing assessment, 168–69
Breath sounds, 216–17
Brown paper bag treatment, 233
Brown-Séquard's syndrome, 427
Bruit, 153
Brunacini, Alan, 530
BS (blood sugar), 277–78, 279
BSI (body substance isolation), 15, 92, 163, 342
Burns, 396–406, 500
  chemical, 401–2
  classifications of, 397–98
  electrical, 402–4
  epidemiology and prevention, 396–97
  inhalation, 401
  pathophysiology, assessment, and types of, 397–99
  radiation exposure, 404–6
  thermal, 399–401
BVM (bag-valve-mask resuscitator), 108–9, 137–39, 488

CAD (computer aided dispatch) system, 196
CAD (coronary artery disease), 73–74
Calcium, 69–70
Call volume, 519
Calm and orderly demeanor, 188
Cancer, 72–73
CAPECHO, 174
Capillary refill time, 169
Capnography, 142
Cardiac enzyme testing, 247
Cardiac muscle, 456
Cardiac tamponade, 252
Cardiac valves, 234
Cardiogenic shock, 251–52
Cardiology, 234–52
  diagnostic tests, 247
  dysrhythmias, 245–46, 482–83
  ECG, 241–45
  electrical therapy, 246–47
  etiology of chest pain, 238–40
  general treatment, 247–48
  history, 240–41
  pathophysiology of vascular disorders, 248–50
  physical examination, 247
  physiology, 234–38
  reperfusion therapy, 247
Cardiomyopathies, 73
Carpopedal spasm, 217
Cartilaginous joints, 456
Catacholamines, 10
CE (continuing education), 22
Cellular adaptation, 60
Cellular communication device, 199
Cellular environment, 64
Cellular immunity, 358
Cellular injury, 62, 63–64
Cellular metabolism impairment, 77
Central cord syndrome, 427
Cerebellum, 413
Cerebral autoregulation, 249
Cerebral neoplasms, 266
Cerebrum, 413
Cervical collar, 139, 181–82
Cervical spine injury, 168
Challenged patients, 502–10
CHD (coronary heart disease), 73–74
Chemical injury, 62
Chemical restraint, 352
Chemoreceptors, 435
CHEMTREC, 562
CHF (congestive heart failure), 228, 250–52
Child abuse and neglect, 477–79
Childbirth. See pregnancy and childbirth
Chloride, 67
Cholinergic receptor, 84
Chronic bronchitis, 220–21
Chronotropism, 236
Circadian rhythms, 3
Circulation assessment, 110
CISM (critical incident stress management), 12–13
Civil Rights Act (Title VII) of 1964, 46
Clandestine drug labs, 571

Claudication, 250
Clawson, Jeff, 18, 196
Clawson's Medical Priority Dispatch® system, 196
Clean accident, 406
Cleaning, 15
Cleft lip, 466
Cleft palate, 466
Clinical decision making, 189–91
Closed fracture, 457
Closed incident, 529
Clotbusters, 247
Clotting systems, 359–60
CNS (central nervous system), 257–59
CO (cardiac output), 435
Combitube®, 579
Comfort care, 47, 513
Common cold, 224
Communication, 24–25, 145–49, 188, 192–200
  electronic, 193, 200
  equipment issues, 198–200
  exchange of information, 192–96
  hospital radio reports, 196–98
  phases of, 192, 193
  verbal, 193, 194
  written, 193
Compartment syndrome, 392
Compensated shock, 383
Complete person, 113
Comprehensive Drug Abuse Prevention and Control Act, 88
Compression-ventilation ratio, 111
Concealment, 572, 573
Concussion, 260, 415
Conductivity, 236
Confidentiality, 47, 208
Confined-space rescues, 548–50
Congenital bleb, 232
Congenital heart defects, 482
Consent, 44, 46, 50, 56
Consolidated action plan, 532
Contained incident, 529
Contamination, 561
Continuing incident, 529
CONTOMS program, 574
Contra-coup brain injury, 260
Controlled Substance Act of 1970, 88
Contusion, 260, 391, 415, 418, 419
Conversion ratios, 101–2
COPD (chronic obstructive pulmonary disease), 220–21, 493
Cover, 573
CPR (cardiopulmonary resuscitation), 104, 108, 110–12
CQI (continuous quality improvement), 26, 29
Cranial nerves, 257, 258, 413
Cricoid pressure, 140
Crime scene awareness, 47–48, 374–75, 567–75
  clandestine drug labs, 571
  CONTOMS program, 574
  domestic violence, 571–72
  hazard awareness control and avoidance, 567–69
  large crowds, 570

preserving evidence, 574–75
responses involving motor vehicles, 569–70
street gangs, 570–71
tactical EMS, 573–74
tactics for safety and patient care, 572–73
violent scenes, 570
Critical thinking, 190–91
Crush injuries, 392, 395
Crying, in infants, 117
CSF (cerebrospinal fluid), 254–55, 261
Cullen's sign, 451
Cultural diversity, 508–9
CUPS format, 170, 487–88
Cushing's syndrome, 287–88
Cushing's triad, 274
Cystitis, 367

DAI (diffuse axonal injury), 415, 417
DAN®, 337
DCAP-BTLS, 174
DCI (decompression illness), 336
DDC (defensive driving course), 54
DEA (Drug Enforcement Agency), 88
Death and dying, 13–14, 515
bathroom as location of, 177
leading causes of, 32–33, 475
pronouncement of, 107
Decompensated shock, 383
Decon, 563–65
Degenerative disk disease, 429
Delegation of authority, 43
Demand-valve, 139
Dementia, 259
Depression, 353, 477, 495–96
Dermatomes, 422
Descending nerve tracts, 421–22
Developmental disability, 506
Dextrose, 279, 284
Diabetes mellitus, 277–80, 496
Diagnosis, 60
Diagnosis-based curricula, 171
Dialysis, 306–7
Diarrhea, 472
Diet, 1–2
Diffusion, 213
Digital communication, 199
Digital intubation, 141–42
Directive No. 6000.10, 18
Dirty accident, 406
Disease. See also under individual diseases
analyzing risk, 72
causes, 60, 72–75
defined, 59
familial, 72
genetic, 72
Disease transmission prevention, 14–16
body substance isolation, 15
exposure, 15, 16
periodic risk assessments, 15–16
protection from air- or blood-borne pathogens, 15
types of pathogens, 15
warning signs of diseases, 15–16

Disentanglement, 543, 544
Disinfection, defined, 15
Dislocation, 458–59, 462–63
Disorder, 59
Dispatch and field time milestones, 195
Distress, 8
Diving emergencies, 335–38
Dizziness, 176, 384
DKA (diabetic ketoacidosis), 281–83
DNAR (do not attempt resuscitation) order, 56, 106–7
DNR (do not resuscitate) order, 47, 106
Documentation, 201–10
abbreviations, 203
medical word parts, 205–8
of procedures, 209
reasons for, 201–2
special situations, 209–10
terms and planes, 204
Doll's eye maneuver, 269
Domestic violence, 571–72
Dopaminergic receptor, 84–85
Doppler ultrasound, 154–55
DOT-KKK-A-1822 Federal Ambulance Specifications, 18
DOT-KKK-1822D Federal Ambulance Specifications, 517
Down syndrome, 466–67, 506
DPE (detailed physical examination), 179–81
DPL (diagnostic peritoneal lavage), 305
Drills, 534–36
Drowning, 334
Drowning machine effect, 546
Drug-induced anemia, 73
Drugs. See pharmacology
Due regard, 52, 523
Duplex communication device, 198
Duty to act, 42
Dysplasia, 61
Dysrhythmias, 245–46

Early release, of patients, 33
ECF (extracellular fluid), 64, 65
ECG (electrocardiogram), 241–45
Echoing, 198
Edema, 66–67, 155
Education, 54
EGTA (esophageal-gastric tube airway), 141
Einthoven's triangle, 244
Electrical shock, 403
Electro-mechanical disassociation, 238
Emancipated minor, 44–45
EMD (emergency medical dispatcher), 18, 23, 196
Emergency Medical Services Systems Act, 18
Emergency (television program), 18
Emotional disorder, 347
Emotional impairment, 506–7
Empathy, 23
Emphysema, 220–21
Empty-nest syndrome, 123
EMS Act, 40
EMS-C (Emergency Medical Services for Children) Act, 18

EMS Command, 532
EMS providers
certification, 20, 54
comparison of levels, 21
identification, 50
injury prevention activities, 34–39
leadership activities, 36–37
licensure, 20, 54
off duty, 46
recertification, 20–21
registration, 20
specific roles of, 26–27, 30, 537–38
EMS systems
components of, 20
continuing education, 22
defined, 19–20
ethics, 22
history of development, 17–19
national issues affecting, 27–29
national organizations with role in, 19
professionalism, 22
standard-setting groups for, 19
EMT-Basic, 5, 112
EMT Code of Ethics, 57–58
Endocrinology, 276–89
Endomeritis, 367
Endometriosis, 367
Endotrol® tube, 143
End-tidal CO2 (colormetric) device, 142, 156
Endurance, 3
Enhanced 911 system, 195
Enteral drug administration, 95, 96, 99
Environmental emergencies, 324–39
EOA (esophageal obturator airway), 141
Epidemiology, 32–34
Epinephrine, 221, 283, 293, 294, 382
Epipen®, 293
Epistaxis, 410
Erectile dysfunction, 309
Error of commission or omission, 42
Escape plan, 568
Eschar formation, 399
Escharotomy, 399
Esophageal intubation detector, 143
ETC (esophageal tracheal combitube), 579
Ethics, 22, 49
allocating scarce resources, 55
definitions and concepts, 55–58
ethical decisions, 55–56
global concepts, 56
Etiology, 59
ET tube, 140, 142, 143, 473
Eustress, 8
EVOC (Emergency Vehicle Operator Course), 54
Exacerbation, 60
Exercise, 3
Extubation, 140
Eye assessment, 268–69
Eye injuries, 408–9
Eye response, 268

Facsimile (fax), 199–200
False imprisonment, 43
False instrument filing, 46
FAS (fetal alcohol syndrome), 469
FBAO (foreign body airway obstruction), 106, 110–11, 131
FCC (Federal Communications Commission), 196
FDA (Food and Drug Administration), 88
Febrile seizures, 483–84
Federal Food, Drug, and Cosmetic Act of 1938, 88
Fetal circulation, 464–65
Fetal development, 464
Fetal distress, 470
Fibrinolysis, 360
Fibrous joints, 456
Fight-or-flight response, 191
Financial impairment, 509–10
First-party caller, 195
Flail segment, 438–39
Flu, 224, 345
Fluid wave test, 305
Focal injuries, 415
Focused examination, 159, 172, 174–75
Focused history, 146, 172, 174
FOIA (Freedom of Information Act), 49–50
Food poisoning, 323
Four cardinal rules of priority dispatching, 195
Fractures, 261, 415–16, 417–18, 419, 437–38, 457–58, 460
Frontal lobotomy, 254
Frostbite, 333–34
Frostnip, 333
FSLA (Fair Labor Standards Act), 51
Fundus, measuring, 371–72
Furosemide, 229

Gallbladder disease, 304
Gallstones, 74
Gangs, 570–71
GAS (general adaptation syndrome), 8–9
Gastric distention, 135
Gastric ulcers, 345
Gastroenteritis, 345
Gastroenterology, 296–307
    assessment, 301–6
    epidemiology, 296–98
    major conditions, 299–300
    pathophysiology, 298–301
GCS (Glasgow Coma Scale), 182, 183, 268, 417
Geriatrics, 491–501
    abuse of elderly, 500
    alcohol and substance abuse, 496–97
    anatomy and physiology, 491–92
    assessment, 500–501
    bone diseases, 497
    common diseases of elderly, 492–96
    demographics, 492
    medication problems, 497–98
    resources, 498–99
    trauma, 499–500
Gerontology, 491

GI bleed, 298–99, 496
GI devices, 514–15
Glaucoma, 270
Global MED-NET®, 148
Glucagon, 284
Glucose, 279
Glucose meter, 279
Glycogen, 283
Good Samaritan law, 42
Gout, 74
Governmental immunity, 44
Governmental obstruction, 46
Granulocytes, 357
Gray matter, 256, 421
Grey-Turner's sign, 451
Grieving, 13, 515
Growth spurt, 120
Guaiac test, 303
GU devices, 514–15
Guidelines 2000, 104–12, 578–79, 580, 581, 583, 584–85
Gynecology and obstetrics, 363–75
    focused history and physical exam, 369–74
    management, 375
    physiology, 363–69
    sexual abuse, 374–75

HACE (high-altitude cerebral edema), 339
Hand washing, 342
Hantavirus, 346
HAPE (high-altitude pulmonary edema), 339
Harrison Narcotic Act of 1914
Hazardous materials, 557–66
    initial isolation and protective action distances, 559
    management, 565–66
    personal protective equipment and decon, 563–65
    physiology, 562–63
    placards and initial response guides, 560
    regulations and guidelines, 558–62
    terminology, 557–58
Headache, 266
Head and facial trauma, 407–19, 500
    anatomy and physiology, 409–10, 412–16
    assessment, 410–11, 416–18
    categories, 414
    incidence, 407–9, 412
    management, 411–12, 418–19
Health, 1
Health Care Power of Attorney, 47
Health care professional, 22
Health history, 145–49
    challenges to getting information, 148–49
    defined, 146
    interviewing, 147–48
    OPQRST, 146
    purpose of, 146
    questions, 146
    SAMPLE, 146
Hearing impairments, 502–3

Heart sounds, 234–36
Heat illness, 327–30
    fever, 329, 472
    heat cramps, 328
    heat exhaustion, 328
    heat stroke, 328–29
Helmets, 432, 538
HELP position, 545
Hematochromatosis, 73
Hematocrit, 305, 356–57
Hematologic conditions, 361–62
Hematology, 355–62
Hematoma, 391, 418
Hematopoietic system, 355
Hemoglobin, 356–57
Hemophilia, 73
Hemorrhage and shock, 75–76, 380–87, 393–94
Hemostatic mechanism, 358–59
Hemothorax, 443
Hepatitis, 343–44
Hepatojugular reflux, 155, 303
Hernias, 473
Hernieated intervertebral disk, 429
HHNC (hyperosmolar hyperglycemia nonketotic coma), 280
High-angle rescues, 553–54
High-permeability pulmonary edema, 227–28
High-pressure pulmonary edema, 227–28
Highway Safety Act, 18
HIV (human immunovirus), 345
Home-care patients, 511–15
Home health care providers, 512
Homeostasis, 276–77, 325
Hospice, 512
Household measurement system, 100, 101
HPV (human papilloma virus), 344
HTN (hypertension), 248, 494
Humane restraints, 47
Human life span development, 113–28
    adolescence, 120–22
    comparison of stages, 125–28
    infancy, 114–17
    principles and concepts, 113–14
    school-age children, 119–20
    toddlers and preschool children, 117–19
Humoral immunity, 358
Huntington's disease, 75
Hydrocephalus, 255
Hydrophobia, 345
Hyperbaric chamber therapy, 401
Hyperbaric O2 therapy, 338
Hyperglycemia, 280–81
Hypernatremia, 68
Hyperplasia, 61
Hypersensitivity, 81, 85
Hypertensive emergency, 248
Hypertrophic scar formation, 390
Hypertrophy, 60–61
Hyperventilation, 217, 233, 261
Hypoglycemia, 283–85, 472
Hyponatremia, 68
Hypothermia, 330–33, 472

Hypothyroidism, 286–87
Hypovolemic shock, 384–85
Hypoxemia, 130
Hypoxia, 130
Hypoxic heart, 246

Iatrogenic disorder, 60, 86
IBS (irritable bowel syndrome), 304
IC, 532
ICF (intracellular fluid), 64, 65
ICS, 530
ILCOR (International Liaison Committee on Resuscitation), 582
Illness prevention. *See* injury prevention
Immune system, 77–82, 290
    B-cell lymphocyte, 78
    cell-mediated response, 78
    cellular interactions, 78
    characteristics, 77–78
    deficiencies, 81–82
    defined, 77
    in elderly, 79
    in fetus or neonate, 78–79
    immunoglobulin, 78
    inflammation response, 79–80, 81–82
    stress and, 79
    wound healing, 80
Immunizations, 3
Immunologic injury, 63
IMS (incident management system), 529–32
Incidence, of injury or illness, 32
Incident report, 48
Index of suspicion, 378–79
Infants
    development of, 114–17, 126–28
    milestones, 116, 128
    normal reflexes, 115
    vital signs, 114, 126
Infectious and communicable diseases, 340–46, 483, 509
Infectious injury, 62
Inflammatory injury, 63
Inflammatory process, 357–58
Influenza (flu), 224, 345
Injurious genetic factors, 63
Injurious nutritional imbalances, 63
Injury, 33
Injury prevention, 5
    community and, 5
    contemplation for, 5
    EMS provider's role in, 34–39
    family and, 5
    handling hostile situations, 6
    implementation of, 38
    lifting patients, 6
    meditation for, 5
    peers and, 5
    personal time for, 5
    resources for, 38–39
    safety equipment and supplies, 8
    safety in rescue situations, 6
    vehicle operation, 6–8
Inspection, 151–52
Integrated communications plan, 530–31

Interstitial fluid, 65–66
Interviewing, 147–49
Intracranial hemorrhage, 416
Involuntary commitment, 46
Involuntary regulation of respiration, 131
Ipecac, 314
IPPB (intermittent positive-pressure breathing), 139
IQ (intelligence quotient), 506
Irreversible shock, 383
Ischemia, 238, 239, 241
Isoimmunity, 81
Isotonic fluid volume, 68

Jaundice, 472
JVD (jugular vein distention), 155

Kefauver-Harris Amendment, 88
Kehr's sign, 451
KE (kinetic energy), 378–79
Keloid scar formation, 390
Korotkoff's sounds, 154
Krulak, Charles C., 57
Kübler-Ross, Elizabeth, 13
Kussmaul's sign, 247

Labor, 372
Lactose intolerance, 304
Larrey, Jean, 17
Laryngeal edema, 131
Laryngeal spasm, 131
Laryngectomy, 137
Laryngoscopy, 140
Latex, 294–95
LeFort classifications, 409
Left ventricular end-diastolic pressure, 250
Legal issues, 40–54. *See also under specific legal terms*
    administrative hearing, 41
    appellate court, 41
    civil litigation process, 43–44
    defendant, 41
    definitions and concepts, 40–51
    for dispatch agencies, 46
    driving an emergency vehicle, 51–54
    grand jury, 41
    jury of peers, 41
    maintenance of records, 44
    plaintiff, 41
    punitive damages, 48
    res ipsa loquitur, 43
    settling out of court, 42
    subpoena, 51
    trial court, 41
    types of law, 40–41
Leukocytes, 357, 358
Leukotriene blockers, 222
Levine's sign, 247
Libel, 43
Life expectancy, 123, 492
Life span, 123
Lightning injuries, 404
Limbic system, 257
Living will, 46
LMA (laryngeal mask airway), 141, 579

Local communication systems, 194–95
LOC (level of consciousness), 166–67, 273, 413
Low back pain, 428–29
Lung cancer, 225–27
Luxation, 458
Lyme disease, 345
LZ (landing zone), 528

Magnesium, 70–71, 222
Malpractice, 47, 48
Manic-depressive disorder, 75
Marfan's syndrome, 249
MAST/PASG (military antishock trousers/pneumatic antishock garment), 306, 386–87, 452
MCI (multiple casualty incident), 166, 209, 529–30, 532–33
MD (muscular dystrophy), 75
Meconium, 470
Medical Command, 532
Medical Direction, 23, 25–26
MedicAlert® Foundation, 148
Medical monitoring, 566
Medical patients, 172–77
Medical Practice Act, 43
Medication administration, 91–103, 473
    abbreviations used in, 98–99
    accountability and obligation, 91–92
    documentation, 92
    dosages and calculations, 100–103
    general precautions, 92–93
    injection sites, 97–98
    needle and syringe sizes, 96–97
    packaging of emergency drugs, 102–3
    principles and procedures, 93–100
    routes for, 95–96, 99–100
    six rights of, 92
Meninges, 255–56, 413–14
Meningitis, 345
Menopause, 492
Menstrual cycle, 363–65
Mental illness, 505–6
Mental impairment, 506–7
Mental retardation, 506
Metabolic acidosis, 71, 212
Metabolic alkalosis, 71, 212
Metaplasia, 61–62
Metric system, 100, 101
Middle meningeal artery, 412
MI (myocardial infarction), 228
Minimum data set, 201
Minute volume, 168
Mitral valve prolapse, 73
Mittelschmerz, 367
Modeling, 119x
MODS (multiple organ dysfunction syndrome), 76–77
MOI (mechanism of injury), 24, 161, 165, 376, 378–79, 408, 423–24, 435
Monocytes, 357
Morals, 55, 120
Morbidity, 32
Morgan Lenses®, 402
Morphine sulphate, 229
Morris, Gary, 530

Mortality, 32
Motor function, testing, 271–72
MS-ABC, 167, 168
MS (mental status), 166–67
MS (multiple sclerosis), 75
Multiplex communication device, 198–99
Muscle movement disorders, 270
Muscle tone, 272
Musculoskeletal trauma, 455–63
    assessment, 460–61
    epidemiology, 455
    management, 461–63
    pathophysiology, 457–60
    physiology, 455–57
Myelin, 257
Myocardial contusion, 445–46
Myocardial rupture, 446
Myxedema, 286–87

NAERG *(North American Emergency Response Guidebook)*, 559–60
NALS (neonatal advanced life support), 471
Narcotic depression, 469–70
Narrow complex SVT, 583
Nasal airways, 133–34
Nasal cannula, 137
Nasotracheal intubation, 143
National Formulary, 87
National SAFE KIDS Campaign, 479
Nature of illness, 165
Nausea, 176
Near drowning, 334–35
Needle cricothyrotomy, 144
Needle-stick injuries, 342
Neglect. *See* child abuse and neglect
Negligence, 41–42
    contributory, 43
    gross, 42
    per se, 43
Neonatalogy, 464–73
    anatomy and physiology, 464–65
    assessment and management, 469–71
    emergencies, 471–73
Neoplasia, 62
Neoplasm, 225–27
Neurological posturing, 167, 273
Neurology, 253–75
    focused neurological assessment, 267–75
    nervous system disorders, 257–59
    neurological emergencies, 261–67
    physiology, 253–57
    terminology, 253
    traumatic brain injury, 259–61
Neurons, 256–57
NHTSA (National Highway Traffic Safety Administration), 18, 34, 36
Nicotine, 5
Nightingale, Florence, 17
911 system, 195
Nitrogen narcosis, 336
Nitroglycerin, 229, 248
Nitrox, 337
Nonadherent dressing, 394

Noninvasive ventilation, 139–40
Non-rebreather mask, 137
Nonsterile dressing, 394
Norephinephrine, 382
Nosebleed, 411
Nosocomial disorder, 60
NPO (nothing by mouth), 305
NREMT (National Registry of EMTs), 18, 20
Nursing homes, 499
Nutrition, 1–2

Obesity, 74, 504–5
Obstetrics. *See* gynecology and obstetrics
Obstructive airway disease, 217–23
Occlusive disease, 248
Occlusive dressing, 394
Ongoing assessment, 171, 189–91
Open-ended questions, 147
Open fracture, 457
Open incident, 529
Open pneumothorax, 441
Ophthalmoscope, 156
OPQRST, 146, 172, 240
Oral airways, 133
Organ donors, 47
Orphan Drug Act, 89
Orthostatic hypotension, 384
Orthostatic vital sign changes, 177
OSHA (Occupational Safety and Health Administration), 50–51, 558
Osmosis, 65
Osmotic diuresis, 281
Osteoarthritis, 497
Osteoporosis, 497
Otoscope, 156
Out-of-hospital care, 50, 56
Overdose, 311, 316–17, 476, 585
Overload, 250
Overpressurization injuries, 335–38
Oxygenation, 129
Oxygen tanks, safety considerations for, 136
Oxyhemoglobin saturation curve, 211–12

Pacemaker, 246–47
Pacemaker cells, 237
Page, Jim, 18
Pagers, for EMS communication, 199
Paget's disease, 497
Palliative care, 512–13
Palpation, 151–52, 153–54
Paraplegia, 505
Parasympatholytic drugs, 222
Parenteral drug administration, 95, 96, 99
Parenting, 118–19
Parkinson's disease, 494
PAR (primary area of responsibility), 519
Partial pressure
Pathogenesis, 59
Pathological fracture, 458
Pathology, 59
Pathophysiology, 59–82
    abnormal fluid accumulations, 66–67

    acid-base balance, 71
    causes of disease, 60, 72–75
    cells and cell injury, 60–64
    concerns at cellular level, 75–77
    definitions and concepts, 59–60
    fluid and electrolyte balance, 67–71
    fluid and water balance, 64–66
    immune system, 77–82
    percentage of body fluids by age and gender, 65
    types of tissues, 60
Patient advocacy, 24
Patient assessment, 158–61
Patient-care flow charts, 191
Patient Self-Determination Act, 47
Pattern recognition, 185–86
PCC (Poison Control Center), 310
PEA algorithm, 582
Peak flow meters, 217
Peak load, 519
Pediatrics, 474–90
    anatomy and physiology, 474–75
    assessment, 485–88
    child abuse and neglect, 477–79
    continuing education, 490
    injuries and injury prevention, 479
    management, 488–90
    medical emergencies, 479–85
    poisonings, toxins, and substance abuse, 476
    suicide and psychiatric problems, 476–77
    trauma, 475
Peer review, 22
Pepper spray, 402
PE (pulmonary embolism), 230–32, 493
Percent, defined, 102
Percussion, 151
Perfusion, 213, 381, 382–83, 414
Pericardial tamponade, 444–45
Permission-to-treat, 46
Pertinent negative, 210
PFDs (personal flotation devices), 539
pH, defined, 71
Pharmaceutics, 83
Pharmacodynamics, 83
Pharmacokinetics, 83–84
Pharmacology, 83–90
    definitions and concepts, 83–86
    drug nomenclature, 86–90
    drug schedules, 88
    forms of drugs, 89
Phlebitis, 250
Phobias, 350
Phone-fast rule, 108
Phone-first rule, 108
Phosphate, 70
Physical examination techniques, 150–57
    assessment skills, 150–51
    equipment, 151
    general appearance of patient, 151
    head-to-toe method, 152
Physical fitness, 2–3
PID (pelvic inflammatory disease), 365–66

Pierre Robin syndrome, 466
Plague, 346
Plasma, 65–66
Platelets, 358
Platinum Ten Minutes, 379
Pleuritic chest pain, 231
PMH (past medical history), 146–47
PND (paroxysmal nocturnal dyspnea), 251
Pneumonia, 223–24, 481, 493
Pneumoperitoneum, 453
Pneumoscrotum, 453
PNI (psychoneuroimmunology), 9–10
PNS (peripheral nervous system), 257
Poisoning, 311–16, 476, 498, 562–63
Poison Prevention Act, 35
Polymedication, 266
Polypharmacology, 266
Positive pressure breathing, 229–30, 488
Post-incident critique, 536
Potassium, 68–69
PPE (personal protective equipment), 538–40, 563–65
Pregnancy and childbirth, 367–69, 371–74, 468–69
Prehospital care report (PCR), 26, 44, 48, 201–10
Prejudice, 5–6
Preload, 250
Premenstrual syndrome (PMS), 363, 365
Preschool children
    changes in body systems, 118
    development of, 117–19, 126–28
    milestones, 118, 128
    vital signs, 117, 126
Pressure dressing, 393
Pressure sores, 499–500
Preventative Health and Health Services Block Grant, 18
Prinzmetal's angina, 240–41
Profession, defined, 22
Professionalism, 22–25
    appearance and personal hygiene, 23
    defined, 22
    delivery of service, 24
    image, 22
    integrity, 22
    on and off duty, 25
    patient advocacy, 24
    self-confidence, 23
    self-motivation, 23
    teamwork and diplomacy, 23–24
    time-management skills, 23
Prognosis, 60
Protective custody, 45
Protester facial, 402
Protocols, 25–26, 191
PTL (pharyngeotracheal lumen airway), 141
Pulmonary and respiratory disorders, 211–33
    chronic versus acute, 211–13
    general assessment, 213–17
    life-threatening signs of, 214

pathophysiology, 213
Pulmonary circulation, 129
Pulmonary contusion, 443–44
Pulmonary edema, 227–30
Pulmonary thromboembolism, 230–32
Pulse check, 110
Pulse deficit, 234
Pulseless ventricular tachycardia, 582
Pulse oximetry, 142, 156–57
Pulsus alternans, 234
Pulsus paradoxus, 134, 234
Pupil assessment, 269–70
Pure Food and Drug Act of 1906, 87
Pursed-lip breathing, 215

Q-T syndrome, 73
Quadriplegia, 505
Queue time, 195

Rabies, 345
Radiating pain, 240
Radiation exposure, 404–6
Radio systems, 196–99
Rales, 216–17
Rapid extrication, 433
Rapid takedown technique, 433
Rapid trauma assessment, 171
Rapid trauma exam, 179
RAS (reticular activating system), 257, 413
Reciprocal socialization, 116
Reciprocity, 21
Record tampering, 46
Reentry, 237–38
Referred pain, 239–40
Reflex arc, 257
Refractory period, 237
Regurgitation, 176
Remission, 60
Renin-angiotensin-aldosterone mechanism, 67–68
Reportable collisions, 522
Rescue awareness and operations, 537–56
    extended care assessment and environmental issues, 555–56
    hazardous atmospheres, 548–50
    hazardous terrain rescue and packaging, 553–55
    highway operations and vehicle rescue, 550–53
    personal protective equipment, 538–40
    phases of rescue operation, 541–44
    role of EMS provider, 537–38
    safety procedures, 540–41
    water rescues, 544–48
Rescue plan, 541, 542
Research, 29–31
Reserve capacity, 520
Respiration, 435
Respiratory acidosis, 71
Respiratory alkalosis, 71
Respiratory disorders. See pulmonary and respiratory disorders
Respiratory distress, 134–44, 481
    assessing patient's breathing, 134

causes of, 134
    protective reflexes, 134
    respiratory patterns, 134–35
Respiratory rate, 130
Responsiveness, of patient, 174
Restraints, 352
Retrograde intubation, 142
Reye's syndrome, 484–85
Rhabdomyolysis, 392
Rheumatic fever, 72
Rh factor, 369
Rib fractures, 437–38
Right-sided heart failure, 215
RMA (refusal of medical assistance), 45, 56
RSI (rapid sequence induction), 144

Safar, Peter, 18
Safety, 6–8. See also injury prevention
Safety zones, 562
Salmonella, 345
SAMPLE, 146, 240
SBS (shaken baby syndrome), 478
Scaffolding, 116–17
Scalp, 412
Scene choreography, 166, 187
Scene size-up, 162–71
Schizophrenia, 75
School-age children
    development of, 119–20, 126–28
    milestones, 128
    reasoning processes, 120
    vital signs, 119, 126
SCI (spinal cord injury), 420–33
    anatomy and physiology, 421–22
    assessment, 422–25
    epidemiology, 420
    management, 430–33
    nontraumatic spinal conditions, 428–29
    traumatic, 425–28
SCIWORA (spinal cord injury without radiographic abnormalities), 426, 479
Scope of practice, 43, 49
SCUBA (self-contained underwater breathing apparatus), 335
Second-party caller, 196
Secure scene, 163
Seizure, 264–65, 472
Self-rescue techniques, 547
Sellick's maneuver, 140
Selye, Hans, 8–9
Sensory function, testing, 272
Sexual abuse, 374–75, 478
Sexual development, 120–21
Sexual harassment, 50
Sexual trauma, 453–54
Sharps, 93
Sherley Amendment, 87
Shipping papers, 561
Shock. See hemorrhage and shock
Sibling rivalry, 118
SIDS (sudden infant death syndrome), 484
Silent AMIs, 239, 278
Simple pneumothorax, 440–41

Singular command, 531
Sirens, proper use of, 523, 568
Six cardinal positions of gaze, 270–71
Six *R*s, 191
Skeletal muscle, 456
Skin assessment, 169–70
Skin lesions, 389–90
Skin turgor, 155
Skull, 412
Skull fracture, 261, 415–16, 417–18, 419
Slander, 43
Sleep, 4
Small volume nebulizer, 137
Smith, Edwin, 17
Smoking, 4–5
Smooth muscle, 456
Snacks, 2
Sniffing position, 140
Social clock, 122
Social distance, 6
Sodium, 67
Sodium-potassium pump, 66–67
Soft spots, 474
Soft tissue trauma, 388–95
SOPs (standard operating procedures), 7, 24, 522–23, 540
Span of control, 532
Special rescue operations, 544
Speech, 271
Speech impairments, 504
Spina bifida, 467
Spinal cord transection, 427
Spinal cord tumors, 429
Spinal immobilization, 423, 430–32
Spinal nerves, 422
Spironolactone, 229
Splenectomy, 225
Splints, 461, 463
Spondylolysis, 429
Spontaneous pneumothorax, 232–33
Sprain, 458, 460
Staging, 533
Standard of care, 49
Standing orders, 191
Starling's law of the heart, 236
START (simple triage and rapid treatment), 534
Status asthmaticus, 219
Status epilepticus, 265
Statute of limitations, 44
STDs (sexually transmitted diseases), 309, 366
Sterile dressing, 394
Sterile technique, 93
Sterilization, 15
Sternal fracture, 439
Steroids, 222, 261, 433
Stethoscope, 153
Stings. *See* bites and stings
Stokes® basket, 554–55
Strainer, 546
Stress, 8–13
Stress fracture, 458
Stroke, 262–63, 483, 584
Stroke volume, 381–82
Subluxation, 458
Substance abuse, 316–17, 496–97

Substance dependence, 316
Suctioning, 132–34
Suicide, 352—53, 476–77, 499
Surfactant, 472
Survival pack, 540
Swift-water rescue teams, 546
Symptomatic bradycardias, 582
Syncope, 177, 241, 265, 384
Syndrome, 60
Synovial joints, 456
System status management, 520

Tactical EMS, 573–74
Tactile intubation, 141–42
TB (tuberculosis), 344–45
Teachable moment, 33
Team leader-patient care provider concept, 187
Tear gas, 402
Telephones, for EMS communication, 199
Television, effect on children, 119
Temperature, body, 157, 272, 501
10-codes, 197
Tension pneumothorax, 232–33, 441–42
Terbutaline, 221
Terminal drop hypothesis, 125
Terminal illness, 509, 515
Testicular torsion, 454
Tetanus, 394
Thalidomide, 468
Thermal regulation, 326–27
Thiamine, 284
Third collision, 379
Third-party caller, 196
Thoracic trauma, 434–48
    anatomy and physiology, 435–36
    assessment, 43537
    epidemiology, 434
    injury patterns, 435
    specific chest injuries, 437–48
Thyroid disease, 285–87, 496
Thyroid storm, 285
Thyrotoxicosis, 285–86
TIA (transient ischemic attack), 261–62, 263
Tiered response, 520
Tilt test, 303–4
Titer, 343
TLCV (translaryngeal cannula ventilation), 144
Toddlers
    changes in body systems, 118
    development of, 117–19, 126–28
    milestones, 118, 128
    vital signs, 117, 126
Tolerance, 316
Tonicity, 67
Tonsils, 467–68
Towler, John, 12
Toxicology, 310–23, 585
    assessment and management, 311–16
    bites and stings, 323
    common drugs involved in emergencies, 317–22

food poisoning, 323
    statistics on emergencies, 310–11
Toxidrome, 313
Transcellular fluid, 64
Transected trachea, 410
Transfer of command, 532
Transtracheal jet insufflation, 144
Trauma, 170–71. *See also under individual types*
    blunt, 379, 408, 450
    epidemiology, 376–77
    focused history and physical examination, 178–84
    patient assessment, 178–82
    penetrating, 379, 408, 450
    special considerations, 183–84
    systems, 377–78
Trauma Care Systems Planning and Development Act, 19
Trauma centers, 182–83, 377
Trauma registry, 377
Trauma score, 182–83
Traumatic asphyxia, 448
Trench rescues, 550
Trending, 161, 189
Triage, 533–34
Trimix, 337
Trismus, 110
True medical emergency, 52
Trunked communication device, 199
Turnout gear, 539
Twins, 465

Unconscious patients, 273
Under-pressurization illness, 338–39
Unified command, 531
Universal precautions, 342
URI (upper-respiratory infection), 224–25
Urology, 299–300, 307–9
Urticaria, 291
U.S. Pharmacopoeia, 87

Vaccinations, 341–42
VADs (vascular access devices), 513–14
Vaginal bleeding, 366–67
Vaginal insufflation syndrome, 453
Vehicle operation, 6–8
Ventilation, 129, 135–36, 213, 435
Vertigo, 176
Viagra®, 309
Virulence, 62
Visual impairments, 503–4
Voluntary regulation of respiration, 131
Vomiting, 176, 472

Webb, Jack, 18
Wellness, 1
White matter, 256, 421
Withdrawal, 316–17
Wound healing, 390
WPW (Wolff-Parkinson-White) syndrome, 246

Years of productive life, 33

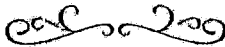

THE GARDENER & THE GRILL

THE BOUNTY OF THE GARDEN MEETS THE SIZZLE OF THE GRILL

KAREN ADLER & JUDITH FERTIG

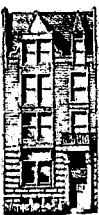

RUNNING PRESS
PHILADELPHIA · LONDON

Published by Running Press,
A Member of the Perseus Books Group

Books published by Running Press are available at special discounts for bulk purchases in
the United States by corporations, institutions, and other organizations. For more information,
please contact the Special Markets Department at the Perseus Books Group, 2300 Chestnut Street,
Suite 200, Philadelphia, PA 19103, or call (800) 810-4145, ext. 5000, or e-mail
special.markets@perseusbooks.com.

ISBN 978-0-7624-4111-2
Library of Congress Control Number: 2011925839
E-book ISBN 978-0-7624-4499-1

9   8   7   6   5   4   3   2
Digit on the right indicates the number of this printing

Cover and interior design by Amanda Richmond
Edited by Kristen Green Wiewora
Typography: Archive, Chronicle, and Clarendon

Running Press Book Publishers
2300 Chestnut Street
Philadelphia, PA 19103-4371

Visit us on the web!
www.runningpresscooks.com

TO GRILLERS & GARDENERS
EVERYWHERE.

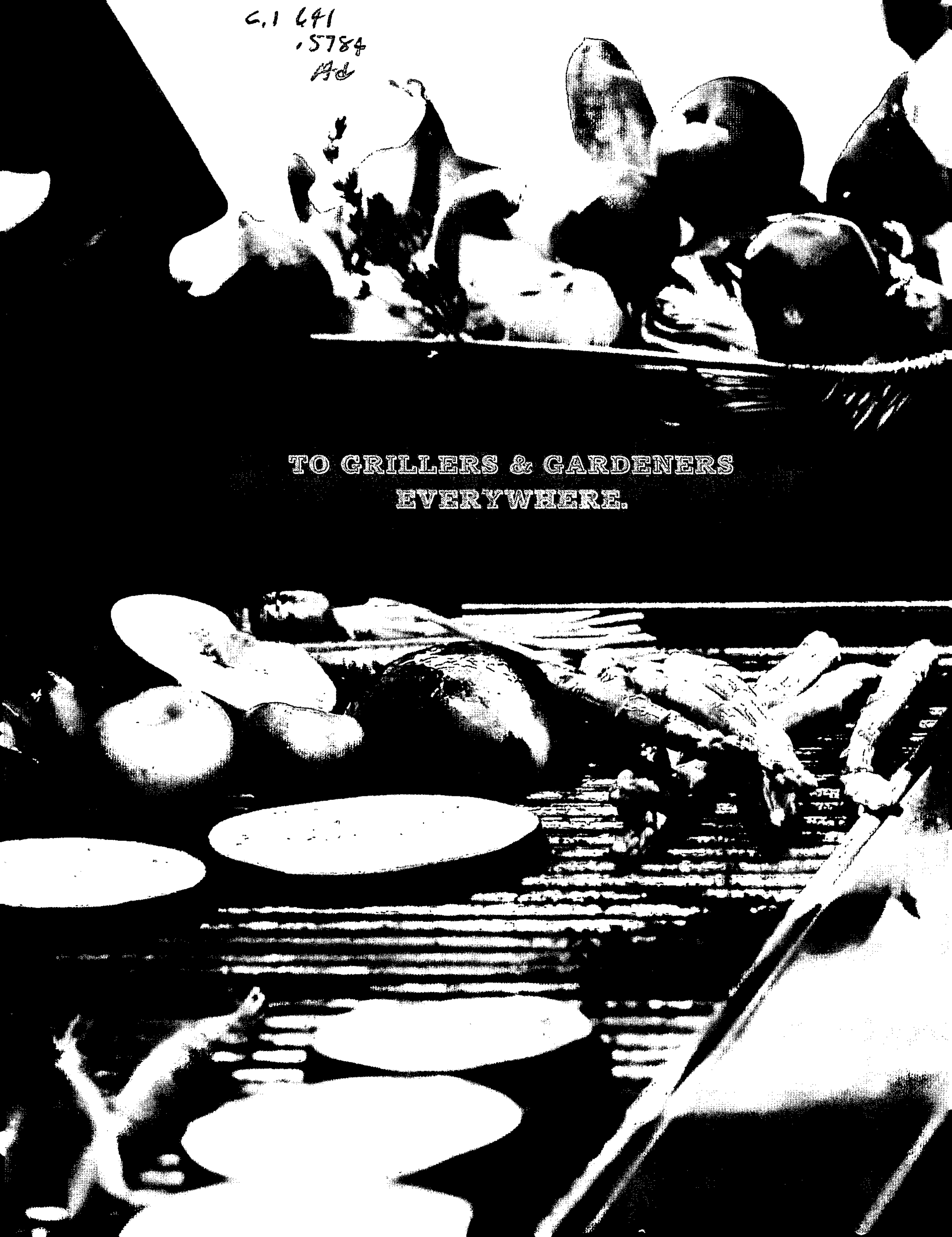

TABLE OF CONTENTS

Acknowledgments ...5

Introduction ...6

Specialty Grilling Techniques ...8

CHAPTER 1:
Pantry ...10

CHAPTER 2:
Appetizers ...46

CHAPTER 3:
Sandwiches, Flatbreads & Pizzas ...78

CHAPTER 4:
Soup & Salad ...106

CHAPTER 5:
Meat, Poultry & Fish ...134

CHAPTER 6:
Vegetable Sides ...158

CHAPTER 7:
Fruits & Desserts ...186

Index ...214

ACKNOWLEDGMENTS

WE ARE DELIGHTED WITH HOW THIS BOOK HAS GROWN. Just like our gardens as they lay dormant in seed packets or in the dark earth, the black and white words that we wrote as text and recipes have sprung to life with food styling and colorful photography. Special thanks are in order to our wonderful editor Kristen Green Wiewora and our designer Amanda Richmond along with all the other good folks at Running Press and Perseus Books Group. We'd like to also thank Sonya Harris who has worked with Karen for many years. Sonya—it is delightful to have you selling one of our books!

Karen thanks her husband Dick whose passion for tomatoes keeps their summer lively as they discuss the right way to get the best flavor and the most yield from their many plants. They both are glad to have Rocky and Lady, their English Pointers, who keep the squirrels at a distance.

Judith is hoping that her grand-dog Mimi can muster enough bark (she's a miniature dachshund) to help her win the squirrel battle, too.

We'd like to thank Lisa and Sally Ekus, our agents, who found a good home for this book. And, of course, we thank all the many talented gardeners and grillers who inspire us every year.

INTRODUCTION

Our story is of two women who love to cook, and especially grill. We remember fondly the wonderful dishes that we have prepared in our lifetimes and think, "Can that dish be as good on the grill—or even better?" And then we set about tweaking our favorites for grilling.

We both love to garden. We love the look of our gardens (most of the time). We talk about what we will do next season differently and what new crop we want to try. But we both garden differently.

Karen's garden mimics the French "potager" (raised-bed in a pattern) style with an emphasis—a BIG EMPHASIS—on tomatoes of every type. She also grows herbs, fruits, and vegetables.

Judith's garden is more edible landscaping and container gardening with baby turnips, rhubarb, melons, Italian plum tomatoes, and baby lettuces amongst the pear trees, raspberries, roses, and lavender.

Even though our garden types and plantings differ, we're both on the same page—grilling makes garden-fresh foods taste great.

Gardening and grilling are all about having foods you like. You might grow pots of patio tomatoes because you love having your own fresh-picked and heirloom varieties for pennies, rather than buying them for exorbitant (but deserving) dollars per pound. Or you might grow fava beans because they're difficult to find fresh in the pod in your area. Likewise, you grill foods because the combination of high heat and outdoor cooking yields a super-concentrated flavor that you just can't get in the kitchen.

When you grill, the high heat brings the natural sugars in foods to the surface, where they caramelize. Grilling makes foods taste fuller, richer, and meatier—even without any meat. The first time we grilled a head of romaine, cut in half lengthwise, we were amazed at how we could taste the crunchy lettuce as well as the slight char of the grill. When you want fresh and healthy foods with more depth of flavor, grilling from the garden makes perfect sense.

As activities, gardening and grilling also complement each other. While gardening can be solitary and even meditative, grilling is social. When you plant or weed or water, you're concentrating. Maybe you're gardening with a friend or spouse, but you're probably not carrying on a lively conversation. If you ask friends to come over to help you weed, you won't get many takers.

Yet when you grill, you might be entertaining guests outdoors or at least anticipating the wonderful meal to come, where the conversation could be lively. Family and friends will bring the food to grill outside, offer to take a turn with the grill tongs, or carry platters of grilled vegetables to the table. When you fire up the grill, you've got a reason for an outdoor party.

"Garden to grill" cooking emphasizes sustainability, freshness, taste, color, and texture. Grilling from the garden also gives you twice the sense of accomplishment—first from growing your own food, and secondly, from making it taste so good.

It doesn't get any fresher than picking ears of corn, and grilling them a few minutes later, slathered with a flavored butter. Mmmmm.

Grilling gives even familiar vegetables a new and exciting makeover. For example, once you harvest a large head of broccoli, the plant keeps producing side shoots. These shoots are delicious grilled, then served with a dipping sauce as an appetizer or side dish. You get a larger yield, creatively interpreted in a new dish. If you're interested in something more unique, you might want to try purple sprouting broccoli, an English heirloom of the "cut and come again" variety.

Herbs from your garden can go into condiments, marinades, sauces, and vinaigrettes that add an easy "wow" factor to simple grilled foods such as hamburgers, chicken, steaks, fish, shellfish, pork tenderloin or chops, and lamb.

Grilling is a very easy way to cook vegetables and fruits to retain their color and flavor. A simple brush of olive oil and a sprinkle of salt are all you need. It's amazing how vibrantly green and full-flavored grilled asparagus can be—even as a leftover, eaten the day after you've grilled it. Fruits can be directly grilled or planked, grilled on garden skewers (like branches of rosemary or lavender), or served with grilled pound cake.

With more and more people talking about "farm to table," we think it's time for "garden to grill to table." That said, it's important to keep things simple. We're going for techniques that are easy for beginners but satisfying enough for the experienced gardener and griller. We've also included some gardening tips, especially as they address the area around your outdoor kitchen or grill.

So, let's grab our garden trowels and our grill tongs and get busy.

SPECIALTY GRILLING TECHNIQUES

OMETIMES, TO GET A CERTAIN FLAVOR AND TEXTURE FROM foods, you'll want to go beyond basic grilling. Your grill can perform many of the same cooking functions as your indoor stovetop and oven, such as searing, stir-frying, planking, and roasting. The grill just gives the food you cook outdoors more flavor.

By moving the food away from the fire, keeping the grill lid closed instead of open, adding wood or herbs to the fire, and using a grill gadget like a grill wok or plank, you can increase the versatility of your grill and your own barbecue repertoire. Here are the specialty techniques you can try in *The Gardener and the Grill*:

GRILL ROASTING. Grill roasting is cooking food away from the fire, with the grill lid closed, for a longer time than simple indirect grilling. Grill-roasted foods cook through and scorch, but do not get grill marks or char. Vegetables usually take about 15 to 45 minutes; a grill-roasted whole chicken takes about 90 minutes. This technique works well for whole peppers, stuffed vegetables, whole baby carrots, cauliflower slices, fingerling potatoes, root vegetables, and whole chicken or fish. Wood-roasting takes this technique a step further; you add wood to the fire, producing an additional smoky flavor.

INDIRECT GRILLING. Indirect grilling is cooking food away from the fire, with the grill lid closed, for a short time, usually under 15 minutes. Most often in this book, we ask you to prepare an indirect fire in your grill—a fire on one side and no fire on the other—so you can get good grill marks on foods on the hot side with the grill lid up, then transfer them to finish cooking on the indirect side, with the grill lid up or down, depending on the recipe. This allows more delicate dishes like Grilled Salmon in Corn Husks (page 151) or grilled pizzas and flatbreads to get good flavor from the fire without getting burned.

PLANKING. Planking is placing foods on a flat piece of hardwood—usually cedar, maple, oak, alder, apple, or hickory—then placing the planked food on the grill grates. Planked food like butternut squash or salmon cook and gently burnish on the indirect or no-heat side with the grill lid closed for anywhere between 20 to 40 minutes.

PLANK-ROASTING. When you want planked foods to be scorched instead of gently burnished, as for Plank-Roasted Pear Salad with Blue Cheese and Walnuts (page 112), you place the plank over direct heat. You close the grill lid and plank for a shorter time (so your plank doesn't burn up), about 12 to 15 minutes.

SMOKING. Smoking adds the flavor of smoldering hardwood to food. You start with an indirect fire, add wood to the fire, place the food on the indirect side, and smoke with the grill lid closed. Smoking usually takes anywhere from 20 to 60 minutes for foods in this book, and is wonderful for garlic, onions, peppers, potatoes, tomatoes, and soft cheeses like fresh chevre.

STIR-GRILLING. Just as you would use a metal wok to stir-fry on your stovetop, so you can use a metal grill wok—one with perforations to let the grill flavor reach the food—on your grill. As for a stir-fry, you want a lean protein (beef, fish, chicken, shrimp, tofu) and possibly also a mixture of colorful vegetables cut in small pieces and usually marinated ahead of time. Because the grill wok has holes in it, you pour the marinated foods into the grill wok placed in the sink or outside on the grass, so you don't have a mess. The grill wok goes over direct heat and you use long-handled grill spatulas or wooden utensils to stir the food as it grills. Your food will have the flavor of the grill, some scorching, but few grill marks. Depending on how hot your fire is and how quickly your food is getting done, you can leave the grill lid open for less heat or close it for more heat. Stir-grilling usually takes between 15 and 30 minutes.

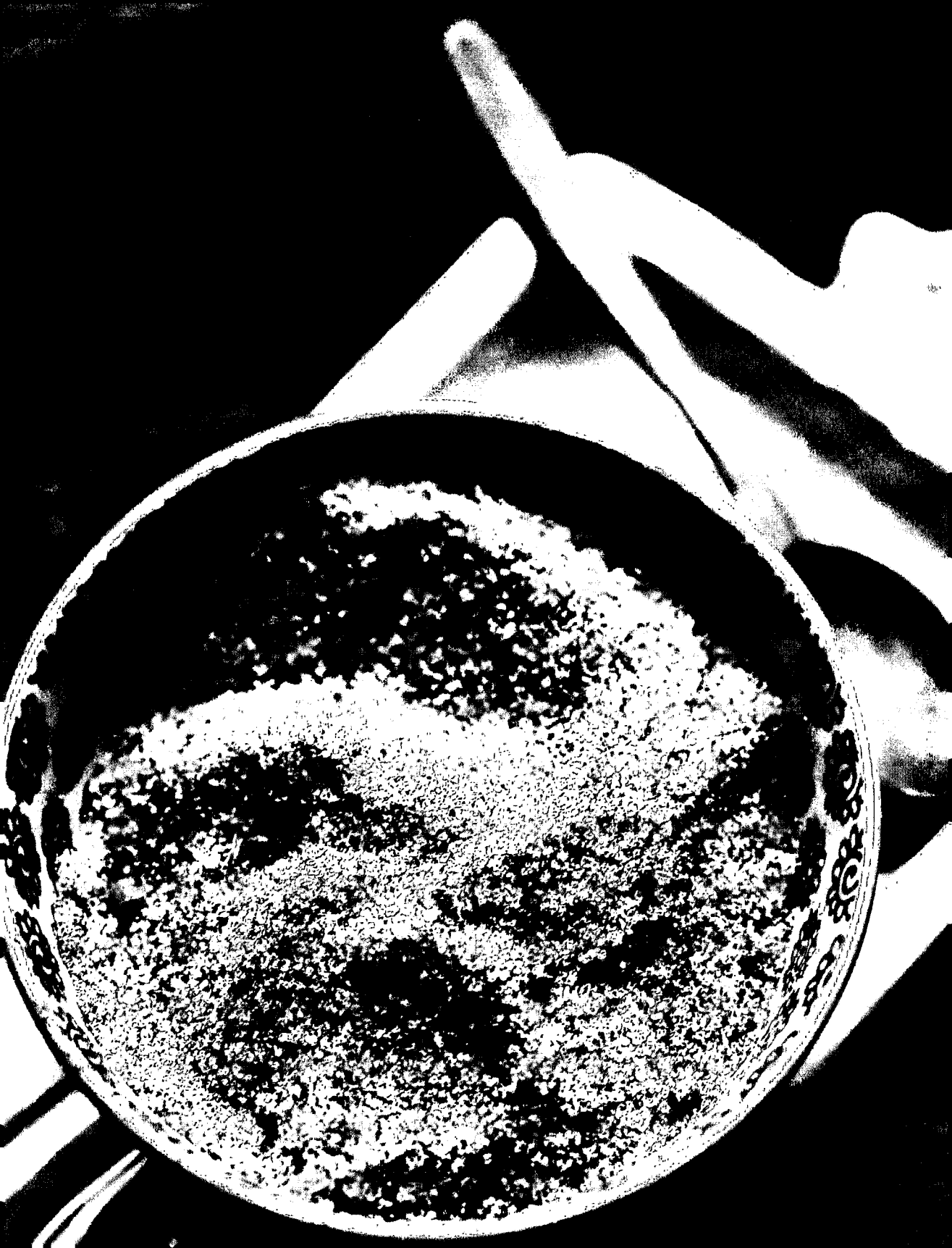

PANTRY

THE GARDENER'S PANTRY ALMOST ALWAYS CONTAINS OILS, vinegars, sweeteners, and seasonings for turning fresh-picked herbs, vegetables and fruits into seasonal dishes. After harvest, the pantry traditionally reflects the bounty of the garden with jams, jellies, and other preserved foods like corn relish or canned tomatoes. But the gardener who also grills has two other types of pantries.

One is a repertoire of easy, make-in-minutes marinades, "drizzles," vinaigrettes, flavored butters, and sauces that help marry fresh garden flavors with the sizzle of the grill. Over high heat, vegetables and fruits need a little moisture. So, we like versatile mixtures that can do triple duty: marinating before grilling, basting during grilling and/or saucing after grilling. After all, we've got gardens that demand our attention, too!

Chimichurri (page 26), the classic South American sauce, is a great example. It's a flavorful marinade for stir-grilled vegetables and skewered foods, a delicious baste for grilled chicken and meats, a fabulous planking sauce for fish fillets, and a wonderful finishing sauce. And you can make it from what you grow in your garden.

If you've lavished care on certain plants in your garden, as the French do, you'll want to serve them with something worthy—a French-style sauce, of course. And we've got buttery, creamy sauces (including a Blender Hollandaise, page 36) that transform humble to "oh, my!" And what doesn't taste better with a dollop of an aioli, we ask you?

The second pantry resides in the freezer, where the gardener can preserve grilled foods. When your garden is going crazy and you've got more than you can eat or give away, grill or smoke your garden harvest, then freeze for later use. See The Gardener's Grill Pantry (page 28) and The Gardener's Smoke Pantry (page 33) for techniques. Frozen assets allow you to bring in the taste of the grill, all year long, in sandwiches, soups, pastas, and sauces. End-of-the-Garden Sauce (page 45) is the epitome of this idea.

We'll be using these recipes throughout the book, but feel free to mix and match a vinaigrette, drizzle, or sauce with other vegetables, fruits, fish, chicken, lamb, beef, or pork as you see fit and as your garden grows.

Seasoning Salt ...13

Red Hot Blackened Seasoning ...14

Toasted Sesame-Soy Marinade and Dressing ...15

Ginger Vinaigrette ...16

Lemon Caesar Vinaigrette ...17

Gardening and Grilling with an Asian Accent ...18

Fresh Basil Vinaigrette ...20

Chipotle Vinaigrette ...22

Satay-Style Peanut Dipping Sauce ...23

Branching Out ...24

Three-Citrus Drizzle for Fruit ...25

Chimichurri Sauce ...26

Rosemary, Garlic, and Lemon Baste ...27

The Gardener's Grill Pantry ...28

Béarnaise Butter ...29

Butter Up! ...30

Italian Parmesan Grilling Paste ...31

Garlic Chive Pesto ...32

The Gardener's Smoke Pantry ...33

Smoked Garlic and Cilantro Cream Sauce ...34

Smoked Poblano Cream Sauce ...35

Blender Hollandaise ...36

Mustard Seed Sauce ...37

Grilled Green Onion Mayonnaise ...38

Lemon-Garlic Aioli ...39

Quick-To-Fix Aioli ...40

Creamy Blue Cheese Dressing ...41

Romesco Sauce ...42

Grill-Roasting Peppers ...43

Tzatziki ...44

End-of-the-Garden Sauce ...45

USE THIS MIXTURE AS A FLAVORFUL ADDITION TO THE VEG-etables and meats of your choice. It is a wonderful addition to Char-Grilled Salmon and Baby Squash (page 150) or Grilled Caesar Sirloin (page 153). It's also a wonderful gourmet gift from the kitchen.

SEASONING SALT

MAKES 1¼ CUPS

1 cup sea salt
2 tablespoons paprika
1 teaspoon parsley flakes
1 teaspoon dried chives
1 teaspoon black pepper
½ teaspoon dried
    marjoram leaves
½ teaspoon celery seed
½ teaspoon curry powder
½ teaspoon garlic powder
¼ teaspoon red pepper

Combine all of the ingredients in a glass jar and cover with a tight-fitting lid. Shake to blend. This keeps for several months in the pantry.

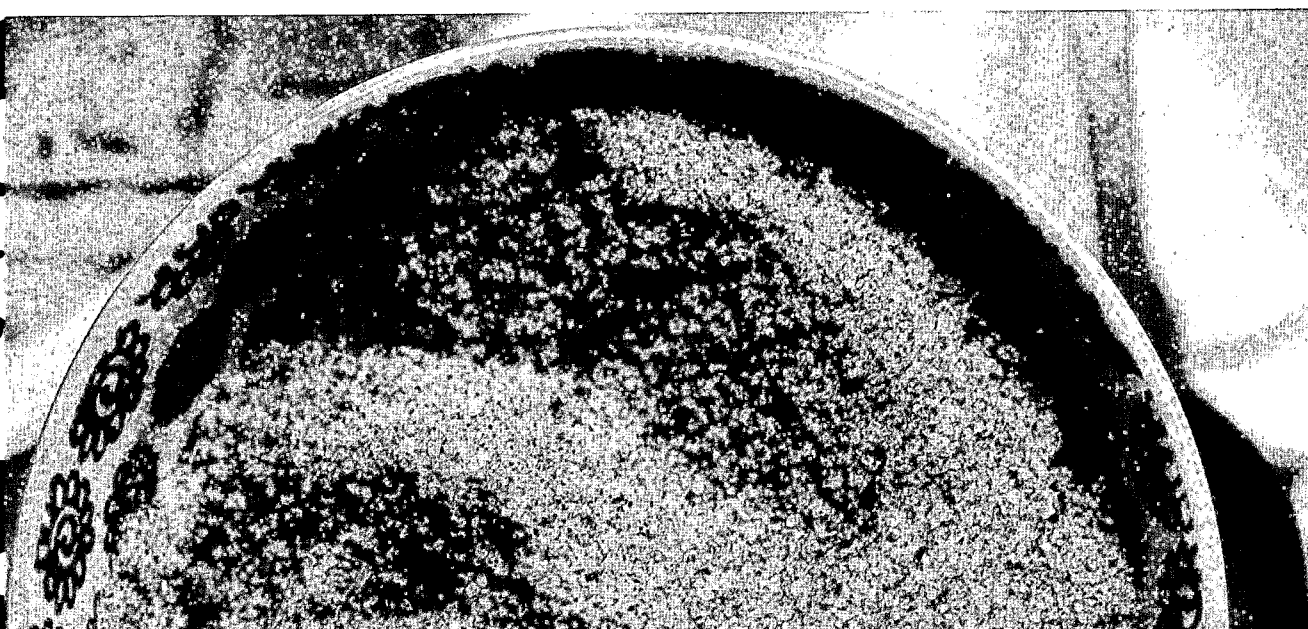

ES, THIS IS HOT, BUT THE ADDITION OF DRIED HERBS GIVES it lots of flavor. If you want to add a kiss of smoke, substitute smoked paprika for one quarter to one half of the regular paprika. Sprinkle this over grilled vegetables. Also adds zing to soups, stews, pasta dishes, sandwiches like The Blackened Fish Po' Boy (page 90), and tacos like Baja Fish Tacos (page148).

RED HOT BLACKENED SEASONING

MAKES ABOUT 1¼ CUPS

½ cup paprika

3 tablespoons garlic salt

2 tablespoons granulated onion

1 tablespoon dried oregano

1 tablespoon dried basil

1½ teaspoons dried thyme

1½ tablespoons black pepper

1½ tablespoons white pepper

1 tablespoon cayenne pepper

Combine all of the ingredients in a glass jar and cover with a tight-fitting lid. Shake to blend. This keeps for several months in the pantry.

THIS IS THE BEST ASIAN-STYLE MARINADE FOR VEGETABLES and is sublime on our Grilled Asparagus Salad (page 111). A simple combination of slivered onions (any kind), beans or peas, cherry or grape tomatoes, and a colorful mix of pepper strips marinated for 30 minutes then stir-grilled (see page 9) over a charcoal fire becomes a whole meal with noodles or rice as a base. Grilled Corn, Tomato, and Red Onion Salad (page 114) is perfect for this marinade, too.

TOASTED SESAME-SOY MARINADE and DRESSING

MAKES ABOUT 1½ CUPS

½ cup olive oil

½ cup grapefruit juice

¼ cup soy sauce

2 tablespoons toasted sesame oil

2 tablespoons packed brown sugar

2 teaspoons grated fresh ginger

1 teaspoon red pepper flakes

Combine all of the ingredients in a glass jar and cover with a tight-fitting lid. Shake to blend. This keeps in the refrigerator for about 5 days.

ITH A WHOPPING 3 TABLESPOONS OF FRESHLY GRATED ginger, this recipe packs a load of flavor. It is a versatile marinade or dressing for grilled greens, squash, asparagus, beans, broccoli, tomatoes, and just about whatever you grow in your garden. Try it on Charred Green Beans with Lemon Verbena Pesto (page 165) for an additional layer of flavor. Use it with poultry, pork, and seafood, too.

GINGER VINAIGRETTE

MAKES 1 CUP

3 tablespoons chicken or
  vegetable stock

3 tablespoons fresh lime
  juice

3 tablespoons grated
  fresh ginger

2 tablespoons finely
  chopped shallots

1 tablespoon honey

1 tablespoon soy sauce

1 garlic clove, minced

2 tablespoons olive oil

Combine all of the ingredients in a glass jar and cover with a tight-fitting lid. Shake to blend. This keeps in the refrigerator for about 5 days.

THIS HAS MORE CITRUS AND LESS GARLIC THAN THE TRAD-
itional Caesar dressing and is wonderful on grilled greens or salads or on
vegetables, fish, shellfish, chicken, or pork—before or after grilling. Use this for
a lighter dressing on the Grilled Summer Slaw with Gorgonzola Vinaigrette
(page 119). Drizzle this on a platter of fresh pasta with grilled vegetables.
Anchovy paste is available in metal tubes at better grocery stores and gourmet
shops, or you can buy canned anchovies and mash them with a fork.

LEMON CAESAR VINAIGRETTE

**MAKES ABOUT
1 CUP**

$^2/_3$ cup extra-virgin olive
  oil

3 tablespoons fresh lemon
  juice

2 tablespoons anchovy
  paste

1 tablespoon white wine
  vinegar

1 tablespoon grated
  lemon zest

1 garlic clove, minced

Combine all the ingredients in a small bowl. Use
a hand-held blender to emulsify. Alternatively,
combine in a food processor and pulse until fully
blended. Store in the refrigerator for up to 1 week.

GARDENING AND GRILLING
WITH AN ASIAN ACCENT

LIKE ANY OTHER FOOD, ASIAN INGREDIENTS TASTE BEST FRESH. Some of these plants come from tropical climates, so they do well outdoors in the summer. When the weather turns cold, transfer them to pots and bring them indoors to a sunny window.

- **BASIL.** Thai basil is the most-used variety used in marinades, bastes, sauces, and curries.

- **EDAMAME.** Fresh soybeans in their pods can be grilled, then the pods popped open and the tender beans dipped in flaked salt.

- **EGGPLANT.** Japanese eggplants are smaller and cylindrical; they can be brushed with oil and grilled whole. Turn them often to cook evenly.

- **GREEN ONIONS.** Sow green onions every week during the growing season (called "succession planting") so you have fresh green onions for longer.

- **LEMONGRASS.** A tropical grass with a citrus aroma and flavor, lemongrass plants are available at garden nurseries.

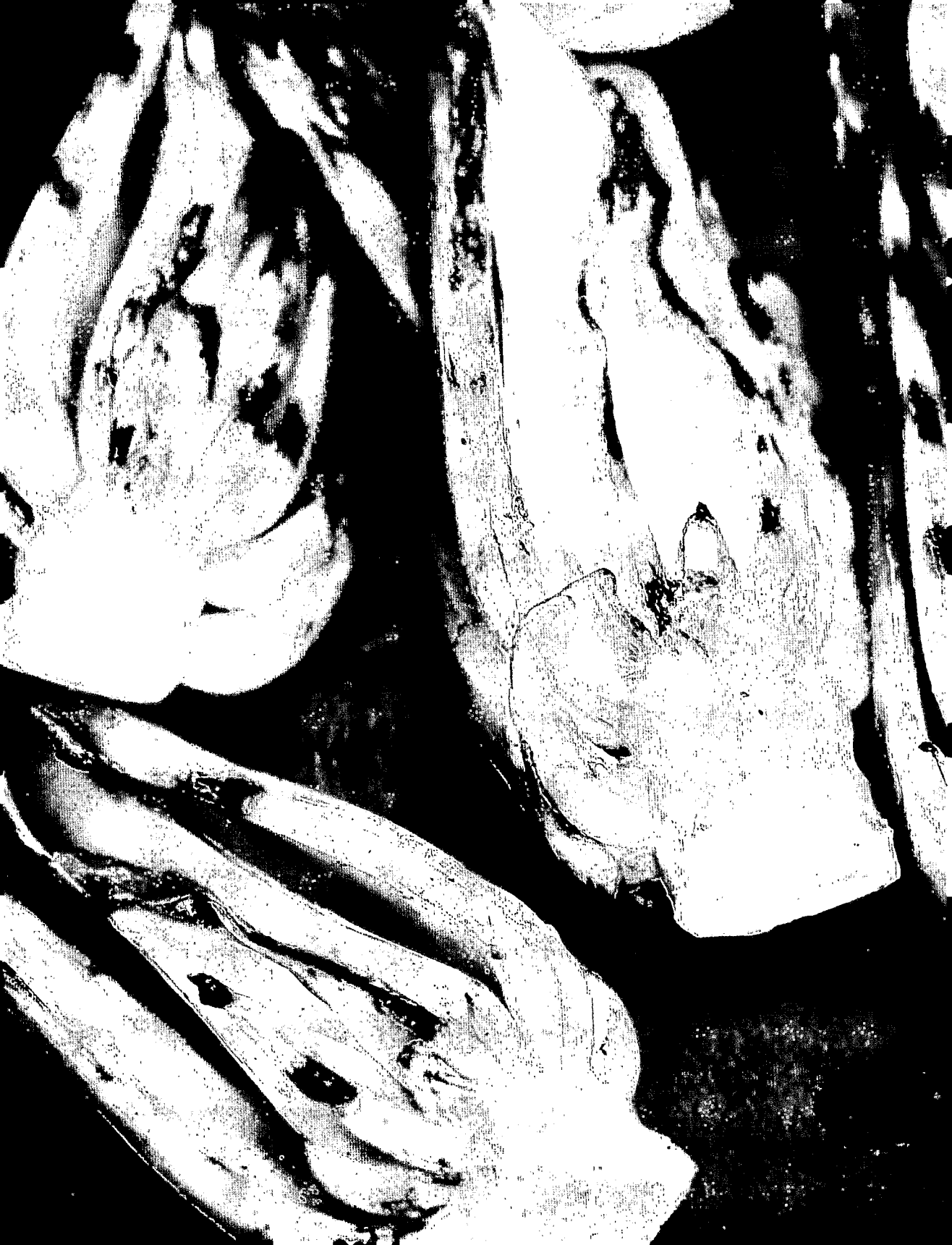

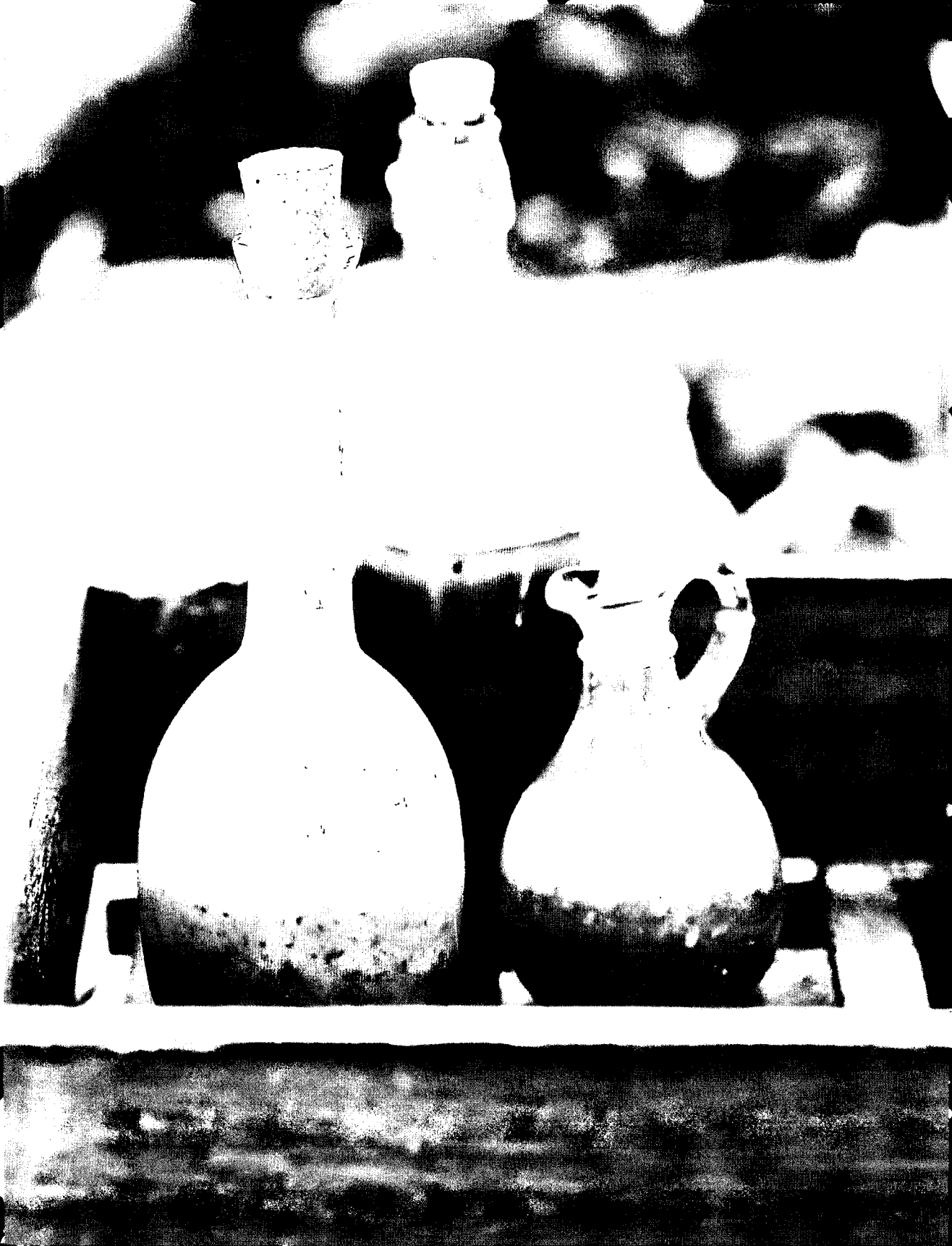

WHEN FRESH BASIL IS LUXURIANT AND AROMATIC IN YOUR garden or at the farmers' market, use it to make this addictive vinaigrette. You'll need a very large bunch (or three to four packages from the grocery store) to make one cup chopped basil, but this luscious vinaigrette is worth it. Because basil can discolor quickly, make this right before serving. Then spoon it over Blistered Summer Squash, Peppers, and Scallions with Goat Cheese (page 183).

FRESH BASIL VINAIGRETTE

**MAKES ABOUT
2 CUPS**

1½ cups extra virgin
  olive oil

½ cup fresh lemon juice
  (from 3 to 4 lemons)

2 garlic cloves, minced

1 tablespoon Dijon
  mustard

1 cup finely chopped fresh
  basil

Fine kosher or sea salt and
  freshly ground black
  pepper to taste

Combine all the ingredients in a bowl. Use a hand held blender to emulsify. Alternatively, combine in a food processor and pulse until fully blended. Use as soon as you make it.

THIS IS SO BEAUTIFULLY BALANCED THAT, EVEN IF YOU ARE NOT a fan of Southwestern spices, you'll like this vinaigrette. It is great as a marinade, baste, or drizzle for any vegetables that you want to give some kick. When you've had your fill of plain sliced tomatoes, try Grilled Goat Cheese Tomato Slices with Baby Greens (page 118) with this spicy vinaigrette.

CHIPOTLE VINAIGRETTE

MAKES ABOUT 1 CUP

3 tablespoons sherry vinegar

1 tablespoon balsamic vinegar

2 garlic cloves, peeled

2 canned chipotle chiles in adobo sauce (or more to taste), chopped, plus 2 tablespoons adobo sauce

½ teaspoon fine kosher or sea salt

⅔ cup olive oil

Freshly ground black pepper to taste

In a food processor or blender, combine the vinegars, garlic, chipotles, adobo sauce, and salt and process until smooth. With the motor running, add the olive oil in a slow, steady stream through the feed tube until incorporated. Season with pepper and pulse to blend. Use immediately or pour into a glass jar and cover with a tight-fitting lid. This keeps in the refrigerator for 5 days.

SERVE THIS INDESCRIBABLY YUMMY SAUCE WITH RAW OR grilled vegetables like asparagus, zucchini sticks, red pepper strips, carrots, and broccoli, as well as pita chips. It is also makes a great marinade for vegetables, poultry, pork, fish, and shellfish. Grilled Baby Bok Choy with Fresh Ginger-Soy Sauce (page 122) marries beautifully with this dipping sauce.

SATAY-STYLE PEANUT DIPPING SAUCE

MAKES 2 CUPS

$\frac{1}{2}$ cup soy sauce

$\frac{1}{2}$ cup rice wine vinegar

$\frac{1}{2}$ cup chunky peanut
  butter

$\frac{1}{3}$ cup chopped cilantro

2 tablespoons dark honey

1 tablespoon toasted
  sesame oil

1 tablespoon freshly grated
  ginger

Zest and juice of 1 lime

2 garlic cloves, minced

$\frac{1}{2}$ teaspoon red pepper
  flakes

Combine all ingredients and mix well. To use as a marinade, pour the sauce over meat or vegetables and marinate for 30 to 60 minutes in the refrigerator. For serving as a dipping sauce, refrigerate until ready to serve.

BRANCHING OUT

HARDY HERB AND PLANT STEMS FROM YOUR GARDEN CAN MAKE sturdy—and aromatic—skewers for foods of all kinds destined for the grill. These woody stems can also be tossed onto a charcoal fire for a lovely aroma, or the leafy fronds of the herbs can be used as basting brushes, too. To use plants as skewers, try piercing the meat or vegetable first with the tip of a metal skewer or sharp knife to make threading easier.

Here are a few that ardent gardeners and grillers love:

- BASIL STEMS become woody in the late summer, especially if you cut the plants back frequently. The stems can hold small Roma tomatoes and cubes of mozzarella for a Caprese salad on a stick.

- LAVENDER PLANTS get woody after blossoming, so when it's time to trim the plant back, choose thick branches. Strip off the leaves, and thread fish, lamb, or chicken alternating with vegetables like yellow squash or zucchini pieces. Lavender branches also add an aromatic flavor to sweet pitted cherries just briefly sizzled on the grill and served with frozen yogurt or ice cream.

- LEMONGRASS, a tropical plant which can be dug up and brought indoors to a sunny window in winter, features tough canes with an aromatic citrus flavor. Simply cut off a length of lemongrass, strip off the leaves, and thread the foods onto the stem. Lemongrass pairs well with Thai or other Asian marinades.

- LEMON VERBENA grows as a small bush. Its branches are plentiful. Thread the vegetables of your choice and insert a lemon verbena leaf in between them.

- ROSEMARY varieties like Tuscan rosemary, which fans out as it grows and develops tough stems, make great skewers for vegetables, chicken, and lamb. Strip off the fresh leaves and use them in a rosemary-flavored marinade or drizzle.

THE LIVELY TARTNESS OF CITRUS MARRIES WITH SAVORY herbs and onions for a unique savory-sweet dressing for grilled fruit like Grilled Persimmons with Three-Citrus Drizzle (page 208). It is a great marinade, too. If you are lucky enough to have fresh citrus growing in your garden, grate a little bit of the zest of these fruits into the recipe.

THREE-CITRUS DRIZZLE for FRUIT

MAKES 2 CUPS

½ cup fresh orange juice

¼ cup fresh lemon juice

¼ cup fresh lime juice

1 tablespoon fresh basil
   leaves

1 tablespoon fresh snipped
   onion or garlic chives

2 tablespoons finely
   chopped red onion

1 cup olive oil

Salt and freshly ground
   pepper to taste

Combine the juices, basil, chives, and onion in a blender or food processor. Slowly add the olive oil while the motor is running to emulsify. Season with salt and pepper and pour into a glass jar and cover with a tight-fitting lid. Keeps in the refrigerator for 2 or 3 days.

THIS TRADITIONAL MARINADE FROM ARGENTINA WILL WAKE up your grilled foods. It is versatile as a side sauce with dishes like Grilled Turkey Breast over Winter Greens with Warm Cranberry Vinaigrette (page 142). Drizzle it as a finishing sauce over grilled vegetable platters, pasta, fish, beef, poultry, and even French-Style Grilled Potato Salad (page 115).

CHIMICHURRI SAUCE

**MAKES ABOUT
3 CUPS**

1 cup olive oil

1 cup sherry vinegar

1 cup chopped flat-leaf
  parsley

$\frac{1}{4}$ cup chopped fresh
  oregano

$\frac{1}{4}$ cup chopped yellow
  onion (1 small onion)

6 garlic cloves, minced

2 teaspoons cayenne
  pepper

1 teaspoon black pepper

$\frac{1}{2}$ teaspoon sea salt

Combine all of the ingredients and mix well. Store in a glass jar for up to 2 weeks in the refrigerator.

LOOSER THAN A PASTE, THIS IS A WONDERFULLY AROMATIC basting sauce or drizzle to use on garden vegetables, beef, pork, chicken, or leg of lamb before, during, and after grilling. Try it on High-Heat Grilled Romaine Salad (page 109). You'll also love this brushed on bread or pizza dough. Make extra to drizzle over grilled asparagus, greens, tomatoes, and more. For the best texture, use a mortar and pestle. You also may use a food processor.

ROSEMARY, GARLIC, and LEMON BASTE

MAKES ABOUT ⅔ CUP

1 tablespoon finely
  chopped fresh rosemary

½ teaspoon fine kosher or
  sea salt

2 garlic cloves, minced

½ cup olive oil

Zest and juice of 1 lemon

Freshly ground black
  pepper to taste

If using a mortar and pestle, combine the rosemary, salt, and garlic in the mortar and grind into a fine paste with the pestle. Drizzle in the olive oil and grind again. Add the lemon zest and juice, grind, and taste. Add more salt, if desired, and season with pepper.

Alternatively, combine the rosemary, salt, and garlic in a food processor and pulse just to chop into a paste. Add the olive oil and pulse again. Add the lemon zest and juice and pulse, then season with salt and pepper as needed.

The baste will keep in the refrigerator for up to 1 week.

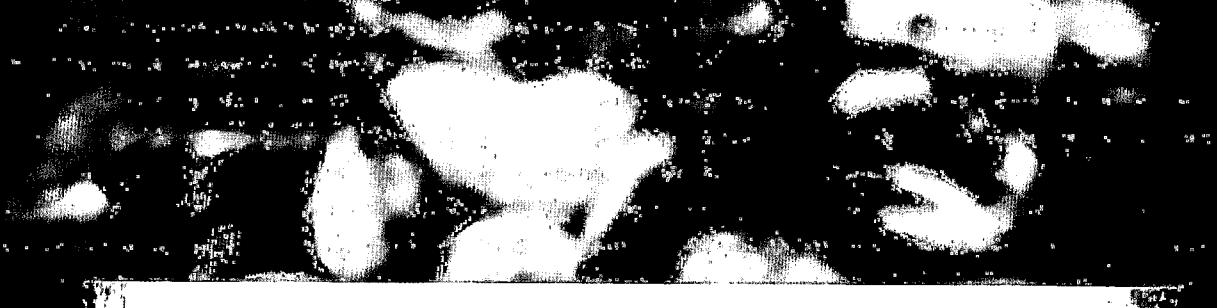

THE GARDENER'S GRILL PANTRY

GRILL FOR LEFTOVERS, THEN FREEZE THEM FOR LATER USE.
Simply brush prepared vegetables with olive oil, season to taste, then grill
over a medium-hot fire until they have good grill marks. Let cool, then chop if
you like and place in freezer containers, marking the date, quantity, and type
of vegetable. When you want to use them, simply thaw and then use on sandwiches or in soups, pastas, or sauces. Tomatoes, with their high water content,
do better smoked than grilled for freezing.

Here are specific techniques for common garden vegetables:

- **ASPARAGUS.** Chop grilled spears and freeze.
- **BELL OR CHILE PEPPERS.** Grill whole peppers, then quarter, stem,
  seed, and freeze.
- **CORN.** Cut grilled kernels from the cob and freeze.
- **EGGPLANT.** Cut into 1-inch thick horizontal slices to grill. Leave as
  slices or chop, then freeze.
- **ONIONS.** Grill green or bulb onions whole; grill round onions in slices.
  Chop grilled onions and freeze.
- **YELLOW SUMMER SQUASH.** Cut into 1-inch thick horizontal slices
  to grill. Leave as slices or chop, then freeze.
- **ZUCCHINI.** Cut into 1-inch thick horizontal slices to grill. Leave as slices
  or chop, then freeze.

IF YOU ARE A FAN OF BÉARNAISE SAUCE, YOU MUST TRY THIS very simple butter. Spread it on a bread crouton to top a cup of Smoked Tomato Bisque (page 128) or add a couple of pats of béarnaise butter to Grilled Spring Platter of Asparagus and Leeks (page 161). Serve it at room temperature with grill-roasted potatoes (page 8), grilled bread, asparagus, poultry, or steaks. The recipe halves easily for a smaller yield, but why not make the whole recipe and label, date, and freeze the other half so it is at the ready?

BÉARNAISE BUTTER

MAKES 2 CUPS

1 cup (2 sticks) unsalted butter, at room temperature

2 tablespoons chopped shallots

1 tablespoon white wine vinegar

2 tablespoons chopped fresh tarragon leaves

¼ teaspoon sea salt

½ teaspoon hot sauce or to taste

In a medium-sized bowl, combine all of the ingredients and stir together with a fork. You can either spoon it into a ramekin or small bowl for serving, or shape into a roll, wrap in waxed paper, and chill. This butter an also be stored in the freezer for up to 3 months: wrap it tightly in a layer of waxed paper, then in layers of plastic wrap and aluminum foil.

BUTTER UP!

ADDING GARDEN GOODIES TO SOFTENED BUTTER IS AN EASY WAY to add flavor to grilled breads, vegetables, fish, shellfish, steak, chicken, or lamb. Simply mash all ingredients together in a bowl or process until smooth in a food processor.

To 1 cup (2 sticks) unsalted butter add:

- $\frac{1}{2}$ cup chopped fresh mint, $\frac{1}{2}$ teaspoon red pepper flakes, and $\frac{1}{2}$ teaspoon grated lemon zest to make Hot Pepper Mint Butter

- $\frac{1}{4}$ cup freshly grated Parmesan cheese, 2 tablespoon anchovy paste, 2 teaspoons Dijon mustard, 1 teaspoon Worcestershire sauce, 2 minced garlic cloves, and grated zest of 1 lemon to make Caesar Butter

- 8 smoked Roma tomatoes (page 33) that have been peeled, seeded, and chopped; $\frac{1}{2}$ cup finely chopped basil; and salt to taste to make Smoked Summer Tomato Basil Butter

- 4 smoked garlic cloves, $\frac{1}{2}$ cup chopped fresh herbs (Italian parsley, basil, oregano, chives, and/or cilantro), and salt to taste to make Herbed Smoked Garlic Butter

- 2 finely chopped jalapeño or serrano peppers, 2 minced garlic cloves, and $\frac{1}{2}$ teaspoon ground chipotle pepper to make a Southwest Butter

- $1\frac{1}{2}$ tablespoons smoked paprika, 2 minced garlic cloves, and 2 teaspoons lime zest to make Smoked Paprika Butter

- 1 tablespoon capers, 2 minced garlic cloves, 2 teaspoons lemon zest to make Caper Butter

- 2 ounces crumbled blue cheese, 2 tablespoons chopped Italian parsley, and 2 crisp pieces of bacon crumbled to make Blue Cheese Bacon Butter

- 3 tablespoons chopped sun-dried tomatoes and 4 ounces goat cheese to make Sun-Dried Goat Cheese Butter

THIS IS A LOVELY THICK PASTE THAT IS GREAT FOR MARINATING vegetables for the grill wok or basket. To use it, combine thick slices of fresh garden onion, peppers, summer squash, tomatoes, and green beans, about 6 cups total, in a large re-sealable plastic bag and add the paste. Marinate, and then grill in a basket over a hot fire. It is delicious brushed on boneless chicken breasts, pork chops, and even nice, thick steaks before grilling. Use one to two tablespoons of paste for each chicken breast, pork chop, or steak. Substitute this recipe for the butter in Brussels Sprouts with Feta Garlic Butter (page 178).

ITALIAN PARMESAN GRILLING PASTE

**MAKES ABOUT
1½ CUPS**

½ cup grated Parmesan
  cheese

¼ cup olive oil

¼ cup red wine vinegar

2 tablespoons dried basil

2 tablespoons dried
  oregano

1 tablespoon seasoned
  pepper

4 garlic cloves, minced

Combine all ingredients and apply to vegetables, poultry, beef, or pork. Store the paste in a glass jar covered with a tight-fitting lid. Keeps in the refrigerator for up to 3 to 4 days.

ONCE GARDENERS ADD GARLIC CHIVES TO THEIR PLOTS, WATCH out! These flat slender leaves are packed with garlic aroma and are wildly prolific. If you are courageous enough to deal with its growth, then you will have the abundance of chives to make this superb pesto. It is a brilliant emerald green and doesn't brown like basil pesto. Mix and match other herbs with the chives like basil, lemon balm, and a little bit of mint. Use it as a spread on sandwiches for Panini Caprese (page 85) or Grilled Garden Loaf (page 81).

GARLIC CHIVE PESTO

MAKES ABOUT 1 CUP

2 cups chopped fresh garlic chives

½ cup toasted walnuts

1 garlic clove, crushed or roughly chopped

¾ cup regular or extra virgin olive oil

½ cup freshly grated Parmesan or Romano cheese

Kosher or sea salt and freshly ground black pepper to taste

In a food processor, process the chives, walnuts, and garlic until they form a smooth paste. With the processor running, drizzle in the olive oil in a slow, steady stream until the pesto solidifies. Add the Parmesan and season to taste with salt and pepper, pulsing just to combine. Use immediately or spoon into a small jar with a tight-fitting lid. This pesto will keep in the refrigerator for about 7 to 10 days or in the freezer for up to 6 to 9 months.

Variation:

For Basil Pesto, substitute fresh packed basil leaves for chives and toasted pine nuts for walnuts.

THE GARDENER'S SMOKE PANTRY

SMOKE FOR LEFTOVERS, THEN FREEZE THEM FOR LATER USE.
You'll need to prepare a hot fire on one side of your grill for indirect cooking and have wood chips or chunks smoldering (see page 9 for how-to). Simply brush prepared vegetables with olive oil, season to taste, then place them in a disposable aluminum pan on the indirect (or no-heat) side of the grill. Cover and smoke until the vegetables have softened, have a good smoky aroma, and a burnished appearance (see page 9 for timing). Let cool, then chop if you like, and place in freezer containers, marking the date, quantity, and type of vegetable. When you want to use them, simply thaw and then use on sandwiches or in soups, pastas, or sauces. Asparagus, eggplant, yellow squash, and zucchini are better grilled than smoked.

Here are specific techniques for common garden vegetables:

- **BELL OR CHILE PEPPERS.** Smoke whole peppers, then quarter, stem, seed, and freeze.
- **CORN.** Cut smoked kernels from the cob and freeze.
- **GARLIC.** Peel and thread whole cloves onto skewers. Or smoke a whole garlic bulb until soft, then squeeze out smoked garlic cloves and remove papery covering. Freeze softened garlic cloves.
- **ONIONS.** Smoke whole, round onions. Chop grilled onions and freeze.
- **TOMATOES.** Smoke whole until softened, then peel and seed before freezing.
- **WINTER SQUASH.** Cut in half or quarter, and scoop out seeds. Brush cut sides with olive oil, season, and place cut-side down in the pan. Scoop out softened, smoked squash and freeze.

IMAGINE A CHAR-GRILLED FLANK STEAK SURROUNDED BY freshly picked and grilled onions, drizzled with the flavors of smoky garlic, cream, and cilantro. Heaven! It also tastes great with grilled chicken, pork, steak, or shellfish marinated in a combination of 6 tablespoons olive oil, 3 tablespoons fresh lime juice, and garlic salt to taste. Pair this with Flank Steak with Grilled Peppers and Onions (page 156).

SMOKED GARLIC and CILANTRO CREAM SAUCE

MAKES ABOUT 2½ CUPS

2 cups heavy cream

½ cup fresh cilantro leaves, plus more for garnish

3 tablespoons fresh lime juice

½ teaspoon kosher or sea salt

6 garlic cloves, smoked (see page 9)

In a blender or food processor, combine all the ingredients and process until smooth.

Transfer the puree to a medium-size saucepan over medium-high heat and cook until the sauce begins to bubble. Serve immediately.

THIS FABULOUSLY EASY SAUCE (IT'S A BEURRE BLANC-STYLE sauce) is great with grilled vegetables, skirt steak, pork tenderloin, or a chicken dish like Skewered Chicken Saltimbocca (page 137). If you can't find a fresh poblano, substitute a jalapeño.

SMOKED POBLANO CREAM SAUCE

**MAKES ABOUT
1½ CUPS**

1 poblano chile, smoked

2 cups heavy cream or evaporated milk

½ cup (1 stick) unsalted butter, cut into pieces

Kosher or sea salt and freshly ground black pepper to taste

Combine the poblano and cream in a medium-size, heavy saucepan and simmer over medium heat until reduced to 1 cup, about 15 minutes.

Strain the mixture, discard the chile, and return the cream to the pan over low heat. Whisk in the butter, one piece at a time, until you have a smooth sauce. Season with salt and pepper and serve immediately.

ERVE THIS WONDERFUL ALL-PURPOSE SAUCE ON GRILLED vegetables, fish, chicken, or that breakfast classic, eggs Benedict. Make up a batch and take your breakfast al fresco with grilled potatoes and onions, charred asparagus, and scrambled eggs on the grill, drizzled with this hollandaise: sublime. Serve a dollop of this on the Grilled Asparagus Salad (page 111).

BLENDER HOLLANDAISE

MAKES ABOUT 1½ CUPS

6 large egg yolks

2 tablespoons fresh lemon juice

1 teaspoon dry mustard

1 cup (2 sticks) unsalted butter, melted and kept warm

¼ teaspoon cayenne pepper, or to taste

Fine kosher or sea salt to taste

Place the egg yolks, lemon juice, and mustard in a blender or food processor and process until smooth. Drizzle in the hot melted butter, pulsing on low speed, until the sauce thickens. Add the cayenne and season with salt. Keep warm in the top of a double boiler or transfer to a stainless steel bowl and set over a pan of hot, not boiling, water until ready to serve.

THIS STIRS TOGETHER IN SECONDS AND IS SO GOOD; YOU'LL always want to have a jar of it in your refrigerator. It is a great dipping sauce for the Grilled Spring Platter of Asparagus and Leeks (page 161).

MUSTARD SEED SAUCE

MAKES ABOUT 1½ CUPS

½ cup Dijon mustard

½ cup whole-grain mustard

½ cup mayonnaise

1 tablespoon lemon juice

1 tablespoon fresh chopped dill

1 teaspoon Worcestershire sauce

½ teaspoon ground white pepper

Combine all of the ingredients in a glass bowl and whisk to blend. Keeps refrigerated for up to 2 weeks.

WHEN YOU'RE ALREADY GRILLING OTHER VEGETABLES, GRILL some green or bulb onions while you're at it. Use them right away in this recipe—delicious on a Blackened Fish Po' Boy, page 90—or chop them up and freeze for later use.

GRILLED GREEN ONION MAYONNAISE

**MAKES ABOUT
⅔ CUP**

8 green onions, scallions,
 or small bulb onions

Olive oil, for brushing

Salt and pepper to taste

⅓ cup mayonnaise

Grated zest and juice of
 1 lemon

2 teaspoons chopped
 fresh basil

Prepare a medium-hot fire in your grill. Place a perforated grill rack over the grill grate. Brush the onions with olive oil and season with salt and pepper.

Place the scallions on the perforated grill rack and grill, turning every minute or so, until the onions get good grill marks. Let cool.

Chop the onions and combine with mayonnaise, lemon zest, lemon juice, and basil until well blended. Serve right away or cover and refrigerate for up to 3 days.

SERVE THIS CREAMY MAYONNAISE AS A DIPPING SAUCE FOR grilled broccoli, asparagus, and zucchini. It is luscious with Flame-Licked Tomatoes on the Stem (page 124) and is a great color contrast, too. It is lovely drizzled over a platter of grilled vegetables and over your favorite grilled fish, shellfish, or poultry. It has the flavor of aioli, without the preparation. Several other flavor combinations follow this recipe in the Quick-To-Fix Aioli recipes (page 40).

LEMON-GARLIC AIOLI

MAKES ABOUT 1 CUP

1 cup mayonnaise

2 tablespoons lemon zest

2 tablespoons lemon juice

2 garlic cloves, minced

1 teaspoon ground white
  pepper

Fine kosher or sea salt to
  taste

Combine all the ingredients in a small bowl, whisking to blend. This mayonnaise will keep, covered, in the refrigerator for up to 2 weeks.

QUICK-TO-FIX AIOLI

IF YOU LIKE BIG FLAVOR AND QUICK RESULTS AIOLI FITS THE ticket. Shortcut aioli is delicious when you use a good-quality store-bought mayonnaise, plus it has a longer shelf life in the refrigerator than from-scratch aioli.

TO 1 CUP LEMON-GARLIC AIOLI (PAGE 39), ADD:

- 2 tablespoons prepared horseradish to make Horseradish Aioli (great on grilled potatoes, onions, steak, or smoked or rotisserie beef sandwiches)

- $\frac{1}{2}$ cup finely chopped roasted red peppers (homemade, see page 43, or from a jar) to make Roasted Red Pepper Aioli (a great vegetable dipping sauce)

- 1 smoked tomato (see page 9), peeled, seeded, and chopped, to make Smoked Tomato Aioli (for grilled bread, vegetables, poultry, and fish)

- $\frac{1}{2}$ cup finely chopped fresh herbs to make Fresh Herb Aioli (for grilled sandwiches, mushrooms, asparagus, broccoli, chicken, and fish)

- 2 tablespoons homemade or prepared pesto to make Pesto Aioli (delicious on fresh or grilled tomatoes and pasta)

- 1 or 2 canned chipotle chiles, chopped or to taste for Spicy Chipotle Aioli (it gives ordinary grilled vegetables a kick)

- 1 tablespoon sun-dried tomato paste and 2 tablespoons chopped fresh basil to make Sun-Dried Tomato Basil Aioli (for grilled vegetables, pastas, seafood, and dolloped on grilled veggie pizzas)

- 2 to 3 tablespoons Dijon mustard to make Dijon Aioli (for grilled vegetable platters and seafood)

- 2 to 3 tablespoons chopped cucumber, 1 teaspoon chopped jalapeño pepper, and 2 ounces crumbled feta cheese for a spicy Greek Aioli (great on tomatoes, grilled bread, and as a dipping sauce for a platter of grilled vegetables)

- Change the lemon juice and zest to another citrus fruit to make Orange, Lime, or Grapefruit Aioli

THIS WONDERFULLY PUNGENT BLUE CHEESE DRESSING MAKES a great dipping sauce for grilled chicken wings or raw or grilled vegetables. It's also superb spooned over a platter of grilled romaine like High-Heat Grilled Romaine Salad (page 109), radicchio, and Napa cabbage.

CREAMY BLUE CHEESE DRESSING

**MAKES ABOUT
4 CUPS**

2 cups sour cream

8 ounces good-quality blue
cheese, such as Maytag,
crumbled

$^2/_3$ cup mayonnaise

3 tablespoons cider vinegar

1 teaspoon red pepper
flakes

Onion salt, celery salt,
and Worcestershire
sauce to taste

Combine all the ingredients in a medium-size bowl, whisking to blend. For the best results, cover and let the flavors develop in the refrigerator for 24 hours before serving chilled. This dressing will keep, covered, in the refrigerator for up to 2 weeks.

A CLASSIC SPANISH SAUCE THICKENED WITH BREAD AND GROUND almonds, Romesco tastes wonderful on grilled vegetables and seafood. It can be substituted for the marinara for the Char-Grilled Eggplant with Grilled Marinara (page 176) and is a great spread for Grilled Chicken Ciabatta with Romesco and Baby Greens (page 86). To toast almonds, sprinkle them on a baking sheet and toast in a 350°F oven for 15 minutes or until lightly browned.

ROMESCO SAUCE

MAKES 2 CUPS

½ cup toasted slivered almonds

2 Grill-Roasted Red Bell Peppers (page 43) or jarred roasted red bell peppers, roughly chopped

2 garlic cloves, minced

1 slice white bread (crust removed), toasted and crumbled

1 tablespoon roughly chopped fresh flat-leaf parsley

½ teaspoon red pepper flakes

⅓ cup red wine vinegar

⅔ cup extra-virgin olive oil

In a food processor, grind the almonds. Add roasted peppers, garlic, bread, parsley and hot pepper flakes. Blend until it becomes a paste. Add the vinegar and pulse to blend. With the motor running, gradually pour the olive oil through the feed tube in a steady stream until the mixture thickens like mayonnaise. Season to taste with salt and black pepper.

Store in a covered container in the refrigerator for up to 3 days.

GRILL-ROASTING PEPPERS

THE DIFFERENCE BETWEEN A GRILLED BELL PEPPER AND A GRILL-roasted bell pepper is texture and grilling time. Grilled peppers retain crispness as well as their skins and take just a few minutes to lightly char. Grill-roasted peppers are cooked whole for a longer time and have the stem, seeds, and skin removed. (For more on grill-roasting, see page 8.)

Grill-roasting peppers just takes one extra step. Brush whole red, green, yellow, purple, or orange bell peppers with olive oil and season with salt and pepper. Grill over a medium-hot fire, turning every few minutes, until they have good grill marks on all sides. Remove the peppers from the grill, place them in a paper or plastic bag, close the bag and let them steam until they're cool enough to handle. Then stem, seed, and remove the skin. Use right away, cover and refrigerate for up to 3 days or freeze for up to 3 months.

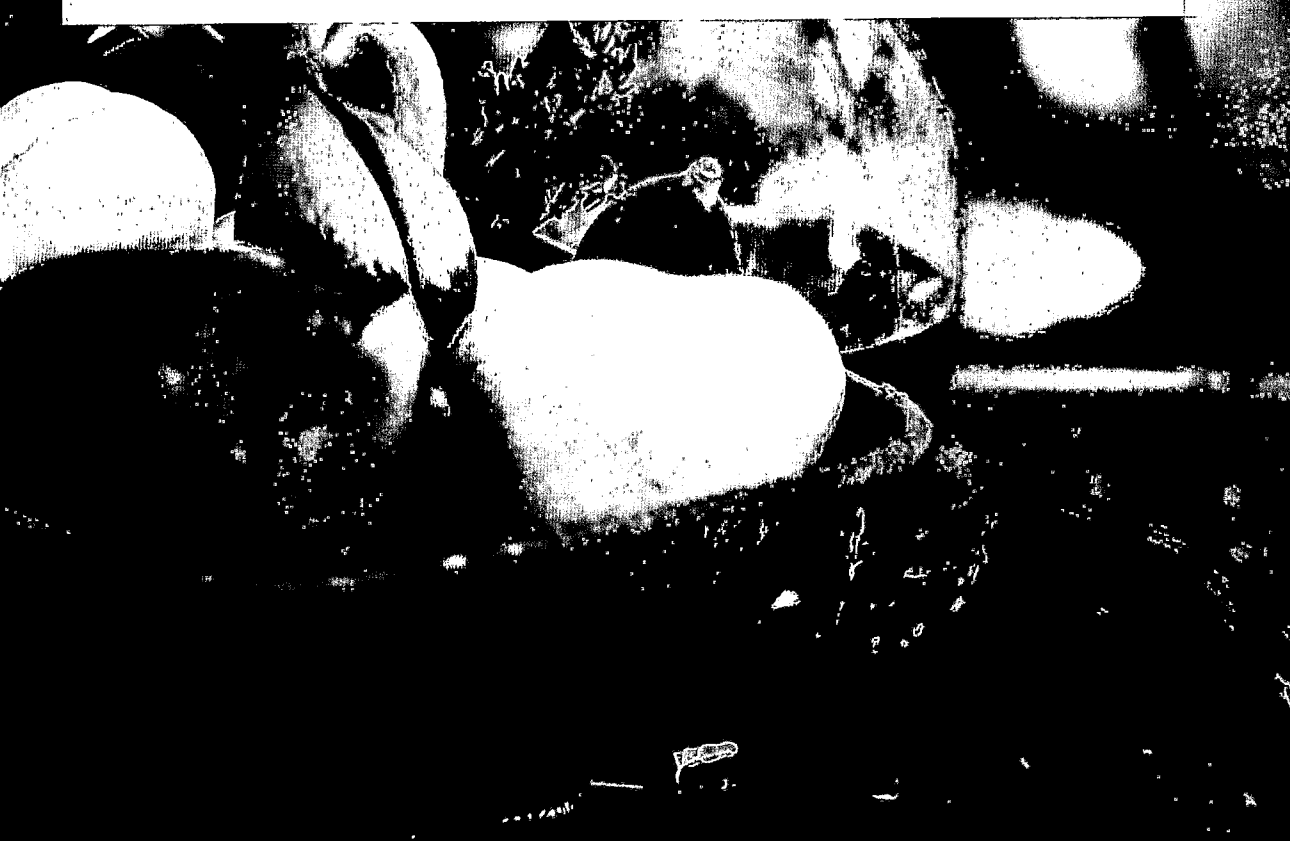

FRESH PITA BREAD, BRUSHED WITH OLIVE OIL AND GRILLED, tastes even more fabulous when served with this Greek yogurt sauce, enlivened with garlic, cucumber, and dill. It is a wonderfully cool and refreshing dipping sauce to add to a platter of grilled summer vegetables too.

TZATZIKI

MAKES 4 CUPS

3 cups Greek yogurt, drained

1 medium-size cucumber, peeled, seeded, and finely shredded

4 large garlic cloves, minced

2 tablespoons olive oil

½ teaspoon dill

Fine kosher or sea salt and freshly ground black pepper to taste

Place the yogurt in a medium-size bowl. Blot the shredded cucumber with paper towels to remove as much moisture as possible. Stir the cucumber, garlic, olive oil, and dill into the yogurt. Season with salt and pepper. Use immediately, or spoon into a covered container and store in the refrigerator up to 3 days.

FOR GARDENERS IN THE MIDWEST, SEPTEMBER PROVIDES THE last abundance of tomatoes, onions, and peppers. This is a classic combination for a vibrant chunky garden tomato sauce. This recipe could easily be renamed Grilled Marinara! Use it as a guideline; it has a lot of flexibility.

END-OF-THE-GARDEN SAUCE

MAKES 8 TO 10 CUPS OR MORE

10 tomatoes, sliced thickly (about 4 pounds)

10 assorted green, red, yellow, orange, or purple bell peppers, quartered and seeded (about 4 pounds)

5 onions, peeled and sliced thickly

1 cup chopped fresh assorted herbs like parsley, chives, and oregano

Prepare a hot fire in your grill.

Place the vegetables over the hot fire and grill for 5 to 10 minutes until charred and soft. You may need to do this in several batches depending on how many vegetables you have to grill.

Let the vegetables cool and rub off some of the skin from the tomatoes and peppers. Core and seed the peppers.

Place batches of grilled vegetables in a food processor and pulse to chop. Have at least one batch of the vegetables processed into a puree. Combine all of the chopped and pureed vegetables in a large bowl. Add the fresh herbs and season to taste with salt and black pepper. Serve the sauce hot or cold. Store sauce in a covered dish in the refrigerator for up to 1 week; the sauce can also be frozen for up to 6 months.

Variation:

After the vegetables are grilled, transfer them to a stockpot to continue to simmer over a medium-low flame. Add garlic, sautéed mushrooms, and more herbs, for a full flavored sauce.

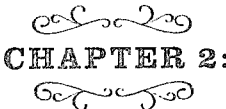

CHAPTER 2:

APPETIZERS

WHETHER YOU LIVE IN AN APARTMENT WITH A SMALL OUTDOOR space, a house with a yard, or a country place with acres and acres, you can go from garden to grill to great appetizers in minutes. With a brush of oil and a sprinkle of seasoning, many vegetables can be quickly grilled or slowly smoked to perfection. All you need to accompany them is grilled bread—French baguettes, artisan rye, flat pita, or airy ciabatta—to soak up all the delicious juices and sauces.

Many garden goodies like fava beans and edamame in the pod, asparagus, bell or chile peppers, and fingerling potatoes can simply be harvested, rinsed, dried, brushed, and grilled. Larger vegetables like eggplant, zucchini and yellow squash can be sliced lengthwise for easy turning on the grill. Greens such as chard make great wrappings for bundled cheeses and other ingredients.

As gardeners and grillers, we try to take advantage of good fortune and good weather by harvesting and grilling more than we really need for a meal. Leftover grilled vegetables (see The Gardener's Grill Pantry (page 28) can be easily frozen to up to 3 months to star later on in dips, spreads, or other appetizers.

Grill-Toasted Bruschetta with Four Seasons Toppings ...49

Goat Cheese with Spring Garlic and Herb Topping ...50

Smoked Summer Tomato Basil Butter ...50

Grilled Autumn Apple and Blue Cheese Topping ...52

Rustic Winter White Bean Spread ...52

**Gardening and Grilling
with a Mediterranean Accent** ...53

Charred Eggplant and Tarragon Spread ...54

Grilled Rye Bread with Boursin and Spring Radishes ...55

French Garden Radish Plate with Grilled Onion Butter ...56

Container Gardens ...58

Crostini with Smoked and Grilled Vegetable Dip ...59

Planked Butternut Squash, Sage, and Brie ...60

Soft Corn Tortillas with Rajas and Queso ...61

A Gardener's Pound ...62

Prosciutto-Wrapped Asparagus Spears ...64

Fire-Roasted Fava Beans in the Pod with Sheep's Milk Cheese ...65

Grill-Roasted Edamame in the Pod ...66

Growing Edamame ...66

Flame-Licked Fingerlings with Romesco Sauce ...68

Grill-Roasted Tomatillo Salsa ...70

Fire-Roasted Pepper Dip ...72

Grilled Zucchini and Yellow Squash Stacks
with Feta and Black Olives ...73

Mesquite-Smoked Jalapeño Poppers ...74

Chard-Wrapped Goat Cheese on the Grill ...75

Tuscan Polenta Platter with Sizzling Peppers,
Onions, and Mushrooms ...76

Grilled Polenta with Stir-Grilled Garlic Greens ...77

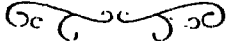

THIS HUMBLE APPETIZER CAN BE ELEVATED TO STAR STATUS by brushing it with olive oil, rubbing it with garlic cloves, then sizzling it on the grill. The toppings are likewise simple and make the most of what's fresh in the garden. Serve the bread in a basket with bowls of topping alongside so that your guests can help themselves (and the bread won't get soggy that way).

GRILL-TOASTED BRUSCHETTA
with FOUR SEASONS TOPPINGS

MAKES 6 SERVINGS

Six ½-inch-thick slices country bread, such as sourdough, Italian, or French boule

Olive oil, for brushing

1 large garlic clove, peeled and cut in half

Bruschetta Topping of choice (four recipes follow)

Prepare a hot fire in your grill.

Brush both sides of the bread with olive oil, and then rub the garlic clove halves over one side of the bread.

Grill the bread directly over the fire, turning once, for 2 to 3 minutes total, or until the bread has turned golden and has good grill marks. Place the bread on a platter and serve with the topping of your choice. Serve immediately.

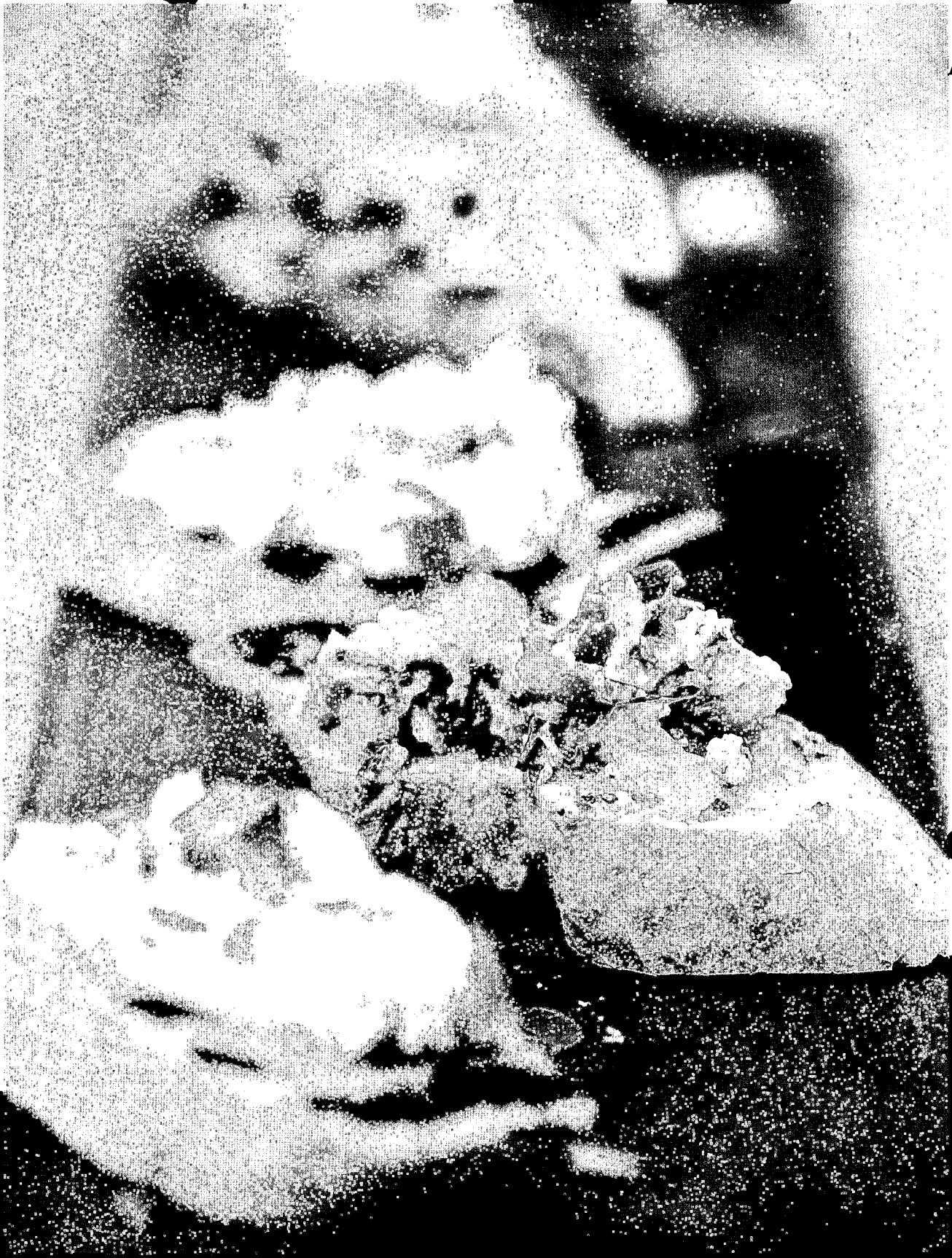

GOAT CHEESE *with* SPRING GARLIC *and* HERB TOPPING

MAKES ABOUT 1 CUP

6 ounces fresh goat cheese, at room temperature

1 garlic clove, minced

½ cup finely chopped mixed fresh herbs, such as tarragon, flat-leaf parsley, and chives

Kosher or sea salt and freshly ground black pepper to taste

Mash all the ingredients together in a small bowl. (You can prepare this 2 to 3 days in advance and store it, covered, in the refrigerator.) Serve at room temperature.

SMOKED SUMMER TOMATO BASIL BUTTER

MAKES ABOUT 2 CUPS

2 large smoked tomatoes (see page 9), peeled, seeded, and chopped

1 cup (2 sticks) unsalted butter, room temperature

½ cup chopped fresh basil

Kosher or sea salt to taste

Whisk all the ingredients together in a small bowl. (You can prepare the butter 2 to 3 days in advance and store it, covered, in the refrigerator.) Bring to room temperature before serving.

GRILLED AUTUMN APPLE
and BLUE CHEESE TOPPING

MAKES 6 SERVINGS

2 large apples, peeled, cored, and cut in half lengthwise

Olive oil, for brushing

1 cup crumbled blue cheese

Brush the apple halves with olive oil and, at the same time you grill the bread, grill the apples over the fire, turning once, until the apples are golden and have good grill marks. Slice the apples and serve on the grilled bread, topped with the crumbled blue cheese.

RUSTIC WINTER
WHITE BEAN SPREAD

**MAKES ABOUT
1½ CUPS**

1½ cups cooked shell beans, such as cannellini, or one 15-ounce can cannellini beans, rinsed and drained

3 garlic cloves, chopped

Juice of 1 lemon (about 3 tablespoons)

½ cup freshly torn basil leaves

¼ cup extra-virgin olive oil

Freshly ground black pepper

In a large bowl, combine all of the ingredients and toss to blend. Serve at room temperature.

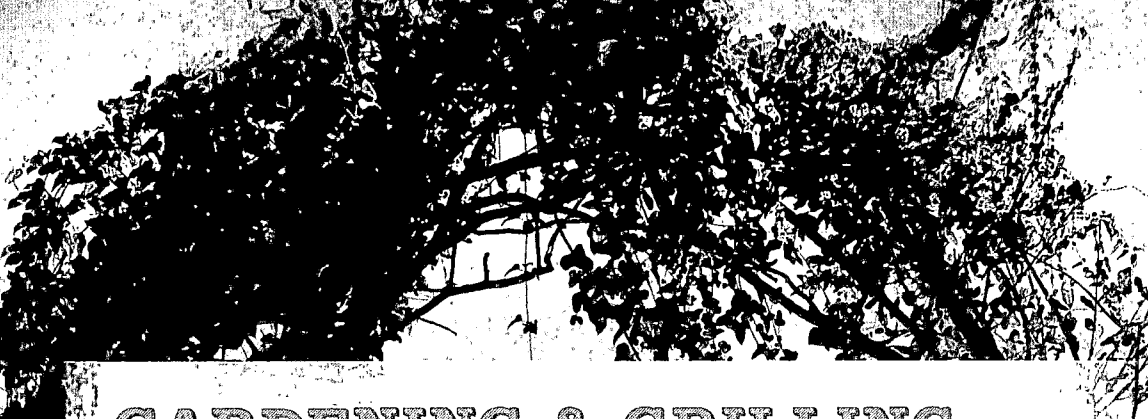

GARDENING & GRILLING
WITH A MEDITERRANEAN ACCENT

THE FOODS OF MEDITERRANEAN GARDENS LOVE HOT SUMMERS—and the grill! They're great to simply grill or to transform into dips or spreads to serve with grilled flatbreads of all kinds.

- **CUCUMBER.** Fresh sliced cucumber adds fresh crunch to a meze or casual meal centered around a grilled flatbread, a dip or spread, and lots of other small dishes.

- **CUMIN.** Native to Egypt, this low-growing plant is grown for its seed and used to flavor flatbreads, dips, and vegetable dishes.

- **EGGPLANT.** Glossy purple eggplants can be sliced horizontally and then grilled.

- **GARLIC.** The whole head of garlic can be placed on the grill and charred or smoked indirectly; it adds dimensions of flavor to anything savory.

- **OREGANO.** Beautiful cascading branches of oregano can garnish a platter of grilled vegetables, and the tiny leaves add a punch of flavor to sauces.

- **ROSEMARY.** Fresh leaves flavor marinades, bastes, grilled flatbreads and vegetables, and sauces. Sturdy stems, stripped of their leaves, can be used as skewers.

DARK, TANGY, AND SMOKY, THIS MIDDLE EASTERN-INSPIRED spread tastes even better when paired with pita bread hot from the grill. It can also be served with strips of red bell pepper, zucchini, or yellow summer squash.

CHARRED EGGPLANT
and TARRAGON SPREAD

MAKES 8 SERVINGS

2 eggplants
   (about 2½ pounds)
¾ cup olive oil, divided,
   plus more for brushing
8 pieces pita bread
1 tablespoon kosher salt
4 garlic cloves, minced
2 tablespoons fresh or 1
   teaspoon dried tarragon
¼ teaspoon freshly ground
   black pepper
1 teaspoon granulated
   sugar

Prepare a hot fire in your grill.

Trim the ends of the eggplants and cut lengthwise into ½-inch-thick slices. Brush both sides with ¼ cup of the olive oil and grill 3 to 4 minutes per side, turning once, until they are nicely charred with good grill marks. Brush the pita bread all over with olive oil. Grill for 1 to 2 minutes per side, turning once, or until it is nicely charred with good grill marks. Keep warm.

Place the grilled eggplant in a food processor. Add the salt, garlic, tarragon, black pepper, and sugar, processing until smooth and well blended. With the machine running, drizzle in the remaining ½ cup olive oil through the feed tube to make a smooth spread. This spread keeps, covered, in the refrigerator for up to 2 days.

TENDER-CRISP SPRING RADISHES ARE JUST 1 INCH IN DIAMETER and a delightful addition to the garden and the table. They love cool weather, growing and mature in about 4 to 8 weeks, depending on the variety. Easter Egg radishes, in purple, pink, and red, look and taste wonderful in this recipe.

GRILLED RYE BREAD *with* SOFT CHEESE *and* SPRING RADISHES

MAKES 4 SERVINGS

4 slices good rye bread, cut into ½-inch-thick slices

Olive oil, for brushing

1 (5-ounce) package Boursin or soft goat cheese

12 to 14 small spring radishes

Kosher or sea salt

Prepare a hot fire in your grill.

Brush both sides of the rye bread with olive oil. Grill the bread directly over the fire, turning once, for 2 to 3 minutes total, or until the bread has begun to char with good grill marks. Serve the bread on a platter with the cheese and the fresh radishes. Offer kosher or sea salt in a small bowl, served on the side.

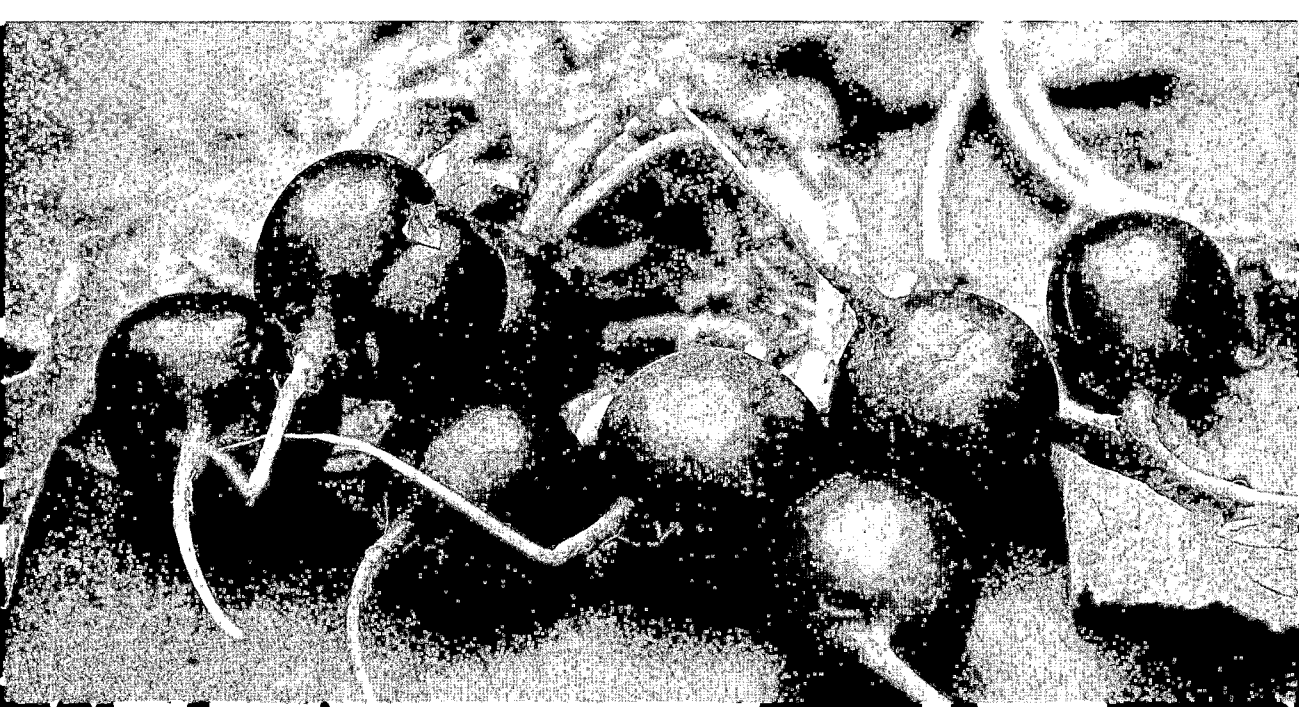

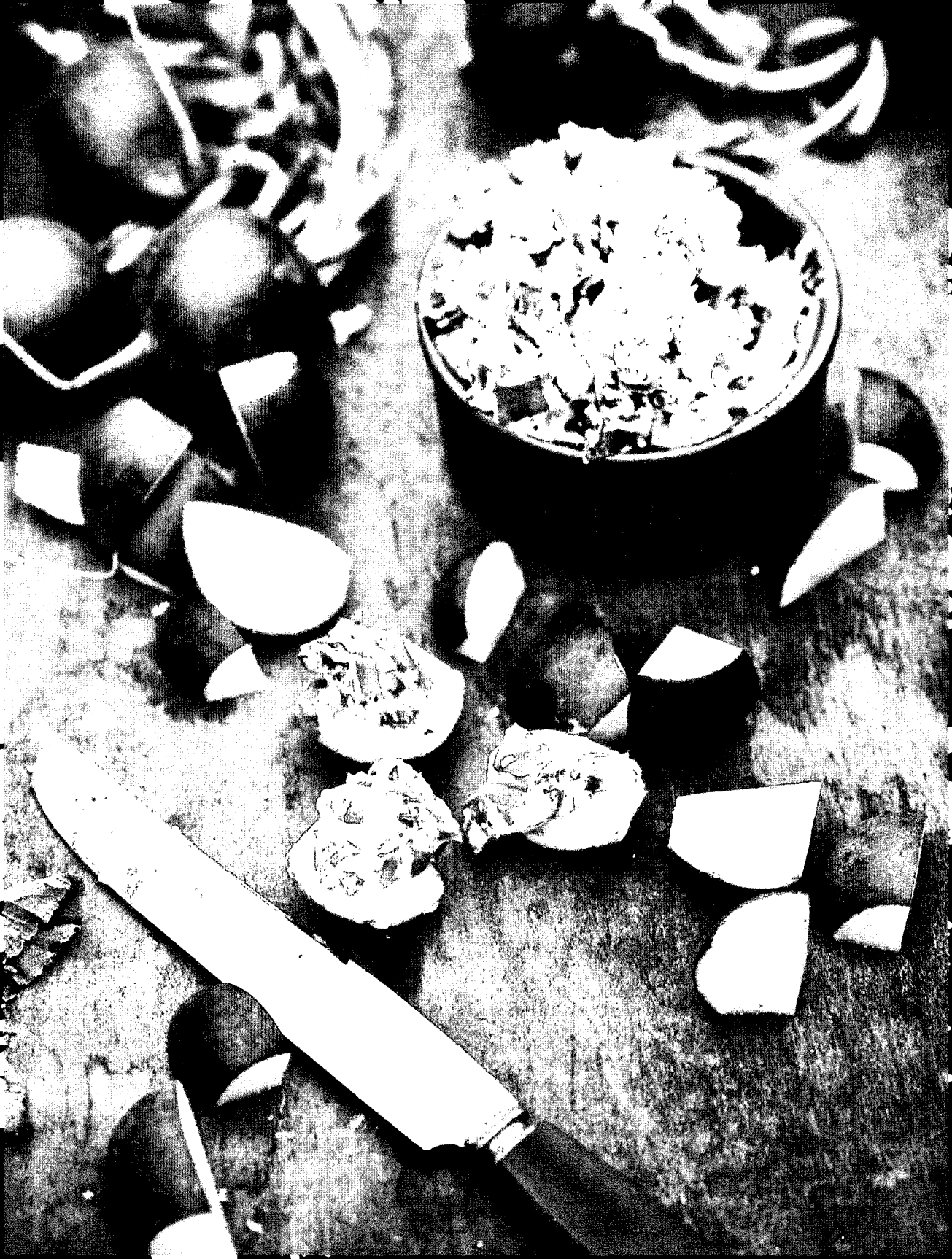

SPREAD OUT A FLORAL TABLECLOTH OUTDOORS AND SERVE this appetizer with a Provençal rosé or a glass of sparkling wine. The radishes can be fresh plucked and quickly rinsed, with the warmth and smell of the earth still lingering. You can make Grilled Onion Butter a couple of days ahead.

FRENCH GARDEN RADISH PLATE
with GRILLED ONION BUTTER

MAKES 6 TO 8 SERVINGS

GRILLED ONION BUTTER

1 small yellow or white onion

$\frac{1}{2}$ cup (1 stick) salted butter, at room temperature

1 teaspoon Worcestershire sauce

$\frac{1}{4}$ teaspoon dry mustard

$\frac{1}{4}$ teaspoon freshly ground black pepper

2 tablespoons chopped green onions or chives

RADISH PLATE

1 loaf crusty French bread

24 small radishes

Prepare a hot fire in your grill.

Slice the onion in $\frac{1}{2}$-inch-thick slices. Grill the onion slices directly over the fire for about 3 or 4 minutes per side, until they have good grill marks and have softened. Let the onion slices cool and then chop them.

Combine the butter, Worcestershire sauce, dry mustard, and black pepper until well blended. Add the grilled chopped onion and herbs, stirring to combine. Place the butter in a bowl. Slice the bread and serve it with the radishes and the Grilled Onion Butter.

CONTAINER GARDENS

FROM ROOFTOP TERRACES IN MANHATTAN HIGHRISES TO DOOR- yards in Tuscan hill towns, container gardens can flourish in small spaces. The keys are to use containers that suit your geographic area, good planting soil, plant fertilizer, and plants that do well in small spaces. You can have vegetables and herbs that you love with a miniature garden that pleases the eye.

- **CONTAINERS.** Choose pots of a material that works with your climate. Avoid metal containers in hot climates, terracotta (which can crack if left outside) in cold climates. Make sure the pot has good drainage holes in the bottom and is large enough to allow the plants room to grow.

- **SOIL.** Soil in container gardens can get compacted more easily than that in the garden, so use planting mixtures or good quality dirt mixed with sand for good drainage.

- **FERTILIZER.** Choose natural compost to mix into the soil or follow the package directions on an all-purpose water-soluble plant fertilizer (usually an equal blend of nitrogen, phosphorus, and potassium).

- **PLANTS.** Large containers can include a tall plant (tomato, eggplant, beans, peas, etc.) tied to stakes or a wire frame in the center of the pot. The border can include root vegetables like radishes or turnips in cooler weather, or tender herbs with a shorter growth habit such as Italian parsley, thyme, basil, tarragon, and cilantro in warmer weather. You can also use smaller pots that hold just one herb or plant each, but group them together: a cherry tomato, tomatillo, or jalapeño plant in the largest pot, surrounded by basil, oregano, and cilantro plants in smaller pots.

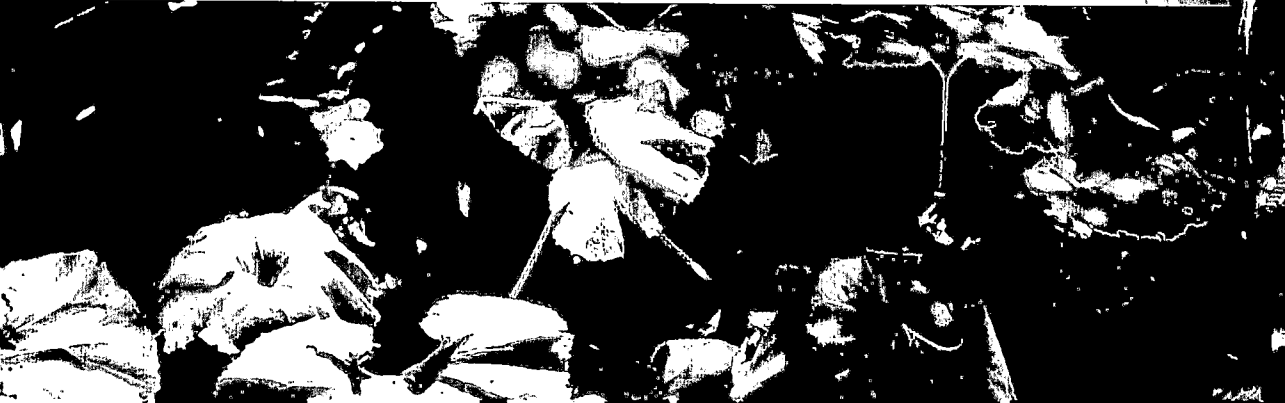

THIS RECIPE IS A GREAT WAY TO USE LEFTOVER SMOKED AND grilled vegetables, thawed from your freezer—see The Gardener's Grill Pantry (page 28) and The Gardener's Smoke Pantry (page 33).

CROSTINI with SMOKED and GRILLED VEGETABLE DIP

1 French baguette, sliced and toasted

2 cups mixed, chopped, grilled and/or smoked vegetables (such as tomato, red bell pepper, eggplant, onion, and jalapeño pepper)

Extra-virgin olive oil and balsamic vinegar to taste

Kosher or sea salt and freshly ground black pepper to taste

Arrange the toasted baguette slices on a platter. In a medium bowl, combine the mixed, chopped vegetables with olive oil and balsamic vinegar to taste. Season with salt and pepper and serve in the middle of the platter.

THIS IS A SUBLIME WAY TO PREPARE WINTER SQUASH AS AN appetizer. The colors are beautiful—burnished orange squash, dark green sage and creamy white cheese.

PLANKED BUTTERNUT SQUASH, SAGE, and BRIE

MAKES 8 TO 10 SERVINGS

1 small butternut squash

Olive oil, for brushing

20-ounce wheel of baby Brie or Camembert

4 sage leaves

Kosher salt and freshly ground white pepper to taste

Crackers or bread, for serving

Prepare a hot fire on one side of your grill for indirect cooking. Soak a baking plank in water for 30 minutes.

Cut the butternut squash into quarters lengthwise and remove the seeds. Using a vegetable peeler, peel the skin. Slice the squash lengthwise into $\frac{1}{2}$-inch-thick slices. Lightly brush with olive oil. Grill directly over the fire for about 4 to 5 minutes per side, turning once, until the squash is just fork tender with good grill marks. Cut the grilled squash into 1-inch bite size pieces.

Place the cheese in the middle of the plank and surround it with the squash. Set on the indirect side of the grill and close the lid. Let it cook for 10 minutes.

In the meantime, stack the 4 sage leaves on top of each other and roll into a cigar shape. Thinly slice the sage. This method is called chiffonade.

After the plank has cooked for 10 minutes, open the grill lid and quickly sprinkle the sage over the squash and cheese. Lightly drizzle all with olive oil and sprinkle with salt and white pepper. Close the lid and let cook for another 10 minutes.

Remove from the grill and serve the planked squash and cheese with a basket of crackers and bread.

S TRIPS OF GRILLED POBLANO PEPPERS AND ONIONS ARE KNOWN as *rajas* or rags. They are a delicious accompaniment to beef dishes of all kinds, as well as filling for corn tacos, as here, as well as sandwiches, burritos, tacos, enchiladas, or quesadillas.

SOFT CORN TORTILLAS
with RAJAS *and* QUESO

MAKES 8 TACOS

RAJAS

4 fresh poblano chiles

Olive oil, for brushing

2 large yellow onions, peeled and cut into ½-inch slices

Kosher or sea salt and freshly ground black pepper to taste

2 cups shredded Monterey Jack cheese (for topping)

SOFT CORN TORTILLAS

1 cup instant corn masa flour

⅛ teaspoon salt

⅔ cup warm water, or more if necessary

Prepare a hot fire in your grill.

Brush the poblanos with olive oil and grill, turning often, until the skins blister and burn. Transfer to a sealable plastic bag and let them steam and soften. Brush the onions with olive oil and grill until you have good grill marks on both sides, about 10 minutes total. Remove the stems, skin, and seeds from the poblanos, and then slice into thin strips. Cut the onion slices in half and break apart with a fork into strands. Combine the poblanos and onions and season to taste. Keep the rajas warm until serving.

To make the tortillas, place the masa flour and salt in a bowl. Stir in the water to make soft dough, adding a little more water if necessary. Divide the dough into 8 portions, forming each portion into a ball. Cover with a damp cloth to deep the dough moist. Place each ball of dough between two unopened plastic sandwich bags, then press to a 5- to 6-inch round in a tortilla press. Preheat an ungreased skillet over medium-high heat. Cook each tortilla for 1 minute on each side until golden in spots. Cover with a damp tea towel until ready to serve.

To serve, divide the rajas evenly between the 8 tortillas and sprinkle ¼ cup cheese on each taco.

WHEN YOUR FRESH ASPARAGUS COMES IN, IT'S A RACE TO harvest the spears every day or so before they get too thick and woody. This is a great dish to showcase your bounty. Like a conga line of sarong-wrapped lovelies, this appetizer sizzles and shimmies on even the plainest of white platters. It's easiest to grill these ganged onto double skewers, turning once, and then finish the dish with a splash of balsamic vinegar.

PROSCIUTTO-WRAPPED
ASPARAGUS SPEARS

MAKES 6 TO 8 SERVINGS

2 pounds fresh asparagus, ends trimmed

4 ounces prosciutto, cut lengthwise into 2-inch strips

Olive oil, for drizzling

Fig balsamic vinegar, for drizzling

Shaved Parmesan cheese, for garnish

Prepare a medium-hot fire in your grill.

Wrap each asparagus spear with a slice of prosciutto. Drizzle the spears with olive oil to lightly coat.

Place the spears perpendicular to the grill rack. Grill until the asparagus is crisp-tender and the prosciutto has blistered, turning often, 8 to 10 minutes. Set the asparagus on a serving platter and splash on the fig balsamic vinegar to taste. Sprinkle with the shaved Parmesan. Serve hot or at room temperature.

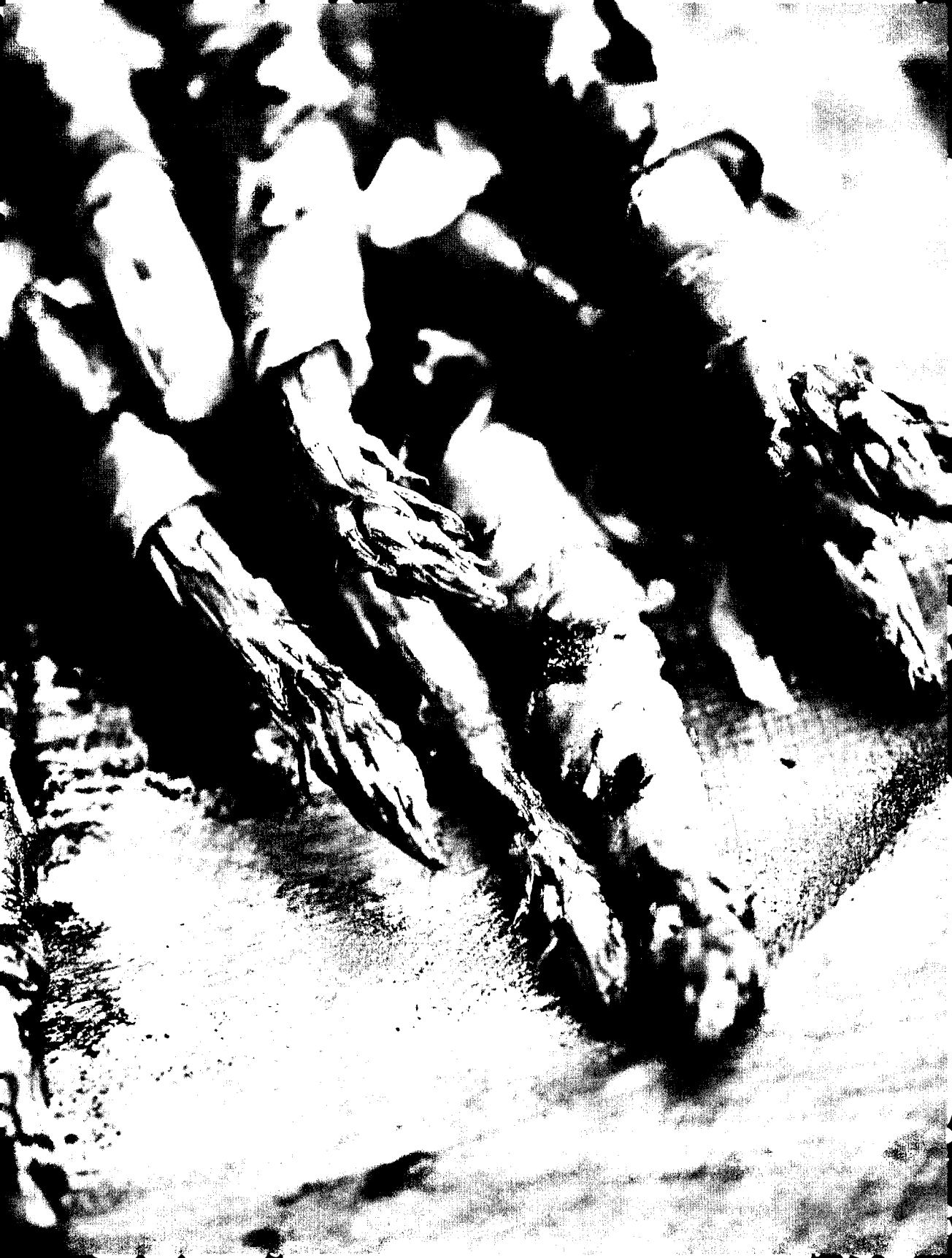

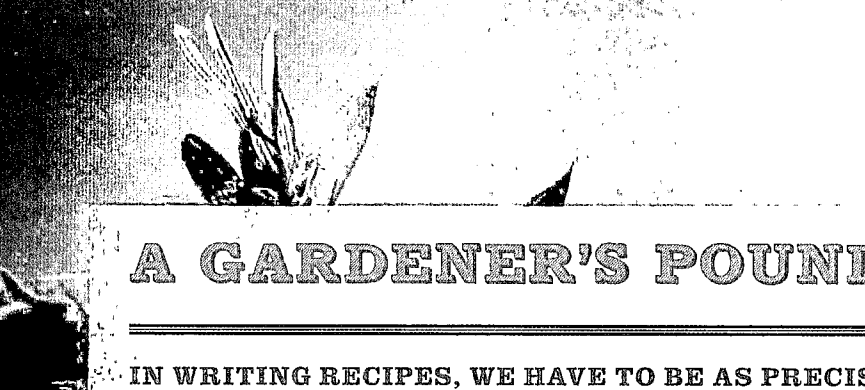

A GARDENER'S POUND

IN WRITING RECIPES, WE HAVE TO BE AS PRECISE AS WE CAN BE, so we call for quantities of asparagus or greens in recipes in weight measurements. Yet if you're harvesting those vegetables from the garden, how can you gauge a pound without a kitchen scale?

Use the following as guidelines for measuring 1-pound increments:

- **ASPARAGUS STALKS:** about what you can encircle with both hands
- **BEANS OR PEAS IN THE POD:** about 4 cups
- **BROCCOLI:** about 1 large crown
- **CHERRY TOMATOES:** about 2 cups
- **LOOSE, LEAFY GREENS (SPINACH):** about 6 cups or handfuls
- **BUNCH GREENS (SWISS CHARD):** about 2 bunches

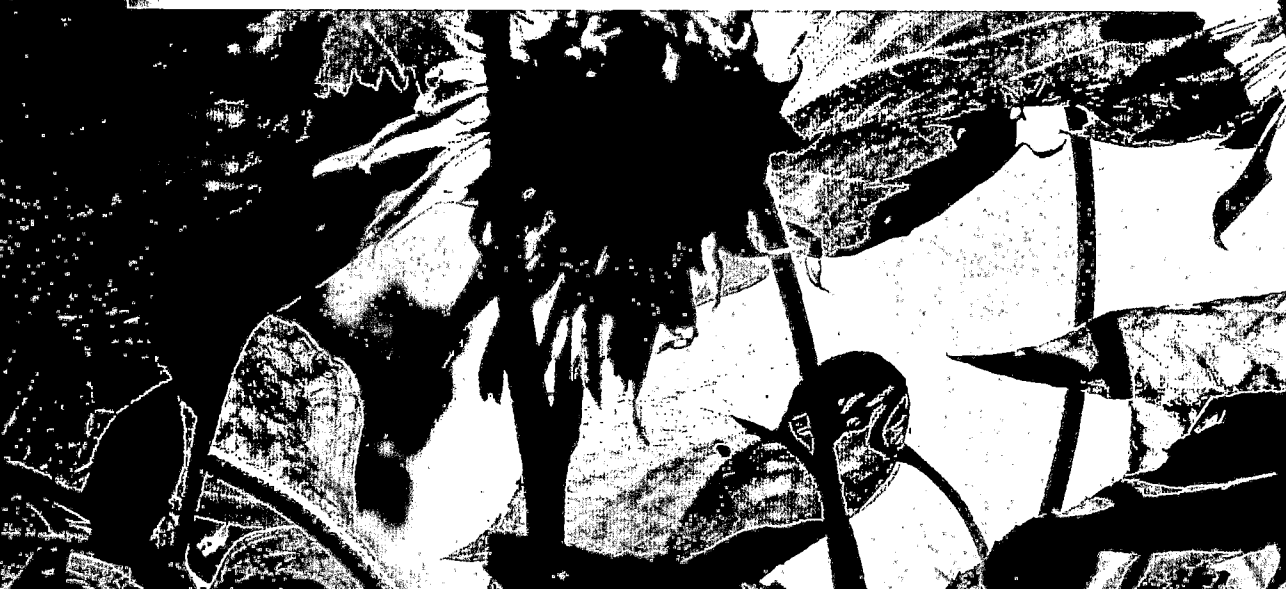

FAVA BEANS ARE A SPRING FAVORITE IN SOUTHERN AND CENTRAL Italy. If you can only find a hard grating pecorino, use Havarti. They are fragrant and delicious as a warm appetizer. Fresh edamame in the pod are also delicious prepared this way.

FIRE-ROASTED FAVA BEANS *in the* POD
with SHEEP'S MILK CHEESE

MAKES 8 SERVINGS

2 pounds fresh unshelled fava beans (about 2 cups shelled beans)

3 tablespoons extra-virgin olive oil

1 tablespoon freshly squeezed lemon juice

1 teaspoon dried leaf oregano

3 tablespoons fresh flat-leaf parsley leaves, snipped with scissors

⅛ teaspoon crushed red peppers (hot red pepper flakes), or to taste

Kosher or sea salt and freshly ground black pepper to taste

8 ounces sliceable sheep's milk cheese such as a pecorino or cow's milk Havarti, cut in small cubes

In a medium bowl, combine all ingredients except the cheese, and toss to blend. Let sit at room temperature for about 15 minutes.

Prepare a hot fire in your grill.

Drain the marinade from the beans and reserve it. Place the beans perpendicular to the grill grates. You may use a grill rack if you like. Grill for about 4 to 5 minutes on each side until blistered. Test for doneness be opening one of the pods. The fava beans should be smooth and creamy when you pop them out of their skins. Set them on a platter and season with salt and pepper. Scatter the cubes of cheese over the beans. Drizzle with the reserved marinade and enjoy.

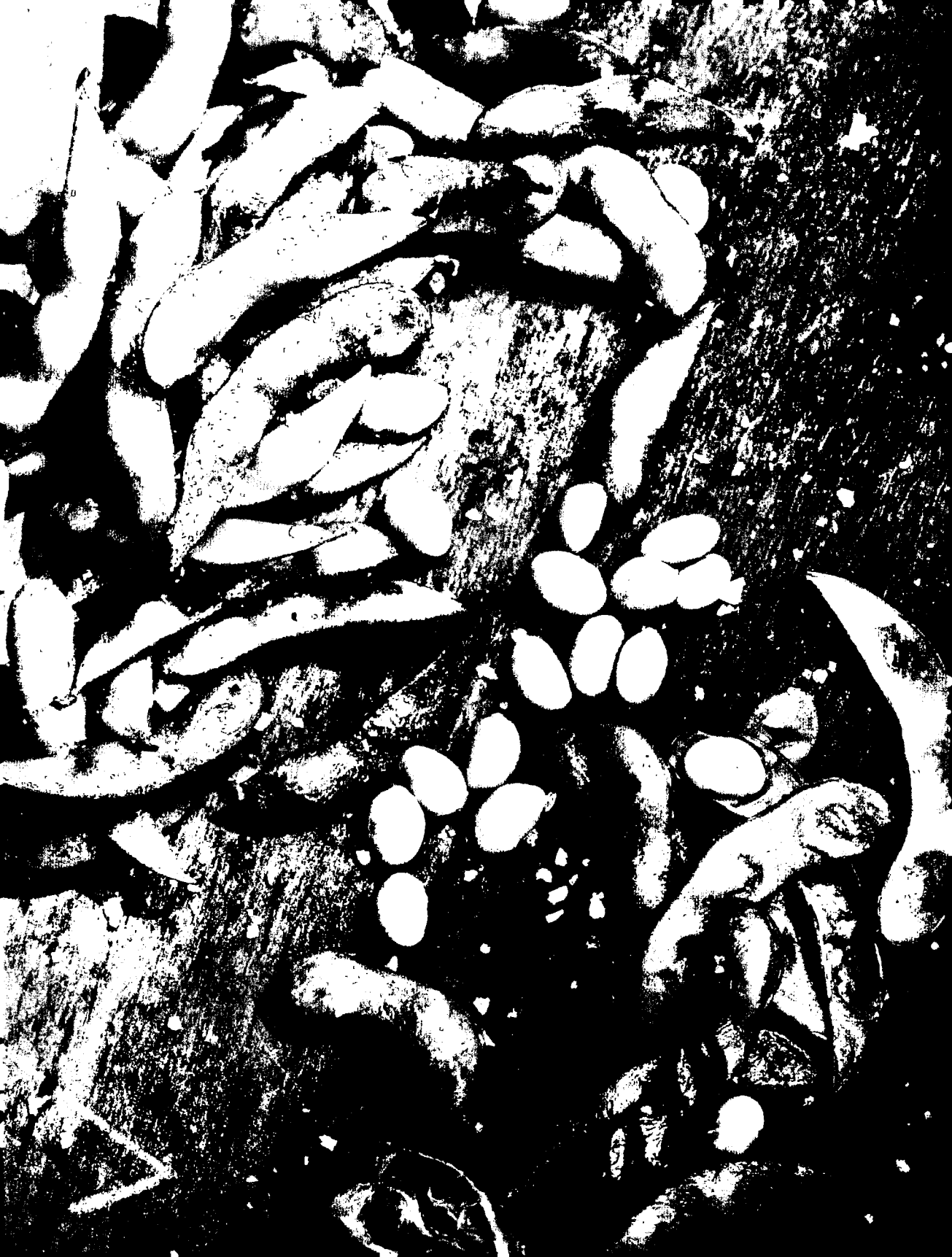

EDAMAME MEANT FOR FRESH EATING CAN BE GRILLED RIGHT in the pod. Serve them on a platter with a small dish of flaked salt.

GRILL-ROASTED EDAMAME in the POD

MAKES 2 TO 4 SERVINGS

1 pound fresh edamame in the pod

1 tablespoon vegetable oil

2 teaspoons toasted sesame oil

Flaked salt for serving

Preheat a grill to medium-high. In a large bowl, toss the edamame pods with the oils. Place them on a perforated grill rack or in a disposable aluminum pan. Arrange them in a single layer on a grill over medium-high heat. Grill-roast (page 8), covered, 4 to 5 minutes, then flip, cover and grill for a few minutes more or until the pods are crisp-tender when pierced with a knife. If you aren't sure when to pull them off, take a pod off the grill, open and taste one of the beans to see if it's ready. To eat, tear open the pods and dip the beans into flaked salt.

GROWING EDAMAME

Although tomatoes, corn, and bell peppers have been gardeners' favorites for generations, edamame or soybeans are quickly claiming their spot. Edamame is the Japanese name for soybeans eaten fresh, rather than dried. You plant them just as you do green beans. After danger of frost, plant the seeds in full sun about 1 inch deep and 2 inches apart. We like to plant them in large pots around a centered wire frame or trellis so the bean stalks can easily be trained upwards as they grow. A cool weather crop like peas, they taste best in the pod in spring or fall. There are about 3 soybeans in each pod; pick them when the soybeans within the pod are young and tender, about $1/2$ inch long.

WHEN YOU HAVE GRILL-ROASTED RED BELL PEPPERS ON HAND (See Grill-Roasting Peppers (page 43) or The Gardener's Grill Pantry (page 28), you can make the flavorful Spanish-style Romesco sauce, which tastes best when made a day or two ahead so the flavors blend together. Then when you grill the fingerlings, you've got a quick and delicious appetizer. If you like, grill fresh fish fillets at the same time, and you have a whole meal.

FLAME-LICKED FINGERLINGS
with ROMESCO SAUCE

MAKES 8 SERVINGS

2 pounds fingerling
  potatoes

Olive oil, for drizzling

Kosher salt and freshly
  ground pepper to taste

1 recipe Romesco Sauce
  (page 42)

Prepare a hot fire in your grill.

Drizzle the fingerling potatoes with olive oil and season with salt and pepper.

Grill the fingerlings in a perforated grill basket or an aluminum pan with holes in it. Place over the hot fire and close the grill lid. After about 3 or 4 minutes, open the grill and toss the potatoes. Close the lid again and repeat the tossing in about another 3 or 4 minutes. Cook until the potatoes are tender when pierced with a fork.

Serve the grilled fingerlings on a platter with a bowl of the Romesco sauce set in the middle for dipping.

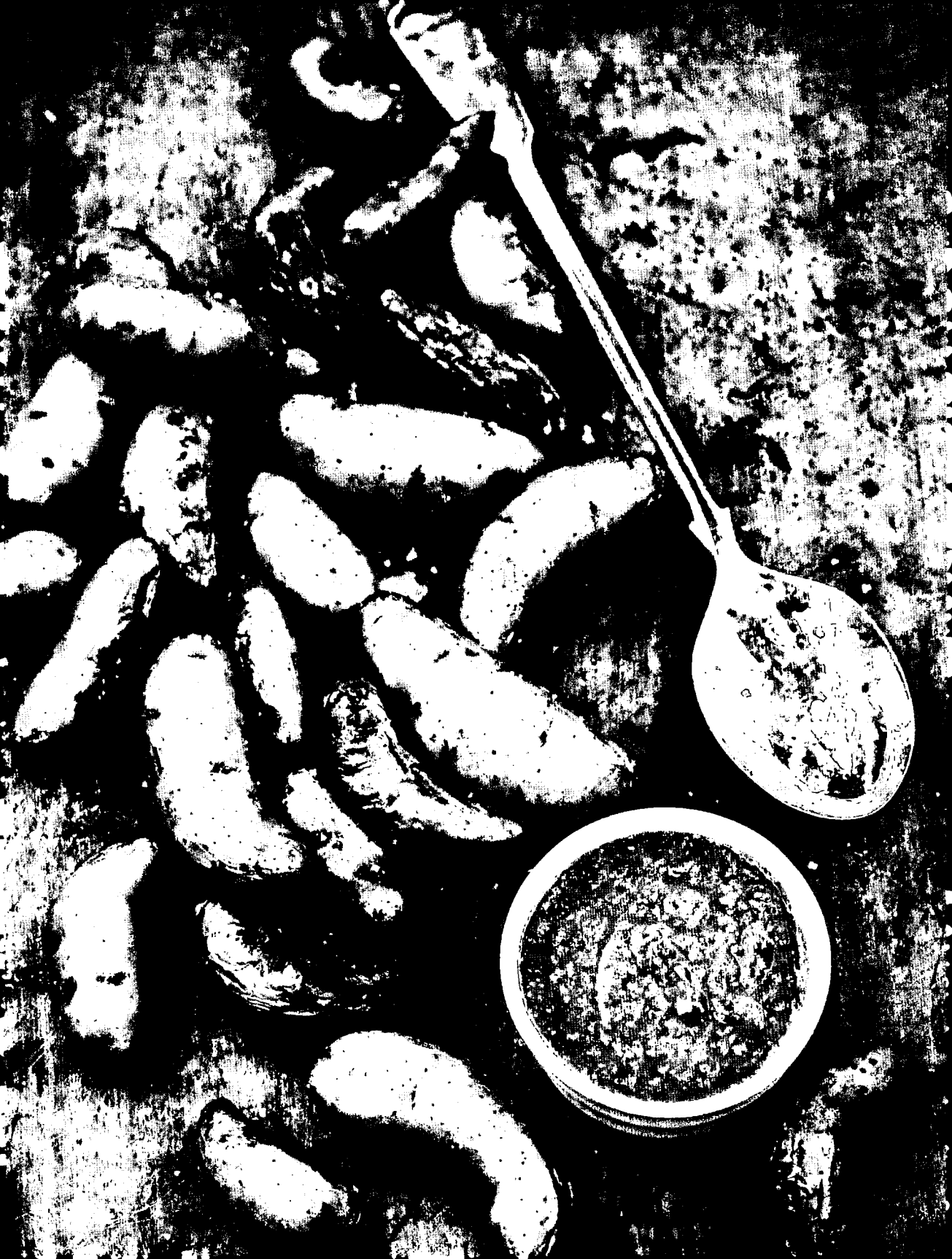

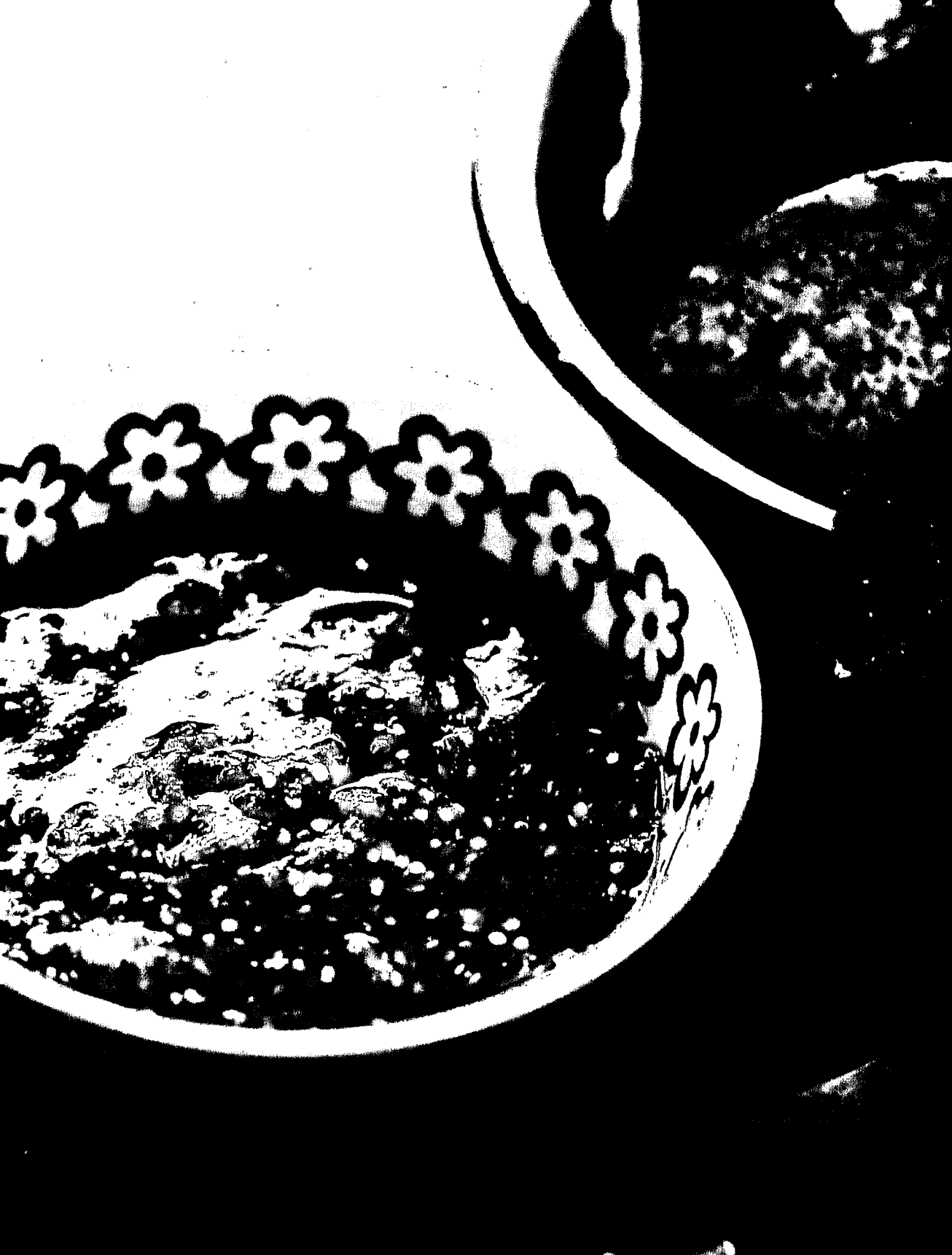

IF YOU CAN GROW TOMATOES, YOU CAN GROW THEIR SMALLER, green cousins, tomatillos. Sharp and citrus-tasting, tomatillos are most often used to make a fresh salsa usually served with chips or chicken, pork, and fish. Tomatillos have papery husks that enclose the small fruits; remove the husks before using.

GRILL-ROASTED TOMATILLO SALSA

MAKES ABOUT 2 CUPS

Vegetable oil, as needed

1½ pounds fresh tomatillos

½ cup freshly chopped cilantro

1 jalapeño pepper, stemmed and seeded

⅓ cup fresh lime juice

Kosher or sea salt to taste

Prepare a medium-hot fire in your grill. Oil a perforated grill rack and place on the grill grates.

Remove the husks from the tomatillos and discard. Arrange the tomatillos on the perforated grill rack in a single layer. Cover and grill-roast (see page 8), turning once until lightly browned, about 20 minutes. Let cool.

In a blender or food processor, place the cooled tomatillos, cilantro, jalapeño, and lime juice. Process until somewhat smooth. Add salt to taste. Will keep, covered, in the refrigerator for up to 3 days.

WE LOVE THIS SAUCE ON GRILLED FISH AND POULTRY. JARS OF roasted red peppers from the grocery store are good fallback as a high-flavor convenience food when the garden crop runs out.

FIRE-ROASTED PEPPER DIP

MAKES ABOUT 2 CUPS

2 large red bell peppers or one 12-ounce jar roasted red peppers, drained

3 tablespoons olive oil, plus more for brushing

½ cup finely chopped pitted kalamata or niçoise olives

½ cup fresh lemon juice (3 to 4 lemons)

2 tablespoons balsamic vinegar

2 teaspoons capers, drained

2 teaspoons anchovy paste

Fine kosher or sea salt and freshly ground black pepper to taste

Prepare a hot fire in your grill.

Brush the peppers with olive oil, and grill them, turning with tongs, on all sides until charred. Remove the peppers from the grill and place them in a paper bag to steam. When the peppers are cool enough to handle, transfer to a cutting board. Remove the papery skin and slice lengthwise. Remove the stem and seeds and discard.

Combine the red peppers, olives, lemon juice, vinegar, capers, and anchovy paste in a food processor and process until fairly smooth. With the machine running, drizzle the olive oil through the feed tube in a steady stream until the sauce solidifies. Season with salt and pepper. Use immediately or spoon into a medium-size jar with a tight-fitting lid. This sauce will keep in the refrigerator for up to 3 days or in the freezer for up to 6 months.

AS A TAPAS- OR MEZE-STYLE APPETIZER WITH GRILLED BREAD or as a side dish, this dish makes the most of two vegetables that can be bland if cooked another way. Before you go out to the grill, make the filling. If you like, add a dipping sauce of your favorite garlicky vinaigrette. All you need with this is a loaf of good, crusty bread. Yum!

GRILLED ZUCCHINI and YELLOW SQUASH STACKS with FETA AND BLACK OLIVES

MAKES 4 SERVINGS

FETA-OLIVE-LEMON FILLING

1 cup (8 ounces) crumbled feta cheese

1 tablespoon olive oil

1 clove garlic, minced

$\frac{1}{2}$ cup finely chopped pitted kalamata or niçoise olives

2 tablespoons finely chopped green onions (white part with some of the green)

1 teaspoon grated lemon zest

ZUCCHINI AND SQUASH STACKS

1 large Japanese eggplant, ends trimmed and sliced lengthwise into $\frac{1}{2}$-inch-thick strips

1 medium-size zucchini, ends trimmed and sliced lengthwise into $\frac{1}{2}$-inch-thick strips

1 medium-size yellow summer squash, ends trimmed and sliced lengthwise into $\frac{1}{2}$-inch-thick strips

Olive oil, for brushing

Fine kosher or sea salt and freshly ground black pepper to taste

Prepare a hot fire in your grill.

Combine the filling ingredients in a bowl until well blended. Set aside. Brush the eggplant, zucchini, and yellow summer squash slices with olive oil and season with salt and pepper to taste. Place on a baking sheet to transfer to the grill.

Grill the vegetable slices for 3 to 4 minutes on one side, or until they have good grill marks

While the slices are still warm from the grill, spread each eggplant slice with some of the feta filling, top with a yellow squash slice, spread with more filling, then top with a zucchini slice to create a stack. Cut each stack into 1-inch pieces, spear with a toothpick, and arrange on a platter. Serve warm or at room temperature.

DAPTED FROM A RECIPE BY ARDIE DAVIS, KNOWN IN BARBECUE circles as Remus Powers, Ph.B., these little bites are addictive. This technique works for smaller peppers of all kinds, so make this recipe when you have plenty in the garden. You can use a special metal chile pepper rack or simply reuse a cardboard egg carton to hold the peppers upright as they smoke. While your poppers are smoking, get some weeding or watering done.

MESQUITE-SMOKED JALAPEÑO POPPERS

MAKES 12

½ cup mesquite wood chips

1 (8-ounce) package cream cheese, softened

½ cup shredded sharp cheddar cheese

12 large jalapeño or other mildly hot chile peppers (red or green), cored and seeded (about 1½ pounds)

6 thin slices smoked bacon, cut in half (twelve 4-inches pieces)

Prepare a medium-hot fire on one side of your grill for indirect cooking. If you have a charcoal grill, soak the wood chips in water for 30 minutes before smoking; if you have a gas grill, place dry wood chips in your grill's metal smoker box or fashion an aluminum foil packet, enclose the dry chips, and poke holes in the top of the foil.

Combine the cream cheese and cheddar until well blended. Stuff the peppers with this mixture. Wrap a half slice of bacon over the top of each stuffed jalapeño and secure with a toothpick. Place the stuffed and wrapped peppers in an egg carton or metal popper rack.

When ready to grill, drain then scatter the soaked wood chips on the charcoal fire, replace the grill rack, and place the peppers on the indirect (or no-fire) side. For a gas grill, place the packet of dry wood chips in the back of a gas grill over direct heat; place the peppers on the indirect (or no-fire) side. Close the lid and smoke for 1 hour and 15 minutes or until the bacon has crisped and the peppers have a burnished appearance and a smoky aroma.

RAINBOW SWISS CHARD IS ONE OF THE MOST BEAUTIFUL VEG-etables to grow in your garden, chock-full of great vitamins and minerals. This recipe works well with other cheeses, too, like Monterey Jack, Gouda, or even cheddar.

CHARD-WRAPPED
GOAT CHEESE *on the* GRILL

MAKES 8 SERVINGS

8 large chard leaves, stem end trimmed

8 ounces goat cheese

8 teaspoons walnut pieces, toasted

8 thin slices prosciutto

Kosher salt and freshly ground black pepper to taste

Balsamic vinegar for drizzling

Lay the leaves on your work counter, ribbed side up. On each leaf, place 1 ounce of goat cheese topped with 1 teaspoon of toasted walnuts. Fold the stem end up over the cheese. Then fold the sides of the leaves towards the middle. Continue to roll the packet up like a burrito. Wrap with prosciutto and secure with toothpicks. The leaf packets can be done a day ahead before grilling.

Prepare a hot fire in your grill.

Place the chard packets on the hot fire. Grill for about 4 to 6 minutes per side, until browned with good grill marks.

Place the chard packets on a platter and season with salt and pepper and drizzle with balsamic vinegar. Serve immediately.

GRILL THE VEGETABLES FIRST, THEN BRING THEM INSIDE AND make the polenta so it's thick and creamy when you serve them all together. With a glass of red wine, this is Tuscan comfort food. If you can't find polenta, you can substitute corn grits; most grocery stores carry the Bob's Red Mill brand.

TUSCAN POLENTA PLATTER
with SIZZLING PEPPERS, ONIONS, and MUSHROOMS

MAKES 4 SERVINGS

3 tablespoons olive oil

1 garlic clove, minced

2 large onions, peeled and cut into 1-inch thick slices

2 red or yellow bell peppers

2 green bell peppers

4 large portabello mushrooms (about 8 ounces), stemmed

Kosher or sea salt and freshly ground black pepper to taste

¼ cup chopped Italian parsley

ASIAGO POLENTA

6 cups vegetable or chicken stock

1 cup quick cooking polenta or cornmeal

1 cup freshly grated Asiago cheese (about 6 ounces)

Fine kosher or sea salt and freshly ground black pepper to taste

Prepare a hot fire in your grill.

In a small bowl, combine the olive oil and garlic, Brush all the vegetables with some of the garlic olive oil; reserve the rest. Grill, turning occasionally, until the onions and mushrooms have good grill marks and the peppers are charred on all sides. Bring inside to a cutting board. Stem, peel, and seed the peppers. Coarsely chop all the vegetables and season with salt and pepper; keep warm.

To make the polenta, in a large pot over medium-high heat, bring the stock to a boil. Sprinkle in the polenta in a steady stream, whisking constantly. Continue cooking and whisking for 5 minutes. When the polenta has bubbled into a thick mass, whisk in the Asiago cheese. Season with salt and black pepper to taste. To serve, spoon the polenta onto each plate, top with the grilled vegetables, drizzle with the remaining garlic oil, and sprinkle with Italian parsley.

THIS SUPER-EASY ENTRÉE COULD MAKE FLEXITARIANS (PEOPLE who eat both vegetarian and meat/fish/poultry diets) out of the most die-hard meat eaters. It's robust, colorful, and healthy. (But don't let that put you off!). Lacinato kale (also known as dinosaur kale) has long, thin, more tender leaves ideal for this recipe.

GRILLED POLENTA *with* STIR-GRILLED GARLIC GREENS

MAKES 4 SERVINGS

One 16-ounce package prepared polenta, cut into ½-inch-thick slices

3 tablespoons olive oil, plus more for brushing

2 garlic cloves, minced

¼ teaspoon red pepper flakes

2 bunches Lacinato kale or Swiss chard, tough stems removed and torn into 3-inch pieces

Fine kosher or sea salt and freshly ground black pepper to taste

7 ounces goat cheese

Prepare a medium-hot fire in your grill.

Brush the polenta slices with olive oil and place on a baking sheet. In a small bowl, combine the olive oil, garlic, and red pepper flakes. Place the greens in a large bowl and drizzle with the olive oil mixture. Toss to coat, and then season with salt and pepper to taste. Place the greens in a perforated grill wok for stir-grilling (see page 9).

Place the grill wok on the grill grates and toss the greens with wooden paddles or grill spatulas until they are wilted and slightly browned. Remove from the grill and set aside. Place the polenta slices on the grill grates and grill for 2 to 3 minutes per side, turning once, or until you get good grill marks. Spread the cheese over each warm polenta slice and top with the wilted greens.

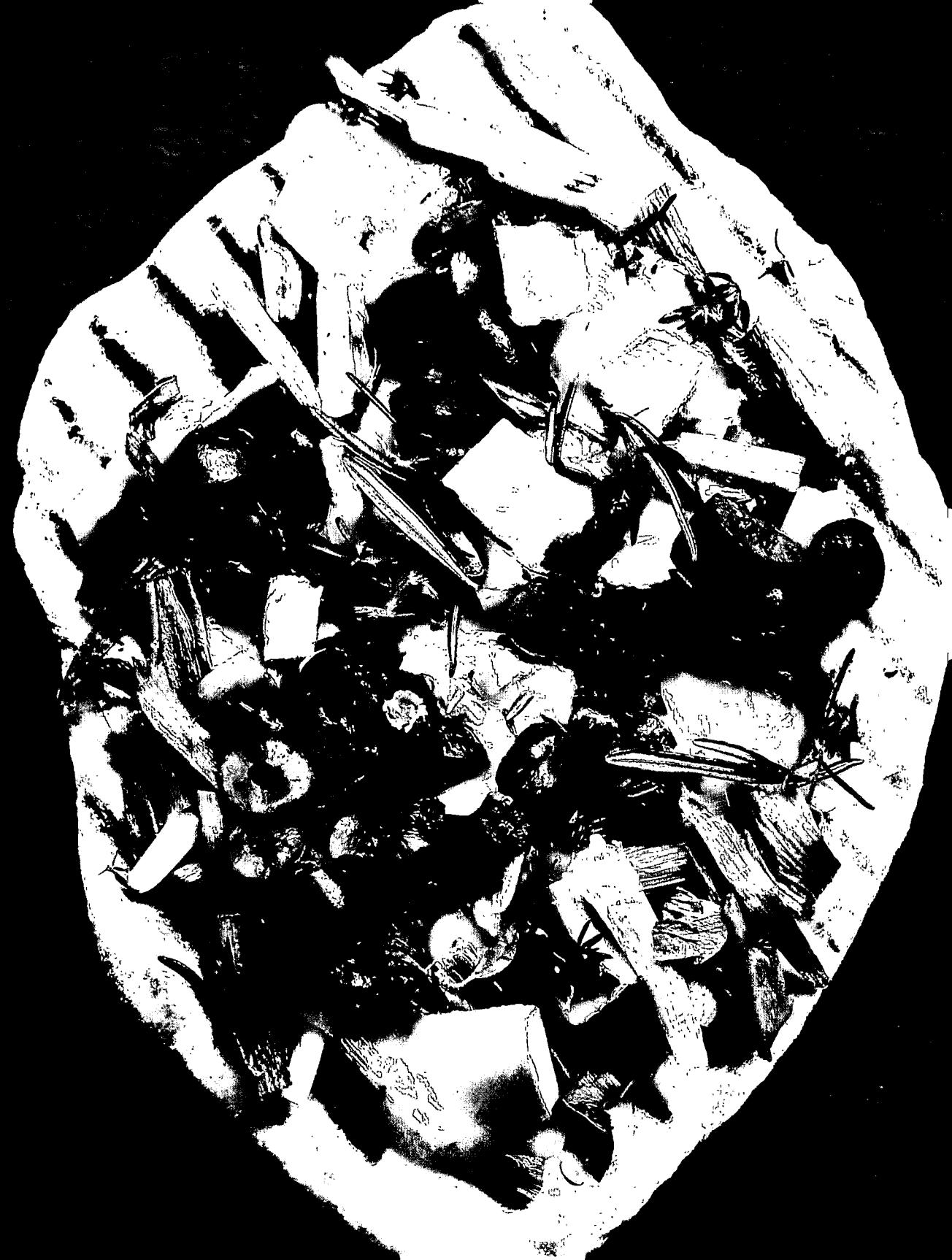

CHAPTER 3:

SANDWICHES, FLATBREADS & PIZZAS

SANDWICHES, FLATBREADS, AND PIZZAS ARE A GARDENER AND griller's friend. They make garden goodies go a long way, are easy to make, and universally enjoyed. They appeal to meat lovers, vegetarians, and vegans alike. And they're terrific for entertaining. Grill individual pizzas, flatbreads, or sandwiches and let guests choose their own toppings or fillings.

To grill a sandwich, pizza, or flatbread, you have to start with a base.

For sandwiches, that's usually a sturdy bread of some sort, such as French baguettes, Italian bread, ciabatta, or hard-crust rolls. But you can also get creative with Grilled Green Tomato "Sandwiches" with Herbed Cream Cheese (page 82) or open-face Grilled Pepper Boat "Sandwiches" (page 84) with a garden-inspired filling. For an added punch of flavor, spread the sandwich bread with one of our Quick-To-Fix Aiolis (page 40) or a flavorful compound butter from Butter Up! (page 30).

For flatbreads, you can use store-bought pita breads and pizza dough, or make your own easy Stir-Together Flatbread and Pizza Dough (page 94). Flatbreads cook on the grill much like pancakes—when the bubbles start to rise through the dough, it's time to turn them on the grill. You can roll out ovals of dough for flatbreads, then fold them over a garden filling—try Herb-Stuffed Afghan Flatbread (page 96), which is traditionally served with grilled, skewered foods like beef, lamb, or vegetables.

Although sandwiches can be thick, enclosed with aluminum foil, and grilled until warmed through, flatbreads and pizzas need to be thin to cook thoroughly on the grill. That means no deep dish, no heavy toppings. Yet you get just as much flavor with a lighter toppings and the sizzle of the grill.

As an added interest, you can replicate what upscale pizzerias do and serve each hot-off-the-grill pizza or flatbread with a frill of fresh greens placed in the center.

We find that it's easiest to put everything on large baking sheets and take it out to the grill at once—a griller's *mise en place*. That way, you can grill a topping, chop on the baking sheet, and grill the flatbreads without running back and forth into the house.

Grilled Garden Loaf ...81

Grilled Green Tomato "Sandwiches" with Herbed Cream Cheese ...82

Grilled Pepper Boat "Sandwiches" ...84

Panini Caprese ...85

Grilled Chicken Ciabatta with Romesco and Baby Greens ...86

Wood-Grilled Burger with Chive Pesto, Grilled
Fresh Tomatoes, and Provolone ...88

Stir-Grilled Italian Sausage, Peppers, and Onion Hoagies ...89

Blackened Fish Po' Boy with Grilled Green Onion Mayonnaise ...90

Grilled Pita Bread with Grilled Baba Ganoush ...92

Make it Meze ...94

Stir-Together Flatbread and Pizza Dough ...94

How to Grill Flatbreads and Pizzas ...95

Herb-Stuffed Afghan Flatbread ...96

Poppy Seed Naan ...97

Gardening and Grilling with an Italian Accent ...98

Pizza Primavera ...99

Wood-Grilled Spring Onion, Brie, and Kalamata Olive Pizza ...100

Kale, Potato, and Chorizo Pizza ...102

Char-Grilled Baby Summer Squash Pizza ...104

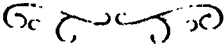

THIS EASY SANDWICH MAKES FOR A GREAT CASUAL MEAL—AND it's even easier if you have grilled red bell peppers, zucchini, or yellow squash (see The Gardener's Grill Pantry, page 28) in your refrigerator or freezer. Feel free to substitute herbed cream cheese for goat cheese, other types of tomatoes or peppers, or fresh cucumber slices for the grilled zucchini or yellow summer squash. This recipe is a blueprint for using what's fresh in your garden.

GRILLED GARDEN LOAF

SERVES 4 TO 6

Olive oil, for brushing

1 large red bell pepper

2 small zucchini or yellow summer squash, trimmed and cut lengthwise into 1-inch-thick slices

Salt and freshly ground black pepper to taste

1 large loaf fresh Italian or French bread

3 tablespoons Chive or Basil Pesto (page 32) or prepared pesto, or more to taste

9 ounces soft goat cheese

3 large tomatoes (about 1 pound), cored and thinly sliced

½ cup pitted and sliced black olives, such as kalamata

½ cup chopped jarred marinated artichoke hearts

Prepare a medium-hot fire in your grill.

Brush the red bell pepper and zucchini strips with olive oil and season with salt and pepper. Grill on both sides until the vegetables have good grill marks. Stem and seed the pepper. Chop the vegetables into 1-inch pieces.

Cut the Italian bread in half lengthwise and turn the top half over so that the crust side is on the counter. With your fingers or a fork, hollow out about one-third of the top half of the bread and discard or reserve for another use. Brush the bottom half with more olive oil, then spread the pesto and goat cheese on it. Layer on the grilled vegetables, tomatoes, olives, and artichoke hearts. Season with pepper to taste. Brush the hollowed top half of the bread with olive oil and place on top of the sandwich fillings. Wrap well in heavy foil.

Grill the sandwich, covered, turning once, until heated through, 20 to 25 minutes. Cut into quarters and serve warm or at room temperature.

IF YOU LIKE FRIED GREEN TOMATOES, YOU'LL LOVE THEM GRILLED. There is no breading and very little oil, but plenty of tangy flavor. You can make the sandwiches by spreading the creamy filling between two grilled tomato slices or you can serve a platter of the grilled tomatoes with grilled bread and the Herbed Cream Cheese on the side.

GRILLED GREEN TOMATO "SANDWICHES" with HERBED CREAM CHEESE

SERVES 6

HERBED CREAM CHEESE

One (8-ounce) package cream cheese, at room temperature

1 garlic clove, minced

2 tablespoons chopped fresh basil

1 tablespoon snipped fresh chives

TOMATOES

4 large green tomatoes (about 1½ pounds), sliced ¾-inch thick (to make 12 slices)

Olive oil, for brushing

2 teaspoons Seasoning Salt (page 13) or kosher salt

Ground black pepper

Prepare a medium-hot fire in your grill. Place a well-oiled perforated grill rack over direct heat.

In a bowl, blend the cream cheese, garlic, basil, and chives together until smooth. Set aside.

Brush the tomato slices with olive oil on both sides and season with seasoning salt and pepper. Place the slices on a baking sheet and bring out to the grill with the bowl of Herbed Cream Cheese and a knife for spreading.

Grill all of the tomatoes on one side for about 3 minutes with the lid open, then flip and grill on the other side for 3 minutes more, or until the tomatoes have good grill marks.

Remove the tomato slices from the grill and allow to cool slightly on the baking sheet. Spread Herbed Cream cheese on half of the slices, top with a second slice, and set the sandwiches on a platter. Serve the sandwiches hot, with oozing cream cheese filling.

Variation:

Grill all of the tomato slices as above and top each grilled tomato with a dollop of the cream cheese and serve open-faced.

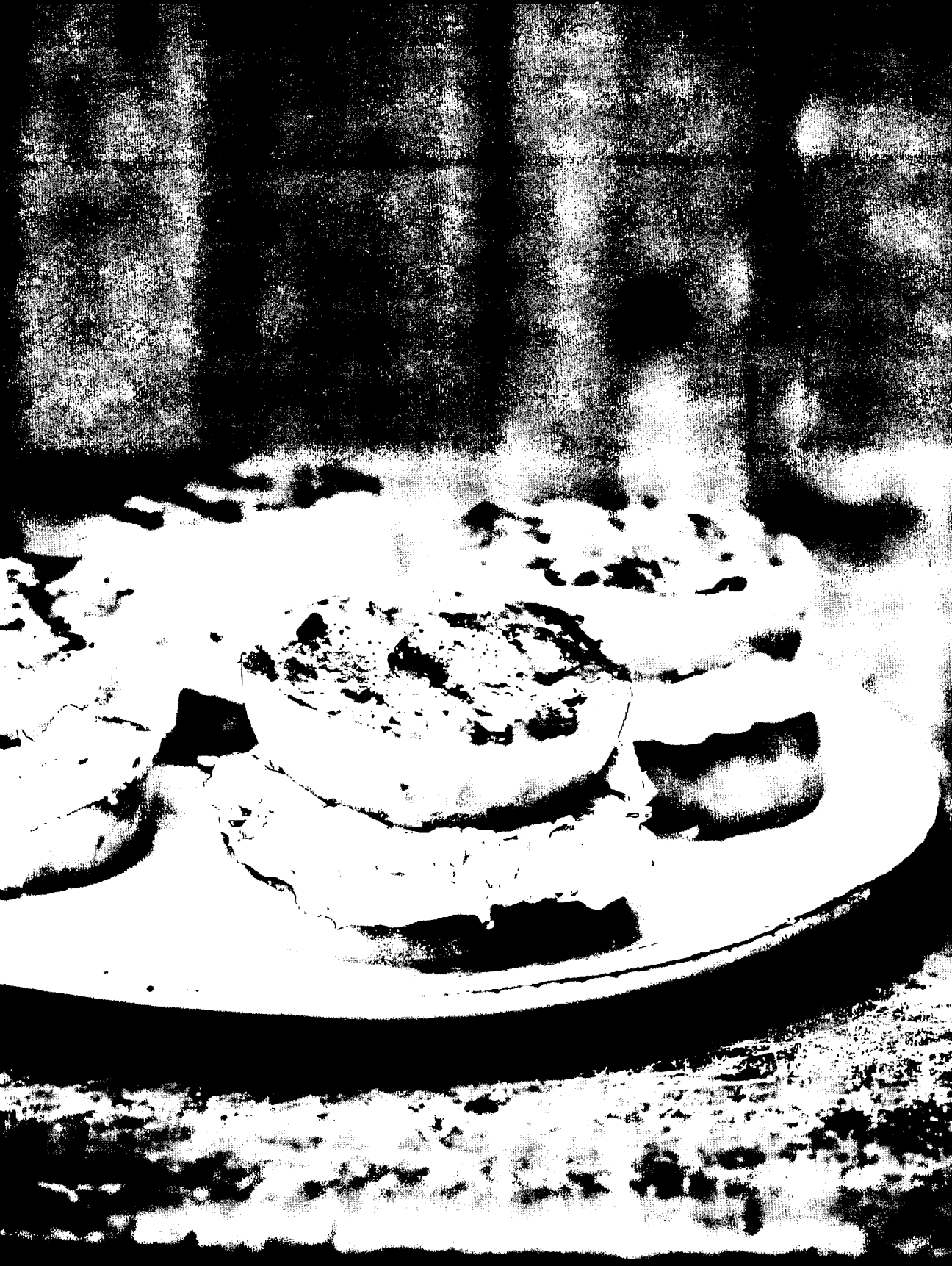

THESE OPEN-FACED, BOAT-SHAPED SANDWICHES—WITH A GRILLED bell pepper as "bread"—are a fresh take on the concept. If your bell peppers are only of a medium size, use 4 and cut them in half instead of quarters.

GRILLED PEPPER BOAT "SANDWICHES"

SERVES 4

2 large yellow, orange, or red bell peppers, stemmed, seeded and quartered

Olive oil, for brushing and drizzling

1 recipe Herbed Cream Cheese (page 82)

½ cup finely chopped fresh yellow, orange, or red tomato

¼ cup chopped Italian parsley

Prepare a medium-hot fire in your grill.

Place a well-oiled perforated grill rack over direct heat.

Brush the skin side of each pepper with olive oil. Dollop a spoonful of Herbed Cream Cheese in each pepper boat. Transfer the boats to the perforated grill rack, cover, and grill until the bottoms are scorched and the cheese has melted, 4 to 5 minutes. Serve sprinkled with tomato and parsley and a drizzle of olive oil. Serve hot with a knife and fork.

HOMEGROWN TOMATOES WITH THE BEST QUALITY MOZZARELLA and fresh-from-the-garden basil combine in the quintessential salad of the summer. They're also wonderful in these on-the-grill pressed sandwiches. To make panini on the grill, simply use aluminum foil-covered bricks to press them down.

PANINI CAPRESE

SERVES 4

8 slices Italian bread, ½-inch-thick

3 large red tomatoes, cut into ½-inch-thick slices

Kosher salt and freshly ground black pepper to taste

1 small red onion, sliced very thinly

8 slices mozzarella cheese

¼ cup large fresh basil leaves

½ cup Basil Pesto (page 32) or prepared pesto

Extra-virgin olive oil, for brushing

Prepare a medium-hot fire in your grill.

Brush each side of bread with the olive oil. Lay 4 slices of bread on a cookie sheet.

For each sandwich, place a layer of tomatoes and season to taste with salt and pepper. Then layer some red onion slices, mozzarella, and basil. Spread the remaining 4 slices of bread with the pesto and lay on top of the sandwich.

Set the sandwiches on the grill over the fire. Wrap bricks in aluminum foil and place one on top of each sandwich to weigh them down. Grill for about 3 or 4 minutes, then turn. Weigh down with the bricks again and cook another 3 to 4 minutes until the bread is a nice golden brown. Cut in half and serve warm.

WE'VE ALL BEEN SUBJECT TO SOME DISAPPOINTING VARIATION on the grilled chicken sandwich. Been there, done that. Here's a fresh take— grilled chicken on wonderful artisan ciabatta bread with a flavorful Spanish Romesco Sauce (made from your own Grill-Roasted Red Bell Peppers, page 43). A *paillard*, or chicken breast pounded thin, only takes minutes to cook on a hot grill. Use a vegetable peeler to shave Manchego or Parmesan for the sandwich.

GRILLED CHICKEN CIABATTA *with* ROMESCO *and* BABY GREENS

SERVES 4

2 loaves ciabatta or 4 cia-battini (ciabatta rolls), sliced in half lengthwise

Olive oil, for brushing

Fine kosher or sea salt and freshly ground black pepper to taste

4 boneless, skinless chicken breasts, pounded to a 1/2-inch thickness

1/2 recipe Romesco Sauce (page 42)

Small wedge (about 4 ounces) of Manchego or Parmesan cheese for shaving

2 cups baby greens

Prepare a hot fire in your grill.

Brush the cut sides of the ciabatta with olive oil. Brush the chicken breasts with olive oil on both sides and season with salt and pepper.

Grill the chicken, turning once, for 5 minutes total. Grill the ciabatta, cut sides down, until it has good grill marks, 1 to 2 minutes.

Slather all the grilled sides of the ciabatta with the Romesco. Place the chicken breasts on the bottom half of the bread, shave some Manchego cheese over the chicken, then top with baby greens and the top half of the bread. If you're using a loaf of ciabatta, you'll have 2 chicken breasts on each loaf, so cut each loaf in half horizontally. If you're using ciabattini, you'll use 1 breast for each roll. Serve immediately.

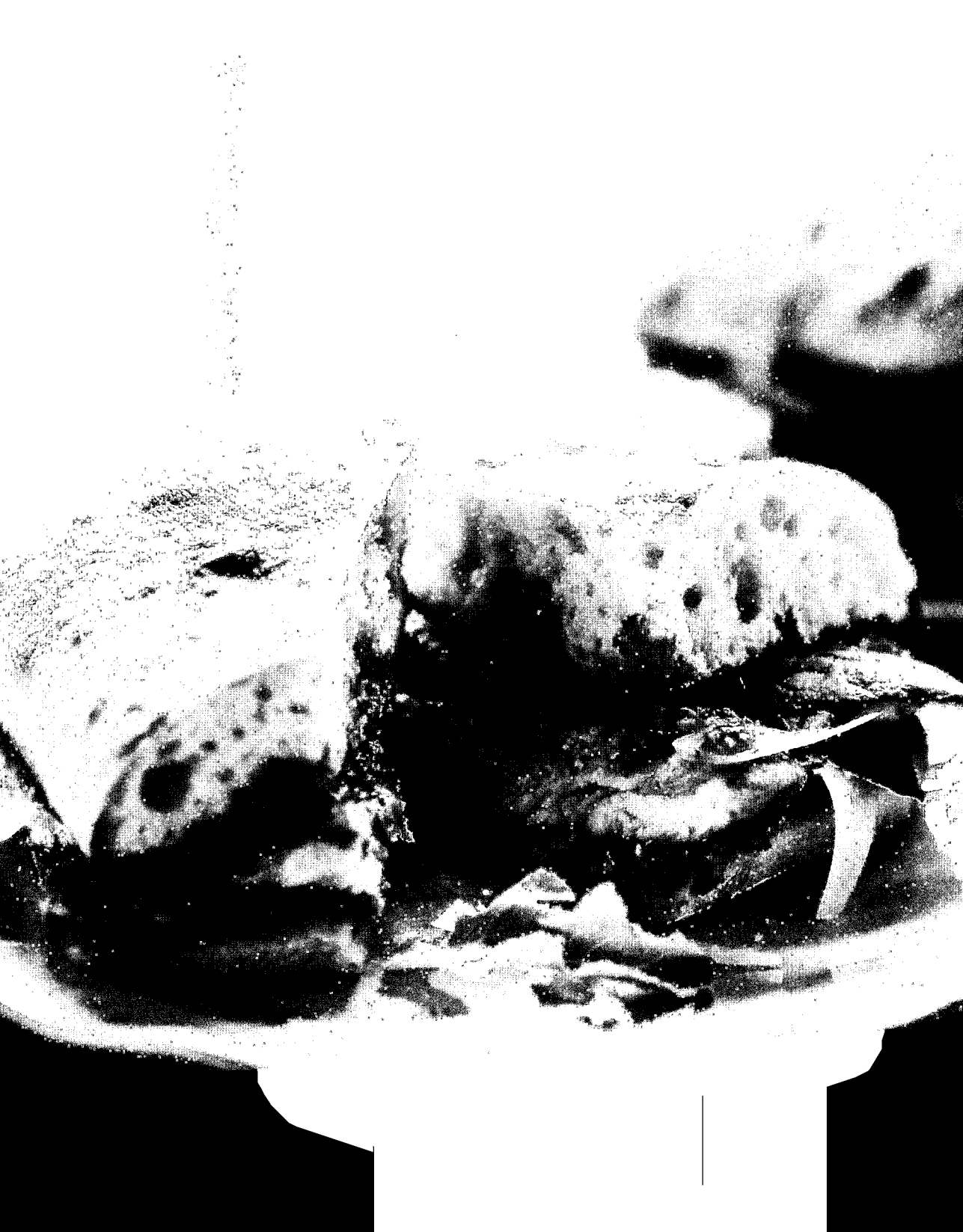

ALL THAT PLANTING, WEEDING, AND WATERING CAN MAKE A gardener hungry. This big juicy burger satisfies that hunger. It gets triple-grill flavor from the grilled burger, the wood smoke, and the grilled sliced tomato, too.

WOOD-GRILLED BURGER
with CHIVE PESTO, GRILLED FRESH TOMATOES, and PROVOLONE

SERVES 4

⅓ cup moistened wood chips or dry wood pellets

2 large, fresh tomatoes, sliced 1-inch thick

Olive oil, for brushing

1 pound ground chuck, formed into four 1-inch-thick patties

Fine kosher or sea salt and freshly ground black pepper to taste

4 slices provolone

4 seeded hamburger buns, kaiser rolls, or ciabattini

1 recipe prepared Garlic Chive Pesto (page 32)

Prepare a hot fire in your grill. Oil a perforated grill rack and place on the grill. If using a charcoal grill, throw moistened wood chips or dry wood pellets directly on the coals right before you want to grill. If using a gas grill, enclose the wood chips or pellets in a foil packet with holes poked in the top; place the packet on the grill grate over the heat source. You're ready to grill when you've seen the smoke from the smoldering wood and the fire is hot.

Brush the tomato slices with olive oil on both sides. Season the patties and tomatoes with salt and pepper.

Grill the tomato slices on the prepared perforated grill rack for 3 to 4 minutes, turning once, or until the tomatoes sizzle and begin to have grill marks. Transfer to a plate.

Grill the burgers directly on the grate, covered, turning once, for 7 minutes total for medium. During the last 2 minutes of grilling, top each burger with a slice of provolone and close the lid.

Slather the cut sides of each bun with Garlic Chive Pesto. Place each burger on the bottom half of a bun and top with the grilled tomato slices. Top with the top portion of the bun and serve immediately.

ITALIAN SAUSAGE IS SO FLAVORFUL THAT A LITTLE CAN GO A long way, as in these hoagies. No matter whether the Italian sausage is pork, turkey, or TVP, you'll get rave reviews.

STIR-GRILLED ITALIAN SAUSAGE, PEPPERS, and ONION HOAGIES

SERVES 4

8 ounces Italian sausage links, cut into 1-inch slices

2 cups bell pepper slices, including red, yellow, or green (about 2 whole peppers)

1 large red onion, cut into 8 wedges

2 tablespoons olive oil

4 Italian hoagie or hard crust rolls, cut in half horizontally

1 cup prepared marinara-style pasta sauce

Prepare a medium-hot fire in your grill. Oil the interior and exterior of a grill wok. In a zipper-top plastic bag, combine the sausage, peppers, and onion. Drizzle with the olive oil and toss to coat.

Place the grill wok on the grill grate over the heat. Dump the contents of the bag into the prepared grill wok and stir-grill (see page 9), tossing with wooden paddles every 2 minutes or so, for 15 minutes, or until the vegetables have browned and softened and the sausage is done. Fill the hoagie rolls with the sausage and vegetables, then drizzle each with marinara sauce. Serve immediately.

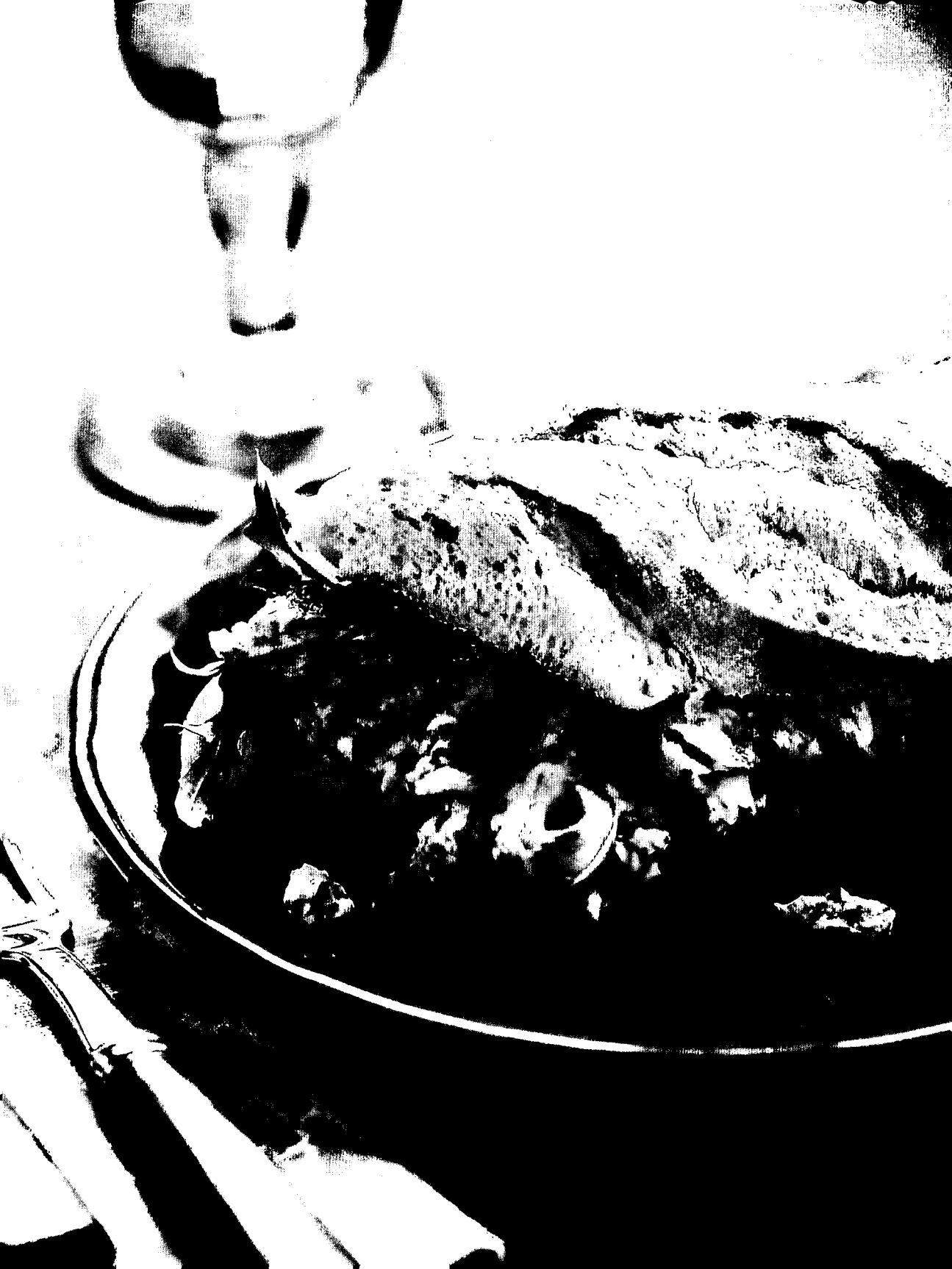

IF YOU'VE NEVER GRILLED FISH BEFORE, FARM-RAISED CATFISH is a great one to get you started. Farm-raised catfish is available year 'round. It's a mildly sweet, firm-textured fish that holds together well on the grill. You can also use halibut, haddock, mahi mahi, or cod. Pick whatever greens you have going in the garden, and you've got a meal in one.

BLACKENED FISH PO' BOY *with* GRILLED GREEN ONION MAYONNAISE

SERVES 4

Four 6- to 8-ounce farm-raised catfish fillets or other medium-textured fish fillets

1 tablespoon olive oil

1 tablespoon Red Hot Blackened Seasoning (page 14)

1 recipe Grilled Green Onion Mayonnaise (page 38)

Four 6-inch baguettes or two longer ones, cut in half lengthwise

2 cups chopped arugula or mesclun greens

Prepare a hot fire in your grill.

Rinse the catfish fillets and pat dry. Brush with olive oil, and sprinkle with the Red Hot Blackened Seasoning.

Grill the catfish for about 3 to 4 minutes on each side, turning once. Transfer the grilled catfish to a flat surface and cut the fish into chunks with a fork. To serve, lightly spread some Grilled Green Onion Mayonnaise on the cut sides of each baguette. Sprinkle $\frac{1}{2}$ cup of the arugula on top of each piece, followed by the fish. Serve immediately with a wedge of lemon.

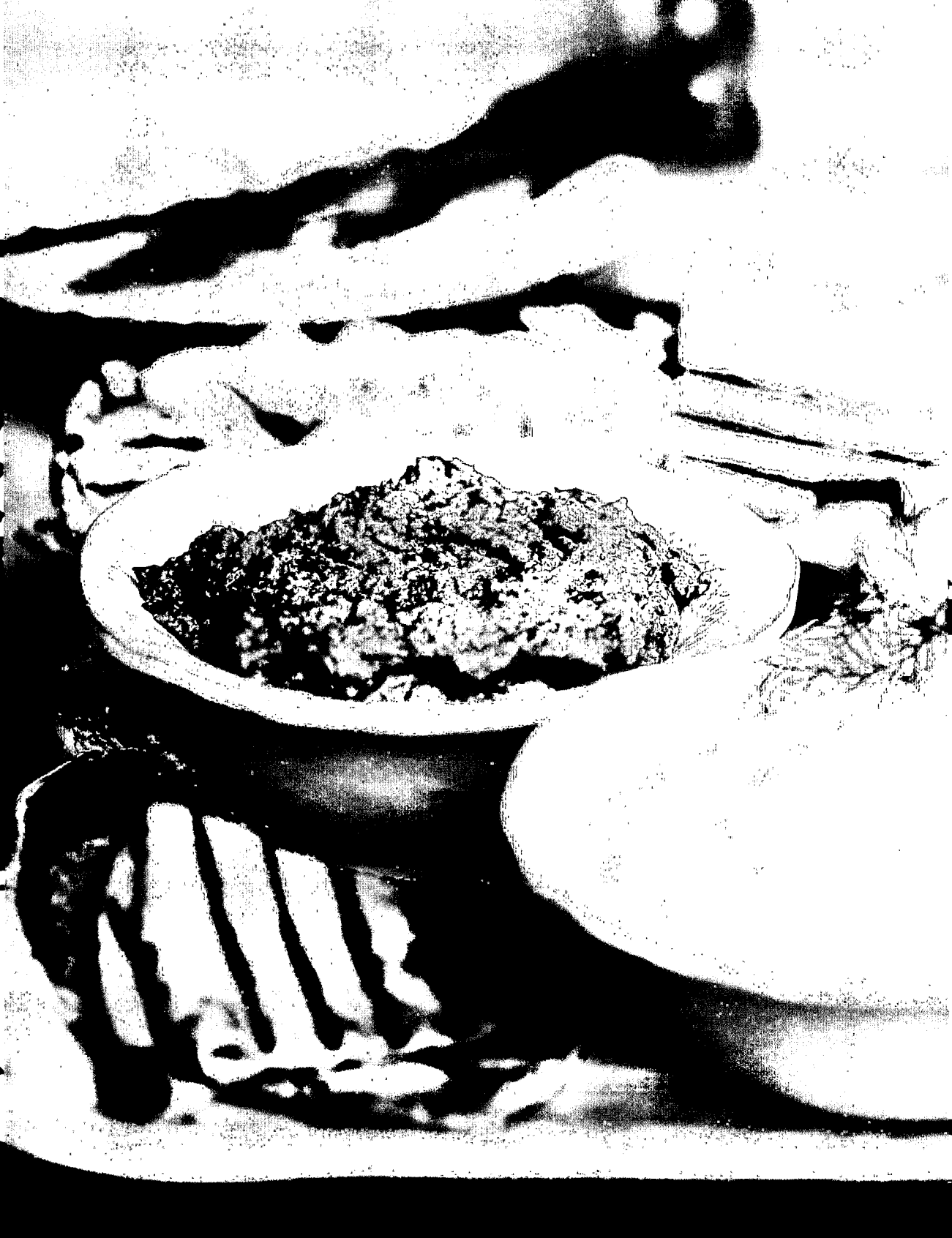

GRILLED PITA BREAD, THE CLASSIC MIDDLE EASTERN FLATBREAD, just needs a brush of olive oil and a few minutes on the grill to taste great. Enjoy it with hummus, Tzatziki (page 44), or this grilled eggplant and red bell pepper spread.

GRILLED PITA BREAD
with GRILLED BABA GANOUSH

SERVES 4

8 large pita bread rounds, brushed with olive oil on both sides

GRILLED BABA GANOUSH

1 large eggplant, ends trimmed and cut lengthwise into 1-inch-thick slices

1 large red bell pepper

2 tablespoons olive oil, plus more for brushing

¼ cup fresh cilantro sprigs

2 garlic cloves

2 tablespoons freshly squeezed lemon juice, or more to your taste

1 teaspoon ground cumin

¼ teaspoon ground coriander

¼ teaspoon cayenne pepper, or more to your taste

Fine kosher or sea salt to taste

Prepare a hot fire in your grill.

Brush the pita breads with olive oil on both sides. Grill the pita breads, turning once, until they have good grill marks, about 2 to 3 minutes total. Cover with foil, and keep warm.

To make the baba ganoush, brush the eggplant slices and red bell pepper with olive oil. Grill the eggplant slices, turning once, until you have good grill marks and the eggplant is tender, 8 to 10 minutes total. Grill the red pepper, turning several times, until it is blackened and blistered all over, 10 to 15 minutes total. Add the grilled eggplant slices to the food processor. Carefully stem and cut the pepper in half; remove the seeds and charred skin, and place the pepper halves in the food processor.

Add the 2 tablespoons olive oil, cilantro, garlic, lemon juice, cumin, coriander, and cayenne pepper and puree until smooth. Add salt to taste and adjust the flavors with more lemon juice, salt, and cayenne pepper if desired. To serve, cut the grilled pita into wedges with kitchen scissors and serve around a bowl of the spread.

MAKE IT MEZE

TURN GRILLED FLATBREAD AND ACCOMPANYING DIPS OR SPREADS into the casual meal known as *meze*, sort of Middle Eastern *tapas*. Serve them with olives, cucumber slices, fresh greens, and cherry tomatoes. Or grill other vegetables or make Grilled Zucchini and Yellow Squash Stacks with Feta and Black Olives (page 73) or Chard-Wrapped Goat Cheese on the Grill (page 75) as *meze* offerings. You can even slice and grill the feta-like haloumi cheese—simply brush $\frac{1}{2}$-inch slices with olive oil and grill for a minute or so on each side until the cheese has grill marks. Set everything out on the table on platters and in bowls and let everyone serve themselves.

STIR-TOGETHER FLATBREAD AND PIZZA DOUGH

USING INSTANT OR BREAD MACHINE YEAST, WHICH DOESN'T HAVE to be proofed in water first, is the key to this easy, no-knead dough. It's great for pizzas or flatbreads on the grill. Allow 1 hour for rising time.

MAKES 1 POUND DOUGH FOR 4 INDIVIDUAL PIZZAS OR FLATBREADS

$1\frac{1}{4}$ teaspoons salt

2 teaspoons instant or bread machine yeast

1 cup lukewarm water

1 teaspoon honey

1 tablespoon olive oil

In a medium bowl, stir the flour, salt and yeast together. Combine the water, honey and olive oil and stir into the flour mixture. Cover the bowl with plastic wrap and let sit at room temperature (72°F) until doubled in bulk, about 1 hour. Cover and refrigerate for up to 3 days. Bring to room temperature before rolling out.

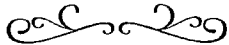

HOW TO GRILL FLATBREADS AND PIZZAS

USE EITHER HOMEMADE STIR-TOGETHER FLATBREAD AND Pizza Dough (opposite page) or 1 pound of prepared pizza or bread dough. Transfer the dough to a floured surface and divide into fourths. Flour a rolling pin or your hands and roll or pat each portion of dough into an oval.

To grill as plain flatbread, prepare a medium-hot fire in your grill. Brush the top side of each dough oval with olive oil. Grill over direct medium-high heat until you see the dough starting to bubble like a pancake, about 2 to 3 minutes, and the bottoms have good grill marks. Turn, quickly brush with more oil, and grill for 1 more minute or until the other side has good grill marks. Serve hot.

To grill as flatbreads or pizzas with toppings, prepare a hot fire on one side of in your grill for indirect cooking. Brush the top side of each dough oval with olive oil. Grill over direct heat until you see the dough starting to bubble like a pancake, about 2 to 3 minutes, and the bottoms have good grill marks. Brush the top side with olive oil and flip the pizza, using tongs, onto a baking sheet. Quickly spoon the topping of your choice over the pizza. Using a grill spatula, place it on the indirect or no-heat side of the fire. Cover and grill for 5 minutes or until the topping is bubbly.

TRADITIONALLY, AFGHAN FOODS WERE COOKED OVER A WOOD and charcoal fire, so the backyard grill is perfect for this flatbread. These grilled half-ovals make a rustic appetizer on their own, or can be a wonderful accompaniment to grilled vegetable, lamb, chicken or beef skewers. Wrap the warm flatbread around the foods on the skewer to help slide them off. Then eat the flatbread and skewered foods like a soft taco.

HERB-STUFFED AFGHAN FLATBREAD

SERVES 4

1 recipe Stir-Together Flatbread and Pizza Dough (page 94) or 1 pound frozen pizza or bread dough, thawed

1 small jalapeño or serrano pepper, seeded and finely chopped

1 cup finely chopped green onions (about 12 green onions)

1 cup finely chopped fresh cilantro

4 teaspoons fine kosher or sea salt

Olive oil, for brushing

While the dough is rising, combine the jalapeño, green onions, cilantro and salt in a medium bowl. Transfer the mixture to a sieve placed over a bowl and let drain for 15 minutes.

Meanwhile, prepare a medium-hot fire in your grill.

Transfer the dough to a floured surface and divide into fourths. Flour a rolling pin or your hands and roll or pat each portion of dough into a $\frac{1}{2}$-inch-thick oval. Place one-quarter of the jalapeño mixture on half of each oval, leaving a $\frac{1}{2}$-inch border around the edge. Brush the perimeter of each oval with water and fold over, pressing the edges together. Brush the surface of each flatbread with olive oil.

Grill for 3 to 4 minutes per side, turning once, until the bread is golden and has some grill marks.

TRADITIONALLY COOKED IN NORTHERN INDIA OVER A CHAR-coal fire in a *tandoor*, a cone-shaped ceramic oven (sort of like a chiminea), these flatbreads also take well to the gardener's grill. Brush these with melted butter instead of olive oil before grilling, and while you're at it, grill up some vegetables for accompaniments. The poppy seeds add a little crunch and a handsome appearance. Poppy Seed Naan is delicious served with Fire-Roasted Fava Beans in the Pod with Sheep's Milk Cheese (page 65), Charred Eggplant and Tarragon Spread (page 54), or your favorite prepared chutney.

POPPY SEED NAAN

SERVES 4

1 recipe Stir-Together Flatbread and Pizza Dough (page 94) or 1 pound frozen pizza or bread dough, thawed

$\frac{1}{4}$ cup ($\frac{1}{2}$ stick) unsalted butter, melted

2 tablespoons poppy seeds

Prepare a medium-hot fire in your grill.

Transfer the dough to a floured surface and divide into fourths. Flour a rolling pin or your hands and roll or pat each portion of dough into a $\frac{1}{2}$-inch-thick oval. Brush each flatbread on both sides with melted butter and sprinkle with poppy seeds.

Place naan on grill, close the lid and grill for about 2 to 3 minutes per side, turning once, until naan is puffed and golden and has a few grill marks. Serve warm, with chutney.

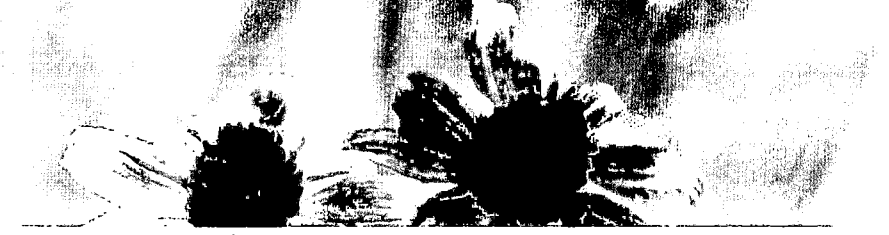

GARDENING AND GRILLING WITH AN ITALIAN ACCENT

IF YOU LOVE TO ADD THE SIZZLE OF THE GRILL TO ITALIAN FOODS, there's no better way to get the freshest than to grow them yourself. Here's a partial list of herbs and vegetables you might want to include in your garden:

- **BASIL.** Genovese (from Genoa) basil is the classic Italian basil variety and the best for pesto.

- **BROCCOLI.** Broccoli is delicious grilled or stir-grilled; try even more colorful varieties like the apple-green Romanesco or purple sprouting broccoli.

- **FAVA BEANS.** A favorite in springtime; grill them in the pod.

- **FLORENCE FENNEL.** Grows like celery and can be grilled or stir-grilled.

- **GARLIC.** Plant this pungent root vegetable between mid-September and the end of November, whenever the soil cools to 60 degrees in your area. It will be ready for harvesting in the late spring.

- **ONIONS.** Look for cipollini onions, small onions that can be grilled, stir-grilled, or smoked, then drizzled with balsamic vinegar.

- **OREGANO.** Fresh oregano is more delicate in flavor than dried.

- **TOMATOES.** Plum- and pear-shaped, cherry, and beefsteak varieties; an heirloom like Rosso Sicilian. Tomatoes are delicious grilled, stir-grilled, or smoked.

- **ZUCCHINI.** Black Beauty is the standard green zucchini; also try Golden Zucchini or yellow summer squash for grilling or stir-grilling.

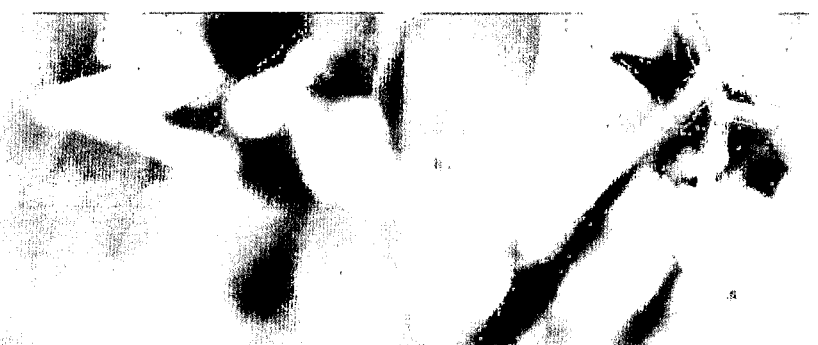

I T'S HARD TO BELIEVE THAT AMERICANS WERE BASICALLY CLUE-less about pesto until the 1970s PBS program, *The Romagnoli's Table*. That cooking show took viewers beyond spaghetti and meatballs to dishes like pasta primavera, tossed with freshly made pesto and spring vegetables. Today, we can marry the flavors of the grill with the early garden harvest in this memorable pizza.

PIZZA PRIMAVERA

SERVES 4

8 ounces fresh asparagus (about 1 small handful of spears), trimmed

Olive oil, for brushing

1 recipe Stir-Together Flatbread and Pizza Dough (page 94) or 1 pound frozen pizza or bread dough, thawed

All-purpose flour, for sprinkling

1/2 cup Basil Pesto (page 32) or prepared pesto

1/2 cup shelled fresh peas or frozen and thawed baby peas

8 ounces fresh goat cheese, sheep's milk cheese or other soft cheese

Freshly ground black pepper

Divide the dough into four equal parts and press or roll each piece into an 8-inch circle. Sprinkle flour on two large baking sheets and place two rounds of dough on each sheet.

Prepare a hot fire on one side of your grill for indirect cooking.

Brush the asparagus with olive oil and grill on the direct heat side, turning often, until they're slightly charred. Quickly chop into 1-inch pieces. To grill directly on the grill grate, brush one side of each pizza with olive oil and place, oiled side down, on the direct heat side. Grill for 1 to 2 minutes, or until you see the dough starting to bubble. Brush the top side with olive oil and flip each pizza, using tongs, onto a baking sheet. Quickly spread each pizza with a fourth of the pesto, then spoon on a fourth of the grilled asparagus and peas, and dollops of goat cheese. Using a grill spatula, place it on the indirect side of the fire. Cover and grill for 4 to 5 minutes or until the cheese is has slightly melted. Sprinkle with black pepper and serve hot.

KISS OF SMOKE DEEPENS AND ENRICHES THE FLAVORS IN this pizza, which goes well with a glass of red wine or a craft beer.

WOOD-GRILLED SPRING ONION, BRIE, and KALAMATA OLIVE PIZZA

SERVES 4

1 recipe Stir-Together Flat-bread and Pizza Dough (page 94) or 1 pound frozen pizza or bread dough, thawed

All-purpose flour, for sprinkling

1 cup moistened wood chips or dry wood pellets

1 large bunch spring bulb onions, trimmed

Olive oil, for brushing and drizzling

1 pound brie, cut into $\frac{1}{2}$-inch pieces, rind on

1 cup brine- or oil-cured kalamata olives, drained, pitted and coarsely chopped

2 teaspoons fresh thyme, oregano, or rosemary leaves

Divide the dough into four equal parts and press or roll each piece into an 8-inch circle. Sprinkle flour on two large baking sheets and place two rounds of dough on each sheet.

Prepare a hot fire on one side of your grill for indirect cooking. If using a charcoal grill, throw moistened wood chips directly on the coals right before you want to grill. If using a gas grill, enclose the wood chips in a foil packet with holes poked in the top; place the packet on the grill grate over the heat source. You're ready to grill when you've seen the smoke from the smoldering wood and the fire is hot.

Brush the onions with olive and grill on the direct heat side, turning often, until they're slightly charred. Quickly chop the onions.

To grill directly on the grill grate, brush one side of each pizza with olive oil and place, oiled side down, on the direct heat side. Grill for 1 to 2 minutes, or until you see the dough starting to bubble. Brush the top side with olive oil and flip the pizza, using tongs, onto a baking sheet. Quickly spoon a fourth of the grilled onions, brie, olives, and thyme over each pizza. Using a grill spatula, place each pizza on the indirect side of the fire. Cover and grill for 4 to 5 minutes or until the cheese has slightly melted. Serve hot.

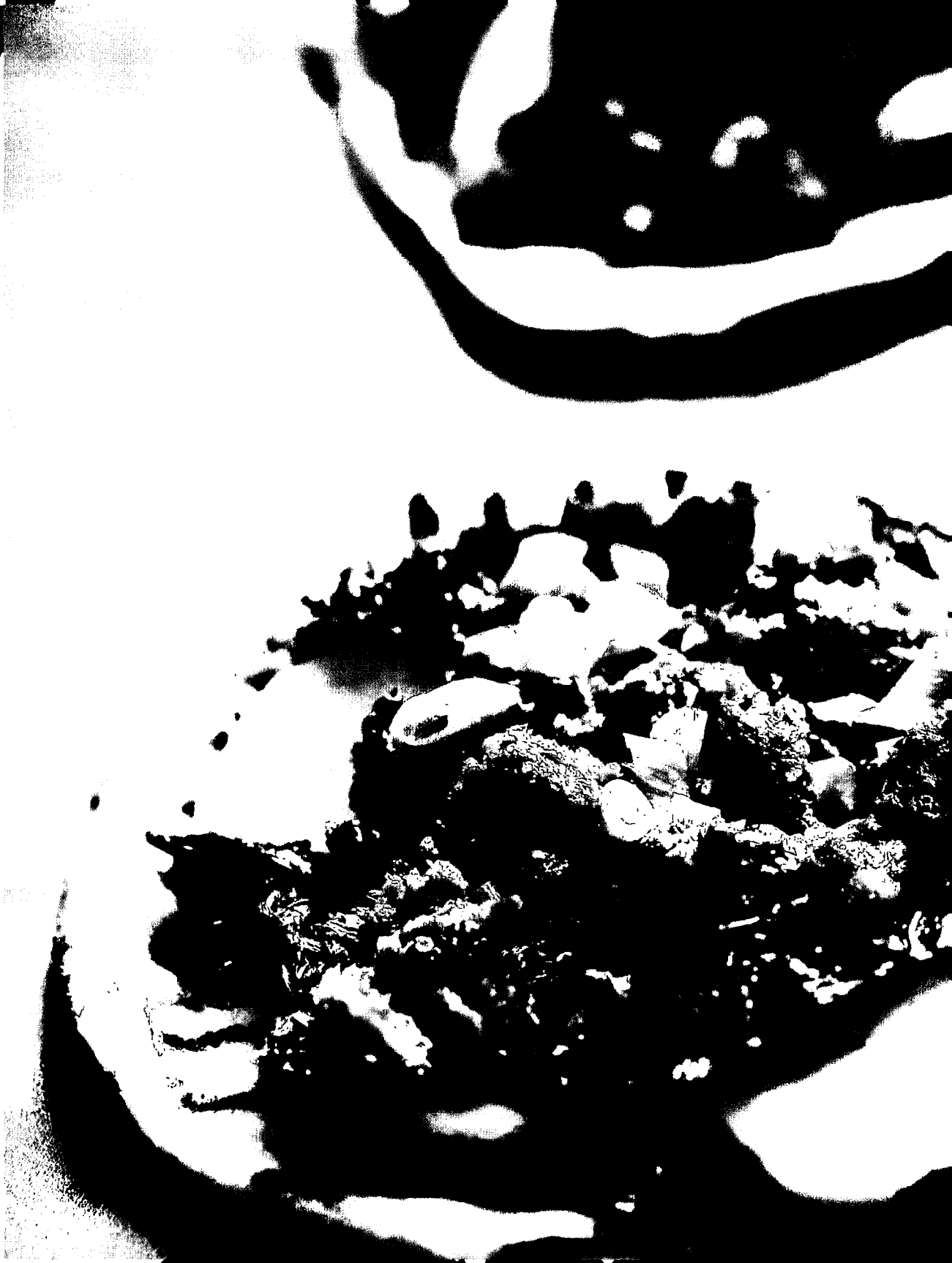

HEARTY WITHOUT BEING HEAVY, THIS PIZZA TAKES KALE AND onions from the garden and adds chorizo or other spicy sausage for an accent. Boil the new potatoes for about 15 minutes, until tender. Use vegetarian chorizo, if you'd like.

KALE, POTATO, and CHORIZO PIZZA

SERVES 4

1 recipe Stir-Together Flatbread and Pizza Dough (page 94) or 1 pound frozen pizza or bread dough, thawed

All-purpose flour, for sprinkling

8 kale leaves

Olive oil, for brushing and drizzling

8 ounces cooked and crumbled chorizo, Portuguese, or other spicy sausage

4 new potatoes, cooked and sliced thinly

½ cup chopped green onion (about 6 green onions, white and light green parts)

Coarse black pepper

Divide the dough into four equal parts and press or roll each piece into an 8-inch circle. Sprinkle flour on two large baking sheets and place two rounds of dough on each sheet.

Prepare a hot fire on one side of your grill for indirect cooking. Oil a perforated grill rack and place over direct heat.

Brush the kale with olive oil. Grill leaves for 1 minute on each side or until slightly charred and softened. Quickly trim off the bottom of the stalk and strip the leaves from the stems. Finely chop the leaves and set aside.

To grill directly on the grill grate, brush one side of each pizza with olive oil and place, oiled side down, on the direct heat side. Grill for 1 to 2 minutes, or until you see the dough starting to bubble. Brush the top side with olive oil and flip each pizza, using tongs, onto a baking sheet. Quickly brush with more olive oil, then spoon on a fourth of the sliced potato and grilled kale. Sprinkle with sausage and green onion. Drizzle with olive oil and season with pepper. Using a grill spatula, place each pizza on the indirect side of the fire. Cover and grill for 4 to 5 minutes or until the kale has slightly wilted and the topping is hot. Serve hot.

IF YOU'RE A VETERAN GARDENER, YOU KNOW HOW IT GOES WITH zucchini, patty pan, or summer squash. If you don't pick them small before it rains, by the next day the squash have doubled in size and are not nearly as tasty. So, when it's summer squash season, try to pick these vegetables young—about 4 to 6 inches long for cylindrical squash and about 2 to 3 inches wide for patty pans. Grill, then chop them to top this delicious pizza. Try to use both green and yellow squash, if you can, for a more colorful dish.

CHAR-GRILLED
BABY SUMMER SQUASH PIZZA

SERVES 4

1 recipe Stir-Together Flat-bread and Pizza Dough (page 94) or 1 pound frozen pizza or bread dough, thawed

All-purpose flour, for sprinkling

4 baby summer squash, such as zucchini, yellow summer squash, or patty pan

Olive oil, for brushing

Salt to taste

1 teaspoon lemon pepper seasoning

½ cup grated Romano or Asiago cheese

½ cup finely chopped fresh basil

Divide the dough into four equal parts and press or roll each piece into an 8-inch circle. Sprinkle flour on two large baking sheets and place two rounds of dough on each sheet.

Prepare a hot fire on one side of your grill for indirect cooking. Oil a perforated grill rack and place over direct heat.

In a bowl, toss the squash with olive oil. Transfer the squash to the perforated grill rack and grill, turning often, until they're slightly charred and softened, 15 to 20 minutes. Quickly chop into 1-inch pieces and sprinkle with salt and lemon pepper seasoning.

To grill directly on the grill grate, brush one side of each pizza with olive oil and place, oiled side down, on the direct heat side. Grill for 1 to 2 minutes, or until you see the dough starting to bubble. Brush the top side with olive oil and flip each pizza, using tongs, onto a baking sheet. Quickly brush with more olive oil, and then spoon on a fourth of the grilled squash and sprinkle with cheese. Using a grill spatula, place each pizza on the indirect side of the fire. Cover and grill for 4 to 5 minutes or until the cheese is has slightly melted. Top with fresh basil and serve hot.

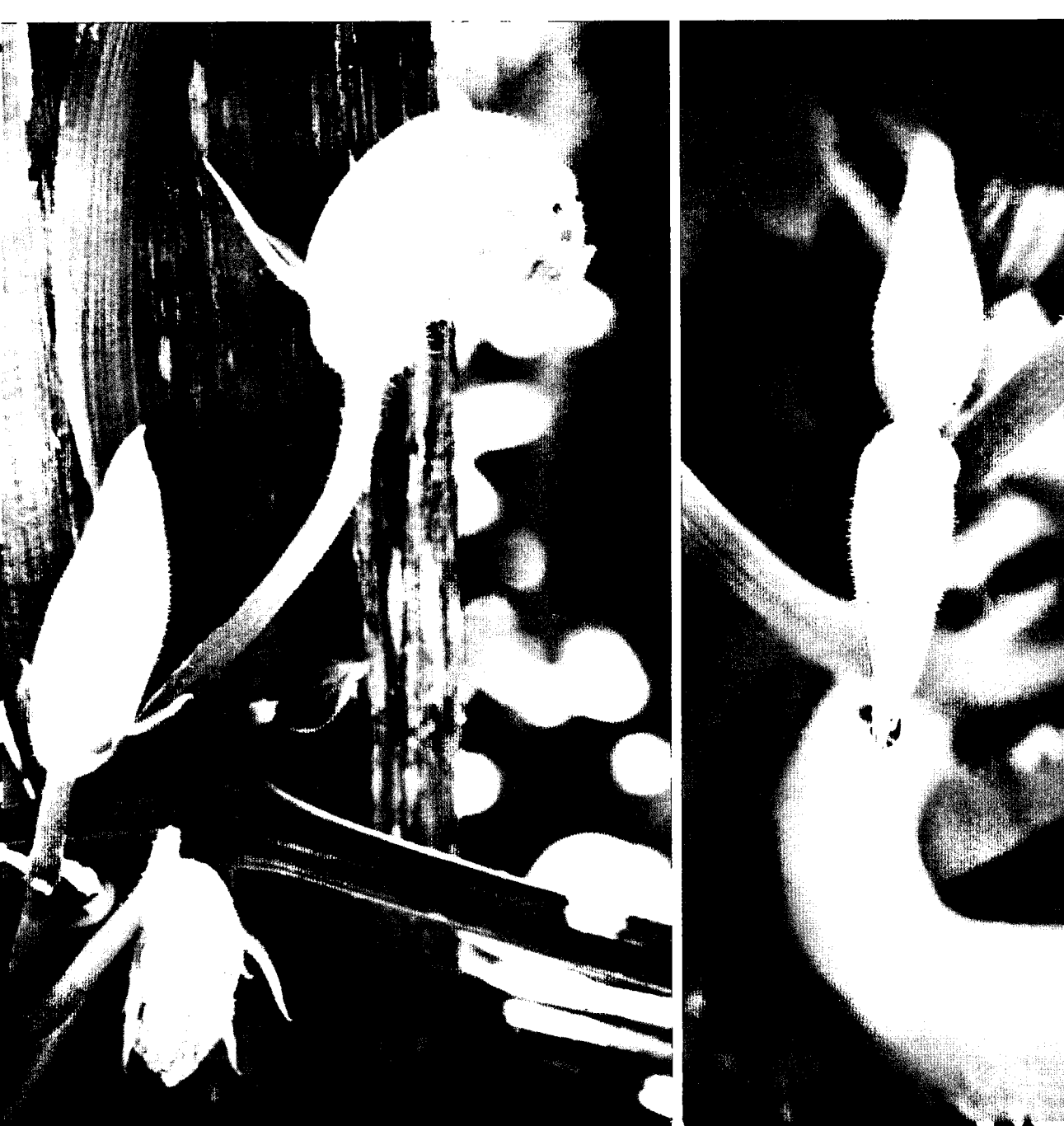

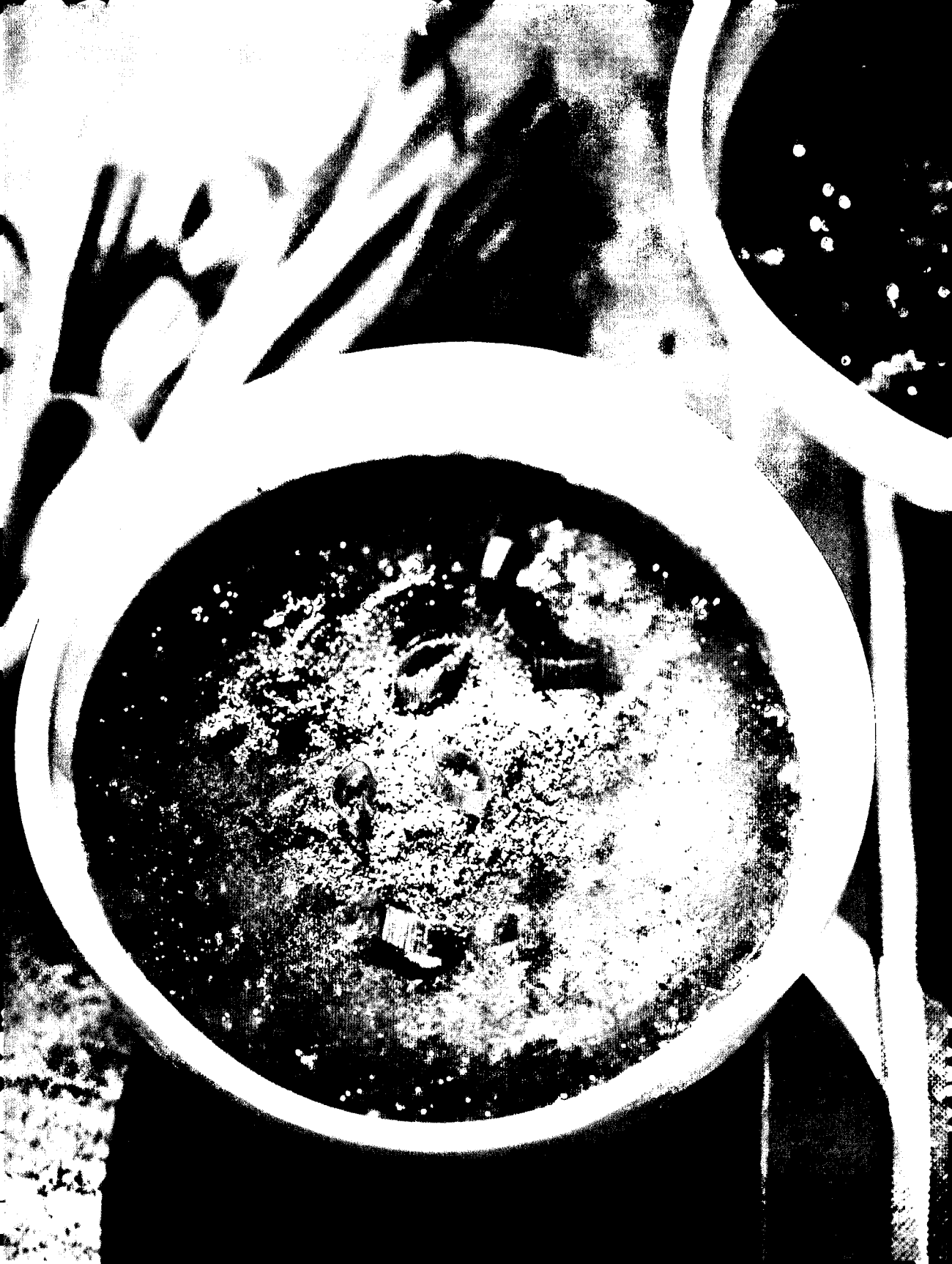

CHAPTER 4

SOUP & SALAD

SALADS AND SOUPS PROVIDE A CULINARY CANVAS FOR BOTH THE gardener and the griller.

A signature salad generally comprises several key ingredients: cool and crisp or grilled-and-still-crisp greens; a fresh-tasting dressing; and bite-size fruits, nuts, vegetables, or cheeses that add flavor, texture, and interest. Adding a grilled protein—like chicken, beef, shrimp, tuna, or tofu—turns a salad into a main course.

A stellar soup, made from grilled or smoked ingredients, has that extra nuance of flavor that evokes home and hearth—just what you want a soup to do. To round out a soup meal, add oven-toasted or grilled bread so you can soak up every last delicious drop.

Throughout this book, we suggest barbecuing more food than you really need for one meal. That's because grilling once so you can eat twice—or three times—is a really efficient way to get more mileage out of hours spent tending garden plants or even 10 minutes grilling vegetables over a hot fire. Your outdoor grill can become the twenty-first century version of the old summer kitchen: a place where you turn the garden's bounty into preserved foods for future meals. These garden goods won't be canned, however. They're destined for the freezer, and will hold perfectly until you're ready to use them. Most grilled or smoked foods can be cooled to room temperature, stored in labeled plastic freezer bags, and kept as frozen assets for up to 6 months.

Although you can certainly grill or smoke all the main ingredients for this chapter's recipes right before you want to serve them, the dishes here also represent creative ways to use and enjoy your grilled leftovers.

High-Heat Grilled Romaine Salad ...109

Grilled Greens ...110

Grilled Asparagus Salad ...111

Plank-Roasted Pear Salad with
Blue Cheese and Walnuts ...112

Grilled Corn, Tomato, and Red Onion Salad ...114

French-Style Grilled Potato Salad ...115

A Griller's Garden of Greens ...116

Grilled Goat Cheese Tomato Slices with Baby Greens ...118

Grilled Summer Slaw with Gorgonzola Vinaigrette ...119

Grilled Radicchio and Brussels Sprouts
with Hot Bacon Dressing ...120

Grilled Baby Bok Choi with Fresh Ginger-Soy Sauce ...122

Flame-Licked Tomatoes on the Stem ...124

Grilled Corn and Chicken Chowder ...125

Grilled Gazpacho ...126

Smoked Tomato Bisque ...128

Red Curry-Coconut Soup with
Grilled Vegetables and Shrimp ...130

Smoked & Smashed Sweet Potato Soup ...132

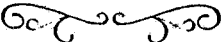

I T'S THE BEST OF ALL POSSIBLE WORLDS—LETTUCE WITH A FRESH crunch, but the flavor of the grill. That's what you get when you grill romaine, a lettuce that is just the right mixture of sturdy and leafy to withstand searing heat. Make sure you cut, rinse, and dry the romaine at least 30 minutes for optimum grill marks and crispness. If too much moisture is in the leaves, the lettuce will steam and wilt. Set a double layer of kitchen towels on the counter and lay lettuce cut-side down to drain. Use another dry towel to pat moisture off the top.

HIGH-HEAT GRILLED ROMAINE SALAD

SERVES 4

2 hearts of romaine,
  halved, rinsed, and dried

Olive oil, for brushing

Fine kosher or sea salt and
  freshly ground black
  pepper to taste

Rosemary, Garlic, and
  Lemon Baste (page 27)

Romano or Parmesan
  cheese shavings for
  garnish

Prepare a hot fire in a grill.

Brush the cut side of the romaine halves with olive oil and season with salt and pepper. Grill on the cut sides only until the leaves are browned and sizzled on the outside edges and the lettuce has great caramelized grill marks, 3 to 4 minutes total.

Place the halves on a platter or on 4 individual plates. Spoon the dressing over the cut sides and shave some cheese on top for a delicious garnish. Serve at once.

VARIATION:

Change the flavors of dressing to make this a classic Caesar with bottled Caesar dressing, or serve bacon, tomatoes, and avocado on the side and spoon Creamy Blue Cheese Dressing (page 41) over the top.

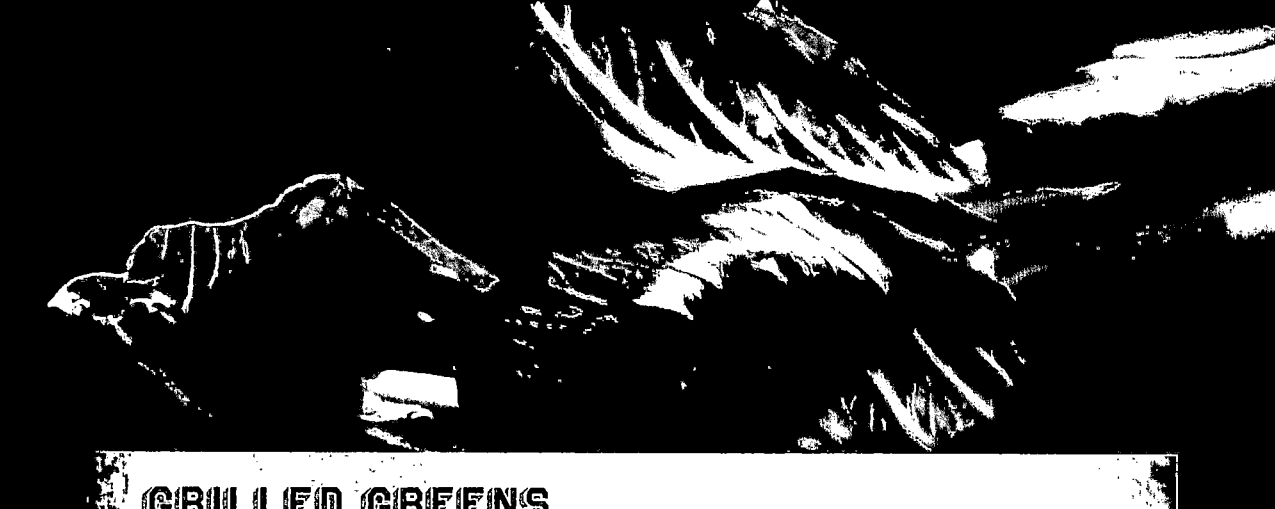

GRILLED GREENS

WHY NOT GRILL GREENS? AS WITH ANY OTHER FOOD, GRILLING adds a touch of caramelization, which means flavor. You get some char on the outside leaves, while the inside leaves remain tender and crisp. Choose greens that form heads, such as red or green cabbage, radicchio, and fennel bulbs. You can also use greens with large, sturdy leaves such as Swiss chard or kale. Greens that grow in small tender leaves, such as arugula, oak leaf, or the mix known as mesclun, will steam and wilt (or fall through the grill grates) rather than char.

The trick to grilling great greens is a hot fire, vigilance, and long-handled, spring-loaded spatulas for quick turning. Brush the cut sides of heading greens or the leaves of sturdy greens with oil, then grill until you get good grill marks, turning as necessary. Watch carefully so the greens don't burn; always keep the grill lid open.

When you've got the hang of grilling greens, you can make a signature garden appetizer or casual entrée. Wrap large, sturdy leaves of Swiss chard, mustard greens, or kale—blanched first in boiling, salted water for a minute until limp—around small rounds of fresh chèvre, sheep's milk cheese, or brie. Simply brush the packets with flavorful vinaigrettes such as Citrus Caesar (000), Fresh Basil (000), or Chipotle (000) and grill, turning once, until the cheese softens and melts. Serve the packets hot, drizzled with more vinaigrette.

O MAKE SURE YOU DON'T LOSE ANY SPEARS THROUGH THE grill grates, thread asparagus crosswise onto two parallel skewers, leaving space between the spears. Prepare this recipe during the height of asparagus season, from April through June, for the most flavorful results. You can also use Toasted Sesame-Soy Marinade and Dressing (page 15), Chipotle Vinaigrette (page 22), or Fresh Basil Vinaigrette (page 20) for a change of pace. If you don't have a kitchen scale, two pounds asparagus is about what you can encircle with your hands, twice, or about 30 medium spears.

GRILLED ASPARAGUS SALAD

SERVES 4 TO 6

2 pounds asparagus,
  trimmed

12 thin slices prosciutto

1 cup Ginger Vinaigrette
  (page 16), separated

6 cups mixed garden
  greens

2 hard-boiled eggs, sliced

Prepare a medium-hot fire in your grill.

Wrap 12 spears of the asparagus with the slices of prosciutto. Lay the rest of the asparagus in a shallow glass dish and drizzle with $\frac{1}{4}$ cup of the Ginger Vinaigrette. Set aside.

Place all of the asparagus on the grill rack, perpendicular to the grate. Grill for 8 to 10 minutes, turning often, until asparagus is tender-crisp and the prosciutto is crispy. Set all the cooked asparagus back in the glass dish and toss in the vinaigrette.

In a large salad bowl, toss the greens and sliced cooked eggs with $\frac{1}{4}$ to $\frac{1}{2}$ cup of the vinaigrette. Divide salad equally among 4 or 6 plates and arrange asparagus atop the salad, dividing the prosciutto-wrapped spears evenly among the plates.

VARIATION:

For a delicious appetizer, place the grilled asparagus, both the plain and prosciutto-wrapped, attractively on a large platter. Serve it with a bowl of Blender Hollandaise (page 36) for dipping.

GARDENERS WHO ALSO GROW PEAR TREES SOON LEARN TO pick pears before they're fully ripe. If left on the tree, pears ripen from the inside out, so will be mushy in the middle by the time the exterior is soft. So, pick them when they're firm, but just starting to turn a yellowish green. Then let them fully mature in the refrigerator. Bartlett pears only need a day or two in the cold, while Bosc and Anjou pears need about two weeks.

PLANK-ROASTED PEAR SALAD *with* BLUE CHEESE *and* WALNUTS

SERVES 4 TO 8

4 large, ripe Anjou or Bartlett pears (about 2 pounds)

2 tablespoons unsalted butter, melted

2 tablespoons wildflower or other amber honey

½ cup crumbled blue cheese, such as Maytag or Point Reyes

Fresh thyme sprigs for garnish

4 cups mixed salad greens

¼ cup Lemon Caesar Vinaigrette (page 17)

Prepare a hot fire in your grill.

Cut the pears in half lengthwise, leaving the stem intact. Using a sturdy teaspoon or a melon baller, remove the core from each half. Place the pear halves on a baking sheet, cut side up. If necessary, trim the pears so they lie flat without rocking.

In a bowl, mix the melted butter and honey. Brush the honey mixture over the cut surface of the pears. Sprinkle the pears with the crumbled blue cheese.

Place the planks on the grill grate and close the lid. When the planks start to smoke and pop, after 3 to 5 minutes, open the lid and, using grill tongs, turn the planks over. Quickly place the pear halves on the planks, cut side up. Cover and plank-roast for 12 to 15 minutes, or until the pears are scorched around the edges and the cheese has melted. Garnish with thyme sprigs and serve alongside mixed greens tossed with Lemon Caesar Vinaigrette.

Variation: Planking-Roasting in the Oven Preheat the oven to 450°F. Place the pears on planks and roast in the center of the oven for 12 to 15 minutes, or until the pears are scorched around the edges.

SOUP & SALAD

CONSIDER THIS A BASIC BLUEPRINT FOR A TASTY SUMMER salad. Use whatever garden bounty you have or enhance it with a myriad of other ingredients, such as grilled peppers, squash, or green onions; olives and artichoke hearts; or smoked peppers and yellow onions. If you like, grill the corn and the onions, but not the tomatoes. Lay fresh tomato slices on a platter and top with the grilled corn kernels, onion slivers, and everything else. Drizzle with either the basil vinaigrette included in this recipe or the Lemon Caesar Vinaigrette (page 17).

GRILLED CORN, TOMATO, and RED ONION SALAD

SERVES 4 TO 6

2 or 3 ears sweet corn, shucked

3 large ripe tomatoes, sliced ½-inch-thick (2 or 3 slices per person)

Olive oil, for brushing

1 small red onion, very thinly sliced

12 fresh basil leaves

1 to 2 tablespoons Fresh Basil Vinaigrette (page 20)

Prepare a hot fire in your grill.

Brush the ears of corn and tomato slices lightly with olive oil.

Grill the corn for about 5 to 6 minutes, turning it to char all over. Let the tomato slices grill on the one side only for about 3 minutes, and then remove.

To serve, divide the tomatoes equally among 4 to 6 plates. Cut the corn off the cob and scatter the kernels and onion slivers evenly over the plates. Stack the basil leaves one on top of the other and slice thinly, then sprinkle over each salad. Spoon 1 or 2 tablespoons of the Fresh Basil Vinaigrette over each salad.

F YOU GROW YOUR OWN POTATOES, YOU KNOW HOW FABULOUS their flavor is compared to store-bought. Make this French-style potato salad with whatever potatoes you grow: new, russet, and fingerlings will all work. Make the potato slices as uniform as possible for even cooking, and then just grill them on both sides until fork-tender. When warm, potatoes absorb flavorings very readily, so dress this salad hot off the grill. Change it up to a Southwest-style potato salad by dressing it with the Chipotle Vinaigrette (page 22) or an Argentinean-style dish with Chimichurri Sauce (page 26) spooned over it.

FRENCH-STYLE
GRILLED POTATO SALAD

SERVES 6 TO 8

2 pounds garden potatoes, peeled if you prefer

2 tablespoons plus $\frac{1}{4}$ cup olive oil, divided

1 bunch green onions, finely chopped

$\frac{1}{4}$ cup chopped flat-leaf parsley

3 tablespoons tarragon vinegar

1 garlic clove, minced

Kosher or sea salt and freshly ground black pepper to taste

Sprigs of tarragon for garnish

Prepare a hot fire in your grill.

Cut the potatoes into $\frac{1}{4}$-inch-thick slices and place in a grill basket or wok. Set the basket over a baking sheet for less mess while you dress the potatoes. Lightly drizzle the potato slices with 2 tablespoons of olive oil and toss to coat. Place the basket of potatoes directly over the fire. Grill for about 15 to 20 minutes, tossing occasionally; until the slices are just fork tender and still hot.

Arrange the potato slices in a shallow casserole or bowl. Top with the onion and parsley. Whisk the tarragon vinegar, the remaining $\frac{1}{4}$ cup olive oil, and minced garlic together, and drizzle over all. Season with salt and pepper to taste. Cover and let stand at room temperature until ready to serve. Garnish with sprigs of fresh tarragon.

A GRILLER'S GARDEN OF GREENS

AS A GARDENER OR A VEGETABLE ENTHUSIAST, YOU HAVE A WIDE choice of greens, both the sturdy kind destined for the grill and the tender varieties that help make up a delicious salad base. Greens do best during the cooler growing seasons of spring and fall, so you sow seed or plant seedlings when the soil is somewhat cool. Colorful heading greens like rainbow chard can make a wonderful border, while tender leafing greens, like the mix known as mesclun, can be sown around large potted plants so you can easily pick greens for salads.

- **CABBAGE.** Cabbage is easy to grow in spring or fall and makes a tasty addition to your salad repertoire. The growth habits of different types of cabbage plants (whether they prefer full or partial sun, or how many days to maturity) also give you more versatility in how and where you plant them.

- **BRUSSELS SPROUTS.** These miniature cabbages grow on a stalk and help add structure to a fall garden. Savvy gardeners know that sprouts left on the stalk in the garden until after the first freeze take on a nuttier flavor and are none the worse for wear.

- **GREEN OR RED CABBAGE.** The tougher, frilled outer leaves and globe-shaped head made this plant ideal for a border. English edible landscapers like to plant round cabbages interspersed with spicy lavender around white roses.

- **NAPA OR SAVOY CABBAGE.** This type of cabbage has a cylindrical shape. Try it as a border in the garden or as row crop.

- **CHINESE AND AUTUMN TORCH HYBRID CABBAGES.** These tall stalks with leafy heads grow quickly in almost any soil. They look similar to broccolini, and their creamy texture tastes a bit like Brussels sprouts.

- **DWARF BOK CHOY AND TOY CHOI HYBRIDS.** Super quick to grow in just 30 days, these tiny bunches of white stalks and tender green leaves are a gardener's favorite.

- **RADICCHIO.** The smaller purple-red heads of radicchio make it ideal for planting in a container garden or as edible landscaping. Pair it with complementary blue flowering or contrasting lime green-colored plants.

- **HEADING LETTUCES AND GREENS.** Some greens just naturally form a head or a loose bunch, take longer to grow, and stand up well to the grill. These varieties include romaine or cos, Swiss or rainbow chard, Lacinato or Dinosaur kale.

- **LOOSE-LEAF LETTUCES.** Other greens grow more as individual leaves, which you pick one by one, as they grow quickly. These varieties include arugula, Amish deer tongue, lollo rossa, oak leaf, heirloom and bronze-tinged Grandpa Admire's lettuce, and dark red mascara. These more tender greens are too delicate for the grill, but remain fresh and crisp on your plate or in a bowl. Toss fresh leaf lettuces with vinaigrette or dressing before you top them with hot foods from the grill.

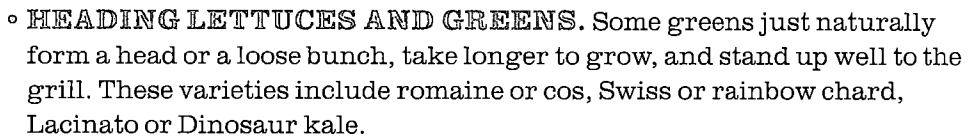

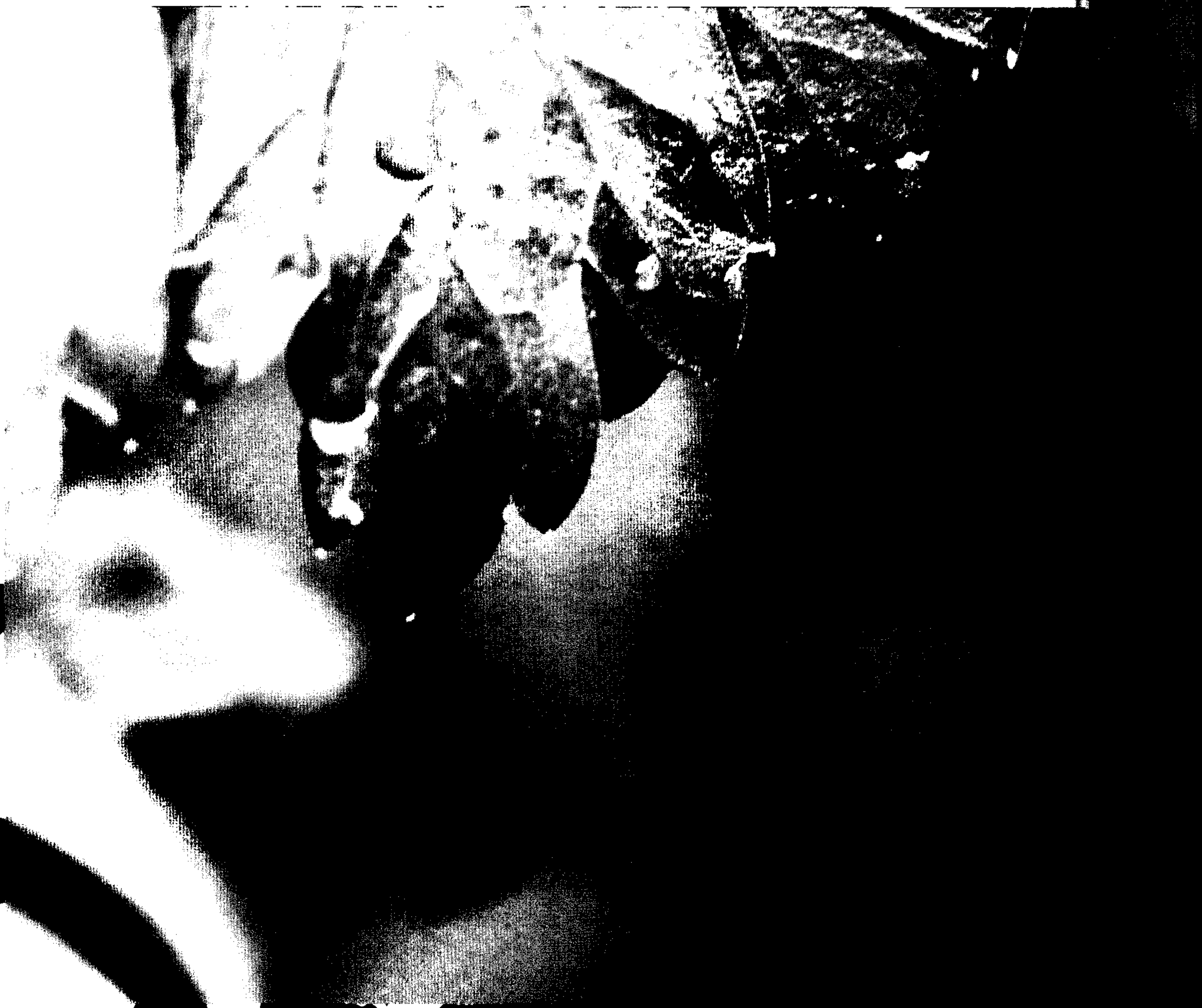

SOFT, WARM GOAT CHEESE WITH THE FLAVOR OF THE GRILL IS a perfect accompaniment to the tender greens from your garden. Dress the leaves sparingly so that their freshness and flavor isn't overwhelmed by the vinaigrette. Try the Chipotle Vinaigrette (page 22) for a Southwest twist.

GRILLED GOAT CHEESE TOMATO SLICES *with* BABY GREENS

SERVES 4

4 thick slices beefsteak tomatoes or similar

Olive oil, for brushing

6 ounces fresh goat cheese

4 cups salad greens

4 to 6 tablespoons Lemon Caesar Vinaigrette (page 17)

8 cherry or grape tomatoes, red or yellow or both

Prepare a hot fire in your grill. Lightly brush the tomato slices with olive oil.

Divide the cheese into 4 small rounds about ½-inch thick. Place one round of cheese atop each of the 4 tomato slices. Place the tomatoes (cheese side up) on the hot grill. Grill on the one side only for about 3 minutes, and then remove.

When ready to serve, toss the greens with the vinaigrette and divide among 4 plates. Top each with a goat cheese-topped tomato slice and garnish with additional cherry or grape tomatoes.

GRILLED COLESLAW? YOU BET! GRILLED CABBAGE WEDGES acquire terrific flavor while retaining their crunchiness. Dress the coleslaw right before serving, as the dressing makes the cabbage wilt.

GRILLED SUMMER SLAW
with GORGONZOLA VINAIGRETTE

SERVES 8 TO 10

8 green onions, tops
   trimmed

1 large head cabbage, tough
   outer leaves removed,
   cored and cut into 8
   wedges

¾ cup vegetable oil, plus
   more for brushing

8 ounces Gorgonzola
   cheese, crumbled

2 garlic cloves, minced

⅓ cup apple cider vinegar

1 teaspoon celery seeds

1 teaspoon kosher or
   sea salt

½ teaspoon freshly ground
   black pepper

¼ teaspoon dry mustard

Prepare a hot fire in your grill.

Brush the green onions and cut sides of cabbage with oil. Grill the green onions on one side for 2 to 3 minutes and remove to a platter. Grill the wedges of cabbage for about 4 or 5 minutes on each cut side, turning once (a total of 8 to 10 minutes) until they have good grill marks on both sides.

Finely chop the grilled cabbage and coarsely chop the green onions. Combine them in a large bowl. Let cool, then stir in half of the Gorgonzola. In another bowl, whisk together the remaining ¾ cup vegetable oil, the garlic, vinegar, celery seeds, salt, pepper, and mustard. Add the remaining Gorgonzola and stir to blend. Pour the dressing over the cabbage mixture and toss to coat. Serve at once.

VARIATIONS:

Grill an assortment of greens and cabbages like Napa or Chinese cabbage, radicchio or fennel. Add chopped tomatoes and grilled corn to make a colorful vegetable slaw. You can even add grilled carrots and peppers.Make it Greek-style slaw by adding crumbled feta cheese instead of the blue cheese, chopped cured olives, and a half-and-half mixture of Tzatziki (page 44) and Lemon Caesar Vinaigrette (page 17) instead of the apple cider vinaigrette given here.

THIS COLORFUL FALL SALAD HAS THE HEARTY FLAVOR YOU WANT when the weather turns crisp.

GRILLED RADICCHIO and BRUSSELS SPROUTS with HOT BACON DRESSING

SERVES 4

HOT BACON DRESSING

4 slices thick-cut bacon, chopped

½ cup apple cider vinegar

3 tablespoons balsamic vinegar

3 tablespoons water

1½ teaspoons sugar

1 teaspoon salt

½ teaspoon white pepper

½ teaspoon celery seed

RADICCHIO AND BRUSSELS SPROUTS

1 pound (about 20) Brussels sprouts, halved, rinsed, and patted dry

Olive oil, for brushing

2 heads radicchio, halved, rinsed, and patted dry

1 red onion, cut into ¼-inch-thick slivers

2 ounces crumbled cheese like feta, blue, or goat cheese

Prepare a hot fire on one side of your grill for indirect cooking.

For the dressing, fry the chopped bacon in a medium skillet until crisp. Add the vinegars and water and heat until boiling. Lower the heat to medium and add the sugar, salt, white pepper, and celery seed, stirring well for about 2 or 3 minutes or until the sugar dissolves. Set the pan aside and keep warm.

Place the Brussels sprouts in a large bowl and lightly drizzle with olive oil and toss. Place the Brussels sprouts in an oiled grill basket or grill wok. Set it on a baking tray.

Lightly brush the cut sides of the radicchio with olive oil and set on the baking tray, too, and take out to the grill.

Set the grill basket filled with Brussels sprouts directly over the fire. Toss the sprouts every few minutes and grill until they are tender when pierced with a fork, about 10 to 15 minutes, then move the basket of sprouts to the indirect side of the grill. Place the radicchio, cut-side down, over direct heat and grill until you have good grill marks, about 4 minutes.

To serve, arrange the radicchio and Brussels sprouts on a platter. Sprinkle with the onion and spoon the Hot Bacon Dressing over all. Serve at once.

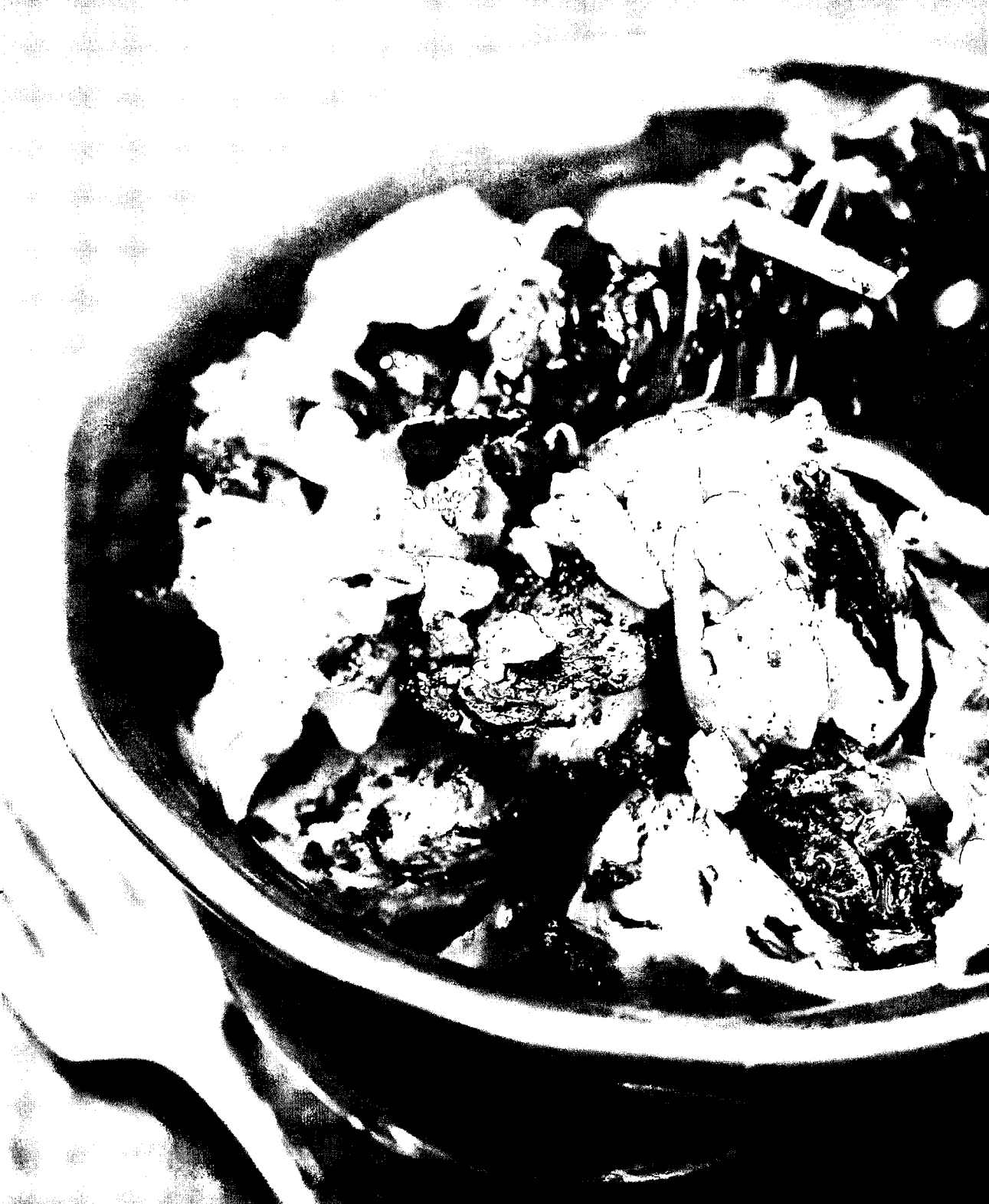

LATE SPRING OR EARLY SUMMER IS WHEN THESE DWARF HEADS of bok choy (also known as pak choi) are tender and sweet. The sturdy leafy stalks are perfect for breaking apart and serving with a dipping sauce like Satay-Style Peanut Dipping Sauce (page 23). The Fresh Ginger-Soy sauce is so versatile. Try it with grilled asparagus, eggplant, and zucchini.

GRILLED BABY BOK CHOY
with FRESH GINGER-SOY SAUCE

SERVES 4

2 small heads bok choy, trimmed and halved lengthwise

FRESH GINGER SOY SAUCE

¼ cup (½ stick) unsalted butter, melted

2 tablespoons olive oil

2 teaspoons soy sauce

2 teaspoons fresh ginger, minced

1 garlic clove, minced

Prepare a medium-hot fire in your grill. Rinse the bok choy, drain well, and pat dry.

To make the Ginger-Soy Sauce, whisk together the melted butter, olive oil, soy sauce, ginger, and garlic.

Brush the bok choy with the sauce and place cut side down directly over the fire. Grill for about 10 minutes. Baste the leaves and turn, continuing to grill for about another 10 minutes until the bok choy is fork-tender. Serve with any remaining sauce.

SOMETIMES THE SIMPLEST INGREDIENTS AND PREPARATION are the best, as with these tomatoes on the stem lightly brushed with olive oil then laid over the fire to sizzle and warm. If you feel especially creative, present the grilled tomatoes atop plates "painted" with pale yellow aioli, deep green Chive or Basil Pesto (page 32), and dark balsamic vinegar: simply use a small brush or a squeeze bottle. Serve with Grill-Toasted Bruschetta (page 49) or crusty artisan bread to mop it all up. If you're a gardener interested in heirloom tomatoes, seek out Hartman's Yellow Gooseberry Tomatoes, a yellow cherry tomato that you can grow from seed.

FLAME-LICKED TOMATOES *on the* STEM

SERVES 6

2 pounds small, ripe tomatoes, like cherry, grape,
currant, cherry Roma, or
small cluster tomatoes,
on the vine or stem (cut
into clusters for easy
grilling)

Olive oil, for brushing

³⁄₄ cup Lemon-Garlic Aioli
(page 39)

6 tablespoons Chive or
Basil Pesto (page 32)

4 teaspoons balsamic
vinegar

Prepare a hot fire in your grill.

Lightly brush the bottoms of the tomatoes with olive oil. Place each stem of tomatoes over the hot fire so that the flames from the fire lick the bottom of the tomatoes. Grill for 2 or 3 minutes to get some char on the tomatoes. Remove from the fire and set aside. (The tomatoes are ready to serve as a side or with a salad of your choice at this point.)

To make painted plates, choose 6 white plates and smear each plate with a brushstroke of 2 table-spoons aioli, a brushstroke of 1 tablespoon pesto, and a drizzle of 1 teaspoon balsamic vinegar. Set the stem of grilled tomatoes on each plate and serve with additional aioli, vinaigrette, and vinegar with crusty bread.

THE FLAVOR OF GARDEN-FRESH CORN COMES THROUGH IN THIS hearty chowder. You can grill the tomatoes and bell pepper right along with the corn, of course, but in this recipe, we want you to think about "frozen assets," previously grilled or smoked vegetables from The Gardener's Grill Pantry (page 28) and The Gardener's Smoke Pantry (page 33).

GRILLED CORN and CHICKEN CHOWDER

SERVES 8 TO 10

6 ears sweet corn

5 tablespoons olive oil, divided

1 cup heavy whipping cream

1 yellow onion, chopped

2 garlic cloves, minced

6 cups chicken stock

1 large chopped grilled or smoked tomato (page 9) (about 1 cup)

2 chopped grilled, grill-roasted, or smoked red bell peppers (pages 8-9) (about 1 cup)

1 (8-ounce) grilled or smoked chicken breast, chopped

1 tablespoon freshly chopped flat-leaf parsley

1 teaspoon ground cumin

½ teaspoon hot sauce

Kosher salt and freshly ground black pepper to taste

6 slices crisp cooked bacon, crumbled

1 cup grilled corn kernels

Prepare a hot fire in your grill. Lightly brush the corn with 2 tablespoons of the olive oil. Place on the hot grill and cook for about 6 to 8 minutes, turning every 2 minutes to get good grill marks on the corn. Let cool. Cut kernels off the cobs. Place one-third of the corn kernels in a food processor. Add 1 cup cream and pulse until smooth. Set aside.

Heat the remaining 3 tablespoons of olive oil in a large pot over medium-high heat. Add the onion and garlic and sauté for about 5 minutes until tender. Add the chicken stock, tomatoes, peppers, chicken, parsley, cumin, and hot sauce. Simmer for about 30 minutes, and then season with salt and pepper. To serve, ladle the soup into bowls and garnish with crumbled bacon and grilled corn.

IF YOU LOVE GAZPACHO, YOU'LL REALLY LOVE THIS VERSION, with the fresh taste of tomatoes from your garden and the flavor of the grill. You can also use smoked tomatoes in this recipe. You can garnish this soup with any of the following toppings: chopped cucumber and green onions, halved cherry tomatoes, chopped cilantro, or a dollop of sour cream.

GRILLED GAZPACHO

SERVES 8

4 large beefsteak tomatoes, sliced

2 red bell peppers, stemmed, seeded, and cut in half lengthwise

1 large red onion, sliced

2 tablespoons plus ½ cup extra-virgin olive oil, divided

¼ cup red wine vinegar

2 tablespoons Worcestershire sauce

1 teaspoon kosher salt

1 teaspoon hot pepper sauce

1 tablespoon butter

1½ cups breadcrumbs

Prepare a hot fire in your grill. Brush beefsteak tomatoes, red peppers, and red onion with 2 tablespoons of olive oil. Grill for 8 to 10 minutes, turning once, until the tomatoes have some char but are still firm and the peppers and onions are nicely charred on all sides. Transfer the grilled vegetables to a food processor and pulse until finely chopped. Add the remaining ½ cup of extra-virgin olive oil, vinegar, Worcestershire, salt, and hot pepper sauce; purée until smooth. Serve immediately or refrigerate until chilled.

For the garnish, heat the butter in a large skillet until foamy. Add breadcrumbs and toast, stirring often, until nicely browned.

To serve, ladle the gazpacho into bowls, then top with the breadcrumbs and other garnishes.

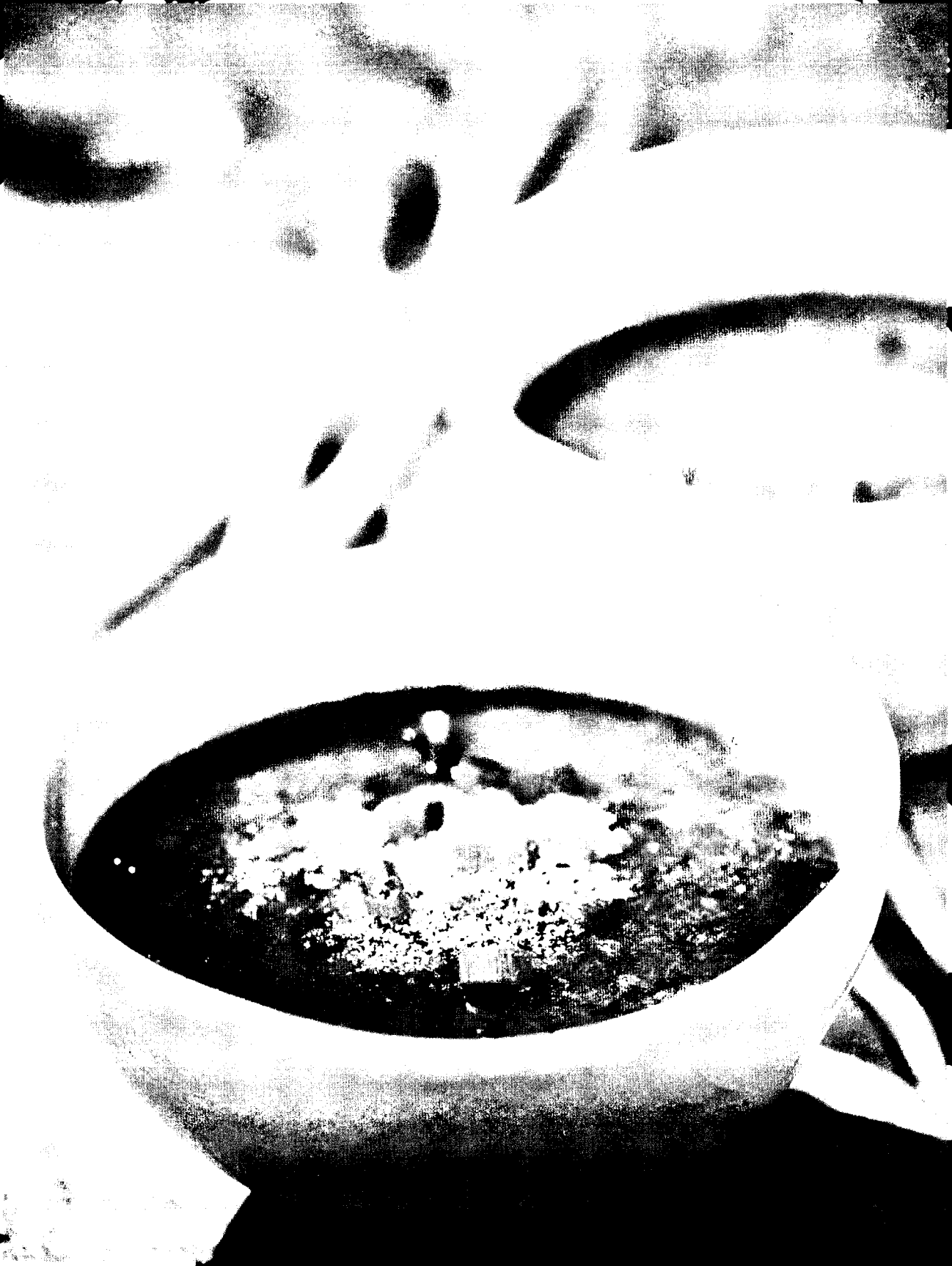

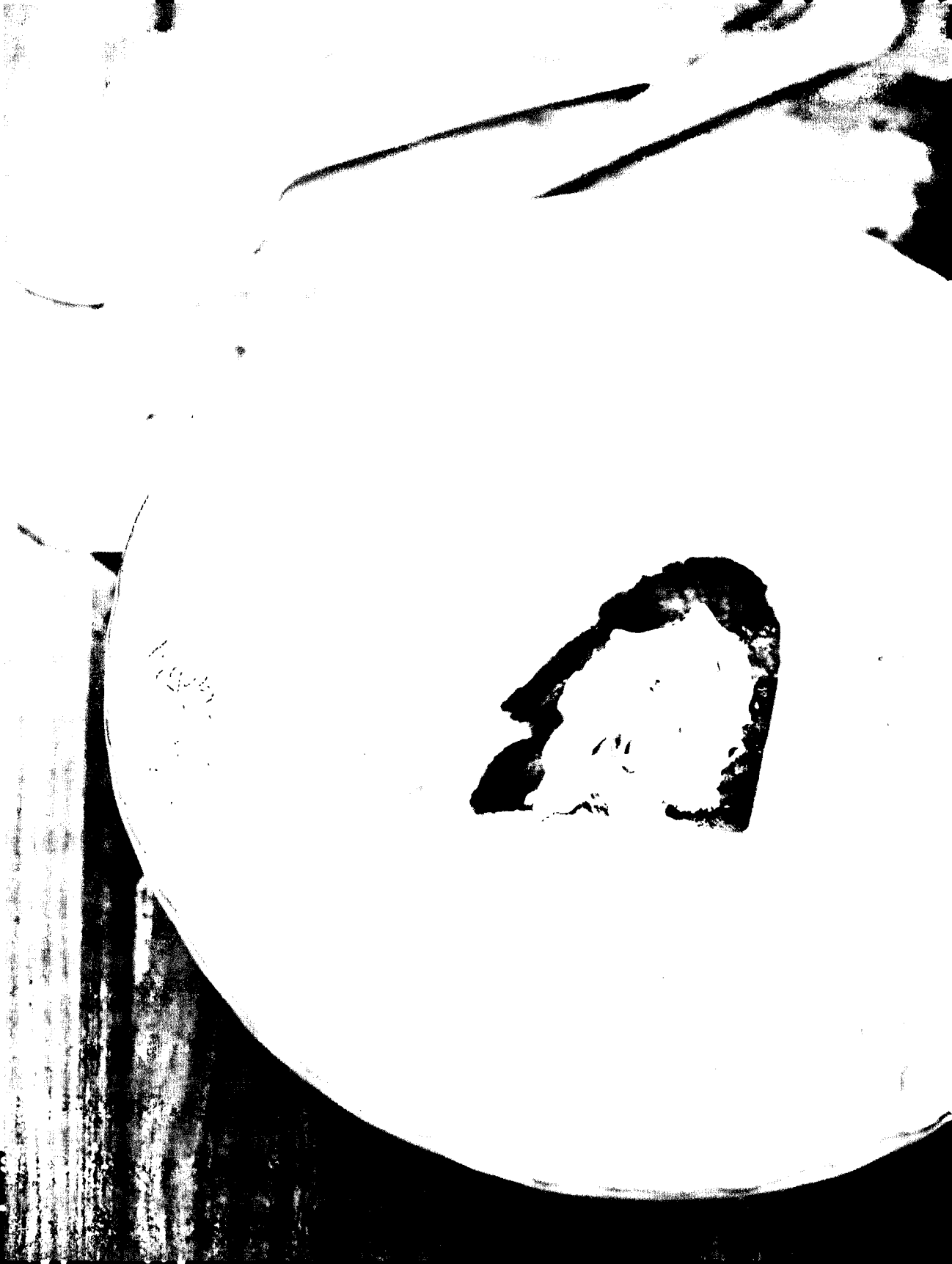

$\mathbb{S}$MOKE TWICE THE TOMATOES FOR THIS RECIPE AND FREEZE and date the extras so you have them the next time you want to make this wonderful soup. Smoked tomatoes also star in Smoked Summer Tomato Basil Butter (page 50), which is delicious slathered on bread or tossed with hot pasta. Add a dollop of Béarnaise Butter (page 29) on a toasted piece of bread to float atop the soup.

SMOKED TOMATO BISQUE

SERVES 4

1 cup moistened wood chips or dry wood pellets

8 plum tomatoes (about 3 pounds)

2 cups chicken stock

1 cup heavy whipping cream

4 ounces goat cheese, crumbled

2 tablespoons fresh lemon juice

Kosher salt and freshly ground black pepper to taste

1 cup chopped fresh basil

Prepare a hot fire on one side of your grill for indirect cooking. Oil a perforated grill rack and place on the grill. For a charcoal grill, throw moistened wood chips or dry wood pellets directly on the coals right before you want to grill. For a gas grill, enclose the wood chips or pellets in a foil packet with holes poked in the top; place the packet on the grill grate over the heat source.

When you see the first wisp of smoke from the wood, place the tomatoes on the indirect or no-heat side of the grill. Close the lid and smoke for about 30 minutes, or until skin starts to peel back from the tomatoes and they have a good, smoky aroma. Let cool, then peel, and chop.

In a large saucepan, heat the chicken stock and cream over medium heat, stirring constantly until just beginning to boil. Add the goat cheese and stir until melted. Add the smoked tomatoes and lemon juice; cook until heated through. Season to taste with salt and pepper.

To serve, ladle the soup into bowls and garnish with fresh basil.

THIS THAI-STYLE SEAFOOD SOUP IS RELATIVELY EASY TO PREPARE and perfect for using leftover grilled vegetables and shrimp from a previous dinner. If you like, substitute grilled chicken for the shrimp. Red curry paste, a mildly hot mixture ground from chiles and aromatic ingredients such as lemongrass and the tuber galangal, is available in the Asian section of the grocery store. If you grow ginger and lemongrass in pots, you can just dig up a little of the fresh ginger root and snip off a lemongrass stalk for this recipe. Likewise, snow peas, a cooler weather crop, are easy to harvest and use here.

RED CURRY-COCONUT SOUP *with* GRILLED VEGETABLES AND SHRIMP

SERVES 6

1 tablespoon vegetable oil

½-inch piece of fresh ginger, sliced

1 lemongrass stalk, sliced into 1-inch pieces

1 tablespoon red curry paste, or more to taste

4½ cups chicken stock

1 cup coconut milk

½ cup heavy whipping cream

1 cup snow or sugar snap peas

1 pint grape or cherry tomatoes

1 cup green onions cut on the diagonal into 1-inch pieces (about 12 green onions)

4 ounces fresh mushrooms, sliced

Prepare a hot fire in your grill.

While the grill is heating, heat the oil in a large saucepan over high heat. Add the ginger, lemongrass, and red curry paste and sauté for about 1 minute or until fragrant. Add the chicken stock, coconut milk, and cream and bring to a boil. Reduce the heat and simmer for 15 to 20 minutes until the soup is slightly reduced.

While the soup is simmering, combine the snap peas, tomatoes, green onions, mushrooms, water chestnuts, and shrimp in a grill basket or wok set on top of a baking sheet. Drizzle the oil over all and toss to coat and take out to the grill. Place the basket directly over the hot fire. Grill for about 10 to 12 minutes, turning often, until the vegetables are warmed through and shrimp is just opaque. Bring inside.

Remove the ginger and lemongrass from the

1 (8-ounce) can water chestnuts, drained and sliced

½ pound medium shrimp, peeled and deveined

2 to 3 tablespoons vegetable oil

Zest and juice of 1 lime, or more to taste

Kosher or sea salt to taste

Hot sauce to taste

Thai basil, shredded, for garnish

soup with a slotted spoon. Add the grilled vegetable and shrimp mixture and the lime zest and juice. Simmer for 5 more minutes. Season to taste with salt and hot sauce. To serve, ladle the soup into bowls and garnish with shredded Thai basil.

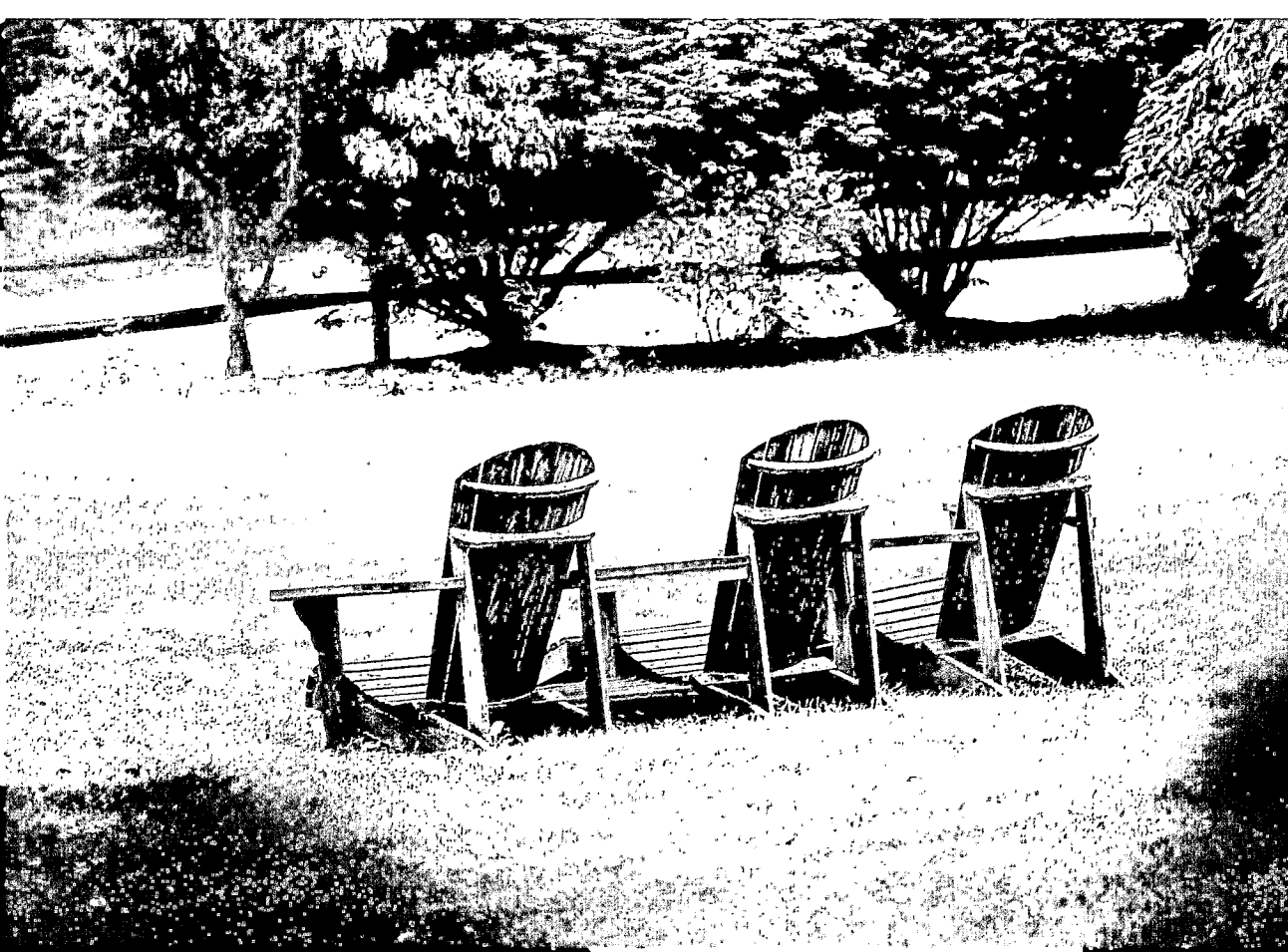

WHEN YOU STILL HAVE SOME SWEET POTATOES IN YOUR COLD cellar, make this creamy, golden soup to feed body and soul. By par-cooking the sweet potatoes first, you cut the time they need to smoke on the grill. Take this soup in insulated containers to a tailgate party, then add a fresh rosemary branch to each mug as an aromatic swizzle stick.

SMOKED and SMASHED
SWEET POTATO SOUP

SERVES 4

4 large sweet potatoes

2 red onions, chopped

6 cloves garlic, chopped

Olive oil, for drizzling

Kosher or sea salt and freshly ground black pepper to taste

4 fresh rosemary branches, plus more for garnish

1 cup moistened wood chips or dry wood pellets

4 cups vegetable or chicken broth

Prick the sweet potatoes all over with a fork. Microwave on high for 8 to 10 minutes or until partially cooked but not soft. Peel the potatoes and cut into 1-inch pieces. Combine the sweet potato, onion, and garlic in a 9 x 13-inch disposable aluminum pan. Drizzle with olive oil and season with salt and pepper. Tuck the rosemary branches in amongst the vegetables.

Prepare a hot fire on one side of your grill for indirect cooking. For a charcoal grill, throw moistened wood chips or dry wood pellets directly on the coals right before you want to grill. For a gas grill, enclose the wood chips or pellets in a foil packet with holes poked in the top; place the packet on the grill grate over the heat source.

When you see the first wisp of smoke from the wood, place the potatoes, onions, and garlic on the indirect or no-heat side of the grill. Close the lid and smoke for about 1 hour, turning the mixture once or twice, until the potatoes are fork tender and have a smoky aroma.

In a large pot, combine the vegetable broth and the sweet potato mixture. Mash with a potato masher or puree with an immersion blender until somewhat smooth. Bring to a boil over medium-high heat, stirring occasionally, then reduce the heat and simmer for 15 minutes. Season to taste. To serve, ladle the soup into mugs and garnish each with a rosemary branch as a stirrer.

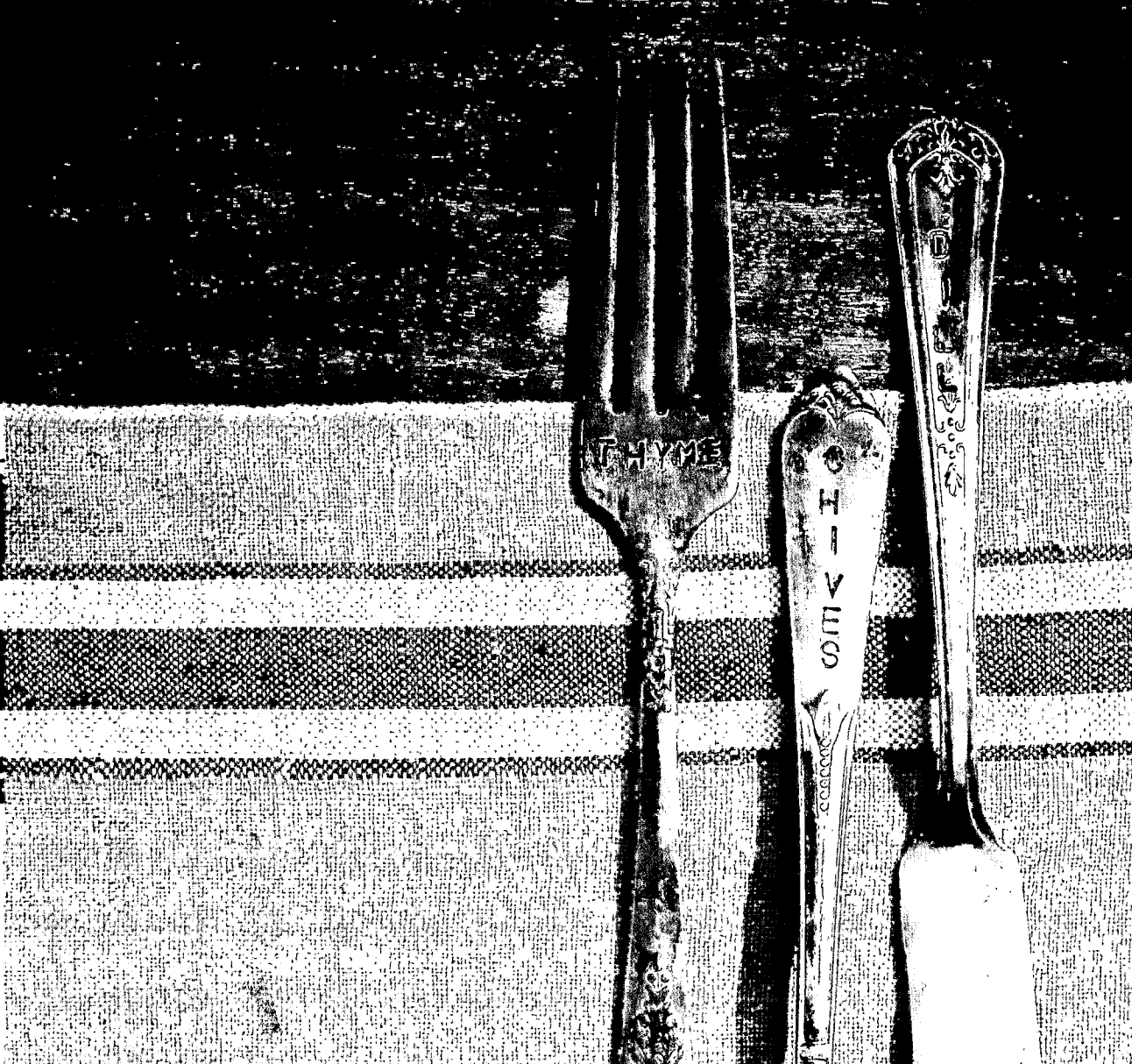

CHAPTER 5

MEAT, POULTRY & FISH

WHEN YOU'VE GOT A GARDEN GOING AND THE GRILL FIRED UP, dinner is only minutes away. A few fresh-picked vegetables and fruits, snipped herbs, and tender cuts of poultry, pork, beef, fish, and shellfish can all combine for a meal worth celebrating. At the very least, you can add a handful of fresh greens to each plate, top them with something grilled, and drizzle the plate with garden-fresh vinaigrette.

Choose thin, tender, boneless cuts of chicken, turkey, pork, or beef to cook as quickly as the vegetables do. Boneless chicken or turkey breast, boneless chicken thighs, pork tenderloin, and boneless steaks all grill well with vegetables.

You can easily substitute firm tofu for any of the chicken, turkey, pork, or beef cuts; simply brush the tofu with olive oil, season to taste, and grill, turning once, until the tofu has good grill marks. Tofu is already "cooked," so you're just adding the grill flavor.

Chicken, turkey, pork, and sausage of all kinds should be completely cooked through to a temperature of 160 to 165°F. Remember that the meat's internal temperature will continue to rise by about 5 degrees after you take it off the grill. Thin cuts are difficult to judge by temperature; it's just as easy to cut into the middle to check doneness. The juices should run clear.

Beef steaks, on the other hand, can be easily checked with a grill or instant-read thermometer. Just remember that the temperature will continue to rise by about 5 degrees after you take the steak off the grill. So, if you like your steak rare (125°F), pull it off the grill when the internal temperature reaches 120°F. Let the steak rest for about 5 to 10 minutes; this also helps keep the juices from running out of the steak when it's cut.Fish fillets and shellfish cook quickly. Fish cooks in about 10 minutes per inch of thickness over a hot fire, turning once. Most fish fillets are about $3/4$ inch thick in the thickest part, so they take about 7 to 8 minutes total to grill. By turning fish fillets only once (and preferably with a wide fish spatula), you keep the delicate fish from falling apart on the grill. If you've never grilled a fish fillet before, practice on a less expensive, but still delicious, farm-raised catfish fillet.

If you have a large grill, you can do the meat on one side and the vegetables on the other. If you have a small grill, it's best for food safety reasons to grill the vegetables first.

Skewered Chicken Saltimbocca ...137

Chicken Paillard and Baby Green Beans
with Mustard Seed Sauce ...138

A Raised Garden Bed ...139

Tandoori Turkey Burgers with
Grilled Red Onions and Tomatoes ...140

Grilled Turkey Breast over Winter Greens with
Warm Cranberry Vinaigrette ...142

Brats with Grilled Kale and Horseradish Butter ...143

Grilled Pork Tenderloin with Fresh Fig Skewers ...144

Wood-Grilled Shrimp and Yellow Peppers ...146

Peppered Tuna with Grilled Peach, Red Bell Pepper,
and Onion Relish ...147

Baja Fish Tacos ...148

Char-Grilled Salmon and Baby Squash ...150

Grilled Salmon in Corn Husks ...151

South-of-the-Border Garden ...152

Grilled Caesar Sirloin ...153

Blackened Beef with Thai Chile Noodles
and Baby Bok Choy ...154

Flank Steak with Grilled Peppers and Onions ...156

Kansas City Strip Steaks with
Parmesan Grilled Vegetables ...157

TRADITIONALLY, SALTIMBOCCA MEANS A THIN CUT OF VEAL AND fresh sage leaves that are wrapped in prosciutto and cooked in a skillet. This grilled version with chicken gives you the flavor of the traditional recipe, but grilled on skewers. You'll need 8 pre-soaked wooden skewers or flat metal skewers to make this. The sage leaves and red onion add just the right touch of garden fresh flavor.

SKEWERED CHICKEN SALTIMBOCCA

SERVES 4

1 pound boneless, skinless chicken breasts, cut into 16 chunks

4 slices prosciutto, each slice cut lengthwise into 4 long pieces

12 large sage leaves

4 small red onions, peeled and quartered (about 1½ pounds)

Olive oil, for brushing and drizzling

2 large lemons, quartered

4 cups baby greens

Prepare a medium-hot fire in your grill.

Wrap a piece of prosciutto around each chicken piece. Slide each prosciutto-wrapped chicken piece onto a skewer, followed by a sage leaf, and a single quarter of red onion. Repeat so that each skewer begins and ends with a piece of chicken. Lightly brush the skewers with olive oil.

Place the skewers perpendicular to the grill grates over the fire. Grill for about 15 minutes, turning every 2 or 3 minutes, until chicken is firm and cooked through.

To serve, place a cup of baby greens on each plate and place the skewers on the greens. Drizzle with olive oil and fresh lemon juice.

HIS RECIPE IS ACTUALLY FRENCH "FAST FOOD." ONCE YOU TRY grilling a chicken breast this simple way, you'll be amazed at how juicy and delicious it is! A *paillard* is a thin piece of boneless, skinless chicken breast, veal, or pork tenderloin. On a hot grill, a *paillard* will take a total of 10 minutes per inch of thickness to cook. So, if you cut and pound a boneless, skinless chicken breast to a $\frac{1}{2}$-inch thickness, you can grill it in $2\frac{1}{2}$ minutes per side, or 5 minutes total. It makes sense to serve it with equally fast side dishes, such as baby green beans drizzled with Mustard Seed Sauce (page 37), Rosemary, Garlic, and Lemon Baste (page 27), or with a dollop of the aioli of your choice (page 40).

CHICKEN PAILLARD *and* BABY GREEN BEANS *with* MUSTARD SEED SAUCE

SERVES 4

4 boneless skinless chicken breast halves (about $1\frac{1}{2}$ pounds)

Olive oil, for brushing and drizzling

1 pound baby green beans

Fine kosher or sea salt and freshly ground black pepper to taste

1 recipe Mustard Seed Sauce (page 37)

Prepare a hot fire in your grill.

To make paillards, slice the chicken breasts in half through the middle so that they are half of their original thickness. Place 2 chicken breast pieces between 2 sheets of parchment paper and quickly pound with a meat cleaver or a rolling pin until the pieces are about $\frac{1}{2}$-inch thick. Brush the paillards on both sides with olive oil.

Place the baby green beans in a perforated grill wok or basket and lightly drizzle with olive oil.

Grill the beans first placing the wok directly over the fire and tossing every 2 minutes until they are slightly charred, about 6 to 8 minutes total cooking time. Then remove the wok.

Grill the chicken paillards directly over the fire for $2\frac{1}{2}$ minutes per side, turning once.

To serve, place the chicken and beans on each plate and season to taste with salt and pepper. Spoon over the Mustard Seed Sauce or sauce of your choice.

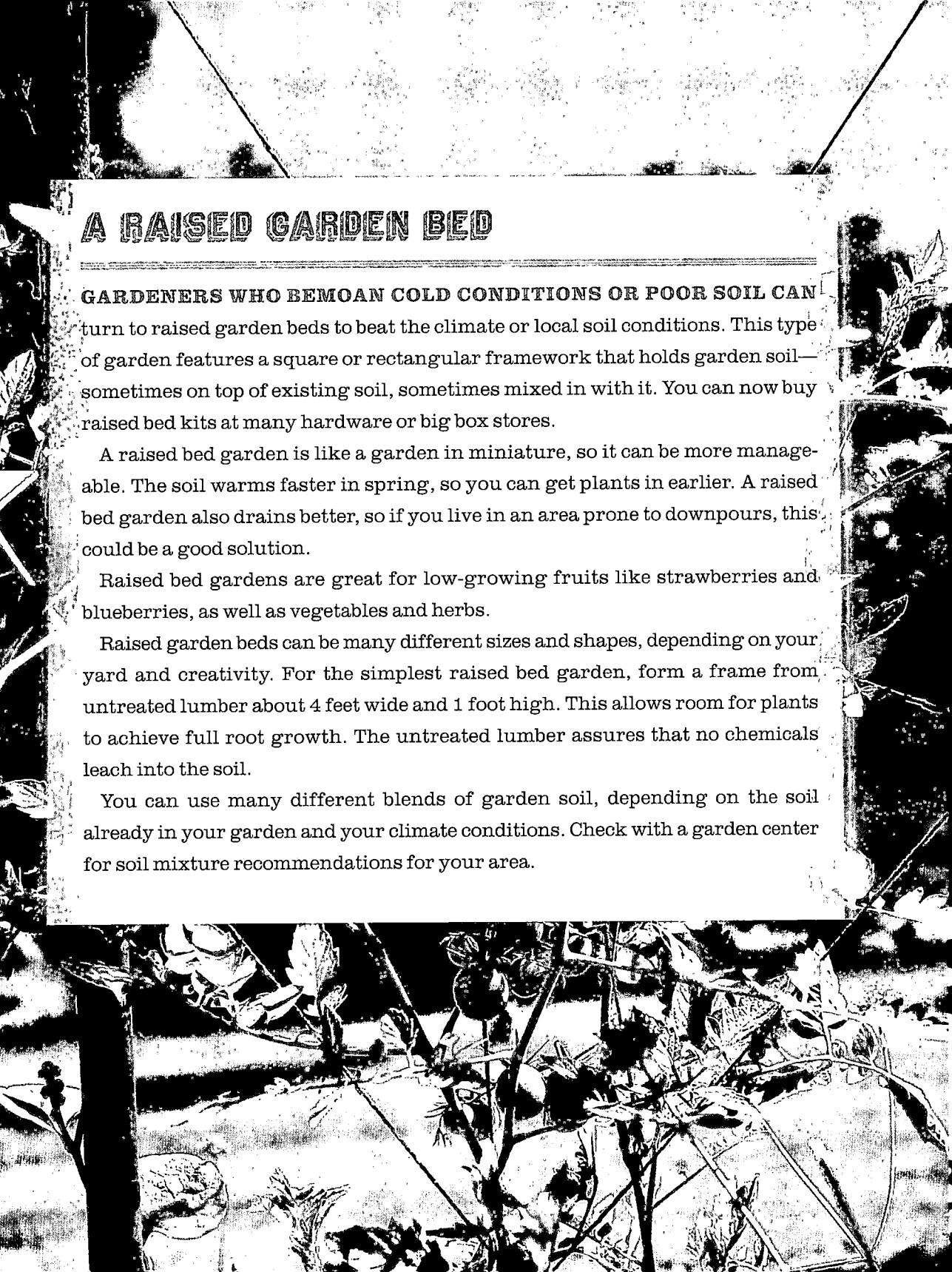

A RAISED GARDEN BED

GARDENERS WHO BEMOAN COLD CONDITIONS OR POOR SOIL CAN turn to raised garden beds to beat the climate or local soil conditions. This type of garden features a square or rectangular framework that holds garden soil— sometimes on top of existing soil, sometimes mixed in with it. You can now buy raised bed kits at many hardware or big box stores.

A raised bed garden is like a garden in miniature, so it can be more manageable. The soil warms faster in spring, so you can get plants in earlier. A raised bed garden also drains better, so if you live in an area prone to downpours, this could be a good solution.

Raised bed gardens are great for low-growing fruits like strawberries and blueberries, as well as vegetables and herbs.

Raised garden beds can be many different sizes and shapes, depending on your yard and creativity. For the simplest raised bed garden, form a frame from untreated lumber about 4 feet wide and 1 foot high. This allows room for plants to achieve full root growth. The untreated lumber assures that no chemicals leach into the soil.

You can use many different blends of garden soil, depending on the soil already in your garden and your climate conditions. Check with a garden center for soil mixture recommendations for your area.

THIS LEANER, HEALTHIER BURGER IS JUICY AND DELICIOUS, too. You can serve the grilled onions and tomatoes both as a topping for the burgers and as a vegetable side dish. If you have any leftover onions and tomatoes, chop them together with sprigs of fresh cilantro and a squeeze of lime juice to make a great grilled salsa. Serve the burgers with a super-simple cumin yogurt sauce.

TANDOORI TURKEY BURGERS *with* GRILLED RED ONIONS *and* TOMATOES

SERVES 4

TURKEY BURGERS

1 pound ground turkey

¼ cup fine, dry breadcrumbs

2 tablespoons plain yogurt

1 teaspoon turmeric

1 teaspoon ground coriander

1 teaspoon ground cumin

1 teaspoon fine kosher or sea salt

CUMIN YOGURT SAUCE

½ cup plain yogurt

½ teaspoon ground cumin

Kosher or sea salt and freshly ground black pepper to taste

TOPPINGS

2 large red onions, thickly sliced

2 large beefsteak tomatoes, thickly sliced

Prepare a medium-hot fire in your grill.

In a large bowl, combine the ground turkey, breadcrumbs, yogurt, turmeric, coriander, cumin, and salt until well blended. Form into four ¾-inch-thick patties.

For the cumin yogurt sauce, combine the yogurt and cumin together in a bowl until smooth. Season to taste with salt and pepper.

Toss the shredded lettuce and cilantro in a bowl and set aside.

Lightly brush the sliced onions, tomatoes, and cut side of the hamburger buns with olive oil and season with salt and pepper. Grill the patties, onions, and tomatoes directly over the fire. Grill the tomatoes for about 2 to 3 minutes on each side. Turn the burgers once after 7 to 8 minutes, then grill for another 7 to 8 minutes, or until the burgers are no longer pink inside and an instant-read thermometer registers 160°F in the center of each patty.

4 seeded hamburger buns

Olive oil, for brushing

Kosher or sea salt and freshly ground black pepper to taste

1 cup shredded lettuce

2 tablespoons chopped fresh cilantro

Grill the onions for about 8 to 9 minutes, turning once halfway through the cooking time, or until softened and slightly charred. During the last minutes of grilling, toast the buns, cut sides down, directly over the fire.

To serve, place a patty on each bun. Top with a slice of grilled onion, tomato, and $\frac{1}{4}$ cup lettuce mixture and a dollop of yogurt sauce. Serve the extra grilled onion and tomato slices on the side.

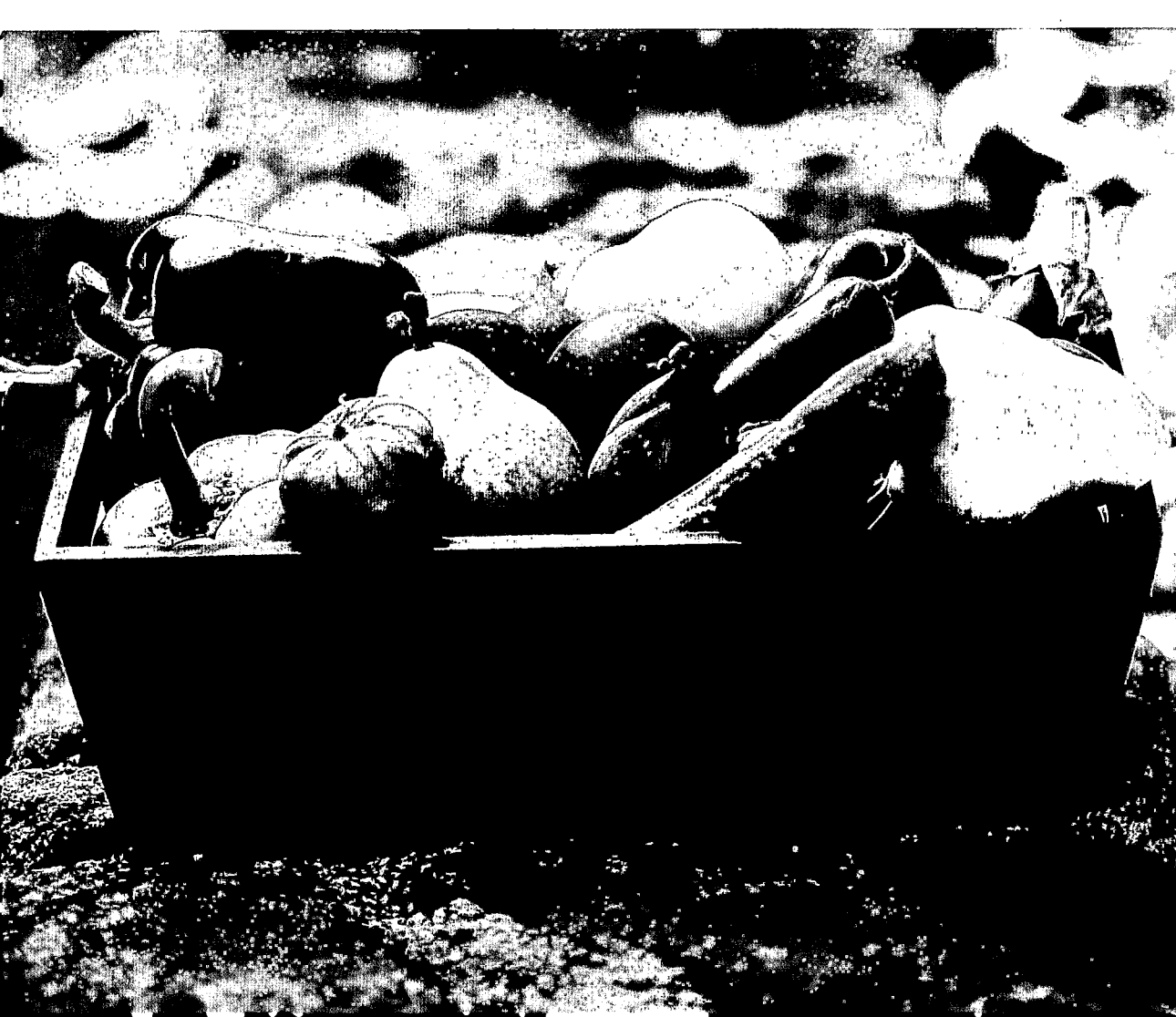

TURKEY BREAST TENDERLOIN STEAKS, CUT ½-INCH THICK, grill like chicken paillard—quickly and easily. For turkey, however, it's best to use a medium to medium-hot fire, as it tends to dry out faster than chicken at higher temperatures. Serve the grilled turkey with an assortment of winter garden greens like spinach, arugula, watercress, tat soi, and kale. Spoon the warm cranberry vinaigrette over all for a delicious twist on tradition. The vinaigrette keeps in the refrigerator for up to 2 weeks.

GRILLED TURKEY BREAST over WINTER GREENS with WARM CRANBERRY VINAIGRETTE

SERVES 4

TURKEY

Four 4- to 6-ounce turkey breast tenderloin steaks, ½-inch-thick

Olive oil, for rubbing

Fine kosher or sea salt and freshly ground black pepper to taste

4 cups assorted tender baby winter greens, such as spinach, tat soi, or kale, torn into small pieces if necessary

WARM CRANBERRY VINAIGRETTE

1½ cups fresh cranberries, picked over and rinsed

¼ cup sugar

3 tablespoons cider vinegar

3 tablespoons orange juice

Prepare a medium to medium-hot fire in your grill. Rub the steaks with olive oil, season with salt and pepper, and set aside.

For the cranberry vinaigrette, heat the cranberries, sugar, and vinegar in a saucepan over medium heat until the cranberries pop, about 5 to 7 minutes. Remove from the heat and add the orange juice, vegetable oil, Dijon mustard, garlic, red pepper flakes, and cinnamon, whisking to blend well. The vinaigrette can be thinned with additional orange juice or vinegar if it is too thick.

Place the turkey steaks directly over the fire and grill for 12 to 15 minutes, turning once, until no longer pink when cut in the center and the internal temperature reads 160°F (the temperature will continue to rise after it comes off the grill). Tent the turkey steaks with foil and allow them to rest for 5 to 10 minutes.

3 tablespoons vegetable oil

1 teaspoon Dijon mustard

1 garlic clove, minced

$\frac{1}{4}$ teaspoon red pepper flakes

$\frac{1}{4}$ teaspoon cinnamon

To serve, place the greens on each plate, top with the grilled turkey, and spoon the warm cranberry vinaigrette over all.

THE FALL GARDENER ENJOYS THE PLEASURES OF COOL WEATHER greens, root vegetables, and orchard fruits. Hearty fare like brats are wonderful served with kale and zesty horseradish butter. A combination of green and purple kale leaves is prettiest for this dish. If you like, switch out the sausage of your choice for the brats.

BRATS *with* GRILLED KALE *and* HORSERADISH BUTTER

SERVES 4

HORSERADISH BUTTER

$\frac{1}{2}$ cup (1 stick) unsalted butter, softened so it can be stirred with a fork

1$\frac{1}{2}$ tablespoons fresh horseradish

2 teaspoons grainy mustard

SAUSAGE AND KALE

12 large kale leaves, washed and dried (preferably a mix of green and purple)

Olive oil cooking spray

4 bratwurst or other link sausages

4 slices of good-quality pumpernickel bread

Prepare a medium-hot fire in your grill.

Combine the butter, horseradish, and grainy mustard and set aside. Spray both sides of the kale leaves with olive oil.

Grill the sausage, turning every 4 minutes, until cooked through, about 12 minutes or a little more, depending on the diameter of the sausage. Grill the kale leaves 1 to 2 minutes per side until leaves are browned in spots and the edges are browned and slightly wilted.

Arrange kale leaves on the plate and top with a bratwurst. Serve the Horseradish Butter and pumpernickel bread on the side.

FIG TREES LOVE WARMER CLIMATES. BUT, FOR THE ADVENTUROUS northern gardener, the best way to grow figs is in a container that can be placed outdoors in warm weather and then brought indoors to winter. The best variety for a container is the Petite Negri fig, a small- to medium-sized black fruit with sweet, red flesh. If you have great weather, Mission figs are superb.

GRILLED PORK TENDERLOIN
with FRESH FIG SKEWERS

SERVES 4

One (1 to 1¼ pounds) pork tenderloin or center-cut pork filet

2 tablespoons olive oil, plus more for brushing

Fine kosher or sea salt and freshly ground black pepper to taste

4 long rosemary branches or wooden skewers, soaked in water for at least 15 minutes

12 small ripe figs

4 ounces goat cheese

2 teaspoons honey

1½ teaspoons finely chopped fresh rosemary

Prepare a hot fire in your grill. Brush the tenderloin with the olive oil and season with salt and pepper.

Remove the skewers from the water. Pierce the figs through the middle with a metal skewer or ice pick to make a hole. Then thread 3 figs onto each rosemary or wooden skewer. Lightly brush the figs with olive oil.

Place the pork tenderloin directly over the fire. Grill for 2 to 3 minutes per side (the center-cut pork loin filet for 5 to 7 minutes per side), turning a quarter turn at a time, until an instant-read meat thermometer inserted in the thickest part registers 140°F for medium and the meat is juicy and slightly pink in the center.

At the same time, place the skewered figs over the fire, turning several times and cooking for about 5 to 6 minutes until they are heated through. When they're caramelized and soft, remove the skewers from the heat and keep warm.

Let the pork rest for about 5 minutes, and then cut on the diagonal into 1- to 2-inch-thick slices.

To serve, arrange 3 slices of pork with a skewer of figs on each plate, all topped with crumbled goat cheese, ½ teaspoon honey, and chopped rosemary.

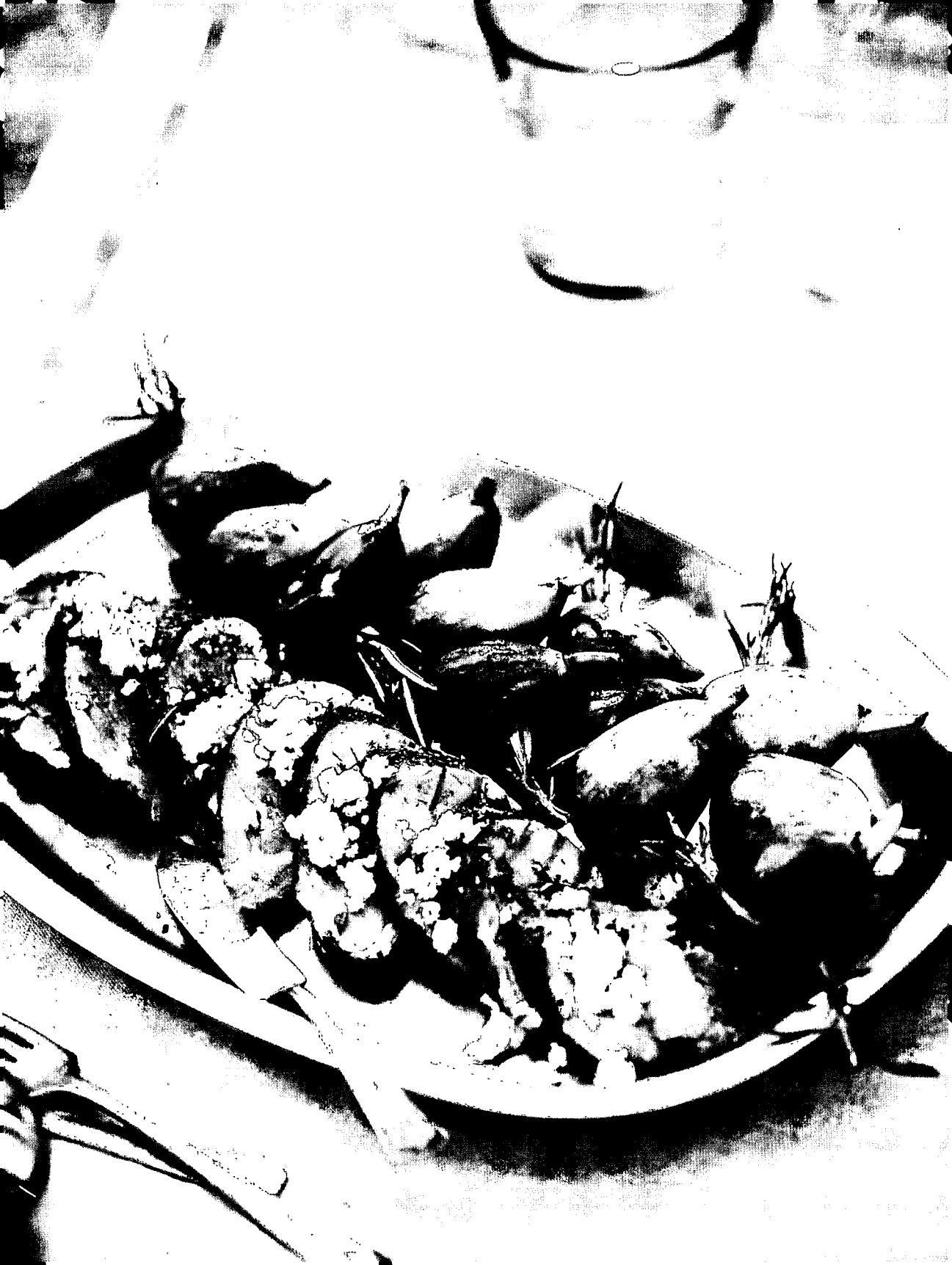

WRAPPING SHRIMP WITH A SPINACH LEAF HELPS TO KEEP IT tender and moist. For contrasting color, wrap half of the shrimp and leave the other half unwrapped for dark green and pink against the golden yellow of the peppers. Mesquite, oak, or pecan wood lend a smoky flavor to this dish.

WOOD-GRILLED SHRIMP
and YELLOW PEPPERS

SERVES 4

½ cup moistened wood chips or dry wood pellets

1½ pounds large shrimp (18-20 count), peeled and deveined

30 medium-size spinach leaves

2 yellow, red, or orange bell peppers, stemmed, seeded, and cut into quarters

¼ cup olive oil

Kosher or sea salt and freshly ground black pepper to taste

Prepare a hot fire on one side of your grill for indirect cooking.

Wrap each shrimp loosely with a large spinach leaf. Place the shrimp in a disposable aluminum pan. Lightly season with sea salt and pepper, and then drizzle lightly with olive oil.

For a charcoal grill, throw ½ cup moistened wood chips or dry wood pellets directly on the coals right before you want to grill. For a gas grill, enclose the wood chips or pellets in a foil packet with holes poked in the top; place the packet on the grill grate over the heat source.

When you see the first wisp of smoke from the wood, place the shrimp on the indirect side of the heat and the peppers on the direct side. Close the lid and grill for 8 minutes. Open the lid and turn the peppers. Grill for another 8 minutes, then open the lid and transfer the peppers to the indirect side. Close the lid and grill for 15 to 20 minutes more, or until the shrimp are cooked through and they have a pleasant smoky aroma.

To serve, cut the peppers into strips, arrange on plates, and top with the shrimp.

SERVE THIS PEPPERY TUNA AND REFRESHING PEACH RELISH with grilled sweet corn.

PEPPERED TUNA *with* GRILLED PEACH, RED BELL PEPPER, *and* ONION RELISH

SERVES 4

PEPPERED TUNA

Four 8-ounce tuna steaks, 1 inch thick

$\frac{1}{4}$ cup extra virgin olive oil

1 teaspoon sea salt

4 teaspoons freshly ground black pepper

FRESH PEACH AND ONION RELISH

3 ripe peaches (about 1$\frac{1}{2}$ pounds), peeled, halved, and pitted

1 red bell pepper, halved, stemmed, and seeded

1 red onion, peeled and sliced $\frac{1}{2}$-inch thick

$\frac{1}{3}$ cup vegetable oil

2 tablespoons white wine vinegar

2 tablespoons fresh lime juice

1 tablespoon chopped fresh mint

1 tablespoon honey

2 garlic cloves, minced

Prepare a hot fire in your grill. Lightly rub the tuna steaks with the olive oil and season generously with salt and pepper. Lightly brush the peaches, red pepper, and onions with olive oil. Set aside.

In a large bowl, combine the vegetable oil, vinegar, lime juice, mint, honey, and garlic, stirring to blend. Set aside.

Grill the fruit and vegetables first, directly over the fire for about 7 to 10 minutes until they all have nice grill marks. Grill the tuna directly over the fire for about 3 minutes per side for rare (do not overcook). Remove from the grill and tent the fish with aluminum foil to keep warm.

Chop the grilled peaches, pepper, and onion. Stir the vinaigrette, then add the chopped fruit and vegetables to the dressing and stir to blend.

To serve, spoon the relish with its juices onto each plate. Top with the tuna and serve immediately.

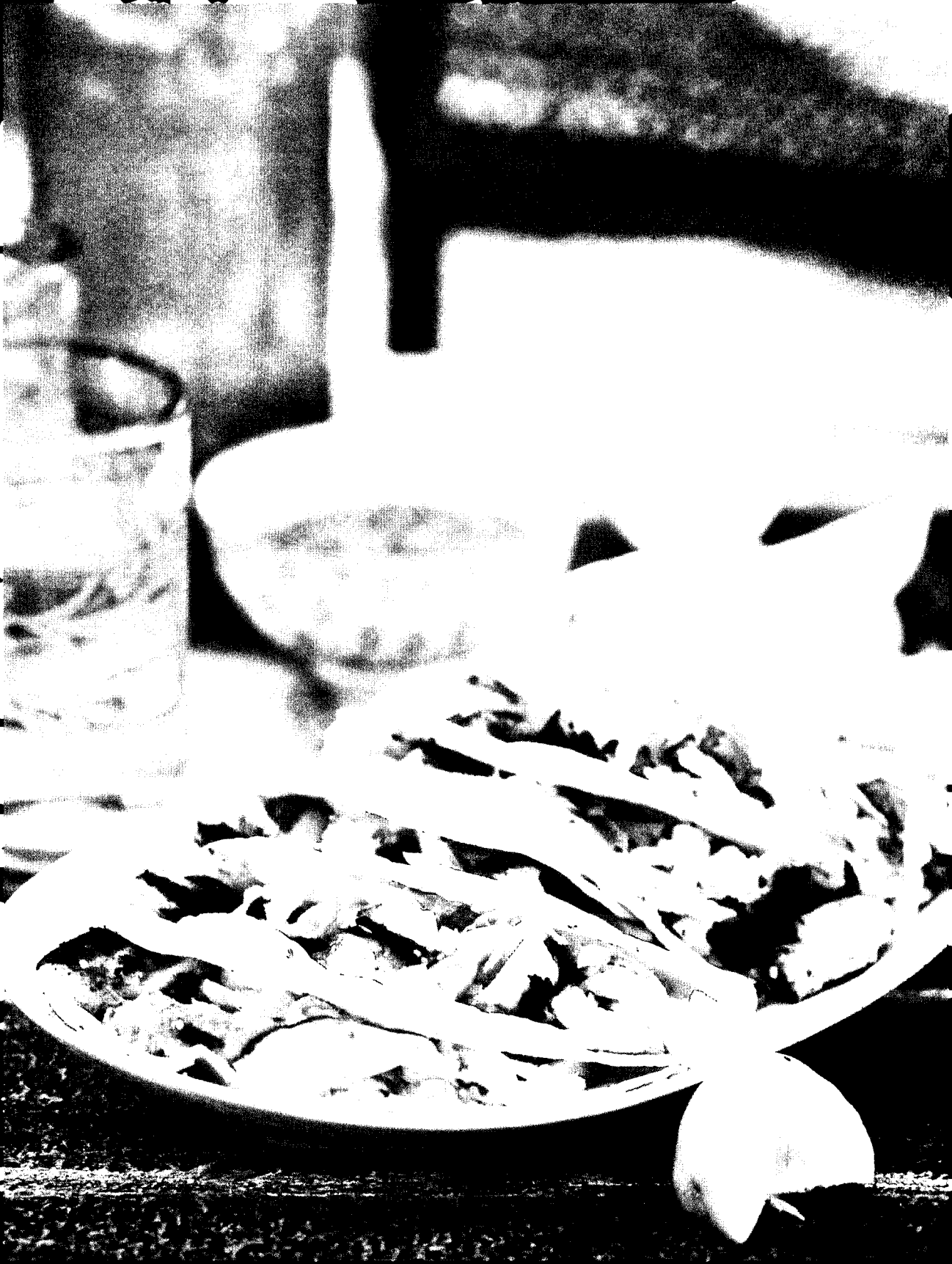

ISH TACOS DON'T GET ANY BETTER THAN THIS. THE RED HOT Blackened Seasoning (page 14) makes $1\frac{1}{2}$ cups, but for this recipe you only need $\frac{1}{4}$ cup. So make a half recipe or better yet, start using it to give some zip to sauces, vinaigrettes, soups, stews, and other grilled vegetables and meats. If you like, serve the tacos with Grilled Corn-in-the-Husk with Ancho-Lime Butter (page 175). Grill the "flesh," or cut side of the fish first (not the skin side) because it is more delicate. Then turn the fish, and finish on the skin side, which has more connective tissue, and will hold together better on the grill.

BAJA FISH TACOS

SERVES 4

GRILLED NAPA CABBAGE SLAW

1 large head Napa cabbage, cut in half lengthwise

Vegetable oil, for brushing

1 cup assorted baby greens

8 green onions, chopped (white and green parts)

$\frac{1}{4}$ cup tarragon vinegar

$\frac{1}{4}$ cup sour cream

$\frac{1}{2}$ cup freshly squeezed lemon juice

$\frac{1}{2}$ teaspoon fine kosher or sea salt

BAJA FISH

$1\frac{1}{2}$ pounds mahi mahi, catfish, halibut, or other mild white fish

$\frac{1}{4}$ cup Red Hot Blackened Seasoning (page 14)

8 flour tortillas, for serving

8 lemon wedges, for serving

$1\frac{1}{2}$ cups salsa, for serving

Prepare a hot fire in your grill.

Brush the cut sides of the Napa cabbage with oil. Coat the fish fillets with the Red Hot Blackened Seasoning.

Grill the cabbage, cut side down, directly over the fire for 2 to 3 minutes or until the cabbage has good grill marks. Remove from the grill.

Grill the fish directly over the fire, flesh side down first, for 4 to 5 minutes per side, or 10 minutes per inch of thickness. Turn only once to grill the skin side, halfway through grilling.

To make the slaw, thinly slice the grilled cabbage and place in a large bowl. Stir in the greens and green onions. In a small bowl, combine the vinegar, sour cream, lemon juice, and salt to make a dressing. Pour the dressing over the cabbage mixture and toss to blend.

To assemble the tacos, place some of the grilled fish on each tortilla. Top with about $\frac{1}{3}$ cup of the slaw and roll up, soft taco-style. Serve with a lemon wedge and a small ramekin of salsa.

SALMON PAIRED WITH AN ASSORTMENT OF BABY SQUASH, SUCH as zucchini, patty pan, and yellow crookneck, can all grill at the same time. The salmon, yellow, and green color combination pleases the gardener, while the griller will love the flavor from the fire. To finish this dish with a final kick, dollop on Spicy Chipotle Aioli (page 40) or compound butter. Pour a glass of crisp, chilled Pinot Grigio, and life is good.

CHAR-GRILLED SALMON
and BABY SQUASH

SERVES 6

Six 6-ounce salmon fillets, skin on

¼ cup olive oil, divided

Seasoning Salt (page 13) to taste

1 pound assorted whole baby squash, such as zucchini, patty pan, and yellow crookneck

Spicy Chipotle Aioli (page 40)

Prepare a hot fire in your grill.

Lightly coat the salmon fillets with about 2 tablespoons of the olive oil and sprinkle the flesh side with the Seasoning Salt. In a bowl, toss the baby squash with the remaining 2 tablespoons of olive oil and Seasoning Salt to taste.

Grill the salmon, flesh (lighter in color) side down, for about 5 minutes. Turn once and grill for another 5 minutes. At the same time, place the squash on a perforated grill rack and grill, turning, until the squash have browned slightly and are crisp tender, 6 to 8 minutes total.

Serve hot, with a dollop of the aioli on top of the fish or on the side.

I N THIS RECIPE, THE CORNHUSKS WRAP THE SALMON AND CHOPPED
vegetables like a special gift. Make the job a little easier by doing the prep work
in the morning and keep refrigerated until ready to grill later. Other fish fillets
like catfish, halibut, and red snapper, along with shellfish like shrimp and smaller
bay scallops, can be substituted for the salmon. Choose other seasonal vegetables
and herbs from the garden to top the fish in the corn husks.

GRILLED SALMON in CORN HUSKS

SERVES 4

4 ears of corn, with the
 husks on

Four 6-ounce skinless
 salmon fillets

4 green onions, chopped

¼ cup seeded and chopped
 red bell pepper

4 teaspoons capers,
 drained

¼ cup (½ stick) unsalted
 butter, cut into 4 tablespoon portions

4 sprigs fresh thyme

Kosher or sea salt and
 freshly ground black pepper to taste

Peel back the husk and remove the silk from the
corn. Break off the corncob at the base, leaving the
husk attached. With a sharp knife, slice the kernels
off 2 of the ears. Combine the kernels with the green
onions, red pepper, and capers in a bowl. Set aside
the other 2 ears. Prepare a hot fire on one side of
your grill for indirect cooking.

Fold back a few of the leaves of each corn husk and
place a salmon fillet in each. Top each fillet with one
quarter of the corn mixture. Top with 1 tablespoon
butter and a sprig of thyme. Season with salt and
pepper to taste. Tie the husk closed so it completely
encloses the salmon, using strips of the corn husk
or kitchen twine. (This can be done earlier in the day
and kept refrigerated until ready to grill.)

When ready to grill, place the packets on the grill
directly over the fire and grill for 5 minutes. Move
to the indirect side and continue to cook for another
6 to 7 minutes with the grill lid closed.

Serve the corn husk packets by folding back the
top of the corn husk to display the salmon inside.

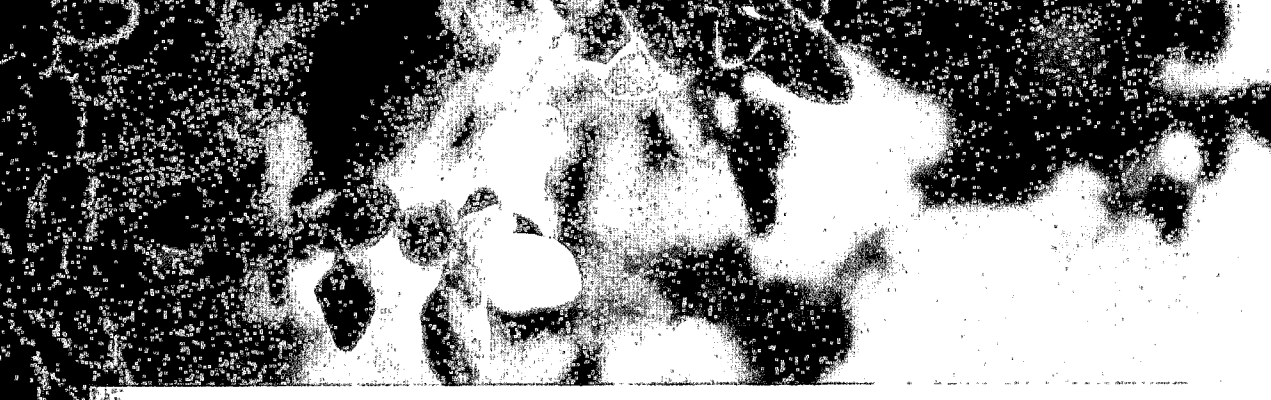

SOUTH-OF-THE-BORDER GARDEN

IF YOU LOVE FAJITAS, TACOS, OR OTHER MEXICAN DISHES, GROWING your own peppers, tomatoes, and herbs can lend the dishes you love more authentic flavors. In pots on a patio or in a garden plot, these plants love the sun. Herbs such as cilantro and *epazote* (Mexican oregano) make even the simplest salsa or bean dish even better. Fresh-picked chile peppers of all kinds can be cut into strips or stuffed and grilled; chile peppers are also delicious smoked for sauces like Smoked Poblano Cream Sauce (page 35). Tomatoes are the essential ingredient for fresh and cooked salsas. Small, tart tomatillos are green tomatoes encased in a stiff husk often used for a green *salsa verde* served with chicken and fish.

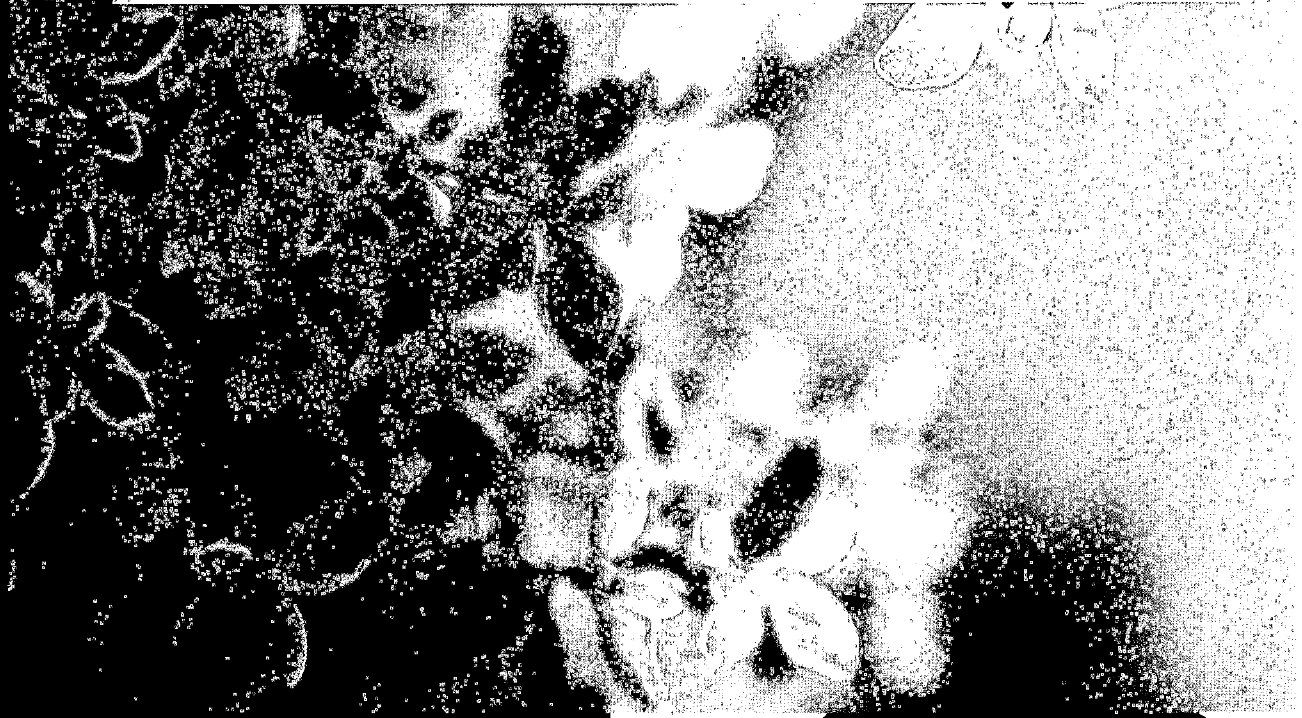

KNOWN AS TAGLIATA, THIS ITALIAN VERSION OF A PERFECTLY grilled, thick steak is served sliced over a bed of arugula. We also like it served alongside grilled romaine and atop a bunch of fresh garden arugula. Save some of the salad dressing to drizzle over the steak.

GRILLED CAESAR SIRLOIN

SERVES 4

High-Heat Grilled
  Romaine Salad (page
  109)

1½ pounds boneless sirloin
  steak, 2 inches thick

Extra-virgin olive oil, for
  brushing

Seasoning Salt (page 13)

4 cups loosely packed
  arugula

1 small wedge (about 4
  ounces) Parmigiano-
  Reggiano

Prepare a hot fire in your grill.

Prepare the romaine for grilling.

Brush the steak with olive oil and sprinkle with the Seasoning Salt to taste.

First grill the steak directly over the hot fire for about 4 minutes, turn and cook for another 4 minutes for rare. Remove from the grill and let rest for 5 minutes.

While steak is resting, grill the romaine.

Place 1 cup of arugula on each of 4 dinner plates. Slice the steak and place the slices on top of the greens. Set a half head of grilled romaine beside the sliced steak. Drizzle with the dressing. Pass the wedge of Parmesan, with a cheese parer or vegetable peeler, at the table and let everyone shave his or her own cheese onto the *tagliata* and grilled romaine.

BOK CHOY, A MEMBER OF THE CABBAGE FAMILY, IS EXCELLENT grilled. For a Japanese version, use Toasted Sesame-Soy Marinade and Dressing (page 15) to marinate the steak, brush the bok choy, and dress soba noodles in place of Thai Chile Noodles.

BLACKENED BEEF *with* THAI CHILE NOODLES *and* BABY BOK CHOY

SERVES 4

THAI CHILE NOODLES

¼ cup olive oil

1 tablespoon chile oil (available at Asian markets), optional

¼ cup seasoned rice vinegar

2 tablespoons chopped fresh mint leaves

2 tablespoons chopped fresh cilantro leaves

1 small chile pepper of your choice, seeded and minced

1 garlic clove, minced

8 ounces rice noodles or linguine, cooked according to package directions

¼ cup chopped, roasted peanuts

BOK CHOY AND STEAK

2 teaspoons toasted sesame oil

2 tablespoons vegetable oil

8 whole baby bok choy or 2 large heads bok choy, cut into quarters

One 12-ounce, 1½-inch-thick boneless top sirloin steak

2 tablespoons Red Hot Blackened Seasoning (page 14)

Fine kosher or sea salt to taste

To make the noodles, combine the olive oil, chile oil, vinegar, herbs, chile, and garlic in a large bowl. Toss the cooked noodles with the dressing. Sprinkle on the peanuts and toss again. Set aside.

Prepare a hot fire in your grill.

Combine the sesame and vegetable oils in a small bowl. Brush the bok choy with this mixture, then the steak. Sprinkle the Blackened Seasoning on the beef.

Grill the steak for 3½ to 4 minutes per side for medium-rare (130°F), or 5 minutes per side for medium (140°F). Grill the bok choy for 2 to 3 minutes per side, turning once, or until you have good grill marks and the vegetables have begun to soften.

Slice the steak thinly. Place a serving of noodles in 4 bowls and top with the steak and bok choy. Serve immediately.

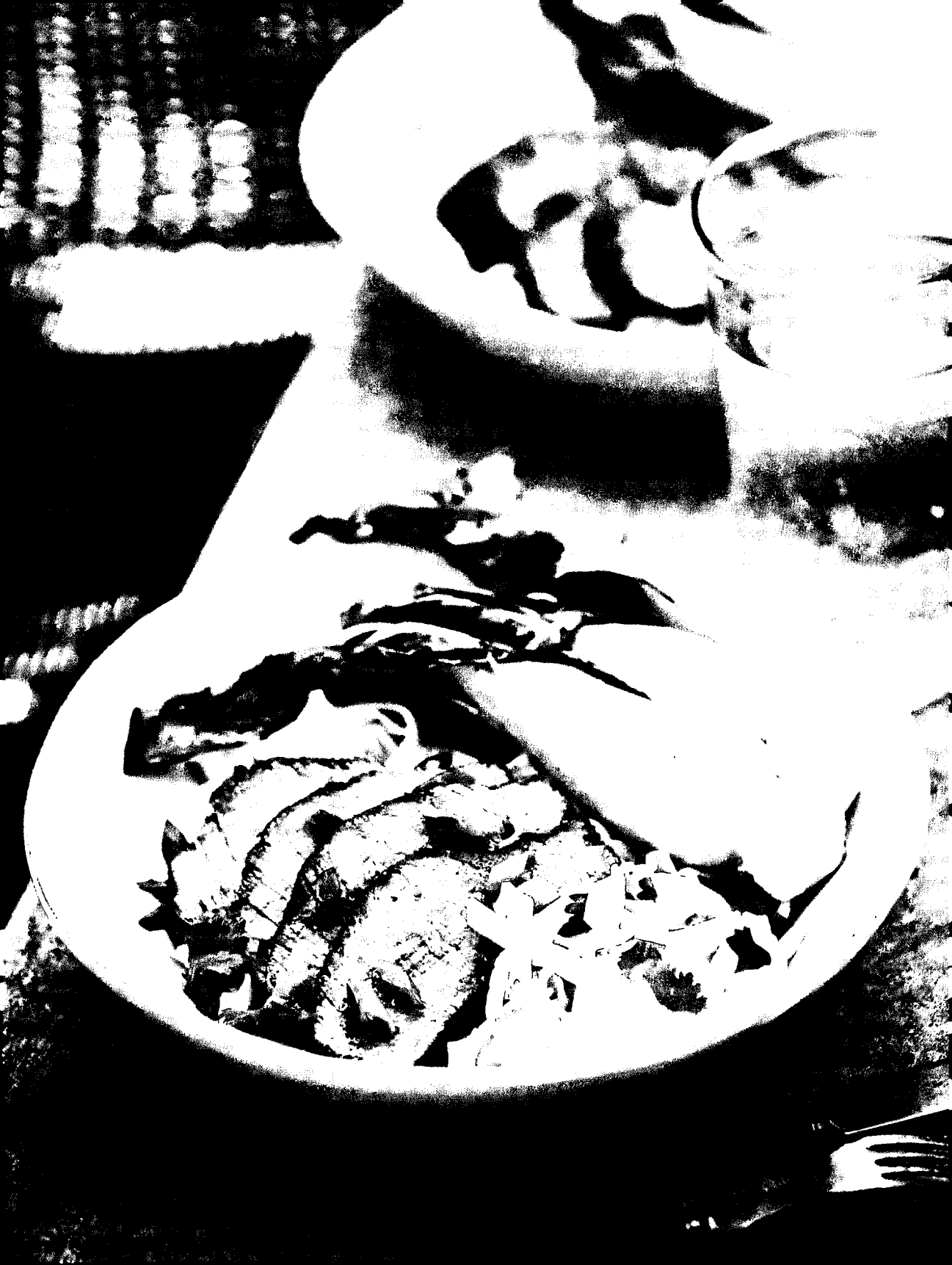

THIS SOPHISTICATED VERSION OF STEAK FAJITAS, TOPPED WITH Smoked Garlic and Cilantro Cream Sauce (page 34) at the end, makes your taste buds do a hat dance. For more color, texture, and eye-appeal, cut the peppers and onions into quarters instead of slivers. Flank steak can be chewy, so tenderize it one of three ways: by marinating it for several hours in Chipotle Vinaigrette (page 22) or bottled Italian vinaigrette, by pounding the steak with a meat tenderizer or mallet, or asking the butcher at the meat counter to run it through the cuber for you. If you like, warm some flour tortillas, wrapped in foil, on the grill to help mop up all the delicious juices and sauce.

FLANK STEAK with GRILLED PEPPERS and ONIONS

SERVES 4

1 cup Chipotle Vinaigrette (page 22) or bottled Italian dressing, divided

1½ pounds flank, skirt, hangar, flat iron, or western griller steak

2 bell peppers, or assorted peppers, seeded and quartered

1 large yellow or white onion, peeled and quartered

Smoked Garlic and Cilantro Cream Sauce (page 34)

Place ½ cup of the dressing and the steak in a resealable plastic bag and refrigerate for at least 1 hour or up to 8 hours.

Place ½ cup of the dressing and the peppers and onion in a separate sealable plastic bag and refrigerate for about 1 hour.

Prepare a hot fire in your grill.

Remove the steak from the marinade and pat dry. Grill for 2 to 3 minutes per side for medium-rare or an internal temperature of 130°F. Let the steak rest for 5 minutes while you grill the peppers and onions directly over the fire for 5 to 8 minutes, turning as needed, or until softened and slightly charry.

To serve, slice the steak against the grain, on the diagonal, and at a 45-degree angle, into slices about ¼-inch thick. Arrange the slices of beef with the grilled peppers and onions on the side. Spoon the warm Smoked Garlic and Cilantro Cream Sauce over all.

SUMMER COOKOUT CAN EASILY GO BEYOND BURGERS. YOU might enjoy the vegetables so much, you almost forget about the steak.

KANSAS CITY STRIP STEAKS *with* PARMESAN GRILLED VEGETABLES

SERVES 4 OR MORE

4 Kansas City strip steaks

Coarse kosher or sea salt and freshly ground black pepper to taste

2 red or yellow bell peppers, quartered and seeded

2 large red onions, peeled and quartered

2 zucchini, sliced ½-inch thick

1 cup cherry or grape tomatoes

Italian Parmesan Grilling Paste (page 31)

Prepare a hot fire in your grill.

Season the steaks with salt and pepper.

Place the vegetables in a grill wok or basket and the steaks directly on the grill and cook directly over the fire. Grill the vegetables for about 12 to 15 minutes, tossing every 2 or 3 minutes. Spoon 5 or 6 tablespoons of the cheese mixture over the vegetables the last 5 minutes of cooking.

Grill the steaks for 10 to 15 minutes for medium-rare (130°F), to medium (140°F) or until the steaks are done to your liking.

Serve each steak with a side of the vegetables and set the remaining Parmesan paste in a bowl on the side for diners to add to their steaks if they desire.

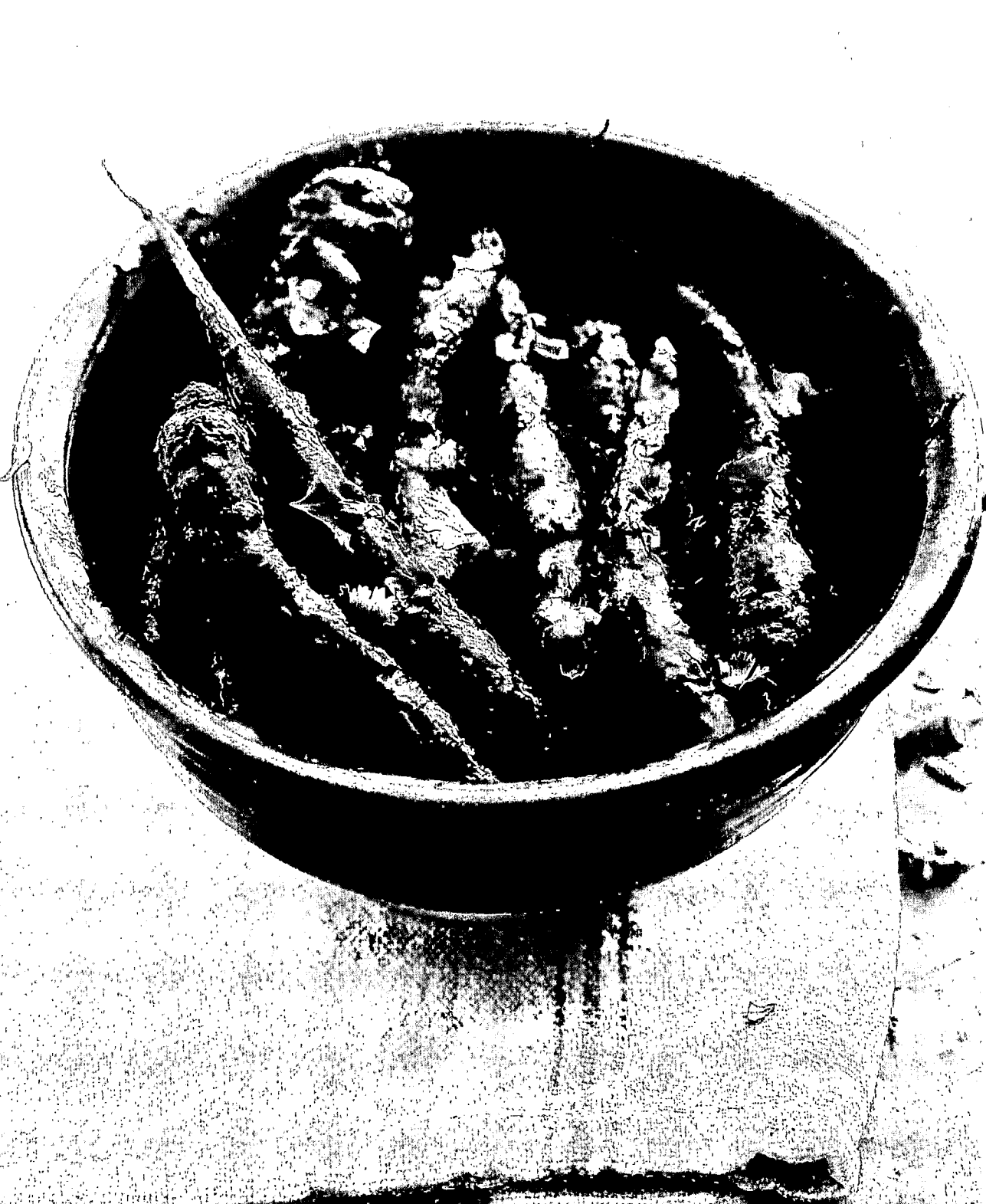

CHAPTER 6

VEGETABLE SIDES

GARDENERS KNOW THAT VEGETABLES PICKED FROM THEIR OWN gardens have a color and flavor far superior to any bought in a store. Grillers know that vegetables keep their vivid colors and flavors better when they're grilled rather than steamed or boiled. The good news for both gardeners and grillers is that vegetables cook fast, taste fresh, and need a minimum of flavor enhancers when they're grilled. Sometimes all you really need is a brush of olive oil and a sprinkle of salt and pepper to have a simply grilled, great-tasting vegetable. If you want to make grilled vegetables the star of the show, however, a sauce or drizzle makes a great finish to the dish.

To grill vegetables, there are a few techniques that are easy to master. First, brush them with olive oil to keep them from sticking to the grill grates. Use a perforated grill rack if you're worried that a thin vegetable like asparagus or a small one like whole baby pattypan squash or cherry tomatoes could fall through the grill grates.

If you love to cook in a wok indoors, try using a metal grill wok to stir-grill marinated vegetables, sometimes in combination with a protein, for a one-dish meal. A grill wok is a perforated metal grill gadget that you can find at barbecue and grill, culinary, and hardware stores. To use a grill wok, you simply marinate the bite-size pieces of vegetables and protein in a sealable plastic bag. Turn the marinated mixture out into the wok, preferably with the wok placed over a sink or the grass in your backyard so the excess marinade drains away. Then place the wok over direct heat and use wooden paddles or long-handed grill spatulas to turn and stir-grill the food every minute or so with the grill lid up. You can serve stir-grilled dishes over cooked pasta, rice, couscous, or polenta, if you wish.

Larger root vegetables and winter squash are best par-cooked before grilling. Microwave these dense vegetables for a few minutes so that they just finish on the grill. This two-step method keeps them from drying out over the high heat of the grill, as they take longer to get tender than vegetables like asparagus, eggplant, or summer squash. Use the indirect (or no-heat) side of the grill with the lid down so vegetables get scorched and caramelized—essentially roasted—without grill marks from direct-heat grilling.

Whenever possible, grill extra vegetables to have on hand for appetizers, sandwiches, salads, or pasta dishes that you can enjoy during the rest of the week.

Grilled Spring Platter of Asparagus and Leeks ...161

Top Ten Garden Vegetables for the Grill ...162

Charred Green Beans with Lemon Verbena Pesto ...164

Stir-Grilling ...166

Stir-Grilled Sugar Snap Peas and
Tear Drop Tomatoes with Basil ...167

Grilled Baby Beets with Scallions and Lemon Herb Butter ...168

Grilled Purple Sprouting Broccoli with
Garlic Anchovy Dipping Sauce ...169

Brussels Sprouts with Feta Garlic Butter ...170

Cauliflower with Tomatillo Salsa ...171

Rainbow Carrots with Cilantro Chile Drizzle ...172

Vegetable Container Gardening ...174

Grilled Corn-in-the-Husk Ancho Chili Lemon Butter ...175

Char-Grilled Eggplant with Grilled Marinara ...176

Baby Eggplant with Gruyère and Sun-Dried Tomatoes ...177

Grill-Roasted Stuffed Peppers ...178

Stuff It! ...179

Skewered Lemon-Rosemary Cherry Tomatoes ...180

Grill-Roasted Root Vegetables with Smoked Tomato Aioli ...182

Blistered Summer Squash, Peppers,
and Scallions with Goat Cheese ...183

Acorn Squash and Apple Rings with Cider Jus ...184

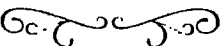

IN WARMER CLIMATES, ASPARAGUS AND LEEKS ARE READY TO harvest around the same time. Wrapping long vegetables with paper-thin slices of prosciutto does several things at once. The "padded" vegetables are easier to grill individually; the prosciutto adds a wonderful salty flavor; and the color contrast of dark pink and green just seems to say "spring." Grilled asparagus and leeks are also delicious when simply drizzled with melted Bearnaise Butter (page 29) instead of being finished with the fig balsamic vinegar and Parmesan.

GRILLED SPRING PLATTER
of ASPARAGUS and LEEKS

SERVES 6

1 pound fresh asparagus

3 medium-sized leeks

2 ounces prosciutto, cut lengthwise into 2-inch pieces

Olive oil, as needed

Fig balsamic vinegar, as needed

Shaved Parmesan cheese

Prepare a medium-hot fire in your grill.

Trim the tough ends off the asparagus. Cut the root ends off the leeks and slice them in half, lengthwise. Rinse the leeks under cold, running water to remove any sand and pat dry.

Wrap about half the asparagus spears and each of the leek halves with a piece of prosciutto. Place them on a baking sheet and drizzle with olive oil to lightly coat.

Place the spears perpendicular to the grill grates (or on a perforated grill rack). Grill, turning often, until the asparagus and leeks are crisp-tender and the prosciutto has blistered, about 8 to 10 minutes. Alternate several spears of asparagus with the leeks on a serving platter and splash on the fig balsamic vinegar, then sprinkle with the shaved Parmesan. Serve hot or at room temperature.

TOP TEN GARDEN VEGETABLES FOR THE GRILL

The ideal garden vegetables for grilling have to be able to stand the high heat, taste delicious when their natural sugars caramelize, and be easy for the griller to handle.

ASPARAGUS. Thicker asparagus does better on the grill. For easier handling, thread wooden skewers, soaked in water for half an hour, through the top and bottom of a line of asparagus spears. This way, you turn them all at once on the grill.

BROCCOLI. Maybe you haven't considered broccoli, but it's delicious on the grill. The secret is to cut the fatter head into long, flatter pieces—or try purple sprouting broccoli, a variety with smaller individual florets.

CABBAGE. Large cabbage kinds (green, red, Napa or Savoy) simply need to be cut into quarters or eighths, smaller cabbages (radicchio, Brussels sprouts) in half. Brush the cut sides with olive oil, then grill until you get good grill marks. Easy.

CORN. Grilled in the husk or with the corn kernels touching the grill grates, corn on the cob tastes great on the grill, especially slathered with a flavored butter.

EGGPLANT. Large, cylindrical eggplants are best sliced lengthwise to grill or, if they're large enough, you can also slice them into large coins. Smaller baby eggplant or long Japanese eggplant varieties can be grilled whole or sliced in half lengthwise.

ONIONS. All members of the onion family do well on the grill. For fat yellow, white, or Bermuda onions, peel and then slice them thickly. If you like, thread them lollipop-style through soaked wooden skewers or simply grill thick slices directly on the grill grates. Scallions or bulb onions can be grilled whole, turning often. Leeks are best sliced in half lengthwise (to more easily rinse out all the grit from the leek) then grilled.

PEPPERS. From bell to chile peppers, these colorful vegetables can be grilled in many different ways. Grill bell or chile peppers whole, then stem, seed, and chop. Slice them and grill them on a perforated grill rack or stir-grill in a grill wok. Or, smoke them on the indirect side of the grill with the lid closed, adding some wood chips, pellets, or chunks to the fire on the direct side.

ROOT VEGETABLES. Vegetables that grow below ground—beets, carrots, parsnips, potatoes, rutabagas, and turnips—need to be par-cooked first in boiling water or in the microwave so that they just finish on the grill.

SUMMER SQUASH. Yellow summer squash and zucchini are best sliced lengthwise, as the long slices are easier to manage on the grill. For stir-grilling, however, they're best sliced into coins or chopped.

TOMATOES. Big beefsteak tomatoes are best grilled whole or as thick slices. Cherry and currant tomatoes take well to skewers or stir-grilling. Meaty Romas are delicious smoked or wood-grilled. Tomatoes on stems can simply be grilled on one side.

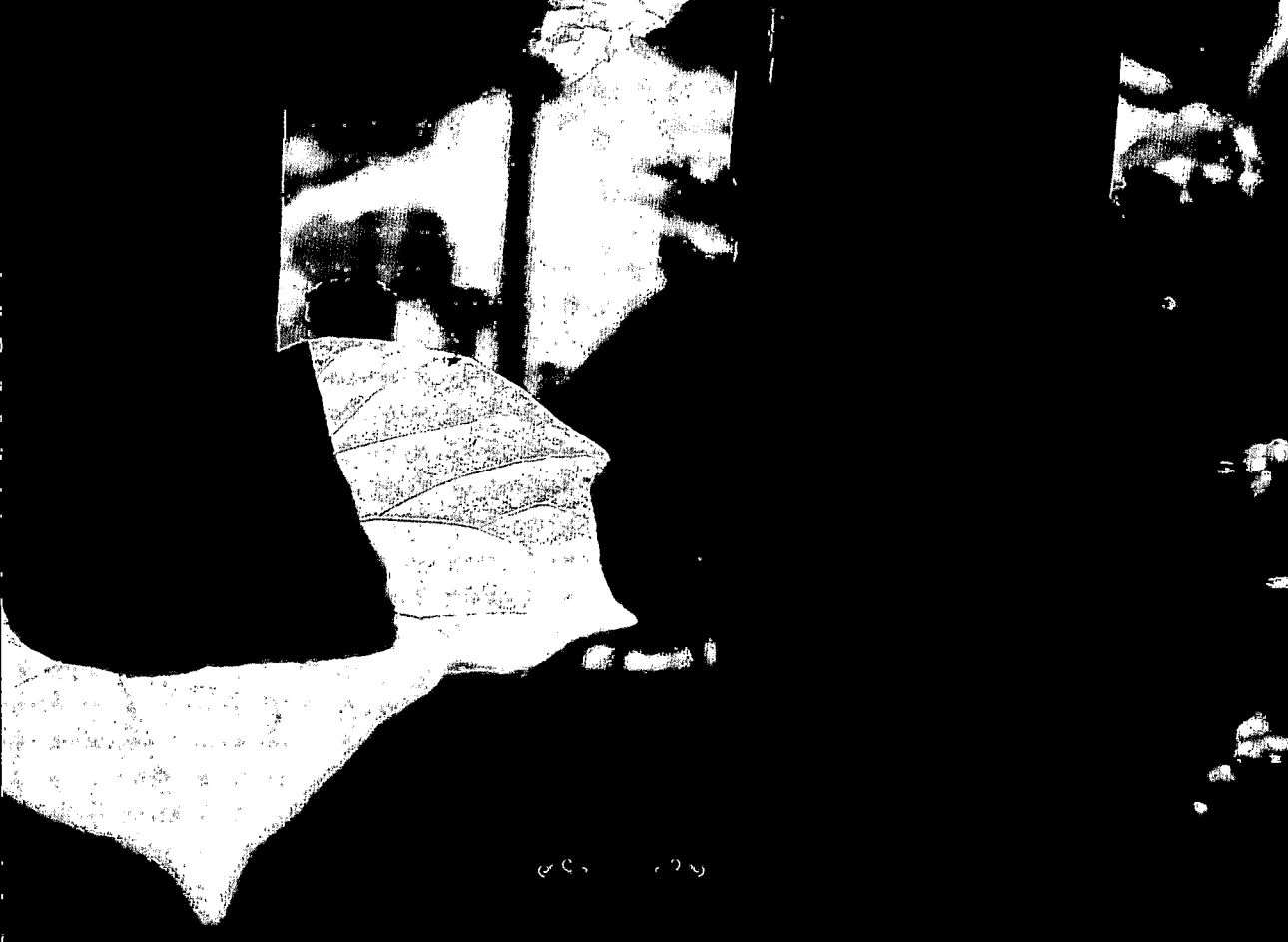

IF YOU GROW POLE BEANS, YOU KNOW THAT AT FIRST GLANCE, you have only a few beans, and then suddenly there is an onslaught. That's when bean varieties like the green Blue Lake or the yellow wax beans can be stir-grilled with a bit of olive oil for a very simple yet satisfying dish to use the surplus of beans. When you're in the mood for a more robust sauce, try this lemony pesto tossed with the grilled beans right before serving. Of course, you can also use Garlic Chive Pesto (page 32) or the Italian Parmesan Paste (page 31).

CHARRED GREEN BEANS
with LEMON VERBENA PESTO

SERVES 2 TO 4

GREEN BEANS
1½ pounds slender green
  beans
2 teaspoons olive oil

LEMON VERBENA PESTO
1 cup fresh lemon verbena
  leaves (substitute fresh
  lemon balm leaves)
2 garlic cloves
¼ cup grated Parmesan
  cheese
¼ cup pine nuts or English
  walnuts
½ cup olive oil
Fine kosher or sea salt and
  freshly ground black
  pepper to taste

Prepare a hot fire in your grill.

Toss the beans with olive oil and place in a perforated grill basket or wok set on a baking sheet.

For the Lemon Verbena Pesto, combine the lemon verbena, garlic, cheese, and nuts in a food processor and pulse to puree. Slowly add the olive oil with the processor running until the mixture thickens and emulsifies, about 1 minute. Season to taste with salt and pepper. The pesto will keep in the refrigerator for 7 to 10 days or it may be frozen for up to 3 months.

Place the grill wok or basket directly over the fire and stir-grill tossing the beans with wooden paddles or grill spatulas until crisp-tender, about 5 to 8 minutes. Transfer the grilled beans to a large bowl and toss with about ¼ cup of the Lemon Verbena Pesto or to taste.

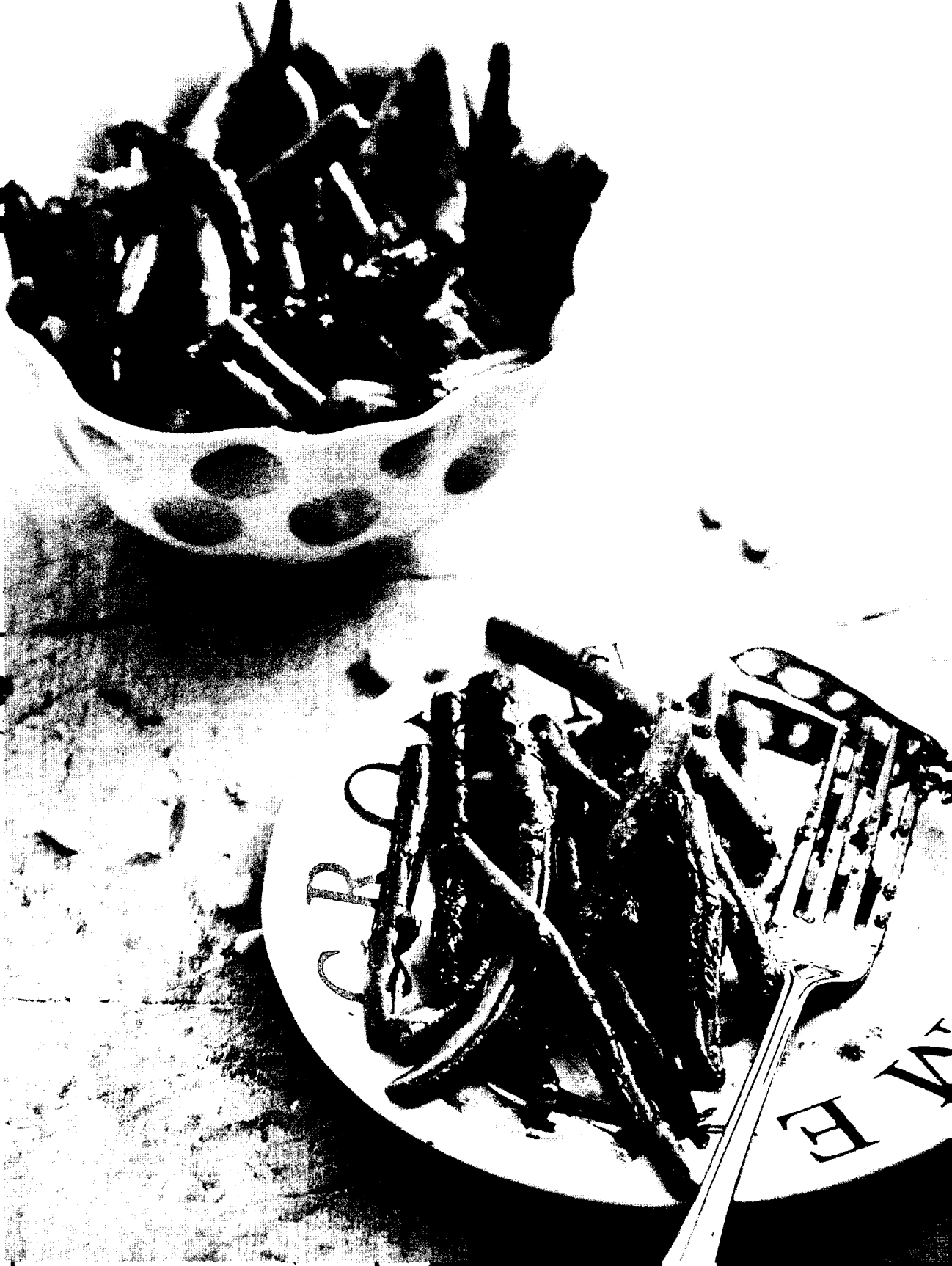

STIR-GRILLING

STIR-GRILLING—PLACING MARINATED OR SEASONED VEGETABLES in a perforated metal grill wok over the grill grates, then stirring and cooking until all the food is crisp-tender—is a barbecue technique tailor-made for the gardener. All you need is a variety of vegetables (about a handful of each), cut so that they're of fairly similar size, and good vinaigrette. When your vegetable crops are just coming in, or ending their season, stir-grilling comes to the rescue when you don't have enough of any one thing to make a full vegetable dish.

Vary the colors in a stir-grilled dish with a little red from cherry tomatoes or red bell peppers, some green from beans, scallions, sugar snap peas, or herbs, a hint of yellow from wax beans or summer squash, and purple from purple sprouting broccoli or eggplant.

You can also add a variety of marinated vegetables like artichoke hearts, olives, red or yellow bell peppers, large caper berries, peperoncinis and such to add a nice piquant flavor to the other stir-grilled vegetables.

Tender seafood like shrimp and scallops that both cook quickly, as well as chunks or strips of tender meats like chicken breast, pork tenderloin, or beef tenderloin can be added to make a tasty stir-grilled meal. These dishes are great served over couscous, pasta, or rice, too.

THIS GRILL-WOK RECIPE COMBINES TEXTURE, COLOR, AND TASTE at its best! Variations abound depending on what is in season. In late summer, switch out the sugar snap peas for green beans or summer squash. If you like peppers add yellow, red, and green bell pepper strips or add jalapeño or banana peppers to make it spicy: whatever you add, just think colorful.

STIR-GRILLED SUGAR SNAP PEAS and TEAR DROP TOMATOES with BASIL

SERVES 4

1 pound sugar snap peas or snow peas, strings removed

1 cup red tear drop or cherry tomatoes

1 cup yellow tear drop or Sungold tomatoes

1 red onion, sliced

1 cup Toasted Sesame-Soy Marinade and Dressing (page 15)

1 tablespoon extra-virgin olive oil, plus more as needed

1 cup loosely packed fresh basil sprigs

Fine kosher or sea salt and freshly ground black pepper to taste

Place the sugar snap peas, tomatoes, and onion in a sealable plastic bag. Add the marinade, seal, shake to coat everything, and marinate for 30 to 45 minutes in the refrigerator.

Prepare a hot fire on the indirect side of your grill.

Oil a perforated grill wok or basket. Place it over the sink and pour the vegetables and marinade into the wok and drain the marinade into the sink. Set the wok on top of a baking sheet to carry it out to the grill, then place the wok directly over the fire. Stir-grill 6 to 8 minutes, using two long-handled wooden spoons to toss the mixture. Quickly tuck sprigs of basil into the vegetable mixture and move the wok to the indirect side of the grill. Drizzle with extra-virgin olive oil and close the lid. Cook for another 4 to 5 minutes. Serve hot or at room temperature.

WHEN WE THINK OF BEETS, IT'S USUALLY THE FAMILIAR DETROIT Dark Red variety. But gardeners who grow beets can have varieties they can't always find at the farmer's market or grocery store, such as the pink and white striped Chioggia, the golden beet, or sweeter hybrid beet varieties like Red Ace, Big Red, or Avenger. Grilling beets is not much different than roasting, but it has more flavorful results. We've added spring scallions to this mix for a ruby red, green, and white array of colors. For grilling, choose the largest scallions or bulb onions.

GRILLED BABY BEETS *with* SCALLIONS *and* LEMON HERB BUTTER

SERVES 4

VEGETABLES

12 baby beets, about 1 inch in diameter, scrubbed and trimmed, leaving 2 inches of green tops

16 scallions (green onions), roots and tops trimmed with white and long green leaves intact

LEMON-HERB BUTTER

$1/2$ cup (1 stick) unsalted butter, at room temperature

2 teaspoons fresh lemon juice

2 tablespoons chopped fresh herbs (such as dill, oregano, thyme, or parsley)

2 garlic cloves, minced (optional)

Fine kosher or sea salt and freshly ground black pepper to taste

Prepare a hot fire in your grill.

Bring a large pot of water to boil, and parboil the beets for 10 to 15 minutes, or until tender enough to pierce with a fork. Drain the beets, rinse in cold water, and pat dry.

In a small saucepan over medium heat, melt the butter and add the lemon juice, herbs, and garlic, stirring to blend.

Place beets and scallions on a perforated grill rack. Brush beets and scallions with the butter mixture and sprinkle with salt and pepper to taste. Reserve half of the remaining butter mixture and take the rest of the butter out to the grill. Place the grill rack directly over the hot fire. Grill the beets, basting with the melted butter and turning occasionally, until they are brown and crunchy on the outside and soft on the inside, about 8 to 10 minutes. Grill the scallions, turning once, until they have good grill marks, about 4 minutes. Serve the beets drizzled with Lemon Herb Butter.

GARDENERS ON BOTH SIDES OF THE ATLANTIC ARE STARTING to enjoy a new variety of broccoli that grows in purple sprouts rather than green crowns. The frequent growth helps guard against the cabbageworm that seems to hide in the stems of green broccoli, surprising the gardener who is rinsing the vegetable after harvest. Whether you grow purple sprouting, the green Calabrese, broccolini, broccoli raab or rapini, or the lime green, cauliflower-like Romanesco broccoli, they all taste great off the grill with this dipping sauce or a dollop of Blender Hollandaise (page 36).

GRILLED PURPLE SPROUTING BROCCOLI
with GARLIC ANCHOVY DIPPING SAUCE

SERVES 4

GARLIC ANCHOVY DIPPING SAUCE

1 teaspoon anchovy paste or mashed, canned anchovy fillets

1 tablespoon Dijon mustard

2 tablespoons fresh lemon juice

1 garlic clove, minced

1 teaspoon chopped fresh rosemary leaves

1 tablespoon minced fresh flat-leaf parsley

6 tablespoons olive oil

BROCCOLI

2 bunches purple sprouting broccoli, broccolini or broccoli raab; or 1 head Calabrese or Romanesco broccoli (about 2$\frac{1}{2}$ pounds)

Olive oil, as needed

Fine kosher or sea salt and freshly ground black pepper to taste

For the dipping sauce, whisk together the anchovy paste, mustard, lemon juice, garlic, rosemary, parsley, and olive oil. Set aside.

Prepare a medium-hot fire in your grill.

Place the broccoli sprouts on a baking sheet. If using crowns or heads of broccoli, slice the broccoli lengthwise into long slices about 1 to 2 inches thick and place on a baking sheet. Brush with olive oil and season to taste with salt and pepper.

Grill directly over the fire, turning once, until you have good grill marks, and the broccoli is crisp-tender, about 5 to 8 minutes.

Serve with the dipping sauce.

I F YOU'VE NEVER GROWN BRUSSELS SPROUTS BEFORE, GIVE THEM a try. They are so unique-looking with their tall stalks: they seem to have little green clusters of ornaments on them. Brussels sprouts can also be sliced in half and stir-grilled in a perforated grill wok or basket directly over a hot fire: you can blanch them first or not. The Italian Parmesan Paste (page 31) is perfect for the stir-grilling method.

BRUSSELS SPROUTS
with FETA GARLIC BUTTER

SERVES 4

1 ½ pounds small Brussels
  sprouts, trimmed

2 tablespoons unsalted
  butter

1 garlic clove, minced

¼ cup crumbled fresh
  feta cheese

2 tablespoons water or
  milk (optional)

Prepare a hot fire in your grill. Soak wooden skewers in water for 30 mintutes.

Bring a pot of water to the boil over high heat. Add the Brussels sprouts and blanch until they are barely tender when pierced with a fork, about 2 minutes. Transfer the sprouts to a bowl of ice water to stop the cooking. Remove the sprouts from the water and pat dry.

In a small saucepan, melt the butter and add the garlic and cheese, stirring over low heat until the mixture is smooth. Add water or milk to thin, if needed.

Thread the Brussels sprouts onto the skewers and brush with the butter mixture. Place the skewers directly over the fire. Turn the skewers frequently, basting continuously with butter mixture until the sprouts are tender, about 8 to 10 minutes.

Serve hot or at room temperature with any remaining sauce.

THIS INTRIGUING FLAVOR COMBINATION IS UNIQUE WITH THE grilled flavors of both the cauliflower and the tomatillos. The pale green tomatillo sauce couldn't be prettier drizzled down the center of the creamy and charred cauliflower "steaks." It is a perfect side dish served with scallops or shrimp, or it can be a main vegetarian course.

CAULIFLOWER with GRILL-ROASTED TOMATILLO SALSA

SERVES 4

1 large head cauliflower, cored and green leaves removed

Olive oil

Fine kosher or sea salt to taste

1 recipe Grill-Roasted Tomatillo Salsa (page 70)

Prepare a hot fire on the indirect side of your grill.

Cut the cauliflower from top to bottom into 1-inch thick slices and place on a baking sheet. Brush the cauliflower with olive oil and salt to taste. Place the cauliflower slices on the indirect or no-heat side of the grill. Close the lid and grill-roast for 20 minutes, turning once or twice, until the cauliflower slices still hold together but are tender when pierced with a paring knife.

To serve, shingle the cauliflower slices on each plate and spoon with Grill-Roasted Tomatillo Salsa.

CARROTS MAKE GREAT CONTAINER GARDEN PLANTS OR FERN-like borders in the garden. And they grow in different shapes (round, thin and long, or cylindrical) and colors (pale yellow, orange, dark pink, and purple). For grilling, we like the Rainbow Hybrid or the traditional Nantes cylindrical orange carrot. Just pick the carrots when they're about 4 to 5 inches long, scrub off the garden soil, and trim back the tops a bit. Then, brush them with olive oil and grill. The Cilantro Chile Drizzle highlights the sweet flavor of this garden favorite.

RAINBOW CARROTS
with CILANTRO CHILE DRIZZLE

SERVES 4

CILANTRO CHILE DRIZZLE

1 cup coarsely chopped
  fresh cilantro leaves and
  tender stems

1 canned chipotle chile in
  adobo sauce

1 large garlic clove

$\frac{1}{3}$ cup seasoned rice wine
  vinegar

$\frac{1}{3}$ cup fresh lime juice

2 tablespoons honey

$\frac{2}{3}$ cup canola oil

Fine kosher or sea salt to
  taste

CARROTS

2 bunches baby carrots
  (about 16), trimmed, with
  2 inches of the green tops

1 tablespoon olive oil

Fine kosher or sea salt to
  taste

2 tablespoons chopped
  fresh cilantro to garnish

For the Cilantro Chile Drizzle, combine the cilantro, chile, garlic, rice wine vinegar, lime juice, honey, and oil in a food processor and process until emulsified. Season with salt to taste. Transfer to a jar with a lid. The drizzle will keep, covered, in the refrigerator for up to 1 week.

Prepare a hot fire on the indirect side of your grill.

Place the carrots in a 9 x 13-inch disposable aluminum pan, drizzle with olive oil, and salt to taste.

Place the carrots on the indirect (or no-heat) side of the grill and close the lid. Grill carrots for 15 to 20 minutes or until the carrots are crisp-tender when pierced with a knife in the thickest part.

To serve, drizzle the carrots with the Cilantro Chile Drizzle and sprinkle with chopped cilantro.

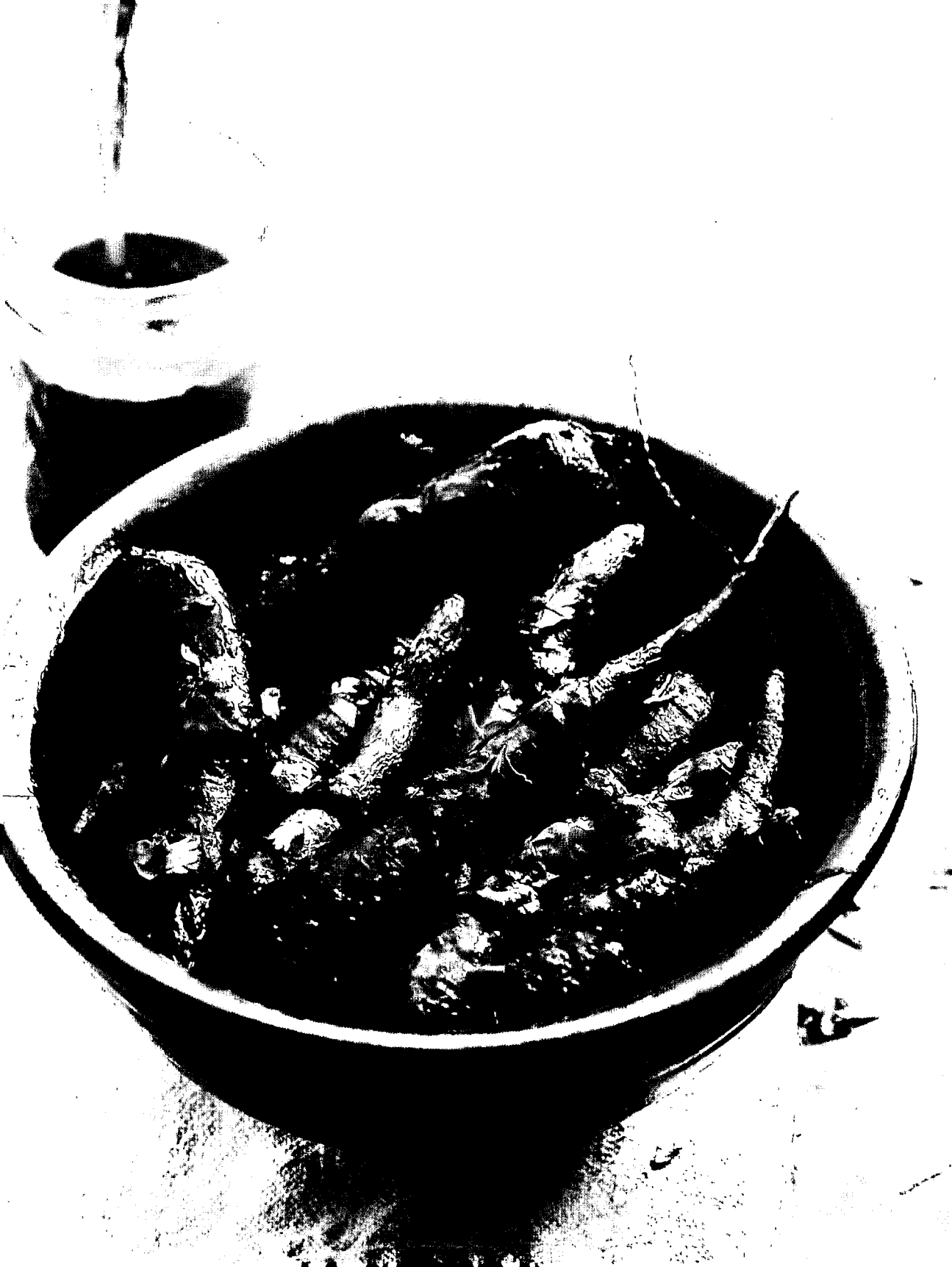

VEGETABLE CONTAINER GARDENING

IF YOU HAVE LIMITED GARDENING SPACE OR JUST LOVE THE IDEA of edible landscaping, you can create container gardens that feature your favorite vegetables, flowers, and herbs.

Start with a pot that has drainage holes (sometimes you have to drill these out yourself) and good potting soil. Find a metal hoop or support that can hold a climbing vegetable and will fit in your pot. Plant a climbing vegetable in the center of the pot, then plant low-growing herbs, root vegetables, or flowers along the perimeter of the pot.

Here are a few possible combinations:

- French filet beans or haricots verts as a center climber, surrounded by carrots and tarragon.
- Baby purple eggplant as a center climber, surrounded by purple basil and yellow marigolds.
- Yellow tear drop tomato as a center climber, surrounded by Genovese basil and radicchio.
- Gypsy peppers as a center climber, surrounded by cilantro and dwarf zinnias.
- Sugar snap peas as a center climber, surrounded by turnips and pansies.

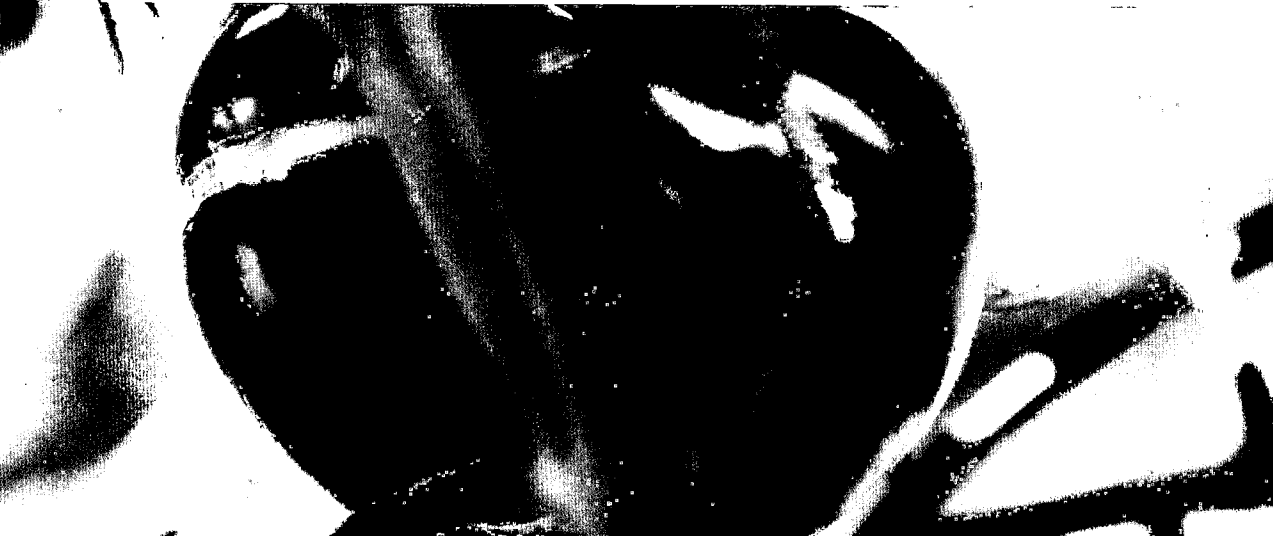

IF YOU WANT YOUR SWEET CORN TO STAY VERY TENDER BUT HAVE a gentle flavor of the grill, then grilling corn in the husk is the way to go. Sweet corn varieties such as Silver Queen, Purdue Super Sweet, Peaches and Cream, or the heirloom Country Gentleman taste fabulous with this treatment.

GRILLED CORN-IN-THE-HUSK
with ANCHO-LIME BUTTER

SERVES 6

6 ears sweet corn, in the husk

1 garlic clove, minced

$^1\!/_4$ cup ($^1\!/_2$ stick) unsalted butter, at room temperature

$^1\!/_2$ teaspoon ground ancho chile powder

$^1\!/_2$ teaspoon grated lime zest

Fine kosher or sea salt to taste

Peel back the corn husks, taking care not to pull them off. Remove the corn silks and pull husks back over the corn, tying the husks securely with kitchen string or part of a corn husk to enclose the ear in the husk. Soak the corn in cold water for 15 minutes. Drain well.

For the ancho lime butter, stir the garlic, butter, ancho chile, and lime zest together in a bowl until well blended. Add salt to taste. Set aside.

Prepare a hot fire in your grill.

Grill the corn directly over the heat, turning often, until the husks are slightly charred and you can see steam rising from the ears, about 10 minutes. Let cool slightly and remove the string.

To serve, pull the husks back and brush the kernels with the Ancho Lime Butter.

IF YOU'VE EVER MADE EGGPLANT PARMIGIANA ON THE STOVE-top, you know that eggplant seems to soak up olive oil like a sponge when you fry it. On the grill, this doesn't happen if you brush the eggplant with olive oil right before it goes over the flame. Try dark purple Black Magic or Black Beauty or striped purple and white Sicilian varieties.

CHAR-GRILLED EGGPLANT
with GRILLED MARINARA SAUCE

SERVES 4

EGGPLANT

2 medium eggplants, like Black Magic, Black Beauty, or Sicilian white or purple (about 2 pounds total)

Fine kosher or sea salt to taste

$1/2$ cup extra-virgin olive oil

GRILLED MARINARA SAUCE

3 cups chopped fresh tomatoes

2 garlic cloves, minced

$1/2$ cup chopped fresh basil

$1/4$ cup extra-virgin olive oil

Fine kosher or sea salt to taste

Trim off the ends of the eggplants, but do not peel. Cut lengthwise into $1/2$-inch slices and lightly salt. Place in colander and let drain for at least 30 minutes to remove excess water. Pat dry.

Meanwhile, prepare a hot fire on the indirect side of your grill.

Place the eggplant slices on a baking sheet. Brush the slices with extra-virgin olive oil on both sides.

For the Grilled Marinara, combine the tomatoes, garlic, basil, and extra-virgin olive oil in a 9 x 13-inch disposable aluminum pan. Season with salt to taste.

Place the tomato mixture on the indirect or no-heat side of the grill and arrange the eggplant slices on the direct heat side. Grill the eggplant turning once, until tender, about 10 minutes. Stir the marinara so it warms through.

To serve, arrange the eggplant slices on plates and top with the Grilled Marinara.

SMALLER EGGPLANT VARIETIES, WHICH MAKE GREAT PLANTS FOR a container garden, also work well on the grill. Use smaller and rounder Baby or Indian or more cylindrical Japanese varieties. For best results, oil the eggplant right before you grill it. This dish is so full of flavor it could easily be an entrée.

BABY EGGPLANT *with* GRUYÈRE *and* SUN-DRIED TOMATOES

SERVES 4

4 small eggplants (about 2 pounds total)

Fine kosher or sea salt to taste

1 garlic clove, finely minced

1/2 cup extra-virgin olive oil

2 tablespoons dried crumbled oregano

1/2 cup chopped sun-dried tomatoes

1/2 cup shredded Gruyère

Trim both ends off the eggplants, but do not peel. Cut lengthwise in half and lightly salt. Place in a colander and let drain for at least 30 minutes to remove excess water. Pat dry.

Prepare a medium-hot fire in your grill.

In a bowl, combine the garlic, olive oil, and oregano. Brush the mixture on both sides of the eggplant halves. Place the eggplant on a baking sheet to take out to the grill.

Grill the eggplant, turning once, until tender, about 10 minutes. Place grilled eggplant on a platter and immediately sprinkle with the sun-dried tomatoes and cheese.

Serve hot.

BACON, ARTISAN BREAD, TOMATOES, AND CHEDDAR COME together for a fabulously easy filling for garden-fresh bell peppers. When you add a little wood to the fire, it gives these peppers the taste of centuries-old hearth cooking.

GRILL-ROASTED STUFFED PEPPERS

SERVES 4

1 cup wood chips or dry wood pellets

4 medium red, yellow, orange, and purple bell peppers (any assortment), stemmed and seeded

8 slices apple- or hickory-smoked bacon, diced

1 bunch green onion, chopped

2 cups cubed artisan bread, such as ciabatta, Italian, hearth, or sourdough

2 cups diced canned tomatoes with juice

1 cup grated sharp cheddar

2 tablespoons chopped fresh flat-leaf parsley

Prepare a hot fire on the indirect side of your grill. If you have a charcoal grill, soak the wood chips in water for 30 minutes before smoking; if you have a gas grill, place dry wood chips in a foil packet, and poke holes in the top of the foil. Oil a deep disposable aluminum baking pan.

Trim the bottoms of the peppers so they sit flat and place them in the prepared baking pan. In a skillet over medium-high heat, cook the bacon until crisp. Remove with a slotted spoon to paper towels and roughly chop. Drain all but about 1 tablespoon of bacon fat from the skillet and sauté the green onions until softened, about 4 minutes. Stir in the bread, tomatoes, cheese, and reserved bacon until the bread is moistened and the mixture is well blended. Spoon the mixture into the peppers.

When ready to grill, drain then scatter the soaked wood chips on the charcoal fire, and replace the grill rack. For a gas grill, place the packet of dry wood chips in the back over direct heat.

When you see the first wisp of smoke from the wood, place the pan of vegetables on the indirect or no-heat side of the grill. Close the lid and grill until the top of the filling is bubbling and burnished, about 30 minutes.

Serve topped with the chopped flat-leaf parsley.

STUFF IT!

THE WOOD-FIRED, OUTDOOR OVEN OF THE VILLAGE IS A PEASANT tradition that still continues throughout Europe. The baker bakes his breads there, then as the bread comes out and the fire dies down a bit, the villagers bring their garden vegetables stuffed with savory fillings to cook. Basically, any vegetable that you can hollow out can be stuffed and grilled directly or indirectly to deliciousness. Large beefsteak tomatoes and bell peppers can be trimmed on their bottoms to sit flat. Long vegetables like zucchini, summer squash, chile peppers, and eggplant can be cut lengthwise, scooped out, and stuffed. As a nod to the village baker tradition, use artisan or hearth-style breads like sourdough or French bread in the stuffing.

F YOU GROW ROSEMARY, USE PIECES OF THE STURDY STALKS FOR the skewers. Rosemary skewers can also be purchased at some grocery stores. Use whatever small ripe tomatoes you can harvest from your garden. Small Romas and cluster tomatoes are perfectly fine for this recipe as are red and yellow grape tomatoes.

SKEWERED LEMON-ROSEMARY CHERRY TOMATOES

SERVES 4

1 pint mixed cherry and grape tomatoes

4 sweet onions, peeled and cut into chunks

$^1/_4$ cup chopped fresh rosemary leaves

$^1/_2$ cup olive oil

$^1/_4$ cup fresh lemon juice

Fine kosher or sea salt and freshly ground black pepper to taste

Thread the cherry tomatoes and onions alternately on pre-soaked wooden skewers. Place skewered vegetables in a large, shallow baking dish. Combine rosemary, olive oil, lemon juice, and seasonings and pour over vegetables, coating well. Marinate at room temperature for at least 30 minutes, turning two or three times.

Prepare a hot fire in your grill.

When ready to grill, place skewered vegetables directly over the fire.

Grill for about 3 to 5 minutes, basting frequently with the marinade until the vegetables are slightly charred.

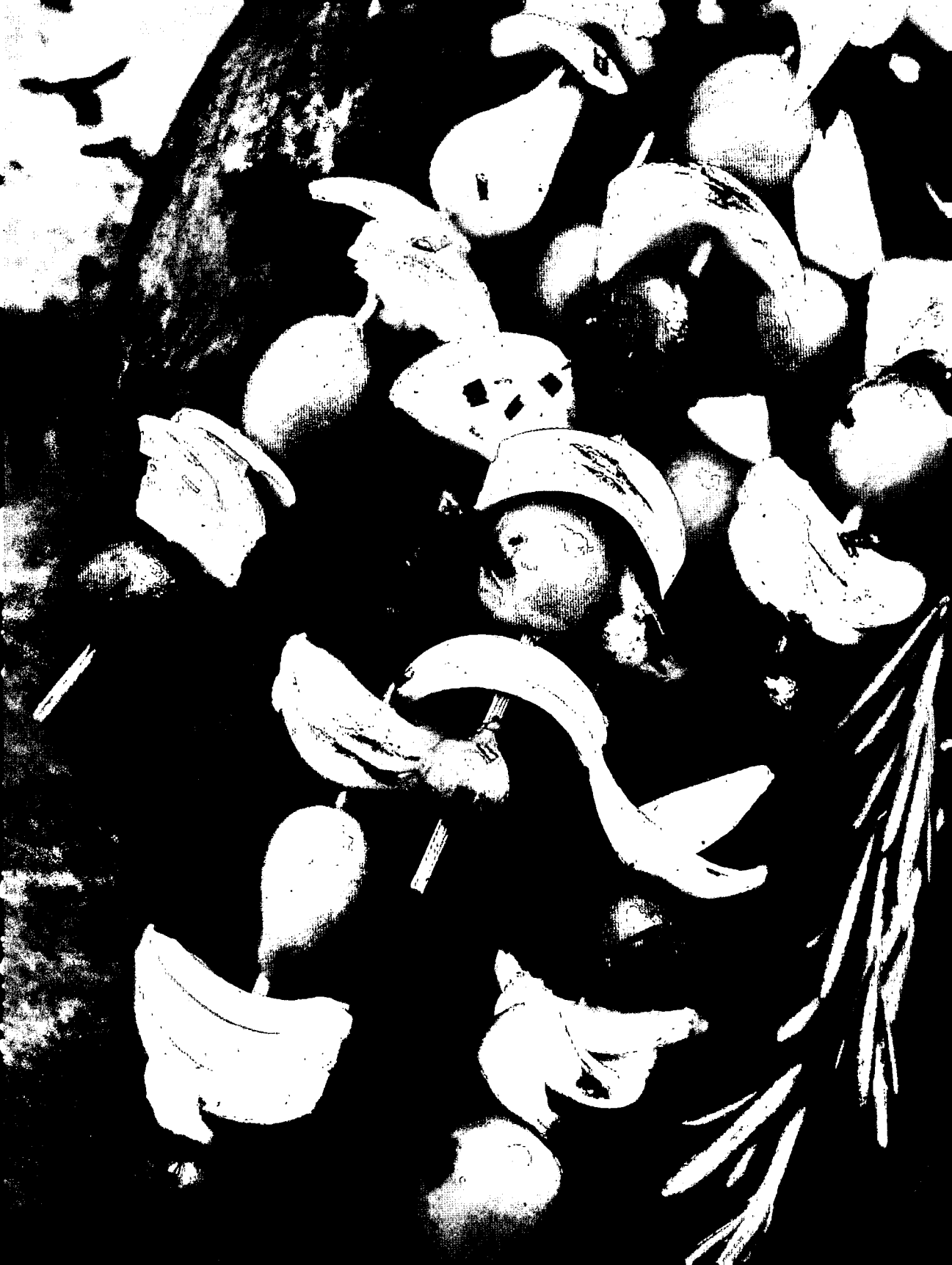

ADDING A LITTLE WOOD TO THE FIRE ADDS THE FLAVOR OF THE hearth cooking to this peasant dish from the south of France. Use a mixture of root vegetables for color, flavor, and texture. An aioli is simply a garlic mayonnaise, but this one is a little milder and smokier from the smoked garlic.

GRILL-ROASTED ROOT VEGETABLES
with SMOKED TOMATO AIOLI

SERVES 6 TO 8

1 cup oak or apple wood chips

4 pounds mixed root vegetables such as sweet and russet potatoes, carrots, parsnips, rutabaga, and turnips

Olive oil

Coarse kosher or sea salt and freshly ground black pepper to taste

1 recipe Smoked Tomato Aioli (page 40)

Prepare a medium-hot fire on the indirect side of your grill. Soak wood chips in water for 30 minutes.

Bring a large pot of water to a boil. Scrub the vegetables. Leaving the skin on the potatoes, cut them into 2-inch chunks. Peel carrots, parsnips, turnips, and rutabaga. Slice the carrots and parsnips lengthwise into 1-inch thick slices. Cut the turnips and rutabaga into 2-inch chunks. Par-cook the vegetables into the boiling water for 10 minutes, and then remove with a slotted spoon to a 9 x 13-inch disposable aluminum pan. Drizzle the vegetables with olive oil and season with salt and pepper.

For a charcoal grill, throw wood chips directly on the coals right before you want to grill. For a gas grill, enclose the wood chips or pellets in a foil packet with holes poked in the top; place the packet on the grill grate over the heat source.

When you see the first wisp of smoke from the wood, place the vegetables on the indirect (or no-heat) side of the grill. Close the lid and smoke until the vegetables are tender, about 1 hour, replenishing the wood chips or pellets as necessary.

To serve, place a dollop of Smoked Tomato Aioli on each serving of vegetables.

WHEN ZUCCHINI AND YELLOW SUMMER SQUASH ARE READILY available, give this dish a try: select the smallest, firmest squash. Choose a variety of whole bell peppers to turn this platter of grilled food into a rainbow of colors. Try a variety of hot peppers, such as banana, serrano, jalapeño, etc. For company, put the vegetables on a platter and serve with a duo of dressings. We suggest Chimichurri Sauce (page 26) and Lemon Caesar Vinaigrette (page 17).

BLISTERED SUMMER SQUASH, PEPPERS, and SCALLIONS with GOAT CHEESE

SERVES 4

2 bunches green onions

8 small zucchini

8 small yellow summer squash

6 bell peppers in assorted colors

8 assorted hot peppers, or more to taste (optional)

3 to 4 tablespoons olive oil

Fine kosher or sea salt and freshly ground black pepper to taste

1½ cups (12 ounces) crumbled goat cheese

Prepare a hot fire in your grill.

Place the green onions, zucchini, yellow summer squash, bell peppers, and, if using, hot peppers on a baking sheet and drizzle with the olive oil, turning to coat everything lightly. Season with salt and pepper to taste.

Place the vegetables over the hot fire and grill, turning them several times until they are charred on the outside and cooked through to your liking, about 15 to 20 minutes.

Place the vegetables on a platter and sprinkle with the crumbled goat cheese. For a spectacular presentation, arrange a row of the green onions, then a row of the green charred zucchini, followed by the yellow summer squash and the peppers. Serve hot or at room temperature.

GOLDEN DELICIOUS APPLES WORK GREAT FOR QUICK GRILLING because they're naturally sweeter with a softer texture than apples like Jonathan or Granny Smith. This dish goes well with turkey, chicken, pork tenderloin, or chops on the grill.

ACORN SQUASH and APPLE RINGS WITH CIDER JUS

SERVES 4

CIDER JUS

1 cup apple cider or juice

2 tablespoons unsalted butter

1 tablespoon bourbon or rum (optional)

Fine kosher or sea salt and ground white pepper to taste

SQUASH AND APPLES

4 Golden Delicious apples, tops and bottoms trimmed off

2 acorn squash, halved horizontally, seeds removed, and microwaved on high for 8 minutes

For the Cider Jus, bring the cider to a boil over high heat in a saucepan. Let it cook for 10 to 15 minutes or until it has reduced to $\frac{1}{2}$ cup. Remove from the heat and whisk in the butter and bourbon, if using. Season to taste. Transfer $\frac{1}{3}$ cup to a small ramekin and reserve.

Prepare a hot fire in your grill. Oil a perforated grill rack.

While the grill is heating, slice the partially cooked squash into $\frac{3}{4}$-inch slices and place on a baking sheet. Brush each slice with a little of the jus and season to taste with salt and pepper. Slice each apple into 4 horizontal slices, then remove the core in each slice. Place the apple rings on the baking sheet and brush each with a little of the jus.

At the grill, place the apple rings on the prepared grill rack. Place the rack on the grill grate and grill with the lid closed for about 2 to 3 minutes on each side, or until you have good grill marks and the apple rings "give" when gently squeezed with grill tongs. Transfer the apple rings to the baking sheet and place the squash slices on the grill rack. Close the lid and grill for 4 minutes on each side, or until the squash has good grill marks and is tender when pierced with a paring knife.

To serve, arrange the squash and apple on each plate and drizzle with the ramekin of reserved jus.

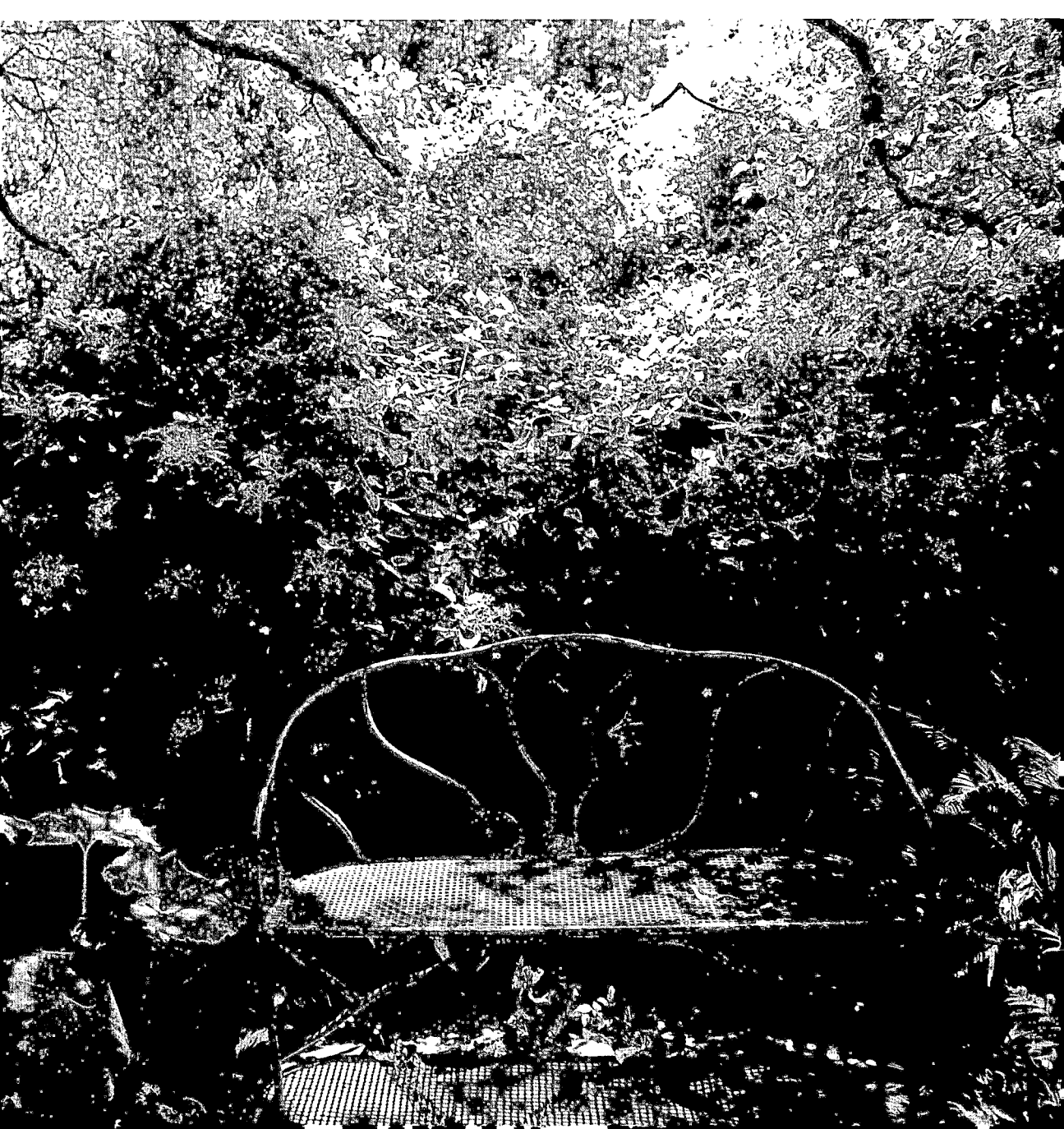

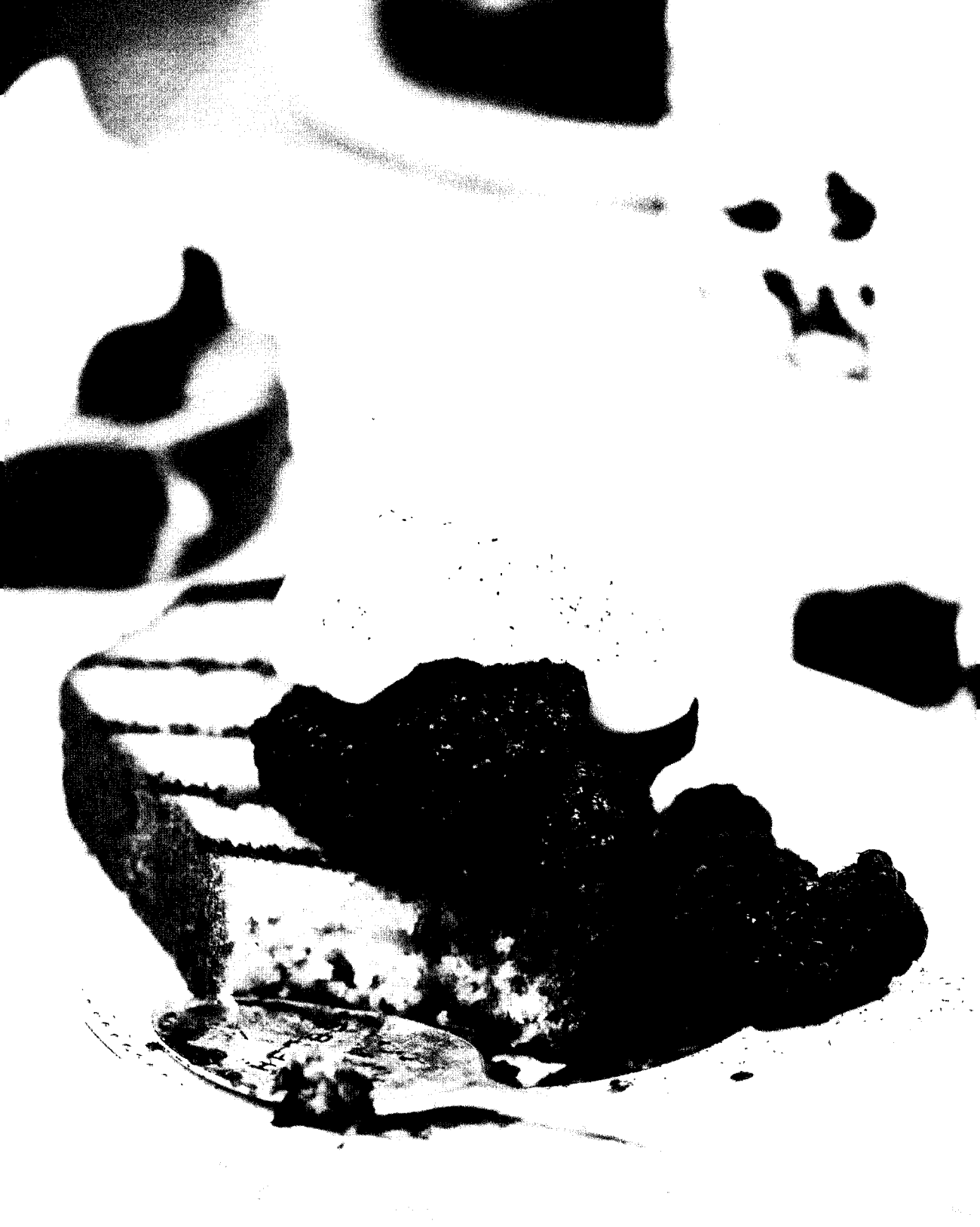

CHAPTER 7

FRUITS & DESSERTS

FRESH-PICKED FRUIT FROM YOUR GARDEN AND THE HEAT OF THE grill can be a fabulous combination. Grilling fruit intensifies its flavor and sweetness. The look of grilled fruit is appealing, too, with deep brown grill marks showing caramelization and a rustic appearance.

You don't want fruit to be overcooked and mushy, so use ripe, firm fruit. Underripe fruit is not a good choice, as it does not have optimum flavor.

Size matters when grilling fruit. Large fruit, halved or cut into wedges, may be fine placed directly on the grill grates, but if the fruit is smaller, skewer it or use a grill rack, wok, or basket.

Naturally soft fruits, such as apricots, peaches, pears, plums, figs, and nectarines, are best grilled cut in half. If you're using skewers or a grill rack, wok, or basket, some of these fruits can be grilled in thick slices. Firmer fruits, such as apples, melon slices with the rind on, and oranges, lemons, limes, and grapefruit with the rind on can be cut in half, sliced, or cut into wedges for grilling. Peeled melon slices or wedges are delicious wrapped in prosciutto. Clusters of grilled grapes make a wonderful addition to a cheese platter. Even strawberries threaded onto skewers can be quickly grilled.

The simplest way to prepare whole or cut fruit for grilling is cook it naked over the fire. If you like, you can brush it with mild olive oil (not extra-virgin), grapeseed oil, or other vegetable oil. Melted butter is also delicious; it won't have time to burn, because you grill fruit for only a few minutes per cut side.

Smaller fruits like cherries and berries take well to skewering, planking, or stirgrilling, so they don't disappear through the grill grates.

For a finishing touch, sprinkle your grilled fruit with colorful edible flowers (see Sidebar page 202). If you grow them yourself, you know they're fine to use.

Planked Brie with Grilled Apricot Jam ...189

Grilled Grapefruit with Brown Sugar Rum Butter ...190

Top Ten Garden-Grown Fruits for the Grill ...192

Grilled Grape & Cheese Board ...193

Companion Plants ...194

Skewered Strawberry and Marshmallow S'mores ...196

Warm Honeyed Blackberries with Grilled Pound Cake ...199

Grill-Roasted Rhubarb and Strawberries
with Lemony Crème Fraîche ...200

Grilled Cantaloupe Rings with Vanilla Bean Ice Cream ...201

Edible Flowers ...202

Grilled Peaches with Lemon Balm Gremolata ...204

Planked Peaches and Blueberries with Amaretto Sauce ...206

Stir-Grilled Nectarines & Plums with Sweet Wine Drizzle ...207

Grilled Persimmons with Three-Citrus Drizzle ...208

Grill-Baked Apples with Cinnamon Nut Stuffing ...209

Rosemary and Sugar-Spice-Rubbed Apple Slices ...210

Plank-Roasted Pears with
Blue Cheese and Balsamic Honey ...211

Grilled Pears with Honey-Cinnamon Crème Fraîche ...213

FRESHLY GRILLED APRICOTS ADD TEXTURE AND EYE-APPEAL to this recipe that can be served as an appetizer or as a dessert. The plank does double duty as the cooking vessel and the serving platter.

PLANKED BRIE *with* GRILLED APRICOT JAM

SERVES 8 TO 10

¼ cup sweet white wine

¼ cup apricot preserves or chutney

1 wheel (8 or 10 ounces) baby brie or Camembert

6 apricots, halved and pitted

1 French baguette, sliced for serving

Soak a grilling plank in water for at least 1 hour. Prepare a hot fire on one side of your grill for indirect cooking.

In a small saucepan, bring wine and apricot preserves to a simmer over medium-low heat. Remove from heat and keep warm.

Place brie on the plank and set the plank on the indirect side of the grill.

Set a grill rack directly over the fire and place the apricot halves on the rack. Grill the apricots for about 3 to 4 minutes on each side or until they have good grill marks. Arrange the apricots on top of the cheese. Close the lid and plank for about 20 minutes, or until cheese is soft and warmed through.

Serve the planked cheese and apricots with the warm apricot mixture spooned over the top with slices of baguette on the side.

IN TEXAS AND SOUTHERN CALIFORNIA, GARDENERS CAN SIMPLY go outside and pick citrus fruit from their own trees. Oranges and grapefruit can be cut in half and placed cut side down directly over the grill fire, or brushed with a little melted butter, and grilled, cut side only. Lemons and limes, cut in half, can be grilled on the cut side only and served as flavorful garnish for both savory and sweet dishes. The benefits of grilling? Citrus fruits take on the flavor of the grill and are actually juicier.

GRILLED GRAPEFRUIT *with* BROWN SUGAR RUM BUTTER

SERVES 4

2 grapefruit, halved and
  seeded

BROWN SUGAR
RUM BUTTER

2 tablespoons unsalted
  butter

2 tablespoons packed
  brown sugar

2 tablespoons dark rum

2 easpoons freshly
  squeezed lime juice

½ teaspoon ground
  cinnamon

Prepare a medium-hot fire in your grill.

In a small saucepan, melt butter over medium heat. Remove from heat and add brown sugar, rum, lime juice and cinnamon; stirring to blend. Set aside.

Place the grapefruit cut side down directly over the fire. Grill for about 4 to 5 minutes until it is warm and has good grill marks. Quickly use a serrated knife to section the grapefruit.

Serve grilled grapefruit halves in a small bowls with the Brown Sugar Rum Butter spooned over the top.

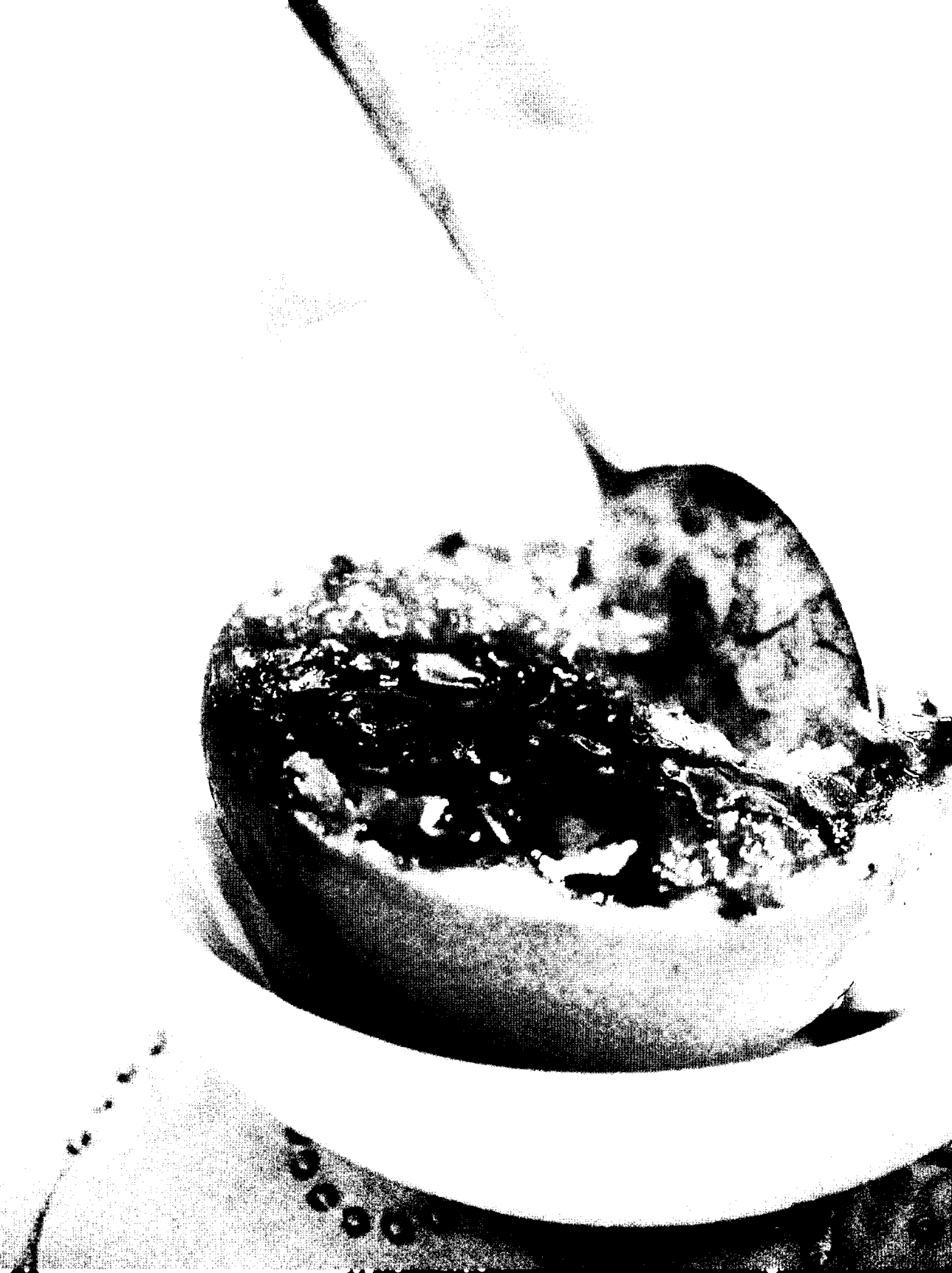

TOP TEN GARDEN-GROWN
FRUITS FOR THE GRILL

GARDENERS CAN GROW MANY TYPES OF FRUITS, FROM BERRIES TO orchard fruits, and most of them work well on the grill. Even small, homegrown berries can be scattered fresh over grilled fruit, then served with ice cream or frozen yogurt. Here are ten fruits that you can grow in your garden and that translate well to the grill.

- **APPLES.** Golden Delicious apples, cut into slices and then cored, are naturally sweet and stand up well to the heat of the grill, softening quickly without drying out. Other types of apples such as Jonathan and Granny Smith can be stuffed, then roasted, over indirect heat.

- **BERRIES.** Strawberries do well on skewers and only need a minute or two; turn them once on the grill. Smaller fruits such as blueberries and blackberries can be stir-grilled in a basket with other fruits or scattered over a planked cheese on the grill.

- **CHERRIES.** Pitted first, sweet cherries also do well on skewers over the grill grates. Turn once.

- **CITRUS.** Grapefruit, oranges, lemons and limes can be cut in half, then grilled cut-side down until the natural sugars caramelize.

- **FIGS.** Grilled whole or cut in half, sweet figs do well as appetizers or desserts.

- **GRAPES.** Grill a whole cluster of grapes, until the grapes have good grill marks, then turn with tongs to grill the other side.

- **MELON.** There's more to melon that just eating it raw. Try grilling slices of cantaloupe or honeydew to bring out their sweetness.

- **PEARS.** Juicy ripe-but-still-firm pears take to grilling and planking for salads and desserts.

- **PERSIMMONS.** Japanese persimmons, especially the Fuyu variety, can be cut in half and grilled so their sweet, bland flavor gets a little boost.

- **STONE FRUITS.** Apricots, peaches, plums, and nectarines—fruits that have a stone or pit in the center—do well cut in half, pitted, and grilled.

HOMEGROWN TABLE GRAPE VARIETIES INCLUDE SEEDLESS RED Concord and white Himrod. But, any variety, preferably seedless, will work for this autumn garden recipe. The 8-ounce wedges of cheese will serve twice as many people as we suggest. We like the larger wedges because they look better on the plank. Any leftover cheese can be stored in the refrigerator for later use.

GRILLED GRAPE & CHEESE BOARD

SERVES 12

1 bunch seedless green
  grapes (about 8 ounces)

1 bunch seedless red grapes
  (about 8 ounces)

2 tablespoons olive oil

One 8-ounce wedge Parme-
  san cheese

One 8-ounce wedge
  Cheddar cheese

1 French baguette, sliced,
  for serving

Soak a grilling plank in water for at least 1 hour. Prepare a medium-hot fire on one side of your grill for indirect cooking.

Lightly brush the grapes with olive oil and set aside.

Place the cheeses on the plank with the largest cut side of the wedges on the plank. Place the plank on the indirect side of the grill and close the lid. Plank for 15 to 20 minutes, or until the cheddar cheese is beginning to ooze. Remove the plank and grill the grapes directly on the medium-hot side of the grill, turning the bunches often, until the grapes are scorched and blistered, about 4 minutes total. Arrange the grapes around the cheeses on the plank and serve with a basket of baguette slices.

COMPANION PLANTS

SOME VEGETABLES, FRUITS, AND HERBS—PLANTED TOGETHER— bring out the best in each other, just like people. Sometimes these plant "buddies" attract beneficial insects or naturally repel others. Some provide missing nutrients, shade, or climbing support. Plant leeks with your tomatoes or apple trees? Yes! Basil with your petunias? You bet. They all grow better together. Consider growing friends together in a container garden or plan them together in an edible landscape. Or take the traditional Native American approach and plant the "three sisters" together: corn, beans, and squash.

- **ALLIUMS** (onions, garlic, leeks, shallots, and chives) help fruit trees, nightshades (tomatoes, peppers, potatoes), brassicas (cabbage, broccoli, kohlrabi, kale), and carrots. Alliums protect against the carrot fly and slugs.

- **ASPARAGUS** helps tomatoes, and vice versa. Each helps protect against the other's most common pests.

- **BASIL** helps tomatoes, peppers, oregano, asparagus, and petunias by warding off whitefly.

- **BEANS** help strawberries, corn, spinach, lettuce, rosemary, summer savory, dill, carrots, the broccoli family, beets, radish, and cucumbers by providing shade, a cooler micro-climate, and more nitrogen in the soil.

- **BORAGE** helps everything, especially strawberries, cucumbers, and tomatoes, because it attracts bees and adds trace minerals to the soil.

- **CARAWAY** helps strawberries by loosening compacted soil.

- **CARROTS** help tomatoes, alliums (onions and chives), and lettuce by deterring pests.

- **CHIVES** (green onions) help apples, carrots, tomatoes, and brassicas (broccoli, cabbage, mustard greens) by improving growth and flavor.

- **GARLIC** helps apple trees, pear trees, roses, cucumbers, peas, lettuce, and celery by repelling aphids and other pests. It also provides sulfur, a natural fungicide.

- **LEEKS** help apple trees and celery by repelling pests.

- **LOVAGE** helps almost all plants by improving their health and flavor.

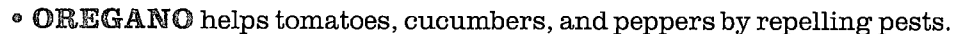

- **OREGANO** helps tomatoes, cucumbers, and peppers by repelling pests.

- **MARIGOLDS** help most plants, especially tomatoes, peppers, cucumber, and broccoli, by acting as a natural insect repellent.

- **NASTURTIUMS** help melons, apple trees, tomatoes, cucumbers, beans, broccoli, cabbage, and radishes by attracting pests away from your crop.

- **SUNFLOWER** helps tomatoes and corn increase their yield.

- **TARRAGON** helps by enhancing the growth and flavor of vegetables planted near it.

- **WINTER SQUASH** helps corn and beans by providing cover for the root system and protection from weeds.

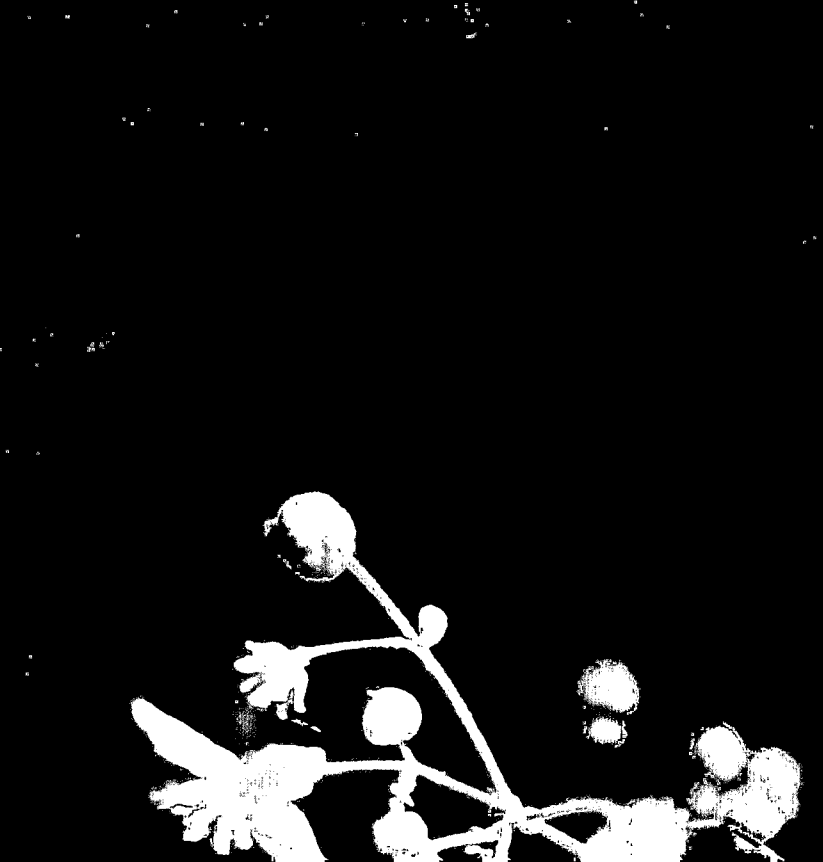

BACKYARD GARDEN STRAWBERRIES ARE OFTEN SMALLER THAN store-bought, so be the judge of how many strawberries you need for the skewers. Or even simpler, grill strawberries on a grill rack until a bit charred and warmed through and spoon atop frozen yogurt or ice cream.

SKEWERED STRAWBERRY &
MARSHMALLOW S'MORES

SERVES 4

12 medium-sized
    strawberries

8 large marshmallows

8 slices French baguette

Olive oil, for brushing

One (4-ounce) bar dark
    chocolate, cut into 8
    pieces

¼ teaspoon coarse kosher
    or sea salt

Prepare a medium-hot fire on one side of your grill. Thread the strawberries and marshmallows alternately on 4 skewers (if using wooden skewers, presoak them). Lightly brush the slices of bread with olive oil.

Place the skewers directly over the fire and grill for about 4 or 5 minutes until the marshmallows have browned.

At the same time, grill one side of the bread. Turn the slices over and move to the indirect side of the grill. Place a piece of chocolate on each slice and sprinkle with a pinch of coarse salt. Remove from the grill when the chocolate is soft but still holds its shape.

Serve the skewers with the grilled bread for a grown-up version of s'mores.

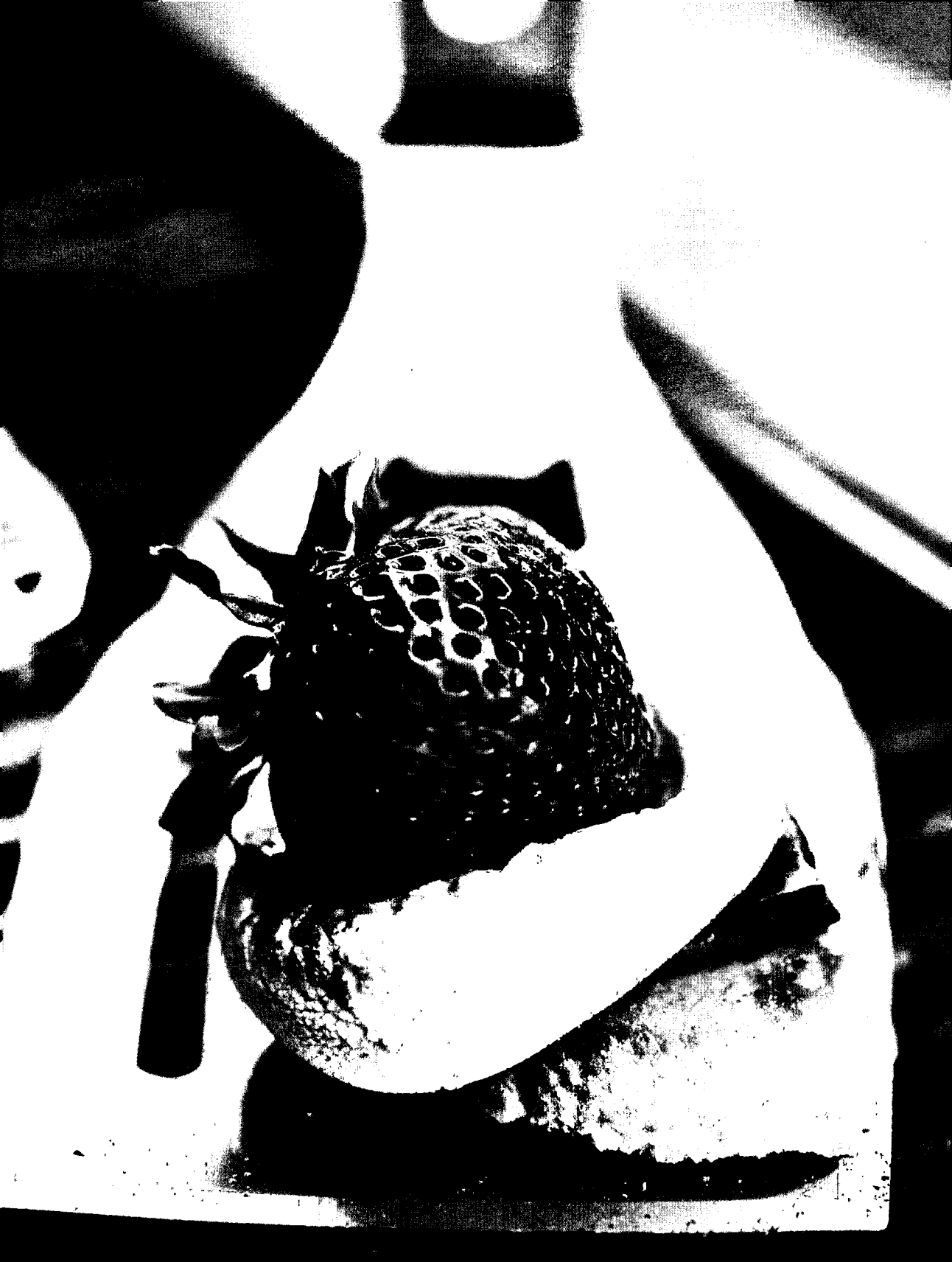

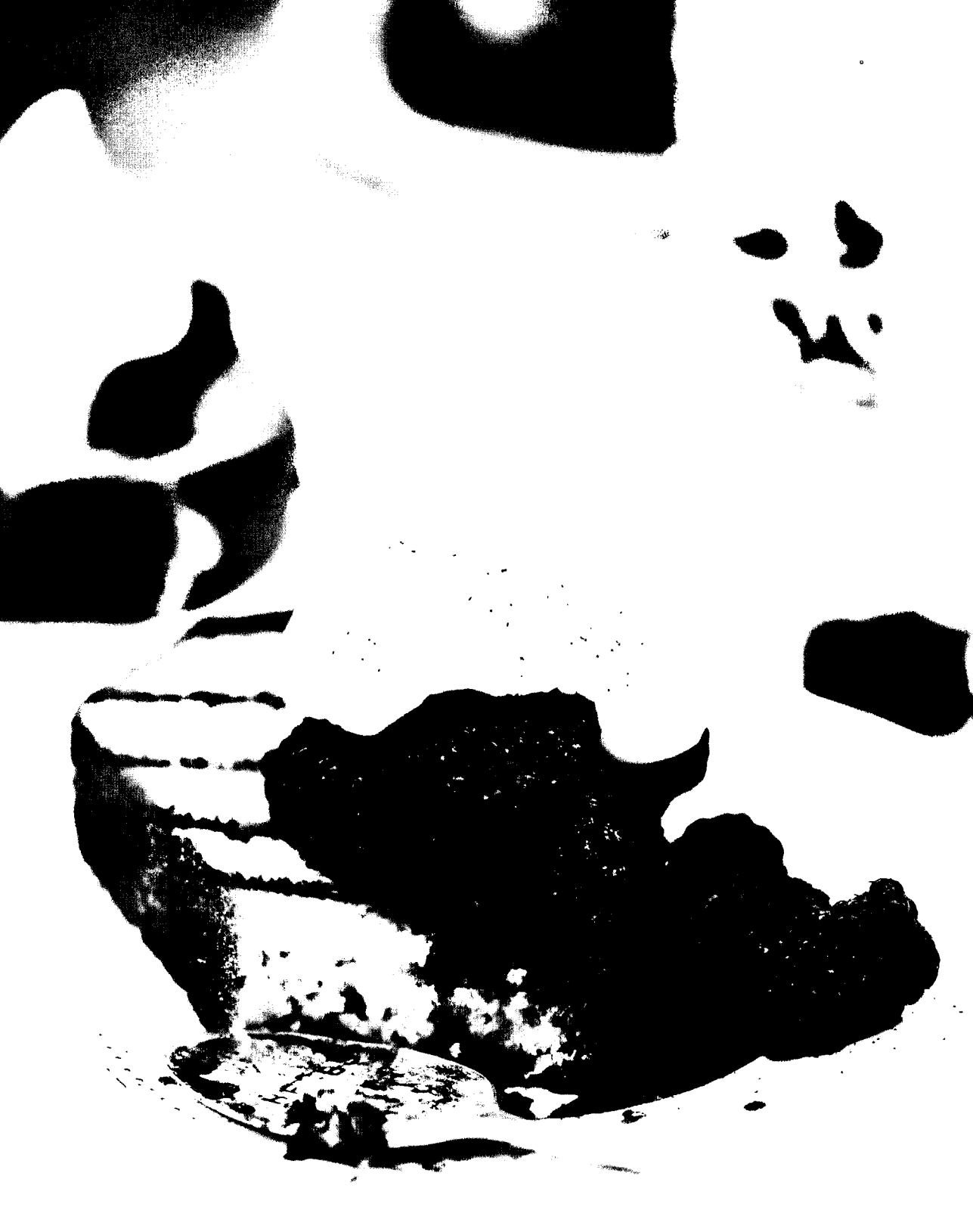

THOUGH THE BERRIES AREN'T GRILLED, THE SAUCE IS COOKED on the grill, along with the grilled slices of pound cake. The butter content in the pound cake is enough to keep it from sticking to the grill grates, so you do not need to brush the slices with oil or butter. The Lemony Crème Fraîche (page 200) or the Honey-Cinnamon Crème Fraîche (page 213) would be a delicious topping instead of the whipped cream.

WARM HONEYED BLACKBERRIES with GRILLED POUND CAKE

SERVES 4

1 cup heavy whipping cream

4 cups blackberries

6 tablespoons honey, divided

Juice of $\frac{1}{2}$ lemon

1 teaspoon ground cinnamon, plus more for sprinkling

4 (1-inch) slices of pound cake

Prepare a hot fire in your grill. Whip the cream with an electric mixer or a whisk until it holds medium peaks, about 5 to 7 minutes. Set aside.

In a heavy saucepan that can be used on the grill or on a grill side burner, combine the blackberries, 4 tablespoons honey, lemon juice, and cinnamon.

Set the saucepan over the heat and stir to blend, cooking until the mixture begins to bubble.

At the same time, grill the pound cake slices for about 3 to 4 minutes per side until they get good grill marks.

Stir 2 tablespoons of the remaining honey into the whipped cream with a light touch.

To serve, set a slice of grilled pound cake on each plate. Spoon the warmed berries over the cake and top with the honeyed whipped cream. Sprinkle with cinnamon and serve.

RHUBARB, STRAWBERRIES, AND LEMON HAVE A NATURAL AFFI-
nity for each other. For a wonderful spring dessert, combine them all in
this dish.

GRILL-ROASTED RHUBARB
and STRAWBERRIES with
LEMONY CRÈME FRAÎCHE

SERVES 4

LEMONY CRÈME FRAÎCHE

1 cup heavy whipping
cream

1 cup sour cream

$\frac{1}{4}$ cup honey, plus more to
taste

Grated zest of $\frac{1}{2}$ lemon

Juice from $\frac{1}{2}$ lemon

FRUIT

Olive oil, as needed

4 stalks rhubarb, sliced
into 1-inch pieces

1 pint strawberries,
cleaned, stemmed, and
cut in half (reserve 4
whole berries for gar-
nish)

In a bowl, stir together the cream, sour cream, and
honey. Cover and let stand for at least 1 hour or up
to 4 hours until it thickens. Add the lemon zest and
juice and stir to blend. Taste and add more honey if
you would like it to be sweeter.

Prepare a medium-hot fire on one side of your
grill for indirect cooking.

Lightly oil a disposable 9 x 13-inch aluminum
pan. Combine the rhubarb with $1\frac{1}{2}$ cups of the
Lemony Crème Fraîche in the pan. Place the pan on
the indirect side, close the lid, and grill-roast (see
page 8) the rhubarb for 10 minutes. Stir in the
strawberries. Close the lid and grill-roast for 6 to 8
minutes or until the rhubarb is tender and the
strawberries warmed through. Spoon the mixture
into bowls and serve with a dollop of the remaining
Lemony Crème Fraîche and garnish with a whole
strawberry.

LIKE MOST OF OUR FRUIT RECIPES FOR THE GRILL, THIS ONE begins with delicious fruit. So make sure your melon is sweet and ripe.

GRILLED CANTALOUPE RINGS
with VANILLA BEAN ICE CREAM

SERVES 4

1 cantaloupe or honeydew
  melon

2 tablespoons packed
  brown sugar

4 scoops vanilla bean ice
  cream

Prepare a hot fire in your grill.

Slice the cantaloupe in half and remove the seeds. Slice off the bottom of each half to the flesh. Slice each half in two circles.

Place cantaloupe rings directly over the fire and grill for about 3 or 4 minutes until they have charred grill marks. Turn the slices over and sprinkle the rings with $\frac{1}{2}$ tablespoon of brown sugar. Grill for about 3 or 4 more minutes.

To serve, set a slice of grilled cantaloupe on a dinner plate. Place a scoop of ice cream in the middle.

EDIBLE FLOWERS

EVERY DAY DURING THE GROWING SEASON, YOUR GARDEN IS A palette of possibilities. If you plant pansies, daylilies, and roses, you have an instant, colorful garnish. Even if you don't plant edible flowers on purpose, you might have them anyway, if you think creatively. Consider the peppery nasturtium, anise-flavored white chive blossoms, and the pale blue flowers of herbs like rosemary. They add a jolt of color and oftentimes a burst of flavor, too. Make sure any blossoms or flowers you use come from chemical- and pesticide-free gardens or even better, grow your own. Sprinkle edible flowers, whole or petals snipped with kitchen shears, over grilled dishes, from appetizers and flatbreads to vegetables, main dishes, and fruit-based desserts.

- **BASIL.** Different varieties produce either bright white, pale pink, or soft lavender flowers. Use them in salads, soups, sandwiches, pastas, and even with fruit.
- **BEE BALM.** Also known as wild bergamot, the red flowers have a minty flavor.
- **BORAGE.** The star-shaped flowers are a pretty cornflower blue and taste a bit like cucumber.
- **CHIVE.** Blossoms are beautiful white and lavender colors. Use them in salads and soups.
- **CHERVIL.** This small white flower has a slight anise flavor. Sprinkle it on salads.
- **DAYLILY.** They have a slightly sweet and mild vegetal flavor. Use the petals to garnish grilled fruit.
- **FENNEL.** Yellow flowers with a mild anise taste are best used with fruits and as a garnish for an entrée.
- **SCENTED GERANIUM.** The flower will taste like the variety; that is, a lemon-scented geranium has a lemon-scented flower. Use the petals to garnish desserts and drinks.
- **LAVENDER.** The flowers have sweet floral notes. Use them as a garnish to any of the fruit dishes.

- **MARIGOLD.** Sprinkle on soups, pastas, rice dishes, and salads. The flower petals look beautiful in herb butters.

- **MINT.** The cone-shaped flowers are pretty snipped with a bit of the leaves for flavor and garnish in salads, desserts, and lamb dishes.

- **NASTURTIUM.** The jewel-tone colors of this peppery flower are one of the most colorful additions to salads or to garnish savory or sweet dishes.

- **PANSY.** The petals have a sweet, mild flavor. They are a colorful garnish for desserts, both green and fruit salads, and soups.

- **PEA BLOSSOMS.** The flowers are usually white or a pale pink and taste sweet and crunchy like peas. Use them to garnish a stir-grilled dish.

- **ROSE.** The flavors of roses range from strawberries to green apples depending on the variety. Sprinkle the petals on salads and desserts or add to butter for a perfume-like flavor.

- **ROSEMARY.** The flower is a mild version of the leaf. Use it in pasta dishes, salads, vinaigrettes, and with entrees.

- **SAGE.** The flowers are tube-like spikes and have a subtle sage flavor. They are delicious with beans and corn.

- **SQUASH BLOSSOMS.** The flavor of these flowers is like a mild tasting squash. They are trumpet-shaped and can be stuffed with goat cheese and served as an appetizer or garnish for salads and entrées.

- **VIOLET.** This also includes Johnny jump-ups and violas with colors from violet to yellow to pale peach and apricot. Garnish salads, sandwiches, and desserts with these petals.

- **WINTER SAVORY.** The flowers are hot and peppery, making them a perfect garnish for anything that needs a zing of pepper.

THIS RECIPE IS VERY SIMPLE, YET FULL OF FLAVOR. A TRADITIONAL gremolata has parsley, lemon zest, and garlic, but this is a sweeter version, delicious with fruit. If you don't have lemon balm in your garden, substitute mint and add more lemon zest. If you use a Microplane grater, you get the flavorful yellow part of the lemon rind without the bitter white pith. By chopping the herbs with the lemon zest, the flavors blend together better.

GRILLED PEACHES
with LEMON BALM GREMOLATA

SERVES 4

$\frac{1}{4}$ cup packed lemon balm
  leaves

1 tablespoon packed mint
  leaves

$\frac{1}{2}$ teaspoon lemon zest

Pinch kosher or sea salt

4 peaches, halved and
  pitted

Prepare a medium-hot fire in your grill.

Chop the lemon balm, mint, and lemon zest together until very fine. Sprinkle a pinch of salt over the leaves and chop again. Set aside in a small bowl.

Place the peach halves cut side down on the grill. Grill for 4 to 6 minutes, turning once, until the peaches are tender and blistered.

To serve, place 2 peach halves in each bowl and sprinkle the Lemon Balm Gremolata over all.

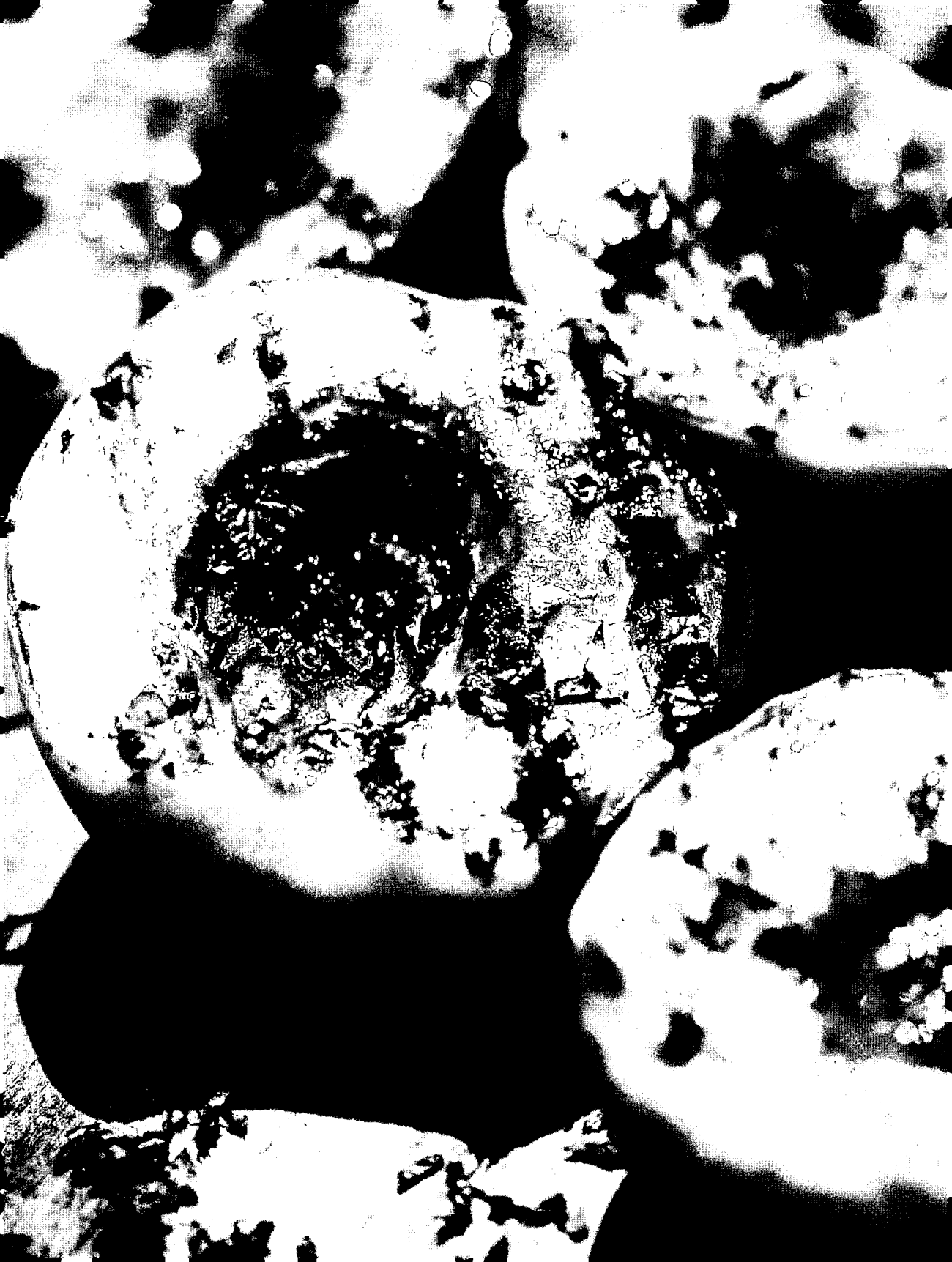

A DELICIOUS, JUICY PEACH IS ONE OF SUMMER'S SPECIAL TASTES. Nectarines substitute beautifully for this recipe, as well as raspberries or blackberries along with or instead of the blueberries.

PLANKED PEACHES and BLUEBERRIES with AMARETTO SAUCE

SERVES 4

AMARETTO SAUCE

3 ounces ($\frac{3}{4}$ stick)
  unsalted butter

6 tablespoons amaretto or
  other almond liqueur

Pinch kosher or sea salt

FRUIT

4 peaches, halved and
  pitted

1 pint blueberries

Prepare a medium-hot fire in your grill.

In a small saucepan, melt butter over medium heat. Remove from heat and stir in the amaretto and salt. Keep warm.

Brush peaches all over with the buttery sauce. Place them cut-side down on the grill. Grill for 4 to 6 minutes, turning and basting once, until peaches are tender and blistered.

To serve, place 2 peach halves in each bowl and divide the berries between them. Spoon any remaining Amaretto Sauce over all.

APANESE PLUM VARIETIES GROW WELL IN WARMER CLIMATES where they aren't susceptible to late frost or freezes. Black Beauty is a purplish-black skinned plum with a yellow flesh. Combine it with a red-fleshed plum like Burgundy for contrast. Fantasia nectarines have gold and crimson skin and yellow flesh. The colors in this dish are just gorgeous.

STIR-GRILLED NECTARINES & PLUMS
with SWEET WINE DRIZZLE

SERVES 4

2 nectarines, like Fantasia, halved, seeded, and sliced

4 to 6 plums, like Black Beauty or Burgundy, halved, pitted, and sliced

¼ cup honey

¼ cup sweet wine, red or white

Prepare a hot fire in your grill.

Place the fruit in a perforated grill wok and set aside. In a small saucepan, heat the honey and stir in the wine. Keep warm.

To stir-grill (see page 9), place the grill wok directly over the fire and toss the fruit with wooden paddles or grill spatulas until it is heated through and a bit charred, about 6 to 8 minutes.

To serve, spoon fruit into 4 bowls and drizzle with the warm honey-wine mixture.

THE BEST OVERALL JAPANESE VARIETY OF PERSIMMON FOR eating and grilling is the Fuyu. They are short, squat, pumpkin-shaped and sweetly mellow in flavor. Eat it fresh like an apple, peeled and sliced, and grill it like an apple, too, but with the skin on.

GRILLED PERSIMMONS
with THREE-CITRUS DRIZZLE

SERVES 4

4 Fuyu persimmons, sliced
  and seeded

1 cup Three-Citrus Drizzle
  for Fruit (page 25),
  divided

Prepare a hot fire in your grill.

Place the fruit in a perforated grill wok on top of a baking sheet and spoon $\frac{1}{2}$ cup of the drizzle over the fruit; toss to coat.

Place the grill wok directly over the fire and toss the persimmon slices with wooden paddles or grill spatulas until they are heated through and blistered, about 6 to 8 minutes.

Serve the persimmon slices in bowls and spoon additional Three-Citrus Drizzle for Fruit over them.

THERE ARE SO MANY VARIETIES OF APPLES FROM EACH GROWING zone to choose from. If you have more than one kind of apple, experiment with doing both to see which you like the best. Grilled apples take on the flavor of the hearth, reminiscent of the old village wood-fired oven. They're delicious for breakfast (so make a double batch). For dessert, serve them hot off the grill, with a scoop of vanilla or cinnamon ice cream. If you have a nut tree, use what's native and in your own back yard.

GRILL-BAKED APPLES
with CINNAMON NUT STUFFING

SERVES 4

4 orchard apples, any firm
  variety

½ cup (1 stick) unsalted
  butter, softened enough
  to combine with a fork

1 cup packed light or dark
  brown sugar

1 tablespoon ground
  cinnamon

½ cup chopped walnuts
  or pecans

Prepare a hot fire on one side of your grill for indirect cooking.

Core the apples, but do not cut all the way through.

Combine the butter, brown sugar, and cinnamon in a small bowl with a fork until well blended. Stir in the nuts. Fill the apples with the stuffing and place on a grill rack.

Place the rack on the indirect side of the grill and close the lid. Grill for 20 to 30 minutes or until the apples are tender when pierced with a knife. Serve warm.

JUST ABOUT ANY VARIETY OF APPLES WORKS IN THIS RECIPE, the slices coated with this fragrant, sweet, and spicy rub. For an extra oomph, drizzle them with a good caramel sauce for dessert. They are a great accompaniment to pork or chicken, too.

ROSEMARY *and* SUGAR-SPICE-RUBBED APPLE SLICES

SERVES 4

3 or 4 medium-size orchard apples, cored and sliced

¼ cup packed brown sugar

1 tablespoon ground cinnamon

½ teaspoon freshly grated nutmeg

½ teaspoon finely chopped fresh rosemary leaves

Prepare a hot fire in your grill.

Place the fruit in a perforated grill wok on top of a baking sheet and set aside.

Combine the sugar, cinnamon, nutmeg, and rosemary and sprinkle half of the mixture over the fruit.

Place the grill wok directly over the fire and toss the apple slices with wooden paddles or grill spatulas until they are heated through and blistered, about 6 to 8 minutes. Sprinkle the apples with the remaining rub and serve warm.

WHETHER YOU SERVE THIS AS A DESSERT WITH A GLASS OF port or over dressed greens as a salad, you'll savor the extra flavor that plank-roasting over high heat gives this mild fruit. You'll scorch one side of the plank, then turn it over and place the fruit on the scorched side. You'll put the plank of fruit right over the fire in this recipe, so make sure you soak your plank the full hour.

PLANK-ROASTED PEARS with BLUE CHEESE and BALSAMIC HONEY

SERVES 4

2 large, ripe Anjou or Bartlett pears, halved with stem intact

2 tablespoons balsamic vinegar

2 tablespoons wildflower or other amber honey

½ cup crumbled blue cheese

Fresh thyme sprigs for garnish

Soak 1 cedar, alder, or oak grilling plank for 1 hour in water. Prepare a hot fire in your grill.

Using a sturdy teaspoon or a melon baller, remove the core from each pear half. Place the pear halves on a baking sheet.

In a bowl, mix together the vinegar and honey. Lightly brush the honey mixture over the cut side of the pears. Spoon the blue cheese crumbled into the center of each pear half. Take the baking sheet out to the grill.

Place a water-soaked wood plank on the grill grate and close the lid. When the plank starts to smoke and pop, after 3 to 5 minutes, open the lid. Using grill tongs, quickly turn the plank and place the pear halves on the plank, cut side up. Cover and plank-roast (see page 9) for 10 to 12 minutes, or until the pears are scorched around the edges.

Drizzle with remaining honey mixture, garnish with thyme sprigs, and serve warm.

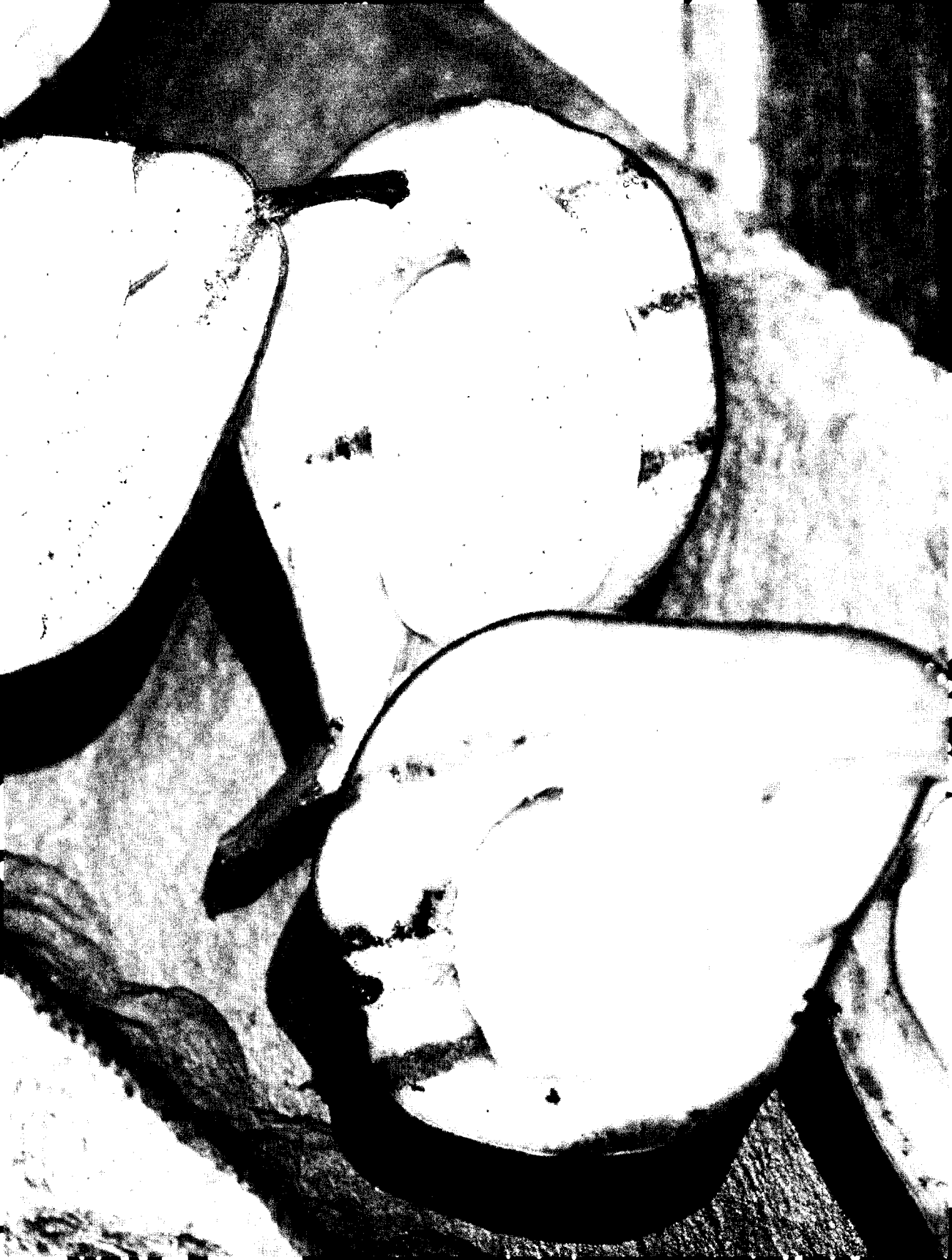

RILLED PEARS ARE DELICIOUS SERVED WITH BLUE CHEESE (see Plank-Roasted Pears with Blue Cheese and Balsamic Honey, page 211 or Plank-Roasted Pear Salad with Blue Cheese and Walnuts, page 112), but they're also great with this easy sauce, made with wildflower honey that the bees make in early summer.

GRILLED PEARS *with*
HONEY-CINNAMON CRÈME FRAÎCHE

SERVES 4

½ cup sour cream

½ cup heavy whipping cream

2 tablespoons wildflower honey

2 teaspoons ground cinnamon

4 pears, halved and cored

In a bowl, stir together the sour cream, cream, honey, and cinnamon. Cover and let stand for at least 1 hour or up to 4 hours until it thickens.

Prepare a medium-hot fire in your grill.

Place the pear halves cut-side down on the grill. Grill for 4 to 6 minutes, turning once, until the pears are tender and blistered.

To serve, place 2 pear halves in each bowl and spoon the crème fraîche on top. Serve warm.

INDEX

Note: Page references in *italics* indicate photographs.

A

Aioli
flavor variations, 40
Lemon-Garlic, 39
Alliums, companion plants for, 194
Almonds
Romesco Sauce, 42
Amaretto Sauce, 206
Ancho-Lime Butter, 175
Anchovy Garlic Dipping Sauce, 169
Appetizers
Chard-Wrapped Goat Cheese on the Grill, 75
Charred Eggplant and Tarragon Spread, 54
Crostini with Smoked and Grilled Vegetable
Dip, 59
Fire-Roasted Fava Beans in the Pod with
Sheep's Milk Cheese, 65
Fire-Roasted Pepper Dip, 72
Flame-Licked Fingerlings with Romesco
Sauce, 68, *69*
French Garden Radish Plate with Grilled
Onion Butter, *56, 57*
Grilled Baba Ganoush, *92, 93*
Grilled Polenta with Stir-Grilled Garlic
Greens, 77
Grilled Rye Bread with Soft Cheese and Spring
Radishes, 55
Grilled Zucchini and Yellow Squash Stacks
with Feta and Black Olives, 73
Grill-Roasted Bruschetta with Four Seasons
Toppings, 49
Grill-Roasted Edamame in the Pod, *66, 67*
Grill-Roasted Tomatillo Salsa, *70,* 71
Mesquite-Smoked Jalapeño Poppers, 74
Planked Brie with Grilled Apricot Jam, 189
Planked Butternut Squash, Sage, and Brie, 60
Prosciutto-Wrapped Asparagus Spears, 62, *63*
Soft Corn Tortillas with Rajas and Queso, 61
Tuscan Polenta Platter with Sizzling Peppers,
Onions, and Mushrooms, 76
Apple(s)
Grill-Baked, with Cinnamon Nut Stuffing, 209
Grilled Autumn, and Blue Cheese Topping, 52
grilling, 192
Rings and Acorn Squash with Cider Jus, 184–
185, *185*
Slices, Rosemary and Sugar-Spice-Rubbed,
210
Apricot(s)
Grilled, Jam, Planked Brie with, 189
grilling, 192
Arugula
Grilled Caesar Sirloin, 153
Asian flavors, 18
Asparagus
companion plants for, 194
grilled, freezing, 28
Grilled, Salad, 111
grilling, 162
and Leeks, Grilled Spring Platter of, 161
measuring without a scale, 64
Pizza Primavera, 99
Spears, Prosciutto-Wrapped, 62, *63*

B

Bacon
Blue Cheese Butter, 30
Dressing, Hot, Grilled Radicchio and Brussels
Sprouts with, 120, *121*
Grill-Roasted Stuffed Peppers, 178–179
Mesquite-Smoked Jalapeño Poppers, 74
Basil
companion plants for, 194
edible flowers from, 202
Fresh, Vinaigrette, *20,* 21
Italian varieties, 98
Panini Caprese, 85
Pesto (var.), 32
Smoked Summer Tomato Butter, 30, *50,* 51
Stir-Grilled Sugar Snap Peas and Tear Drop
Tomatoes with, 167
Sun-Dried Tomato Aioli, 40
Thai, for Asian recipes, 18
woody stems, for skewers, 24
Baste, Rosemary, Garlic, and Lemon, 27
Bean(s). *See also* Green Beans
companion plants for, 194
fava, grilling, 98
Fava, in the Pod, Fire-Roasted, with Sheep's
Milk Cheese, 65
grilling and serving edamame, 18
Grill-Roasted Edamame in the Pod, *66, 67*

growing edamame, 67

measuring without a scale, 64

White, Spread, Rustic Winter, 52

Béarnaise Butter, 29

Bee balm, edible flowers from, 202

Beef

best cuts for grilling, 135

Blackened, with Thai Chile Noodles and Baby Bok Choy, 154, *155*

checking doneness, 135

Flank Steak with Grilled Peppers and Onions, 156–157

Grilled Caesar Sirloin, 153

Kansas City Strip Steaks with Parmesan Grilled Vegetables, 157

Wood-Grilled Burger with Chive Pesto, Grilled Fresh Tomatoes, and Provolone, 88

Beets, Baby, Grilled, with Scallions and Lemon Herb Butter, 168

Berries

grilling, 192

Grill-Roasted Rhubarb and Strawberries with Lemony Crème Fraîche, 200

Planked Peaches and Blueberries with Amaretto Sauce, 206

Skewered Strawberry & Marshmallow S'mores, 196, *197*

Warm Cranberry Vinaigrette, 142

Warm Honeyed Blackberries with Grilled Pound Cake, *198*, 199

Blackberries

grilling, 192

Warm Honeyed, with Grilled Pound Cake, *198*, 199

Blender Hollandaise, 36

Blueberries

grilling, 192

and Planked Peaches with Amaretto Sauce, 206

Blue Cheese

Bacon Butter, 30

and Balsamic Honey, Plank-Roasted Pears with, 211

Dressing, Creamy, 41

and Grilled Autumn Apple Topping, 52

Grilled Summer Slaw with Gorgonzola Vinaigrette, 119

and Walnuts, Plank-Roasted Pear Salad with, *112*, 113

Bok Choy

Baby, and Thai Chile Noodles, Blackened Beef with, 154, *155*

Baby, Grilled, with Fresh Ginger-Soy Sauce, *122*, 123

growing, 116

Borage

companion plants for, 194

edible flowers from, 202

Brats with Grilled Kale and Horseradish Butter, 143

Breads. *See also* Flatbreads; Pizza

Crostini with Smoked and Grilled Vegetable Dip, 59

Grill-Roasted Bruschetta with Four Seasons Toppings, 49

Pita, Grilled, with Grilled Baba Ganoush, *92*, 93

Rye, Grilled, with Soft Cheese and Spring Radishes, 55

Broccoli

grilling, 162

measuring without a scale, 64

Purple Sprouting, Grilled, with Garlic Anchovy Dipping Sauce, 169

varieties of, 98

Bruschetta, Grill-Roasted, with Four Seasons Toppings, 49

Bruschetta Toppings

Goat Cheese with Spring Garlic and Herb, *50*, 51

Grilled Autumn Apple and Blue Cheese, 52

Rustic Winter White Bean Spread, 52

Smoked Summer Tomato Basil Butter, *50*, 51

Brussels Sprouts

with Feta Garlic Butter, 170

growing, 116

and Radicchio, Grilled, with Hot Bacon Dressing, 120, *121*

Burgers

Tandoori Turkey, with Grilled Red Onions and Tomatoes, 140–141

Wood-Grilled, with Chive Pesto, Grilled Fresh Tomatoes, and Provolone, 88

Butter

Ancho-Lime, 175

Béarnaise, 29

Feta Garlic, 170

flavored, recipes for, 30

Grilled Onion, *56*, 57

Horseradish, 143

Lemon-Herb, 168

Smoked Summer Tomato Basil, *50*, 51

C

Cabbage
  Chinese and autumn torch hybrid, growing, 116
  Grilled Summer Slaw with Gorgonzola Vinaigrette, 119
  grilling, 162
  growing, 116
  Napa, Grilled, Slaw, 149
  napa or savoy, growing, 116
  red or green, growing, 116
Caesar Butter, 30
Cake, Grilled Pound, Warm Honeyed Blackberries with, *198, 199*
Cantaloupe Rings, Grilled, with Vanilla Bean Ice Cream, 201
Caper Butter, 30
Caraway, companion plants for, 194
Carrots
  companion plants for, 194
  Rainbow, with Cilantro Chile Drizzle, 172, *173*
Cauliflower with Grill-Roasted Tomatillo Salsa, 171
Chard-Wrapped Goat Cheese on the Grill, 75
Charred Eggplant and Tarragon Spread, 54
Cheese. *See also* Blue Cheese; Goat Cheese; Parmesan
  Baby Eggplant with Gruyère and Sun-Dried Tomatoes, 177
  Char-Grilled Baby Summer Squash Pizza, 104–105
  Cream, Herbed, Grilled Green Tomato "Sandwiches" with, 82, *83*
  Feta Garlic Butter, 170
  Greek Aioli, 40
  & Grilled Grape Board, 193
  Grilled Zucchini and Yellow Squash Stacks with Feta and Black Olives, 73
  Grill-Roasted Stuffed Peppers, 178–179
  Mesquite-Smoked Jalapeño Poppers, 74
  On the Grill, Chard-Wrapped Goat, 75
  Panini Caprese, 85
  Planked Brie with Grilled Apricot Jam, 189
  Planked Butternut Squash, Sage, and Brie, 60
  Sheep's Milk, Fire-Roasted Fava Beans in the Pod with, 65
  Soft, and Spring Radishes, Grilled Rye Bread with, 55
  Soft Corn Tortillas with Rajas and Queso, 61
  Wood-Grilled Burger with Chive Pesto, Grilled Fresh Tomatoes, and Provolone, 88
  Wood-Grilled Spring Onion, Brie, and Kala-

mata Olive Pizza, 100, *101*
Cherries, grilling, 192
Chervil, edible flowers from, 202
Chicken
  best cuts for grilling, 135
  checking doneness, 135
  Grilled, Ciabatta with Romesco and Baby Greens, 86, *87*
  and Grilled Corn Chowder, 125
  Paillard and Baby Green Beans with Mustard Seed Sauce, 138
  Skewered, Saltimbocca, 137
Chile peppers
  Blackened Beef with Thai Chile Noodles and Baby Bok Choy, 154, *155*
  Chipotle Vinaigrette, 22
  Cilantro Chile Drizzle, 172, *173*
  grilled, freezing, 28
  grilling and smoking, 152
  Mesquite-Smoked Jalapeño Poppers, 74
  smoked, freezing, 33
  Smoked Poblano Cream Sauce, 35
  Soft Corn Tortillas with Rajas and Queso, 61
  Southwest Butter, 30
  Spicy Chipotle Aioli, 40
Chimichurri Sauce, 26
Chipotle Vinaigrette, 22
Chive(s)
  companion plants for, 194
  edible flowers from, 202
  Pesto, Garlic, 32
Chocolate
  Skewered Strawberry & Marshmallow S'mores, 196, *197*
Choi hybrids, growing, 116
Chowder, Grilled Corn and Chicken, 125
Cilantro
  Chile Drizzle, 172, *173*
  Herb-Stuffed Afghan Flatbread, 96
  and Smoked Garlic Cream Sauce, 34
Coconut-Red Curry Soup with Grilled Vegetables and Shrimp, 130–131
Container gardens, 58
Corn
  Grilled, and Chicken Chowder, 125
  grilled, freezing, 28
  grilling, 162
  Husks, Grilled Salmon in, 151
  -in-the-Husk, Grilled, with Ancho-Lime Butter, 175
  smoked, freezing, 33
  Tomato, and Red Onion, Grilled, Salad, 114

Cranberry Vinaigrette, Warm, 142
Cream Cheese
    Herbed, Grilled Green Tomato "Sandwiches"
        with, 82, *83*
    Mesquite-Smoked Jalapeño Poppers, 74
Crème Fraîche
    Honey-Cinnamon, Grilled Pears with,
        212, 213
    Lemony, 200
Crostini with Smoked and Grilled Vegetable
    Dip, 59
Cucumbers
    serving ideas, 53
    Tzatziki, 44
Cumin, flavoring with, 53
Cumin Yogurt Sauce, 140
Curry, Red, -Coconut Soup with Grilled
    Vegetables and Shrimp, 130–131

D
Daylily petals, garnishing with, 202
Desserts
    Grill-Baked Apples with Cinnamon Nut
    Stuffing, 209
    Grilled Cantaloupe Rings with Vanilla Bean
        Ice Cream, 201
    Grilled Grape & Cheese Board, 193
    Grilled Grapefruit with Brown Sugar Rum
        Butter, 190, *191*
    Grilled Peaches with Lemon Balm Gremolata,
        204, *205*
    Grilled Pears with Honey-Cinnamon Crème
        Fraîche, *212,* 213
    Grilled Persimmons with Three-Citrus
        Drizzle, 208
    Grill-Roasted Rhubarb and Strawberries with
        Lemony Crème Fraîche, 200
    Planked Brie with Grilled Apricot Jam, 189·
    Planked Peaches and Blueberries with
        Amaretto Sauce, 206
    Plank-Roasted Pears with Blue Cheese and
        Balsamic Honey, 211
    Rosemary and Sugar-Spice-Rubbed Apple
        Slices, 210
    Skewered Strawberry & Marshmallow
    S'mores, 196, *197*
    Stir-Grilled Nectarines & Plums with Sweet
        Wine Drizzle, 207
    Warm Honeyed Blackberries with Grilled
        Pound Cake, *198,* 199
Dips and spreads

aioli flavor variations, 40
    Basil Pesto (var.), 32
    Charred Eggplant and Tarragon Spread, 54
    Chive Pesto, 32
    Creamy Blue Cheese Dressing, 41
    Crostini with Smoked and Grilled Vegetable
        Dip, 59
    Fire-Roasted Pepper Dip, 72
    Garlic Anchovy Dipping Sauce, 169
    Grilled Baba Ganoush, *92,* 93
    Grilled Green Onion Mayonnaise, 38
    Grill-Roasted Tomatillo Salsa, *70,* 71
    Lemon-Garlic Aioli, 39
    Lemon Verbena Pesto, 164, *165*
    Mustard Seed Sauce, 37
    Romesco Sauce, 42
    Satay-Style Peanut Dipping Sauce, 23
    Tzatziki, 44
Dressings
    Blue Cheese, Creamy, 41
    Chipotle Vinaigrette, 22
    Fresh Basil Vinaigrette, *20,* 21
    Ginger Vinaigrette, 16
    Lemon Caesar Vinaigrette, 17
    Three-Citrus Drizzle for Fruit, 25
    Toasted Sesame–Soy, 15

E
Edamame
    grilling and serving, 18
    growing, 67
    in the Pod, Grill-Roasted, *66,* 67
Eggplant
    Baby, with Gruyère and Sun-Dried
        Tomatoes, 177
    Char-Grilled, with Grilled Marinara
        Sauce, 176
    Charred, and Tarragon Spread, 54
    grilled, freezing, 28
    Grilled Baba Ganoush, *92,* 93
    Grilled Zucchini and Yellow Squash Stacks
        with Feta and Black Olives, 73
    grilling, 53, 162
    Japanese, grilling, 18

F
Fennel
    edible flowers from, 202
    Florence, about, 98
Fig(s)
    grilling, 192

Skewers, Fresh, Grilled Pork Tenderloin with, 144, *145*

Fish. *See also* Shellfish
Blackened, Po'Boy with Grilled Green Onion Mayonnaise, *90,* 91
Char-Grilled Salmon and Baby Squash, 150
Garlic Anchovy Dipping Sauce, 169
Grilled Salmon in Corn Husks, 151
grilling, 135
Peppered Tuna with Grilled Peach, Red Bell Pepper, and Onion Relish, 147
Tacos, Baja, *148,* 149

Flatbread and Pizza Dough, Stir-Together, 94

Flatbreads
breads for, 79
Grilled Pita Bread with Grilled Baba Ganoush, *92,* 93
grilling, 95
Herb-Stuffed Afghan, 96
Poppy Seed Naan, 97

Florence fennel, about, 98

Flowers, edible, 202–203

French Garden Radish Plate with Grilled Onion Butter, *56,* 57

French-Style Grilled Potato Salad, 115

Fruit. *See also* Berries; *specific fruits*
choosing, for grilling, 187
preparing for grilling, 187
Three-Citrus Drizzle for, 25
top ten, for the grill, 192

G

Gardening and grilling notes
with Asian flavors, 18
best greens for grilling, 116–117
creating container gardens, 58, 174
creating raised garden beds, 139
edible flowers, 202–203
flavored aioli, 40
flavored butters, 30
freezing grilled vegetables, 28
freezing smoked vegetables, 33
grilling flatbreads and pizza, 95
grilling greens, 110
grilling stuffed vegetables, 179
grill-roasting peppers, 43
growing companion plants, 194–195
growing edamame, 67
herbal skewers, 24
with Italian flavors, 98
with Mediterranean flavors, 53

meze, ideas for, 94
with south-of-the border flavors, 152
specialty grilling techniques, 8–9
stir-grilling, 166
Stir-Together Flatbread and Pizza Dough, 94
top ten fruits for grilling, 192
top ten vegetables for grilling, 162–163
vegetable container gardens, 174
vegetable measuring guidelines, 64

Garlic
Anchovy Dipping Sauce, 169
companion plants for, 194
Feta Butter, 170
flavoring with, 53
-Lemon Aioli, 39
planting and harvesting, 98
Rosemary, and Lemon Baste, 27
Smoked, and Cilantro Cream Sauce, 34
smoked, freezing, 33
Smoked, Herbed Butter, 30

Gazpacho, Grilled, 126, *127*

Geraniums, scented, garnishing with, 202

Ginger
Fresh, Soy Sauce, *122,* 123
Vinaigrette, 16

Goat Cheese
Blistered Summer Squash, Peppers, and Scallions with, 183
Chard-Wrapped, on the Grill, 75
Grilled Garden Loaf, 81
Grilled Polenta with Stir-Grilled Garlic Greens, 77
Pizza Primavera, 99
Smoked Tomato Bisque, *128,* 129
with Spring Garlic and Herb Topping, *50,* 51
Sun-Dried Tomato Butter, 30
Tomato Slices, Grilled, with Baby Greens, 118

Grains. *See* Polenta

Grapefruit
Aioli, 40
Grilled, with Brown Sugar Rum Butter, 190, *191*
grilling, 192

Grape(s)
Grilled, & Cheese Board, 193
grilling, 192

Greek Aioli, 40

Green Beans
Baby, and Chicken Paillard with Mustard Seed Sauce, 138
Charred, with Lemon Verbena Pesto, 164, *165*

Green Onion(s)

Grilled, Mayonnaise, 38
growing, 18
Herb-Stuffed Afghan Flatbread, 96
Greens
Baby, Grilled Goat Cheese Tomato Slices
with, 118
Brats with Grilled Kale and Horseradish
Butter, 143
bunched, measuring without a scale, 64
Grilled Asparagus Salad, 111
Grilled Caesar Sirloin, 153
Grilled Radicchio and Brussels Sprouts with
Hot Bacon Dressing, 120, *121*
grilling, tips for, 110
heading, varieties of, 117
High-Heat Grilled Romaine Salad, 109
Kale, Potato, and Chorizo Pizza, *102,* 103
loose, leafy, measuring without a scale, 64
Plank-Roasted Pear Salad with Blue Cheese
and Walnuts, *112,* 113
Stir-Grilled Garlic, Grilled Polenta with, 77
varieties of, 116–117
Winter, with Warm Cranberry Vinaigrette,
Grilled Turkey Breast over, 142–143
Wood-Grilled Shrimp and Yellow Peppers,
146
Grill roasting, description of, 8

H
Ham. *See* Prosciutto
Herb(s). *See also specific herbs*
Fresh, Aioli, 40
Herbed Cream Cheese, Grilled Green Tomato
"Sandwiches" with, 82, *83*
Herbed Smoked Garlic Butter, 30
herb stems used as skewers, 24
for Southwestern flavor, 152
and Spring Garlic, Goat Cheese with,
Topping, *50,* 51
-Stuffed Afghan Flatbread, 96
Hollandaise, Blender, 36
Honeyed Blackberries, Warm, with Grilled
Pound Cake, *198,* 199
Horseradish Aioli, 40
Horseradish Butter, 143

I
Indirect grilling, description of, 8
Italian flavors, 98
Italian Parmesan Grilling Paste, 31

K
Kale
Grilled, and Horseradish Butter, Brats with,
143
Potato, and Chorizo Pizza, *102,* 103

L
Lavender
edible flowers from, 202
woody stems, for skewers, 24
Leeks
and Asparagus, Grilled Spring Platter of, 161
companion plants for, 194
Lemon Balm Gremolata, Grilled Peaches with,
204, *205*
Lemongrass
about, 18
woody stems, for skewers, 24
Lemon(s)
Caesar Vinaigrette, 17
-Garlic Aioli, 39
grilling, 192
-Herb Butter, 168
Lemony Crème Fraîche, 200
Rosemary, and Garlic Baste, 27
-Rosemary Cherry Tomatoes, Skewered, 180,
181
Three-Citrus Drizzle for Fruit, 25
Lemon Verbena
Pesto, 164, *165*
stems, for skewers, 24
Lettuce
Grilled Caesar Sirloin, 153
heading, varieties of, 117
High-Heat Grilled Romaine Salad, 109
loose-leaf, growing, 117
Lime(s)
Aioli, 40
-Ancho Butter, 175
grilling, 192
Three-Citrus Drizzle for Fruit, 25
Lovage, companion plants for, 194

M
Main dishes
Baja Fish Tacos, *148,* 149
Blackened Beef with Thai Chile Noodles and
Baby Bok Choy, 154, *155*
Brats with Grilled Kale and Horseradish
Butter, 143
Char-Grilled Salmon and Baby Squash, 150

Chicken Paillard and Baby Green Beans with Mustard Seed Sauce, 138
Flank Steak with Grilled Peppers and Onions, 156–157
Grilled Caesar Sirloin, 153
Grilled Pork Tenderloin with Fresh Fig Skewers, 144, *145*
Grilled Salmon in Corn Husks, 151
Grilled Turkey Breast over Winter Greens with Warm Cranberry Vinaigrette, 142–143
Kansas City Strip Steaks with Parmesan Grilled Vegetables, 157
Peppered Tuna with Grilled Peach, Red Bell Pepper, and Onion Relish, 147
Skewered Chicken Saltimbocca, 137
Tandoori Turkey Burgers with Grilled Red Onions and Tomatoes, 140–141
Wood-Grilled Shrimp and Yellow Peppers, 146
Marigolds
  companion plants for, 195
  garnishing with, 203
Marinades
  Chimichurri Sauce, 26
  Chipotle Vinaigrette, 22
  Ginger Vinaigrette, 16
  Italian Parmesan Grilling Paste, 31
  Satay-Style Peanut Dipping Sauce, 23
  Three-Citrus Drizzle for Fruit, 25
  Toasted Sesame–Soy, 15
Marshmallow & Skewered Strawberry S'mores, 196, *197*
Mayonnaise
  aioli flavor variations, 40
  Grilled Green Onion, 38
  Lemon-Garlic Aioli, 39
Meat. *See* Beef; Pork
Mediterranean flavors, 53
Melon
  Grilled Cantaloupe Rings with Vanilla Bean Ice Cream, 201
  grilling, 192
Meze, ideas for, 94
Mint
  edible flowers from, 203
  Hot Pepper Butter, 30
Mushrooms
  Peppers, and Onions, Sizzling, Tuscan Polenta Platter with, 76
  Red Curry-Coconut Soup with Grilled Vegetables and Shrimp, 130–131
Mustard

Dijon Aioli, 40
Seed Sauce, 37

N

Naan, Poppy Seed, 97
Nasturtiums
  companion plants for, 195
  garnishing with, 203
Nectarines
  grilling, 192
  & Plums, Stir-Grilled, with Sweet Wine Drizzle, 207
Noodles, Thai Chile, and Baby Bok Choy, Blackened Beef with, 154, *155*
Nuts. *See* Almonds; Walnuts

O

Olive(s)
  Black, and Feta, Grilled Zucchini and Yellow Squash Stacks with, 73
  Fire-Roasted Pepper Dip, 72
  Grilled Garden Loaf, 81
  Kalamata, Brie, and Wood-Grilled Spring Onion Pizza, 100, *101*
Onion(s). *See also* Green Onion(s)
  cipollini, grilling, 98
  End-of-the-Garden Sauce, 45
  Grilled, Butter, *56,* 57
  grilled, freezing, 28
  grilling, 162
  Kansas City Strip Steaks with Parmesan Grilled Vegetables, 157
  Peppers, and Mushrooms, Sizzling, Tuscan Polenta Platter with, 76
  Peppers, and Stir-Grilled Italian Sausage Hoagies, 89
  and Peppers, Grilled, Flank Steak with, 156–157
  Red, and Tomatoes, Grilled, Tandoori Turkey Burgers with, 140–141
  Red, Corn, and Tomato, Grilled, Salad, 114
  Red Bell Pepper, and Peach, Grilled, Relish, 147
  Skewered Chicken Saltimbocca, 137
  smoked, freezing, 33
  Soft Corn Tortillas with Rajas and Queso, 61
  Spring, Wood-Grilled, Brie, and Kalamata Olive Pizza, 100, *101*
Orange(s)
  Aioli, 40
  grilling, 192

Three-Citrus Drizzle for Fruit, 25
Oregano
    Chimichurri Sauce, 26
    companion plants for, 195
    flavoring dishes with, 53
    fresh, about, 98

P
Pansies, garnishing with, 203
Paprika
    Red Hot Blackened Seasoning, 14
    Smoked, Butter, 30
Parmesan
    Caesar Butter, 30
    Grilled Grape & Cheese Board, 193
    Grilled Vegetables, Kansas City Strip Steaks
        with, 157
    Grilling Paste, Italian, 31
Parsley
    Chimichurri Sauce, 26
Paste, Grilling, Italian Parmesan, 31
Peach(es)
    Grilled, with Lemon Balm Gremolata,
        204, *205*
    grilling, 192
    Planked, and Blueberries with Amaretto
        Sauce, 206
    Red Bell Pepper, and Onion, Grilled, Relish,
        147
Peanut Dipping Sauce, Satay-Style, 23
Pear(s)
    Grilled, with Honey-Cinnamon Crème
        Fraîche, *212,* 213
    grilling, 192
    Plank-Roasted, Salad with Blue Cheese and
        Walnuts, *112,* 113
    Plank-Roasted, with Blue Cheese and
        Balsamic Honey, 211
Pea(s)
    blossoms, garnishing with, 203
    measuring without a scale, 64
    Pizza Primavera, 99
    Red Curry-Coconut Soup with Grilled
        Vegetables and Shrimp, 130–131
    Sugar Snap, and Tear Drop Tomatoes, Stir-
        Grilled, with Basil, 167
Peppered Tuna with Grilled Peach, Red Bell
Pepper, and Onion Relish, 147
Pepper(s). *See also* Chile peppers
    End-of-the-Garden Sauce, 45
    Fire-Roasted, Dip, 72

grilled, freezing, 28
Grilled Baba Ganoush, *92,* 93
Grilled Garden Loaf, 81
Grilled Gazpacho, 126, *127*
Grilled Pepper Boat "Sandwiches," 84
grilling, 162–163
Grill-Roasted Stuffed, 178–179
grill-roasting, directions for, 43
Kansas City Strip Steaks with Parmesan
    Grilled Vegetables, 157
Onions, and Mushrooms, Sizzling, Tuscan
    Polenta Platter with, 76
and Onions, Grilled, Flank Steak with, 156–
    157
Red Bell, Peach, and Onion, Grilled, Relish,
    147
Roasted Red, Aioli, 40
Romesco Sauce, 42
smoked, freezing, 33
Stir-Grilled Italian Sausage, and Onion Hoa-
    gies, 89
Summer Squash, and Scallions, Blistered,
    with Goat Cheese, 183
Yellow, and Shrimp, Wood-Grilled, 146
Persimmons
    Grilled, with Three-Citrus Drizzle, 208
    grilling, 192
Pesto
    Aioli, 40
    Basil (var.), 32
    Chive, 32
    Lemon Verbena, 164, *165*
Pizza
    Char-Grilled Baby Summer Squash, 104–105
    grilling, 95
    Kale, Potato, and Chorizo P, *102,* 103
    pizza dough and flatbreads for, 79
    Primavera, 99
    Wood-Grilled Spring Onion, Brie, and Kala-
        mata Olive, 100, *101*
Pizza and Flatbread Dough, Stir-Together, 94
Planking, description of, 8–9
Plank-roasting, description of, 9
Plums
    grilling, 192
    & Nectarines, Stir-Grilled, with Sweet Wine
        Drizzle, 207
Poblano Cream Sauce, Smoked, 35
Polenta
    Grilled, with Stir-Grilled Garlic Greens, 77
    Platter, Tuscan, with Sizzling Peppers,
        Onions, and Mushrooms, 76

Poppy Seed Naan, 97
Pork. *See also* Bacon; Prosciutto; Sausage(s)
  best cuts for grilling, 135
  checking doneness, 135
  Tenderloin, Grilled, with Fresh Fig Skewers,
    144, *145*
Potato(es)
  Flame-Licked Fingerlings with Romesco
    Sauce, 68, *69*
  Grilled, Salad, French-Style, 115
  Kale, and Chorizo Pizza, *102*, 103
  Sweet, Smoked and Smashed, Soup, 132–133
Poultry. *See* Chicken; Turkey
Prosciutto
  Chard-Wrapped Goat Cheese on the Grill, 75
  Grilled Asparagus Salad, 111
  Grilled Spring Platter of Asparagus and
    Leeks, 161
  Skewered Chicken Saltimbocca, 137
  -Wrapped Asparagus Spears, 62, *63*

R
Radicchio
  and Brussels Sprouts, Grilled, with Hot Bacon
    Dressing, 120, *121*
  growing, 116
Radish(es)
  Plate, French Garden, with Grilled Onion
    Butter, *56,* 57
  Spring, and Soft Cheese, Grilled Rye Bread
    with, 55
Red Curry-Coconut Soup with Grilled Vegeta-
  bles and Shrimp, 130–131
Red Hot Blackened Seasoning, 14
Relish, Grilled Peach, Red Bell Pepper, and
  Onion, 147
Rhubarb and Strawberries, Grill-Roasted, with
  Lemony Crème Fraîche, 200
Romesco Sauce, 42
Rosemary
  edible flowers from, 203
  flavoring with, 53
  Garlic, and Lemon Baste, 27
  -Lemon Cherry Tomatoes, Skewered, 180, *181*
  and Sugar-Spice-Rubbed Apple Slices, 210
  woody stems, for skewers, 24
Roses, garnishing with, 203

S
Sage
  edible flowers from, 203

Skewered Chicken Saltimbocca, 137
Salads
  Flame-Licked Tomatoes on the Stem, 124
  Grilled Asparagus, 111
  Grilled Baby Bok Choy with Fresh Ginger-
    Soy Sauce, *122,* 123
  Grilled Corn, Tomato, and Red Onion, 114
  Grilled Goat Cheese Tomato Slices with Baby
    Greens, 118
  Grilled Potato, French-Style, 115
  Grilled Radicchio and Brussels Sprouts with
    Hot Bacon Dressing, 120, *121*
  Grilled Summer Slaw with Gorgonzola
    Vinaigrette, 119
  High-Heat Grilled Romaine, 109
  Plank-Roasted Pear, with Blue Cheese and
    Walnuts, *112,* 113
Salmon
  and Baby Squash, Char-Grilled, 150
  Grilled, in Corn Husks, 151
Salsa, Grill-Roasted Tomatillo, *70,* 71
Salt, Seasoning, 13
Sandwiches. *See also* Burgers
  Blackened Fish Po'Boy with Grilled Green
    Onion Mayonnaise, *90,* 91
  breads for, 79
  Grilled Chicken Ciabatta with Romesco and
    Baby Greens, 86, *87*
  Grilled Garden Loaf, 81
  Grilled Green Tomato "Sandwiches" with
    Herbed Cream Cheese, 82, *83*
  Grilled Pepper Boat "Sandwiches," 84
  Panini Caprese, 85
  Stir-Grilled Italian Sausage, Peppers, and
    Onion Hoagies, 89
Satay-Style Peanut Dipping Sauce, 23
Sauces
  Amaretto, 206
  Basil Pesto (var.), 32
  Blender Hollandaise, 36
  Chimichurri, 26
  Chive Pesto, 32
  Cilantro Chile Drizzle, 172, *173*
  Cumin Yogurt, 140
  Dipping, Garlic Anchovy, 169
  Dipping, Satay-Style Peanut, 23
  End-of-the-Garden, 45
  Fresh Ginger-Soy, *122,* 123
  Grilled Marinara, 176
  Honey-Cinnamon Crème Fraîche, *212,* 213
  Lemon-Garlic Aioli, 39
  Lemon Verbena Pesto, 164, *165*

Lemony Crème Fraîche, 200
Mustard Seed, 37
Romesco, 42
Rosemary, Garlic, and Lemon Baste, 27
Smoked Garlic and Cilantro Cream, 34
Smoked Poblano Cream, 35
Tzatziki, 44
Sausage(s)
Brats with Grilled Kale and Horseradish
Butter, 143
checking doneness, 135
Italian, Stir-Grilled, Peppers, and Onion
Hoagies, 89
Kale, Potato, and Chorizo Pizza, *102,* 103
Scallions
and Lemon Herb Butter, Grilled Baby Beets
with, 168
Summer Squash, and Peppers, Blistered, with
Goat Cheese, 183
Seafood. *See* Fish; Shellfish
Seasonings
Red Hot Blackened Seasoning, 14
Seasoning Salt, 13
Shellfish
grilling, 135
Red Curry-Coconut Soup with Grilled
Vegetables and Shrimp, 130–131
Wood-Grilled Shrimp and Yellow Peppers,
146
Shrimp
and Vegetables, Grilled, Red Curry-Coconut
Soup with, 130–131
and Yellow Peppers, Wood-Grilled, 146
Skewers, herbal, 24
Slaws
Grilled Napa Cabbage, 149
Grilled Summer, with Gorgonzola Vinai-
grette, 119
Smoked Paprika Butter, 30
Smoked Poblano Cream Sauce, 35
Smoked Garlic and Cilantro Cream Sauce, 34
Smoked Summer Tomato Butter, 30
Smoking, description of, 9
S'mores, Skewered Strawberry & Marshmallow,
196, *197*
Soups
Grilled Corn and Chicken Chowder, 125
Grilled Gazpacho, 126, *127*
Red Curry-Coconut, with Grilled Vegetables
and Shrimp, 130–131
Smoked and Smashed Sweet Potato, 132–133
Smoked Tomato Bisque, *128,* 129

South-of-the-border flavors, 152
Southwest Butter, 30
Soybeans, fresh. *See* Edamame
Soy-Ginger Sauce, Fresh, *122,* 123
Spinach
measuring without a scale, 64
Wood-Grilled Shrimp and Yellow Peppers,
146
Squash
Acorn, and Apple Rings with Cider Jus, 184–
185, *185*
Baby, and Salmon, Char-Grilled, 150
Baby Summer, Char-Grilled, Pizza, 104–105
blossoms, cooking with, 203
Butternut, Sage, and Brie, Planked, 60
Grilled Garden Loaf, 81
summer, grilling, 163
Summer, Peppers, and Scallions, Blistered,
with Goat Cheese, 183
winter, companion plants for, 195
winter, par-cooking before grilling, 159
winter, smoked, freezing, 33
Yellow, and Zucchini, Grilled, Stacks with
Feta and Black Olives, 73
yellow summer, grilled, freezing, 28
Stir-grilling, description of, 9, 166
Strawberry(ies)
grilling, 192
and Rhubarb, Grill-Roasted, with Lemony
Crème Fraîche, 200
Skewered, & Marshmallow S'mores, 196, *197*
Sunflowers, companion plants for, 195
Sweet Potato, Smoked and Smashed, Soup, 132–
133
Swiss chard
Chard-Wrapped Goat Cheese on the Grill, 75
measuring without a scale, 64

T
Tacos, Baja Fish, *148,* 149
Tandoori Turkey Burgers with Grilled Red
Onions and Tomatoes, 140–141
Tarragon
Béarnaise Butter, 29
and Charred Eggplant Spread, 54
companion plants for, 195
Three-Citrus Drizzle for Fruit, 25
Toasted Sesame–Soy Marinade and Dressing, 15
Tomatillo(s)
Grill-Roasted, Salsa, *70,* 71
for salsas, 152
Tomato(es)

Cheery, Skewered Lemon-Rosemary, 180, *181*
cherry, measuring without a scale, 64
Corn, and Red Onion, Grilled, Salad, 114
End-of-the-Garden Sauce, 45
Flame-Licked, on the Stem, 124
Fresh, Grilled, Chive Pesto, and Provolone,
    Wood-Grilled Burger with, 88
Goat Cheese Slices, Grilled, with Baby
    Greens, 118
Green, Grilled, "Sandwiches" with Herbed
    Cream Cheese, 82, *83*
Grilled Gazpacho, 126, *127*
Grilled Marinara Sauce, 176
grilling, 163
Grill-Roasted Stuffed Peppers, 178–179
Kansas City Strip Steaks with Parmesan
    Grilled Vegetables, 157
Panini Caprese, 85
and Red Onions, Grilled, Tandoori Turkey
    Burgers with, 140–141
for salsas, 152
Smoked, Aioli, 40
Smoked, Bisque, *128,* 129
smoked, freezing, 33
Smoked Summer, Basil Butter, *50,* 51
Smoked Summer, Butter, 30
Sun-Dried, and Gruyère, Baby Eggplant with,
    177
Sun-Dried, Basil Aioli, 40
Sun-Dried, Goat Cheese Butter, 30
Tear Drop, and Sugar Snap Peas, Stir-Grilled,
    with Basil, 167
varieties of, 98
Tortillas
    Baja Fish Tacos, *148,* 149
    Soft Corn, with Rajas and Queso, 61
Tuna, Peppered, with Grilled Peach, Red Bell
Pepper, and Onion Relish, 147
Turkey
    best cuts for grilling, 135
    Breast, Grilled, over Winter Greens with
    Warm Cranberry Vinaigrette, 142–143
    Burgers, Tandoori, with Grilled Red Onions
        and Tomatoes, 140–141
    checking doneness, 135
Tuscan Polenta Platter with Sizzling Peppers,
Onions, and Mushrooms, 76
Tzatziki, 44

V
Vegetable(s). *See also specific vegetables*
    grilled, freezing, 28
    grilling techniques, 159
    measuring without a scale, 64
    par-cooking before grilling, 159
    Parmesan Grilled, Kansas City Strip Steaks
        with, 157
    root, grilling, 163
    Root, Grill-Roasted, with Smoked Tomato
        Aioli, 182
    and Shrimp, Grilled, Red Curry-Coconut
        Soup with, 130–131
    smoked, freezing, 33
    Smoked and Grilled, Dip, Crostini with, 59
    stir-grilling, 159
    top ten, for the grill, 162–163
Vinaigrettes
    Chipotle, 22
    Cranberry, Warm, 142
    Fresh Basil, *20,* 21
    Ginger, 16
    Lemon Caesar, 17
Violets, garnishing with, 203

W
Walnuts
    and Blue Cheese, Plank-Roasted Pear Salad
        with, *112,* 113
    Chard-Wrapped Goat Cheese on the Grill, 75
    Chive Pesto, 32
    Grill-Baked Apples with Cinnamon Nut
        Stuffing, 209
Winter savory flowers, garnishing with, 203

Y
Yogurt
    Sauce, Cumin, 140
    Tzatziki, 44

Z
Zucchini
    grilled, freezing, 28
    Grilled Garden Loaf, 81
    Kansas City Strip Steaks with Parmesan
        Grilled Vegetables, 157
    varieties of, 98
    and Yellow Squash, Grilled, Stacks with Feta
        and Black Olives, 73